EVIDENCE-BASED ORTHOPAEDICS

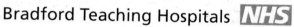

EVIDENCE-BASED ORTHOPAEDICS

The Best Answers to Clinical Questions

James G. Wright, MD, MPH, FRCSC

Professor, Departments of Surgery, Public Health Sciences, and Health Policy, Management and Evaluation, University of Toronto; Surgeon-in-Chief, Chief of Perioperative Services, and Robert B. Salter Chair of Paediatric Surgical Research, Hospital for Sick Children; Toronto, Ontario, Canada

SECTION EDITORS

Henry Ahn, MD, FRCSC
Department of Surgery, Division of Orthopaedic Surgery, University of Toronto; Specialist, Adult Spinal Disorders and Trauma, Division of Orthopaedic Surgery, St. Michael's Orthopaedic Associates, St. Michael's Hospital; Toronto, Ontario, Canada

Brent Graham, MD, MSc, FRCSC
Assistant Professor, Department of Surgery, Divisions of Orthopaedic Surgery and Plastic Surgery, University of Toronto; Director, Hand Program, University Health Network; Toronto, Ontario, Canada

Andrew Howard, MD, MSc, FRCSC
Associate Professor, Department of Surgery, University of Toronto; Pediatric Orthopaedic Surgeon, Department of Orthopaedic Surgery, The Hospital for Sick Children; Director, Office of International Surgery, University of Toronto; Toronto, Ontario, Canada

Hans J. Kreder, MD, MPH, FRCSC
Associate Professor, Departments of Orthopaedic Surgery and Health Policy, Management, and Evaluation, University of Toronto; Marvin Tile Chair and Chief, Division of Orthopaedics, Program Chief, Holland Musculoskeletal Program, Sunnybrook Health Sciences Centre; Adjunct Scientist, Institute for Clinical Evaluative Sciences; Toronto, Ontario, Canada

Johnny Tak-Choy Lau, MD, MSc, FRCSC
Assistant Professor, Department of Surgery, University of Toronto; Consultant Orthopaedic Surgeon, Department of Surgery, University Health Network, Toronto Western Division; Toronto, Ontario, Canada

Sheldon S. Lin, MD
Associate Professor, Department of Orthopaedic Surgery, New Jersey Medical School, University of Medicine and Dentistry of New Jersey; Newark, New Jersey, USA; Chief of Foot and Ankle, North Jersey Orthopedic Institute, Newark, New Jersey, USA

Nizar N. Mahomed, MD, ScD, FRCSC
Associate Professor, Smith and Nephew Chair in Orthopaedic Surgery Research, Department of Surgery, University of Toronto; Director, Musculoskeletal Health and Arthritis Program, Department of Surgery, University Health Network; Toronto, Ontario, Canada

Daniel Whelan, MD, MSc, FRCSC
Assistant Professor, Department of Surgery, University of Toronto; Orthopaedic Staff Surgeon, Department of Surgery, St. Michael's Hospital, Toronto, Ontario, Canada

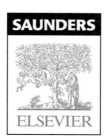

SAUNDERS

ELSEVIER

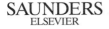

SAUNDERS
ELSEVIER

1600 John F. Kennedy Blvd.
Ste 1800
Philadelphia, PA 19103-2899

EVIDENCE-BASED ORTHOPAEDICS: THE BEST ANSWERS
TO CLINICAL QUESTIONS

ISBN: 978-1-4160-4444-4

NOTICE

Knowledge and best practice in this field are constantly changing. As new research and experience broaden our knowledge, changes in practice, treatment and drug therapy may become necessary or appropriate. Readers are advised to check the most current information provided (i) on procedures featured or (ii) by the manufacturer of each product to be administered, to verify the recommended dose or formula, the method and duration of administration, and contraindications. It is the responsibility of the practitioner, relying on their own experience and knowledge of the patient, to make diagnoses, to determine dosages and the best treatment for each individual patient, and to take all appropriate safety precautions. To the fullest extent of the law, neither the Publisher nor the Editors assumes any liability for any injury and/or damage to persons or property arivsing out of or related to any use of the material contained in this book.

The Publisher

Library of Congress Cataloging-in-Publication Data

Evidence-based orthopaedics : the best answers to clinical questions / [edited by] James G. Wright.
— 1st ed.
    p. ; cm.
Includes bibliographical references.
ISBN 978-1-4160-4444-4
1. Orthopedics–Miscellanea. 2. Evidence-based medicine. I. Wright, James G. (James Gardner), 1957-
[DNLM: 1. Orthopedic Procedures–methods. 2. Evidence-Based Medicine–methods.
WE 190 E935 2009]
RD732.E95 2009
616.7–dc22

2008034472

Publishing Director: Kim Murphy
Developmental Editor: John Ingram, Faith Brody
Project Manager: Mary Stermel
Designer: Steve Stave
Marketing Manager: Catlina Nolte

Printed in the United States of America

Last digit is the print number: 9 8 7 6 5 4 3 2 1

This book is dedicated to all of the orthopaedic surgeons who work so hard to do the right thing for their patients.

Foreword

I am honored to be invited by Dr. Wright to write the foreword to this precedent-setting textbook. Over the last decade the discipline of orthopaedic surgery has advanced primarily because of a much more substantial emphasis on evidence-based decision making in clinical practice. Many orthopaedic journals have focused on the quality of study design in the articles that they have published, and have encouraged authors to pursue higher-level studies. Although there are many questions related to musculoskeletal care that, because of the rarity of the disease or the uniqueness of the clinical circumstances, will never be subjected to randomized controlled trials, many important clinical questions in orthopaedics can be addressed with well-designed Level II and III studies. Although the older orthopaedic literature was replete with reports of retrospective case series, and many book chapters and podium presentations simply reflected the opinion of the author or presenter, much more reliable information is now becoming available on many important clinical questions. This textbook presents a rich sampling of this higher-level evidence in a concise and easy-to-read format that is focused on specific areas of clinical interest. The authors have done an outstanding job of culling the critical studies from the literature and providing the reader with useful clinical insights. Dr. Wright and his collaborators are to be congratulated on providing a compendium of clinically important information that will enable us all to advance the quality of the care of our patients based on scientific principles.

James D. Heckman, MD
Boston, Massachusetts
November 20, 2007

Contributors

SECTION EDITORS

Henry Ahn, MD, FRCSC
Department of Surgery, Division of Orthopaedic Surgery, University of Toronto, Toronto, Ontario, Canada; Specialist, Adult Spinal Disorders and Trauma, Division of Orthopaedic Surgery, St. Michael's Orthopaedic Associates, St. Michael's Hospital, Toronto, Ontario, Canada
Spinal Topics

Brent Graham, MD, MSc, FRCSC
Assistant Professor, Department of Surgery, Divisions of Orthopaedic Surgery and Plastic Surgery, University of Toronto, Toronto, Ontario, Canada; Director, Hand Program, University Health Network, Toronto, Ontario, Canada
Upper Extremity Topics

Andrew Howard, MD, MSc, FRCSC
Associate Professor, Departments of Surgery, University of Toronto, Toronto, Ontario, Canada; Paediatric Orthopaedic Surgeon, Department of Orthopaedic Surgery, The Hospital for Sick Children, Toronto, Ontario, Canada; Director, Office of International Surgery, University of Toronto, Toronto, Ontario, Canada
Pediatric Topics

Hans J. Kreder, MD, MPH, FRCSC
Associate Professor, Departments of Orthopaedic Surgery and Health Policy, Management, and Evaluation, University of Toronto, Toronto, Ontario, Canada; Marvin Tile Chair and Chief, Division of Orthopaedics, Program Chief, Holland Musculoskeletal Program, Sunnybrook Health Sciences Centre, Toronto, Ontario, Canada; Adjunct Scientist, Institute for Clinical Evaluative Sciences, Toronto, Ontario, Canada
Trauma Topics

Johnny Tak-Choy Lau, MD, MSc, FRCSC
Assistant Professor, Department of Surgery, University of Toronto, Toronto, Ontario, Canada; Consultant Orthopaedic Surgeon, Department of Surgery, University Health Network, Toronto, Western Division, Toronto, Ontario, Canada
Foot and Ankle Topics

Sheldon S. Lin, MD
Associate Professor, Department of Orthopaedic Surgery, New Jersey Medical School, University of Medicine and Dentistry of New Jersey, Newark, New Jersey, USA
Foot and Ankle Topics

Nizar N. Mahomed, MD, ScD, FRCSC
Associate Professor, Smith and Nephew Chair in Orthopaedic Surgery Research, Department of Surgery, University of Toronto, Toronto, Ontario, Canada; Director, Musculoskeletal Health and Arthritis Program, Department of Surgery, University Health Network, Toronto, Ontario, Canada
Arthroplasty Topics

Daniel Whelan, MD, MSc, FRCSC
Assistant Professor, Department of Surgery, University of Toronto, Toronto, Ontario, Canada; Orthopaedic Staff Surgeon, Department of Surgery, St. Michael's Hospital, Toronto, Ontario, Canada
Sports Medicine Topics

CONTRIBUTORS

Masahiko Akiyama, MD, DMSC
Clinical Fellow, University of Toronto, Toronto, Ontario, Canada; Clinical Fellow, St. Michael's Hospital, Toronto, Ontario, Canada
What Is the Optimal Method of Managing a Patient with Cervical Myelopathy?

Isam Atroshi, MD, PhD
Associate Professor of Orthopaedics, Department of Clinical Sciences, Lund University, Lund, Sweden; Consultant Hand Surgeon, Department of Orthopaedics, Hassleholm and Kristianstad Hospitals, Hassleholm, Sweden
What Is the Evidence for a Cause-and-Effect Linkage Between Occupational Hand Use and Symptoms of Carpal Tunnel Syndrome?

Terry S. Axelrod, MD, MSc, FRCS(C)
Professor, Department of Surgery, Division of Orthopaedic Surgery, University of Toronto, Toronto, Ontario, Canada; Staff Surgeon, Division of Orthopaedic Surgery, Sunnybrook Health Sciences Centre, Toronto, Ontario, Canada
When Is It Safe to Resect Heterotopic Ossification?

David Backstein, MD, Med, FRCSC
Associate Professor, Director of Undergraduate Education, Department of Surgery, University of Toronto, Toronto, Ontario, Canada; Orthopaedic Surgery, Mount Sinai Hospital, Toronto, Ontario, Canada
What Are the Facts and Fiction of Minimally Invasive Hip and Knee Arthroplasty Surgery?

A. Kursat Barin, MSc
McCaig Centre for Joint Injury and Arthritis Research,
Department of Physiology and Biophysics,
University of Calgary, Calgary, Alberta, Canada
What Is the Role for Hip Resurfacing Arthroplasty?

S. Samuel Bederman, MD, MSc, FRCSC
Research Fellow, Division of Orthopaedic Surgery,
Department of Surgery, University of Toronto,
Toronto, Ontario, Canada; Research Fellow, Child
Health Evaluative Sciences, The Hospital for Sick
Children Research Institute, Toronto, Ontario,
Canada
Do Bone Morphogenetic Proteins Improve Spinal Fusion?

Caleb Behrend, MS
David Geffen School of Medicine at the University of
California, Los Angeles, Los Angeles, California, USA
What Is the Best Treatment for Plantar Fasciitis?

Gregory K. Berry, MD
Assistant Professor, Orthopaedic Surgery, McGill
University, Montreal, Quebec, Canada; Staff,
Orthopaedic Trauma, McGill University Medical
Center, Montreal, Quebec, Canada
Humeral Shaft Fractures: What Is the Best Treatment?

Mohit Bhandari, MD, MSc, FRCSC
Associate Professor, Canada Research Chair,
McMaster University, Hamilton, Ontario, Canada
*Are Bone Substitutes Useful in the Treatment and Prevention
of Nonunions and in the Management of Subchondral
Voids?; Femoral Neck Fractures: When Should a Displaced
Subcapital Fracture Be Replaced versus Fixed?; Femoral
Shaft Fractures: What Is the Best Treatment?*

Paul Binhammer, MSc, MD, FRCS(C)
Assistant Professor, University of Toronto, Toronto,
Ontario, Canada; Head, Division of Plastic Surgery,
Sunnybrook Health Sciences Centre, Toronto,
Ontario, Canada
*What Is the Best Treatment for Acute Injuries of the
Scapholunate Ligament?*

Piotr A. Blachut, MD, FRCSC
Clinical Professor, Division of Orthopaedic Trauma,
Department of Orthopaedics, University of British
Columbia, Vancouver, British Columbia, Canada;
Subunit Director, Division of Orthopaedic Trauma;
Department of Orthopaedics, Vancouver General
Hospital, Vancouver, British Columbia, Canada
Tibial Diaphyseal Fractures: What Is the Best Treatment?

Thomas E. Brown, MD
Associate Professor, Orthopaedic Surgery, University
of Virginia, Charlottesville, Virginia, USA
*Total Hip Replacement: Hybrid versus Uncemented:
Which Is Better?*

Richard Brull, MD, FRCPC
Assistant Professor, Department of Anesthesia,
University of Toronto, Toronto, Ontario, Canada;
Staff Anesthesiologist, Director, Regional
Anesthesia Fellowship Program, Toronto
Western Hospital, University Health Network,
Toronto, Ontario, Canada
*Regional Anesthesia for Total Hip and Knee Arthroplasty:
Is It Worth the Effort?*

Dianne Bryant, BSc, BA, MSc, PhD
Assistant Professor, University of Western Ontario,
London, Ontario, Canada; Assistant Professor,
London Health Sciences Centre, London, Ontario,
Canada
*Multiligament Knee Injury: Should Surgical Reconstruction Be
Acute or Delayed?*

Richard E. Buckley, MD, FRCSC
Associate Professor, University of Calgary, Calgary,
Alberta, Canada; Head, Orthopedic Trauma,
Foothills Medical Center, Calgary, Alberta,
Canada
*What Is the Best Treatment for Displaced Intra-Articular
Calcaneus Fractures?*

Rebecca Carl, MD
Fellow, Non-Operative Orthopaedics, Orthopaedics
and Rehabilitation, University of Wisconsin
Hospitals and Clinics, Madison, Wisconsin, USA
What Is the Best Treatment for Forearm Fractures?

Dominic Carreira, MD
Orthopedic Surgery, Foot and Ankle, Hip Arthroscopy,
and Sports Medicine Specialist, Fort Lauderdale,
Florida, USA
*What Is the Best Treatment for Injury to the Tarsometatarsal
Joint Complex?*

Steven Casha, MD, PhD, FRCSC
Assistant Professor, Division of Neurosurgery,
Department of Clinical Neurosciences, University
of Calgary, Calgary, Alberta, Canada; Neurosurgeon,
Foothills Medical Center, Calgary, Alberta,
Canada
*Should Patients with Acute Spinal Cord Injuries Receive
Steroids?*

Denise Chan, BSc, MBT
Research Coordinator, University of Calgary Division
of Health Sciences, Calgary, Alberta, Canada
*Autograft Choice in Anterior Cruciate Ligament Reconstruction:
Should It Be Patellar Tendon or Hamstring Tendon?*

Vincent W. S. Chan, MD, FRCPC
Professor, Department of Anesthesia, University
of Toronto, Toronto, Ontario, Canada; Staff
Anesthesiologist, Head, Regional Anesthesia
and Pain Management Program, Toronto Western
Hospital, University Health Network, Toronto,
Ontario, Canada
*Regional Anesthesia for Total Hip and Knee Arthroplasty: Is It
Worth the Effort?*

Neal C. Chen, MD
Clinical Fellow, Department of Orthopaedics, Hand
and Upper Extremity Service, Massachusetts
General Hospital, Boston, Massachusetts, USA
*What Is the Best Treatment for Displaced Fractures of the
Distal Radius?*

Christine J. Cheng, MD, MPH
Clinical Assistant Professor, Department of
Orthopaedics, University of Missouri–Kansas
City, Kansas City, Missouri, USA; Kansas City Bone
and Joint Clinic, Overland Park, Kansas, USA
What Is the Best Management of Digital Triggering?

Christopher P. Chiodo, MD
Clinical Instructor, Department of Orthopaedic Surgery, Harvard Medical School, Boston, Massachusetts, USA; Chief, Division of Foot and Ankle Surgery, Department of Orthopedic Surgery, Brigham and Women's Hospital, Boston, Massachusetts, USA
> *What Is the Best Treatment of Displaced Talar Neck Fractures?*

Kevin C. Chung, MD, MS
Professor of Sugery, Section of Plastic Surgery, University of Michigan Health System, Ann Arbor, Michigan, USA
> *What Are the Best Diagnostic Tests for Complex Regional Pain Syndrome?*

Katie N. Dainty, MSc, CRPC
Program Manager, Centre for Health Services Sciences, Sunnybrook Health Sciences Centre, Toronto, Ontario, Canada
> *Autograft Choice in Anterior Cruciate Ligament Reconstruction: Should It Be Patellar Tendon or Hamstring Tendon?*

Tim R. Daniels, MD, FRCSC
Associate Professor, Full-time Faculty, University of Toronto, Ontario, Canada; Full-time Staff Position, St. Michael's Hospital, University of Toronto, Ontario, Canada
> *What Is the Best Treatment for End-Stage Ankle Arthritis?*

J. Roderick Davey, MD, FRCSC
Associate Professor of Surgery, University of Toronto, Toronto, Ontario, Canada; Associate Director of Social Services, Head, Division of Orthopaedic Surgery, University Health Network; Medical Director, Operating Rooms, Toronto Western Hospital, Toronto, Ontario, Canada
> *What Is the Role of Antibiotic Cement in Total Joint Replacement?*

Luciano Dias, MD
Professor, Orthopaedic Surgery, Feinberg School of Medicine, Northwestern University, Chicago, Illinois, USA; Medical Director, Motion Analysis Center, Children's Memorial Hospital, Chicago, Illinois, USA
> *What Is the Optimal Treatment for Spine and Hip in Myelomenigocele?*

Frederick R. Dietz, MD
Professor, Department of Orthopaedic Surgery, University of Iowa Hospitals and Clinics, Iowa City, Iowa, USA
> *What Is the Best Treatment for Idiopathic Club Foot?*

Christopher C. Dodson, MD
Fellow, Sports Medicine and Shoulder Service, Hospital for Special Surgery, New York, New York, USA
> *Is There a Role for Arthroscopy in the Treatment of Knee Osteoarthritis?*

Lori A. Dolan, PhD
Assistant Research Scientist, Department of Orthopaedics and Rehabiliation, University of Iowa, Iowa City, Iowa, USA
> *Best Treatment for Adolescent Idiopathic Scoliosis: What Do Current Systematic Reviews Tell Us?*

Michael J. Dunbar, MD, FRCSC, PhD
Associate Professor of Surgery, Director of Orthopaedic Research, Dalhousie University, Halifax, Novia Scotia, Canada; Consultant Orthopaedic Surgeon, QEII Health Sciences Centre, Halifax, Novia Scotia, Canada
> *When Should a Unicompartmental Knee Arthroplasty Be Considered?*

Warren R. Dunn, MD, MPH
Assistant Professor, Orthopaedics and Rehabilitation, General Internal Medicine and Public Health, Vanderbilt University Medical Center, Nashville, Tennessee, USA
> *Are Anterior Cruciate Ligament Injuries Preventable?*

Marcel F. Dvorak, MD, FRCSC
Head, Division of Spine, Department of Orthopaedics, University of British Columbia, Vancouver, British Columbia, Canada; Combined Neurosurgical and Orthopaedic Spine Program, Vancouver General Hospital, Vancouver, British Columbia, Canada; Cordula and Gunther Paetzold Chair in Spinal Cord Injury Clinical Research, International Collaboration on Repair Discoveries, Vancouver Coastal Health Research Institute, Vancouver, British Columbia, Canada
> *What Is the Optimal Treatment for Thoracolumbar Burst Fractures?*

Mark E. Easley, MD
Professor, Orthopaedic Surgery, Duke University Medical Center, Duke Health Center, Durham, North Carolina, USA
> *What Is the Best Treatment for Hallux Valgus?*

Peter Faris, PhD
Department of Community Health Sciences, University of Calgary, Calgary, Alberta, Canada
> *What Is the Role for Hip Resurfacing Arthroplasty?*

Paul Vincent Fearon, BSc (Hons), MB, Bch, BAO, FRCC (Tr and Orth), MD
Consultant, Orthopaedic Trauma Surgeon, Department of Orthopaedic Trauma, Newcastle General Hospital, Newcastle upon Tyne, United Kingdom
> *What Is the Best Treatment for Pilon Fractures?*

Michael G. Fehlings, MD, PhD, FRCSC, FACS
Professor, Krembil Chair in Neural Repair and Regeneration, Department of Surgery, Division of Neurosurgery, University of Toronto, Toronto, Canada; Medical Director, Krembil Neuroscience Center, Head, Spinal Program, Toronto Western Hospital, Toronto, Ontario, Canada
> *Is Neuromonitoring Beneficial During Spinal Surgery?*

Nicole L. Fetter, MD
Resident, Harvard Combined Orthopaedic Residency Program, Massachusetts General Hospital, Boston, Massachusetts, USA
> *What Is the Best Treatment of Displaced Talar Neck Fractures?*

Joel A. Finkelstein, MD, FRCS(C)
Associate Professor, University of Toronto, Toronto, Ontario, Canada; Spine Section Head, Division of

Orthopaedics, Sunnybrook Health Sciences Centre, Toronto, Ontario, Canada
What Is the Ideal Surgical Treatment for an Adult Patient with a Lytic Spondylolisthesis?

Charles G. Fisher, MD, MHSc, FRCSC
Assistant Professor, Department of Orthopaedics, University of British Columbia, Vancouver, British Columbia, Canada
What Is the Optimal Treatment for Thoracolumbar Burst Fractures?

John M. Flynn, MD
Associate Professor of Orthopaedic Surgery, University of Pennsylvania School of Medicine, Philadelphia, Pennsylvania, USA; Associate Chief of Orthopaedic Surgery, The Children's Hospital of Philadelphia, Philadelphia, Pennsylvania, USA
What Is the Best Treatment for Femoral Fractures?

Eric Francke, MD
Eastern Carolina University, Brody School of Medicine, Greenville, North Carolina, USA; Orthopaedic Surgery, Pitt County Memorial Hospital, Greenville, North Carolina, USA
Should Patients Undergoing Decompression for a Grade 1 Degenerative Spondylolisthesis Also Have an Instrumented Fusion?

Julio Cesar Furlan, MD, MBA, MSc, PhD
Associate Research Scientist, Toronto Western Research Institute, Toronto, Ontario, Canada
Is Neuromonitoring Beneficial During Spinal Surgery?

Robert D. Galpin, MD, FRCSC
Clinical Professor of Orthopaedic Surgery, University at Buffalo, Buffalo, New York, USA; Chief of Orthopaedics, Women and Children's Hospital of Buffalo, Buffalo, New York, USA
What Is the Best Treatment for Wrist Fractures?

Rajiv Gandhi, MD, FRCSC
Orthopaedic Surgeon, Toronto Western Hospital, University Health Network, Toronto, Ontario, Canada
What Is the Role of Antibiotic Cement in Total Joint Replacement?; What Is the Role of Computer Navigation in Hip and Knee Arthroplasty?

Donald S. Garbuz, MD, MHSc, FRCSC
Assistant Professor and Head, Division of Lower Limb Reconstruction and Oncology, Department of Orthopaedics, University of British Columbia, Vancouver, British Columbia, Canada
Should the Patella be Resurfaced in Total Knee Replacement?; How Do You Make a Diagnosis of an Infected Arthroplasty?

Ahmer K. Ghori, BA
Medical Student, University of Michigan School of Medicine, University of Michigan, Ann Arbor, Michigan, USA
What Are the Best Diagnostic Tests for Complex Regional Pain Syndrome?

J. Robert Giffin, MD, FRCSC
Fowler Kennedy Sport Medicine Clinic, University of Western Ontario, London, Ontario, Canada
Multiligament Knee Injury: Should Surgical Reconstruction Be Acute or Delayed?

Howard Ginsberg, BASc, MD, PhD, FRCSC
Assistant Professor, Department of Surgery and Institute of Biomaterials and Biomedical Engineering, University of Toronto, Toronto, Ontario, Canada; Neurosurgeon, St Michael's Hospital, Toronto, Ontario, Canada
What Is the Optimal Method of Managing a Patient with Cervical Myelopathy?

Mark Glazebrook, MSc, PhD, MD, FRCS(C)
Assistant Professor, Dalhousie University, Halifax, Nova Scotia, Canada; Orthopaedic Consultant, Queen Elizabeth II Health Sciences Center, Halifax, Nova Scotia, Canada
What Is the Best Treatment for Achilles Tendon Rupture?

Jennifer Goebel, BA
Clinical Research Coordinator, Division of Orthopaedic Surgery, The Children's Hospital of Philadelphia, Philadelphia, Pennsylvania, USA
What Is the Best Treatment for Femoral Fractures?

Andreas H. Gomoll, MD
Instructor, Orthopaedic Surgery, Harvard Medical School, Boston, Massachusetts, USA; Associate Orthopaedic Surgeon, Cartilage Repair Center, Brigham and Women's Hospital, Boston, Massachusetts, USA
What Is the Best Treatment for Chondral Defects in the Knee?

Philippe Grondin, MD
University of Montreal, Montreal, Quebec, Canada
What Are the Indications for Surgery, and What Is the Best Surgical Treatment for Chronic Lateral Epicondylitis?

Abha A. Gupta, MD, MSC, FRCPC
Assistant Professor, Department of Pediatrics, University of Toronto, Toronto, Ontario, Canada; Staff Oncologist, The Hospital for Sick Children, Toronto, Ontario, Canada
What Is the Best Treatment of Malignant Bone Tumors in Children?

Raphael C. Y. Hau, MBBS, FRACS
Clinical Fellow, Department of Orthopaedics, University of British Columbia, Vancouver, British Columbia, Canada; Clinical Fellow, Division of Lower Limb Reconstruction and Oncology, Vancouver General Hospital, Vancouver, British Columbia, Canada; Consultant Orthopaedic Surgeon, Department of Orthopaedics, The Northern Hospital, Melbourne, Victoria, Australia; Consultant Orthopaedic Surgeon, Department of Orthopaedics, Box Hill Hospital, Melbourne, Victoria, Australia
Should the Patella Be Resurfaced in Total Knee Replacement?

Robert H. Hawkins, MD, FRCS(C)
Clinical Professor of Orthopaedics, University of
British Columbia, Vancouver, British Columbia,
Canada; Attending Surgeon, Vancouver General
Hospital, Vancouver, British Columbia, Canada
What Is the Best Surgical Treatment for Cuff Tear Arthropathy?

Näder Helmy, MD
Department of Orthopaedics, University of Zurich,
Zurich, Switzerland; Consultant, Department
of Orthopaedics, University of Zurich, Balgrist,
Zurich, Switzerland
Tibial Diaphyseal Fractures: What Is the Best Treatment?

Harry Herkowitz, MD
Chairman, Department of Orthopaedic Surgery,
and Fellowship Coordinator for Spine and Sports
Medicine, William Beaumont Hospital, Royal Oak,
Michigan, USA
*Should Patients Undergoing Decompression for a Grade 1
Degenerative Spondylolisthesis Also Have an Instrumented
Fusion?*

John Anthony Herring, MD
Professor, Orthopedic Surgery, University of Texas
Southwestern Medical School, Dallas, Texas, USA;
Chief of Staff, Texas Scottish Rite Hospital for
Children, Dallas, Texas, USA; Staff Surgeon,
Orthopedic Surgery, Children's Medical Center,
Dallas, Texas, USA
Legg–Calve-Perthes Disease: How Should It Be Treated?

**Richard A. Hocking, BSc (Med), MBBS (Hons),
FRACS (orth)**
Visiting Medical Officer, The Canberra Hospital,
Canberra, ACT, Australia
*Which Bearing Surface Should Be Used: Highly Cross-Linked
Polyethylene versus Metal or Metal versus Ceramic on
Ceramic?*

Richard M. Holtby, MBBS, FRCSC
Assistant Professor, University of Toronto, Toronto,
Ontario, Canada; Active Staff, Sunnybrook Health
Sciences Centre, Toronto, Ontario, Canada
Is Arthroscopic Rotator Cuff Repair Superior?

Sevan Hopyan, MD, PhD, FRCSC
Assistant Professor, Department of Surgery, University
of Toronto, Toronto, Ontario, Canada; Orthopaedic
Surgeon, The Hospital for Sick Children, Toronto,
Ontario, Canada
*What Is the Best Treatment of Malignant Bone Tumors in
Children?*

Andrew Howard, MD, MSc, FRCSC
Associate Professor, Department of Surgery,
University of Toronto; Pediatric Orthopaedic
Surgeon, Department of Orthopaedic Surgery, The
Hospital for Sick Children; Director, Office of
International Surgery, University of Toronto,
Toronto, Ontario, Canada
*Can We Prevent Children's Fractures?; How Should We Treat
Elbow Fractures in Children?*

Jason L. Hurd, MD
Fellow, Shoulder and Elbow Surgery, New York
University Hospital for Joint Diseases, New York,
New York, USA
*What Is the Best Treatment for Complex Proximal Humerus
Fractures? What Are the Main Determinants of Outcome
after Arthroplasty?*

R. John Hurlbert, MD, PhD, FRCSC, FACS
Associate Professor, Department of Clinical
Neurosciences, University of Calgary, Calgary,
Alberta, Canada; Division of Neurosurgery, Foothills
Hospital and Medical Center, Calgary, Alberta, Canada
Should Patients with Acute Spinal Cord Injuries Receive Steroids?

Heidi Israel, PhD
Assistant Research Professor, Department of
Orthopaedic Surgery, St. Louis University School
of Medicine, St. Louis, Missouri, USA
*What Is the Best Way to Prevent Heterotopic Ossification after
Acetabular Fracture Fixation?*

Richard J. Jenkinson, MD, FRCS(C)
Orthopaedic Surgery Associate, Sunnybrook Health
Sciences Center, Toronto, Ontario, Canada
Acetabular Fractures: Does Delay to Surgery Influence Outcome?

Jesse B. Jupiter, MD
Hansjörg-Wyss AO Professor of Orthopaedic
Surgery, Harvard Medical School, Boston,
Massachusetts, USA; Director, Hand and Upper
Extremity Service, Massachusetts General
Hospital, Boston, Massachusetts, USA
*What Is the Best Treatment for Displaced Fractures of the
Distal Radius?*

Michael O. Kelleher, FRCS, MD
RCSI Neurosurgery Lecturer, The Royal College of
Surgeons in Ireland, Dublin, Ireland; Neurosurgery
Lecturer, Beaumont Hospital, Dublin, Ireland
Is Neuromonitoring Beneficial During Spinal Surgery?

Mininder S. Kocher, MD, MPH
Associate Professor of Orthopaedic Surgery,
Harvard Medical School/Harvard School of Public
Health, Boston, Massachusetts, USA; Associate
Director, Division of Sports Medicine, Department
of Orthopaedic Surgery, Children's Hospital
Boston, Boston, Massachusetts, USA
How Do You Best Diagnose Septic Arthritis of the Hip?

Hans J. Kreder, MD, MPH, FRCSC
Associate Professor, Departments of Orthopaedic
Surgery and Health Policy, Management, and
Evaluation, University of Toronto, Toronto,
Ontario, Canada; Marvin Tile Chair and Chief,
Division of Orthopaedics, Program Chief, Holland
Musculoskeletal Program, Sunnybrook Health
Sciences Centre, Toronto, Ontario, Canada;
Adjunct Scientist, Institute for Clinical Evaluative
Sciences, Toronto, Ontario, Canada
*What Is the Role of Splinting for Comfort?; How Does Surgeon
and Hospital Volume Affect Patient Outcome after
Traumatic Injury?; Acetabular Fractures: Does Delay to
Surgery Influence Outcome?*

Paul R. T. Kuzyk, BSc, MASc, MD, FRCS(C)
Clinical Fellow, St. Michael's Hospital, University of Toronto, Toronto, Ontario, Canada
Hip Dislocation: How Does Delay to Reduction Affect Avascular Necrosis Rate?; Combined Fractures of the Hip and Femoral Shaft: What Is the Best Treatment Method?; Intracapsular Femoral Neck Fracture: How Does Delay in Surgery Affect Complication Rate?; Should You Save or Substitute the Posterior Cruciate Ligament in Total Knee Replacement?

Johnny Tak-Choy Lau, MD, MSc, FRCSC
Assistant Professor, Department of Surgery, University of Toronto, Toronto, Ontario, Canada; Consultant Orthopaedic Surgeon, Department of Surgery, University Health Network, Toronto Western Division, Toronto, Ontario, Canada
What Is the Best Treatment for End-Stage Hallux Rigidus?

Constance M. Lebrun, MDCM, MPE, CCFP
Associate Professor, Faculty of Physical Education and Recreation, Faculty of Medicine and Dentistry, University of Alberta, Edmonton, Alberta, Canada; Director, Glen Sather Sports Medicine Clinic, University of Alberta, Edmonton, Alberta, Canada
What Are the Best Diagnostic Criteria for Lateral Epicondylitis?

Ross K. Leighton, BSc, MD, FRCSC, FACS
Professor of Surgery, Department of Surgery, Dalhousie University, Halifax, Nova Scotia, Canada; President, District Medical Staff Association, QEII Health Sciences Centre, Halifax, Nova Scotia, Canada
Are Bone Substitutes Useful in the Treatment and Prevention of Nonunions and in the Management of Subchondral Voids?; Supracondylar Femoral Fractures: Is a Locking Plate or a Nail Better?

André Leumann, MD
Foot and Ankle Clinic, Orthopaedic Department, University Hospital of Basel, Basel, Switzerland
What Is the Best Treatment for Ankle Osteochondral Lesions?

Isador Lieberman, MD, MBA, FRCS
Professor of Surgery, Cleveland Clinic Lerner College of Medicine, Cleveland, Ohio, USA; Chairman, Medical Interventional and Surgical Spine Center, Cleveland Clinic Florida, Weston, Florida, USA
Vertebral Augmentation: What Is the Role of Vertebroplasty and Kyphoplasty?

Allan S. L. Liew, MD, FRCSC
Assistant Professor, Surgery, University of Ottawa, Ottawa, Ontario, Canada
Subtrochanteric Femoral Fractures: Is a Nail or Plate Better?

Sheldon S. Lin, MD
Associate Professor, Department of Orthopaedic Surgery, New Jersey Medical School, University of Medicine and Dentistry of New Jersey, Newark, New Jersey, USA; Chief of Foot and Ankle, North Jersey Orthopedic Institute, Newark, New Jersey, USA
What Is the Best Treatment for Posterior Tibial Tendonitis?

Robert Litchfield, MD, FRCSC
Associate Professor, Department of Surgery, University of Western Ontario, London, Ontario, Canada; Medical Director, Fowler Kennedy Sport Medicine Clinic, London Health Sciences Centre, London, Ontario, Canada
Open versus Arthroscopic Repair for Shoulder Instability: What's Best?

Randall T. Loder, MD
Garceau Professor of Othopaedic Surgery, Vice Chairman, Department of Orthopaedic Surgery, Indiana University School of Medicine, Indianapolis, Indiana, USA; Chief of Orthopaedic Surgery, James Whitcomb Riley Hospital for Children, Indianapolis, Indiana, USA
What Is the Optimal Treatment for Slipped Capital Femoral Epiphysis?

Marcella A. W. Maathuis, MD
Medical Student, University of Groningen, Groningen, the Netherlands
Acetabular Fractures: Does Delay to Surgery Influence Outcome?

Joy C. MacDermid, PT, PhD
McMaster University School of Rehabilitation Science, McMaster University, Hamilton, Ontario, Canada; Co-Director, Clinical Research, Hand and Upper Limb Centre, St. Joseph's Health Centre, London, Ontario, Canada; New Investigator, Canadian Institute of Health Research, Canada
What Is the Optimal Rehabilitative Approach to Post-Traumatic Elbow Stiffness?

Steven J. MacDonald, MD, FRCSC
Associate Professor, Division of Orthopaedic Surgery, University of Western Ontario London, London, Ontario, Canada
Which Bearing Surface Should Be Used: Highly Cross-Linked Polyethylene versus Metal or Metal versus Ceramic on Ceramic?

Nizar N. Mahomed, MD, ScD, FRCSC
Associate Professor, Smith and Nephew Chair in Orthopaedic Surgery Research, Department of Surgery, University of Toronto; Director, Musculoskeletal Health and Arthritis Program, Department of Surgery, University Health Network; Toronto, Ontario, Canada
What Is the Role of Computer Navigation in Hip and Knee Arthroplasty?

Jacquelyn Marsh, BHSc
Health and Rehabilitative Science, University of Western Ontario, London, Ontario, Canada
Multiligament Knee Injury: Should Surgical Reconstruction Be Acute or Delayed?

Robert G. Marx, MD, MSc, FRCSC
Associate Professor, Orthopedic Surgery, Weill Medical College of Cornell University, New York, New York, USA; Associate Professor, Public Health, Weill Medical College of Cornell University, New York, New York, USA; Associate Attending Orthopedic Surgeon, Sports Medicine and Shoulder Service, Hospital for Special Surgery, New York, New York, USA; Director, Foster Center for Clinical

Outcome Research, Hospital for Special Surgery, New York, New York, USA
Is There a Role for Arthroscopy in the Treatment of Knee Osteoarthritis?

Bassam A. Masri, MD, FRCSC
Professor and Chairman, Department of Orthopaedics, University of British Columbia, Vancouver, British Columbia, Canada; Head, Department of Orthopaedics, Vancouver General and University of British Columbia Hospitals, Vancouver, British Columbia, Canada
Should the Patella Be Resurfaced in Total Knee Replacement?; How Do You Make a Diagnosis of an Infected Arthroplasty?

Steven J. McCabe, MD, MSc
Director of Decision Sciences, School of Public Health and Information Sciences, University of Louisville, Louisville, Kentucky, USA; Louisville Arm and Hand, Norton Healthcare, Louisville, Kentucky, USA
What Is the Best Surgical Procedure for Cubital Tunnel Syndrome?

Mark McCarthy, MSI
University of Minnesota Medical School, Duluth, Minnesota, USA
Total Hip Replacement: Hybrid versus Uncemented: Which Is Better?

Stuart A. McCluskey, MD, PhD, FRCPC
Assistant Professor, Anesthesia, University of Toronto, Toronto, Ontario, Canada; Medical Director, Perioperative Blood Conservation Program, Anesthesia and Pain Management, Toronto Western Hospital, University Health Network, Toronto, Ontario, Canada
What Blood Conservation Techniques for Total Joint Arthroplasty Work?

Jenny McConnell, B App Sci (Phty), Grad Dip, Man Ther, M Biomed Eng
Visiting Senior Fellow, Sports Medicine, University of Melbourne, Melbourne, Victoria, Australia; Director, McConnell and Clements Physiotherapy, Sydney, NSW, Australia
What Are Effective Therapies for Anterior Knee Pain?

Michael D. McKee, MD, FRCS(C)
Associate Professor, Department of Surgery, Division of Orthopaedics, University of Toronto, St. Michael's Hospital, Toronto, Ontario, Canada
What Is the Optimal Treatment of Displaced Midshaft Clavicle Fractures?; Fracture Healing: How Strong is the Effect of Smoking on Bone Healing?; Supracondylar Humeral Fractures: Is Open Reduction and Internal Fixation or Primary Total Elbow Arthroplasty Better in Poor Quality Bone?

Greg A. Merrell, MD
Indiana Hand Center, Indianapolis, Indiana, USA
What Is the Best Surgical Treatment for Early Degenerative Osteoarthritis of the Wrist?

William Mihalko, MD, PhD
Associate Professor, Department of Orthopaedic Surgery, Department of Mechanical and Aerospace Engineering, University of Virginia, Charlottesville, Virginia, USA; University of Virginia Health Science Center, Department of Orthopaedic Surgery, University of Virginia, Charlottesville, Virginia, USA
Total Hip Replacement: Hybrid versus Uncemented: Which Is Better?

Tom Minas, MD, MS
Associate Professor, Orthopaedic Surgery, Harvard Medical School, Boston, Massachusetts, USA; Director, Cartilage Repair Center, Orthopaedic Surgery, Brigham and Women's Hospital, Boston, Massachusetts, USA
What Is the Best Treatment for Chondral Defects in the Knee?

Shashank Misra, MBBS, DNB
Clinical Fellow, University of Toronto, Toronto, Ontario, Canada
Is Arthroscopic Rotator Cuff Repair Superior?

Kyle A. Mitsunaga, MD
Resident Physician, Department of Orthopaedic Surgery, University of California at Davis, Sacramento, California, USA
What Is the Best Method of Rehabilitation after Flexor Tendon Repair in Zone II: Passive Mobilization or Early Active Motion? What Is the Best Suture Configuration for Repair of Flexor Tendon Lacerations?

Berton R. Moed, MD
Professor and Chairman, Department of Orthopaedic Surgery, St. Louis University School of Medicine, St. Louis, Missouri, USA; Chief, Department of Orthopaedic Surgery, St. Louis University Hospital, St. Louis, Missouri, USA
What Is the Best Way to Prevent Heterotopic Ossification after Acetabular Fracture Fixation?

Nicholas G. Mohtadi, MSc
University of Calgary Division of Health Sciences, Calgary, Alberta, Canada
Autograft Choice in Anterior Cruciate Ligament Reconstruction: Should It Be Patellar Tendon or Hamstring Tendon?

Mohamed Maged Mokhimer, FRCS, Tr&Orth, MCh
Toronto University, Toronto, Ontario, Canada; St. Michael's Hospital, Orthopedic Surgery, Toronto, Ontario, Canada
What Is the Best Treatment for End-Stage Ankle Arthritis?

Mark S. Myerson, MD
Director, Institute for Foot and Ankle Reconstruction, Mercy Medical Center, Baltimore, Maryland, USA
What Is the Best Treatment for Injury to the Tarsometatarsal Joint Complex?

Unni G. Narayanan, MBBS, MSc, FRCSC
Assistant Professor, Department of Surgery, University of Toronto, Toronto, Ontario, Canada; Scientist, Bloorview Research Institute; Pediatric Orthopaedic Surgeon, The Hospital for Sick Children, Toronto, Ontario, Canada
What Is the Best Treatment for Ambulatory Cerebral Palsy?

Kenneth Noonan, MD
Associate Professor of Pediatric Orthopedics, Department of Orthopaedics and Rehabilitation,

University of Wisconsin, Madison, Wisconsin, USA; Department of Orthopaedics, St. Mary's Hospital, Madison, Wisconsin, USA; Department of Orthopaedics, Meriter Hospital, Madison, Wisconsin, USA
What Is the Best Treatment for Forearm Fractures?

Shahryar Noordin, MBBS, FCPS
Senior Instructor, Division of Orthopaedics, Department of Surgery, Aga Khan University, Karachi, Pakistan; Consultant Orthopaedic Surgeon, Aga Khan University, Karachi, Pakistan; Former Clinical Fellow, Paediatric Orthopaedic Surgery, The Hospital for Sick Children, University of Toronto, Toronto, Ontario, Canada
Muscular Dystrophy: How Should It Be Treated?

Peter J. O'Brien, MD, FRCSC
Associate Professor, Department of Orthopaedics, Faculty of Medicine, University of British Columbia, Vancouver, British Columbia, Canada; Head, Division of Orthopaedic Trauma, Department of Orthopaedics, Vancouver Coastal Health Authority, Vancouver, British Columbia, Canada
Damage Control Trauma Care: Does It Save Lives or Make No Difference?; What Is the Best Treatment for Pilon Fractures?

Brad A. Petrisor, MSc, MD, FRCSC
Assistant Professor, McMaster University, Hamilton, Ontario, Canada; Orthopaedic Trauma Surgeon, Hamilton Health Sciences, General Hospital, Hamilton, Ontario, Canada
What Is the Relation Between Malunion and Function for Lower Extremity Tibial Diaphyseal Fractures?

Stephen Pinney, MD, FRCSC
Associate Professor, Clinical Orthopaedics, Chief, Foot and Ankle Services, Department of Orthopaedics, University of California, San Francisco, San Francisco, California, USA
What Is the Best Treatment for Posterior Tibial Tendonitis?

Rudolf W. Poolman, MD, PhD
Consultant Orthopaedic Surgeon, Onze Lieve Vrouwe Gasthuis, Teaching Hospital with the University of Amsterdam, Amsterdam, The Netherlands
Femoral Shaft Fractures: What Is the Best Treatment?

James Powell, MD, FRCSC
Associate Clinical Professor, Department of Surgery, University of Calgary, Calgary, Alberta, Canada
What Is the Role for Hip Resurfacing Arthroplasty?

Atul Prabhu, MD
Assistant Professor, Anesthesia, University of Toronto, Toronto, Ontario, Canada; Medical Director, Perioperative Blood Conservation Program, Anesthesia and Pain Management, Toronto Western Hospital, University Health Network, Toronto, Ontario, Canada
What Blood Conservation Techniques for Total Joint Arthroplasty Work?

G Arun Prasad, MBBS, DA, FRCA
Clinical Fellow, Department of Anesthesia, Toronto Western Hospital, University Health Network, Toronto, Ontario, Canada; Specialist Registrar,
Stoke School of Anesthesia, Stoke on Trent, United Kingdom
Regional Anesthesia for Total Hip and Knee Arthroplasty: Is It Worth the Effort?

Quanjun Qui, MD, MS
Assistant Professor, Department of Orthopaedic Trauma, Adult Reconstruction, University of Virginia School of Medicine, Charlottesville, Virginia, USA
Total Hip Replacement: Hybrid versus Uncemented: Which is Better?

Y. Raja Rampersaud, MD, FRCSC
Assistant Professor, Divisions of Orthopaedics and Neurosurgery, Chairman, University of Toronto Spine Group, University of Toronto, University Health Network, Toronto, Ontario, Canada
Do Bone Morphogenetic Proteins Improve Spinal Fusion?

John S. Reach, Jr, MD, MSc
Director of Foot and Ankle Orthopaedic Surgery, Orthopaedic Surgery and Rehabilitation, Yale University School of Medicine, New Haven, Connecticut, USA
What Is the Best Treatment for Hallux Valgus?

Bill Regan, MD, FRCSC
Associate Professor, Department of Orthopaedics, University of British Columbia, Vancouver, British Columbia, Canada; Head, Division of Upper Extremity Surgery, Department of Orthopaedics, University of British Columbia, Vancouver, British Columbia, Canada; Associate Head, Department of Orthopaedics, University of British Columbia, Vancouver, British Columbia, Canada
What Are the Indications for Surgery, and What Is the Best Surgical Treatment for Chronic Lateral Epicondylitis?

Andreas Roposch, MD, MSc, FRCS
Honorary Reader in Orthopaedic Surgery and Clinical Epidemiology, Institute of Child Health, University College London, London, United Kingdom; Consultant Orthopaedic Surgeon, Department of Orthopaedic Surgery, Great Ormond Street Hospital for Sick Children, London, United Kingdom
What Is the Best Treatment for Developmental Dysplasia of the Hip?

Thomas A. Russell, MD
Department of Orthopaedic Surgery, Campbell Clinic, University of Tennessee, Memphis, Tennessee, USA
Are Bone Substitutes Useful in the Treatment and Prevention of Nonunions and in the Management of Subchondral Voids?

Khaled Saleh, MD, MSc, FRCSC, FACS
Professor, Department of Orthopaedic Surgery, Division Head, Adult Reconstructive Surgery, Fellowship Director, Adult Reconstruction, Professor, Department of Public Health Sciences, University of Virginia Health System, Charlottesville, Virginia, USA
Total Hip Replacement: Hybrid versus Uncemented: Which Is Better?

David W. Sanders, MD, MSc, FRCSc
Associate Professor, Department of Orthopaedic
Surgery, University of Western Ontario, London,
Ontario, Canada; Orthopaedic Surgeon, London
Health Sciences Centre, London, Ontario, Canada
Mangled Extremity: Are Scoring Systems Useful?

Emil H. Schemitsch, MD, FRCS(C)
Professor of Surgery, University of Toronto,
Toronto, Ontario, Canada; Head, Division of Or-
thopaedic Surgery, St. Michael's Hospital, Toronto,
Ontario, Canada
*Hip Dislocation: How Does Delay to Reduction Affect Avascular
Necrosis Rate?; Combined Fractures of the Hip and Femoral
Shaft: What Is the Best Treatment Method?; Intracapsular
Femoral Neck Fracture: How Does Delay in Surgery Affect
Complication Rate?; Should You Save or Substitute the
Posterior Cruciate Ligament in Total Knee Replacement?*

Ralph Schoeniger, MD
Orthopaedic Trauma Fellow, University of British
Columbia, Vancouver, British Columbia, Canada;
Attending, Department of Orthopaedic Surgery,
Spital Bern-Ziegler, Berne, Switzerland
*Damage Control Trauma Care: Does It Save Lives or Make No
Difference?*

Lew Schon, MD
Assistant Professor of Orthopaedic Surgery,
Department of Orthopaedic Surgery, The Johns
Hopkins University, Baltimore, Maryland, USA;
Director of Foot and Ankle Services, Department of
Orthopaedic Surgery, The Union Memorial Hospital,
Baltimore, Maryland, USA; Active Staff, Part-time,
Department of Orthopaedic Surgery, Johns Hopkins
Medical Institutions, Baltimore, Maryland, USA;
Clinical Associate Professor of Orthopaedic Surgery,
Department of Orthopaedic Surgery, Georgetown
University School of Medicine, Washington, DC
What Is the Best Treatment for a Charcot Foot and Ankle?

Fintan Shannon, MD
Fowler Kennedy Sport Medicine Clinic, University of
Western Ontario, London, Ontario, Canada
*Open versus Arthroscopic Repair for Shoulder Instability:
What's Best?*

Meena Shatby, MD
Orthopedic Foot and Ankle Fellow, Orthopedic
Surgery, Union Memorial Hospital, Baltimore,
Maryland, USA
What Is the Best Treatment for a Charcot Foot and Ankle?

Alexander Siegmeth, MD, FRCS (Tr & Orth)
Fellow, Adult Reconstruction, Department of
Orthopaedics, Vancouver General Hospital,
Vancouver, British Columbia, Canada
How Do You Make a Diagnosis of an Infected Arthroplasty?

Krzysztof Siemionow, MD
Resident, Orthopaedic Surgery, Cleveland Clinic,
Cleveland, Ohio, USA
*Vertebral Augmentation: What Is the Role of Vertebroplasty
and Kyphoplasty?*

Lyndsay Somerville, BSc, MSc
Health and Rehabilitative Science, University of
Western Ontario, London, Ontario, Canada
*Multiligament Knee Injury: Should Surgical Reconstruction Be
Acute or Delayed?*

Nelson Fong SooHoo, MD
Assistant Professor, Department of Orthopaedic
Surgery, UCLA School of Medicine, Los Angeles,
California, USA
What Is the Best Treatment for Plantar Fasciitis?

David John Garth Stephen, MD, FRCS(C)
Associate Professor, Department of Surgery,
University of Toronto, Toronto, Ontario, Canada;
Director of Orthopaedic Trauma, Department of
Surgery, Sunnybrook Health Sciences Centre,
Toronto, Ontario, Canada
*What Is the Appropriate Timing of Prophylactic Stabilization
of Osseous Metastases?; Acetabular Fractures: Does Delay
to Surgery Influence Outcome?*

Vineeta T. Swaroop, MD
Instructor of Clinical Orthopaedic Surgery, North-
western University Feinberg School of Medicine,
Chicago, Illinois, USA; Attending Pediatric
Orthopaedic Surgeon, Rehabilitation Institute of
Chicago, Chicago, Illinois, USA
*What Is the Optimal Treatment for Hip and Spine in
Myelomenigocele?*

Robert M. Szabo, MD, MPH
Professor of Orthopaedic Surgery, Professor of
Plastic Surgery, University of California at Davis
School of Medicine, Sacramento, California, USA;
Chief, Hand and Upper Extremity Service, Univer-
sity of California at Davis Health Care System,
Sacramento, California, USA
*What Is the Best Method of Rehabilitation after Flexor Tendon
Repair in Zone II: Passive Mobilization or Early Active
Motion? What Is the Best Suture Configuration for Repair
of Flexor Tendon Lacerations?*

Tim Theologis, MD, MSc, PhD, FRCS
Honorary Senior Clinical Lecturer, Clinical Medicine,
University of Oxford, Oxford, United Kingdom;
Consultant Orthopaedic Surgeon, Nuffield Ortho-
paedic Centre and Oxford Children's Hospital,
Oxford, United Kingdom
*What Is the Best Treatment for Growth Plate Injuries?; What Is
the Best Treatment for Hip Displacement in Nonambulatory
Patients with Cerebal Palsy?*

Kelly Trask, MSc
Research Engineering Associate, Department of Or-
thopaedic Surgery, QEII Health Sciences Centre,
Halifax, Nova Scotia, Canada
*Are Bone Substitutes Useful in the Treatment and Prevention
of Nonunions and in the Management of
Subchondral Voids?; Supracondylar Femoral Fractures: Is a
Locking Plate or a Nail Better?*

Hans-Joerg Trnka, MD
Department of Orthopaedics, University Clinic of
  Vienna, Vienna, Austria; Department of Surgery,
  Krankenhaus Gottlicher Heiland, Vienna, Austria;
  Fusszentrum Wien, Vienna, Austria
  What Is the Best Treatment for Hallux Valgus?

Victor Valderrabano, MD, PhD
Foot and Ankle Clinic, Orthopaedic Department,
  University Hospital of Basel, Basel, Switzerland
  What Is the Best Treatment for Ankle Osteochondral Lesions?

**Andrew Wainwright, BSc (Hons), MB, ChB, FRCS
(Tr and Orth)**
Honorary Senior Lecturer, Nuffield Department of
  Orthopaedics, University of Oxford, Oxford,
  United Kingdom; Consultant Orthopaedic Surgeon,
  Paediatric Orthopaedics, Nuffield Orthopaedic
  Centre, Oxford, United Kingdom
  *What Is the Best Treatment for Growth Plate Injuries?; What Is
    the Best Treatment for Hip Displacement in Nonambulatory
    Patients with Cerebal Palsy?*

Donald Weber, MD, BSc, FRCSC
Associate Clinical Professor, Chief, Department of
  Orthopaedic Surgery, University of Alberta,
  Edmonton, Alberta, Canada
  What Is the Best Treatment for Open Fractures?

Stuart L. Weinstein, MD
Ignacid V. Ponseti Chair and Professor of Orthopaedic
  Surgery, University of Iowa, Iowa City, Iowa, USA
  *Best Treatment for Adolescent Idiopathic Scoliosis: What Do
    Current Systematic Reviews Tell Us?*

Arnold-Peter C. Weiss, MD
Professor and Assistant Dean of Medicine
  (Admissions), Department of Orthopaedics,
  The Warren Albert Medical School of Brown
  University, Providence, Rhode Island, USA; Hand
  Surgeon, Orthopaedics, Rhode Island Hospital,
  Providence, Rhode Island, USA
  *What Is the Best Surgical Treatment for Early Degenerative
    Osteoarthritis of the Wrist?*

Iris Weller, MSc, PhD
Assistant Professor, Institute of Medical Science,
  Department of Surgery, Rehabilitation Science,
  Public Health Sciences, University of Toronto,
  Toronto, Ontario, Canada; Epidemiologist, Holland
  Muscoloskeletal Program, Sunnybrook Health
  Sciences Centre, Toronto, Ontario, Canada
  *Does the Type of Hospital in Which a Patient Is Treated Affect
    Outcomes in Orthopedic Patients?*

Daniel Whelan, MD, MSc, FRCS(C)
Assistant Professor, Department of Surgery, University
  of Toronto, Toronto, Ontario, Canada; Orthopaedic
  Staff Surgeon, Department of Surgery, St. Michael's
  Hospital, Toronto, Ontario, Canada

  *Autograft Choice in Anterior Cruciate Ligament Reconstruction:
    Should It Be Patellar Tendon or Hamstring Tendon?; Should
    First-Time Shoulder Dislocators Be Stabilized Surgically?*

R. Baxter Willis, MD, FRCSC
Professor, Department of Surgery, University of
  Ottawa, Ottawa, Ontario, Canada; Chief of Surgery,
  Children's Hospital of Eastern Ontario, Ottawa,
  Ontario, Canada
  *What Is the Best Treatment for Anterior Cruciate Ligament
    Injuries in Skeletally Immature Individuals?*

Praveen Yalamanchili, MD, FRCSC
Resident, Department of Orthopaedic Surgery,
  University Hospital, New Jersey Medical School,
  Newark, New Jersey, USA
  What Is the Best Treatment for Posterior Tibial Tendonitis?

Suzanne Yandow, MD
Department of Pediatric Orthopaedics,
  Dell's Children's Hospital, Austin, Texas, USA
  What Is the Best Treatment for Simple Bone Cysts?

Albert J. M. Yee, MD, MSc, FRCSC
Associate Professor, Department of Surgery, University
  of Toronto, Toronto, Ontario, Canada; Active Staff,
  Division of Orthopaedic Surgery, Sunnybrook Health
  Sciences Centre, Toronto, Ontario, Canada
  *What Is the Optimal Treatment for Degenerative Lumbar
    Spinal Stenosis?*

Erik L. Yeo, MD, FRCPC
Associate Professor, Division of Haematology,
  Department of Medicine, University of Toronto,
  Toronto, Ontario, Canada; Director of Thrombosis,
  Toronto General Hospital, University Hospital
  Network, Toronto, Ontario, Canada
  *Should Thromboprophylaxis Be Used for Lower Limb Joint
    Replacement Surgery?*

Alastair Younger, MB, ChB, FRCSC, MSc, ChM
Clinical Associate Professor, Division of Lower
  Extremity Reconstruction and Oncology,
  Department of Orthopaedics, University of British
  Columbia, Vancouver, British Columbia, Canada;
  Director, British Columbia's Foot and Ankle Clinic,
  Providence Health Care, St. Paul's Hospital,
  Vancouver, British Columbia, Canada
  What Is the Best Treatment for Recurrent Ankle Instability?

Joseph D. Zuckerman, MD
Walter A. L. Thompson Professor and Chair,
  Orthopaedic Surgery, New York University
  School of Medicine, New York, New York, USA;
  Surgeon-in-Chief, NYU Hospital for Joint Diseases,
  New York, New York, USA
  *What Is the Best Treatment for Proximal Humeral Fractures?
    What Are the Main Determinants of Outcome after
    Arthroplasty?*

Contents

An Introduction to Evidence-Based Orthopaedics

JAMES G. WRIGHT, MD, MPH, FRCSC

Evidence-based medicine has been defined as "the conscientious, explicit, and judicious use of the current best evidence in making decisions about the care of individual patients. The practice of evidence-based medicine means integrating individual clinical expertise with the best available external clinical evidence from systematic research."[1] More recently, evidence-based medicine has been described as the "integration of best research evidence with clinical expertise and patient values."[2]

These definitions are consistent with most orthopedic surgeons' practice. Surgeons rely on evidence in making clinical decisions. Surgeons often critically appraise the surgical literature and integrate the evidence with their clinical expertise to make decisions with their patients. Surgeons, however, may not perform evidence-based medicine in a systematic fashion and may struggle with what constitutes the best evidence. The purpose of this chapter is to introduce the principles of evidence-based practice, to briefly describe the practical steps of evidence-based practice, and to discuss what constitutes the "best" evidence.

The evidence cycle has been conceptualized as the five As: (1) assess, (2) ask, (3) acquire, (4) appraise, and (5) apply.[2–4] *Assess* refers to the clinical situation such as a child in the office or a young adult in the trauma room. *Ask* refers to the inevitable questions: What is wrong with this patient (diagnosis)? What is the likely outcome for this patient (prognosis)? How can we intervene to improve the outcome (therapeutics)? *Acquire* refers to gathering the information necessary to make clinical decisions. Sources of information include training, past experience, colleagues, experts, textbooks, the Internet, practice guidelines, systematic overviews, and the surgical literature. *Appraise* refers to critically appraising the information to develop a set of possible options. *Apply* refers to the final step of deciding with the patient which option to apply.

In addressing clinical questions, a useful acronym is PICO (Patients, Intervention, Comparison, and Outcome): what patients are of concern, what treatment is proposed, what are the alternatives, and what are the outcomes.[4,5] For example, in a 70-year-old healthy woman with a displaced subcapital fracture (Patient), is hemiarthroplasty (Intervention) better than reduction and internal fixation (Comparison) for long-term function (Outcome)? For every clinical question, however, there may be multiple treatment options and multiple possible outcomes and/or complications. To arrive at the best decision, you must answer all these questions.

Acquiring the evidence is a critical step. Although for some questions, training, experience, clinical experts, and colleagues may all agree (e.g., hip fractures in healthy patients require operative treatment), for many clinical decisions, opinions vary on the appropriate surgical option. Thus, other sources of information must guide treatment decisions. Textbooks are convenient but may be out of date or suffer the biases of the individual author. Practice guidelines, if current, comprehensive, systematic, and evidence based, may be a rapid approach to useful treatment recommendations.[6] However, practice guidelines may not be available or evidence based. Systematic overviews, such as the Cochrane database,[7] may address some clinical questions. The Cochrane database, however, relies almost exclusively on randomized trials and, therefore, does not provide answers for most orthopedic questions. When these sources of information are not available, the surgical literature may be the only source for the "best" evidence.

Acquiring the appropriate surgical literature raises multiple issues including which databases should be used, which years should be accessed, what languages should be searched, and how the search strategy should be constructed.[8]

In general, Medline is a good start, but a comprehensive search strategy should also include other databases such as Embase. Because the quality of literature has improved with time, and for feasibility reasons, searches are often restricted to the last 20 years. The quality of the literature does not appear to depend on the language of publication. Therefore, searches should not be restricted to English, but inevitably will be limited by translation ability. Finally, the search strategy should be developed with a librarian or evidence analyst.

Determining the best evidence is the most controversial aspect of evidence-based practice. If all evidence is in agreement, then determining the "best" literature is unnecessary. However, individual studies frequently contradict; therefore, the evidence must be evaluated to determine which study or studies provide the best answer. The determination of the best literature is usually based on the design of the study and the absence of bias.

In a few circumstances, case series have provided major advances in orthopedics. For example, John Charnley's[9] original publication on cemented total hip arthroplasty was so obviously superior to prior techniques that a randomized trial was not needed. In recent times, Ponseti's[10] treatment of clubfoot is so obviously superior to extensive clubfoot release that a randomized trial is not needed. However, in most clinical conditions, case series do not provide definitive answers. The multitude of case series in orthopedics has led to many treatment options with little clear direction for surgeons and patients.

Several aspects of study design make the results more credible. Levels of evidence are a rapid approach to evaluating study quality.[11] The first step in assigning a level of evidence is to determine the primary research question. The second step is to determine the study type: therapeutic, prognostic, diagnostic, and economic or decision analyses. The third step is to assign a level from I to V. Levels of evidence, used throughout this book, are simple methods that rely on the general principles that controlled are generally better than uncontrolled, prospective are generally better than retrospective, and randomized are generally better than nonrandomized studies.[12] Levels of evidence have been shown to be reliable, but the reliability is dependent on the level of research training.[13] Grades of recommendation, based on levels of evidence, summarize a body of literature.[14,15] Although several have been described,[16] *Journal of Bone and Joint Surgery American* (JBJS) assigns a grade A for good evidence (consistent Level I evidence), grade B for fair evidence (consistent Levels II and III evidence), grade C for poor evidence (consistent Levels IV and V evidence), and grade I (for insufficient or conflicting evidence). The JBJS levels of evidence and grade of recommendations are used in this book (Tables I–1 and I–2). Levels of evidence and grades of recommendation, however, provide only a simplistic measure of study quality. For example, a well-done, prospective Level II study may be of better or equal quality to a poorly performed randomized, controlled trial.[17,18] A full critical appraisal is necessary to completely evaluate a study.

Although beyond the scope of this chapter,[19] a complete critical appraisal must consider several critical elements of study design to reduce bias. First, the study population must be explicitly defined. Without this step, surgeons will be uncertain to whom the study results apply. Second, important baseline characteristics of the study population must be collected. Such information is needed to interpret differences in outcome between the treatment and comparison groups. Third, the study must specify why patients were treated in a particular fashion. For example, if sicker and older patients predominantly receive nonoperative treatment, surgery will always have better outcomes. Ensuring patients are similar in every way other than treatment received is the rationale for randomization. Fourth, randomization, if performed, must ensure that treatment assignment is not known. For example, alternate days or hospital numbers are inappropriate means of randomization because treating physicians who know treatment assignment may direct patients to particular treatments. Fifth, the interventions must be applied in a consistent, explicit, standardized, and proficient manner. Sixth, all patients need to be followed up or accounted for. Seventh, the patient, assessor, and ideally also the surgeon and analyst should be blind to the treatment received. Eighth, the sample size and statistical analysis plan needs to be developed in advance of study initiation. Ninth, patients' outcomes must be analyzed according to the treatment they were assigned (not the treatment they actually received). This principle of analyses, called *intention to treat,* is controversial. However, patients who do not comply with treatment recommendations are different than those who do; therefore, analysis by treatment actually received will lead to biased estimates of treatment effectiveness. Several formal methods are available to evaluate the quality of a clinical trial and the completeness of reporting. The Consolidated Standards of Reporting Trials (CONSORT) criteria are the most commonly used but are not ideal for surgical trials.[20,21] The more recently developed Checklist to Evaluate a Report of a Nonpharmacologic Trial (CLEAR NPT) criteria are more appropriate for surgical trials.[22]

The number of randomized trials in orthopedics is relatively low.[23] Evidence-based medicine relies almost exclusively on methodologically rigorous randomized trials, so how do surgeons make decisions without randomized trials? Although randomized trials or meta-analysis generally represent the best evidence, well-done nonrandomized trials may provide the same or sometimes even better evidence.[18,19] Furthermore, no single study definitively answers any clinical question. The editors of this book assert that controlled studies are probably a minimum requirement for best evidence, and that uncontrolled studies, or case series, seldom answer a clinical question definitively.

It would be apparent to most readers that the time required to identify all appropriate literature exceeds the capacity of busy surgeons. Furthermore, detailed critical analyses, assessment of bias, and interpretation of statistical analyses would be difficult for most surgeons. This book has used the evidence cycle and thereby will hopefully address, using the "best" evidence, those clinical questions of interest to surgeons. As the quality of studies continues to improve in orthopedics, surgeons will be increasingly required to use the principles of evidence-based orthopedics to identify the best evidence to make decisions with patients.

TABLE 1–1. Grades of Recommendation for Summaries or Reviews of Orthopedic Surgical Studies

A: Good evidence (Level I studies with consistent findings) for or against recommending intervention
B: Fair evidence (Level II or III studies with consistent findings) for or against recommending intervention
C: Poor-quality evidence (Level IV or V studies) not allowing a recommendation for or against intervention
I: There is insufficient evidence to make a recommendation

TABLE 1–2. Levels of Evidence for Primary Research Question

Types of Studies

	THERAPEUTIC STUDIES—INVESTIGATING THE RESULTS OF TREATMENT	PROGNOSTIC STUDIES—INVESTIGATING THE EFFECT OF A PATIENT CHARACTERISTIC ON THE OUTCOME OF DISEASE	DIAGNOSTIC STUDIES—INVESTIGATING A DIAGNOSTIC TEST	ECONOMIC AND DECISION ANALYSES—DEVELOPING AN ECONOMIC OR DECISION MODEL
Level I	• High-quality, randomized, controlled trial with statistically significant difference or no statistically significant difference but narrow confidence intervals • Systematic review* of Level I randomized, controlled trials (and study results were homogeneous†)	• High-quality, prospective study‡ (all patients were enrolled at the same point in their disease with ≥80% follow-up of enrolled patients) • Systematic review* of Level I studies	• Testing of previously developed diagnostic criteria in series of consecutive patients (with universally applied reference "gold" standard) • Systematic review* of Level I studies	• Sensible costs and alternatives; values obtained from many studies; multiway sensitivity analyses • Systematic review* of Level I studies
Level II	• Lesser-quality, randomized, controlled trial (e.g., <80% follow-up, no blinding, or improper randomization) • Prospective‡ comparative study§ • Systematic review* of Level II studies or Level I studies with inconsistent results	• Retrospective¶ study • Untreated control subjects from a randomized, controlled trial • Lesser-quality prospective study (e.g., patients enrolled at different points in their disease or <80% follow-up) • Systematic review* of Level II studies	• Development of diagnostic criteria on basis of consecutive patients (with universally applied reference "gold" standard) • Systematic review* of Level II studies	• Sensible costs and alternatives; values obtained from limited studies; multiway sensitivity analyses • Systematic review* of Level II studies
Level III	• Case–control study¶ • Retrospective¶ comparative study§ • Systematic review* of Level III studies	• Case–control study¶	• Study of nonconsecutive patients (without consistently applied reference "gold" standard) • Systematic review* of Level III studies	• Analyses based on limited alternatives and costs; poor estimates • Systematic review* of Level III studies
Level IV	Case series	Case series	• Case–control study¶ • Poor reference standard	• No sensitivity analyses
Level V	Expert opinion	Expert opinion	Expert opinion	Expert opinion

A complete assessment of the quality of individual studies requires critical appraisal of all aspects of the study design.
*A combination of results from two or more prior studies.
†Studies provided consistent results.
‡Study was started before the first patient enrolled.
§Patients treated one way (e.g., with cemented hip arthroplasty) compared with patients treated another way (e.g., with cementless hip arthroplasty) at the same institution.
¶Study was started after the first patient enrolled.
¶Patients identified for the study on the basis of their outcome (e.g., failed total hip arthroplasty), called *cases*, are compared with those who did not have the outcome (e.g., had a successful total hip arthroplasty), called *controls*.
**Patients treated one way with no comparison group of patients treated another way.
Adapted from material published by the Centre for Evidence-Based Medicine, Oxford, United Kingdom (for more information, see www.cebm.net).

REFERENCES

1. Sackett DL, Rosenberg WM, Gray JA, et al: Evidence based medicine: What it is and what it isn't. BMJ 312:71–72, 1996.
2. Sackett DL, Richardson WS, Rosenberg W, et al: Evidence-based medicine. How to practice and teach EBM, 2nd ed. London: Churchill Livingstone, 2000.
3. Guyatt GH, Rennie D, The Evidence-Based Medicine Working Group: Users' guides to the medical literature: A manual for evidence-based clinical practice. Chicago, AMA Press, 2002.
4. Poolman RW, Kerkhoffs GM, Struijs PA, et al: Don't be misled by the orthopaedic literature: Tips for critical appraisal. Acta Orthop Scand 78:162–171, 2007.
5. Richardson WS, Wilson MD, Nishikawa J, Haward RS: The well-built clinical question: A key to evidence-based decisions. ACP J Club 123:A12–A13, 1995.
6. National Guideline Clearinghouse on line: Available at: www.guideline.gov
7. The Cochrane Collaboration on line: Available at: www.cochrane.org
8. Center for Evidence-Based Medicine on line: Available at: www.cebm.net
9. Charnley J, Cupic Z: The nine and ten year results of the low-friction arthroplasty of the hip. Clin Orthop Relat Res 95:9–25, 1973.
10. Ponseti IV: Treatment of congenital club foot. J Bone Joint Surg Am 74:448–454, 1992.
11. Wright JG: A practical guide to assigning levels of evidence. J Bone Joint Surg Am 89:1128–1130, 2007.
12. Wright JG, Swiontkowski MF, Heckman JD: Introducing levels of evidence to the journal. J Bone Joint Surg Am 85-A:1–3, 2003.
13. Bhandari M, Swiontkowski MF, Einhorn TA, et al: Interobserver agreement in the application of levels of evidence to scientific papers in the American volume of the Journal of Bone and Joint Surgery. J Bone Joint Surg Am 86-A:1717–1720, 2004.
14. Wright JG, Einhorn TA, Heckman JD: Grades of recommendation. J Bone Joint Surg Am 87:1909–1910, 2005.
15. Wright JG: Revised grades of recommendation for summaries or reviews of orthopaedic surgical studies. J Bone Joint Surg Am 88-A:1161–1162, 2006.
16. Guyatt G, Schuneman HG, Cook DJ, et al: Grades of recommendation for antithrombotic agents. Chest 119(suppl):3–7, 2001.
17. Concato J, Horwitz RI: Beyond randomised versus observational studies. Lancet 363:1660–1661, 2004.
18. Concato J, Shah N, Horwitz RI: Randomized, controlled trials, observational studies, and the hierarchy of research designs. N Engl J Med 342:1887–1892, 2000.
19. Haynes RB, Sackett DL, Guyatt GH: Clinical epidemiology: How to do clinical practice research with CDROM, 3rd ed. Philadelphia, Lippincott Williams & Wilkins, 2005.
20. Moher D, Schulz KF, Altman D, CONSORT Group: (Consolidated Standards of Reporting Trials): The CONSORT statement: Revised recommendations for improving the quality of reports of parallel-group randomized trials. JAMA 285:1987–1991, 2001.
21. Altman DG, Schulz KF, Moher D, et al: The revised CONSORT statement for reporting randomized trials: Explanation and elaboration. Ann Intern Med 134:663–694, 2001.
22. Boutron I, Moher D, Tugwell P, et al: A checklist to evaluate a report of a nonpharmacological trials (CLEAR NPT) was developed using consensus. J Clin Epidemiol 58:1233–1240, 2005.
23. Bhandari M, Richards RR, Sprague S, Schemitsch EH: The quality of reporting of randomized trials in the Journal of Bone and Joint Surgery from 1988 through 2000. J Bone Joint Surg Am 84:388–396, 2004.

SPINAL TOPICS

Should Patients with Acute Spinal Cord Injuries Receive Steroids?

Steven Casha, MD, PhD, FRCSC and R. John Hurlbert, MD, PhD, FRCSC, FACS

The annual incidence of spinal cord injuries (SCIs) is estimated between 11.5 and 53.4 per 1 million people,[1–8] and prevalence is estimated at around 700 SCI cases per 1 million people in the United States.[9] These injuries are characterized by high mortality and morbidity rates. In those individuals who survive to arrive at an acute care institution, mortality rates range between 4.4% and 16.7%.[3,5,8] These survivors typically experience prolonged hospitalization in acute care hospitals and rehabilitation centers.[8,10] Patients are typically young (mean and median ages ranging in the late 20s and early 30s) and male (80–85% of patients).[8] Approximately 45% of patients experience a complete neurologic injury with no detectable neurologic function below the level of the lesion.[11] Fifty-five percent of patients are injured between C1 and C7-T1.[8] Hospital admissions of a week or longer are necessary for approximately 10% of patients with SCI every year because of complications including pressure sores, autonomic dysreflexia, pneumonia, atelectasis, deep venous thrombosis, and renal calculi.[12–14] Spasticity and pain also add significantly to neurologic disability in 25% of patients.[12] Long-term reduced life expectancy is largely accounted for by pneumonia, pulmonary emboli, and septicemia. Furthermore, the financial burden of managing these injuries both to the individual and to society is enormous. The estimated cost to the United States for care of all patients with SCI in 1990 was $4 billion.[8]

Accordingly, therapies that limit the extent of neurologic dysfunction after SCI (neuroprotection) or that improve recovery of function (neuroregeneration and neuroaugmentation) would have a huge impact on this patient population. Significant research interest in these strategies has identified many potential therapeutic targets in animal models. Of these, several have been applied to high-quality human investigations. Unfortunately, none has been proved effective in humans. The American Association of Neurological Surgeons and Congress of Neurological Surgeons Joint Section on Disorders of the Spine and Peripheral Nerves' 2002 *Guidelines for the Management of Acute Cervical Spine and Spinal Cord Injury*[15] specifically recognizes methylprednisolone and GM-1 ganglioside as options for treatment in patients with acute SCI. However, these options were qualified "without demonstrated clinical benefit" in the case of GM-1 ganglioside

and with "evidence suggesting harmful side effects" that is more consistent than any suggestion of clinical benefit in the case of methylprednisolone. Tirilazad and naloxone have also been studied in humans but without any evidence of efficacy to warrant inclusion in the guidelines.

This chapter attempts to critically review the evidence for use of methylprednisolone and other corticosteroids in the treatment of human SCI. The discussion focuses on human studies; a wealth of animal studies that preceded the study of these medications in humans is beyond the scope of this chapter.

METHYLPREDNISOLONE AND OTHER CORTICOSTEROIDS IN SPINAL CORD INJURY

Steroids in various forms have been used in the treatment of SCI for many years. Historically, the rationale for the use of corticosteroids in the management of neural trauma extended from their use in decreasing edema in the management of brain tumors. In addition, their anti-inflammatory effect was thought to be beneficial to the secondary injury pathophysiology of SCI. Studies in dogs supported these hypotheses and demonstrated a modest improvement in neurologic outcome with steroid treatment and a modified anti-inflammatory response.[16] Subsequently, other animal studies have provided support for improved neurologic recovery after SCI in animal models when methylprednisolone is administered and have provided evidence for inhibition of lipid peroxidation, protection of energy metabolism, reduced post-traumatic ischemia, maintenance of neurofilament structure, and decreased post-traumatic ionic shifts.[17]

The role of steroids in human SCI management became more rigorously considered after publication of the Second National Acute Spinal Cord Injury Study (NASCIS II). Unfortunately, the initial enthusiasm for an apparent positive effect of methylprednisolone in SCI demonstrated by NASCIS II has not stood up to the extensive scrutiny that ensued.[18–21] However, despite significant criticism, this medication continues to be prescribed by many physicians, and a 2002 study suggests that most practitioners prescribe it because of peer pressure or fear of litigation, rather than a firm belief that it is indeed efficacious.[22]

The first NASCIS study compared low- (100 mg/day × 10 days) and high-dose (1000 mg/day × 10 days) methylprednisolone, and did not include a placebo group.[23] It failed to demonstrate a difference between the doses tested. The high-dose group exhibited an increased risk for complications. That study was followed by a randomized, controlled trial comparing a 24-hour protocol (30 mg/kg methylprednisolone bolus followed by 5.4 mg/hg/hr until 24 hours) with placebo in NASCIS II.[24,25] The dose selected in NASCIS II was greater than that of the original study because of further animal work that suggested a therapeutic threshold of 30 mg/kg.[25] NASCIS II concluded that improved neurologic recovery was seen when the methylprednisolone treatment protocol was initiated within 8 hours of injury. That study was then followed by NASCIS III, which compared patients randomized to the 24-hour NASCIS II protocol with those randomized to a 48-hour protocol (5.4 mg/kg/hr methylprednisolone after the 30-mg/kg bolus).[26,27] That study concluded that patients for whom therapy was initiated within 3 hours did not gain any benefit from extending treatment to 48 hours, whereas those for whom therapy was initiated between 3 and 8 hours did benefit further. No benefit has been shown if therapy is initiated beyond 8 hours in NASCIS II.

Both the NASCIS II and NASCIS III trials were well designed and executed. However, closer scrutiny demonstrates that the primary analyses of methylprednisolone treatment effect were negative in both studies. The stated conclusions were based on post hoc analyses that suggested minor treatment effects on motor scores at 1 year and when therapy was initiated in the 8- and 3- to 8-hour windows identified in NASCIS II and III, respectively (statistical probability was slightly greater than 0.05 for 1-year motor scores in the NASCIS III 48-hour steroid group). None of the sensory scores was different between treatment groups in either study.

Several concerns have arisen regarding the post hoc analyses of NASCIS II and III. The left-sided motor scores were not published but reported "similar" to right-sided scores. Thus, half the available data were excluded. The statistical analyses failed to correct for multiple statistical comparisons, and it is unclear whether the repeated-measures design was considered. More than 65 methylprednisolone-related *t* tests were performed in NASCIS II, and more than 100 *t* tests in NASCIS III. There was, therefore, a high likelihood of type I error (erroneously detecting a statistical difference that does not exist) through random chance. The rationale for an 8-hour subanalysis (NASCIC II) is unclear. It has been claimed that this subgroup was selected based on median time to treatment. However, by definition, 50% of patients should have initiated treatment before the median time of treatment initiation. In fact, only 38% of patients (183/487) were included in this post hoc analysis. The justification for the 3- and 8-hour windows in NASCIS III is similarly obscure. Other observations raise concern about imposing these artificial time-related stratifications. For example, in NASCIS II, the incompletely injured placebo group when separated into <8- and >8-hour gr-oups differs in recovery, with the latter group showing improved recovery comparable with the <8-hour incompletely injured methylprednisolone group.[17] This implies that these patients could be treated with placebo beyond 8 hours and a similar result to treatment with methylprednisolone initiated within 8 hours can be expected. Finally, another common criticism of the NASCIS studies has been the lack of outcomes assessing functional recovery meaningful to the patient's expected activities.

In addition to the NASCIS studies, Otani and colleagues[28] published a prospective, randomized trial investigating the NASCIS II methylprednisolone dosing protocol. The investigators were not blinded to treatment, and the control group was allowed to receive alternate steroids at the physicians' discretion. Of 158 patients entered, 117 were analyzed. The primary outcome measures (American Spinal Injury Association [ASIA] motor and sensory scores) were not different between treatment groups. Post hoc analyses suggested that more patients improved on the NASCIS II steroid regimen compared with control patients. However, for a greater number of steroid-treated patients to improve, the fewer control patients who also improved must have demonstrated a larger magnitude of recovery (because overall ASIA motor and sensory scores were no different between groups). Thus, such post hoc analyses become difficult to interpret in the face of a negative overall effect.

A retrospective study with concurrent case controls also suggested a benefit with corticosteroid administration.[29] This study investigated the use of dexamethasone initiated within 24 hours of injury with the specific dose left to the discretion of the attending physicians. Length of follow-up was not specified, and a new but unvalidated neurologic grading system was used for outcome assessment. This study reports that the percentage of patients who improved was significantly greater in the steroid-treated group. However, there was a much greater mortality rate within the control group, suggesting a selection bias to more severely injured patients in the control arm. The magnitude of the mortality rate is also a concern and suggests that the study population may not be representative and that the results are not generalizable.

A randomized, controlled trial designed to examine the potential therapeutic benefit of nimodipine (a calcium channel antagonist) included an NASCIS II methylprednisolone regimen and a placebo group.[30,31] This study, which included approximately 25 patients in each group, failed to show any difference between any of four groups (placebo, nimodipine, methylprednisolone, methylprednisolone and nimodipine) using ASIA scores and ASIA grade outcomes. However, this study was remarkable for an increase in infectious complications in the methylprednisolone group.

Most recently, the data from the five randomized trials of methylprednisolone (NASCIS, NASCIS II, NASCIS III, Otani and colleagues,[28] and Pointillart and coworkers[31]) were subject to a meta-analysis and concluded that high-dose methylprednisolone given within 8 hours of acute SCI is safe and modestly effective. This article estimated a treatment effect of 4.1 motor score points (from ASIA score) over placebo treatment (using the NASCIS II 24-hour protocol). The findings and limitations of the individual articles included in this review are discussed earlier in this chapter (Table 1–1).

It must also be recognized that corticosteroid administration comes with increased risk for several potential adverse events including pneumonia, sepsis, and steroid-induced myopathy, all of which may negatively impact outcome in patients with SCI, potentially overshadowing any unproven beneficial effect.[32] Galandiuk and colleagues[33] demonstrate that patients with SCI treated with corticosteroids exhibited a greater rate of pneumonia (79% vs. 50% with placebo treatment) and required a longer hospital stay (44.4 vs. 27.7 days with placebo treatment). Matsumoto and coauthors[34] specifically investigated the complication rate in patients treated with the NASCIS II protocol compared with placebo in a small randomized trial. They found a nonstatistically significant trend to greater complication rates with steroid treatment overall, but a significant difference in respiratory and gastrointestinal complications. The majority of these complications were pneumonia and gastric ulcer, respectively. NASCIS II did not find an increased complication rate with steroid treatment, but NASCIS III reported a greater rate of sepsis and pulmonary complications particularly with the 48-hour infusion. The Corticosteroid Randomization after Significant Head Injury (CRASH) trial investigated the use of a corticosteroid regimen similar to that used in NASCIS II in the setting of closed head injury.[35] It demonstrated increased mortality with steroid use in that population. One must certainly recognize the possibly of an increased mortality risk in patients with SCI as well. However, it must also be noted that Sauerland and colleagues[36] performed a large meta-analysis review of approximately 2500 patients treated with preoperative high-dose steroids (>15 mg/kg methylprednisolone) and found no evidence of increased risk for gastrointestinal bleeding, wound complications, pulmonary complications, or death. They suggest that some reports that claim increased complication rates with high-dose steroid use were subject to selection bias.

CONCLUSIONS

In summary, although well-designed and executed studies have been performed, they have failed to demonstrate convincingly a beneficial effect of methylprednisolone or other corticosteroids in the management of SCI. Post hoc analyses have been used to argue a small effect on motor function in three randomized trials. However, all of these analyses contain significant flaws rendering conclusions of efficacy dubious. These observations have led two national organizations to publish guidelines recommending methylprednisolone administration as a treatment option rather than as a standard of care or recommended treatment (Table 1–2).[15,37]

TABLE 1–1. Human Clinical Trials in Spinal Cord Injury Investigating Methylprednisolone and Other Corticosteroids

AUTHOR	YEAR	DESIGN	AGENT	REPORTED RESULT
Bracken et al.[23] (NASCIS I)	1984	Prospective, randomized, double blind	Methylprednisolone	Negative
Bracken et al.[24,25] (NASCIS II)	1990, 1992	Prospective, randomized, double blind	Methylprednisolone	Positive
Bracken et al.[26,27] (NASCIS III)	1997, 1998	Prospective, randomized, double blind	Methylprednisolone	Positive
Otani et al.[28]	1994	Prospective, randomized, no blinding	Methylprednisolone	Positive
Pointillart et al.[31]	2000	Prospective, randomized, blinded	Methylprednisolone	Negative
Kiwerski[29]	1993	Retrospective, concurrent case–control	Dexamethasone	Positive

TABLE 1–2. Summary of Recommendations

STATEMENT	LEVEL OF EVIDENCE/GRADE OF RECOMMENDATION	REFERENCES
1. Corticosteroids are a treatment option in the management of acute spinal cord injury without proven benefit.	A	23–25, 28, 30, 31
2. Corticosteroids used in the setting of acute spinal cord injury increase complications.	A	23, 26, 30, 31, 33, 34

*Although data are available from level 1 publications, this item was not the main focus of these articles and the studies were not necessarily powered to address this issue.

REFERENCES

1. Botterell EH, Jousse AT, Kraus AS, et al: A model for the future care of acute spinal cord injuries. Can J Neurol Sci 2:361–380, 1975.
2. Gjone R, Nordlie L: Incidence of traumatic paraplegia and tetraplegia in Norway: A statistical survey of the years 1974 and 1975. Paraplegia 16:88–93, 1978.
3. Kraus JF, Franti CE, Riggins RS, et al: Incidence of traumatic spinal cord lesions. J Chronic Dis 28:471–492, 1975.
4. Kraus JF: A comparison of recent studies on the extent of the head and spinal cord injury problem in the United States. J Neurosurg Suppl:S35–43, 1980.
5. Kraus JF: Injury to the head and spinal cord. The epidemiological relevance of the medical literature published from 1960 to 1978. J Neurosurg Suppl:S3–10, 1980.
6. Kurtzke JF: Epidemiology of spinal cord injury. Exp Neurol 48:163–236, 1975.
7. Minaire P, Castanier M, Girard R, et al: Epidemiology of spinal cord injury in the Rhone-Alpes Region, France, 1970-75. Paraplegia 16:76–87, 1978.
8. Tator CH: Epidemiology and general characteristics of the spinal cord-injured patient. In Tator CH, Benzel EC (eds): Contemporary management of spinal cord injury: From impact to rehabilitation. Park Ridge, IL, The American Association of Neurological Surgeons Publications Committee, 2000, pp 15–19.
9. Harvey C, Rothschild BB, Asmann AJ, Stripling T: New estimates of traumatic SCI prevalence: A survey-based approach. Paraplegia 28:537–544, 1990.
10. Tator CH, Duncan EG, Edmonds VE, et al: Complications and costs of management of acute spinal cord injury. Paraplegia 31:700–714, 1993.
11. Tator CH, Duncan EG, Edmonds VE, et al: Changes in epidemiology of acute spinal cord injury from 1947 to 1981. Surg Neurol 40:207–215, 1993.
12. Johnson RL, Gerhart KA, McCray J, et al: Secondary conditions following spinal cord injury in a population-based sample. Spinal Cord 36:45–50, 1998.
13. Krause JS: Aging after spinal cord injury: An exploratory study. Spinal Cord 38:77–83, 2000.
14. McKinley WO, Jackson AB, Cardenas DD, DeVivo MJ: Long-term medical complications after traumatic spinal cord injury: A regional model systems analysis. Arch Phys Med Rehabil 80:1402–1410, 1999.
15. Pharmacological therapy after acute cervical spinal cord injury. Neurosurgery 50:S63–72, 2002.
16. Ducker TB, Hamit HF: Experimental treatments of acute spinal cord injury. J Neurosurg 30:693–697, 1969.
17. Zeidman SM, Ling GS, Ducker TB, Ellenbogen RG: Clinical applications of pharmacologic therapies for spinal cord injury. J Spinal Disord 9:367–380, 1996.
18. Nesathurai S: Steroids and spinal cord injury: Revisiting the NASCIS 2 and NASCIS 3 trials. J Trauma 45:1088–1093, 1998.
19. Coleman WP, Benzel D, Cahill DW, et al: A critical appraisal of the reporting of the National Acute Spinal Cord Injury Studies (II and III) of methylprednisolone in acute spinal cord injury. J Spinal Disord 13:185–199, 2000.
20. Hurlbert RJ: Methylprednisolone for acute spinal cord injury: An inappropriate standard of care. J Neurosurg 93:1–7, 2000.
21. Short DJ, El Masry WS, Jones PW: High dose methylprednisolone in the management of acute spinal cord injury—a systematic review from a clinical perspective. Spinal Cord 38:273–286, 2000.
22. Hurlbert RJ, Moulton R: Why do you prescribe methylprednisolone for acute spinal cord injury? A Canadian perspective and a position statement. Can J Neurol Sci 29:236–239, 2002.
23. Bracken MB, Collins WF, Freeman DF, et al: Efficacy of methylprednisolone in acute spinal cord injury. Jama 251:45–52, 1984.
24. Bracken MB, Shepard MJ, Collins WF Jr, et al: Methylprednisolone or naloxone treatment after acute spinal cord injury: 1-year follow-up data. Results of the second National Acute Spinal Cord Injury Study. J Neurosurg 76:23–31, 1992.
25. Bracken MB, Shepard MJ, Collins WF, et al: A randomized, controlled trial of methylprednisolone or naloxone in the treatment of acute spinal-cord injury. Results of the Second National Acute Spinal Cord Injury Study. N Engl J Med 322:1405–1411, 1990.
26. Bracken MB, Shepard MJ, Holford TR, et al: Administration of methylprednisolone for 24 or 48 hours or tirilazad mesylate for 48 hours in the treatment of acute spinal cord injury. Results of the Third National Acute Spinal Cord Injury Randomized Controlled Trial. National Acute Spinal Cord Injury Study. Jama 277:1597–1604, 1997.
27. Bracken MB, Shepard MJ, Holford TR, et al: Methylprednisolone or tirilazad mesylate administration after acute spinal cord injury: 1-year follow up. Results of the third National Acute Spinal Cord Injury randomized controlled trial. J Neurosurg 89:699–706, 1998.
28. Otani K, Abe H, Kadoya S: Beneficial effect of methylprednisolone sodium succinate in the treatment of acute spinal cord injury. Sekitsui Sekizui J 7:633–647, 1994.
29. Kiwerski JE: Application of dexamethasone in the treatment of acute spinal cord injury. Injury 24:457–460, 1993.
30. Petitjean ME, Pointillart V, Dixmerias F, et al: Medical treatment of spinal cord injury in the acute stage. Ann Fr Anesth Reanim 17:114–122, 1998.
31. Pointillart V, Petitjean ME, Wiart L, et al: Pharmacological therapy of spinal cord injury during the acute phase. Spinal Cord 38:71–76, 2000.
32. Tator CH: Review of treatment trials in human spinal cord injury: Issues, difficulties, and recommendations. Neurosurgery 59:957–987, 2006.
33. Galandiuk S, Raque G, Appel S, Polk HC Jr: The two-edged sword of large-dose steroids for spinal cord trauma. Ann Surg 218:419–427, 1993.
34. Matsumoto T, Tamaki T, Kawakami M, et al: Early complications of high-dose methylprednisolone sodium succinate treatment in the follow-up of acute cervical spinal cord injury. Spine 26:426–430, 2001.
35. Roberts I, Yates D, Sandercock P, et al: Effect of intravenous corticosteroids on death within 14 days in 1000 adults with clinically significant head injury (MRC CRASH trial): Randomised placebo-controlled trial. Lancet 364:1321–1328, 2004.
36. Sauerland S, Nagelschmidt M, Mallmann P, Neugebauer EA: Risks and benefits of preoperative high dose methylprednisolone in surgical patients: A systematic review. Drug Saf 23:449–461, 2000.
37. Hugenholtz H, Cass DE, Dvorak MF, et al: High-dose methylprednisolone for acute closed spinal cord injury—only a treatment option. Can J Neurol Sci 29:227–235, 2002.

Chapter 2

Should Patients Undergoing Decompression for a Grade 1 Degenerative Spondylolisthesis Also Have an Instrumented Fusion?

HARRY HERKOWITZ, MD AND ERIC FRANCKE, MD

BACKGROUND

Degenerative spondylolisthesis, spondylolisthesis with an intact neural arch, typically affects patients older than 40 years. The disorder is three times more common in people of African descent, and is four to six times more common in female than male individuals.[1] The cause of degenerative spondylolisthesis is thought to derive from a combination of degenerative disc disease and facet arthritis in the presence of ligamentous laxity. Degenerative spondylolisthesis most commonly affects the L4-L5 level. The natural history of degenerative spondylolisthesis was reviewed in Matsunaga and colleagues'[2] study, which followed a group of 40 patients over an average of 8.25 years (Level of Evidence 4). This study demonstrates that the conditions of only 10% of patients deteriorated clinically and were a subset of a group of patients who did not demonstrate progression of the spondylolisthesis. In this study, progression of the slip was found in 30% of patients, all of whom were asymptomatic. A majority of these of patients exhibited some improvement in their clinical symptoms over time. In Matsunaga and colleagues'[3] long-term follow-up study, progressive slip was found in 34% of 145 nonsurgically managed patients at a minimum of 10 years (Level of Evidence 4). At the beginning of the study, 75% of patients were neurologically normal and remained so at final follow-up. Patients with neurologic symptoms comprised 34% of the patient population, and 84% of this group experienced neurologic deterioration with a resultant poor outcome.[3] Several studies have demonstrated a lack of correlation between spondylolisthesis progression and clinical deterioration.[4,5]

The clinical presentation of symptomatic degenerative spondylolisthesis is similar to spinal stenosis and includes axial back pain, leg pain, or both. The axial component of degenerative spondylolisthesis involves increasing back pain with extension, which distinguishes it from degenerative disc pain that involves increasing pain with flexion. The leg pain caused by degenerative spondylolisthesis may exhibit a radicular component or a neurogenic claudication component, or both. The radicular component exhibits a dermatomal pattern, is often unilateral, and more frequently involves the nerve root traversing the level of the spondylolisthesis. A degenerative spondylolisthesis at L4-L5 produces compression in the lateral recess, which can produce an L5 radiculopathy, manifested by sensory changes in the lateral thigh, lateral calf, and dorsum of foot, as well as extensor hallucis longus motor weakness. A degenerative spondylolisthesis will also anatomically narrow the neural foramen at the level of the slip, thereby compressing the exiting nerve root. As such, a degenerative spondylolisthesis at L4-L5 can also produce an L4 radiculopathy. This is manifested by sensory changes in the anterior thigh and knee extending to the anterior leg and tibialis anterior motor weakness. Neurogenic claudication involves weakness, paresthesias, or pain that typically extends from the thighs into the legs in a nondermatomal distribution and is secondary to central stenosis. The symptoms of neurogenic claudication increase with ambulation or standing because of decreased spinal canal cross-sectional area in lumbar extension leading to nerve root compression.[6] The symptoms of neurogenic claudication are improved with lumbar flexion, which increases the canal cross-sectional area.[7] Neurogenic claudication may be bilateral or unilateral with pain typically being the predominant symptom. Foraminal, lateral recess, and central stenosis leading to radicular pain or neurogenic claudication in the setting of spinal stenosis are exacerbated by concomitant degenerative spondylolisthesis, which contributes to the compressive effect. Physical examination of patients with a degenerative spondylolisthesis often de-monstrates normal or hypermobility of the lumbar spine. This has been suggested to be secondary to general ligamentous laxity thought to predispose these patients to degenerative spondylolisthesis.

The diagnosis of degenerative spondylolisthesis is confirmed with a radiographic examination of the lumbar spine that includes a standing lateral radiograph.[8] A standing lateral radiograph will demonstrate the presence of a spondylolisthesis that is not detected in 15% of patients with supine films alone.

Flexion/extension films of the lumbar spine may demonstrate dynamic instability at the level of spondylolisthesis. Computed tomography (CT), with or without myelography, has traditionally been used to further evaluate degenerative spondylolisthesis associated with spinal stenosis. CT gives excellent detail of the source of compression and the osseous pathology. Magnetic resonance imaging (MRI) has been used to further evaluate the source of nerve root compression including disc pathology, facet joint synovial cysts, and ligamentum flavum hypertrophy. An MRI scan may fail to demonstrate a degenerative spondylolisthesis that may be reduced with the patient supine. The "Open Facet Sign" on MRI involves increased T2 signal in the facet joints that are subluxed open. The "Open Facet Sign" may indicate instability in the absence of a visible spondylolisthesis, and ideally the MRI would have been preceded by a standing lateral radiograph of the lumbar spine. More recently, the upright MRI has been developed to further identify soft-tissue pathology with the patient in the standing position. Spondylolisthesis is typically measured in millimeters from the posterior inferior corner of the cephalad vertebra to the posterior superior corner of the caudal vertebra.[9] The Meyerding classification of spondylolisthesis provides a simple quantification system for the degree of spondylolisthesis. The Meyerding classification of spondylolisthesis describes the percentage of forward translation of the cephalad vertebral body relative to the end plate of the caudal vertebrae. A grade 1 slip is 0% to 25%, a grade 2 slip is 26% to 50%, a grade 3 slip is 51% to 75%, a grade 4 slip is 76% to 100%, and a grade 5 slip is greater than 100%.[10] Although the Meyerding classification system was traditionally used to describe isthmic spondylolisthesis, it can also be applied to degenerative spondylolistheses. As such, translation secondary to degenerative spondylolisthesis can be objectively quantified on a standing lateral lumbar radiograph. Unfortunately, the radiographic differentiation between normal motion and symptomatic instability is more problematic. Clinically significant radiographic instability of the lumbar spine is difficult to distinguish from the reference range of translation seen between motion segments in the lumbar spine.[11,12] The importance of identifying clinically significant instability on an upright radiograph secondary to degenerative spondylolis-thesis is essential to selecting the appropriate treatment.

TREATMENT

The initial conservative management for symptomatic degenerative spondylolisthesis with associated low back and/or leg pain is limited rest, nonsteroidal anti-inflammatory medications, and physical therapy (Level of Evidence 5). Physical therapy should involve flexion-based exercises and back strengthening, and progress toward an aerobic regimen to maintain the patient's weight within ideal parameters (Level of Evidence 5). Epidural steroid injections can also be used in the treatment of degenerative spondylolisthesis with the goal of relieving leg pain (Level of Evidence 5). After all conservative measures have failed an adequate trial, operative intervention may be considered if the patient continues to experience a significant reduction in quality of life.

The classic surgical indications as described by Herkowitz and Kurz[13] for degenerative spondylolisthesis are persistent or recurrent leg pain despite a minimum of 3 months of conservative treatment, progressive neurologic deficit, significant reduction in the quality of life, and confirmatory imaging studies concordant with the clinical findings[14] (Level of Evidence 5). The options for surgical intervention include decompression alone, decompression and posterolateral fusion with or without instrumentation, or anterior or posterior interbody fusion. The focus of this chapter is to review the literature and evidence available to answer the question, "Should patients undergoing decompression for a grade 1 degenerative spondylolisthesis also have an instrumented fusion?"

EVIDENCE

A meta-analysis of the role of decompression without fusion for the treatment of degenerative spondylolisthesis reviewed 11 articles published from 1970 to 1993.[15] The studies reviewed included a nonrandomized retrospective study, two randomized prospective studies, and eight nonrandomized, retrospective, and uncontrolled studies[16] (Level of Evidence 4). This study included 216 patients and found that 69% had a satisfactory result, 31% had an unsatisfactory result, and 31% had progression of the spondylolisthesis. This meta-analysis reviewed the literature regarding decompression without fusion only. Another retrospective study reviewed surgeon-reported outcomes of decompression without fusion for degenerative spondylolisthesis. This study examined a group of 290 patients with an average age of 67 years and suggested similar results.[17] This study was limited to patients with a stable spondylolisthesis that was defined as a slip with less than 4-mm translation and less than 12 degrees of angulation on flexion-extension lateral lumbar radiographs. The average follow-up was 10 years with 69% of patients having excellent results, 13% with good results, 12% with fair results, and 6% with poor results. It was concluded in this group of elderly patients with a stable degenerative spondylolisthesis that a decompression without fusion was a successful procedure with an 82% rate of excellent or good results (Level of Evidence 4).

Another retrospective study reviewed a group of 49 elderly patients with an average age of 68 years with symptomatic degenerative spondylolistheses who underwent decompression without fusion (Level of Evidence 4). These patients all had stable slips on flexion-extension radiographs and were followed for an average of 3.7 years. Clinical instability is defined as the loss of the ability of the spine under physiologic loads to maintain relationships between vertebrae in such a way that there is neither initial nor subsequent damage to the spinal cord or nerve roots; in addition, there is no development of incapacitating deformity or severe pain.[18] Gross clinical instability should be suspected whenever there is 4.5 mm of translation or 22 degrees of relative sagittal plane angulation on lateral radiographs.[19] This study reported 73.5% excellent or good results with 10% of patients eventually needing an instrumented fusion. The previously referenced studies recommend that, in older patients with stable spondylolistheses, decompression without fusion avoids the significant potential morbidity and mortality related to a fusion procedure in this age group.[14,20–22]

The role of noninstrumented fusion in the treatment of degenerative spondylolisthesis with instability is generally accepted as beneficial. A meta-analysis reviewing the results of noninstrumented fusions for degenerative spondylolisthesis included a total of six publications.[15] This study found a satisfactory clinical outcome in 90% of patients undergoing decompression with a noninstrumented fusion, and 86% of patients achieved arthrodesis. The fusion rate varied significantly between the studies from 30% to 100%. When this group of patients who underwent decompression and fusion were compared with the group of patients who underwent decompression alone, they had statistically significantly better clinical outcomes (Level of Evidence 3).

Herkowitz and Kurz[13] performed a prospective and randomized study that compared decompression alone with decompression with noninstrumented fusion in patients with L3-L4 and L4-L5 degenerative spondylolisthesis and associated stenosis. This study demonstrated a statistically significant difference between 44% satisfactory outcomes in the decompression group compared with 96% satisfactory outcomes in the decompression and fusion group. The proportion of excellent outcomes was also significantly greater at 44% for the decompression and arthrodesis group compared with 8% for the decompression alone group ($P = 0.0001$). This result was independent of the variables of age, sex, preoperative disc height, extent of decompression, or success of achieving a solid arthrodesis. In fact, 36% of the arthrodesis group experienced development of a pseudoarthrosis, but all of these patients had an excellent or good result. In the group of patients who underwent decompression alone, there was a significant increase ($P = 0.02$) in the progression of spondylolisthesis. This randomized, prospective study demonstrated better clinical outcomes in patients who underwent in situ fusions for degenerative spondylolisthesis with concomitant stenosis (Level of Evidence 1).

The role of fusion in patients with a degenerative spondylolisthesis was investigated by Lombardi and colleagues[22a], who completed a study that involved 47 patients who underwent decompression with or without fusion (Level of Evidence 3). These results showed that the patients who underwent a radical decompression faired poorly, and those who received a fusion fared the best. The poor results with decompression without fusion were attributed to the progression of the spondylolisthesis or persistent instability, or both, at the level of the spondylolisthesis. Another smaller study that supported the addition of fusions to decompressive procedures for degenerative spondylolisthesis found that in patients who underwent decompression alone, 45% had good results and 55% had fair or poor results in a group of 11 patients. This was compared with the finding of 63% good results with an arthrodesis and decompression in a group of eight patients.[23]

A multicenter historical cohort study of 2684 patients with degenerative spondylolisthesis reviewed spinal fusion using pedicle screw instrumentation and found solid arthrodesis in 89% of patients who underwent instrumented fusion and only 70% of patients without instrumentation[24] (Level of Evidence 3). The clinical outcomes for the instrumented fusion group were also better relative to the noninstrumented fusion group in this study. A recent comprehensive literature review of lumbar and lumbosacral fusions from 1979 to 2000 reported a trend in increasing instrumented fusions.[25]

A prospective randomized study compared noninstrumented, semirigid, and rigid instrumented fusions in 124 patients at 1 year after surgery.[26] A subset of 56 patients was treated for degenerative spondylolisthesis, and this group achieved a radiographic fusion rate of 65% for the noninstrumented group, 50% for the semirigid instrumentation group, and 86% for the rigid instrumentation group. This study demonstrated a trend toward better clinical outcomes in the group that underwent instrumented fusions that achieved 95% good results compared with 89% for the semirigid instrumentation group and 71% of the noninstrumented group (Level of Evidence 2). A retrospective review of 30 patients undergoing decompression and instrumented fusion for degenerative spondylolisthesis used both radiographic evaluation of arthrodesis and clinical outcomes as measured by the Short Form-36 (SF-36) and patient questionnaire.[27] This study demonstrated that both the rate of fusion and the rate of patient satisfaction was 93% despite a 43% complication rate (Level of Evidence 5).

A prospective and randomized study divided a group of patients with degenerative spondylolisthesis into those who received no fusion, noninstrumented posterolateral fusion, and instrumented posterolateral fusion.[28] This study demonstrated significantly improved fusion rates, functional outcomes, and sagittal alignment in the instrumented posterolateral fusion group relative to the other groups. This study also showed that slip progression correlated with a poorer outcome in a subgroup of 10 patients who underwent decompression with noninstrumented fusion. The functional outcome was improved in only 30% of patients, and 70% had a progression in their spondylolisthesis that correlated with a poorer outcome (Level of Evidence 1). Another study that examined posterolateral fusion for unstable spondylolisthesis demonstrated that instrumentation significantly improved the functional outcomes if a decompression was performed[29] (Level of Evidence 3). Other comparisons between the instrumented and noninstrumented groups, including fusion rates, did not show significant differences. A meta-analysis of the literature on degenerative spondylolisthesis found that of patients who underwent decompression without arthrodesis, 69% had a satisfactory outcome.[3] Progression of the spondylolisthesis was noted in the majority of patients in this study. The addition of arthrodesis increased the satisfactory outcome to 90%, with 86% achieving a solid fusion. This meta-analysis also reported a strong trend with increasing fusion rates with instrumentation that did not affect clinical outcomes (Level of Evidence 3).

A prospective and randomized study of 68 patients with degenerative spondylolisthesis and stenosis compared decompression and noninstrumented arthrodesis with decompression and segmental transpedicular instrumented arthrodesis. At an average follow-up of 2 years, there was a significantly greater fusion rate of 83% in the instrumented group compared with the noninstrumented group, which had a fusion rate of 45%.[30] Despite the increased fusion rate in the instrumented fusion group relative to the noninstrumented group, there was no significant difference in clinical outcomes with 86% compared with 76% good/excellent outcomes, respectively, at the 2-year time point. Interestingly, a comparison of outcomes at an average follow-up of 7 years and 8 months for 47 patients from both the noninstrumented and instrumented fusion groups demonstrated a significant difference in clinical outcome.[31] With this longer follow-up, these two groups of patients exhibited excellent and good clinical outcomes in 86% of patients who experienced development of a solid arthrodesis, but in only 56% of those who experienced development of a pseudoarthrosis. The group of patients who had a solid arthrodesis was reported to have significantly less back pain and a better functional outcome relative to the group of patients who had a pseudoarthrosis. A clear benefit was demonstrated regarding the effects of achieving a solid arthrodesis after decompression for degenerative spondylolisthesis. As such, it was inferred that because instrumented fusions result in a greater rate of arthrodesis and because arthrodesis results in improved long-term clinical outcomes, instrumented fusions produce better long-term clinical outcomes in the treatment of degenerative spondylolisthesis (Level of Evidence 2).

RECOMMENDATIONS

First and foremost, an adequate trial of nonsteroidal anti-inflammatory medications, physical therapy, and epidural steroid injections is indicated before surgical intervention (Level of Evidence 5). The symptoms caused by degenerative spondylolisthesis are multifactorial and are related to the degree and location of associated stenosis and instability. The stenosis is addressed with decompression, which should be thorough and decompress all clinically symptomatic stenotic areas. The exiting and/or traversing nerve roots affected by foraminal or lateral recess stenosis, or both, should be thoroughly decompressed. The pars interarticularis must be undercut to open up the foramen and adequately decompress the exiting nerve root. The facet must be undercut to the pedicle to adequately decompress the traversing nerve root. Resection of the pars, more than 50% of each facet joint, or an entire facet increases the risk for iatrogenic instability. Central stenosis addressed with multilevel bilateral laminectomies increases the risk for iatrogenic instability.

The majority of more recent literature supports decompression with arthrodesis for the treatment of degenerative spondylolisthesis secondary to improved clinical outcomes with successful arthrodesis (grade B). Furthermore, the literature demonstrates that arthrodesis augmentation with transpedicular instrumentation increases the rate of successful fusion (grade A). As such, instrumented arthrodesis for degenerative spondylolisthesis leads to improved clinical outcomes (grade B). The use of instrumentation to augment the arthrodesis should be tailored to the extent of the decompression and the amount of preoperative instability. In the presence of gross instability on preoperative flexion-extension radiographs and in the presence of an aggressive decompression with the associated risks for iatrogenic instability, the immediate stability afforded by an instrumented fusion warrants its increased morbidity, time, and expense (grade B). Furthermore, young and active patient populations with instability and good bone stock are more appropriate surgical candidates for instrumented fusions than are older and sedentary populations with stable degenerative spondylolistheses and poor bone stock. In conclusion, the question "Should patients undergoing decompression for a grade 1 degenerative spondylolisthesis also have an instrumented fusion?" can be answered from the available literature. It can be concluded that because instrumentation increases arthrodesis rates and achieving arthrodesis improves long-term clinical outcomes, instrumented fusions in certain patient populations should also improve long-term clinical outcomes in the surgical management of degenerative spondylolisthesis.[32-34]

Summary of Recommendations		
STATEMENT	**LEVEL OF EVIDENCE/GRADE OF RECOMMENDATION**	**REFERENCE**
1. Decompression for degenerative sponylolisthesis has better outcomes when performed with fusion	A	13
2. Rates of fusion are increased with instrumentation	A	30
3. Decompression for degenerative sponylolisthesis has better outcomes when performed with instrumented fusions in certain patient populations	B	28, 31

REFERENCES

1. Rosenberg NJ: Degenerative spondylolisthesis. Predisposing factors. J Bone Joint Surg Am 57:467–474, 1975.
2. Matsunaga S, Sakou T, Morizono Y, et al: Natural history of degenerative spondylolisthesis: Pathogenesis and natural course of the slippage. Spine 15:1204–1210, 1990.
3. Matsunaga S, Ijiri K, Hayashi K: Nonsurgically managed patients with degenerative spondylolisthesis: A 10- to 18-year follow-up study. J Neurosurgery 93(2 suppl):194–198, 2000.
4. Grob D, Humke T, Dvorak J: Degenerative lumbar spinal stenosis decompression with and without arthrodesis. J Bone Joint Surg Am 77:1036–1041, 1995.
5. Cinotti G, Pstacchini F, Fassari F, et al: Predisposing factors in degenerative spondylolisthesis: A radiographic and CT study. Int Orthop 21:337–342, 1997.
6. Katz J, Dalgas M, Stucki G, et al: Degenerative lumbar spinal stenosis: Diagnostic value of the history and physical examination. Arthritis Rheum 38:1236–1241, 1995.
7. Inufusa A, An HS, Lim TH: Anatomic changes of the spinal canal and intervertebral foramen association with flexion-extension movement. Spine 21:2412–2420, 1996.
8. Bendo J, Ong B: Importance of correlating static and dynamic imaging studies in diagnostic degenerative lumbar spondylolisthesis. Am J Orthop 30:247–250, 2001.
9. O'Brien MF, Kuklo TR, Blanke KM, Lenke LG: Spinal Deformity Study Group. Radiographic Measurement Manual. Medtronic Sofamore Danek USA, Inc., 2004.
10. Meyerding HW: Spondylolisthesis. J Bone Joint Surg 13:39–48,1931.
11. Hayes MA, Howard TC, Gruel CR, et al: Roentgenographic evaluation of lumbar spine flexion-extension in asymptomatic individuals. Spine 14:327–331, 1989.
12. Boden SD, Wiesel SW: Lumbosacral segmental motion in normal individuals: Have we been measuring instability properly? Spine 5:571–576, 1990.
13. Herkowitz HN, Kurz LT: Degenerative lumbar spondylolisthesis with spinal stenosis: A prospective study comparing decompression with decompression and intertransverse progressive arthrodesis. J Bone Joint Surg Am 73:802–808, 1991.
14. Turner JA, Ersek M, Herron L, et al: Patient outcomes after lumbar spinal fusions. JAMA 268:907–911, 1992.
15. Mardjetko S, Connolly P, Shott S: Degenerative lumbar spondylolisthesis: A meta-analysis of the literature, 1970-1993. Spine 19(20 suppl):2256S–2265S, 1994.
16. Johnson K, Uden A, Rosen I: The effect of decompression on the natural course of spinal stenosis: A comparison of surgically treated and untreated patients. Spine 16:615–619, 1991.
17. Epstein N, Epstein J: Decompression in the surgical management of degenerative spondylolisthesis: Advantages of a conservative approach in 290 patients. J Spinal Disord 11:116–122, 1998.
18. White AA III, Panjabi MM: Clinical Biomechanics of the Spine, 2nd ed. Philadelphia, JB Lippincott, 1990.
19. Neumann P, Nordwal A, Osvalder A: Traumatic instability of the lumbar spine: A dynamic in vitro study of flexion distraction injury. Spine 20:1111–1121, 1995.
20. Oldridge N, Yuan Z, Stoll J, Rimm A: Lumbar spine surgery and mortality among medicare beneficiaries, 1986. Am J Public Health 84:1292–1298, 1994.
21. Deyo R, Ciol M, Cherkin D, et al: Lumbar spinal fusion: A cohort study of complications, reoperations, and resource use in the medicare population. Spine 18:1463–1470, 1993.
22. Deyo R, Cherkin D, Loeser J, et al: Morbidity and mortality in association with operations of the lumbar spine. J Bone Joint Surg Am 74:536–543, 1992.
22a. Lombardi JS, Wiltse LL, Reynolds JB, Widell EH, Spencer C: Treatment of degenerative spondylolisthesis. Spine 10:821–827, 1985.
23. Feffer H, Wiesel S, Cuckler JM, Rothman RH: Degenerative spondylolisthesis: To fuse or not to fuse. Spine 10:287–289, 1985.
24. Yuan HA, Garfin SR, Dickman CA, et al: A historical cohort study of pedicle screw fixation in thoracic, lumbar, and sacral spinal fusions. Spine 19(20 suppl):2279–2296, 1994.
25. Bono CM, Lee CK: Critical analysis of trends in fusion for degenerative disc disease over the past 20 years: Influence of techniques on fusion rate and clinical outcome. Spine 29:455–463, 2004.
26. Zdeblick T: A prospective randomized study of lumbar fusion. Spine 18:983–991, 1993.
27. Nork SE, Serena SH, Workman KL, et al: Patient outcomes after decompression and instrumented posterior spinal fusion for degenerative spondylolisthesis. Spine 24:561–569, 1999.
28. Bridwell K, Sedgewick T, O'Brien M, et al: The role of fusion and instrumentation in the treatment of degenerative spondylolisthesis with spinal stenosis. J Spinal Disord 6:467–472, 1993.
29. Thomsen K, Christensen FB, Eiskjaer SP, et al: The effect of pedicle screw instrumentation on functional outcome and fusion rates in posterolateral lumbar spinal fusion: A prospective, randomized clinical study. Spine 22:2813–2822, 1997.
30. Fischgrund JS, Mackay M, Herkowitz HN, et al: Degenerative lumbar spondylolisthesis with spinal stenosis: A prospective, randomized study comparing decompressive laminectomy and arthrodesis with and without spinal instrumentation. Spine 22:2807–2812, 1997.
31. Kornblum MB, Fischgrund JS, Herkowitz HN, et al: Degenerative lumbar spondylolisthesis with spinal stenosis. Spine 29:726–734, 2004.
32. McLain RF: Instrumented fusion for degenerative spondylolisthesis, is it necessary. Spine 29:170, 2004.
33. Phillips FM: The argument for noninstrumented posterolateral fusion for patients with spinal stenosis and degenerative spondylolisthesis. Spine 29:170–172, 2004.
34. Fischgrund JS: The argument for instrumented posterolateral for patients with spinal stenosis and degenerative spondylolisthesis. Spine 29:173–174, 2004.

Vertebral Augmentation: What Is the Role of Vertebroplasty and Kyphoplasty?

Isador Lieberman, MD, MBA, FRCS and Krzysztof Siemionow, MD

Osteoporosis is a disorder characterized by decreased bone density, disruption of trabecular architecture, and increased susceptibility to fractures. There are approximately 700,000 vertebral body compression fractures (VCFs) occur in the United States each year.[1] Approximately 70,000 of those result in hospitalization, with an average hospital stay per patient of 8 days.[2] The lifetime risk for a clinically evident vertebral fracture among postmenopausal white women older than 50 years has been estimated at about 16%, whereas the lifetime risk in white men is about 5%.[3] Clinical evidence shows that, if untreated, up to 20% of patients with a prior VCF are likely to have an additional VCF within the same year.[4] The diagnosis of a single osteoporotic VCF increases the risk for subsequent fractures by a factor of 5. Patient population studies suggest an increased mortality rate in patients with osteoporotic VCFs that correlates with the number of fractured vertebrae.[1] A benign natural history has long been assumed for osteoporotic VCFs, but up to 30% of those who are symptomatic and seek treatment do not respond adequately to nonsurgical treatment.[5,6]

VERTEBRAL AUGMENTATION

Currently, vertebral augmentation can be performed using either a vertebroplasty or kyphoplasty technique. They are both used in the treatment of osteoporotic vertebral fractures, and these methods should not be considered mutually exclusive. They are both minimally invasive procedures used in the treatment of symptomatic osteoporotic VCFs. The objective of any vertebral augmentation technique is to restore strength and stiffness to the fractured vertebral body with the injection of cement.

Historically, "percutaneous vertebroplasty" was conceived in France in 1984 to reduce pain from symptomatic vertebral hemangiomas.[7] A cervical vertebra was injected with acrylic cement during open surgery to strengthen the vertebral body. An analgesic effect was noted, and indications for the technique expanded to include both neoplastic disease and osteoporotic compression fractures through a percutaneous insertion of cannulas into the vertebral body, through which cement was injected.

The "kyphoplasty" technique was developed later in 1997; it is a minimally invasive technique that helps restore vertebral body height before cement augmentation.[8] It involves inserting inflatable bone tamps, through percutaneously placed cannulas, into the vertebral body under fluoroscopic guidance. Once inflated, the bone tamps push up on the end plates, helping to reduce the loss of vertebral body height while creating a cavity for the bone cement.

The traditional indications for vertebral augmentation are progressive collapse of a vertebral body and intractable pain. Either a transpedicular or extrapedicular approach is used to reach the vertebral body. Contraindications to vertebral augmentation are systemic pathology such as sepsis, prolonged bleeding times, or cardiopulmonary pathology, which would preclude the safe completion of the procedure. Other relative contraindications include patients presenting with neurological signs or symptoms, nonosteolytic infiltrative spinal metastases, vertebral height collapse of more than 60%, burst fractures, or vertebral bodies with deficient posterior cortices[9,10] (Tables 3–1 and 3–2).

REVIEW OF THE LITERATURE

A review of Ovid and PubMed conducted in April 2007 using the search terms "kyphoplasty," "vertebroplasty," and "outcomes" revealed 722 vertebroplasty-related articles and 250 kyphoplasty-related articles. Of that group, 152 articles included both techniques. Most balloon kyphoplasty and vertebroplasty studies are grade 4, single-center, and single-arm studies of a prospective or retrospective nature.

Several reports with higher levels of evidence have been published. However, no blinded randomized trials have compared either technique against medical management. One was a multicenter prospective study of kyphoplasty.[11] Two were concurrently controlled prospective studies comparing kyphoplasty with nonsurgical management.[12,13] There were two concurrently controlled prospective studies,[14,15] and one nonconcurrently controlled study comparing vertebroplasty with nonsurgical management.[16] Several studies compared kyphoplasty and vertebroplasty. However, most were nonconcurrent comparisons,[17–19]

TABLE 3–1. Efficacy of Kyphoplasty in Reducing Pain in Osteoporotic Vertebral Compression Fracture

AUTHORS	PATIENTS (N)	NUMBER OF VERTEBRAL BODIES	PATIENTS WITH GOOD TO EXCELLENT PAIN RESPONSE (%)	PAIN REDUCTION (VISUAL ANALOGUE SCALE)	STUDY DESIGN/GRADE OF EVIDENCE
Majd et al.[31]	222	360	89		Retrospective/B
Grafe et al.[13]	40	73	77.5	−1.8	Prospective/B
Garfin et al.[12]	100	136	90	−4.5	Prospective/A
Khanna et al.[32]	314	875	ODI (−12.6)		Prospective/B
Theodorou et al.[44]	15	24	100		Retrospective/B
Wong et al.[45]	85	143	94		Retrospective/B
Wilhelm et al.[46]	34	56		−4.3	Prospective/B
Phillips et al.[47]	29	61	95.6	−8	Prospective/B
Crandall et al.[48]	47	86	93.5	−3	Prospective/B
Berlemann et al.[49]	24	27	95		Prospective/B
Hillmeier et al.[50]	102	102	99	−6.9	Retrospective/B
Gaitanis et al.[51]	47	49	95.5		Prospective/B
Total	1059	1992			

ODI, Oswestry Disability Index.

TABLE 3–2. Efficacy of Vertebroplasty in Reducing Pain in Osteoporotic Vertebral Compression Fractures

AUTHORS	PATIENTS (N)	NUMBER OF VERTEBRAL BODIES	PATIENTS WITH GOOD TO EXCELLENT PAIN RESPONSE (%)	PAIN REDUCTION (VISUAL ANALOGUE SCALE)	STUDY DESIGN/GRADE OF EVIDENCE
Jensen et al.[52]	29	47	90		Retrospective/B
Martin et al.[53]	9		77.7		Retrospective/B
Cortet et al.[54]	16	20	88	−6	Prospective/B
Cyteval et al.[55]	20	23	90		Prospective/B
O'Brien et al.[56]	6	6	83		Retrospective/B
Barr et al.[57]	38	70	95		Retrospective/B
Grados et al.[58]	25	34	96	−4.3	Retrospective/B
Heini et al.[59]	17	45	100	−4.3	Prospective/B
Maynard et al.[60]	27	35	93	−7.4	Retrospective/B
Amar et al.[61]	97	258	63		Retrospective/B
Moreland et al.[62]	35	53	89		Retrospective/B
Kaufmann et al.[63]	75	122		−7.5	Retrospective/B
McGraw et al.[64]	100	156	97	−6.9	Prospective/B
Peh et al.[65]	37	48	97		Retrospective/B
Kallmes et al.[66]	41	63		−8	Retrospective/B
Zoarski et al.[67]	30	54	96		Prospective/B
Gaughen et al.[68]	48	84	95	−7.6	Retrospective/B
Nakano et al.[69]	16	17	100	−7.7	Retrospective/B
Ryu et al.[70]	159	347	87		Retrospective/B
Perez-Higueras et al.[71]	13	27	92	−8	Prospective/B
Evans et al.[72]	245	554		−5	Retrospective/B
Jang et al.[73]	16	16	88	−4.7	Retrospective/B
Diamond et al.[74]	55	71	96		Prospective/B
Peh et al.[75]	18	19	77		Retrospective/B
Gangi et al.[76]	187	289	78		Retrospective/B
Brown et al.[77]	90	186	86		Retrospective/B
Chen et al.[78]	70	87	86	−4.4	Retrospective/B
Winking et al.[79]	38	66	92	−5.2	Prospective/B
Legroux-Gerot et al.[80]	16	21	75	−3.5	Prospective/B
Alvarez et al.[81]	101	151		−4.5	Prospective/B

and two were unclear.[20,21] Several meta-analyses compared kyphoplasty and vertebroplasty,[22–24] and there were also several meta-analyses of only kyphoplasty or only vertebroplasty.[25–28]

SYSTEMATIC REVIEW OF VERTEBRAL AUGMENTATION OUTCOMES

Taylor et al[23] performed a systematic review and metaregression to compare the efficacy and safety of balloon kyphoplasty and vertebroplasty for the treatment of VCFs, and to examine the prognostic factors that predict outcome. They found Level III evidence to support both balloon kyphoplasty and vertebroplasty as effective therapies in the management of patients with symptomatic osteoporotic VCFs refractory to conventional medical therapy. However, balloon kyphoplasty appeared to offer a better adverse event profile.

In a follow-up study, the authors concluded that in direct comparison with conventional medical management, patients undergoing kyphoplasty experienced superior improvements in pain, functionality, vertebral height, and kyphotic angle at least up to 3 years after the procedure. Reductions in pain with kyphoplasty appeared to be greatest in patients with newer fractures. The authors concluded that balloon kyphoplasty appeared to be more effective than medical management of osteoporotic VCFs and as least as effective as vertebroplasty.[26]

Hulme[22] conducted a systematic review of 69 studies in the literature. The objective of the review was to evaluate the safety and efficacy of vertebroplasty and kyphoplasty using the data presented in published clinical studies, with respect to patient pain relief, restoration of mobility and vertebral body height, complication rate, and incidence of new adjacent vertebral fractures. A large proportion of subjects had some pain relief, including 87% with vertebroplasty and 92% with kyphoplasty. Vertebral height restoration was possible using kyphoplasty (average, 6.6 degrees) and for a subset of patients using vertebroplasty (average, 6.6 degrees). Cement leaks occurred for 41% and 9% of treated vertebrae for vertebroplasty and kyphoplasty, respectively. New fractures of adjacent vertebrae occurred for both procedures at rates that are greater than the general osteoporotic population but approximately equivalent to the general osteoporotic population that had a previous vertebral fracture. The authors concluded that the problem with stating definitively that vertebroplasty and kyphoplasty are safe and effective procedures was the lack of comparative, blinded, randomized, clinical trials.[22]

In a review of cumulative data from 1279 vertebral bodies treated with kyphoplasty and 2729 vertebral bodies treated with vertebroplasty, Hadjipavlou and researchers[30] found that the mean good to excellent pain response was reported by 90% of patients treated with vertebroplasty and 95.6% of patients treated with kyphoplasty. Vertebroplasty was associated with a 29% rate of cement leakage compared with 8.4% for kyphoplasty. The rate of epidural leakage was 10.7% with vertebroplasty and 1.2% for kyphoplasty. The series included VCF secondary to osteoporosis and tumor.[29]

DOES VERTEBRAL AUGMENTATION IMPROVE OUTCOME IN PATIENTS WITH VERTEBRAL COMPRESSION FRACTURES?

In a prospective, nonrandomized, "intention-to-treat" study, Diamond and investigators[14] treated 126 consecutive patients (39 men and 87 women; ages 51–95 years) with acute osteoporotic vertebral fractures. Eighty-eight patients were treated by percutaneous vertebroplasty and 38 by conservative therapy. The primary outcome measure was change in the patients' pain score and level of function at 24 hours, 6 weeks, 6 to 12 months, and 24 months after therapy. Secondary outcome measures were occurrence of new clinical or radiological vertebral

fractures and survival at 2 years. Outcomes in patients treated with vertebroplasty showed greater reduction in visual analogue pain scores, faster return to normal function, and lower rates of hospitalization when compared with those treated conservatively ($P < 0.001$ for the comparison of all variables at 24 hours). Lower pain scores persisted in the group treated with vertebroplasty at 6 weeks ($P < 0.001$), but no differences between the two groups were evident at 12 and 24 months. In the group treated with vertebroplasty, compared with the control group, the rates of new vertebral fractures and death showed no significant difference. The authors concluded that the analgesic benefit of percutaneous vertebroplasty and the low complication rates suggest that cement augmentation is a useful therapy for acute painful osteoporotic vertebral fractures.[14]

Alvarez and colleagues[15] performed a prospective study consisting of 101 consecutive patients who underwent vertebroplasty and 27 patients who refused operative treatment and were managed conservatively. Patients who elected for vertebroplasty as a treatment of their fractures had significantly more pain and functional impairment before the procedure than the patients in the conservative group ($P < 0.001$). Vertebroplasty demonstrated a rapid and significant relief of pain and improved the quality of life.[15]

Majd and researchers[30] prospectively followed 222 osteoporotic patients with 360 VCFs who were treated with kyphoplasty. Immediate pain relief was reported by 89% of patients at the first follow-up visit. One patient experienced postoperative pain as a result of radiculopathy related to leakage into the foramen. Sixty-nine percent of fractures exhibited restoration of lost vertebral height. Twelve percent (30/254) of the patients required additional kyphoplasty procedures to treat 36 symptomatic, new adjacent and remote fractures.[30]

Studies comparing kyphoplasty with conventional medical treatment found that kyphoplasty consistently improved pain and physical function, with results sustained at 12 months.[12] In addition, the authors found that there were significantly fewer patients with new vertebral fractures of the thoracic and lumbar spine, after 12 months, in the kyphoplasty group than in the group treated medically. Another benefit of the kyphoplasty technique is the restoration of mobility. Garfin and investigators[11] demonstrated that elderly patients with VCFs had rapid, significant, and sustained improvements in back pain, back function, and quality of life after balloon kyphoplasty.

Khanna and colleagues[31] prospectively followed 155 patients with VCFs secondary to osteoporosis and 56 patients with malignant osteolysis for a mean 55.0 weeks after kyphoplasty. The average Owestry Disability Index score decreased by 12.6 points ($P < 0.001$) in the overall group, by 11.8 points ($P < 0.001$) at short-term follow-up, and by

8.6 points ($P < 0.001$) at long-term follow-up. All Health Survey Short Form-36 subscores except for general health and role-emotional showed statistically significant improvement from baseline values at the same time points. No statistically significant difference was found for functional outcome in the osteoporosis and multiple myeloma subgroups.[31]

DOES VERTEBRAL AUGMENTATION RESTORE VERTEBRAL HEIGHT AND SAGITTAL ALIGNMENT?

In a study of vertebroplasty, Jang and coworkers[32] report that the mean anterior vertebral height, as measured on the standing flexion radiographs before operation, improved from 14.8 mm to 21.8 mm with extension of the spine in a series of patients with single fractures. After vertebroplasty, the mean anterior height was 19.8 mm, suggesting that considerable height restoration can be achieved by postural extension and then be preserved by vertebroplasty. Some reports suggest that the age of the fracture is a major determinant in achieving an optimal reduction,[33,34] whereas others demonstrate that significant correction can be achieved even in fractures older than 3 months.[33,35] In a study of kyphoplasty, Crandall and coauthors[33] reported failure of significant correction in 20% of chronic fractures compared with 8% of acute fractures.[33]

Pradhan and colleagues[36] examined the effects of single-level and multilevel kyphoplasty procedures on local and overall sagittal alignment of the spine. The authors found that the majority of kyphosis correction is limited to the vertebral body treated. The majority of height gained after kyphoplasty occurs in the midbody. Higher correction over longer spans of the spine can be achieved with multilevel kyphoplasty procedures, in proportion to the number of levels addressed. The authors felt that it would be unrealistic to expect a one- or two-level kyphoplasty to significantly improve the overall sagittal alignment of the spine.

Shindle and coworkers[37] prospectively followed 25 consecutive patients with a total of 43 osteoporotic VCFs to evaluate the effect of postural changes and balloon inflation on vertebral fracture reduction. Their findings support the concept that many VCFs can be moved with positioning. However, balloon kyphoplasty enhanced the height reduction by an amount equal to or greater than 4.5-fold over the positioning maneuver alone and accounted for more than 80% of the ultimate reduction. The authors concluded that if height restoration is the goal, kyphoplasty is clearly superior in most cases to the positioning maneuver alone.[37]

Voggenreiter has demonstrated that placement of the patient in the prone position displayed a significant spontaneous reduction in deformity of 6.5 degrees ± 4.1 degrees Cobb angle. Inflation of the inflatable bone tamp demonstrated a further reduction of the fracture and a significant improvement of the Cobb angle of 3.4 degrees compared with baseline prone position. After deflation and removal of the inflatable bone tamp and placement of the cement, no significant loss of fracture reduction was seen. Postoperative measurement of the Cobb angle by means of standing radiographs demonstrated a 3.1-degree loss of reduction compared with the intraoperative measurement in prone position after cement application.[38]

DOES VERTEBRAL AUGMENTATION PREDISPOSE TO FURTHER VERTEBRAL COMPRESSION FRACTURES?

Painful osteoporotic compression fractures can be effectively treated with methylmethacrylate vertebral augmentation, but the effect of intervention on the generation of future remote and adjacent fractures remains a topic of debate. A VCF causes a local kyphotic deformity. This deformity moves the center of gravity forward, resulting in an increased forward bending moment. This increases the load on the adjacent vertebrae and predisposes it to fracture. Silverman et al[4] showed that, if untreated, up to 20% of patients with a prior VCF are likely to have an additional VCF within the same year. The authors also reported that 58% of women with one or more fractures had adjacent fractures.[39] The rates of new fracture after cement augmentation procedures are not comparable among patients treated with vertebroplasty (0–52%), kyphoplasty (5.8–36.8%), and conservative approaches (19.2–58%), because of the poor scientific design of the studies. Most are retrospective or nonrandomized prospective reports[29] (Table 3–3).

TABLE 3–3. Literature Regarding Possible Predisposition of Vertebral Augmentation to Further Vertebral Compression Fractures

AUTHORS	PATIENTS (N)	NUMBER OF VERTEBRAL BODIES	PATIENTS WITH NEW FRACTURE	METHOD	STUDY DESIGN/GRADE OF EVIDENCE
Lin et al.[40]	38	96	36%	Vertebroplasty	Retrospective/B
Grafe et al.[12]	40	73	17.5%	Kyphoplasty	Prospective/B
Pflugmacher et al.[42]	42	67	21%	Kyphoplasty	Prospective/B
Harrop et al.[43]	115	225	22.6%	Kyphoplasty	Retrospective/B

Lin and colleagues[40] treated 38 patients with vertebroplasty and found that 14 patients developed new fractures during the follow-up period. Seventy-one percent of patients with secondary fractures had intradiscal leakage of cement. In their study, vertebral bodies adjacent to a disc with leakage of cement had a 58% chance of developing a new fracture compared with 12% of vertebral bodies adjacent to a disc without leakage. The authors concluded that leakage of cement into the disc, by impeding the flexibility, may increase the risk for a secondary fracture in an adjacent vertebral body.[40] Trout and coworkers[44] performed a retrospective review of 86 patients treated with vertebroplasty to identify those who developed adjacent segment fractures.[41] They found that 186 incident fractures developed in these 86 patients. Seventy-seven (41%) of these incident fractures occurred adjacent to treated vertebrae.

Reduction of the kyphotic deformity with kyphoplasty may potentially decrease the risk for new fractures. Two prospective, nonrandomized studies compared kyphoplasty with conservative treatment. Grafe and coworkers[12,13] found that at 12-month follow up, 50% of patients who had been treated conservatively developed secondary fractures, compared with 17.5% of patients who had undergone kyphoplasty.[12,13] Komp and coauthors[12,13] report that at 6-month follow-up examination, the incidence of new fractures in 17 conservatively treated patients was 65%, compared with 37% in 19 patients treated by kyphoplasty.[13,14] However, these were not randomized studies.

Pflugmacher and researchers[42] conducted a 2-year prospective follow-up to evaluate the incidence of adjacent vertebral fractures in patients treated with balloon kyphoplasty. It did not include comparison or control groups. The authors reported an annualized refracture rate of 10%.[42] In 8 patients (21.6%; 5 female and 3 male patients), an adjacent fracture occurred in 11 vertebrae (18.3%) within 3 weeks to 22 months of follow-up (after 22 months, no adjacent fracture occurred). In three patients, the adjacent fractures were asymptomatic. Five patients with symptomatic adjacent fractures (eight vertebrae) were treated again with balloon kyphoplasty.

Harrop and colleagues[43] treated 225 vertebral bodies in 115 patients using the kyphoplasty technique, and patients were followed prospectively. Of those, 26 patients developed 34 subsequent compression fractures. The mean follow-up was 11 months (range, 3–33 months). The incidence of subsequent fracture per procedure per kyphoplasty was 15.1% (34 of 225). The overall incidence rate per patient was 22.6% (26 of 115). Seventeen of the 26 (65%) patients with subsequent fracture had secondary steroid-induced osteoporosis, while only 9 of the 26 (35%) had primary osteoporosis. Therefore, the incidence of postkyphoplasty vertebral compression fractures in patients with primary osteoporosis was 11.25% (9 of 80), and the incidence in patients with steroid-induced osteoporosis was 48.6% (17 of 35). This increased fracture rate in the steroid-dependent patients was significantly greater than in patients with primary osteoporosis ($P < 0.0001$), together with a significantly greater proportion of adjacent fractures (12 of 19 taking steroids; $P = 0.0009$) and remote fractures (7 of 9 taking steroids; $P = 0.027$) compared with the patients with primary osteoporosis.[43]

RECOMMENDATIONS

As the population ages and osteoporosis becomes more prevalent, the incidence of symptomatic vertebral compression fractures will increase. For those with severe pain or progressive collapse, early vertebral augmentation, either kyphoplasty or vertebroplasty, affords excellent early pain relief, early return to function, and some restoration of local sagittal alignment. Recent 2-year follow-up data suggest that the benefits of the procedure persist with time. Table 3–4 provides a summary of recommendations

TABLE 3–4. Summary of Recommendations

STATEMENT	LEVEL OF EVIDENCE/GRADE OF RECOMMENDATION
1. Patients with osteoporotic compression fractures should undergo vertebral augmentation to improve physical function and reduce pain.	B
2. Patients with osteoporotic compression fractures should undergo vertebral augmentation to correct kyphotic deformity.	B
3. Kyphoplasty is less prone than vertebroplasty to cause adjacent-level compression fractures by more effectively restoring the overall spinal balance.	B
4. Kyphoplasty is less prone than vertebroplasty to cause cement extravasation.	B

REFERENCES

1. Cooper C, et al: Incidence of clinically diagnosed vertebral fractures: A population-based study in Rochester, Minnesota, 1985–1989. J Bone Miner Res 7:221–227, 1992.
2. Kim DH, Vaccaro AR: Osteoporotic compression fractures of the spine; current options and considerations for treatment. Spine J 6:479–487, 2006.
3. Melton LJ 3rd, Kallmes DF: Epidemiology of vertebral fractures: Implications for vertebral augmentation. Acad Radiol 13:538–545, 2006.
4. Silverman SL: The clinical consequences of vertebral compression fracture. Bone 13(suppl 2):S27–S31, 1992.
5. Melton LJ 3rd, et al: Epidemiology of vertebral fractures in women. Am J Epidemiol 129:1000–1011, 1989.
6. Wasnich RD: Vertebral fracture epidemiology. Bone 18(3 suppl):179S–183S, 1996.
7. Galibert P, Deramond H, Rosat P, Le Gars D: [Preliminary note on the treatment of vertebral angioma by percutaneous acrylic vertebroplasty]. Neurochirurgie 33:166–168, 1987.
8. Lieberman IH, et al: Initial outcome and efficacy of "kyphoplasty" in the treatment of painful osteoporotic vertebral compression fractures. Spine 26:1631–1638, 2001.
9. Bai B, et al: The use of an injectable, biodegradable calcium phosphate bone substitute for the prophylactic augmentation of osteoporotic vertebrae and the management of vertebral compression fractures. Spine 24:1521–1526, 1999.
10. Cotten A, et al: Percutaneous vertebroplasty: State of the art. Radiographics 18:311–323, 1998.
11. Garfin SR, Buckley RA, Ledlie J: Balloon kyphoplasty for symptomatic vertebral body compression fractures results in rapid, significant, and sustained improvements in back pain, function, and quality of life for elderly patients. Spine 31:2213–2220, 2006.
12. Grafe IA, et al: Reduction of pain and fracture incidence after kyphoplasty: 1-year outcomes of a prospective controlled trial of patients with primary osteoporosis. Osteoporos Int 16:2005–2012, 2005.
13. Komp M, Ruetten S, Godolias G: Minimally invasive therapy for functionally unstable osteoporotic vertebral fracture by means of kyphoplasty: prospective comparative study of 19 surgically and 17 conservatively treated patients. J Miner Stoffwechs 11(suppl 1):13–15, 2004.
14. Diamond TH, et al: Clinical outcomes after acute osteoporotic vertebral fractures: A 2-year non-randomised trial comparing percutaneous vertebroplasty with conservative therapy. Med J Aust 184:113–117, 2006.
15. Alvarez L, et al: Percutaneous vertebroplasty: Functional improvement in patients with osteoporotic compression fractures. Spine 31:1113–1118, 2006.
16. Nakano M, et al: Calcium phosphate cement-based vertebroplasty compared with conservative treatment for osteoporotic compression fractures: A matched case-control study. J Neurosurg Spine 4:110–117, 2006.
17. Fourney DR, Schomer DF, Nader R, et al: Percutaneous vertebroplasty and kyphoplasty for painful vertebral body fractures in cancer patients. J Neurosurg 98:21–30, 2003.
18. Grohs JG, Matzner M, Trieb K, Krepler P: Minimal invasive stabilization of osteoporotic vertebral fractures: A prospective nonrandomized comparison of vertebroplasty and balloon kyphoplasty. J Spinal Disord Tech 18:238–242, 2005.
19. Masala S, Schillaci O, Massari F: MRI and bone scan imaging in the preoperative evaluation of painful vertebral fractures treated with vertebroplasty and kyphoplasty. In Vivo 19:1055–1060, 2005.
20. Pflugmacher R, Kandziora F, Schröder R, et al: [Vertebroplasty and kyphoplasty in osteoporotic fractures of vertebral bodies—a prospective 1-year follow-up analysis]. Rofo 177:1670–1676, 2005.
21. Köse KC, Cebesoy O, Akan B, et al: Functional results of vertebral augmentation techniques in pathological vertebral fractures of myelomatous patients. J Natl Med Assoc 98:1654–1658, 2006.
22. Hulme PA, et al: Vertebroplasty and kyphoplasty: A systematic review of 69 clinical studies. Spine 31:1983–2001, 2006.
23. Taylor RS, Taylor RJ, Fritzell P: Balloon kyphoplasty and vertebroplasty for vertebral compression fractures: A comparative systematic review of efficacy and safety. Spine 31:2747–2755, 2006.
24. Hadjipavlou AG, Tzermiadianos M, Katonis PG, Szpalski M: Percutaneous vertebroplasty and balloon kyphoplasty for the treatment of osteoporotic vertebral compression fractures and osteolytic tumours. J Bone Joint Surg Br 87:1595–1604, 2005.
25. Taylor RS, Fritzell P, Taylor RJ: Balloon kyphoplasty in the management of vertebral compression fractures: An updated systematic review and meta-analysis. Eur Spine J 2007;16:1085–1100.
26. Bouza C, Lopez T, Magro A, et al: Efficacy and safety of balloon kyphoplasty in the treatment of vertebral compression fractures: A systematic review. Eur Spine J 15:1050–1067, 2006.
27. Ploeg WT, Veldhuizen AG, The B, Sietsma MS: Percutaneous vertebroplasty as a treatment for osteoporotic vertebral compression fractures: A systematic review. Eur Spine J 2006;15:1749–1758.
28. Hochmuth K, Proschek D, Schwarz W, et al: Percutaneous vertebroplasty in the therapy of osteoporotic vertebral compression fractures: A critical review. Eur Radiol 16:998–1004, 2006.
29. Hadjipavlou AG, et al: Percutaneous vertebroplasty and balloon kyphoplasty for the treatment of osteoporotic vertebral compression fractures and osteolytic tumours. J Bone Joint Surg Br 87:1595–1604, 2005.
30. Majd ME, Farley S, Holt RT: Preliminary outcomes and efficacy of the first 360 consecutive kyphoplasties for the treatment of painful osteoporotic vertebral compression fractures. Spine J 5:244–255, 2005.
31. Khanna AJ, et al: Functional outcomes of kyphoplasty for the treatment of osteoporotic and osteolytic vertebral compression fractures. Osteoporos Int 17:817–826, 2006.
32. Jang JS, Kim DY, Lee SH: Efficacy of percutaneous vertebroplasty in the treatment of intravertebral pseudarthrosis associated with noninfected avascular necrosis of the vertebral body. Spine 28:1588–1592, 2003.
33. Crandall D, et al: Acute versus chronic vertebral compression fractures treated with kyphoplasty: Early results. Spine J 4:418–424, 2004.
34. Berlemann U, et al: Kyphoplasty for treatment of osteoporotic vertebral fractures: A prospective non-randomized study. Eur Spine J 13:496–501, 2004.
35. Gaitanis IN, et al: Restoring geometric and loading alignment of the thoracic spine with a vertebral compression fracture: Effects of balloon (bone tamp) inflation and spinal extension. Spine J 5:45–54, 2005.
36. Pradhan BB, et al: Kyphoplasty reduction of osteoporotic vertebral compression fractures: Correction of local kyphosis versus overall sagittal alignment. Spine 31:435–441, 2006.
37. Shindle MK, et al: Vertebral height restoration in osteoporotic compression fractures: Kyphoplasty balloon tamp is superior to postural correction alone. Osteoporos Int 17:1815–1819, 2006.
38. Voggenreiter G: Balloon kyphoplasty is effective in deformity correction of osteoporotic vertebral compression fractures. Spine 30:2806–2812, 2005.
39. Silverman SL, et al: The relationship of health-related quality of life to prevalent and incident vertebral fractures in postmenopausal women with osteoporosis: Results from the Multiple Outcomes of Raloxifene Evaluation Study. Arthritis Rheum 44:2611–2619, 2001.
40. Lin EP, et al: Vertebroplasty: Cement leakage into the disc increases the risk of new fracture of adjacent vertebral body. AJNR Am J Neuroradiol 25:175–180, 2004.
41. Trout AT, Kallmes DF, Kaufman TJ: New fractures after vertebroplasty: adjacent fractures occur significantly sooner. AJNR Am J Neuroradiol 27(1):217–223, 2006.
42. Pflugmacher R, Schroeder RJ, Klostermann CK: Incidence of adjacent vertebral fractures in patients treated with balloon

kyphoplasty: Two years' prospective follow-up. Acta Radiol 47:830–840, 2006.

43. Harrop JS, et al: Primary and secondary osteoporosis' incidence of subsequent vertebral compression fractures after kyphoplasty. Spine 2004 29:2120–2125, 2004.

44. Theodorou DJ, Theodorou SJ, Duncan TD, Garfin SR, Wong WH: Percutaneous balloon kyphoplasty for the correction of a spinal deformity in painful vertebral compression fractures. Clin Imaging 26:1–5, 2002.

45. Wong WH, Olan WJ, Belkoff SM: Balloon kyphoplasty. In: Mathis JM, Deramond H, Belkoff SM, eds. Percutaneous vertebroplasty. New York: Springer-Verlag, 2002: 109–124.

46. Wilhelm K, Stoffel M, Ringel F, et al: Preliminary experience with balloon kyphoplasty for the treatment of painful osteoporotic compression fractures. Rofo 177:1690–1696, 2003 (in German).

47. Phillips FM, Ho E, Campbell-Hupp M, et al: Early radiographic and clinical results of balloon kyphoplasty for the treatment of osteoporotic vertebral compression fractures. Spine 28:2260–2267, 2003.

48. Crandall D, Slaughter D, Hankins PJ, Moore C, Jerman J: Acute versus chronic vertebral compression fractures treated with kyphoplasty: early results. Spine J 4:418–424, 2004.

49. Berlemann U, Franz T, Orler R, Heini PF: Kyphoplasty for treatment of osteoporotic vertebral fractures: a prospective non-randomized study. Eur Spine J 13:496–501, 2004.

50. Hillmeier J, Grafe I, Da Fonseca K, et al: The evaluation of balloon kyphoplasty for osteoporotic vertebral fractures: an interdisciplinary concept. Orthopade 33:893–904, 2004 (in German).

51. Gaitanis I, Hadjipavlou AG, Katonis PG, et al: Balloon kyphoplasty for the treatment of pathological vertebral compressive fractures. Eur Spine J 14:250–260, 2005.

52. Jensen ME, Evans AJ, Mathis JM, et al: Percutaneous polymethylmethacrylate vertebroplasty in the treatment of osteoporotic vertebral body compression fractures: technical aspects. AJNR Am J Neuroradiol 18:1897–1904, 1997.

53. Martin JB, Jean B, Sugiu K, et al: Vertebroplasty: clinical experience and followup results. Bone 25(2 Suppl):11–15, 1999.

54. Cortet B, Cotten A, Boutry N, et al: Percutaneous vertebroplasty in the treatment of osteoporotic vertebral compression fractures: an open prospective study. J Rheumatol 26:2222–2228, 1999.

55. Cyteval C, Sarrabère M, Roux JO, et al: Acute osteoporotic vertebral collapse: open study on percutaneous injection of acrylic surgical cement in 20 patients. AJR Am J Roentgenol 173:1685–1690, 1999.

56. O'Brien JP, Sims JT, Evans AJ: Vertebroplasty in patients with severe vertebral compression fractures: a technical report. AJNR Am J Neuroradiol 21:1555–1558, 2000.

57. Barr JD, Barr MS, Lemley TJ, McCann RM: Percutaneous vertebroplasty for pain relief and spinal stabilization. Spine 25:923–928, 2000.

58. Grados F, Depriester C, Cayrolle G, et al: Long-term observations of vertebral osteoporotic fractures treated by percutaneous vertebroplasty. Rheumatology 39:1410–1414, 2000.

59. Heini PF, Wälchli B, Berlemann U: Percutaneous transpedicular vertebroplasty with PMMA: operative technique and early results: a prospective study for the treatment of osteoporotic compression fractures. Eur Spine J 9:445–450, 2000.

60. Maynard AS, Jensen ME, Schweickert PA, et al: Value of bone scan imaging in predicting pain relief from percutaneous vertebroplasty in osteoporotic vertebral fractures. AJNR Am J Neuroradiol 21:1807–1812, 2000.

61. Amar AP, Larsen DW, Esnaashari N, et al: Percutaneous transpedicular polymethylmethacrylat vertebroplasty for the treatment of spinal compression fractures. Neurosurgery 49:1105–1114, 2001.

62. Moreland DB, Landi MK, Grand W: Vertebroplasty: techniques to avoid complications. Spine J 1:66–71, 2001.

63. Kaufmann TJ, Jensen ME, Schweickert P, Marx WF, Kallmes DF: Age of fracture and clinical outcomes of percutaneous vertebroplasty. AJNR Am J Neuroradiol 2001;22:1860–1863.

64. McGraw JK, Lippert JA, Minkus KD, et al: Prospective evaluation of pain relief in 100 patients undergoing percutaneous vertebroplasty: results and follow-up. J Vasc Interv Radiol 13:883–886, 2002.

65. Peh WC, Gilula LA, Peck DD: Percutaneous vertebroplasty for severe osteoporotic vertebral body compression fractures. Radiology 223:121–126, 2002.

66. Kallmes DF, Schweickert PA, Marx WF, Jensen ME: Vertebroplasty in the mid and upper thoracic spine. AJNR Am J Neuroradiol 23:1117–1120, 2002.

67. Zoarski GH, Snow P, Olan WJ, et al: Percutaneous vertebroplasty for osteoporotic compression fractures: quantitative prospective evaluation of long-term outcomes. J Vas Interv Radiol 13:139–148, 2002.

68. Gaughen JR, Jensen ME, Schweickert PA, et al: Relevance of antecedent venography in percutaneous vertebroplasty for the treatment of osteoporotic compression fractures. AJNR Am J Neuroradiol 23:594–600, 2002.

69. Nakano M, Hirano N, Matsura K, et al: Percutaneous transpedicular vertebroplasty with calcium phosphate cement in the treatment of osteoporotic vertebral compression and burst fractures. J Neurosurg Spine 97:287–293, 2002.

70. Ryu KS, Park CK, Kim MC, Kang JK: Dose-dependent epidural leakage of polymethylmethacrylate after percutaneous vertebroplasty in patients with osteoporotic vertebral compression fractures. J Neurosurg Spine 96:56–61, 2002.

71. Perez-Higueras A, Alvarez L, Rossi R, Quinones D, Al-Assir I: Percutaneous vertebroplasty: long-term clinical and radiological outcome. Neuroradiology 44:950–954, 2002.

72. Evans AJ, Jensen ME, Kip KE, et al: Vertebral compression fractures: pain reduction and improvement in functional mobility after percutaneous polymethylmethacrylate vertebroplasty: retrospective report of 245 cases. Radiology 226:366–372, 2003.

73. Jang JS, Kim DY, Lee SH: Efficacy of percutaneous vertebroplasty in the treatment of intravertebral pseudarthrosis associated with noninfected avascular necrosis of the vertebral body. Spine 28:1588–1592, 2003.

74. Diamond TH, Champion B, Clark WA: Management of acute osteoporotic vertebral fractures: a nonrandomized trial comparing percutaneous vertebroplasty with conservative therapy. Am J Med 114:257–265, 2003.

75. Peh WC, Gelbart MS, Gilula LA, Peck DD: Percutaneous vertebroplasty: treatment of painful vertebral compression fractures with intraosseous vacuum phenomena. AJR Am J Roentgenol 180:1411–1417, 2003.

76. Gangi A, Guth S, Imbert JP, Marin H, Dietermann JL: Percutaneous vertebroplasty: indications, technique, and results. Radiographics 23:10, 2003.

77. Brown DB, Glaiberman CB, Sehgal M, Shimony JS: Treatment of chronic symptomatic vertebral compression fractures with percutaneous vertebroplasty. Am J Roentgenol 182:319–322, 2004.

78. Chen LH, Niu CC, Yu SW, et al., Minimally invasive treatment of osteoporotic vertebral compression fracture. Chang Gung Med J 27:261–267, 2004.

79. Winking M, Stahl JP, Oertel M, Schnettler R, Boker DK: Treatment of pain from osteoporotic vertebral collapse by percutaneous PMMA vertebroplasty. Acta Neurochir (Wien) 146:469–476, 2003.

80. Legroux-Gerot I, Lormeau C, Boutry N, et al: Long-term follow-up of vertebral osteoporotic fractures treated by percutaneous vertebroplasty. Clin Rheumatol 23:310–317, 2004.

81. Alvarez L, Pérez-Higueras A, Quinones D, Calvo E, Rossi RE: Vertebroplasty in the treatment of vertebral tumors: postprocedural outcome and quality of life. Eur Spine J 12:356–360, 2003.

What Is the Ideal Surgical Treatment for an Adult Patient with a Lytic Spondylolisthesis?

Joel A. Finkelstein, MD, FRCS(C)

Lytic spondylolisthesis is a condition where many treatment alternatives have been developed. It can be argued that where several treatment choices are described, then none can be entirely satisfactory; alternatively, all may be satisfactory with little differentiation between them aside from surgeon preference. If the latter is the case, then factors such as operative morbidity and cost should enter into the equation for the ideal treatment. This chapter reviews the current literature in evaluation of these treatment options with a view of identifying the ideal treatment for this condition.

NATURAL HISTORY AND CLASSIFICATION

Lytic spondylolisthesis initially must be defined and classified. The focus of this review is on lytic spondylolisthesis in the adult patient. It should be established, however, that the lytic lesion (defect in the pars interarticularis) develops in childhood. The lesion is not present at birth but has been noted in children as young as 4 months. The pathologic lesion occurs from 5.5 to 7 years of age and during increased activity from ages 11 to 16.[1] The prevalence of a lysis is estimated to be 4.4% at age 6 and increases to 6% in adulthood.[2] In skeletally immature individuals, the tendency of lumbosacral slip progression is most likely to occur in adolescents younger than 15 years. The majority of skeletally mature individuals with a mild lumbosacral slip are asymptomatic, and slippage after adulthood is uncommon. In a long-term follow-up study, Osterman and colleagues[3] note that 90% of the slip had occurred by the time the patient was first seen, and when evaluating long-term outcomes, it was difficult to prove the connection between the radiographic findings and pain.

Most adolescents and young adults with spondylolytic spondylolisthesis have no radicular symptoms. When symptoms do occur, it is due to irritation of the exiting nerve root (L5 in a L5-S1 spondylolisthesis). This develops generally after two to three decades and is secondary to disc degeneration with facet arthropathy leading to lateral recess and foraminal stenosis. This compounds the compression of the L5 nerve root caused by the fibrocartilaginous material formed at the edges of the pars defect[4–6] (Fig. 4–1).

When comparing treatment options, it is critical that similar pathologic lesions are being compared. Spinal level involved and degree of slip are clinical features that are important in categorization. L5-S1 accounts for 82% of the occurrences of lytic spondylolisthesis; L4-L5 level is involved in 11% of cases. In contrast with the L5-S1 isthmic lesion, the L4-L5 level is more prone to be unstable and subject to further slip progression in adulthood. Sagittal rotation, shear translation, and axial rotation are all greater at the L4-L5 level with a pars defect.[7] This can accelerate disc degeneration, further compromise mechanical stability, and lead to greater and earlier onset symptoms compared with the L5-S1 level.[3] The L5-S1 level has greater inherent stability, and hence a lower rate of slip progression and symptoms.

Degree of slip (anterior displacement of L5 on S1) is categorized on a scale I to V. Sagittal rotation or slip angle describes the rotational relation between L5 and the sacrum. Higher slip angles commonly create increased lumbosacral kyphosis and are generally associated with higher degree slips. Generally, the spectrum of developmental lytic spondylolisthesis is divided into low and high grades. Low grade encompasses no slip (spondylolysis alone) to less than 50% (grades I and II). High grade is a slip greater than 50% (grades III, IV, V). High- and low-grade slips, although manifestations of the same pathology, require different treatment strategies. Evaluation of these needs to be independent.

HIGH-GRADE SPONDYLOLISTHESIS

High-grade spondylolisthesis is more commonly treated in the adolescent population when the symptoms develop. Few adults are seen with symptomatic severe slips, which were untreated at a younger age. Most studies in adults that include both high- and low-grade spondylolisthesis report no difference in the outcomes; however, the numbers of high-grade slips included are small.[8,9]

Most authors suggest posterior fusion to include L4 to S1. Numerous approaches to fusion are reported; however, low cohort numbers and no comparative study groups are available for critical evaluation of

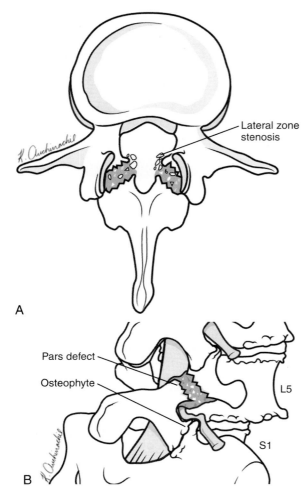

A

B

FIGURE 4–1. *A,* Axial view of vertebrae with bilateral pars defect with fibrocartilage creating lateral zone stenosis. *B,* L5-S1 lateral view demonstrating secondary degenerative changes causing compression of the L5 nerve root at the subarticular and extraforaminal zones.

these various techniques. In summary of the described techniques, these include in situ posterior fusion with instrumentation, transvertebral screws (S1 pedicle screw transgressing the S1 superior end plate to the L5 body), fibular dowels for L5/S1 interbody fusion with L4-S1 instrumentation, titanium cages from either an anterior or posterior approach for interbody L5/S1 fusion, iliac screw supplementation, and L5 vertebrectomy. Good clinical outcomes and fusion rates are described by the advocates of each; however, all studies are class Level IV and V evidence. The role of reduction has inconsistent data to support or refute this, although the risk for neurologic injury is greater with reductions compared with fusions in situ.[10]

LOW-GRADE SPONDYLOLISTHESIS

Greater number and more comprehensive studies are available for low-grade slips in the adult population.

Surgery vs. Conservative Management

In a randomized, controlled study comparing operative versus conservative management, fusion with or without instrumentation compared with an exercise program demonstrated superior clinical outcomes at 2 years. At a longer term, 9-year follow-up, some of the shorter term improvement was lost; however, patients with fusion still classified their global outcome as better than patients receiving conservative treatments.[11,12]

Surgical Techniques

Direct Pars Repair. Direct pars repair is not typically recommended in the adult. In considering this treatment, regardless of the technique chosen, prerequisites are a spondylolysis with no slip, no neurologic symptoms, and a normal magnetic resonance imaging scan at the level of the defect. Degenerative disc disease is the more likely pain generator leading to persistent pain despite a solid pars repair. No Level I, II, or III studies have compared this with nonoperative treatment for back pain. Insufficient evidence is available to suggest that any procedural variation is superior to the next.

Decompression Alone. Decompression alone is not typically recommended for spondylolytic spondylolisthesis. Gill[13] initially described removal of the L5 lamina and pars fibrocartilage to decompress the L5 nerve roots. This "Gill laminectomy" without fusion is not recommended by most authors because of the concern for destabilization, increased slippage, and worsening of back pain. This sentiment is well established through numerous case series.

One case series has reported good results in a select group of patients using a more limited decompression without fusion. When there is minimal back pain and unilateral L5 symptoms and grade 1 spondylolisthesis are present, Weiner and McCulloch[14] describe using a unilateral microsurgical approach to the lateral zone for decompression of the subarticular, foraminal, and extraforaminal structures. As shown in Figure 4–1, the pathoanatomic lesion and compression are lateral. The central portion of the canal is expanded. The fibrocartilaginous mass associated with the pars lesion, facet hypertrophy, and far lateral impingement can all be addressed from this approach.[14] These authors do note that, in the majority of cases of spondylolytic spondylolisthesis, fusion is indicated; however, in this subgroup of patients, a role exists for this therapeutic option.

The decision to perform a decompression in addition to fusion should take into account the presence of neurologic symptoms. In a randomized, controlled trial in patients with minimal or no neurologic symptoms, decompression (Gill's procedure) in addition to posterolateral fusion was compared with a posterolateral fusion alone. The decompression group had a greater rate of pseudarthrosis and unsatisfactory clinical outcomes regardless of the use of instrumentation.[15] A wide decompression may exacerbate the instability and impede fusion rate.

Posterolateral Intertransverse Fusion with or without Instrumentation. Comparing posterolateral intertransverse fusion with and without instrumentation has been evaluated in four randomly controlled trials. In two of these studies, the entire cohort contained patients with a low-grade spondylolytic spondylolisthesis[16,17]; in the other two studies, spondylolytic spondylolisthesis was a subgroup within the study cohort.[18,19] All studies were consistent in their findings in that there were no significant differences between the two groups with respect to functional outcomes and fusion rate.

Interbody Fusion. The addition of an interbody fusion from either a posterior approach (PLIF), transforaminal approach (TLIF), or anterior approach (ALIF) allows for circumferential stability and a biologically superior environment for fusion. The biologic advantage of a PLIF/ALIF/TLIF over a posterolateral fusion is due to the construct being placed under compression along the weight-bearing axis and near the center of rotation. This allows for a blood supply from the adjacent vertebral bodies to the bone graft within the cage. Madan and Boeree,[20] La Rosa and coworkers,[21] and Suk and researchers[22] have performed retrospective comparative studies comparing posterolateral fusion with instrumentation with or without the addition of PLIF. The correction of subluxation, disc height, and foraminal area were maintained better in the PLIF group. However, this did not result in any clinical or functional advantage over the posterolateral fusion/instrumentation group without PLIF.[20] Madan and Boeree[21] found that the group with posterolateral fusion/instrumentation had better clinical outcomes than the PLIF group; however, the latter was more predictable in maintaining correction and achieving union.[21] Suk and researchers[22] found the PLIF condition to have more patients rating their clinical outcome as excellent compared with the posterolateral fusion/instrumentation group.[22]

A recent study (Level III) describes the use of transforaminal lumbar interbody fusion for anterior column support. Lauber and investigators[23] prospectively evaluated TLIF in 20 patients who also underwent a Gill laminectomy and posterolateral fusion with instrumentation. They found improvement in Oswestry Disability Index from a mean score of 20 to 11 at 2-year follow-up. The results were maintained at 4 years. This was not a comparative study; however, TLIF was shown to be a viable treatment alternative, and further study with the more established PLIF is needed in comparing anterior column support/fusion techniques.[23]

Anterior Lumbar Interbody Fusion. There is a lack of evidence to support ALIF alone as a treatment alternative. Direct decompression of the nerve roots is not possible with this approach. It is suggested by these authors however (Level IV evidence), that the provision of stability alone may be adequate in

managing this pathology.[24,25]

In a prospective comparative study, Swan and colleagues[26] compare posterolateral instrumented fusion/decompression with posterolateral instrumented fusion/decompression with ALIF. Clinical and radiologic outcomes at 2 years were superior in the combined anteroposterior group compared with posterior-alone surgery (Level II evidence). Spruit and coworkers[27] and Wang and coauthors[28] in two separate case series also describe good clinical outcomes with ALIF in addition to posterolateral fusion, decompression, and instrumentation. Although these latter studies were methodologically poor (Level IV), they report radiologic outcomes with excellent maintenance of slip reduction at 2- to 3-year follow-up. Together, these studies give evidence in support of the use of anterior interbody support (ALIF) in addition to posterior instrumented fusion and decompression.

RECOMMENDATIONS

Currently, no Level I evidence exists to provide support for any one treatment option over another. For low-grade slips, stability of the L5-S1 level by way of instrumentation and fusion addresses the dynamic component of this disorder. Interbody fusion has been shown to provide better maintenance of reduction and foraminal height. Better clinical outcomes with Level II evidence have been shown using a combined anterior (ALIF) and posterior approach. With posterior-only surgery (PLIF), the current literature is limited to Level III evidence. These have not necessarily shown better clinical outcomes compared with posterolateral fusion/instrumentation alone, but again have shown better radiologic outcomes. It would seem that the advantages of anterior column support and circumferential fusion should be equally apparent by PLIF as with ALIF, but without the need for a secondary surgery in the latter. Better methodologic studies are certainly needed.

It is expected that treatment options will continue to evolve as newer implants and minimally invasive techniques continue to develop. A recent trend is toward TLIF whereby interbody fusion with centering of the implant can be achieved from one side. This may have the potential to allow unilateral approaches for the necessary decompression, and provide anterior and posterior column support. Given the current and developing techniques, only through prospective randomized trials will the optimal surgical treatment be established. Table 4–1 provides a summary of recommendations for the treatment of lytic spondylolisthesis.

TABLE 4–1. Summary of Recommendations

STATEMENT	LEVEL OF EVIDENCE/GRADE OF RECOMMENDATION	REFERENCES
1. Surgery is superior to conservative care in symptomatic patients for both low- and high-grade slips.	A	11, 12
2. The addition of posterior instrumentation does not improve the efficacy of posterolateral fusion (L5-S1).	B	16–19
3. Anterior column support by way of anterior lumbar interbody fusion has been shown to provide superior clinical and radiologic results than posterolateral fusion/decompression with instrumentation alone.	B	26–28
4. Anterior column support by posterior lumbar interbody fusion in addition to posterolateral fusion/decompression and instrumentation has demonstrated inconclusive results.	C	20–22
5. Anterior column support by transforaminal lumbar interbody fusion in addition to postero-lateral fusion/decompression has demonstrated good outcomes.	B	23
6. Decompression alone by way of the "Gill procedure" is not supported. In a select group of patients (no back pain, unilateral leg symptoms, and grade I slip), a unilateral microsurgical approach to the lateral zone for decompression has yielded good results.	B	13–15

REFERENCES

1. Wiltse LL: The etiology of spondylolisthesis. J Bone Joint Surg Am 44-A:539–560, 1962.
2. Fredrickson BE, Baker D, et al: The natural history of spondylolysis and spondylolisthesis. J Bone Joint Surg Am 66:699–707, 1984.
3. Osterman K, Schlenzka D, et al: Isthmic spondylolisthesis in symptomatic and asymptomatic subjects, epidemiology, and natural history with special reference to disk abnormality and mode of treatment. Clin Orthop Relat Res (297):65–70, 1993.
4. Floman Y: Progression of lumbosacral isthmic spondylolisthesis in adults. Spine 25:342–347, 2000.
5. Seitsalo S, Osterman K, et al: Progression of spondylolisthesis in children and adolescents. A long-term follow-up of 272 patients. Spine 16:417–421, 1991.
6. Virta L, Osterman K: Radiographic correlations in adult symptomatic spondylolisthesis: A long-term follow-up study. J Spinal Disord 7:41–48, 1994.
7. Grobler LJ, Novotny JE, Wilder DG, et al: L4-5 isthmic spondylolisthesis. A biomechanical analysis comparing stability in L4-5 and L5-S1 isthmic spondylolisthesis. Spine 19:222–227, 1994.
8. Hanley E, Levy JA: Surgical treatment of isthmic lumbosacral spondylolisthesis. Analysis of variables influencing results. Spine 14:48–50, 1989.
9. Johnson LP, Nasca RJ, Dunham WK: Surgical treatment of isthmic spondylolisthesis. Spine 13:93–97, 1988.
10. Hu S, Bradford DS, Transfeldt E: Reduction of high-grade spondylolisthesis using Edwards instrumentation. Spine 21:367–371, 1996.
11. Ekman PH, Moller H, Hedlund R: The long-term effect of posterolateral fusion in adult isthmic spondylolisthssis: A randomized controlled study. Spine 5:36–44, 2005.
12. Moller H, Hedlund R: Surgery versus conservative management in adult isthmic spondylolisthesis—a prospective randomized study: Part 1. Spine 25:1711–1715, 2000.
13. Gill GG: Long-term follow-up evaluation of a few patients with spondylolisthesis treated by excision of the loose lamina with decompression of the nerve roots without spinal fusion. Clin Orthop Relat Res (182):215–219, 1984.
14. Weiner BK, McCulloch JA: Microdecompression without fusion for radiculopathy associated with lytic spondylolisthesis. J Neurosurg 85:582–585, 1996.
15. Carragee EJ: Single-level posterolateral arthrodesis, with or without posterior decompression, for the treatment of isthmic spondylolisthesis in adults. A prospective, randomized study. J Bone Joint Surg Am 79:1175–1180, 1997.
16. McGuire RA, Amundson GM: The use of primary internal fixation in spondylolisthesis. Spine 18:1662–1672, 1993.
17. Moller H, Hedlund R: Instrumented and noninstrumented posterolateral fusion in adult spondylolisthesis—a prospective randomized study: Part 2. Spine 25:1716–1721, 2000.
18. France JC, Yaszemski MJ, Lauerman WC, et al: A randomized prospective study of posterolateral lumbar fusion outcomes with and without pedicle screw instrumentsation. Spine 24:553–560, 1999.
19. Thomsen K, Christensen FB, Eiskjaer SP, et al: The effect of pedicle screw instrumentation on functional outcome and fusion rates in posterolateral lumbar spinal fusion: A prospective randomized clinical study. Spine 22:2813–2822.
20. Madan S, Boeree NR: Outcome of posterior lumbar interbody fusion versus posterolateral fusion for spondylolytic spondylolisthesis. Spine 27:1536–1542, 2002.
21. La Rosa G, Conti A, et al: Pedicle screw fixation for isthmic spondylolisthesis: Does posterior lumbar interbody fusion improve outcome over posterolateral fusion? J Neurosurg 99(2 suppl):143–150, 2003.
22. Suk SI, Lee CK, et al: Adding posterior lumbar interbody fusion to pedicle screw fixation and posterolateral fusion after decompression in spondylolytic spondylolisthesis. Spine 22:210–220, 1997.
23. Lauber S, Schulte TL, et al: Clinical and radiologic 2-4-year results of transforaminal lumbar interbody fusion in degenerative and isthmic spondylolisthesis grades 1 and 2. Spine 31:1693–1698, 2006.
24. Cheng CL, Fang D, et al: Anterior spinal fusion for spondylolysis and isthmic spondylolisthesis. Long term results in adults. J Bone Joint Surg Br 71:264–267, 1989.
25. Ishihara H, Osada R, et al: Minimum 10-year follow-up study of anterior lumbar interbody fusion for isthmic spondylolisthesis. J Spinal Disord 14:91–99, 2001.

26. Swan J, Hurwitz E, Malek F, et al: Surgical treatment for unstable low-grade isthmic spondylolisthesis in adults: A prospective controlled study of posterior instrumented fusion compared with combined anterior-posterior fusion. Spine J 6:606–614, 2006.

27. Spruit M, Van Jonbergen JPW, et al: A concise follow-up of a previous report: Posterior reduction and anterior lumbar interbody fusion in symptomatic low-grade adult isthmic spondylolisthesis. Eur Spine J 14:828–832, 2005.

28. Wang JM, Kim DJ, et al: Posterior pedicular screw instrumentation and anterior interbody fusion in adult lumbar spondylolysis or grade I spondylolisthesis with segmental instability. J Spinal Disord 9:83–88, 1996.

Chapter 5

What Is the Optimal Treatment for Degenerative Lumbar Spinal Stenosis?

Albert J. M. Yee, MD, MSc, FRCSC

Although it is unclear which factors account for patients who become significantly symptomatic from lumbar spinal stenosis, treatment for this condition is a common component of any spinal clinical practice. In deciding on the optimal treatment for degenerative lumbar spinal stenosis, one must first define the entity that requires treatment. Strictly speaking, spinal stenosis relates to the anatomic structural narrowing of the neural elements of the lumbar spinal canal. Some individuals are born with a morphologically narrowed canal in relation to the general population, and the term *congenital lumbar spinal stenosis* is used. Acquired lumbar spinal stenosis most commonly occurs because of degenerative changes with aging in the presence or absence of a congenitally small canal. It may be associated with other structural degenerative features that include spondylolisthesis. The term *neurogenic claudication* (or *pseudoclaudication*) relates to the constellation of symptoms of activity-related leg pain that is relieved with rest and is spondylogenic in origin because of structural spinal stenosis. Although the exact cause and pathophysiology of the symptoms remain evasive and poorly delineated, multiple factors have been implicated in its pathogenesis. In the era of modern generation imaging techniques, structural degenerative changes including spinal stenosis is prevalent in the general population and in individuals with minimal low back or low-related symptomatology.[1] One must first carefully delineate the patients with symptoms before deciding on what may be the optimal treatment for their conditions. The degenerative process of the lumbar spine (i.e., spondylosis) with or without anatomic structural evidence for spinal stenosis can in itself be a pain generator of back pain in certain individuals, and not all individuals with spinal stenosis experience development of neurogenic claudication. The correlation between structural stenosis and the presence and severity of claudicant symptoms is poor; therefore, the clinical evaluation of a patient is paramount. Many studies reporting results relating to spinal stenosis often use the term interchangeably with neurogenic claudication. Unfortunately, the clinical presentation of symptomatic lumbar spinal stenosis is variable, and many studies group these patients with other patients with low-back–associated symptoms, for example, patients with chronic mechanical low back pain. In addition, leg symptomatology that is spondylogenic has variable presentations, and certain individuals may have primarily radiculopathic or sciatica-like symptomatology relating to structural spinal stenosis without the more classic description of a claudicant pattern. Symptoms can be unilateral or bilateral. Therefore, the comparison of a heterogeneous population of patients is a confounder to the review of literature.

OPTIONS

Acquired degenerative lumbar spinal stenosis is a chronic condition currently without a cure for its underlying pathogenesis. As eluded to in the introduction, a potential myriad of presenting clinical symptoms exists. As such, a variety of options is available for treatment. Because the constellation of symptoms and symptom severity varies considerably from patient to patient and over time in a particular patient, treatment needs to be individualized. The goals of treatment are to relieve pain and to improve physical functioning and activity, thereby positively impacting patient quality of life. This chapter focuses on predominantly *Journal of Bone and Joint Surgery* combined volumes (JBJS) Level I and II evidence, and potential therapeutic options discussed utilize the JBJS Grades of Recommendations. In general, the strength of evidence in literature for the potential therapies that will be discussed is fair or insufficient (grade B or I, respectively) at best. It is clear that additional research and study is warranted to fully endorse some of the available therapies. With a heterogeneous condition such as spinal stenosis, treatment effects are likely specific to patient subgroups. Degenerative lumbar spondylolisthesis with associated lumbar stenosis is discussed elsewhere in this textbook and will not formally form part of this chapter's specific review.

Nonsurgical Treatment (Grade I)

A relative paucity of randomized clinical trials in the support of many of the commonly practiced and reported nonsurgical therapies in lumbar spinal stenosis exists. As such, available recommendations are primarily based on expert opinion rather than on evidence.

Education (Grade I). Many professionals in the practice of medicine consider patient education to be paramount in the success of any recommended therapy. Recent spinal literature has focused on a variety of both nonsurgical and surgical therapies. Although some randomized trials evaluate the effect of educational programs as a therapeutic adjunct in the surgical treatment of patients undergoing lumbar disc decompression surgery, other trials applying educational strategies have grouped heterogeneous populations of patients.[2,3] A relative paucity in recent Level I and II literature evaluating the effects of educational therapy or programs specifically in the treatment of lumbar spinal stenosis exists. Deyo and investigators[4] evaluated the effect of an interactive video program in the decision-making process for patients considering surgical treatment for their lumbar spinal conditions. This prospective, randomized clinical trial at two centers enrolled a heterogeneous population of patients (171 patients with herniated discs, 110 patients with lumbar spinal stenosis, 112 with other diseases). The authors observed a greater rate of surgery in the video group (39% video and booklet vs. 29% booklet alone). However, this was not statistically significant ($P = 0.34$), and the authors indicated that the study was underpowered for their subgroup proportional comparisons in the patients with lumbar spinal stenosis (power analysis post hoc = 12%). The study did not observe a significant effect of the video program on symptomatic and functional results at 3 months and 1 year. In addition, there did not appear to be a significant effect on patient satisfaction with care or their satisfaction with the decision-making process comparing the two randomized groups. Overall study follow-up rate was 88% at 1 year. Compliance in the video program and booklet group was 97% for the video portion and 84% for the booklet portion, respectively, and 97% in the booklet alone group. In a follow-up study evaluating the knowledge gain as assessed by a pretreatment and post-treatment knowledge test, the combination of the interactive video with booklet produced greater knowledge gains than the book alone group in the subgroup of patients with the least knowledge at baseline.[5]

Medications (Grade I). A wide gamut of oral medications is available for the potential treatment of symptomatic lumbar spinal stenosis. These include, among others, nonsteroidal agents, analgesics (narcotic and non-narcotic), and antineuritics (tricyclic antidepressants, anticonvulsants). Although there are many randomized studies of various medications for lower back disorders and low back pain, few have specifically focused on patients with stenosis. Of the few studies that have focused specifically on patients with lumbar stenosis, a couple of randomized studies on the evaluation of calcitonin treatment have been reported.[6–8] Eskola and colleagues[6] performed a randomized, placebo-controlled, double-blind, crossover study in 40 patients with lumbar spinal stenosis with 1-year follow-up demonstrating that calcitonin had beneficial effects on patients'

symptoms without producing significant adverse effects.[6] The investigators observed primarily an analgesic effect with some positive effect on walking distance, although the authors note that the treatment effect was poor in those patients with marked limitation in walking distance caused by neurogenic claudication. Podichetty and coauthors[7] randomized 55 patients with clinical lumbar canal stenosis and pseudoclaudication and pain visual analog scale (VAS) index of greater than or equal to 6 to either placebo or intranasal calcitonin for 6 weeks followed by an open-label 6-week extension during which all patients received active drug. Calcitonin was administered by nasal spray (400 IU daily) at twice the clinical dose typically used for postmenopausal women with osteoporosis. The overall study dropout rate was 22% for reasons relating to study protocol deviations, adverse event reporting, or withdrawal because of lack of perceived efficacy. Rash, erythema, and burning of the face and neck regions severe enough to cause withdrawal from treatment occurred in two patients in the experimental group. At 6 weeks, there was no difference between the two groups in change in pain VAS when compared with baseline. No difference existed between groups in time from the onset of walking to the onset of pain. Patients in both treatment groups reported improvements to their overall walking distance. However, no difference was present between the study groups. There also did not appear to be a significant effect on patient-reported functional outcome measures. The authors conclude that nasal calcitonin is not superior to placebo, and they suggest that the drug does not appear to have a role in the nonoperative treatment of lumbar canal stenosis. The study authors evaluated efficacy primarily at 6 weeks. The open-label phase during the subsequent 6 weeks suggested a trend toward improvement in patients treated with salmon calcitonin during the second phase of the trial, particularly in pain scores and 36-Item Short Form Health Survey (SF-36) results. The authors note that it is possible that the beneficial effects of nasal calcitonin could require a longer preload of drug, and that efficacy may be achieved using a different treatment schedule. In addition, the authors also indicate that the mean walking distance of patients in their study was in the more limited range where efficacy was also not demonstrated in the similar subpopulation of the study that Eskola and colleagues[6] reported.

One of the more recent randomized studies specifically focusing on lumbar spinal stenosis patients evaluated the use of gabapentin, which has been used in the treatment of chronic neuropathic pain. Yaksi and coworkers[9] randomized 55 patients with lumbar spinal stenosis and intermittent neurogenic claudication into 2 groups. Both randomized groups received physical therapy exercises, lumbosacral corset using a steel reinforced bracing design, and pharmacologic treatment with nonsteroidal anti-inflammatory drugs. The treatment group received in addition oral gabapentin administered at a dosage of 900 mg/day and increased weekly in increments of 300 mg up to a total maximal dosage of 2400 mg/day. Patients who experienced side effects (drowsiness and dizziness) were prescribed bed rest and increased oral fluid intake. Study end points to 4 months included objective assessments of walking distance, VAS scores, and proportional methods analysis of motor and sensory deficits within each group and at the end of treatment. At follow-up, both groups demonstrated improvement, with the gabapentin treatment group showing significantly better walking distance and improvements in pain scores and recovery of sensory deficit. Limitations of the study include the length of follow-up and the potential confounder of the placebo effect (Level II).

Therapeutic Exercises (Grade I). Many randomized, controlled trials evaluating therapeutic or rehabilitative exercise programs in lumbar spinal disorders have often used a heterogenous population of patients with chronic low back pain. A small number of patients evaluated represent patients with spinal stenosis for which the severity and extent of neurologic leg symptomatology relative to back pain is poorly characterized. In addition, studies comparing therapeutic exercise with surgery have primarily evaluated fusion surgery as compared with nonsurgical treatment in the management of mechanical low back pain in lumbar spondylosis.[10–12] In lumbar spinal stenosis, some authors have proposed programs that use lumbar flexion exercises with the avoidance of extension exercises because of the spinal canal and neuroforaminal narrowing produced by lumbar extension. General aerobic conditioning and aqua therapy have also been advised in the treatment of these patients. However, limited evidence is available that actually guides the recommendation of one program over another or evaluates the benefit of such programs over natural history alone. In one study by Whitman and colleagues,[13] the authors performed a multicenter, randomized, controlled trial on 58 patients with lumbar spinal stenosis. Patients were randomized to one of two 6-week physical therapy programs. One program consisted of manual therapy, lumbar exercises, and body weight supported treadmill walking, whereas the other program consisted of ultrasound, lumbar flexion exercises, and treadmill walking. Patient-perceived recovery was the primary outcome with secondary measures including Oswestry Disability Index, a numeric pain rating, satisfaction, and the results of the treadmill test. Patients in both randomized groups demonstrated improvements to measured outcome parameters. Perceived recovery was greater for the program consisting of manual therapy, treadmill walking, and exercise (perceived recovery 2.6; confidence interval, 1.8–7.8). Considerations to the study results was follow-up to 1 year and that a subset of patients in each group received additional treatment during the study period consisting of epidural steroid injection, surgery, medications, and/or additional specialty physician consultations (Level II).

Therapeutic Injections (Grade I)

A variety of anesthetics, corticosteroids, or opioids can be injected into various anatomic locations in the lumbar spine. Conflicting results have been reported in the literature on their use in spinal stenosis to allow for recommendation for or against intervention. In Fukusaki and coauthors' study,[14] 53 patients with neurogenic claudication of less than 20 m were randomized to either epidural injection with 8 mL saline ($n = 16$), epidural block with 8 mL of 1% mepivacaine ($n = 18$), or epidural block with 8 mL of 1% mepivacaine and 40 mg methylprednisolone ($n = 19$). There did not appear to be a significant advantage of epidural steroid injection as compared with epidural block with a local anesthetic alone. The study had a relative short follow-up to 3 months. Primary study outcome was walking distance in meters to intractable leg pain as quantified by an independent reviewer. By 1 week, patients in the epidural block with or without steroid groups demonstrated greater walking distances when compared with patients in the saline group. At 1- and 3-month follow-up, patients in the epidural block with or without steroids group had a greater improvement in walking distance compared with before injection. With the sample size, a statistically significant effect comparing the three randomized groups in walking distances after 1 or 3 months of follow-up did not exist. Cuckler and colleagues'[15] randomized study on 73 patients with lumbar radicular pain syndromes caused by either disc herniation or lumbar stenosis did not demonstrate a significant effect of 7 mL methylprednisolone acetate and procaine over 7 mL physiologic saline solution and procaine in the treatment of patients observed for an average of 20 months. Wilson-MacDonald and coworkers'[16] study randomized and compared epidural steroid injection with intramuscular injection with local anesthetic with steroid and observed better improvement in short-term pain relief in the epidural group; however, the long-term benefits or need for subsequent surgery was no different over the long term between groups. The study evaluated 93 randomized patients for a minimum of 2 years. All patients evaluated in the study were considered potential candidates for surgical treatment. Ng and colleagues[17] evaluated 86 randomized patients with unilateral radicular symptoms who received either bupivacaine with methylprednisolone injection ($n = 43$) or bupivacaine alone ($n = 43$). At 3-month follow-up, both groups demonstrated improvement. However, there did not appear to be an added benefit to the use of corticosteroids in pain severity, claudicant walking distance, or patient-derived functional outcome.

Surgical Treatment (B)

The abundance of Level I and II evidence relating to surgery in lumbar spinal stenosis is more focused on variations in surgical techniques than on evaluating the specific efficacy of surgical versus nonsurgical strategies. With the realization that there really is a lack of grade A or consistent grade B evidence for many nonsurgical therapies that are commonly practiced, the mainstay of lumbar spinal stenosis surgery can be more broadly categorized into surgical decompressive techniques with or without adjuvant spondylodesis or spinal fusion. The surgical principles involve decompression of compressive elements in lumbar canal stenosis (overgrown bony facets, ligamentous hypertrophy, disc herniations/extrusions) with or without adjuvant fusion of grossly degenerate levels or those levels with instability. Instability in the context of lumbar spinal stenosis in association with degenerative spondylolisthesis is discussed elsewhere in this textbook and is not included in this chapter (Chapter 4). The results of surgical intervention are generally positive in the relief of neurogenic claudicant symptomatology and patient-related quality of life, although its effect on objective physical parameters of function in the literature has been more variable. The notion that surgery for lumbar stenosis is typically more successful in the relief of claudicant symptomatology versus the relief of mechanical low back pain is generally accepted (Levels IV/V). However, there is a lack of large randomized trials comparing surgery with nonsurgical therapy in a homogeneous population with symptomatic lumbar spinal stenosis. The most recent Cochrane review of published randomized clinical trials for the surgical treatment of degenerative lumbar stenosis has included a review of heterogeneous studies, with seven relating to spondylolisthesis, spinal stenosis, and nerve compression.[18] In reviewing those Class I and II studies that specifically compare surgical with nonsurgical treatment in lumbar stenosis, several reports relate to the long-term results from the Maine Lumbar Spine Study. These studies have compared a prospective cohort of patients treated a priori with either surgery or nonsurgical therapy[19–21] (Level II). In the most recent report of 148 eligible consenting patients who were initially enrolled, 105 were alive after 10 years.[21] Among surviving patients, long-term follow-up of between 8 and 10 years was available for 97 of 123 (79%) patients. As anticipated, patients undergoing surgery had worse baseline symptoms and functional status than those initially treated without surgery. Outcomes at 1 and 4 years favored those patients who underwent initial surgery. After 8 to 10 years, there was no difference comparing treatment groups in the percentage of patients who reported that their back pain was improved (53% vs. 50%, surgical vs. nonsurgical; $P = 0.8$), improvements in predominant symptom of either back or leg pain (54% vs. 42%; $P = 0.3$), and satisfaction with their current status (55% vs. 49%; $P = 0.5$). Leg pain relief and greater back-related functional status continued to favor those initially treated surgically. By 10 years, 23% of surgical patients had undergone at least a second lumbar spine operation, and those patients who required additional surgeries faired worse when compared with those patients who continued with their initial treatment. No difference was reported in outcomes accordant to actual treatment received at 10 years. The study limitations include its observational and nonrandomized design, although baseline differences among treatment groups were considered and adjusted for in the analysis. Surgery in their Maine Lumbar Spine study consisted predominantly but not exclusively of decompressive nonfusion surgery, and the authors were not able to provide substantive clinical details for why subsequent surgeries were required in certain patients and what type of procedure was subsequently required.

Herno and investigators[22] performed a matched-pair study of surgically and nonsurgically treated patients with lumbar spinal stenosis (Level III). A total of 496 patients who underwent surgery between 1974 and 1987, and 57 patients treated conservatively between 1980 and 1987 were evaluated at an average of 4 years after recommended treatment. Sex, age, myelographic findings, major symptom, and duration of symptoms were matched. At follow-up, subjective disability was assessed by Oswestry questionnaire, and functional status was evaluated by clinical examination. No statistical difference was found in outcome between the matched-pair groups, although male patients who underwent surgery fared better when compared with male patients who underwent conservative treatment. Functional status was good in both treatment groups and for both sex groups.

In Amundsen and colleagues' study,[23] a prospective cohort of 100 patients with symptomatic lumbar spinal stenosis was provided surgical or conservative treatment and followed for 10 years (Level II). Nineteen patients with what was considered to be severe symptoms were treated with surgery, 50 patients with moderate symptoms were treated nonoperatively, and 31 patients were randomized to either conservative ($n = 18$) or surgical ($n = 13$) treatment. Patients with an unsatisfactory result from conservative treatment were offered delayed surgery at a median of 3.5 months. The results of patients randomized to surgery were better than for patients randomized to conservative treatment. The treatment results of delayed surgery were similar to that of the initial group. Clinically significant deterioration of symptoms during the final 6 years of the study period was not observed. Patients with significant multilevel pathology did not respond as well as those with primarily single-level pathology. Limitations of the study included a relatively small number of patients randomized and the lack of patient-derived functional outcome measures.

In a more recent study that randomized 94 patients into surgical and nonsurgical groups, Malmivaara and investigators[24] performed a multicenter prospective study evaluating outcome based primarily on assessment of functional disability using the Oswestry Disability Index. Inclusion criteria included back pain with radiation to buttocks or lower limbs, fatigue or loss of sensation in the lower limbs aggravated by walking, persistent pain without progressive neurologic dysfunction, imaging consistent with lumbar stenosis (midsagittal diameter <10 mm^2 or cross-sectional dural area <75 mm^2), and symptoms and signs for longer than 6 months. In the 50 patients randomized to surgery, surgery consisted of decompressive laminectomy of the stenotic segment(s), and in 10 patients, adjuvant transpedicular fusion was performed. The nonsurgical group was followed by a physiatrist who assessed the need for individualized treatment that included medications such as nonsteroidal anti-inflammatories or active/passive physiotherapy programs. Baseline low back or lower limb pain scores, Oswestry Disability Index scores, or walking ability was not significantly different comparing the two randomized groups, although there was a greater proportion of female patients and patients with good perceived health randomized to the surgical group. At 2-year follow-up, patients in both randomized groups reported improvements to their condition. In the 44 patients randomized to the nonoperative group, 4 patients required surgery by 2 years because of persistent symptoms. The authors observed at 2-year follow-up that those patients who underwent initial decompressive surgery reported greater improvement regarding leg pain, back pain, and overall disability when compared with the nonsurgical group. Limitations to the study include the length of follow-up and varying surgery type being performed in the surgical arm. The most recent study by Weinstein et al.[24a] described a randomized study of surgical versus nonsurgical therapy for lumbar spinal stenosis. Surgical candidates with at least 12 weeks of symptoms and spinal stenosis without spondylolisthesis were randomized to decompressive surgery or nonsurgical care. The primary outcomes were bodily pain and physical function on the Medical Outcomes Study 36-item SF36 and modified Oswestry Disability Index at 6 weeks through 2 years. Of the 289 patients enrolled in the randomized cohort and 365 patients enrolled in the observational cohort, there was significant cross-over with 67% of patients randomized to surgery receiving surgery and 43% of patients randomized to nonsurgical care also undergoing surgery by the study 2 year follow-up. The intention-to-treat analysis of the randomized cohort favored surgery on the SF-36 scale for bodily pain with a mean change from baseline of 7.8 points (95% confidence interval, 1.5 to 14.1). The as-treated analysis, adjusted for potential confounders, demonstrated a significant advantage for surgery by 3 months for all primary outcomes that remained significant at 2 years.

In a study on the radiographic severity in lumbar spinal stenosis, Hurri and colleagues[25] reviewed 12-year data on 75 patients with myelographic changes diagnostic for stenosis. The authors observed that the severity of stenosis radiographically predicted disability after adjusting for the effects of age, sex, therapy regimen, and body mass index. Surgical and nonsurgical therapy was not a significant correlate with later disability as quantified by Oswestry Disability Index. Using more recent radiographic imaging, Weiner and investigators[26] prospectively evaluated 27 consecutive patients undergoing isolated surgical decompression at L4-5 for lumbar canal stenosis. Using magnetic resonance imaging (MRI) evaluation of stenosis, the au-

thors observed that a greater than 50% reduction in cross-sectional area or preoperative MRI was more likely to have a successful surgical outcome as quantified by Weiner and Fraser's neurogenic claudication outcome score when compared with those individuals with less than 50% reduction in cross-sectional area.[26] Less consistent evidence has been reported in larger prospective cohort, noncontrolled, surgical series regarding radiographic severity and surgical outcome; although with larger series, one may anticipate a more heterogeneous population of study patients as it pertains to the number of involved lumbar motion segments, and variation in type and extent of lumbar surgery performed.[27,28]

For surgery beyond lumbar spinal decompression, there does not appear to be significant evidence to support or refute the use of adjuvant lumbar fusion in patients undergoing surgery for stenosis in the absence of spondylolisthesis or significant segmental instability. In Grob and coauthors'[29] study, 45 patients were randomized to 1 of 3 treatment groups accordant to the day that patients were admitted to the hospital. The average study follow-up was 28 months, and surgery was performed by a single surgeon. Fifteen patients received lumbar decompressive laminotomy and medial facetectomy, 15 patients received decompression followed by arthrodesis of the most stenotic segment, and 15 patients received decompression followed by arthrodesis of all decompressed spinal levels. Patients in all groups reported improvements in pain and walking distance after surgery. The authors did not observe significant differences in the results among the three groups with regard to the relief of pain, although the study was limited by sample size and also lacked validated patient-derived functional outcome measures. In the prospective multicenter observational study by Katz and colleagues,[28] the authors reviewed 272 patients who underwent lumbar surgery (Level II). The authors acknowledge limitations of this nonrandomized study in terms of the number of participating surgeons and a modest sample size. With this caveat, the authors indicated that the individual surgeon was a more accurate correlate of the decision to perform arthrodesis versus clinical parameters such as spondylolisthesis, that noninstrumented lumbar fusion resulted in greater relief of back pain, and that the costs relating to adjunctive instrumentation in lumbar fusion were not an insignificant consideration.

More recent surgical strategies have included the application of less invasive surgical decompressive techniques, dynamic stabilization techniques as an alternative to lumbar instrumented fusion, and minimally invasive techniques utilizing the concept of affording indirect lumbar spinal decompression. Many of these studies are limited in sample size, heterogeneity of the study population of interest, and lack long-term data. Newer, less invasive surgical strategies have involved modifications to conventional laminectomy and partial facetectomy to balance the degree and extent of bony and soft-tissue dissection/resection necessary to achieve adequate restoration of spinal canal space.[30–32] Several equivalency randomized trials have corroborated in the short term that, in the correct surgical hands, patient outcomes appear to be favorable when compared with conventional laminectomy.[31,32] In Cho and colleagues'[31] study, split-spinous process laminotomy and discectomy were compared with conventional laminectomy (30 patients), with or without discectomy in 70 patients randomized and followed prospectively. The follow-up ranged from 10 to 18 months, with a mean of 15.1 months for the split-spinous process group and 14.8 months for the conventional laminectomy group. There was a shorter mean postoperative duration until ambulation without assistance, a reduction in mean duration of hospital stay, a lower mean creatine phosphokinase-muscular–type isoenzyme level, and a lower VAS score for back pain at 1-year follow-up for the split-spinous process group. Operative time and surgical blood loss, however, were greater for this group. The authors conclude that although the split-spinous process method required more operative time than laminectomy, earlier mobilization and shortened length of stay with reduction in pain and satisfactory neurologic and functional outcomes with the method was an attractive consideration in the context of surgical procedures aimed to address structural lumbar stenosis. In Thome and colleagues'[32] study, 120 consecutive patients with 207 levels of lumbar stenosis (without instability or disc herniation) underwent randomization to bilateral laminotomy, unilateral laminotomy, or laminectomy. Patients were managed for 1 year with visual analogue pain and functional outcome measures (Roland-Morris Scale and SF-36). Complications were lowest in the bilateral laminotomy group, and the authors observed the bilateral laminotomy group to have favorable outcomes when compared with either laminectomy or unilateral laminotomy groups.[32] In addition, there have been short- to intermediate-term randomized studies comparing minimally invasive strategies using indirect lumbar decompressive techniques/devices for patients with stenosis when compared with nonsurgical treatment. In their study, Zucherman and coauthors[33] reviewed the 2-year results of patients randomized to either surgical treatment using the X STOP device or to nonsurgical treatment. The rationale of the device is to increase the interspinous process distance to indirectly decompress the spinal canal positioning the lumbar spine into a relatively more flexed position (minimizing the extent of lumbar extension over the motion segment), which is analogous to the physical therapeutic posturing techniques (e.g., William's flexion program) that may transiently improve patient symptoms relating to lumbar stenosis. One hundred patients were evaluated in the surgical arm and 91 in the control group. The primary measure was the Zurich Claudication questionnaire (ZCQ). At 2 years, experimental patients improved by 45.4% over the mean baseline symptom severity score when compared with 7.4% in the control group. There was greater satisfaction in the treatment group (73.1%) when compared with the control group (35.9%). Observed differences in the ZCQ physical function component favored the treatment group. The control group consisted of an epidural steroid injection after enrollment. Fifty-nine percent of control patients received more than one injection over the study period. Control patients were also prescribed medications and physiotherapy as necessary. Limitations of this study included the lack of comparison with conventional surgical treatment, lack of consistency in the nonsurgical treatment arm, and the study length of follow-up. In their study, Kondrashov and colleagues[34] reviewed a subset of patients who participated in the FDA clinical trial on X STOP and identified 18 patients whose subsequent analysis at 4 years suggested that surgical outcomes were stable as measured by the Oswestry Disability Index. Clearly, longer term follow-up with a larger sample size and validation by independent investigators is warranted before consideration of its use over currently reported strategies. Finally, newer strategies have also included surgical dynamic stabilization utilizing newer implants/devices as a potential alternative to lumbar fusion.[35] Literature on its use has focused primarily on comparisons with conventional techniques of instrumented surgical fusion. The theoretical consideration of dynamic stabilization may have merit as an alternative to lumbar fusion. However, larger randomized series evaluating such technology have coupled the application of these implants/devices to lumbar fusion. Given the lack of high-level evidence with consistent funding to support the use of fusion strategies in general as an adjunct to decompression in lumbar spinal stenosis, future studies evaluating dynamic stabilization require appropriate comparison with surgical decompression without fusion and nonsurgical control subjects. Insufficient evidence exists to support or refute the potential application of many newer surgical strategies in the treatment of lumbar spinal stenosis, and additional studies are required before providing an evidence-based opinion in recommendation(s).

RECOMMENDATIONS

In summary, the strength of evidence according to the JBJS grades of recommendation is insufficient (I) or fair (B) at best for many options that are available to treat patients with symptomatic lumbar spinal stenosis. Many studies have evaluated these patients in the broader context of patients with chronic low back pain. In general, a lack of good evidence (JBJS grade A) exists as it pertains to Level I studies with consistent findings that would guide evidenced-based recommendations for intervention (Table 5–1). Despite anticipated awareness and improvements to evidence-based practice and study design with an increase in Level I studies being reported, much of the current treatment of symptomatic lumbar spinal stenosis is based on expert opinion and medical

Continued on page 36

TABLE 5–1. Review of Level I/II Evidence in the Treatment of Lumbar Spinal Stenosis

OPTION	TYPE	AUTHORS (YEAR OF PUBLICATION)	STUDY TYPE	CONCLUSIONS	JBJS LEVEL OF EVIDENCE	JBJS GRADE OF RECOMMENDATION
Education	Interactive video	Deyo (2000)[4]	RCT	No significant effect of video program on patient satisfaction with care or with decision-making process comparing patients randomized to educational video and booklet or to booklet alone	2	I
Medication	Nasal calcitonin	Eskola (1992)[6]	RCT	Beneficial effect on primarily pain symptoms without adverse side effects	2	I
	Epidural steroids	Podichetty (2004)[7]	RCT	No significant benefit short-term pain or walking distance	2	
		Cuckler (1985)[15]	RCT	No significant effect on lumbar radicular pain caused by disc herniation or lumbar stenosis	2	
		Wilson-MacDonald (2005)[16]	RCT	Better short-term pain relief with epidural steroids, but no significant difference at 2 years	1	
		Fukusaki (1998)[14]	RCT	No significant benefit in walking distances at early term follow-up to 3 months	2	
		Ng (2005)[17]	RCT	No added benefit of steroids at 3 months in pain severity, walking distance, or patient functional outcome	2	
	Methylcoba lamin	Waikakul (2000)[8]	RCT	No difference in randomized to control groups in pain improvement or neurologic signs except neurogenic claudication distance, which was better in the experimental group in follow-up to 2 years	2	
	Gabapentin	Yaksi (2007)[9]	RCT	Gabapentin improves walking distance in the short term (4 months)	2	
Therapeutic exercise		Whitman (2006)[13]	RCT of two physical therapy programs	Perceived recovery was greater for the program with manual therapy, treadmill walking, and exercises	2	I
Surgery	Lumbar spinal decompression	Atlas (1996, 2000, 2005)[19–21]	Prospective observational study	Surgery consisted of decompression in all, with or without fusion (noninstrumented); early outcomes at 1–4 years favored patients undergoing initial surgery versus nonoperative treatment.; however, no difference in outcomes accordant to actual treatment received at 10 years	2	B

Continued

TABLE 5–1. Review of Level I/II Evidence in the Treatment of Lumbar Spinal Stenosis—cont'd

OPTION	TYPE	AUTHORS (YEAR OF PUBLICATION)	STUDY TYPE	CONCLUSIONS	JBJS LEVEL OF EVIDENCE	JBJS GRADE OF RECOMMENDATION
		Malmivaara (2007)[24]	RCT	Surgery consisting of decompression (single or multilevel) with or without fusion (instrumented); at 2 years, patient undergoing initial decompressive surgery reported greater improvement regarding leg pain, back pain, and overall disability when compared with nonsurgical group	1	
		Grob (1995)[29]	RCT	Assessed fusion in conjunction with decompression for stenosis in the absence of spondylolisthesis or significant segmental instability; no significant benefit to additional fusion	2	
		Zucherman (2005)[33]	RCT	Surgical treatment with X STOP compared with nonsurgical arm; greater satisfaction and physical function observed in the surgical arm	2	
		Amundsen (2000)[23]	Prospective cohort with one group (n = 31) randomized	Off the smaller cohort randomized in the study, the surgical group demonstrated greater improvement than the nonsurgical group; study lacks functional outcome measures and reports categoric surgeon and patient rating of surgical outcomes; follow-up to 10 years	2	
		Mariconda (2002)[30]	Prospective comparative study	Single-level or multilevel unilateral laminectomy was compared with conservative therapy; better early improvements in functional and clinical status observed in the surgical group	2	
		Thome (2005)[32]	Randomized comparison of various surgical techniques	Unilateral laminotomy, bilateral laminotomy, and laminectomy compared in the treatment of lumbar stenosis in patients followed for 1 year; patient satisfaction observed to be greater in the bilateral laminotomy group; this group observed to have shorter length of stay and less complications; however, operative time and blood loss greater in the nonlaminectomy groups	2	
		Weinstein (2008)[24a]	RCT	Intent to treat and as-treated analysis demonstrated a significant advantage to decompressive surgery when compared to nonsurgical treatment for symptomatic lumbar spinal stenosis		

JBJS = Journal of Bone and Joint Surgery combined volumes; RCT = randomized, controlled trial.

consensus. Appropriate control arms with consistent and comparable inclusion criteria are required to further strengthen existing literature in this area. Understandably, some of the difficulty in characterizing this condition and ensuring consistency in a homogenous population of study has been described in the introduction. It highlights what many of us encounter in the management of patients with symptomatic lumbar spinal stenosis—a chronic condition with a heterogeneous presentation that changes over time. With this consideration in mind, several themes are available on review of current literature. Symptomatic patients can often be managed through nonsurgical approaches, although insufficient evidence is available to support one specific type of approach over another. It would make inherent sense that patient education is paramount and additional Level I/II studies may further guide strategies that will optimize informing patients of the appropriate knowledge necessary to understand their conditions and treatment options. Many commonly used oral medications have not been convincingly proved effective specifically in the treatment of lumbar stenosis, although some renewed interest in antineuritic medications such as gabapentin warrant further validation and longer term study in patients with symptomatic claudication from spinal stenosis. There is insufficient evidence to substantiate therapeutic exercises over other alternatives in the management of patient-related symptoms apart from the possibly related general health benefits of aerobic conditioning on the cardiovascular system. Epidural steroids are mixed in their results in the literature. The natural history of the condition would appear to be favorable, and nonsurgical therapy in many patients is not necessarily associated with significant clinical deterioration over time. There is a lack of sufficient good evidence and Level I studies to make a strong recommendation of surgery over nonsurgical therapies. It would appear, however, that surgery can be of significant benefit in certain patient subpopulations that require ongoing characterization. As such, fair evidence (JBJS grade B) in the role of surgery in the treatment of persistently symptomatic lumbar stenosis exists. Patients should be appropriately informed that the results of surgery if required at a later stage are not convincingly lessened if a nonsurgical approach is initially chosen. Of the surgical treatment options, insufficient evidence exists to recommend many of the available options beyond a decompressive posterior lumbar procedure. The historical standard of care has been a lumbar laminectomy with or without partial facetectomy. This consideration also needs to be weighed in the context of patients who elect to choose the surgical route because there is an appreciable risk for requiring an additional lumbar procedure over time for their condition, and the results of subsequent lumbar surgical procedures are not as successful as index procedures. Although the structural severity of the stenosis may relate to success of surgery, it is also cautioned that the severity of stenosis radiographically is not a good correlate to patient symptom severity or perceived function. Rapid, progressive neurologic deterioration appears uncommon with any of the available therapies. The optimal timing for surgical intervention in the context among patient symptom severity, structural stenosis severity, and self-perceived quality of life and physical function warrants additional study. In conclusion, until stronger evidence is available for recommending therapeutic intervention in symptomatic lumbar stenosis, treatment for this condition needs to be individualized. Currently, insufficient evidence exists to recommend an optimal treatment regimen for a patient with symptomatic lumbar spinal stenosis.

Summary of Recommendations

STATEMENT	EE O EIDENCE ADE O ECOMMENDATION	E E ENCES
1. There is limited evidence on educational programs directed towards lumbar spinal stenosis patients	1 / I	4
2. There is conflicting evidence on the potential efficacy of medications such as nasal calcitonin and epidural steroids for the treatment of spinal stenosis.	1 / I	2,7,14,15,16,17
3. There may be some potential benefit of gabapentin in improving walking distance in the short term	1 / B	9
4. There is limited evidence on the efficacy of therapeutic exercise in the treatment of symptomatic spinal stenosis	2 / I	13
5. In patients who have failed nonsurgical treatment, decompressive surgery can improve patient symptoms with some evidence that surgery may be associated with better outcomes in the early term when compared to additional nonsurgical treatment in this patient subpopulation. Longer term efficacy studies, however, are warranted.	1 / B	19-21,23, 24,24a, 29, 30,32,33

REFERENCES

1. Boden SD, Davis DO, Dina TS, et al: Abnormal magnetic-resonance scans of the lumbar spine in asymptomatic subjects. A prospective investigation. J Bone Joint Surg Am 72:403–408, 1990.
2. Selkowitz DM, Kulig K, Poppert EM, et al: The immediate and long-term effects of exercise and patient education on physical, functional, and quality-of-life outcome measures after single-level lumbar microdiscectomy: a randomized controlled trial protocol. BMC Musculoskelet Disord 7:70, 2006.
3. Burton AK, Waddell G, Tillotson KM, et al: Information and advice to patients with back pain can have a positive effect. A randomized controlled trial of a novel educational booklet in primary care. Spine 24:2484–2491, 1999.
4. Deyo RA, Cherkin DC, Weinstein J, et al: Involving patients in clinical decisions: Impact of an interactive video program on use of back surgery. Med Care 38:959–969, 2000.
5. Phelan EA, Deyo RA, Cherkin DC, et al: Helping patients decide about back surgery: A randomized trial of an interactive video program. Spine 26:206–212, 2001.
6. Eskola A, Pohjolainen T, Alaranta H, et al: Calcitonin treatment in lumbar spinal stenosis: A randomized, placebo-controlled, double-blind, cross-over study with one-year follow-up. Calcif Tissue Int 50:400–403, 1992.
7. Podichetty VK, Segal AM, Lieber M, et al: Effectiveness of salmon calcitonin nasal spray in the treatment of lumbar canal stenosis: A double-blind, randomized, placebo-controlled, parallel group trial. Spine 29:2343–2349, 2004.
8. Waikakul W, Waikakul S: Methylcobalamin as an adjuvant medication in conservative treatment of lumbar spinal stenosis. J Med Assoc Thai 83:825–831, 2000.
9. Yaksi A, Ozgonenel L, Ozgonenel B: The efficiency of gabapentin therapy in patients with lumbar spinal stenosis. Spine 32:939–942, 2007.
10. Sculco AD, Paup DC, Fernhall B, et al: Effects of aerobic exercise on low back pain patients in treatment. Spine J 1:95–101, 2001.
11. Fritzell P, Hagg O, Wessberg P, et al: 2001 Volvo Award Winner in Clinical Studies: Lumbar fusion versus nonsurgical treatment for chronic low back pain: A multicenter randomized controlled trial from the Swedish Lumbar Spine Study Group. Spine 26:2521–2534, 2001.
12. Brox JI, Sorensen R, Friis A, et al: Randomized clinical trial of lumbar instrumented fusion and cognitive intervention and exercises in patients with chronic low back pain and disc degeneration. Spine 28:1913–1921, 2003.
13. Whitman JM, Flynn TW, Childs JD, et al: A comparison between two physical therapy treatment programs for patients with lumbar spinal stenosis: A randomized clinical trial. Spine 31:2541–2549, 2006.
14. Fukusaki M, Kobayashi I, Hara T, et al: Symptoms of spinal stenosis do not improve after epidural steroid injection. Clin J Pain 14:148–151, 1998.
15. Cuckler JM, Bernini PA, Wiesel SW, et al: The use of epidural steroids in the treatment of lumbar radicular pain. A prospective, randomized, double-blind study. J Bone Joint Surg Am 67:63–66, 1985.
16. Wilson-MacDonald J, Burt G, Griffin D, et al: Epidural steroid injection for nerve root compression. A randomised, controlled trial. J Bone Joint Surg Br 87:352–355, 2005.
17. Ng L, Chaudhary N, Sell P: The efficacy of corticosteroids in periradicular infiltration for chronic radicular pain: A randomized, double-blind, controlled trial. Spine 30:857–862, 2005.
18. Gibson JN, Waddell G: Surgery for degenerative lumbar spondylosis: Updated Cochrane Review. Spine 30:2312–2320, 2005.
19. Atlas SJ, Deyo RA, Keller RB, et al: The Maine Lumbar Spine Study, Part III. 1-year outcomes of surgical and nonsurgical management of lumbar spinal stenosis. Spine 21:1787–1795, 1996.
20. Atlas SJ, Keller RB, Robson D, et al: Surgical and nonsurgical management of lumbar spinal stenosis: Four-year outcomes from the Maine lumbar spine study. Spine 25:556–562, 2000.
21. Atlas SJ, Keller RB, Wu YA, et al: Long-term outcomes of surgical and nonsurgical management of lumbar spinal stenosis: 8 to 10 year results from the Maine lumbar spine study. Spine 30:936–943, 2005.
22. Herno A, Airaksinen O, Saari T, et al: Lumbar spinal stenosis: A matched-pair study of operated and non-operated patients. Br J Neurosurg 10:461–465, 1996.
23. Amundsen T, Weber H, Nordal HJ, et al: Lumbar spinal stenosis: Conservative or surgical management? A prospective 10-year study. Spine 25:1424–1436, 2000.
24. Malmivaara A, Slatis P, Heliovaara M, et al: Surgical or nonoperative treatment for lumbar spinal stenosis? A randomized controlled trial. Spine 32:1–8, 2007.
24a. Weinstein JN, Tosteson TD, Lurie JD, et al: Surgical versus nonsurgical therapy for lumbar spinal stenosis. N Engl J Med 358:818–24, 2008.
25. Hurri H, Slatis P, Soini J, et al: Lumbar spinal stenosis: Assessment of long-term outcome 12 years after operative and conservative treatment. J Spinal Disord 11:110–115, 1998.
26. Weiner BK, Patel NM, Walker MA: Outcomes of decompression for lumbar spinal canal stenosis based upon preoperative radiographic severity. J Orthop Surg 2:3, 2007.
27. Jonsson B, Annertz M, Sjoberg C, et al: A prospective and consecutive study of surgically treated lumbar spinal stenosis. Part II: Five-year follow-up by an independent observer. Spine 22:2938–2944, 1997.
28. Katz JN, Stucki G, Lipson SJ, et al: Predictors of surgical outcome in degenerative lumbar spinal stenosis. Spine 24:2229–2233, 1999.
29. Grob D, Humke T, Dvorak J: Degenerative lumbar spinal stenosis. Decompression with and without arthrodesis. J Bone Joint Surg Am 77:1036–1041, 1995.
30. Mariconda M, Fava R, Gatto A, et al: Unilateral laminectomy for bilateral decompression of lumbar spinal stenosis: A prospective comparative study with conservatively treated patients. J Spinal Disord Tech 15:39–46, 2002.
31. Cho DY, Lin HL, Lee WY, et al: Split-spinous process laminotomy and discectomy for degenerative lumbar spinal stenosis: A preliminary report. J Neurosurg Spine 6:229–239, 2007.
32. Thome C, Zevgaridis D, Leheta O, et al: Outcome after less-invasive decompression of lumbar spinal stenosis: A randomized comparison of unilateral laminotomy, bilateral laminotomy, and laminectomy. J Neurosurg Spine 3:129–141, 2005.
33. Zucherman JF, Hsu KY, Hartjen CA, et al: A multicenter, prospective, randomized trial evaluating the X STOP interspinous process decompression system for the treatment of neurogenic intermittent claudication: Two-year follow-up results. Spine 30:1351–1358, 2005.
34. Kondrashov DG, Hannibal M, Hsu KY, et al: Interspinous process decompression with the X-STOP device for lumbar spinal stenosis: A 4-year follow-up study. J Spinal Disord Tech 19:323–327, 2006.
35. Korovessis P, Papazisis Z, Koureas G, et al: Rigid, semirigid versus dynamic instrumentation for degenerative lumbar spinal stenosis: A correlative radiological and clinical analysis of short-term results. Spine 29:735–742, 2004.

What Is the Optimal Treatment for Thoracolumbar Burst Fractures?

Marcel F. Dvorak, MD, FRCSC, and Charles G. Fisher, MD, MHSc, FRCSC

Despite injury prevention initiatives and safer automobile designs, the incidence of thoracolumbar high-energy trauma remains significant.[1] Burst fractures of the thoracolumbar spine account for approximately 45% of all thoracolumbar trauma cases, and half of these patients remain neurologically intact after injury.[2] The 1990s and 2000s have brought significant technologic advancements, specifically the wide-spread use of pedicle screw fixation in the thoracic spine,[3–7] the design of stiffer and more rigid instrumentation,[3,8,9] the ability to reconstruct the anterior spinal column with expandable cages[10] and biologics,[11] and less invasive spinal surgical approaches.[12] The treatment of thoracolumbar trauma, however, and specifically that of burst fractures, continues to be one of the most controversial areas in spine trauma care despite the high incidence of these injuries and extensive published research.

A well-formulated question provides the foundation for a good systematic review, and this review investigates the variety of treatment options available for thoracolumbar burst fractures and tries to produce guidelines as to which treatment is most effective in producing predictable and safe outcomes for various types of injuries.

OPTIONS

It is important to define the population discussed here. Patients with burst fractures between T10-L2 inclusive, with or without neurologic deficit, who are a minimum age of 16 years are included. The term *burst fracture* refers to a fracture of the vertebral body with fracture lines that extend into the posterior vertebral body wall and result in a separation or widening of the pedicles.[13] Burst fractures may be associated with varying degrees of disruption to the posterior vertebral elements, specifically the facet and laminar complex and the posterior ligamentous complex.[14]

Essentially, two major decisions need to be made by the treating physician: First, and more fundamentally, should the patient be treated with or without surgery? Second, if surgery is to be selected, what approach and technique should be used? Nonoperative care may involve the use of a thoracolumbar sacral orthosis (TLSO), body cast, hyperextension brace, or no orthosis at all, whereas operative treatment may involve

anterior surgery alone, posterior surgery alone, or a combination of both. The posterior surgical fixation options include hook or wire constructs,[7,15,16] short-segment pedicle screw fixation at one level above and one below the fractured vertebra,[3,4,6,7,17] and long-segment fixation, characteristically two or three segments of fixation above and below the fracture.[7,18,19] When the anterior column of the spine is surgically reconstructed, the vertebral body and discs may be approached indirectly through transpedicular bone[3,7,20] or cement augmentation,[21,22] or by an indirect postero-lateral approach. A direct anterior approach facilitates vertebral body resection, decompression of the anterior spinal canal, anterior reconstruction of the vertebra, and also anterior fixation with either plates or screw-rod constructs.[23,24] Prosthetic devices (fixed and expanding cages), as well as autograft and allograft, are the most commonly used anterior vertebral reconstruction options.[10,23–28]

EVIDENCE

Operative versus Nonoperative Treatment

Five Level II studies directly compare operative with nonoperative care for thoracolumbar burst fractures (Table 6–1).[2,29–32] All of these studies include thoracolumbar burst fractures with normal neurology. Some of the fractures included would be described as unstable with significant kyphosis and some degree of posterior ligamentous disruption, though most would be described as stable.

Wood and colleagues[31] recruited 53 patients, 27 of whom were randomized to the nonoperative treatment arm, which contained two forms of nonoperative treatment, either a postural reduction and cast or a hyperextension custom-molded jacket TLSO worn for 12 to 16 weeks. Twenty-six patients were treated by a variety of surgical techniques, either a posterior screw/hook construct and fusion spanning between two to five levels or an anterior vertebrectomy, rib strut graft, and instrumentation. Patients' outcome evaluation included the Medical Outcomes Study 36-Item Short Form Health Survey (SF-36), modified Roland Morris Disability Scale (RMDS) score, Oswestry Questionnaire, visual analogue pain scale (VAS), and a radiographic evaluation. The study does have significant limitations, including a

TABLE 6–1. Thoracolumbar Fractures: Articles Comparing Operative and Nonoperative Treatment

First Author (Year of Publication)	Description	Level of Evidence of Primary Question	Topic and Conclusions
Siebenga (2006)[30]	Prospective randomized trial of posterior short-segment fixation vs. brace treatment for burst fractures with normal neurology	II	34 patients randomized to brace or posterior short-segment instrumentation. Improved pain, disability, and return to work in the surgically treated patients.
Shen (2001)[29]	Prospective (not fully randomized) trial comparing short-segment posterior fixation vs. hyperextension bracing	II	80 patients, 33 treated with posterior short-segment fixation and 47 treated with brace. Operatively treated group had less pain and improved function at 3 and 6 months, but the difference was not sustained to longer term follow-up.
Wood (2003)[31]	Prospective randomized trial comparing various surgical fixation techniques to TLSO bracing	II	47 patients randomized to anterior fixation, posterior fixation, or TLSO bracing. Improved pain and function in the nonoperatively treated group.
Thomas (2006)[32]	Qualitative systematic review	II	Careful review of the literature could not identify evidence of superiority of operative vs. nonoperative treatment for burst fractures without neurologic injury.
Domenicucci (1996)[2]	Prospective comparative study of posterior instrumentation vs. nonoperative treatment	II	31 patients followed prospectively; 20 patients treated with reduction and casting, and 11 patients with posterior fixation.
Rechtine (1999)[34]	Retrospective comparative study	III	235 patients with unstable fractures, half treated with 6 weeks of bedrest and half with surgical fixation. Overall complication rates were similar.
Knight (1993)[33]	Retrospective comparative study	III	22 patients for whom posterior and anterior fixation compared with brace treatment.

TLSO = thoracolumbar sacral orthosis.

lack of standardization, multiple treatment options, outcome measures reported at varying intervals, lack of a priori determination of a primary outcome, no power calculations, and multiple comparisons without statistical adjustment.

A statistically significant difference between operative and nonoperative treatment was observed favoring nonoperative treatment, for physical function ($P = 0.002$) and role physical ($P = 0.003$). Wood and colleagues[31] report an average Roland Disability score of 8.2 for the operative group and 3.9 for the nonoperative group ($P = 0.02$). These authors also used the Oswestry questionnaire, reporting an average score of 20.75 and 10.66 for the surgical and nonsurgical groups, respectively. For both the Roland and Oswestry instruments, a lower score signifies better function.

In contradistinction with Wood and colleagues'[31] study, Siebenga and investigators[30] included a homogeneously defined cohort and carefully standardized treatment of both the operative and nonoperative groups. By randomizing 34 patients to brace treatment and posterior short-segment fixation, Siebenga and investigators[30] showed a significant difference in pain (72 vs. 87 mm; $P = 0.033$), Rolland Morris Disability scores (8.9 vs. 3.1; $P = 0.030$), and return to work (38% vs. 85%; $P = 0.018$), each in favor of operative treatment. The methodology and uniformity of treatment applied to each group make this a strong study, whereas the lack of an a priori power calculation and an a priori description of a primary outcome prevent it from attaining Level I evidence status.

Shen and coauthors[29] attempted to randomize patients to receive short-segment posterior instrumentation and fusion or nonoperative care using a hyperextension brace. Because of recruitment difficulties, some patients were not randomized, and as such, this study should be considered a prospective cohort study. Outcomes were measured by an independent assessor at 1, 3, 6, 12, 18, and 24 months. Also using a VAS, at 2-year follow-up, Shen and coauthors[29] note the VAS to be 1.5 and 1.8 for the nonoperative and operative cohorts, respectively. For the 3- and 6-month follow-up, Shen and coauthors[29] show improved pain in the surgically compared with the brace-treated patients. The authors note a better Greenough low back outcome score in the surgically treated group for up to 6 months, but this effect was not observed with longer follow-up.

The systematic review by Thomas and investigators[32] was performed before the study by Siebenga and colleagues,[30] and concludes that there was no evidence of superiority of operative over nonoperative treatment for neurologically intact thoracolumbar burst fractures. The final of the five Level II studies is a prospective comparative study by Domenicucci and coworkers,[2] which has multiple methodologic flaws, and although it favors surgery for patients with increased radiographic deformity (kyphosis over 20 degrees), issues of power and bias are significant.

Two Level III studies compare operative and nonoperative care (see Table 6–1).[33,34] Rechtine and colleagues'[34] article is thought provoking in that it brings to mind the issues of costs of care, as well as patient preference, and shows that even in severely injured individuals, satisfactory outcomes may be obtained with or without surgery, however, with different treatment approaches, resource implications, costs, and risk.

In addition, a number of Level IV studies show satisfactory outcomes with nonoperative treatment of a variety of these thoracolumbar fractures.[33,35–40] An example of one of these is an article by Mumford and coauthors,[40] who reviewed 41 of 47 patients treated with a variable period of bed rest (range, 7–68 days) followed by a custom-made TLSO for an average of 12 weeks. Inclusion criteria included burst fractures between T11-L5, and the data for each individual patient were reported. For patients treated without surgery, Mumford and coauthors[40] found that 50% of patients had little to no pain at final follow-up, as measured on a Likert Scale.

In summary, strong evidence has been reported to support satisfactory outcomes with both operative and nonoperative treatment. Two Level II studies[29,30] suggest improved outcomes with operative treatment, one of which shows improved outcomes only at 3 and 6 months, and not sustained out to longer follow-up.[29] Wood and colleagues'[31] study has significant enough methodologic defects to make its conclusions nebulous.

Choice of Operative Approach

Specifically looking at the decision to operate from an anterior approach alone, posterior alone, or combined anterior and posterior approaches, two Level II studies[28,41] and six Level III studies[5,7,35,42–44] address this as their primary question (Table 6–2).

Wood and colleagues,[28] in an article that appears to be a subset of a previously reported randomized trial,[31] randomly assigned 43 patients to either anterior partial vertebrectomy and Kaneda or Isola instrumentation or posterior Isola rod-hook stabilization. Unfortunately, the use of posterior rod-hook constructs is likely inferior to the more commonly used pedicle screw-rod systems currently used; thus, the high rate (11/18) of implant-related complications in the posterior surgery group is not that surprising. The generally good clinical outcomes in the anterior surgery group and the low complication rate make this a potentially reasonable option in the neurologically intact thoracolumbar burst fracture that requires surgical treatment.

Esses and coauthors'[41] study strongly favors short-segment posterior fixation over an anterior fixation system (Kostuik–Harrington device) that tended to fail as frequently as the posterior short-segment fixator and required a greater degree of complexity and risk for its insertion.

Two Level III systematic reviews[5,7] compare various surgical approaches and techniques. Though suffering from a lack of high-quality studies in his systematic review, Dickman and coworkers[5] confidently state that segmental pedicle screw fixation of thoracolumbar fractures has a higher fusion rate than do rod-screw constructs or anterior fixation devices. Verlaan and investigators[7] in a meta-analysis of 132 articles divided treatment into 5 categories, including posterior long- and short-segment instrumentation, a mixture of short- and long-segment instrumentation, anterior alone, and combined anterior and posterior fixation. Verlaan and investigators[7] conclude that none of the five techniques reliably maintains alignment, and there is no compelling evidence of the superiority of one of these techniques over another.

Been and Bouma,[42] in a retrospective, comparative study of short-segment posterior fixation, with and without concomitant anterior strut grafting, reported a 21% instrumentation failure rate with the posterior short-segment instrumentation, reduced to 4% when an anterior strut graft is added. In another retrospective comparative study, Danisa and coauthors[43] compared anterior alone (16 patients), posterior alone (27 patients), and combined anterior and posterior (6 patients); even with significant selection bias, there was no significant difference in kyphosis, pain, return to work, or neurologic recovery among the three groups. Danisa and coauthors[43] recommend posterior fixation as the least complex procedure. Briem and colleagues[44] performed a Level III matched-pairs analysis comparing posterior instrumentation alone with combined posterior and anterior fixation. Although the combined anterior and posterior procedure maintained sagittal alignment more effectively than posterior alone, there was no difference in SF-36 between the two groups. The SF-36 likely lacks the sensitivity to detect change that a disease-specific outcome measure would have. Finally, Aligizakis and investigators,[45] in a parallel study of several cohorts, attempted to use the load sharing classification to

TABLE 6–2. Thoracolumbar Fractures: Articles Comparing Operative Approaches (Anterior and Posterior)

First Author (Year of Publication)	Description	Level of Evidence of Primary Question	Topic and Conclusions
Wood (2005)[28]	Prospective randomized study of anterior vs. posterior fusion	II	38 patients randomized to posterior hook-rod construct and anterior decompression fusion. High failure rate with posterior hook rods.
Esses (1990)[41]	Prospective randomized study	II	40 patients comparing anterior and posterior fixation. Posterior thought to be as effective as anterior.
Verlaan (2004)[7]	Qualitative systematic review of Class III and IV studies	III	132 articles were included, and surgical treatment was divided into five categories. No single technique maintained kyphosis correction. Overall low complication rate.
Dickman (1994)[5]	Qualitative systematic review of Class III and IV studies	III	58 articles included in a systematic review demonstrating that pedicle screw fixation was superior to hook rod and had a high fusion rate.
Danisa (1995)[43]	Retrospective comparative study	III	49 patients, 16 anterior alone, 27 posterior alone, six combined anterior and posterior. No difference between groups.
Been (1999)[42]	Retrospective comparative study	III	46 patients comparing combined anterior and posterior with posterior short segment. Posterior short segment had a 21% failure rate.
Briem (2004)[44]	Retrospective comparative study	III	10 patients treated with posterior fixation alone were matched to 10 patients treated with combined anterior and posterior. Improved radiographic outcomes in the combined anterior/posterior patients, but no difference in 36-Item Short Form Health Survey (SF-36).
Aligizakis (2003)[45]	Prospective comparative study	III	30 patients: 21 treated with posterior short segment, three anterior Kaneda, six posterior and anterior combined.

guide the choice of surgical approach and technique. This study[45] reports good outcomes of several selected cohorts where the addition of an anterior approach is based on the numeric score of the load sharing classification. Aligizakis and investigators[45] treated simple burst fractures with posterior alone short-segment instrumentation (21 patients), whereas "complete" burst fractures (three patients with significant vertebral body comminution) were treated with anterior alone Kaneda devices and burst fractures with posterior element distraction (six patients with flexion/distraction injuries) were treated with posterior instrumentation and an anterior load-bearing strut graft.[45]

Choice of Operative Technique

Andress and colleagues[4] report on 50 patients treated with short-segment pedicle screw instrumentation that was routinely removed 9 to 15 months after surgery (Table 6–3). The mean 46-month follow-up included a radiographic evaluation, preinjury (assigned retrospectively after fracture) and postinjury Hanover score, and a seven-point clinical assessment scale. Sanderson and coworkers[46] evaluated a cohort of 28 patients who were treated between 1990 and 1993, using pedicle screw instrumentation two levels above and below without fusion, followed by routine hardware removal 6 to 12 months after surgery. Surgi-

TABLE 6-3. Thoracolumbar Fractures: Articles Describing Operative Techniques

First Author (Year of Publication)	Description	Level of Evidence of Primary Question	Topic and Conclusions
Alanay (2001)[3]	Prospective randomized study of posterior fixation with or without bone grafting	II	20 patients randomized to posterior short-segment fixation with and without transpedicular grafting. No difference in outcome.
Cho (2003)[21]	Prospective randomized study of posterior fixation with or without cement	II	70 patients assigned to posterior short-segment fixation with (20) and without (50) transpedicular cement injection. Better maintenance of alignment and pain control with cement.
Andress (2002)[4]	Retrospective case series	IV	50 patients treated with posterior short-segment fixation and grafting.
Sanderson (1999)[46]	Retrospective case series	IV	28 patients with posterior short-segment fixation without bone grafting.

cal indications were listed as kyphosis greater than 20 degrees and/or greater than 50% loss of anterior vertebral height. In these and other reports of short-segment posterior fixation, the failure rate of the posterior instrumentation has been variously reported as 14%,[46] 17%,[8] 21%,[42] 22%,[21] 50%,[47] and 53%.[17] Despite the popularity and relative surgical simplicity of this technique, the predictable high mechanical failure rate clearly makes it difficult to accept this procedure as the optimal treatment option.

Several attempts have been made to minimize the collapse of the vertebral body and resultant instrument failure, one of these being the addition of transpedicular intracorporeal grafting,[48] and this is the focus of one Level II study[20] and is prominent in a Level III sys-tematic review.[7] Alanay and coworkers[20] randomized 20 consecutive patients to short-segment pedicle instrumentation with or without transpedicular intracorporeal grafting. The technique of transpedicular intracorporeal grafting did not influence the collapse of the fractured vertebra, and this finding was confirmed by Verlaan and investigators[7] in a systematic review of a number of articles. The technique of transpedicular intracorporeal bone grafting can be described confidently as ineffective.

In a novel modification of the short-segment posterior fixation technique, several authors have proposed transpedicular intracorporeal injection of cements.[21,22] In a particularly interesting, prospective, comparative Level II study, Cho and colleagues[21] compare posterior short-segment fixation with and without intracorporeal cement injection. The cement injection was shown to maintain vertebral height and kyphosis correction, whereas a 22% instrumentation failure rate occurred in the group without cement injection. The long-term significance of cement in a vertebral body of a young patient is unknown; thus, this technique must remain experimental.

AREAS OF UNCERTAINTY

Based on the literature reviewed earlier, it is remarkable how our efforts to stratify patients with thoracolumbar burst fractures into subgroups and tailor their treatment remain unclear and ineffective. Most studies treat the 20-year-old laborer in the same way that they treat the 70-year-old adult who falls in the bath. Similarly, classification systems are only now becoming available that guide treatment to some degree.[14] The principal areas where we believe attention should be directed are as follows:

1. What are the costs of operative and nonoperative treatment, and what is the temporal profile and eventual extent of functional recovery with either treatment?
2. What are the variables that would stratify patients with thoracolumbar burst fractures into a group that should be selected for operative as opposed to what appears to be the vast majority that do well with nonoperative treatment?
3. In patients whom physicians believe require surgery, precisely what criteria can be used reliably to select either anterior surgery alone or the addition of anterior structural support to reinforce posterior instrumentation?
4. What is the impact of neurologic impairment on the choice of treatment and surgical technique, timing, and approach?

From individual studies and from several meta-analyses, it appears that the rates of serious complication for even the most extensive surgical treatments are relatively low. Documented neurologic deterioration after baseline assessment, regardless of treatment, is extremely rare,[8,23,42,43,49–54] although one study does report this problem.[13] Further careful consideration of complication rates and patterns is required.

GUIDELINES

Fair evidence exists to recommend nonoperative treatment as an option for the majority of thoracolumbar burst fractures as long as they do not appear to have neurologic impairment, significant posterior element disruption, or a significant deformity (kyphosis over 25–30 degrees, although this is debatable). Level II and III studies have consistently shown satisfactory clinical outcomes with nonoperative treatment in this patient population, and no one has been able to conclusively link the degree of eventual deformity to the quality of clinical outcome. It appears as if it is the achievement of "stability" or healing and not necessarily the alignment of the spine that determines a good clinical outcome.

Superimposed on the earlier fairly consistent and weighty body of literature, there are several recent studies that provide fair evidence that, although nonoperative outcomes appear to be satisfactory, the surgical treatment of thoracolumbar burst fractures may improve pain relief, function, and return to work. The small sample sizes in studies such as Cho and colleagues,[21] Siebenga and investigators,[30] and Shen and coauthors[29] require further study and verification before operative treatment can be strongly considered. Furthermore, the fairly consistent reports of instrumentation-related failure with the most common surgical technique, namely, short-segment posterior fixation, makes the authors uneasy in recommending the abandonment of nonoperative treatment in pursuit of the improved outcomes promised by an operative treatment that has such a high mechanical failure rate.

Satisfactory clinical results have been consistently achieved with acceptable complication rates using several operative approaches and techniques. The criteria on which one selects anterior vertebrectomy graft and plate (or rod) stabilization, posterior short- or long-segment fixation, or a combination of anterior and posterior fixation are not clearly defined. Several statements can be made based on what are fairly consist findings in Level III and IV clinical studies. Posterior instrumentation with pedicle screws provides better fixation than hook constructs.[5] Longer segment instrumentation (two motion segments above and two below the fractured vertebra) will reduce the risk for instrument failure at the bone-screw interface or within the instrumentation itself.[15,47] Short-segment posterior fixation and, to some degree, most operative treatment techniques will fail to maintain the operatively achieved alignment and will drift into kyphosis approximately 10 degrees greater than that achieved at surgery.[7] Kyphosis does not appear to be related to clinical outcome, at least not when it is less than 25 to 30 degrees.[7,55]

Finally, some techniques have been shown not to be associated with satisfactory results, and these include the transpedicular injection of bone[20] or OP-1,[11] anterior fixation utilizing the Slot–Zielke divice,[23] and anterior grafting using bovine bone.[27]

RECOMMENDATIONS

Burst fractures of the thoracolumbar junction are commonly treated surgically despite the fact that the available evidence to justify the additional risks of surgery is minimal. A strong need for properly designed and conducted clinical trials exists. Given the use of multiple-outcome instruments in different studies, it is difficult, if not impossible, to compare or combine results between studies, and thus facilitate a meta-analysis.

For the majority of thoracolumbar burst fractures without neurologic deficit, particularly those where the initial segmental kyphosis is less than 25 or 30 degrees, we would recommend nonsurgical treatment in a TLSO, cast, or other orthosis (Jewett). Some intriguing data suggest that potentially the outcomes of posterior surgical stabilization for these injuries may reduce pain and improve function. However, these studies require confirmation through carefully performed prospective studies of larger patient populations before nonsurgical treatment recommendations can be justified. It is certainly possible that surgery is the treatment of choice for burst fractures at the thoracolumbar junction without neurologic deficit. Surgery theoretically may result in earlier mobilization, and hospital discharge, less initial pain, and faster return to work, an issue of considerable economic relevance.

When the segmental kyphosis is on the order of 25 or 30 degrees, either because of the degree of anterior vertebral body comminution or posterior ligamentous complex incompetence, then surgical treatment is the preferred treatment option, although nonoperative treatment remains an option. The studies by Siebenga and investigators[30] and Shen and coauthors[29] are both well done and suggest improved outcomes with surgery. Therefore, there is likely a place for surgery and experience. Widespread practice would support that surgery would be reserved for higher degrees of kyphosis and posterior ligament injuries (Level V).

In the presence of neurologic injury, it is widespread practice in North America to treat these injuries surgically, either simply stabilizing the fracture with posterior instrumentation or adding a concomitant decompression. Because of the lack of convincing data to favor one surgical approach over another, and the reported high failure rate of short-segment posterior instrumentation, the authors use posterior instrumentation utilizing pedicle screws at two segments above and two below as the most reliable and lowest risk surgical procedure. Posterior stabilization may be followed by reimaging (computed tomography or MRI) to assess the degree of spinal canal occlusion (in the case of neurologic deficit) and vertebral comminution, and the surgeon can use clinical judgment, as well as guidance from the load sharing classification,[45] in deciding when to perform an additional anterior corpectomy and strut grafting.

Summary of Recommendations

STATEMENT	LEVEL OF EVIDENCE/GRADE OF RECOMMENDATION	REFERENCES
1. Stable burst fractures with a kyphotic angle less than 25° can be safely and effectively treated with bracing, casting, or an orthosis	B	31,32
2. Posterior short segment surgical stabilization of stable burst fractures with kyphotic angles less than 25° may reduce pain, improve function, and accelerate return to work	B	21,29,30
3. Posterior instrumentation with rod-screw constructs provides better fixation than rod-hook constructs	B	5
4. Longer segment posterior fixation reduces the risk of instrumentation failure	B	15,47
5. Most fixation techniques, particularly posterior short segment fixation, tend to develop some degree of progressive kyphosis following surgery	B	7
6. Transpedicular bone grafting is not effective at preventing the progressive kyphosis after surgery	B	7,55

REFERENCES

1. Fisher CG, Noonan VK, Dvorak MF: Changing face of spine trauma care in North America. Spine 31:S2–S8, 2006.
2. Domenicucci M, Preite R, Ramieri A, et al: Thoracolumbar fractures without neurosurgical involvement: Surgical or conservative treatment? J Neurosurg Sci 40:1–10, 1996.
3. Alanay A, Acaroglu E, Yazici M, et al: Short-segment pedicle instrumentation of thoracolumbar burst fractures: Does transpedicular intracorporeal grafting prevent early failure? Spine 26:213–217, 2001.
4. Andress HJ, Braun H, Helmberger T, et al: Long-term results after posterior fixation of thoraco-lumbar burst fractures. Injury 33:357–365, 2002.
5. Dickman CA, Yahiro MA, Lu HT, Melkerson MN: Surgical treatment alternatives for fixation of unstable fractures of the thoracic and lumbar spine. A meta-analysis. Spine 19:2266S–2273S, 1994.
6. Kramer DL, Rodgers WB, Mansfield FL: Transpedicular instrumentation and short-segment fusion of thoracolumbar fractures: A prospective study using a single instrumentation system. J Orthop Trauma 9:499–506, 1995.
7. Verlaan JJ, Diekerhof CH, Buskens E, et al: Surgical treatment of traumatic fractures of the thoracic and lumbar spine: A systematic review of the literature on techniques, complications, and outcome. Spine 29:803–814, 2004.
8. Liu CL, Wang ST, Lin HJ, et al: AO fixateur interne in treating burst fractures of the thoracolumbar spine. Chung Hua I Hsueh Tsa Chih (Taipei) 62:619–625, 1999.
9. Wang ST, Ma HL, Liu CL, et al: Is fusion necessary for surgically treated burst fractures of the thoracolumbar and lumbar spine? A prospective, randomized study. Spine 31:2646–2652, 2006.
10. Lange U, Knop C, Bastian L, Blauth M: Prospective multicenter study with a new implant for thoracolumbar vertebral body replacement. Arch Orthop Trauma Surg 123:203–208, 2003.
11. Laursen M, Hoy K, Hansen ES, et al: Recombinant bone morphogenetic protein-7 as an intracorporal bone growth stimulator in unstable thoracolumbar burst fractures in humans: Preliminary results. Eur Spine J 8:485–490, 1999.
12. Oner FC, Dhert WJ, Verlaan JJ: Less invasive anterior column reconstruction in thoracolumbar fractures. Injury 36(suppl 2): B82–B89, 2005.
13. Denis F, Armstrong GWD, Searls K, Matta L: Acute thoracolumbar burst fractures in the absence of neurologic deficit. A comparison between operative and nonoperative treatment. Clin Orthop 189:142–149, 1984.
14. Vaccaro AR, Lehman RA Jr, Hurlbert RJ, et al: A new classification of thoracolumbar injuries: The importance of injury morphology, the integrity of the posterior ligamentous complex, and neurologic status. Spine 30:2325–2333, 2005.
15. Serin E, Karakurt L, Yilmaz E, et al: Effects of two-levels, four-levels, and four-levels plus offset-hook posterior fixation techniques on protecting the surgical correction of unstable thoracolumbar vertebral fractures: A clinical study. Eur J Orthop Traumatol 14:1–6, 2004.
16. Vornanen MJ, Bostman OM, Myllynen PJ: Reduction of bone retropulsed into the spinal canal in thoracolumbar vertebral body compression burst fractures. A prospective randomized comparative study between Harrington rods and two transpedicular devices. Spine 20:1699–1703, 1995.
17. McLain RF, Sparling E, Benson DR: Early failure of short-segment pedicle instrumentation for thoracolumbar fractures. A preliminary report. J Bone Joint Surg Am 75:162–167, 1993.
18. Akbarnia BA, Crandall DG, Burkus K, Matthews T: Use of long rods and a short arthrodesis for burst fractures of the thoracolumbar spine. A long-term follow-up study. J Bone Joint Surg Am 76:1629–1635, 1994.
19. Korovessis P, Baikousis A, Koureas G, Zacharatos S: Correlative analysis of the results of surgical treatment of thoracolumbar injuries with long Texas Scottish rite hospital construct: Is the use of pedicle screws versus hooks advantageous in the lumbar spine? J Spinal Disord Tech 17:195–205, 2004.
20. Alanay A, Acarolu E, Yazici M, et al: The effect of transpedicular intracorporeal grafting in the treatment of thoracolumbar burst fractures on canal remodeling. Eur Spine J 10:512–516, 2001.
21. Cho DY, Lee WY, Sheu PC, et al: Treatment of thoracolumbar burst fractures with polymethyl methacrylate vertebroplasty and short-segment pedicle screw fixation. Neurosurgery 53:1354–1361, 2003.
22. Verlaan JJ, Oner FC, Dhert WJ: Anterior spinal column augmentation with injectable bone cements. Biomaterials 27:290–301, 2006.
23. Been HD: Anterior decompression and stabilization of thoracolumbar burst fractures by the use of the Slot-Zielke device. Spine 16:70–77, 1991.
24. McDonough PW, Davis R, Tribus C, Zdeblick TA: The management of acute thoracolumbar burst fractures with anterior corpectomy and Z-plate fixation. Spine 29:1901–1908, 2004.
25. Dvorak MF, Kwon BK, Fisher CG, et al: Effectiveness of titanium mesh cylindrical cages in anterior column reconstruction after thoracic and lumbar vertebral body resection. Spine 28:902–908, 2003.
26. Schnee CL, Ansell LV: Selection criteria and outcome of operative approaches for thoracolumbar burst fractures with and without neurological deficit. J Neurosurg 86:48–55, 1997.
27. Schultheiss M, Sarkar M, Arand M, et al: Solvent-preserved, bovine cancellous bone blocks used for reconstruction of thoracolumbar fractures in minimally invasive spinal surgery—First clinical results. Eur Spine J 14:192–196, 2005.
28. Wood KB, Bohn D, Mehbod A: Anterior versus posterior treatment of stable thoracolumbar burst fractures without neurologic deficit: A prospective, randomized study. J Spinal Disord Tech 18(suppl):S15–S23, 2005.
29. Shen WJ, Liu TJ, Shen YS: Nonoperative treatment versus posterior fixation for thoracolumbar junction burst fractures without neurologic deficit. Spine 26:1038–1045, 2001.

30. Siebenga J, Leferink VJM, Segers MJM, et al: Treatment of traumatic thoracolumbar spine fractures: A multicenter prospective randomized study of operative versus nonsurgical treatment. Spine 31:2881–2890, 2006.

31. Wood K, Buttermann G, Mehbod A, et al: Operative compared with nonoperative treatment of a thoracolumbar burst fracture without neurological deficit. A prospective, randomized study [erratum appears in J Bone Joint Surg Am 2004 Jun;86-A(6):1283]. J Bone Joint Surg Am 85:773–781, 2003.

32. Thomas KC, Bailey CS, Dvorak MF, et al: Comparison of operative and nonoperative treatment for thoracolumbar burst fractures in patients without neurological deficit: A systematic review. J Neurosurg Spine 4:351–358, 2006.

33. Knight RQ, Stornelli DP, Chan DP, et al: Comparison of operative versus nonoperative treatment of lumbar burst fractures. Clin Orthop Relat Res (293):112–121, 1993.

34. Rechtine IG, Cahill D, Chrin AM: Treatment of thoracolumbar trauma: Comparison of complications of operative versus nonoperative treatment. J Spinal Disord 12:406–409, 1999.

35. Aligizakis A, Katonis P, Stergiopoulos K, et al: Functional outcome of burst fractures of the thoracolumbar spine managed non-operatively, with early ambulation, evaluated using the load sharing classification. Acta Orthop Belg 68:279–287, 2002.

36. Cantor JB, Lebwohl NH, Garvey T, Eismont FJ: Nonoperative management of stable thoracolumbar burst fractures with early ambulation and bracing. Spine 18:971–976, 1993.

37. Chow GH, Nelson BJ, Gebhard JS, et al: Functional outcome of thoracolumbar burst fractures managed with hyperextension casting or bracing and early mobilization. Spine 21:2170–2175, 1996.

38. Hitchon PW, Torner JC, Haddad SF, et al: Management options in thoracolumbar burst fractures. Surg Neurol 49:619–627, 1998.

39. Kraemer WJ, Schemitsch EH, Lever J, et al: Functional outcome of thoracolumbar burst fractures without neurological deficit. J Orthop Trauma 10:541–544, 1996.

40. Mumford J, Weinstein JN, Spratt KF, Goel VK: Thoracolumbar burst fractures. The clinical efficacy and outcome of nonoperative management. Spine 18:955–970, 1993.

41. Esses SI, Botsford DJ, Kostuik JP: Evaluation of surgical treatment for burst fractures. Spine 15:667–673, 1990.

42. Been HD, Bouma GJ: Comparison of two types of surgery for thoraco-lumbar burst fractures: Combined anterior and posterior stabilisation vs. posterior instrumentation only. Acta Neurochir (Wien) 141:349–357, 1999.

43. Danisa OA, Shaffrey CI, Jane JA, et al: Surgical approaches for the correction of unstable thoracolumbar burst fractures: A retrospective analysis of treatment outcomes. J Neurosurg 83:977–983, 1995.

44. Briem D, Lehmann W, Ruecker AH, et al: Factors influencing the quality of life after burst fractures of the thoracolumbar transition. Arch Orthop Trauma Surg 124:461–468, 2004.

45. Aligizakis AC, Katonis PG, Sapkas G, et al: Gertzbein and load sharing classifications for unstable thoracolumbar fractures. Clin Orthop Relat Res (411):77–85, 2003.

46. Sanderson PL, Fraser RD, Hall DJ, et al: Short segment fixation of thoracolumbar burst fractures without fusion. Eur Spine J 8:495–500, 1999.

47. Moon MS, Choi WT, Moon YW, et al: Stabilisation of fractured thoracic and lumbar spine with Cotrel-Dubousset instrument. J Orthop Surg (Hong Kong) 11:59–66, 2003.

48. Knop C, Fabian HF, Bastian L, et al: Fate of the transpedicular intervertebral bone graft after posterior stabilisation of thoracolumbar fractures. Eur Spine J 11:251–257, 2002.

49. Kirkpatrick JS, Wilber RG, Likavec M, et al: Anterior stabilization of thoracolumbar burst fractures using the Kaneda device: A preliminary report. Orthopedics 18:673–678, 1995.

50. Knop C, Bastian L, Lange U, et al: Complications in surgical treatment of thoracolumbar injuries. Eur Spine J 11:214–226, 2002.

51. Ruan D-K, Shen G-B, Chui H-X: Shen instrumentation for the management of unstable thoracolumbar fractures. Spine 23:1324–1332, 1998.

52. Sasso RC, Cotler HB: Posterior instrumentation and fusion for unstable fractures and fracture-dislocations of the thoracic and lumbar spine: A comparative study of three fixation devices in 70 patients. Spine 18:450–460, 1993.

53. Shen W-J, Shen Y-S: Nonsurgical treatment of three-column thoracolumbar junction burst fractures without neurologic deficit. Spine 24:412–415, 1999.

54. Shiba K, Katsuki M, Ueta T, et al: Transpedicular fixation with Zielke instrumentation in the treatment of thoracolumbar and lumbar injuries. Spine 19:1940–1949, 1994.

55. Knop C, Blauth M, Bühren V, et al: [Surgical treatment of injuries of the thoracolumbar transition—3: Follow-up examination. Results of a prospective multi-center study by the "Spinal" Study Group of the German Society of Trauma Surgery]. Unfallchirurg 104:583–600, 2001.

Is Neuromonitoring Beneficial During Spinal Surgery?

Michael O. Kelleher, FRCS, MD, Julio Cesar Furlan, MD, MBA, MSc, PhD, and Michael G. Fehlings, MD, PhD, FRCSC, FACS

Neurologic injury may follow even technically precise spinal surgery. Because neurologic complications after spinal surgery are potentially devastating, the development of preventative strategies, including intraoperative neurophysiologic monitoring, is of significant clinical relevance and great importance for enhancing patient safety.[1] Intraoperative neurophysiologic monitoring is a method used to physiologically monitor the integrity of neural structures and to avoid surgical insults by enabling real-time response and action by the surgical team.

The ideal intraoperative monitoring modality should be highly sensitive and specific to spinal cord or nerve root injury and should also be "user friendly." Currently, no such modality exists that fulfils all of these criteria. Somatosensory-evoked potential (SSEP) monitoring remains the standard test for intraoperative monitoring despite its suboptimal sensitivity to detect all types of neural injury.[2] Despite the advances that have occurred in intraoperative spinal monitoring since the late 1990s, universal acceptance as to the benefit of intraoperative monitoring has not yet occurred.

MONITORING OPTIONS

Numerous neurophysiologic monitoring methods are now available including continuous free running electromyography (EMG), evoked EMG, compound muscle action potentials, rectal and urinary sphincter EMG, motor-evoked potentials (MEPs), SSEPs, and most recently, spinal cord mapping.[1,3–5] None of these tests individually provides a global assessment of cord and root function. However, when multiple modalities are monitored, each one adds selective information that allows the surgical team to assess neural function with enhanced precision. Each of these electrophysiologic approaches has advantages and disadvantages. Hence, the decision regarding the optimal choice of approaches to monitor needs to be individually tailored for each surgery depending on what level of the spine is undergoing surgery and what aspect of neural function is most at risk.

Somatosensory-Evoked Potentials

Early attempts at monitoring relied solely on recording SSEPs. Reports of false-negative outcomes when using only SSEP monitoring illustrated the need for multimodality monitoring.[6–8] SSEPs remain the standard technique for intraoperative monitoring. Newer techniques such as EMG and MEP have been developed and are used as an adjunct to SSEP monitoring.

Motor-Evoked Potentials

Because of the well-reported limitations of SSEP monitoring, the recording of MEPs has been advocated. Myogenic transcranial MEP offers the advantage of assessing the entire length of the corticospinal tract from the cortex to the distal extremity beyond the neuromuscular junction. The most significant issue when recording MEPs is the anesthetic regimen: total intravenous anesthetic without neuromuscular blockade needs to be utilized to provide the optimal environment for recording MEPs. This requires experience on the part of the surgical and anesthetic teams. For example, surgical exposure may be somewhat more challenging and the depth of anesthesia may require closer vigilance.

Electromyography

Spontaneous electromyographic recordings provide real-time data that are sensitive to surgical manipulation or compression.[2] Myotomes are selected for recording based on the operative level and the nerve roots most at risk. Burst or train activity is considered significant and is thought to represent ongoing compression or stretch. Spontaneous EMG is sensitive but not specific.[9] As well as recording spontaneous electromyographic activity, a number of other applications have used electromyographic recordings to determine the proximity of nerve roots. Direct nerve root testing with EMG recording aids in the dissection of nerve roots off intradural tumors especially in the conus region. Triggered EMG has been used to aid in placement of pedicle screws.

EVIDENCE FOR MONITORING

Although the evidence for monitoring continues to evolve, there has been a vast increase in the body of evidence in the published literature that supports many aspects of current monitoring practices. Several authors have reported the results of good-quality studies that demonstrate a benefit when intraoperative monitoring is performed during spinal surgery. Relevant articles from the published literature were assigned a level of evidence as per the *Journal of Bone and Joint Surgery* (JBJS) guidelines.[10] For the purposes of this review, only articles of Level II evidence were available and are discussed.

Evidence for Somatosensory-Evoked Potentials

Most of the earlier literature predominantly evaluated the role of SSEPs alone in spinal surgery. As far back as 1982, Grundy and colleagues[11] reported a study showing that a wake-up test was not necessary provided SSEPs were monitored and stable. The authors prospectively studied the effects of moderate hypotension on 24 patients undergoing spinal fusion with Harrington rod instrumentation. Five of the 24 patients had alterations in their SSEPs and required an intraoperative wake-up test, all of which had normal results.

Epstein and coworkers[12] evaluated the role of SSEPs in cervical surgery by comparing the outcomes of patients who were monitored and operated on over a 3-year period (1989–1991) with those who were not monitored and had been operated on between 1985 and 1989. No instances of quadriplegia in the 100 patients who were monitored versus eight in the 218 who were not monitored were reported. The authors conclude that the reduction of neurologic deficit was attributed in part to early SSEP detection of vascular or mechanical compromise and to the immediate alteration of anesthetic or surgical technique in response to SSEP changes. Kombos and coworkers[13] report similar findings in a prospective evaluation of the impact of SSEP monitoring during anterior cervical surgery. In a prospective study of 100 patients, they deduce that SSEP monitoring was easy to perform and helped to increase the safety during anterior cervical surgery. Monitoring of both cortical and subcortical sites for SSEP responses has been shown to increase the reliability of SSEPs during spinal surgery.[14]

Evidence for Motor-Evoked Potentials

Concerns over false-negative results when using SSEPs alone have led to the proposal of alternative strategies, with either monitoring of MEPs alone or used in combination with other modalities.[6] Hilibrand and investigators[15] analyzed the data of 427 patients who underwent anterior or posterior cervical spine surgery over a 2-year period. Twelve of their patients

had loss of amplitude of MEPs, of which 10 had complete reversal of the loss after prompt intraoperative intervention and the remaining 2 had a new postoperative deficit. The sensitivity and specificity for MEPs was 100% in their series, whereas SSEP had only a sensitivity of 25%, although it was 100% specific. The authors conclude that transcranial MEPs appeared to be superior to conventional SSEPs for identifying evolving motor tract injury during cervical spine surgery.

Difficulties in obtaining and maintaining MEP responses with transcranial stimulation has led some authors to propose direct spinal cord stimulation to obtain neurogenic MEPs in certain pathologies.[16] Komanetsky and colleagues[17] compared two methods of stimulation when obtaining neurogenic MEPs. They prospectively compared spinous process stimulation with percutaneous stimulation in obtaining neurogenic MEPs in 184 patients. Both methods were found to be sensitive to neurologic deficit. When responses were obtained, the percutaneous method was found to be sufficiently reliable to obviate the need for the spinous process method.

Numerous studies have addressed the difficulties in obtaining reliable predictors for postoperative C5 palsy.[18] Tanaka and colleagues[18] evaluated the usefulness of transcranial MEPs for prediction of the occurrence of postoperative C5 palsy after cervical laminoplasty. They prospectively evaluated 62 consecutive patients, three of which developed postoperative transient C5 palsy. No critical decrease in amplitude occurred in any of the 62 patients. Because of this, the authors conclude that postoperative C5 palsy after cervical laminoplasty was not associated with an intraoperative injury (Table 7–1).

Evidence for Electromyography

There are fewer Level I or II evidence articles in the literature that validate the use of intraoperative EMG monitoring in spinal surgery. Dimopoulos and investigators[19] conducted a prospective randomized trial to correlate the findings of intraoperative EMG with immediate postoperative pain in patients undergoing lumbar microdiscectomy (Level II). They found no correlation between intraoperative electromyographic findings and postoperative pain.

Krassioukov and coauthors[20] examined the neurologic outcomes of 61 patients, most of whom were treated for spinal/spinal cord tumours (61%) or adult tethered cord syndrome (25%). Patients underwent multimodal neurophysiologic monitoring with EMG monitoring of the lower-limb muscles, external anal sphincter (EAS), external urethral sphincter (EUS), and lower-limb SSEPs. Spontaneous electromyographic activity was observed in the lower-extremity muscles and/or EAS and EUS in 51 cases (84%). In addition to spontaneously recorded electromyographic activity, electrically evoked EMG activity was also used as an intraoperative adjunct. The presence of electrically evoked EMG activity in structures encountered during

TABLE 7–1. Evidence for Intraoperative Monitoring

YEAR OF PUBLICATION	ARTICLE TITLE	AUTHORS	LEVEL OF EVIDENCE	PATIENTS, N	CONCLUSION
1982	Deliberate hypotension for spinal fusion: prospective randomized study with evoked potential monitoring	Grundy et al.[11]	2	24	Patients subjected to spinal fusion need not be awakened provided SSEPs are monitored and stable.
1993	Evaluation of intraoperative somatosensory-evoked potential monitoring during 100 cervical operations	Epstein et al.[12]	2	100	Monitoring with SSEPs reduced the postoperative neurologic deficit in patients undergoing cervical surgery.
1997	Comparison of the effects of ketamine-midazolam with those of fentanyl-midazolam on cortical somatosensory-evoked potentials during major spine surgery	Langeron et al.[23]	2	20	Both ketamine and fentanyl allowed reliable cortical SSEPs to be obtained.
1998	Neurogenic motor-evoked potentials: A prospective comparison of stimulation methods in spinal deformity surgery	Komanetsky et al.[17]	2	184	Both spinous process–elicited NMEPs and percutaneous-elicited NMEP are sensitive to neurologic deficit.
1999	Comparative study of propofol and midazolam effects on somatosensory evoked potentials during surgical treatment of scoliosis	Laureau et al.[24]	2	30	Use of either propofol or midazolam in scoliosis surgery is appropriate. Preoperative small-amplitude SSEPs may favor propofol.
2000	Low-dose propofol as a supplement to ketamine-based anesthesia during intraoperative monitoring of motor-evoked potentials	Kawaguchi et al.[25]	2	58	With pulse-train stimulation, low-dose propofol can be used as a supplement to ketamine-based anesthesia during monitoring of myogenic MEPs.
2001	Remifentanil- and fentanyl-based anesthesia for intraoperative monitoring of somatosensory-evoked potentials	Samra et al.[26]	2	41	Remifentanil infusion offers quicker recovery from anesthesia and less variability in SSEP morphology.
2002	Effect of sevoflurane/nitrous oxide versus propofol anaesthesia on somatosensory-evoked potential monitoring of the spinal cord during surgery to correct scoliosis	Ku et al.[27]	2	20	Sevoflurane produces a faster decrease and recovery of SSEP amplitude, as well as a better conscious state on emergence than propofol.
2002	Combined monitoring of motor and somatosensory-evoked potentials in orthopaedic spinal surgery	Pelosi et al.[21]	2	97	Combined monitoring with SSEP and MEP is superior to single-modality monitoring.

TABLE 7–1. Evidence for Intraoperative Monitoring—cont'd

YEAR OF PUBLICATION	ARTICLE TITLE	AUTHORS	LEVEL OF EVIDENCE	PATIENTS, N	CONCLUSION
2003	Impact of somatosensory-evoked potential monitoring on cervical surgery	Kombos et al.[13]	2	100	Intraoperative SSEP monitoring is easy to perform and helps to increase safety during anterior cervical surgery.
2004	The effects of propofol, small-dose isoflurane, and nitrous oxide on cortical somatosensory-evoked potential and bispectral index monitoring in adolescents undergoing spinal fusion	Clapcich et al.[29]	2	12	Propofol better preserves cortical SSEP amplitude.
2004	The effects of isoflurane and propofol on intraoperative neurophysiological monitoring during spinal surgery	Chen[28]	2	35	Isoflurane inhibited intraoperative monitoring more than propofol.
2004	Does intraoperative electromyographic monitoring in lumbar microdiscectomy correlate with postoperative pain?	Dimopoulos et al.[19]	2	112	No correlation between intraoperative electromyographic findings and postoperative pain.
2004	Real-time continuous intraoperative electromyographic and somatosensory-evoked potential recordings in spinal surgery: correlation of clinical and electrophysiologic findings in a prospective, consecutive series of 213 cases	Gunnarsson et al.[9]	2	213	In thoracolumbar spine surgery, EMG has a high sensitivity but low specificity. In contrast, SSEPs have a low sensitivity but high specificity.
2004	Multimodality intraoperative monitoring during complex lumbosacral procedures: indications, techniques, and long-term follow-up review of 61 consecutive cases	Krassioukov et al.[20]	2	61	Combined SSEP and EMG and anal/urethral sphincter monitoring is optimal for complex procedures involving the conus medullaris and cauda equina. These modalities influence microsurgical decision making and reduce the risk for perioperative complications.
2004	Comparison of transcranial electric motor and somatosensory-evoked potential monitoring during cervical spine surgery	Hilibrand et al.[15]	2	427	Transcranial electric MEP appears to be superior to conventional SSEP for identifying evolving injury during cervical spine surgery.

TABLE 7–1. Evidence for Intraoperative Monitoring—cont'd

YEAR OF PUBLICATION	ARTICLE TITLE	AUTHORS	LEVEL OF EVIDENCE	PATIENTS, N	CONCLUSION
2005	Effects of isoflurane and propofol on cortical somatosensory-evoked potentials during comparable depth of anaesthesia as guided by bispectral index	Liu et al.[30]	2	60	Propofol causes less suppression of cortical SSEPs, with better preservation of amplitude, and less variability at an equivalent depth of anesthesia.
2005	Combined application of two somatosensory-evoked potential techniques at various recording points for monitoring the onset of stretch spinal injury during rhachial orthomorphia	He et al.[14]	2	104	Monitoring of both cortical and subcortical SSEPs during spinal surgery can increase the reliability.
2006	Intraoperative motor-evoked potential monitoring in scoliosis surgery: comparison of desflurane/nitrous oxide with propofol total intravenous anesthetic regimens	Lo et al.[31]	2	20	Both desflurane and total intravenous anesthetic regimens allow successful intraoperative monitoring. Abductor hallucis is the preferred muscle with a desflurane anesthetic.
2006	Multimodality intraoperative neurophysiologic monitoring findings during surgery for adult tethered cord syndrome: analysis of a series of 44 patients with long-term follow-up	Paradiso et al.[1]	2	44	The combined recording of SSEPs in concert with continuous and evoked EMGs may provide a useful adjunct to complex microsurgery for adult tethered cord syndrome.
2006	Postoperative segmental C5 palsy after cervical laminoplasty may occur without intraoperative nerve injury: a prospective study with transcranial electric motor-evoked potentials	Tanaka et al.[18]	2	62	The development of postoperative C5 palsy after cervical laminoplasty is not associated with intraoperative injury.
2007	Somatosensory- and motor-evoked potential monitoring during spine and spinal cord surgery	Costa et al.[22]	2	52	Combined MEP and SSEP monitoring reliable to detect and prevent injury.

EMG = electromyography; MEP = motor-evoked potential; NMEP = neurogenic motor-evoked potential; SSEP = somatosensory-evoked potential.

microdissection altered the plan of treatment in 24 cases (42%).

Similar findings were reported by Paradiso and colleagues,[1] who examined the use of intraoperative monitoring in tethered cord syndrome. Posterior tibial nerve SSEPs were found to have high specificity, but low sensitivity, for predicting new neurologic deficits. In contrast, continuous EMG showed high sensitivity and low specificity. Evoked EMG accurately identified functional neural tissue.

Multimodality Monitoring

To overcome the limitations of individual monitoring modalities, many teams have explored the value of multimodal monitoring to obtain a more robust real-time assessment of intraoperative neural function. Pelosi and researchers[21] investigated the combined monitoring of MEPs and SSEPs in 126 spinal operations. Combined monitoring was successfully achieved in 104 operations; it was possible only to monitor a single modality in 18 patients (16 SSEPs, 2 MEPs). No response to either modality could be recorded in two patients. The authors report that combined monitoring was superior to single-modality techniques both for increasing the number of patients in whom satisfactory monitoring could be achieved and for improving the sensitivity and predictivity of monitoring.

Gunnarsson and coauthors[9] correlate the clinical and electrophysiologic findings in a prospective, consecutive series of 213 patients. Intraoperative electromyographic activation had a sensitivity of 100% and a specificity of 23.7% for the detection of a new postoperative neurologic deficit. SSEPs had a sensitivity of 28.6% and specificity of 94.7%. The authors conclude that combined intraoperative neurophysiologic monitoring with EMG and SSEP is helpful for predicting and possibly preventing neurologic injury during thoracolumbar spine surgery.

Costa and colleagues'[22] prospective observational study reports on the use of combined multimodal monitoring in a cohort of patients undergoing a variety of spinal procedures. Combined SSEP and MEP monitoring was successfully obtained in 38 of 52 patients (73%), whereas MEPs from at least 1 target muscle were obtained in 12 patients (23%); both SSEPs and MEPs were absent in 2 patients (3.8%). Significant intraoperative changes occurred in one or both modalities in five patients, two of which were transient, whereas three had persistent changes associated with new deficits or worsening of the preexisting neurologic disability. The authors suggested that intraoperative combined monitoring is a safe, reliable, and sensitive method to detect and reduce neurologic injury to the spinal cord. However, there was no comparative group that did not use neuromonitoring.

After comparing transcranial MEPs and SSEP monitoring in a large cohort of patients who underwent cervical spine surgery, Hilibrand and investigators[15] highlight the fact that, although SSEPs were specific, they remain relatively insensitive. In addition, they highlight the need for multimodal monitoring in cervical spine surgery.

Case Example

A 64-year-old man with known ankylosing spondylitis presented with a 6-month history of progressive gait difficulties and impairment of upper-limb fine motor function. His clinical examination confirmed that he had cervical myelopathy. Preoperative imaging (Fig. 7–1A and C) showed that he had marked cord compression on the T2-weighted magnetic resonance imaging. He was electively booked for surgery where he underwent a multilevel cervical laminectomy and instrumented fusion. During the decompression stage of the operation, the surgeon was alerted that the patient had developed spontaneous electromyographic train activity in an upper-limb muscle (see Fig. 7–2A). Shortly after this, the

patient's SSEP responses in all four limbs deteriorated (see Fig. 7–2B). A diagnosis of a presumptive cord injury was made and treatment was instituted with blood pressure elevation and administration of steroids. The patient's SSEP traces in his upper limbs began to recover toward the end of the case. Postoperative imaging showed new high signal changes in the spinal cord (Fig. 7–1B and D). Immediately after surgery, the patient was quadriparetic, legs worse than arms, but his deficit had improved substantially by the time of discharge. The immediate diagnosis and institution of treatment potentially prevented a complete injury and a suboptimal clinical outcome for this patient.

Anesthetic Regimen for Monitoring

Some of the best evidence available in the intraoperative monitoring literature pertains to the optimal anesthetic regimen to use. In 1997, a randomized trial of 20 patients was undertaken to compare the effects of ketamine with those of fentanyl (both combined with midazolam) on cortical SSEP monitoring during major spinal surgery.[23] Cortical SSEP latencies were not significantly affected in either group. The authors conclude that both ketamine and fentanyl allowed the recording of reliable cortical SSEPs, but a longer delay for voluntary postoperative motor assessment was observed in the ketamine group (Level II).

Laureau and colleagues[24] report a prospective, randomized trial comparing the effects of propofol and midazolam in 2 groups of 15 patients undergoing surgery for idiopathic scoliosis. The amplitude of the cortical SSEP responses decreased after induction in both groups; in the midazolam-treated group, the amplitudes were smaller. The most significant finding in the study was that both propofol and midazolam seemed to be acceptable hypnotic agents for total intravenous anesthesia during intraoperative monitoring in the surgical treatment of scoliosis. This study has limitations in that it is difficult to correlate postoperative neurologic deficits and intraoperative monitoring data because no SSEP changes occurred and also because cortical SSEPs were recorded only unilaterally (Level II).

The effects of low-dose propofol as a supplement to ketamine-based anesthesia during intraoperative monitoring of MEPs has been reported by Kawaguchi and coauthors.[25] Intraoperative monitoring of MEPs was performed in 58 patients who underwent elective spinal surgery. Anesthesia was maintained with nitrous oxide-fentanyl-ketamine with or without low-dose propofol. The authors found that low-dose propofol could be effectively used as a supplement to ketamine-based anesthesia during intraoperative monitoring of myogenic MEPs as long as a train of pulses was used for transcranial stimulation. Addition of propofol significantly reduced the ketamine-induced psychedelic effects.

In 2001, Samra and colleagues'[26] study was published comparing remifentanil- and fentanyl-based

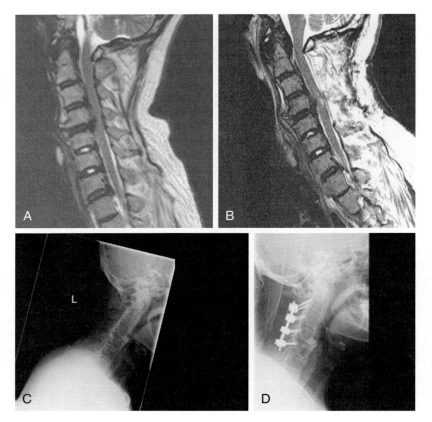

FIGURE 7–1. Preoperative and postoperative T2 magnetic resonance imaging (MRI) and lateral C-spine radiographs. Preoperative T2 MRI *(A)* showing marked cord compression and *(B)* postoperative T2 MRI showing new high-signal change in the cord substance. *C, D,* Preoperative and postoperative plain lateral radiographs.

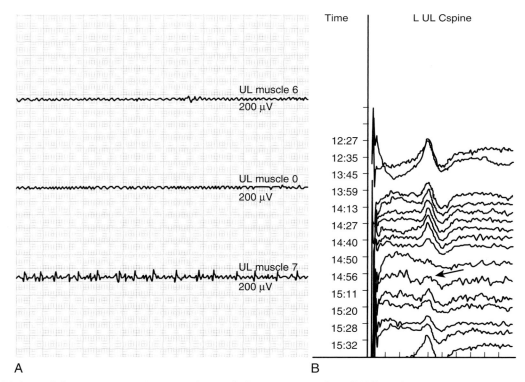

FIGURE 7–2. Multimodality intraoperative recordings of electromyographic (EMG) and somatosensory-evoked potential (SSEP) responses. Intraoperative electromyography showing the run of spontaneous EMG activity before the SSEP deterioration *(A)*. The patient's SSEP tracing is shown at various time points. At 14.56 *(arrow)*, the patient had complete loss of his SSEP responses. Treatment was instituted immediately, and by 15.11, there had begun to be some recovery of the SSEP response.

anesthesia for intraoperative monitoring of SSEPs with special attention to the speed of recovery from the anesthetic. They studied 41 patients who were randomized into 2 groups to receive either remifentanil- or fentanyl-based anesthesia. The authors report that both remifentanil and fentanyl infusion allowed satisfactory monitoring of SSEPs. Remifentanil infusion offers the advantage of quicker recovery from anesthesia and less variability of SSEP morphology.

Ku and coworkers[27] have reported the effect of sevoflurane/nitrous oxide versus propofol anesthesia on SSEP monitoring during scoliosis surgery. They randomized 20 patients into 2 groups to receive either sevoflurane or propofol. Changes in anesthetic concentrations produced little effect on the latency of SSEP, but the effect on the variability of amplitude was significant. The authors conclude that sevoflurane produced a faster decrease and recovery of SSEP amplitude, as well as a better conscious state on waking, than did propofol (Level II).

A number of studies have compared the effects of propofol versus isoflurane on monitoring SSEPs and MEPs intraoperatively.[28–30] Clapcich and investigators[29] randomized 12 patients into 4 groups receiving either variable doses of isoflurane-nitrous oxide combinations or a propofol combination. Chen[28] randomized a group of 35 patients into 2 groups to receive either an isoflurane or a propofol infusion. Liu and coauthors[30] reported a randomized trial of 60 patients who were randomized to receive similar types of infusions. All of the groups reported that both propofol and isoflurane decreased SSEP amplitude while the anesthetic took effect. Propofol caused less suppression of the cortical SSEP responses with better preservation of SSEP amplitude. Chen[28] reports that MEPs were recordable in all patients receiving propofol, but in only 50% of patients receiving isoflurane[28] (Level II).

In 2006, Lo and coauthors'[31] study was published comparing a desflurane-nitrous oxide combination with propofol total intravenous anesthetic regimen. They prospectively randomized 20 patients undergoing scoliosis correction surgery into 2 groups. Reproducible MEP responses were always obtained throughout the procedure. The authors conclude that both desflurane and total intravenous anesthetic with propofol allow successful monitoring. They suggest using abductor hallucis muscle for recording MEPs when using desflurane (Level II).

AREAS OF UNCERTAINTY

Limitations of Current Evidence

All of the articles discussed in the previous section are deemed Level II evidence. No Level I evidence exists to support the use of intraoperative monitoring. Moreover, many of the class II studies are limited by relatively small sample sizes. The lack of validated quantitative methods to assess intraoperative electromyographic changes also poses a limitation in evaluating the literature for this neurophysiologic modality.

With the advancement and development of new anesthetic agents, the question as to which anesthetic regimen is optimal for intraoperative monitoring is likely to be asked many times in the future. The answering of such a question in the presence of clinical equipoise could potentially be deciphered by performing a prospective, randomized, blinded, controlled trial (PRCT).

What is much more challenging, however, is to try and establish a similar level of evidence to support the use of intraoperative neurophysiologic monitoring. The difficulty is that trials on this subject do not lend themselves well to the PRCT type model. Devising any such outcome study, which would include blinding the surgeon, would be ethically unacceptable to those who routinely use intraoperative monitoring.

It appears likely, therefore, that the answers of future questions on whom should be monitored and how they should be monitored will more likely come from well-documented, nonrandomized, prospectively collected studies on large series of patients rather than other types of study design.

Which Spinal Patients Should Be Monitored?

Currently, no universal agreement exists as to which patients should undergo intraoperative monitoring during spinal surgery. The published literature would indicate that patients with a preexisting cord deficit have a greater risk for having a major neurophysiologic alert and are at greater risk for an intraoperative injury.[2,32,33] Given that these patients appear to be at greater risk, it would seem prudent to monitor them.

MEPs are reliable in predicting clinical motor outcome, and their use has altered the surgical approach; for example, gross total resections of intramedullary tumors are more readily attempted as long as MEP data indicate the intact functional integrity of the corticospinal tract.[34]

The applicability and effectiveness of intraoperative monitoring increase with its use and familiarity. Therefore, we recommend that it be used for all spine surgery cases where neurologic compromise is a potential risk. The most effective application of these techniques requires a team-based approach involving the surgical, anesthetic, and monitoring personnel.

What Modalities Are Optimal to Monitor?

Which set of tests is optimal to monitor needs to be individually tailored for each surgery. The choice of what modalities to use is dependent on the preference of the surgeon, the nature and localization of the pathology involved, and the technical feasibility of the modality in the specific context. A good way to select which tests to use is to choose a combination of modalities most specific to the neural tissue at risk during the procedure—MEPs for anterior cord, SSEPs for posterior cord, and EMGs for roots at risk, respectively.

The combined electrophysiologic exploration of motor and sensory potentials has proved to be the most useful tool for monitoring patients during spinal surgery. Combined MEPs and SSEPs (as well as EMG) provide independent and complementary information, and improve spinal cord monitoring. Good practices such as being consistent in its use and keeping a good and constant communication between the monitoring and surgical team are key for its success.

RECOMMENDATIONS

All current electrophysiologic approaches have limitations. Currently, no all-encompassing test exists that can adequately monitor all facets of neural function during spinal surgery. The approach in our unit has been to combine highly specific, though relatively insensitive, electrophysiologic modalities (e.g., SSEPs with highly sensitive but less specific techniques) (e.g., free-running spontaneous EMG activity).[1,9,20] Monitoring of MEPs is reserved for high-risk cases—for example, for patients with a preexisting cord deficit or those undergoing surgery for intramedullary lesions.

The monitoring approach needs to be tailored to each patient depending on the underlying pathology and location. Importantly, the successful application of intraoperative monitoring requires a team-based approach with clear communication among the neurophysiologist, surgeon, and anesthetist. It is our position that multimodal monitoring enables the most comprehensive assessment of neural function during spinal surgery and provides useful feedback to the surgical team, resulting in enhanced patient safety and reduced risk for perioperative neurologic complications.

Based on our expert opinion, attention to such quantitative intraoperative monitoring data may help to minimize postoperative motor deficits by avoiding or correcting excessive spinal cord manipulation, intraoperative hypotension to the spinal cord, and modifying surgical technique during tumor resection (Level V). We also advocate the use of free-running and evoked EMGs when operating in the cervical or lumbar areas. Table 7–2 provides recommendations for intraoperative spinal monitoring (graded as per JBJS guidelines[35]: grade B = fair evidence, Level II or III studies with consistent findings).

TABLE 7–2. Recommendations for Intraoperative Spinal Monitoring

STATEMENT	LEVEL OF EVIDENCE/GRADE OF RECOMMENDATION
1. SSEPs should not be recorded in isolation because of their low sensitivity.	B
2. Spontaneous EMG monitoring is optimal for lesions involving the conus or cauda equina.	B
3. Evoked EMG is beneficial when operating on conus or cauda equina lesions to identify functional neural elements.	B
4. MEPs have a greater accuracy than SSEPs and therefore should be used in high-risk cases.	B

Graded as per *Journal of Bone and Joint Surgery* (JBJS) guidelines[35]: grade B = fair evidence, Level II or III studies with consistent findings.

EMG = electromyography; MEP = motor-evoked potential; SSEP = somatosensory-evoked potential.

REFERENCES

1. Paradiso G, Lee GY, Sarjeant R, et al: Multimodality intraoperative neurophysiologic monitoring findings during surgery for adult tethered cord syndrome: Analysis of a series of 44 patients with long-term follow-up. Spine 31:2095–2102, 2006.
2. Padberg AM, Thuet ED: Intraoperative electrophysiologic monitoring: Considerations for complex spinal surgery. Neurosurg Clin N Am 17:205–226, 2006.
3. Kothbauer KF, Novak K: Intraoperative monitoring for tethered cord surgery: An update. Neurosurg Focus 16:E8, 2004.
4. Quinones-Hinojosa A, Gulati M, Lyon R, et al: Spinal cord mapping as an adjunct for resection of intramedullary tumors: Surgical technique with case illustrations. Neurosurgery 51:1199–1206, 2002.
5. Shi YB, Binette M, Martin WH, et al: Electrical stimulation for intraoperative evaluation of thoracic pedicle screw placement. Spine 28:595–601, 2003.
6. Wiedemayer H, Sandalcioglu IE, Armbruster W, et al: False negative findings in intraoperative SEP monitoring: Analysis of 658 consecutive neurosurgical cases and review of published reports. J Neurol Neurosurg Psychiatry 75:280–286, 2004.
7. Ben-David B, Haller G, Taylor P: Anterior spinal fusion complicated by paraplegia. A case report of a false-negative somatosensory-evoked potential. Spine 12:536–539, 1987.
8. Lesser RP, Raudzens P, Luders H, et al: Postoperative neurological deficits may occur despite unchanged intraoperative somatosensory evoked potentials. Ann Neurol 19:22–25, 1986.
9. Gunnarsson T, Krassioukov AV, Sarjeant R, et al: Real-time continuous intraoperative electromyographic and somatosensory evoked potential recordings in spinal surgery: Correlation of clinical and electrophysiologic findings in a prospective, consecutive series of 213 cases. Spine 29:677–684, 2004.
10. Wright JG, Swiontkowski MF, Heckman JD: Introducing levels of evidence to the journal. J Bone Joint Surg Am 85:1–3, 2003.
11. Grundy BL, Nash CL Jr, Brown RH: Deliberate hypotension for spinal fusion: Prospective randomized study with evoked potential monitoring. Can Anaesth Soc J 29:452–462, 1982.
12. Epstein NE, Danto J, Nardi D: Evaluation of intraoperative somatosensory-evoked potential monitoring during 100 cervical operations. Spine 18:737–747, 1993.
13. Kombos T, Suess O, Da SC, et al: Impact of somatosensory evoked potential monitoring on cervical surgery. J Clin Neurophysiol 20:122–128, 2003.
14. He JM, Tang Y: Combined application of two somatosensory evoked potential techniques at various recording points for monitoring the onset of stretch spinal injury during rhachial orthomorphia. Zhongguo Linchuang Kangfu 9:164–165, 2005.

15. Hilibrand AS, Schwartz DM, Sethuraman V, et al: Comparison of transcranial electric motor and somatosensory evoked potential monitoring during cervical spine surgery. J Bone Joint Surg Am 86:1248–1253, 2004.

16. Accadbled F, Henry P, de Gauzy JS, et al: Spinal cord monitoring in scoliosis surgery using an epidural electrode. Results of a prospective, consecutive series of 191 cases. Spine 31:2614–2623, 2006.

17. Komanetsky RM, Padberg AM, Lenke LG, et al: Neurogenic motor evoked potentials: A prospective comparison of stimulation methods in spinal deformity surgery. J Spinal Disord 11:21–28, 1998.

18. Tanaka N, Nakanishi K, Fujiwara Y, et al: Postoperative segmental C5 palsy after cervical laminoplasty may occur without intraoperative nerve injury: A prospective study with transcranial electric motor-evoked potentials. Spine 31:3013–3017, 2006.

19. Dimopoulos VG, Feltes CH, Fountas KN, et al: Does intraoperative electromyographic monitoring in lumbar microdiscectomy correlate with postoperative pain? South Med J 97:724–728, 2004.

20. Krassioukov AV, Sarjeant R, Arkia H, et al: Multimodality intraoperative monitoring during complex lumbosacral procedures: Indications, techniques, and long-term follow-up review of 61 consecutive cases. J Neurosurg Spine 1:243–253, 2004.

21. Pelosi L, Lamb J, Grevitt M, et al: Combined monitoring of motor and somatosensory evoked potentials in orthopaedic spinal surgery. Clin Neurophysiol 113:1082–1091, 2002.

22. Costa P, Bruno A, Bonzanino M, et al: Somatosensory- and motor-evoked potential monitoring during spine and spinal cord surgery. Spinal Cord 45:86–91, 2007.

23. Langeron O, Lille F, Zerhouni O, et al: Comparison of the effects of ketamine-midazolam with those of fentanyl-midazolam on cortical somatosensory evoked potentials during major spine surgery. Br J Anaesth 78:701–706, 1997.

24. Laureau E, Marciniak B, Hebrard A, et al: Comparative study of propofol and midazolam effects on somatosensory evoked potentials during surgical treatment of scoliosis. Neurosurgery 45:69–74, 1999.

25. Kawaguchi M, Sakamoto T, Inoue S, et al: Low dose propofol as a supplement to ketamine-based anesthesia during intraoperative monitoring of motor-evoked potentials. Spine 25:974–979, 2000.

26. Samra SK, Dy EA, Welch KB, et al: Remifentanil- and fentanyl-based anesthesia for intraoperative monitoring of somatosensory evoked potentials. Anesth Analg 92:1510–1515, 2001.

27. Ku AS, Hu Y, Irwin MG, et al: Effect of sevoflurane/nitrous oxide versus propofol anaesthesia on somatosensory evoked potential monitoring of the spinal cord during surgery to correct scoliosis. Br J Anaesth 88:502–507, 2002.

28. Chen Z: The effects of isoflurane and propofol on intraoperative neurophysiological monitoring during spinal surgery. J Clin Monit Comput 18:303–308, 2004.

29. Clapcich AJ, Emerson RG, Roye DP Jr, et al: The effects of propofol, small-dose isoflurane, and nitrous oxide on cortical somatosensory evoked potential and bispectral index monitoring in adolescents undergoing spinal fusion. Anesth Analg 99:1334–1340, 2004.

30. Liu EH, Wong HK, Chia CP, et al: Effects of isoflurane and propofol on cortical somatosensory evoked potentials during comparable depth of anaesthesia as guided by bispectral index. Br J Anaesth 94:193–197, 2005.

31. Lo YL, Dan YF, Tan YE, et al: Intraoperative motor-evoked potential monitoring in scoliosis surgery: Comparison of desflurane/nitrous oxide with propofol total intravenous anesthetic regimens. J Neurosurg Anesthesiol 18:211–214, 2006.

32. Thuet ED, Padberg AM, Raynor BL, et al: Increased risk of postoperative neurologic deficit for spinal surgery patients with unobtainable intraoperative evoked potential data. Spine 30:2094–2103, 2005.

33. Lee JY, Hilibrand AS, Lim MR, et al: Characterization of neurophysiologic alerts during anterior cervical spine surgery. Spine 31:1916–1922, 2006.

34. Sala F, Palandri G, Basso E, et al: Motor evoked potential monitoring improves outcome after surgery for intramedullary spinal cord tumors: A historical control study. Neurosurgery 58:1129–1143, 2006.

35. Wright JG, Einhorn TA, Heckman JD: Grades of recommendation. J Bone Joint Surg Am 87:1909–1910, 2005.

What Is the Optimal Method of Managing a Patient with Cervical Myelopathy?

Howard Ginsberg, BASc, MD, PhD, FRCSC and Masahiko Akiyama, MD, DMSC

Cervical spondylotic myelopathy (CSM) is the most common cause of spinal cord dysfunction in the elderly and the most common cause of nontraumatic spastic paraparesis and quadriparesis.[1] Although CSM is a common disorder, the treatment of CSM remains controversial in terms of "surgery or conservative management," "surgical indication and timing of surgery," "surgical approach," and "type of surgery." This chapter reviews and discusses evidence-based literature on the optimal management of CSM.

SURGERY VERSUS CONSERVATIVE MANAGEMENT: TIMING OF SURGERY

Knowledge of the natural history of CSM is critical in decision making for treatment of CSM. However, few studies and no Level I evidence studies are available. Early studies on the course of CSM suggest that most patients with myelopathy experience progressive neurological worsening, most commonly with episodic deterioration.[2–4] In contrast, another long-term study of myelopathic patients by Lees and Turner[5] shows that a long period of nonprogression was the rule and progressive deterioration was the exception. A small cohort study of 24 patients, treated by collar immobilization and followed for a mean duration of 6.5 years, found that the conditions of approximately one third of patients improved, one third deteriorated, and one third were stable.[6] Similar results were confirmed by Nurick.[7] In the majority of CSM cases, there is an initial phase of deterioration, followed by a stable period lasting a number of years, during which the degree of disability does not change significantly for those mildly affected. In general, older patients and those with motor deficits are more likely to experience development of progressive deterioration. As a result, Nurick[7] states that surgery should be reserved for those with progressive disability and those older than 60 years. Patients with milder disease may have a better prognosis.[8] However, some authors state that patients treated conservatively show progressive neurologic deterioration.[9,10] In addition, patients with CSM may be at increased risk for spinal cord injury after minor trauma,[11] which supports early intervention for even mildly

symptomatic patients. Few direct comparisons of conservative and operative treatment in patients with myelopathy exist even in the recent literature. A nonrandomized cohort study comparing medical and surgical treatment in 43 patients, 23 of whom were treated without surgery, reported significant worsening of their ability to perform activities of daily living, with worsening of neurologic symptoms.[12] In contrast, 20 surgically treated patients had a significant improvement in functional status and overall pain with improvement also observed in neurologic symptoms. Although this study demonstrates that the results of surgical treatment are better than those of conservative management, it lacks randomization and had significant treatment selection bias. In the 2002 Cochrane review on the role of surgery for cervical myelopathy,[13] one small study reports 49 patients with mild or moderate myelopathy who were randomized to surgery versus conservative treatment. Although age and sex ratios were similar between the two groups, the conservative group had slightly better modified Japanese Orthopaedic Association (mJOA) scores, suggesting a possible bias in treatment allocation. At 6 months, mJOA scores and gait scores were better in the conservatively treated group. But no differences were reported at 2 years. In addition, a subgroup with severe disability improved after surgical intervention.[13] A more recent 3-year, prospective, randomized study of 68 patients with mild-to-moderate nonprogressive CSM did not demonstrate a significant difference in outcomes (mJOA score and self-evaluation) between surgically and nonsurgically treated patients.[14] In addition, timed 10-m walk in the nonsurgical group was significantly better than that in the surgical group. The authors conclude that their results could mean that the conservative approach can treat CSM with a degree of success similar to that of surgery for at least 3 years, supporting rather than proving the "wait and see" strategy.[14] This study failed to prove that surgical intervention has any advantage over conservative management. However, the poor specificity of the mJOA scoring scale, the small number of randomized patients, and relatively short follow-up period for this disorder (3 years) may account for the apparent lack of any lasting beneficial effect of surgery on the natural history of cervical myelopathy. In addition, the potential risk for spinal cord injury after minor trauma, which is impossible to quantify, should be considered when conservative management is selected.

Kadanka and colleagues'[15] more recent study of a subclass analysis demonstrated that the patients with a good outcome in the surgically treated group had a more serious clinical picture (expressed in mJOA score and slower walk). They conclude that surgery is more suitable for patients who are clinically worse and have a spinal canal transverse area of less than 70 mm[2].[15] Once moderate signs and symptoms develop, patients are less likely to improve on their own and would likely benefit from surgical intervention.[16]

One crucial question is what group of patients will experience development of CSM and clinically progress. Bednarik and investigators[17] conducted a prospective cohort study of clinically asymptomatic cervical cord compression cases (66 cases). Patients were managed to determine which patients experienced development of clinical signs of cervical myelopathy. During a median 4-year follow-up period, clinical signs of myelopathy were detected in 13 patients (19.7%). These signs were also associated with symptomatic cervical radiculopathy, electromyographic evidence of an anterior horn lesion, and abnormal somatosensory-evoked potentials.

Little information is available on nonoperative treatment of cervical myelopathy. Cervical collars have been recommended for symptomatic relief but have no effect on long-term outcomes, including neurologic progression. Although a recent study demonstrated the effectiveness of "rigorous" conservative management including 3- or 4-hour cervical traction, cervical orthosis, drug therapy, and exercise therapy,[18] manipulation and traction are generally considered to be contraindicated because of the potential for aggravation of neurologic symptoms.[2]

RECOMMENDATIONS

1. Once moderate signs and symptoms develop, patients are less likely to improve on their own and would likely benefit from surgical intervention (grade C recommendation).
2. Manipulation and traction are not recommended because of the potential risk for aggravation of neurologic symptoms (grade C recommendation).

SELECTION OF THE SURGICAL APPROACH

Selection of the appropriate surgical approach is based on a complete understanding of the factors responsible for the cord dysfunction. Because abnormal radiographic findings are common even in asymptomatic patients,[17,19] clinicians need to be careful to correlate the patient's complaints, physical examination, and imaging results to discern the precise diagnosis. The purpose of surgery is to decompress neural elements,

restore lordosis, and stabilize the spine to prevent additional degeneration at the affected level. Surgery for CSM has been performed by anterior, posterior, and combined approaches; each has unique advantages and disadvantages. The decision of which surgical approach to use is based on multiple factors, including the source of spinal cord compression, the number of vertebral segments involved in the disease process, cervical alignment, the magnitude of coexisting neck pain, patient comorbidities, and the surgeon's familiarity with various techniques. Therefore, the selection of surgical approach remains controversial, especially in patients with multilevel degenerative disease.

In general, primarily ventral pathology causing cord compression, particularly if it is focal rather than contiguous over multiple levels (Fig. 8–1), is best treated via an anterior approach.[20] An anterior approach provides for direct visualization and removal of the offending pathologic lesion without manipulation of the cord. When a neutral or kyphotic cervical sagittal alignment is present, anterior procedures may also serve to restore physiologic lordosis. Restoration of lordosis allows for shifting of the cord dorsally to diminish the effect of anterior compression. After anterior decompression, spinal column stability is restored through segmental arthrodesis, which may have the added benefit of eliminating painful motion from the spondylotic motion segment.[21] In contrast, if the compression is posterior and related primarily to facet hypertrophy or buckling ligamentum flavum, posterior decompression should be considered.[9] However, the optimal surgical approach for the treatment of cervical myelopathy resulting from stenosis at three or more levels remains controversial. In addition to the earlier discussion, some other principles can assist in the selection

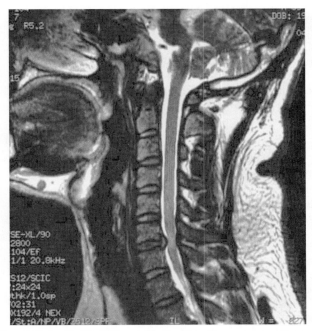

FIGURE 8–1. Sagittal T2-weighted magnetic resonance imaging scan shows a large herniated cervical disc at C6-C7 causing spinal cord compression.

of the appropriate approach, although an element of the surgeon's preference will also be involved.[22] An anterior arthrodesis of three or more motion segments is associated with a greater incidence of nonunion and graft-related problems than one- or two-level procedures.[23–25] A posterior procedure, including laminectomy with or without fusion or laminoplasty, can achieve an indirect decompression and may be an excellent alternative to anterior decompression if the spine is lordotic[21] (Fig. 8–2). If the spine is kyphotic, however, a posterior approach may be contraindicated because the spinal cord cannot displace dorsally from the anterior compressive structures, and a ventral approach is indicated. If the patient's spine is straight, either procedure can be used.[10]

Other considerations include patient's age and overall medical condition. Anterior surgery is more prolonged, and patients with multiple levels will be more likely to have dysphagia and voice problems after surgery; therefore, posterior surgery may be preferable if the alignment is not kyphotic for an older or a high medical risk patient.[22]

Although the optimal selection of surgical approach for CSM involving three or more motion segments in the presence of a lordotic sagittal alignment remains controversial (Fig. 8–3), few comparative studies are available. In 1985, one study compared the results of laminectomy versus corpectomy and anterior cervical discectomy and fusion (ACDF) for the treatment of multilevel CSM, and demonstrated that multilevel corpectomy has a significantly greater rate of recovery and decreased late neurologic deterioration compared with laminectomy.[26] These results disfavor laminectomy mainly because of the well-known sequelae, such as segmental instability, kyphosis, and

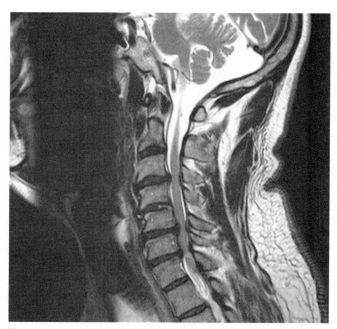

FIGURE 8–3. Sagittal T2-weighted magnetic resonance imaging scan shows multilevel degenerative disease with spondylotic changes at C3-C4 and from C5 to C7 causing spinal cord compression.

perineural adhesions.[27–36] In Japan, relatively poor outcomes associated with cervical laminectomy led to the evolution of laminoplasty, which remarkably reduced the sequelae after laminectomy.[37–40] A radiographic analysis of cervical alignment after laminectomy and laminoplasty in humans demonstrated that segmental kyphosis was present in 33% of laminectomy patients and 6% of laminoplasty patients at an average of 6 years after surgery.[41] A later study compared the results of laminoplasty with subtotal corpectomy[42] and reported that there were no significant differences in either the maximum JOA recovery rate or the final recovery rate for the two procedures. However, a notable difference was the overall incidence rate of complications (29% for corpectomy and 7% for laminoplasty). A similar retrospective study[43] showed that both procedures had similar rates of maintained neurologic improvement, and the disadvantages noted for the two procedures were pseudarthrosis (26%) and asymptomatic adjacent segment degeneration in a majority of patients after corpectomy, and decreased range of motion and axial discomfort (40%) after laminoplasty. A more recent prospective cohort study demonstrated that patients undergoing both procedures enjoyed a similar degree of subjective and objective neurologic improvement, but the incidence of complications was significantly greater for patients in the corpectomy cohort, especially persistent dysphagia and dysphonia.[44] The authors conclude that laminoplasty may be the preferred method of treatment for multilevel cervical myelopathy in the absence of preoperative kyphosis. Another interesting observation of this study was that the laminoplasty cohort tended to require less pain medication at final follow-up than did the multilevel corpectomy cohort.[44]

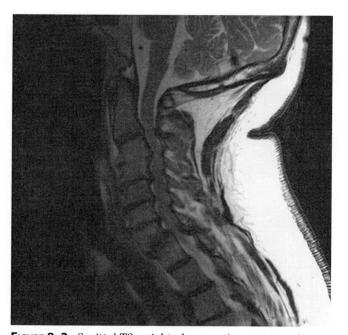

FIGURE 8–2. Sagittal T2-weighted magnetic resonance imaging scan demonstrates multilevel degenerative disease with spondylotic changes spanning from C2 to T1 resulting in spinal canal stenosis.

Surgical indications of the combined approach to CSM are limited. A combined anterior and posterior approach may be considered for the following patients: (1) those with both anterior and posterior compression, which is difficult to treat with a single approach; (2) those with a loss of lordosis (either straightening or kyphosis) in addition to multilevel (three or more disc spaces) severe anterior compression from an osteocartilaginous spur or ossification of posterior longitudinal ligament (OPLL)[45,46]; or (3) those with severe osteoporosis, diabetes, or heavy nicotine use who have a poor rate of spinal fusion with ventral surgery alone.[46] Some studies demonstrate that a single-stage combined procedure maximizes the decompression and reduces the graft-related surgical complications, as well as reducing perioperative complications when compared with staged combined procedures.[45–47]

RECOMMENDATIONS

1. Primarily focal ventral pathology causing cord compression is best treated via an anterior approach (grade C recommendation).
2. If compression is posterior and related primarily to facet hypertrophy or buckling ligamentum flavum, posterior decompression should be considered (grade C recommendation).
3. The optimal surgical approach for the treatment of cervical myelopathy resulting from stenosis at three or more levels remains controversial. If the spine is lordotic or straight, either an anterior or posterior approach can be used; however, if the spine is kyphotic, the posterior approach may be contraindicated (grade C recommendation).
4. The combined procedure may be used for treatment of patients with severe multilevel anterior compression with a kyphotic spine (grade C recommendation).
5. Laminoplasty remarkably reduced the sequelae after laminectomy, such as segmental instability, kyphosis, and perineural adhesions (grade C recommendation).
6. Laminoplasty may be preferable for multilevel cervical myelopathy in the absence of preoperative kyphosis (grade C recommendation).

ANTERIOR APPROACH

Anterior decompression and fusion has been widely applied to the treatment of cervical stenosis resulting from herniated discs, spondylosis, or OPLL. When the pathology occurs at the level of the intervertebral disc, ACDF provides sufficient access to the stenotic focus. Clinical studies have demonstrated that successful arthrodesis can be achieved in 92% to 96% of patients after single-level ACDF with satisfactory clinical results.[21,48–50] Selection of surgical procedure (multilevel discectomy vs. cervical corpectomy) in multilevel pathology is controversial.[51,52] Few studies directly compare multilevel ACDFs and

corpectomy. In general, if compressive lesions are present at the level of the disc only, either a single-level or a multilevel ventral discectomy should be performed. However, if the lesion is behind the vertebral body, a corpectomy should be performed.

The advantage of performing a multilevel ACDF instead of a single-level or multilevel corpectomy and fusion is that with the multilevel discectomy, postdecompression segmental fixation can be achieved by placing screws into the intervening vertebral bodies. It is easier to restore sagittal balance after a multilevel ventral cervical discectomy as opposed to a cervical corpectomy by using this strategy.[53] However, the disadvantage of multilevel ACDFs is that the incidence of nonunion increases with the number of levels being fused, although the rate of neurologic improvement remains high for multilevel ACDFs.[54] The recently reported fusion rate for a one-level ACDF using autograft iliac crest without plating (two graft–host sites) was 96%.[49] This decreased to a 75% fusion rate when a two-level ACDF was performed and to a 56% fusion rate with a three-level ACDF (six graft–host fusion sites).[55]

Corpectomy is an alternate option to improve the fusion rate after multilevel anterior decompression. Only two points must fuse in a corpectomy, as compared with multiple surfaces that must fuse with multilevel ACDFs. The additional advantage of a single-level or multilevel cervical corpectomy is the ability to decompress lesions behind the vertebral bodies.[46] The studies that compared the fusion rate after multilevel ACDF and corpectomy reported the nonunion rate in corpectomy was 7% to 10% compared with 34% to 36% for patients undergoing multilevel ACDFs.[23,25] Based on these factors, corpectomy may be considered preferable to multilevel ACDF, especially in higher-risk patients, such as smokers, patients with diabetes, or revision cases.[21]

The disadvantage of a cervical corpectomy is dislodgement of the graft, which often requires revision. Some reports have documented that the early strut dislocation rate was 8.7% to 21%.[56–58] Various plate designs, including static plates, buttress plates, and more recently, dynamic plates, have been introduced to prevent anterior strut graft dislodgement and to decrease the rate of nonunion after corpectomy.[59–61] However, early experience with static plating with multilevel corpectomies has shown that such plates might increase the incidence of strut graft dislodgement.[24] Early designs of ventral cervical plates were not dynamic and shielded the bone graft from load bearing. Consequently, these designs did not exploit Wolff's law, in which bone heals better when subjected to some loading stress to achieve subsequent fusion.[46] Anterior cervical buttress plates were designed to prevent graft dislodgement whereas allowing for physiologic patterns of force application through the anterior column. However, failure at the implant–host bone interface and subsequent strut graft dislodgement were observed after multilevel corpectomy.[62] Some studies have suggested additional posterior fusion to increase the rate of fusion and decrease the incidence of graft- and implant-related complication.[46,63] A new generation of dynamic anterior plates has been developed to avoid the failures of static and buttress plates. These new plates resolved the stress-shielding problem by providing variable-angle screws, which allow for rotational pivoting at the screw–plate interface or interlocking sliding plates, which allow a certain degree of settling. As a result of this rotational pivoting or settling, these plates allow for increased loads to be placed on the disc space, thereby exploiting Wolff's law to achieve fusion across the disc space or the corpectomy defect.[64] However, no randomized clinical trials or even large matched-cohort studies are available to compare plated versus nonplated cervical corpectomy models. The role of these plates in a multilevel anterior decompression procedure remains inconclusive.

Autograft iliac crest has been widely used for anterior cervical surgery with an excellent fusion rate. However, reported patient morbidity rate with autograft iliac crest was greater than 20%, mainly because of donor site complications, including pain, hernia, and lateral femoral cutaneous nerve injury.[65,66] In addition, limited bone stock and curved shape of the iliac crest are issues when replacing more than two levels with a corpectomy. Allograft is an alternative option to avoid these complicating factors of autograft. However, fusion rates with allograft are generally not as high as autograft. Multiple studies have compared the use of autograft and allograft, which have revealed that autograft is superior to allograft in terms of fusion rate,[50,67–69] time to fuse,[50] and graft collapse.[50,67,69] The introduction of the ventral cervical plate has made the use of allograft more appealing. Ventral cervical plates have decreased subsidence and improved fusion rates,[55,70] which now approach the fusion rate of autograft in ACDF procedures.[71]

Titanium cages are another option for graft. They are readily available, there is no limitation in supply (unlike allograft and autograft), they avoid donor-site morbidity (unlike autograft), and they avoid the risk for infection from a donor cadaver (unlike allograft). When combined with ventral plate fixation, titanium cages perform well biomechanically in resisting flexion, extension, and lateral bending.[72] Recent prospective, randomized studies comparing ACDF with autograft versus titanium cages have demonstrated that ACDF with titanium cage had a lower risk for complications, less requirement for graft harvest,[73] and better clinical outcome of radiculopathy[74] compared with autograft. Fusion rate,[73] subsidence, and flexion deformity[74] are not different between the two groups.

Cervical arthroplasty has recently become another alternative option for treatment of cervical degenerative disc disease (DDD). Cervical disc arthroplasty has the potential of maintaining anatomical disc space height, normal segmental lordosis, and physiologic motion patterns after surgery. These characteristics may reduce or delay the onset of DDD at adjacent cervical spinal motion segments after anterior cervical decompressive surgery,[75–78] although conclusive evidence has yet to be shown. Compared with ACDF, prospective, randomized, clinical trials have demonstrated that cervical disc arthroplasty maintained physiologic segmental mo-

tion, improved clinical outcomes, and reduced rate of secondary surgeries.[75,76,79]

> ## RECOMMENDATIONS
>
> 1. Corpectomy may be preferable to multilevel ACDF, especially in higher-risk patients such as smokers, patients with diabetes, or revision cases (grade C recommendation).
> 2. The role of plates in multilevel anterior decompression procedure still remains inconclusive (grade I recommendation).
> 3. Autograft is superior to allograft in terms of fusion rate, duration to fuse, and graft collapse (grade B recommendation).
> 4. ACDF with a titanium cage is superior to autograft in terms of lower risk for complications, less requirement for graft harvest, and better clinical outcome of radiculopathy (grade A recommendation).
> 5. Cervical arthroplasty maintains physiologic segmental motion, improves clinical outcomes, and reduces rate of secondary surgeries compared with ACDF (grade C recommendation).

POSTERIOR APPROACH

The posterior approach has been most commonly used for the management of cervical myelopathy involving three or more levels. The advantages of the posterior approach are to avoid the technical problems encountered with anterior cervical approach resulting from obesity, a short neck, barrel chest, anterior soft-tissue pathologic lesions, and a previous anterior surgery, as well as to avoid the potential for injury to the esophagus, trachea, and laryngeal nerves.[21] Disadvantages of the posterior approach include iatrogenic cord or root trauma,[80] nerve root dysfunction (especially C5 nerve root),[30,40,81–84] late neurologic deterioration associated with kyphotic deformity,[26,85] and axial symptoms, such as neck pain, stiffness, fatigue, or shoulder discomfort.[86]

Historically, laminectomy has been regarded as the standard posterior procedure for the treatment of multilevel CSM with satisfactory results in a high percentage of patients.[34,35,41,87] However, significant problems were associated with postlaminectomy segmental instability and kyphosis secondary to iatrogenic destabilization of the cervical spine. Also, development of a scar membrane around the dura can cause neurologic worsening in a subset of patients.[34,35,41,87] Some studies have shown that resection of greater than 50% of the facet joint significantly compromises facet strength[88] and results in segmental hypermobility,[50] whereas biomechanically, as little as a 25% facetectomy affects stability after multilevel laminectomy.[89] Another biomechanical study demonstrated that 36% of load transmission was through the anterior (vertebral bodies) columns, whereas 64% was through the posterior columns.[90] Therefore, the posterior neural arch is responsible for most of the load transmission in the cervical spine, and significant loss of integrity of this posterior arch-facet complex can result in instability, causing the weight-bearing axis to shift anteriorly.[91] Kyphosis progresses subsequent to this loss of sagittal balance, which places the cervical musculature at a mechanical disadvantage, requiring constant contractions to maintain upright head posture. This progression causes most of the weight to be borne by the discs and anterior vertebral bodies, which may lead to further degeneration and spondylosis.[92,93]

The addition of posterior cervical fusion with instrumentation is an option that attempts to avoid the development of a postlaminectomy kyphotic deformity.[93–96] Fusion also allows for a more extensive laminectomy and foraminotomy without jeopardizing stability. Recently, lateral mass fixation, involving fixation of a small plate or rod to the lateral masses with screws, has been widely applied.[57,97–101] These devices provide superb flexural stability and resist torsion and extension significantly better than spinous process wiring.[102] The enhanced stability can decrease or eliminate the need for a postoperative orthosis. Disadvantages of these procedures include nonunion, hardware failure, adjacent segment degeneration, high cost, and potential injury to the nerve root and vertebral artery.[103,104]

Laminoplasty, which was developed in Japan in the late 1970s[39] with numerous modification since that time,[38,105–108] is another valid option to avoid the development of a postlaminectomy kyphosis. This procedure, by leaving the dorsal stabilizing structures in situ, is thought to mitigate the development of kyphosis and, with subsequent bone fusion, to stabilize the cervical spine with an improved outcome.[109] However, laminoplasty performed on patients with cervical kyphosis has resulted in less vertebral canal enlargement and functional recovery than those patients with a lordotic alignment. Additional factors associated with inferior outcomes are cord atrophy, long duration of symptoms, advanced age, severe cord compression, and radiculopathy.[110,111] Laminoplasty is not considered a fusion procedure. However, most patients experience a significant loss of subaxial motion after the procedure and some do go on to fusion.[112]

Few prospective comparative studies between the procedures available exist. A study comparing laminectomy and laminoplasty has demonstrated that patients with both procedures improved in gait, strength, sensation, pain, and degree of myelopathy. However, laminoplasty was associated with fewer late complications.[113] Another matched cohort study of laminoplasty and laminectomy with fusion demonstrated that laminoplasty was favorable because of less procedural complications, although patients in both groups showed no statistical difference in improvement of strength, dexterity, sensation, pain, and gait.[103] The high complication rate (9/13 patients) in the laminectomy fusion group, included instrumentation failure, nonunion, and development of myelopathy. In contrast, the laminoplasty group had no complications. This may be biased because of the surgeon's procedural familiarity with laminoplasty, rather than laminectomy with fusion.

RECOMMENDATIONS

Laminoplasty or laminectomy with instrumented posterior cervical fusion is recommended to avoid the development of a postlaminectomy kyphotic deformity (grade C recommendation).

Summary of Recommendations		
STATEMENT	**LEVEL OF EVIDENCE/GRADE OF RECOMMENDATION**	**REFERENCES**
1. Once moderate signs and symptoms develop, patients would likely benefit from surgical intervention.	Grade C	16
2. Manipulation and traction are not recommended because of the potential risk for aggravation of neurologic symptoms.	Grade C	2
3. Primarily focal ventral pathology causing cord compression is best treated via an anterior approach.	Grade C	20
4. If compression is posterior and related primarily to facet hypertrophy or buckling ligamentum flavum, posterior decompression should be considered.	Grade C	9
5. The optimal surgical approach for the treatment of cervical myelopathy resulting from stenosis at three or more levels remains controversial. If the spine is lordotic or straight, either anterior or posterior approach can be used; however, if the spine is kyphotic, the posterior approach may be contraindicated.	Grade C	10
6. The combined procedure may be used for treatment of patients with severe multilevel anterior compression with a kyphotic spine.	Grade C	45-47
7. Laminoplasty remarkably reduced the sequelae after laminectomy.	Grade C	37-40
8. Laminoplasty may be preferable for multilevel cervical myelopathy in the absence of preoperative kyphosis.	Grade C	44
9. Corpectomy may be preferable to multilevel ACDF, especially in higher-risk patients such as smokers, patients with diabetes, or revision cases.	Grade C	21
10. The role of plates in multilevel anterior decompression procedure remains inconclusive.	Grade I	
11. Autograft is superior to allograft in terms of fusion rate, duration to fuse and graft collapse.	Grade B	50, 67-69
12. ACDF with a titanium cage is superior to autograft in terms of lower risk for complications, less requirement for graft harvest, and better clinical outcome of radiculopathy.	Grade A	73,74
13. Cervical arthroplasty maintains physiologic segmental motion, improves clinical outcomes, and reduces rate of secondary surgeries compared with ACDF.	Grade C	75,76,79
14. Laminoplasty or laminectomy with instrumented posterior cervical fusion is recommended to avoid the development of a postlaminectomy kyphotic deformity.	Grade C	38, 93-96, 105-108

REFERENCES

1. Young WF: Cervical spondylotic myelopathy: A common cause of spinal cord dysfunction in older persons. Am Fam Physician 62:1064–1073, 2000.
2. Clarke E, Robinson PK: Cervical myelopathy: A complication of cervical spondylosis. Brain 79:483–510, 1956.
3. Spillane JD, Lloyd GH: The diagnosis of lesions of the spinal cord in association with 'osteoarhritic' disease of the cervical spine. Brain 75:177–186, 1952.
4. Symon L, Lavender P: The surgical treatment of cervical spondylitic myelopathy. Neurology 17:117–127, 1967.
5. Lees F, Turner JW: Natural history and prognosis of cervical spondylosis. Br Med J 2:1607–1610, 1963.
6. Roberts AH: Myelopathy due to cervical spondylosis treated by collar immobilization. Neurology 16:951–954, 1966.
7. Nurick S: The pathogenesis of the spinal cord disorder associated with cervical spondylosis. Brain 95:87–100, 1972.
8. Rao R: Neck pain, cervical radiculopathy, and cervical myelopathy: Pathophysiology, natural history, and clinical evaluation. J Bone Joint Surg Am 84:1872–1881, 2002.
9. Epstein JA, Epstein NE: The surgical management of cervical spinal stenosis, spondylosis, and myeloradiculopathy by means of the posterior approach. In Sherk HH, Dunn EJ, Eismont FJ, et al (eds): The Cervical Spine, 2nd ed. Philadelphia, JB Lippincott, 1989, pp 625–643.
10. McCormick WE, Steinmetz MP, Benzel EC: Cervical spondylotic myelopathy: Make the difficult diagnosis, then refer for surgery. Cleve Clin J Med 70:899–904, 2003.
11. Firooznia H, Ahn JH, Rafii M, Ragnarsson KT: Sudden quadriplegia after a minor trauma: The role of preexisting spinal stenosis. Surg Neurol 23:165–168, 1985.
12. Sampath P, Bendebba M, Davis JD, Ducker TB: Outcome of patients treated for cervical myelopathy: A prospective multicenter study with independent clinical review. Spine 25:670–676, 2000.
13. Fouyas IP, Statham PF, Sandercock PA: Cochrane review on the role of surgery in cervical spondylotic radiculomyelopathy. Spine 27:736–747, 2002.
14. Kadanka Z, Mares M, Bednarik J, et al: Approaches to spondylotic cervical myelopathy: Conservative versus surgical results in a 3-year follow-up study. Spine 27:2205–2210, 2002.
15. Kadanka Z, Mares M, Bednarik J, et al: Predictive factors for spondylotic cervical myelopathy treated conservatively or surgically. Eur J Neurol 12:55–63, 2005.
16. Emery SE: Cervical spondylotic myelopathy: Diagnosis and treatment. J Am Acad Orthop Surg 9:376–388, 2001.
17. Bednarik J, Kadanka Z, Dusek L, et al: Presymptomatic spondylotic cervical cord compression. Spine 29:2260–2269, 2004.
18. Yoshimatsu H, Nagata K, Goto H, et al: Conservative treatment for cervical spondylotic myelopathy: Prediction of treatment effects by multivariate analysis. Spine J 1:269–273, 2001.
19. Boden SD, McCowin PR, Davis DO: Abnormal magnetic-resonance scans of the cervical spine in asymptomatic subjects: A prospective investigation. J Bone Joint Surg Am 72:1178–1184, 1990.
20. Matz PG, Pritchard PR, Hadley MN: Anterior cervical approach for the treatment of cervical myelopathy. Neurosurgery 60(suppl 1):S64–S70, 2007.
21. Edwards CC 2nd, Riew KD, Anderson PA, et al: Cervical myelopathy. Current diagnostic and treatment strategies. Spine J 3:68–81, 2003.
22. Hillard VH, Apfelbaum RI: Surgical management of cervical myelopathy: Indications and techniques for multilevel cervical discectomy. Spine J (6 suppl):242S–251S, 2006.
23. Swank M, Lowery G, Bhat A: Improved arthrodesis with strut-grafting and instrumentation: Multi-level interbody grafting or strut graft reconstruction. Eur Spine J 6:138–143, 1997.
24. Vaccaro AR, Falatyn SP, Scuderi GJ: Early failure of long segment anterior cervical plate fixation. J Spinal Disord 11:410–415, 1998.
25. Hilibrand A, Fye M, Emery S: Improved arthrodesis with strut-grafting after multi-level anterior cervical decompression. Spine 27:146–151, 2002.
26. Yonenobu K, Fuji T, Ono K, et al: Choice of surgical treatment for multisegmental cervical spondylotic myelopathy. Spine 10:710–716, 1985.
27. Butler JC, Whitecloud TS III: Postlaminectomy kyphosis: Causes and surgical management. Orthop Clin North Am 23:505–511, 1992.
28. Cerisoli M, Vernizzi E, Guilioni M: Cervical spine changes following laminectomy: Clinico-radiological study. J Neurosurg Sci 24:63–70, 1980.
29. Crandall PH, Gregorious FK: Long-term follow-up of surgical treatment of cervical spondylotic myelopathy. Spine 2:139–146, 1977.
30. Dai L, Ni B, Yuan W, Jia L: Radiculopathy after laminectomy for cervical compression myelopathy. J Bone Joint Surg Br 80:846–849, 1998.
31. Guigui P, Lefevre C, Lassale B, Deburge A: Static, dynamic changes of the cervical spine after laminectomy for cervical spondylotic myelopathy. Rev Chir Orthop Reparatrice Appar Mot 84:17–25, 1998.
32. Ishida Y, Suzuki K, Ohmori K, et al: Critical analysis of extensive cervical laminectomy. Neurosurgery 24:215–222, 1989.
33. Lonstein JE: Post-laminectomy kyphosis. Clin Orthop 128:93–100, 1977.
34. Mikawa Y, Shikata J, Yamamuro T: Spinal deformity and instability after multilevel cervical laminectomy. Spine 12:6–11, 1987.
35. Morimoto T, Okuno S, Nakase H, et al: Cervical myelopathy due to dynamic compression by the laminectomy membrane: Dynamic MR imaging study. J Spinal Disord 12:172–173, 1999.
36. Sim FH, Suien HJ, Bickel WH, Janes JM: Swan neck deformity following extensive cervical laminectomy. J Bone Joint Surg Am 56:564–580, 1974.
37. Hirabayashi K: Expansive open-door laminoplasty for cervical spondylotic myelopathy [in Japanese]. Jpn J Surg 32:1159–1163, 1978.
38. Kurokawa T, Tsuyama N, Tanaka H, et al: Enlargement of spinal canal by the sagittal splitting of the spinous process. Bessatsu Seikei Geka 2:234–240, 1982.
39. Oyama M, Hattori S, Moriwaki N: A new method of posterior decompression [in Japanese]. Cent Jpn J Orthop Traumat Surg 16:792–794, 1973.
40. Tomita K, Kawahara N, Toribatake Y, Heller JG: Expansive midline T-saw laminoplasty (modified spinous process-splitting) for the management of cervical myelopathy. Spine 23:32–37, 1998.
41. Matsunaga S, Sakou T, Nakansisi K: Analysis of the cervical spine alignment following laminoplasty and laminectomy. Spinal Cord 37:20–24, 1999.
42. Yonenobu H, Hosono N, Iwasaki M, et al: Laminoplasty versus subtotal corpectomy: A comparative study of results in multisegmental cervical spondylotic myelopathy. Spine 17:1281–1284, 1992.
43. Wada E, Suzuki S, Kanazawa A: Subtotal corpectomy versus laminoplasty for multilevel cervical spondylotic myelopathy: A long-term follow-up study of over 10 years. Spine 26:1443–1447, 2001.
44. Edwards CC 2nd, Heller JG, Murakami H: Corpectomy versus laminoplasty for multilevel cervical myelopathy: An independent matched-cohort analysis. Spine 27:1168–1175, 2002.
45. Schultz KD Jr, McLaughlin MR, Haid RW Jr, et al: Single-stage anterior-posterior decompression and stabilization for complex cervical spine disorders. J Neurosurg 93(2 suppl):214–221, 2000.
46. Mummaneni PV, Haid RW, Rodts GE Jr: Combined ventral and dorsal surgery for myelopathy and myeloradiculopathy. Neurosurgery 60(1 suppl 1):S82–S89, 2007.
47. McAfee PC, Bohlman HH, Ducker TB, et al: One-stage anterior cervical decompression and posterior stabilization. A study of one hundred patients with a minimum of two years of follow-up. J Bone Joint Surg Am 77:1791–1800, 1995.
48. Bosacco D, Berman A, Levenberg R: Surgical results in anterior cervical discectomy and fusion using a countersunk interlocking autogenous iliac bone graft. Orthopedics 15:923–925, 1992.

49. Emery SE, Bolesta MJ, Banks MA, Jones PK: Robinson anterior cervical fusion—comparison of the standard and modified techniques. Spine 19:660–663, 1994.

50. Zdeblick TA, Ducker TB: The use of freeze-dried allograft bone for anterior cervical fusions. Spine 16:726–729, 1991.

51. Barnes B, Haid RW, Rodts GE Jr: Multilevel ACDF vs. corpectomy: Significantly better outcomes with corpectomy at 19 month follow-up. Platform presentation at the Congress of Neurological Surgeons Annual Meeting, October 2002, Philadelphia.

52. Emery SE, Bohlman HH, Bolesta MJ, Jones PK: Anterior cervical decompression and arthrodesis for the treatment of cervical spondylotic myelopathy. Two to seventeen-year follow-up. J Bone Joint Surg Am 80:941–951, 1998.

53. Kaiser MG, Haid RW Jr, Subach BR, et al: Anterior cervical plating enhances arthrodesis after discectomy and fusion with cortical allograft. Neurosurgery 50:229–238, 2002.

54. Zhang Z, Yin H, Yang K: Anterior intervertebral disc excision and bone grafting in cervical spondylotic myelopathy. Spine 5:16–19, 1983.

55. Wang JC, McDonough PW, Endow KK, Delamarter RB: Increased fusion rates with cervical plating for two-level anterior cervical discectomy and fusion. Spine 25:41–45, 2000.

56. Whitecloud TS, LaRocca H: Fibular strut graft in reconstructive surgery of the cervical spine. Spine 1:33–43, 1976.

57. Zdeblick TA, Bohlman HH: Cervical kyphosis and myelopathy. Treatment by anterior corpectomy and strut-grafting. J Bone Joint Surg Am 71:170–182, 1989.

58. Macdonald RL, Fehlings MG, Tator CH, et al: Multilevel anterior cervical corpectomy and fibular allograft fusion for cervical myelopathy. J Neurosurg 86:990–997, 1997.

59. An HS, Gordin R, Renner K: Anatomic considerations for plate-screw fixation of the cervical spine. Spine 16:548–551, 1991.

60. Grubb MR, Currier BL, Shih JS: Biomechanical evaluation of anterior cervical spine stabilization. Spine 15:886–892, 1998.

61. Katsuura A, Hakuda S, Imanaka T, et al: Anterior cervical plate used in degenerative disease can maintain cervical lordosis. J Spinal Dis 9:470–476, 1996.

62. Riew KD, Sethi NS, Devney J, et al: Complications of buttress plate stabilization of cervical corpectomy. Spine 24:2404–2410, 1999.

63. Epstein N: Anterior cervical discectomy and fusion without plate instrumentation in 178 patients. J Spinal Disord 13:1–8, 2000.

64. Mummaneni PV, Srinivasan JK, Haid RW, Mizuno J: Overview of anterior cervical plating. Spinal Surg 16:207–216, 2002.

65. Heary RF, Schlenk RP, Sacchieri TA, et al: Persistent iliac crest donor site pain: Independent outcome assessment. Neurosurgery 50:510–517, 2002.

66. Sasso RC, Ruggiero RA Jr, Reilly TM, Hall PV: Early reconstruction failures after multi-level cervical corpectomy. Spine 28:140–142, 2003.

67. An HS, Simpson JM, Glover JM, Stephany J: Comparison between allograft plus demineralized bone matrix versus autograft in anterior cervical fusion: A prospective multicenter study. Spine 20:2211–2216, 1995.

68. Bishop RC, Moore KA, Hadley MN: Anterior cervical interbody fusion using autogenic and allogenic bone graft substrate: A prospective comparative analysis. J Neurosurg 85:206–210, 1996.

69. Floyd T, Ohnmeiss D: A meta-analysis of autograft versus allograft in anterior cervical fusion. Eur Spine J 9:398–403, 2000.

70. Caspar W, Geisler FH, Pitzen T, Johnson TA: Anterior cervical plate stabilization in one- and two-level degenerative disease: Overtreatment or benefit? J Spinal Disord 11:1–11, 1998.

71. Deutsch H, Haid R, Rodts G Jr, Mummaneni PV: The decision-making process: Allograft versus autograft. Neurosurgery 60(suppl):S98–S102, 2007.

72. Kandziora F, Pflugmacher R, Schafer J, et al: Biomechanical comparison of cervical spine interbody fusion cages. Spine 26:1850–1857, 2001.

73. Hacker RJ, Cauthen JC, Gilbert TJ, Griffith SL: A prospective randomized multicenter clinical evaluation of an anterior cervical fusion cage. Spine 25:2646–2654, 2000.

74. Lind BI, Zoega B, Rosen H: Autograft versus interbody fusion cage without plate fixation in the cervical spine: A randomized clinical study using radiostereometry. Eur Spine J 16:1251–1256, 2007.

75. Cummins BH, Robertson JT, Gill SS: Surgical experience with an implanted artificial cervical joint. J Neurosurg 88:943–948, 1998.

76. Goffin J, Van Calenbergh F, van Loon J, et al: Intermediate follow-up after treatment of degenerative disc disease by the Bryan Cervical Disc Prosthesis: Single-level and bi-level. Spine 28:2673–2678, 2003.

77. Mummaneni PV, Haid RW: The future in the care of the cervical spine: Interbody fusion and arthroplasty. J Neurosurg Spine 1:155–159, 2004.

78. Wigfield CC, Gill S, Nelson R, et al: Influence of an artificial cervical joint compared with fusion on adjacent-level motion in the treatment of degenerative cervical disc disease. J Neurosurg 96(1 suppl):17–21, 2002.

79. Goffin J, Casey A, Kehr P, et al: Preliminary clinical experience with the Bryan Cervical Disc prosthesis. Neurosurgery 51:840–847, 2002.

80. Kirita Y: Posterior decompression or the cervical spondylosis and ossification of the posterior longitudinal ligament in the cervical spine [in Japanese]. Surgery 30:287–302, 1976.

81. Kawaguchi Y, Kanamori M, Hirokazu I: Minimum 10-year followup after en block cervical laminoplasty. Presented at the Cervical Spine Research Society, November 30, 2000 to December 2, 2000, Charleston, SC.

82. Yonenobu K, Yamamoto T, Ono K: Laminoplasty for myelopathy: Indications, results, outcome and complications. In Clark (ed): The Cervical Spine, 3rd ed. Philadelphia, 1998, pp 849–864.

83. Yonenobu K, Hosono N, Iwasaki M, et al: Neurologic complications of surgery for cervical compression myelopathy. Spine 16:1277–1282, 1991.

84. Dante SJ, Heary R, Kramer D: Cervical laminectomy for myelopathy. Oper Techn Orthop 6:30–37, 1996.

85. Kaptain GJ, Simmons NE, Replogle RE, et al: Incidence and outcome of kyphotic deformity following laminectomy for cervical spondylotic myelopathy. J Neurosurg 93:1999–2004, 2000.

86. Hosono N, Yonenobu K, Ono K: Neck and shoulder pain after laminoplasty: A noticeable complication. Spine 21:1969–1973, 1996.

87. Snow RB, Weiner H: Cervical laminectomy and foraminotomy as surgical treatment of cervical spondylosis: A follow-up study with analysis of failures. J Spinal Disord 6:245–250, 1993.

88. Raynor RB, Pugh J, Shapiro I: Cervical facetectomy and its effect on spine strength. J Neurosurg 63:278–282, 1995.

89. Nowinski GP, Visarius H, Nolte LP, et al: A biomechanical comparison of cervical laminoplasty and cervical laminectomy with progressive facetectomy. Spine 18:1995–2004, 1993.

90. Pal PP, Cooper HH: The vertical stability of the cervical spine. Spine 13:447–449, 1988.

91. Raynor RB, Moskovich R, Zidel P, Pugh J: Alterations in primary and coupled neck motions after facetectomy. Neurosurgery 21:681–687, 1987.

92. Albert TJ, Vacarro A: Postlaminectomy kyphosis. Spine 23:2738–2745, 1998.

93. Houten JK, Cooper PR: Laminectomy and posterior cervical plating for multilevel cervical spondylotic myelopathy and ossification of the posterior longitudinal ligament: Effects on cervical alignment, spinal cord compression, and neurological outcome. Neurosurgery 52:1081–1088, 2003.

94. Kumar VG, Rea GL, Mervis L, et al: Cervical spondylotic myelopathy—functional and radiographic long-term outcome after laminectomy and posterior fusion. Neurosurgery 44:771–777, 1999.

95. Miyazaki K, Hirohuji E, Ono S: Extensive simultaneous multi-segmental laminectomy and posterior decompression with posterolateral fusion. J Jpn Res Soc 5:167, 1994.

96. Maurer PK, Ellenbogen RG, Eckland J, et al: Cervical spondylotic myelopathy: Treatment with posterior decompression and Luque rectangle bone fusion. Neurosurgery 28:680–683, 1991.

97. Cherney WB, Sonntag VK, Douglas RA: Lateral mass posterior plating and facet fusion for cervical spine instability. Barrow Neurol Inst Q 7:2–11, 1991.

98. Cooper PR, Cohen A, Rosiello A, Koslow M: Posterior stabilization of cervical spine fractures and subluxations using plates and screws. Neurosurgery 23:300–306, 1988.

99. Magerl F, Grob D, Seemann P: Stable dorsal fusion of the cervical spine (C2-Th1) using hook plates. In Kehr P, Weidner A (eds): Cervical Spine, vol 1. New York, Springer-Verlag, 1987, pp 217–221.

100. Roy-Camille R, Saillant G, Mazel C: Internal fixation of the unstable cervical spine by a posterior osteosynthesis with plates and screws. In Cervical Spine Research Society (ed): The Cervical Spine. Philadelphia, JB Lippincott, 1989, pp 390–403.

101. Weidner A: Internal fixation with metal plates and screws. In Cervical Spine Research Society (ed): The Cervical Spine, 2nd ed. Philadelphia, JB Lippincott, 1989, pp 404–421.

102. Sato T: Radiological follow-up of motion in the cervical spine after surgery [in Japanese]. Nippon Seikeigeka Gakkai Zasshi 66:607–620, 1992.

103. Heller JG, Edwards CC 2nd, Murakami H, Rodts GE: Laminoplasty versus laminectomy and fusion for multilevel cervical myelopathy: An independent matched cohort analysis. Spine 26:1330–1336, 2001.

104. Wellman BJ, Follett KA, Traynelis VC: Complications of posterior articular mass plate fixation of the subaxial cervical spine in 43 consecutive patients. Spine 23:193–200, 1998.

105. Hirabayashi K, Watanabe K, Wakano K, et al: Expansive open-door laminoplasty for cervical spinal stenotic myelopathy. Spine 8:693–699, 1983.

106. Kokubun S, Sato T, Ishii Y, Tanaka Y: Cervical myelopathy in the Japanese. Clin Orthop Relat Res 323:129–138, 1996.

107. Nakano N, Nakano T, Nakano K: Comparison of the results of laminectomy and open-door laminoplasty for cervical spondylotic myeloradiculopathy and ossification of the posterior longitudinal ligament. Spine 13:792–794, 1988.

108. Tsuji H: Laminoplasty for patients with compressive myelopathy due to so-called spinal canal stenosis in cervical and thoracic regions. Spine 7:28–34, 1982.

109. Vitarbo E, Sheth RN, Levi AD: Open-door expansile cervical laminoplasty. Neurosurgery 60(suppl 1):S154–S159, 2007.

110. Kohno K, Kumon Y, Oka Y: Evaluation of prognostic factors following expansive laminoplasty for cervical spinal stenotic myelopathy. Surg Neurol 48:237–245, 1997.

111. Lee TT, Manzano GR, Green BA: Modified open-door cervical expansive laminoplasty for spondylotic myelopathy: Operative technique, outcome and predictors of gait improvement. J Neurosurg 86:64–68, 1997.

112. Edwards CC, Heller JG, Silcox DH: "T-saw" laminoplasty for the management of cervical spondylotic myelopathy: Clinical and radiographic outcome. Spine 25:1788–1794, 2000.

113. Kaminsky SB, Clark CR, Traynelis VC: Operative treatment of cervical spondylotic myelopathy and radiculopathy. A comparison of laminectomy and laminoplasty at five year average follow-up. Iowa Orthop J 24:95–105, 2004.

Do Bone Morphogenetic Proteins Improve Spinal Fusion?

S. Samuel Bederman, MD, MSc, FRCSC and Y. Raja Rampersaud, MD, FRCSC

BACKGROUND

Lumbar spinal fusion is a common surgical treatment for many degenerative, traumatic, deformity, and destructive conditions of the lumbar spine. It has been shown to improve outcomes in disabling conditions such as spinal stenosis, degenerative and isthmic spondylolisthesis, and degenerative disc disease (DDD).[1] With advances in diagnostic tools, fusion techniques, subspecialty training, raised patient and physician awareness, and better understanding of the causes and consequences of these disorders, as well as their management, there has been a dramatic increase in overall rates of spinal fusion.[2] Spinal fusion surgery can be technically demanding, surgical costs are high, and complications can be significant.[3] Population-based reoperation rates after spinal fusion in the early 1990s were 10% to 20%.[4,5] Nonunion of the spine is a common reason for pain and reoperation after spinal fusion.[6] Harvesting iliac crest autograft for spinal fusion is another common cause of persistent pain and reduced functional outcome after lumbar spinal fusion surgery.[7–9]

Bone morphogenetic proteins (BMPs), first identified by Urist in 1965,[10] consist of protein components of bone matrix that can be extracted to induce the differentiation of osteoprogenitor cells into bone-producing osteogenic cells, thus stimulating the production of new bone.[11] Further research has been able to identify many different BMPs, of which BMP-2, BMP-6, and BMP-7 appear to have the most important roles.[12]

Earlier preclinical and clinical studies demonstrated that BMPs increase fusion rates. In a comprehensive review, Sandhu suggests that recombinant BMPs can be used as substitutes for autograft, and that in some circumstances, their efficacy for inducing fusion is superior.[13]

The rationale for BMPs in spinal fusion surgery is to avoid the complications of autogenous iliac crest bone graft harvesting, to reduce the risks for nonunion and reoperations, and to improve functional outcomes for patients. The main objective of this systematic review was to determine whether BMPs improve spinal fusion. In particular, do BMPs reduce the risk for nonunion and improve clinical outcomes for patients undergoing lumbar spinal fusion?

SYSTEMATIC REVIEW

From our systematic review (Table 9-1), we identified 75 articles, of which 14 were considered potentially relevant from abstract review. One additional published randomized, controlled trial (RCT) was identified from a manual bibliography search; however, abstract review excluded it based on inadequate length of follow-up.[14] Hand searches of major meeting proceedings identified an additional RCT; however, this study has not yet been submitted for publication. The 14 potentially relevant trials were retrieved in full for data abstraction.[15–28] The baseline characteristics of these trials are presented in Table 9–2. Once all data were abstracted, the trials were then reviewed in an unblinded fashion. It became apparent that many of them included the same randomized patients presented in different publications.

We attempted to consolidate the trials that included the same patients to avoid over-reporting and to obtain mutually exclusive trials. Two trials included patients with DDD who underwent anterior lumbar interbody fusion (ALIF) with tapered cylindrical cages randomized to BMP-2 or autograft.[17,19] One trial included 45 patients at 1 center, whereas the larger of the two reported on 279 patients at 16 investigational sites. Because follow-up was similar in both trials and the smaller trial reported only radiographic outcomes, we decided to include only the larger of the two trials.[17]

Three trials included patients with DDD who underwent ALIF using threaded cortical allografts randomized to BMP-2 or autograft.[18,20,21] The smallest trial reported a pilot series that was reanalyzed in the two other larger studies. Of the larger studies, only one of them reported radiographic outcomes and focused on the healing patterns, whereas the other reported both clinical and radiographic outcomes for the entire cohort. Thus, we included only the larger trial with both clinical and radiographic outcomes.[20]

Two trials of patients with degenerative spondylolisthesis who underwent posterolateral noninstrumented fusion randomized to BMP-7 or autograft were identified.[27,28] One was a longer follow-up (to 24 months) of the same cohort and, therefore, the one only included for analysis.[28] Finally, two trials

TABLE 9–1. MEDLINE and EMBASE Search Strategies

KEYWORD	MEDLINE (1950–2007 WEEK 11)	EMBASE (1980–2007 WEEK 11)
Clinical trials	Clinical trials/ or clinical trials, phase i/ or clinical trials, phase ii/ or clinical trials, phase iii/ or clinical trials, phase iv/ or controlled clinical trials/ or randomized controlled trials/ or multicenter studies/ or cross-over studies/ or double-blind method/ or meta-analysis/ or random allocation/ or single-blind method/ or systematic review$. ti,ab. or ((singl$ or doubl$ or tripl$) adj (mask$ or blind$)).ti,ab. or (blind$ or random$).ti,ab.	Randomized controlled trial/ or ((controlled study/ or comparative study/) and (clinical trial/ or phase 1 clinical trial/ or phase 2 clinical trial/ or phase 3 clinical trial/ or phase 4 clinical trial/ or major clinical study/ or prospective study/)) or "systematic review"/ or randomization/ or double blind procedure/ or single blind procedure/ or triple blind procedure/ or ((singl$ or doubl$ or tripl$) adj (mask$ or blind$)).ti,ab. or (blind$ or random$).ti,ab.
Spinal fusion	Spinal Fusion/ or spondylosyndesis.ti,ab. or spondylodesis.ti,ab. or (spin$ adj2 fusion$).ti,ab.	Exp spine fusion/
Bone morphogenetic protein	Exp Bone Morphogenetic Proteins/ or bone morphogenetic protein.mp or bone morphogenic protein or bone derived growth factor.mp or bmp.mp or osteogenic protein.mp	Bone Morphogenetic Protein/ or bone morphogenetic protein.mp or Bone Morphogenetic Protein 2/ or bone morphogenetic protein 2.mp or Bone Morphogenetic Protein 6/ or bone morphogenetic protein 6.mp or Bone Morphogenetic Protein 9/ or bone morphogenetic protein 9.mp or bmp.mp or bone derived growth factor.mp or osteogenic protein.mp or bone morphogenetic protein$.ti,ab.

TABLE 9–2. Baseline Characteristics of Primary Trials

AUTHOR (YEAR OF PUBLICATION)	DIAGNOSIS	FUSION TYPE	IMPLANT	BMP	OUTCOME	FOLLOW-UP (MONTHS)	INCLUDED
Boden et al. (2000)[15]	DDD	IB	ALIF	BMP-2	C, R	24	Y
Burkus et al. (2002)[18]	DDD	IB	ALIF	BMP-2	C, R	24	N
Boden et al. (2002)[16]	DDD	PL	PS	BMP-2	C, R	12–24	Y
Johnsson et al. (2002)[25]	IS	PL	None	BMP-7	R	12	Y
Burkus et al. (2002)[17]	DDD	IB	ALIF	BMP-2	C, R	24	Y
Burkus et al. (2003)[19]	DDD	IB	ALIF	BMP-2	R	24	N
Vaccaro et al. (2004)[27]	DS	PL	None	BMP-7	C, R	12	N
Haid et al. (2004)[24]	DDD	IB	PLIF	BMP-2	C, R	24	Y
Burkus et al. (2005)[20]	DDD	IB	ALIF	BMP-2	C, R	24	Y
Glassman et al. (2005)[23]	DDD	PL	PS	BMP-2	R	12	N
Vaccaro et al. (2005)[28]	DS	PL	None	BMP-7	C, R	24	Y
Burkus et al. (2006)[21]	DDD	IB	ALIF	BMP-2	R	24	N
Kanayama et al. (2006)[26]	DS	PL	PS	BMP-7	C, R, S	12	Y
Dimar et al. (2006)[22]	DDD	PL	PS	BMP-2	C, R	24	Y

ALIF = anterior lumbar interbody fusion cage; BMP = bone morphogenetic protein; C = clinical outcome; DDD = degenerative disc disease; DS = degenerative spondylolisthesis; IB = interbody fusion; IS = isthmic spondylolisthesis; PL = posterolateral fusion; PLIF = posterior lumbar interbody fusion cages; PS = pedicle screws; R = radiographic outcome; S = surgical exploration for fusion.

of patients with DDD who underwent posterolateral fusion with pedicle screw fixation randomized to BMP-2 or autograft were identified.[22,23] The smaller of the two reported only radiographic results for a single institution of a multicenter trial with 12-month follow-up. The larger trial that included clinical and radiographic outcomes at 24 months for two of the investigating centers was retained for analysis.[22] In all cases of trials that were eliminated, information abstracted was used to complete missing information for those retained. Therefore, our results are reported in detail for the nine "mutually exclusive" trials.[15–17,20,22,24–26,28]

Overall, descriptions of randomization methods were poor. Only one of the nine trials (Burkus and colleagues, 2005[20]) described an adequate method of randomization of subjects. One other trial (Johnsson

and coworkers, 2002[25]) indicated that randomization was blind to patient and surgeon; however, only until the time of surgery. Also, the method of randomization was not discussed to ensure allocation concealment. The other eight trials had unclear or no discussion of randomization methods.

Six of the nine trials had over 24-month follow-up data, and three trials had at least 12-month follow-up data. Four trials had near-complete follow-up with minimal dropouts. One trial (Vaccaro and coauthors, 2005[28]) had incomplete 24-month follow-up data but imputed the missing values with 36-month data. One trial (Haid and colleagues, 2004[24]) had unclear accounting of the final numbers of patients analyzed, although the discrepancy was relatively small. Two trials (Burkus and colleagues, 2002[17]; Burkus and colleagues, 2005[20]) failed to perform intention-to-treat analyses and had removed patients who underwent reoperations from subsequent analyses. One other trial (Dimar and investigators, 2006[22]) had a follow-up rate of less than 67% without a proper account of the dropouts.

Patients and investigators were not blinded to treatment in any of the trials at the time of outcome assessment. Radiologists and orthopedic surgeons who assessed radiographic fusion were blinded in seven of the trials. Two trials (Johnsson and coworkers, 2002[25]; Kanayama and colleagues, 2006[26]) did not mention whether the radiologists were blinded to treatment assignment at the time of their assessment.

Eight of the trials provided validated patient-oriented clinical outcome measures (ODI, 36-Item Short Form Health Survey [SF-36]). Six trials reported both outcome measures, and two of them (Burkus and colleagues, 2002[17]; Kanayama and colleagues, 2006[26]) reported only one (Oswestry Disability Index [ODI]). One trial (Johnsson and coworkers, 2002[25]) had no validated patient-oriented clinical outcome measure. Seven of the nine trials reported on adverse surgical events, and eight of the nine trials reported on the need for reoperation.

Four of the nine trials evaluated interbody fusion, all using BMP-2 in patients with DDD, and five evaluated posterolateral fusions with both BMP-2 and BMP-7 in patients with varying diagnoses. Of the interbody fusions, three utilized an anterior approach with two trials of metal ALIF cages and one using an allograft dowel. The fourth interbody fusion trial investigated posterior lumbar interbody fusion (PLIF) as a stand-alone construct.

Of the five posterolateral fusions, two trials used BMP-2 for patients with DDD in instrumented fusions. The other three trials all used BMP-7. One was in noninstrumented fusions in patients with isthmic spondylolisthesis. Two trials evaluated BMP-7 in posterolateral fusions in patients with degenerative spondylolisthesis, one noninstrumented and one instrumented. Commercial funding sources and/or conflicts of interest were reported for all of the trials. Commercial funding solely designated to research and education was reported in only one of the trials (Kanayama and colleagues, 2006[26]).

EVIDENCE

A summary of our findings is shown in Table 9–3. The evidence is presented for three main clinical applications. The first is BMP-2 in interbody fusion for patients with DDD (four trials). The second application is the use of BMP-2 in posterolateral fusion for patients with DDD (two trials), and the final is the use of BMP-7 in posterolateral fusion for patients with spondylolisthesis (three trials).

Interbody Fusion Using Bone Morphogenetic Protein-2 in Degenerative Disc Disease

Boden and coauthors (2000)[15] investigated the efficacy of recombinant human BMP-2 (rhBMP-2) versus iliac crest autograft in patients with DDD who underwent ALIF using tapered cylindrical threaded fusion cages. Fourteen patients were randomized in a 3:1 ratio (intervention/control ratio). Eleven patients who were randomized to the intervention received 1.5 mg/mL rhBMP-2 on an absorbable collagen sponge giving a total dose of 1.3 or 2.6 mL depending on the cage size. The three control patients received iliac crest autograft bone.

No statistically significant differences were found for clinical or radiographic outcomes. Mean improvement in ODI was found to be greater in rhBMP-2 patients at 24 months (25 points) compared with control subjects (15 points). Clinical success (defined as 15% improvement in preoperative ODI score) improved more rapidly in rhBMP-2 patients than control patients, and at 24 months, 10 of 11 rhBMP-2 patients (91%) had clinical success compared with 2 of 3 control patients (67%). Radiographic evidence of fusion, by plain radiography and computed tomography (CT), also increased more rapidly in rhBMP-2 patients than control patients and at 24 months. All 11 rhBMP-2 patients and 2 of the 3 control patients were considered fused. The one patient who had not fused underwent posterior instrumented fusion at 18 months after the index procedure. No adverse events were found.

In a large multicenter trial, Burkus and colleagues (2002)[17] compared rhBMP-2 with iliac crest autograft

TABLE 9–3. Summary of Results						
FUSION TYPE	**BMP**	**DIAGNOSIS**	**IMPLANT**	**CLINICAL OUTCOME**	**FUSION***	**NUMBER OF STUDIES**
Interbody	BMP-2	DDD	ALIF	0	+	3
	BMP-2	DDD	PLIF†	0	0	1
Posterolateral	BMP-2	DDD	PS/ none	0	+	2
	BMP-7	IS	None	0	0	1
	BMP-7	DS	None	0	0	1
	BMP-7	DS	PS	0	0	1

*0 = no significant benefit; + = some significant benefit.
†Stand-alone PLIF.
ALIF = anterior lumbar interbody fusion; BMP = bone morphogenetic protein; DDD = degenerative disc disease; DS = degenerative spondylolisthesis; IS = isthmic spondylolisthesis; PLIF = posterior lumbar interbody fusion; PS = pedicle screw and rod.

in patients with single-level DDD who underwent ALIF using tapered interbody cages. Two hundred and seventy-nine patients were enrolled in the study. The 143 patients who were randomized to receive rhBMP-2 were given 1.5 mg/mL on an absorbable collagen sponge for a total dose ranging from 4.2 to 8.4 mg depending on the size of the cage used. The 136 control patients received autograft. Intention-to-treat analyses were not performed.

No significant differences in outcomes were detected. Mean improvement in ODI was similar between both groups. There was a 15% improvement from the preoperative ODI in 103 of 122 BMP patients (84.4%) and 89 of 108 controls (82.4%). Radiographic fusion was reported in 120 of 127 BMP patients (94.5%) and 102 of 115 controls (88.7%). At 24 months, 32% of controls still reported discomfort at the graft site. Eleven rhBMP-2 patients (7%) underwent reoperations—two had implant removals for displacement and nine had supplemental fixation, seven for presumed pseudarthrosis and two for persistent pain. Fourteen control patients (10%) underwent supplemental fixation, 12 for presumed pseudarthrosis and two for persistent pain.

Burkus and colleagues (2005)[20] report on the results of a two-part multicenter trial evaluating rhBMP-2 versus iliac crest autograft in another series of patients with single-level DDD who underwent ALIF using threaded cortical allograft bone dowels. A total of 131 patients were enrolled at 13 sites (46 patients in the pilot phase and 85 in the pivotal phase). Seventy-nine patients randomized to rhBMP-2 received 1.5 mg/mL rhBMP-2 on an absorbable collagen sponge giving a total dose between 8.4 and 12 mg depending on the size of dowels. The 52 control patients received autograft. Intention-to-treat analysis was not performed because patients who underwent secondary surgery were removed from subsequent analyses.

Mean improvement in preoperative ODI was significantly greater for rhBMP-2 patients at 3- and 6-month follow-up ($P < 0.03$). At 24 months, mean ODI improvement averaged 33.4 points for the rhBMP-2 group and 27.0 points for control patients ($P < 0.12$). Physical Component score (PCS) of the SF-36 improved 15.7 points for the rhBMP-2 group compared with 11.6 points in control patients at 24 months. Absolute PCSs were significantly better in rhBMP-2 patients than control patients at all postoperative time points including 24 months ($P < 0.015$). Radiographic fusion was reported in 98.5% of rhBMP-2 patients at 24 months compared with 76.1% of control patients ($P < 0.001$). Supplemental fixation was required in two rhBMP-2 patients (3%) and eight control patients (15%).

Haid and colleagues (2004)[24] report the results of multicenter trial evaluating rhBMP-2 versus autograft in patients with DDD undergoing PLIF via a posterior approach. A total of 67 patients were enrolled in this 14-center trial. The trial suspended enrollment prematurely because of concerns about ectopic bone formation posterior to the cages in investigational patients. Thirty-four patients were randomized to

receive 1.5 mg/mL rhBMP-2 on a collagen sponge for total doses between 4 and 8 mg, and 33 patients to iliac crest autograft as control. Follow-up at the 24-month period was 85% of rhBMP-2 patients from enrollment and 91% of control patients.

No statistically significant differences were found between the rhBMP-2 and control groups with respect to ODI or SF-36. However, mean improvements and percentage of patients with a 15-point improvement in preoperative ODI were greater in the rhBMP-2 group. Fusion rates at 24 months were 92.3% of rhBMP-2 patients and 77.8% for control patients. New bone formation extending into the spinal canal or neuroforamina was found in 28 patients (24 rhBMP-2 patients and 4 control patients), although no correlation was found between ectopic bone formation and the development of leg pain. Six patients in each group underwent reoperations. In each group, three patients were at the same level as the index procedure and three were at different levels.

Posterolateral Fusion Using Bone Morphogenetic Protein-2 in Degenerative Disc Disease

Boden and coauthors (2002)[16] assessed the outcome of rhBMP-2 in patients with DDD undergoing instrumented and noninstrumented posterior fusion. Twenty-seven patients were enrolled at six investigational centers. Eleven patients were randomized to receive a total dose of 40 mg rhBMP-2 (concentration, 2.0 mg/mL) on a 60% hydroxyapatite/40% tricalcium phosphate (HA/TCP) granule carrier with pedicle screw and rod instrumentation. Nine patients were randomized to receive the same rhBMP-2 with carrier and no internal fixation, and five additional patients were randomized to iliac crest autograft and pedicle screw fixation. Follow-up was to a minimum of 12 months but up to 24 months for some patients.

At the final follow-up, the mean ODI improvement was greatest in the rhBMP-2 only group (28.7 points; $P < 0.001$) compared with rhBMP-2 with instrumentation and the control group. The rhBMP-2 only group also had significantly greater SF-36 PCS and Bodily Pain scores at early follow-up. At final follow-up, the mean SF-36 Pain Index Subscale for the rhBMP-2 only group (67.9) was better ($P < 0.049$) than rhBMP-2 with instrumentation (39.3) and control patients (38.0). Radiographic fusion was 100% in both rhBMP-2 groups, both significantly greater than the 40% (2/5) observed in the control group ($P < 0.02$ and 0.03). Two patients in the rhBMP-2 with instrumentation underwent reoperation, one for revision decompression and another for evacuation of epidural hematoma, and subsequently decompression at another level. Two patients in the rhBMP-2 only group underwent reoperation, one for revision fusion with an anterior approach and one had a postoperative superficial hematoma that was evacuated.

Dimar and investigators (2006)[22] also compared rhBMP-2 with autograft in patients with DDD undergoing posterior pedicle screw and rod instrumented fusions. From this multicenter randomized trial, 150 patients were enrolled but only 98 of them (65%) were available for review at 2 years after surgery. Of the 98 patients, 53 received a total dose of 40 mg rhBMP-2 (concentration, 2.0 mg/mL) combined with a bovine collagen and an HA/TCP compression-resistant matrix, and 45 patients received autograft bone from the iliac crest. At 2 years follow-up, the mean improvement in ODI for the rhBMP-2 group was 24.5 points compared with 21.4 points in the control group. The mean improvement in SF-36 PCS score was 8.6 and 10.7 points for the rhBMP-2 and control groups, respectively. No clinical improvements were significantly different for the two groups. Radiographic fusion, based on plain radiographs and CT, was observed in 48 of 53 rhBMP-2 patients (90.6%) and 33 of the 45 control patients (73.3%). This difference was found to be significant at the $P < 0.05$ level. Three control patients underwent reoperation for revision of malpositioned screws. No reoperations were reported for the rhBMP-2 group.

Posterolateral Fusion Using Bone Morphogenetic Protein-7 in Spondylolisthesis

Johnsson and coworkers (2002)[25] evaluated the use of recombinant human BMP-7, also termed osteogenic protein-1 (OP-1) in patients with isthmic low-grade spondylolisthesis (no more than 50% vertebral slip) undergoing noninstrumented posterolateral fusion. This trial of 20 patients primarily evaluated outcomes by radiostereometric analysis. The only clinical assessment was subjective back pain; however, the investigators assessed plain radiographic evidence of fusion. Ten patients were randomized to receive 3.5 mg rhOP-1 reconstituted with a bone collagen carrier into a paste for each side of the fusion (total dose, 7 mg). Ten other patients received iliac crest autograft through the initial incision. At 12-month follow-up, fusion (bilateral bridging bone) was observed in 6 of 10 rhOP-1 patients and 8 of 10 control patients. Radiostereometric analysis did not show any significant differences between the groups.

Vaccaro and coauthors (2005)[28] compared OP-1 with autograft in a series of patients with degenerative spondylolisthesis (no more than 50% slip) undergoing decompression and noninstrumented posterolateral fusion. This multicenter trial enrolled 36 patients at five centers and randomized them in a 2:1 ratio (OP-1/control ratio) such that 24 received OP-1 and 12 received iliac crest autograft. OP-1 patients were given 3.5 mg rhOP-1 with 1 g bovine bone collagen and 200 mg carboxymethylcellulose on each side of the fusion (total dose, 7 mg).

Four patients (three OP-1 and one control patient) discontinued the study before the 24-month follow-up. Four additional patients (three OP-1 and one control patient) had incomplete 24-month data; however, their 36-month data were used in the final analyses. The authors found that 17 of 20 OP-1 patients (85%) had a 20% improvement in preoperative ODI compared with 7 of 11 control patients (64%). The mean improvement in SF-36 PCS was 17.4 points compared with a decline of 1.1 points in the control group at 24 months. Radiographic fusion, evaluated by plain radiography for the presence of bilateral bridging bone and absence of instability, was observed in 11 of 20 OP-1 patients (55%) and in 4 of 10 control patients (40%). Radiographic fusion, based entirely on the presence of bridging bone alone, was observed in 15 of 20 OP-1 patients (75%) and 8 of 10 control patients (80%). No patients underwent reoperation at the latest reported follow-up time.

Kanayama and colleagues (2006)[26] also evaluated the use of OP-1 in patients with degenerative spondylolisthesis (no more than 25% slip). These patients underwent pedicle screw instrumentation and posterolateral fusion. Twenty patients were enrolled in this study, and 10 were randomized to receive 3.5 mg OP-1, type I bovine collage, and carboxymethylcellulose per side (total dose, 7 mg). The other 10 patients randomized to control treatment received 5 g HA/TCP mixed with locally harvested autograft bone for each side of the fusion. Clinical and radiographic assessments were made at 12 months, and surgical exploration for fusion and hardware removal was planned when radiographic fusion criteria were met.

The authors found no significant differences in ODI or change from preoperative scores between the two groups. Radiographic fusion, by plain radiographs and CT, was found in seven of nine OP-1 patients. Because of the HA/TCP in control patients, radiographic evidence of bridging bone was difficult; however, 9 of 10 control patients were found to have no instability (the other radiographic criterion for fusion) and, therefore, underwent surgical exploration and hardware removal. Solid arthrodesis was achieved in four of seven OP-1 patients and seven of nine control patients. Histologic assessment of the fusion mass demonstrated viable bone in six of the seven OP-1 patients and all nine control patients.

SUMMARY

From our analysis, neither BMP-2 nor BMP-7 have any significant long-term clinical benefit over iliac crest autograft as assessed by validated clinical outcome measures. Small but significant increases in fusion rates have been shown for BMP-2 both for interbody and posterolateral fusions. In contrast, BMP-7 has not shown significantly improved fusion rates compared with autograft bone.

The radiographic fusion benefit of BMP-2 without a concomitant clinical benefit illustrates the well-known concept of discrepancy between physician-based outcome measures (fusion) and patient-based measures. It would be reassuring to see corresponding results from both of these outcomes. However, this is not the case. The question then arises, how do we resolve differences between patient-based and physician-based outcomes?

The clinical benefit of a definite fusion mass is controversial. Randomized trials of spinal fusions with and without instrumentation found increased rates of fusion but no differences in clinical improvement.[29,30] However, in a study of patients who had noninstrumented fusions, clinical outcomes were superior at longer term follow-up for those with solid fusions compared with those who experienced development of pseudarthroses.[31] Potentially, clinical benefit may not have been realized by the current BMP studies because of short follow-up periods. Negative clinical outcomes associated with pseudarthroses may not become evident for many years.

No definitive evidence of clinical superiority was demonstrated in the use of BMPs compared with autograft. Some of the smaller studies reported clinical superiority, particularly at the earlier follow-up intervals. However, these results were not realized in larger multicenter studies. This may be a reflection of increased variability in patients and patient-selection factors.

Consequently, BMPs may only offer an avenue for eliminating sources of morbidity (i.e., iliac crest bone graft) and improving the reliability of achieving fusion without statistically improving clinical outcomes. Obviating the need to harvest iliac crest autograft, whereas still maintaining a comparable or improved rate of fusion, would have tremendous benefits on its own regarding donor-site pain and other potential complications such as donor-site fracture, infection, and nerve injury. Under these circumstances of outcome equivalency, the use of BMP may still have important and beneficial practical uses.

From an economic consideration, with a safety profile free from adverse events, and a price lower than the cost-equivalent of donor-site morbidity, the use of BMPs may be justifiable. Economic evaluation performed from the payer's perspective (i.e., not accounting for health-related quality of life or lost productivity) has suggested that with obviating donor-site complications and considering other cost offsets, a 3.6% increase in fusion success rate with a $3000 price for BMP would be all that is required to achieve cost neutrality over iliac crest autograft.[32] The authors also suggest that economic analyses accounting from a societal perspective (i.e., accounting for health-related quality of life and lost productivity) would require smaller in-

RECOMMENDATIONS

Our recommendations are summarized in Table 9–4. All of the RCTs were found to be of lesser quality (Level II) with regard to adequacy of random allocation, how patients were accounted for, and blinding to intervention.

Interbody fusion was assessed in four trials that all evaluated the use of BMP-2. Fair evidence (grade B) exists that no significant clinical improvement beyond 6 postoperative months can be attributed to the use of BMP-2 in interbody fusions compared with iliac crest autograft. There is also fair evidence (grade B) that a significant increase in the rate of radiographic fusion can be attributed to the use of BMP-2 in interbody fusions over iliac crest autograft.

Posterolateral fusion was assessed in five trials. In two trials using BMP-2 in patients with DDD with and without spinal instrumentation, we found fair evidence (grade B) to conclude that no significant clinical improvement can be attributed to the use of BMP-2 in posterolateral fusion compared with iliac crest autograft. There is also fair evidence (grade B) that a significant increase in the rate of radiographic fusion can be attributed to the use of BMP-2 over autograft.

From three trials assessing BMP-7 in posterolateral fusion in patients with spondylolisthesis, there is fair evidence (grade B) that no significant clinical improvement and no increase in fusion rate can be attributed to the use of BMP-7 in posterolateral fusion compared with iliac crest autograft bone.

creases in fusion success to achieve similar cost neutrality.

Furthermore, in patients considered high risk for nonunion (heavy smokers, revision surgery, rheumatoid arthritis, other medical comorbidities, etc.), marginal increases in fusion rates of BMP over autograft, even in the absence of clinical improvements, may justify its use.[33]

Conflict of Interest

Y. Raja Rampersaud is a consultant for Medtronic-Sofamor Danek (Surgical Navigation Technologies and Minimal Access Surgical Technologies).

TABLE 9–4. Summary of Recommendations			
FUSION	CLINICAL BENEFIT	FUSION BENEFIT	LEVEL OF EVIDENCE/GRADE OF RECOMMENDATION
Interbody using rhBMP-2	0	+	B
Posterolateral using rhBMP-2	0	+	B
Posterolateral using BMP-7 (OP-1)	0	0	B

BMP = bone morphogenetic protein; OP-1 = osteogenic protein-1; rhBMP-2 = recombinant human BMP-2.

REFERENCES

1. Bambakidis NC, Feiz-Erfan I, Klopfenstein JD, et al: Indications for surgical fusion of the cervical and lumbar motion segment. Spine 30:S2–S6, 2005.
2. Weinstein JN, Lurie JD, Olson PR, et al: United States' trends and regional variations in lumbar spine surgery: 1992-2003. Spine 31:2707–2714, 2006.
3. Katz JN: Lumbar spinal fusion. Surgical rates, costs, and complications. Spine 20:78S–83S, 1995.
4. Martin BI, Mirza SK, Comstock BA, et al: Reoperation rates following lumbar spine surgery and the influence of spinal fusion procedures. Spine 32:382–387, 2007.
5. Hu RW, Jaglal S, Axcell T, et al: A population-based study of reoperations after back surgery. Spine 22:2265–2271, 1997.
6. Lee C, Dorcil J, Radomisli TE: Nonunion of the spine: A review. Clin Orthop 419:71–75, 2004.
7. Robertson PA, Wray AC: Natural history of posterior iliac crest bone graft donation for spinal surgery: A prospective analysis of morbidity. Spine 26:1473–1476, 2001.
8. Goulet JA, Senunas LE, DeSilva GL, et al: Autogenous iliac crest bone grafts. Complications and functional assessment. Clin Orthop Relat Res 339:76–81, 1997.
9. Sasso RC, LeHuec JC, Shaffrey C, et al: Iliac crest bone graft donor site pain after anterior lumbar interbody fusion: A prospective patient satisfaction outcome assessment. J Spinal Disord Tech 18(suppl):S77–S81, 2005.
10. Urist MR: Bone: Formation by autoinduction. Science 150:893–899, 1965.
11. Urist MR, Silverman BF, Buring K, et al: The bone induction principle. Clin Orthop 53:243–283, 1967.
12. Cheng H, Jiang W, Phillips FM, et al: Osteogenic activity of the fourteen types of human bone morphogenetic proteins (BMPs). J Bone Joint Surg Am 85:1544–1552, 2003.
13. Sandhu HS: Bone morphogenetic proteins and spinal surgery. Spine 28:S64–S73, 2003.
14. Mummaneni PV, Pan J, Haid RW, et al: Contribution of recombinant human bone morphogenetic protein-2 to the rapid creation of interbody fusion when used in transforaminal lumbar interbody fusion: A preliminary report. J Neurosurg Spine 1:19–23, 2004.
15. Boden SD, Zdeblick TA, Sandhu HS, et al: The use of rhBMP-2 in interbody fusion cages. Definitive evidence of osteoinduction in humans: A preliminary report. Spine 25:376–381, 2000.
16. Boden SD, Kang J, Sandhu HS, et al: Use of recombinant human bone morphogenetic protein-2 to achieve posterolateral lumbar spine fusion in humans. A prospective, randomized clinical pilot trial: 2002 Volvo Award in Clinical Studies. Spine 27:2662–2673, 2002.
17. Burkus JK, Gornet MF, Dickman CA, et al: Anterior lumbar interbody fusion using rhBMP-2 with tapered interbody cages. J Spinal Disord Tech 15:337–349, 2002.
18. Burkus JK, Transfeldt EE, Kitchel SH, et al: Clinical and radiographic outcomes of anterior lumbar interbody fusion using recombinant human bone morphogenetic protein-2. Spine 27:2396–2408, 2002.
19. Burkus JK, Dorchak JD, Sanders DL: Radiographic assessment of interbody fusion using recombinant human bone morphogenetic protein type 2. Spine 28:372–377, 2003.
20. Burkus JK, Sandhu HS, Gornet MF, et al: Use of rhBMP-2 in combination with structural cortical allografts: Clinical and radiographic outcomes in anterior lumbar spinal surgery. J Bone Joint Surg Am 87:1205–1212, 2005.
21. Burkus JK, Sandhu HS, Gornet MF: Influence of rhBMP-2 on the healing patterns associated with allograft interbody constructs in comparison with autograft. Spine 31:775–781, 2006.
22. Dimar JR, Glassman SD, Burkus JK, et al: Clinical outcomes and radiographic fusion success at 2 years of single-level instrumented posterolateral fusions with recombinant human bone morphogenetic protein-2/compression resistant matrix versus iliac crest bone graft. Spine 31:2534–2539, 2006.
23. Glassman SD, Dimar JR, Carreon LY, et al: Initial fusion rates with recombinant human bone morphogenetic protein-2/compression resistant matrix and a hydroxyapatite and tricalcium phosphate/collagen carrier in posterolateral spinal fusion. Spine 30:1694–1698, 2005.
24. Haid RW, Branch CL, Alexander JT, et al: Posterior lumbar interbody fusion using recombinant human bone morphogenetic protein type 2 with cylindrical interbody cages. Spine J 4:527–539, 2004.
25. Johnsson R, Stromqvist B, Aspenberg P: Randomized radiostereometric study comparing Osteogenic Protein-1 (BMP-7) and autograft bone in human noninstrumented posterolateral lumbar fusion: 2002 Volvo Award in Clinical Studies. Spine 27:2654–2661, 2002.
26. Kanayama M, Hashimoto T, Shigenobu K, et al: A prospective randomized study of posterolateral lumbar fusion using Osteogenic Protein-1 (OP-1) versus local autograft with ceramic bone substitute: Emphasis of surgical exploration and histologic assessment. Spine 31:1067–1074, 2006.
27. Vaccaro AR, Patel T, Fischgrund J, et al: A pilot study evaluating the safety and efficacy of OP-1 Putty (rhBMP-7) as a replacement for iliac crest autograft in posterolateral lumbar arthrodesis for degenerative spondylolisthesis. Spine 29:1885–1892, 2004.
28. Vaccaro AR, Anderson DG, Patel T, et al: Comparison of OP-1 Putty (rhBMP-7) to iliac crest autograft for posterolateral lumbar arthrodesis: A minimum 2-year follow-up pilot study. Spine 30:2709–2716, 2005.
29. Fischgrund JS, Mackay M, Herkowitz HN, et al: Degenerative lumbar spondylolisthesis with spinal stenosis: A prospective, randomized study comparing decompressive laminectomy and arthrodesis with and without spinal instrumentation. Spine 22:2807–2812, 1997.
30. Thomsen K, Christensen FB, Eiskjaer SP, et al: The effect of pedicle screw instrumentation on functional outcome and fusion rates in posterolateral lumbar spinal fusion: A prospective, randomized clinical study. Spine 22:2813–2822, 1997.
31. Kornblum MB, Fischgrund JS, Herkowitz HN, et al: Degenerative lumbar spondylolisthesis with spinal stenosis: A prospective long-term study comparing fusion and pseudarthrosis. Spine 29:726–733, 2004.
32. Ackerman SJ, Mafilios MS, Polly DW Jr: Economic evaluation of bone morphogenetic protein versus autogenous iliac crest bone graft in single-level anterior lumbar fusion: An evidence-based modeling approach. Spine 27:S94–S99, 2002.
33. Govender PV, Rampersaud YR, Rickards L, et al: Use of osteogenic protein-1 in spinal fusion: Literature review and preliminary results in a prospective series of high-risk cases. Neurosurg Focus 13:e4, 2002.

UPPER EXTREMITY TOPICS

Chapter 10

What Is the Best Surgical Procedure for Cubital Tunnel Syndrome?

STEVEN J. MCCABE, MD, MSc

The second most common site of nerve compression in the upper extremity is the ulnar nerve in the region of the cubital tunnel. Until recently, the surgical management of cubital tunnel syndrome was represented in the literature by numerous case series with the authors reporting experience with a specific surgical procedure. Clinical research related to cubital tunnel syndrome answered many important questions about this disorder and its care; however, until recently, there has been only low-quality evidence supporting one type of surgical procedure over others.

In 1989, Dellon[1] advocated a staging system for ulnar nerve compression at the elbow. He reviewed the literature and concluded that severity of compression, a characteristic he used to divide the syndrome into three stages, was an important prognostic factor and should be used to guide surgical management. Parallel to the staging of carpal tunnel syndrome, he divided cubital tunnel syndrome into "mild," "moderate," and "severe" stages. Although it remains unknown whether the stage of compression is an important guide for choice of surgery, if the prognosis of surgical care is related to the severity of compression, then this information would be useful in randomized trials to define the population and ensure balance of treatment groups.

For measurement of the results of cubital tunnel surgery, Kleinman and Bishop[2] have devised a grading system. The domains include "satisfaction," "improvement," "severity of residual symptoms," "work status," "leisure activity," "strength," and "sensibility."

This has been used widely since its introduction, and although it requires some measurement by a trained person, it is recommended for anyone performing clinical research in cubital tunnel syndrome. As a disorder causing symptoms and functional problems in the hand, in clinical research, some patient-oriented method of evaluation of the results of treatment should be used. The use of electrodiagnostic testing to measure the outcome of cubital tunnel surgery may be misleading. It has been reported that electrodiagnostic testing may not be accurate after anterior transposition.[3] In addition, in other forms of nerve compression, electrodiagnostic tests may not return to normal despite good clinical results after surgery. The importance of these measurement issues in the use of electrical testing to evaluate the results of cubital tunnel surgery has not been explored. These concerns add to the importance of patient-oriented measures in outcomes research in cubital tunnel syndrome.

OPTIONS

The surgical options for cubital tunnel syndrome include three main decisions with some variation. The nerve can be decompressed and left in its normal anatomic position. This can be performed with a standard open approach or through a minimal incision method. The epicondyle can be removed in conjunction with release. The nerve can be transposed anterior to the epicondyle into a subcutaneous, an intramuscular, or a submuscular position.

Simple Release

The value of simple release of the ulnar nerve is that it is technically simple to perform and, if successful, causes the least morbidity for the patient. The surgery is of short duration and the postoperative care is simplified requiring no prolonged immobilization. This procedure leaves the nerve in its anatomic position, and therefore reduces the chance of inducing secondary compression by changing the anatomic course of the nerve. The concern with the procedure is that the nerve is left in a position behind the elbow where it can continue to undergo traction with full elbow flexion. Another potential problem is created because the nerve is released from its tethers within its anatomic bed. Theoretically, this increases the potential for subluxation of the nerve with flexion of the elbow. A variation of simple release is to use minimal incisions and some type of "endoscopic" visualization of the procedure. Nathan and colleagues[4] report 89% good or excellent immediate postoperative relief of symptoms using simple decompression of the nerve in 164 nerves in 131 patients. At an average follow-up period of 4.3 years, 79% of patients still reported good or excellent relief.

Epicondylectomy

The nerve is released as in a simple release and a portion of the medial epicondyle is removed to perform medial epicondylectomy. This procedure also leaves the nerve in its anatomic position. By combining a simple release with epicondylectomy, theoretically, when the elbow flexes, the nerve will not snap over the medial epicondyle. A minimal degree of epicondylar excision appears to be as effective as a partial epicondylectomy.[5]

Subcutaneous Transposition

Subcutaneous transposition places the nerve anterior to the axis of flexion of the elbow joint, preventing tension of the nerve by elbow flexion. The theoretic advantage of this procedure is that the nerve is moved out of the site of compromise into a tension-free environment. Compared with the submuscular transposition, the subcutaneous transposition should have a shorter recovery time. Potential problems with the procedure include introducing a new site of compression such as the medial intermuscular septum or fascial septae in the flexor origin. One variation of the procedure is to create a fascial sling for the nerve to prevent it from subluxing back behind the elbow. This sling can also create a site of compression. In thin people, the nerve may not have much coverage in the subcutaneous plane and may be sensitive.

Intramuscular and Submuscular Transposition

For intramuscular and submuscular transposition, the nerve is removed from its anatomic location and placed within[2] or deep to the flexor pronator muscle origin. In this procedure, the nerve is placed anterior to the elbow and is placed within a protective environment. The surgeon may introduce additional sites of compression, and the patient must have a period of postoperative immobilization to allow the flexor origin to heal. One variation is to perform lengthening of the flexor pronator origin to loosen this structure over the nerve. In Dellon's[6] report of submuscular transposition on 121 patients and 161 extremities using the musculofascial lengthening technique, 88% of patients had an excellent or good result with a 7.5% failure rate. In Pasque and Rayan's[7] study, 84% of patients had good or excellent grades after submuscular transposition with a Z lengthening.

EVIDENCE

In an attempt to compare all these procedures, Dellon[1] compiled the literature on each procedure. In his article, he reviewed the previous 90 years of literature and concluded, "This study demonstrates that despite more than 50 reported series of patients treated for ulnar nerve compression at the elbow, a collective experience with more than 2000 patients, there are at present no statistically significant guidelines based on prospective randomized studies for choosing one operative technique over another."[1]

Dellon[1] found that in mild compression, the literature supported nonsurgical management with an expectation of 50% of patients achieving excellent results and almost 100% of patients achieving excellent results with any of the five common surgical procedures. For moderate compression, he noted that the literature suggested the anterior submuscular technique yielded the most excellent results with the least recurrence, and for severe compression, the intramuscular technique yielded the fewest excellent results and the most recurrence.

A meta-analysis of 30 clinical studies from 1945 to 1995 compared patients having nonsurgical management, simple decompression, medial epicondylectomy, subcutaneous, submuscular transposition. Although it appears that none of the studies was a randomized trial, the authors tried to collect information from each patient in each study where possible. The report provides a list of publications evaluating each procedure and is useful to provide historical context to the surgery for cubital tunnel syndrome. Patients were categorized by preoperative staging of severity. Outcomes were scored as "total relief," "improvement," "no change," and "worse." In minimum stage compression, total relief was experienced by 92% having medial epicondylectomy. The remaining groups were small; however, it was noted only 9% of 22 patients had complete relief after subcutaneous transfer. In moderate stage compression, submuscular transposition yielded 80% complete relief, and in severe stage compression, all the procedures faired poorly with simple decompression providing 26% complete relief and no significant differences except medial epicondylectomy, which had the lowest satisfaction rate at 38% and had no patients with complete relief. In this systematic review, more than 450 patients were analyzed with severe compression.[8]

Recently, randomized trials have been used to compare some of the surgical procedures used for cubital tunnel syndrome. In 2005, Bartels and co-workers[9] used a randomized trial to compare the outcome of simple decompression versus anterior subcutaneous transposition.

First, the authors used a survey of neurosurgeons in the Netherlands to determine the most commonly performed procedures. From a single center, 152 patients were randomized by a computer-generated randomization list to simple release or anterior subcutaneous transposition. Inclusion criteria included duration of symptoms greater than 3 months, clinical and electrical criteria, and failure of nonsurgical management. Exclusion criteria included diabetes, arthritis of the elbow, and previous surgery on the symptomatic side, among other factors listed in the article. The exact surgical methods used were not detailed in the article; however, the tendency of the ulnar nerve to sublux was noted and found to have no influence on the result. Preoperative severity of compression was recorded. The authors found no influence of the preoperative grade, the extent of muscle weakness, or the duration of symptoms on the probability of improvement, although the analysis of this was not presented. In addition to neurologic grade noted earlier, outcomes were measured using the SF-36 and a Dutch version of the McGill Pain Questionnaire. The authors state the results of both instruments improve with time with no statistical difference at any follow-up interval. No further statistical detail or data from either instrument are reported. A total of 147 participants were included in the analysis. The results were reported as excellent and good in 65% of simple decompression and 70% of anterior subcutaneous transposition. The complication rate was lower in the simple decompression patients at 9.6% compared with 31.1% in anterior subcutaneous transposition. Eighteen of 152 patients were deemed to have unsuccessful surgical results.

One concern with the methods used in that article is that the surgeon who performed the surgery also evaluated the results. To mitigate this problem, a blinded neurologist randomly selected 30 patients at one postoperative visit for evaluation with a reported reliability greater than 97% for history and physical examination. According to the results, the difference in complications between groups was primarily due to increased loss of sensibility around the scar in the anterior transposition group. The overall clinical results favored the anterior transposition group to a minor degree that could be accounted for by chance. The study had sufficient power to discover a difference of 25%, if present.

This study is a randomized trial of reasonable size. The evidence would have been more powerful if the outcomes were evaluated by a person blinded to the treatment. The "cure rate" favors anterior transposition at 62% compared with 49%; however, this is not statistically significant. More powerful statistical tests could have been used and the reporting of the results could have been clearer (Level I).

In another study, Nabhan and coauthors[10] report on a randomized trial of simple decompression compared with subcutaneous transposition of the ulnar nerve. Sixty-six patients were included and randomized using a sealed envelope method. Patients with previous elbow trauma were excluded. Outcomes were measured by a sensory scale, intrinsic motor strength, pain, and nerve conduction velocity. The surgical procedures are described. After a 6- to 9-month follow-up, there were no significant differences between the two groups. The article does not report how many patients experienced complete relief of symptoms and how many failures occurred in each group (Level II).

Both of these randomized trials failed to show any benefit of transposition of the nerve over simple release. In Bartels and coworkers'[9] report, neither the preoperative severity of compression nor the tendency of the nerve to sublux over the epicondyle had an effect on the outcome. The Nabhan and coauthors'[10] findings are consistent with those of Bartels and coworkers,[9] putting into question the need for transposition of the nerve in patients without trauma or elbow pathology.

Biggs and Curtis[11] compared "ulnar neurolysis" with submuscular transposition in a randomized, controlled trial. In this study, 44 patients were stratified and randomized. Inclusion and exclusion criteria were documented, and the procedures are described in the article. Using the Louisiana State University Medical Center system, the authors note neurologic improvement in 61% of the neurolysis group and 67% of the transposition group. In medium- and high-grade compression, there was no statistically significant difference in the groups, with 82% improving in the neurolysis group and 68% in the transposition group. Although the numbers are small, the simple decompression group had better results in this more severe degree of compression. Three of 21 patients experienced development of wound infection after transposition, and 0 of 23 after neurolysis. The surgery and the postsurgical evaluations were performed by the lead author, so the study could not be considered blinded with regard to measurement of the results of surgery (Level II).

Gervasio and coworkers[12] compared simple decompression versus anterior submuscular decompression in severe cubital tunnel syndrome. Patients were "randomized" based on their hospital reservation number, and one of two surgeons was assigned depending on the procedure. All patients had severe cubital tunnel syndrome, termed *Dellon 3,* or severe compression. Exclusion criteria are presented in the article. Surgical procedures are described. The postoperative evaluations were performed by a blinded neurologist using the Bishop rating system (see earlier). The results showed that both groups improved to a similar degree with no significant differences in electrical or clinical improvement. Eighty percent of patients had a good to excellent outcome with simple decompression, and 82.9% has a good or excellent outcome with submuscular transposition. Simple decompression yielded 54.3% excellent, 25.7% good, and 20% fair results, whereas anterior submuscular transposition gave 51.4% excellent, 31.4% good, and 17.1% fair results (Level II).

Once again, the two trials failed to show any improvement afforded by transposition of the nerve into the submuscular location over simple decompression of the nerve. This was specifically found in severe compression in the trial that Gervasio and coworkers[12] reported. Although that study was not truly randomized, a large proportion of patients with severe compression had good or excellent results after simple decompression.

In a randomized trial of medial epicondylectomy versus anterior transposition in a population of 47 patients, Geutjens and investigators[13] found no difference in the results with regard to two-point discrimination recovery or muscle power. A larger proportion of patients was the same or worse after anterior transposition, and fewer transposition patients would have the procedure again. Patients were randomized using sealed envelopes and had one of the two procedures performed by one of two surgeons. Both surgeons performed both procedures.

Postoperative evaluation was blinded. The statistical methods are not elaborated in the article (Level II).

A nonrandomized comparative study of 56 patients comparing minimal medial epicondylectomy and anterior subcutaneous transposition similarly found that the two procedures produced similar results.[14] The medial epicondylectomy yielded 41% excellent, 45% good, 9% fair, and 5% poor results, whereas the subcutaneous transfer had 41% excellent, 38% good, 18% fair, and 3% poor.

Both studies show no improvement in the results for transposition of the nerve compared with epicondylectomy. Although each of these studies has some methodologic concerns, they are consistent in their results, showing more involved surgery does not produce superior results. Transposition does not appear to add any benefit to a simple release or epicondylectomy, but it does increase the morbidity of the surgery. It is notable for surgeons to remember that these studies excluded patients with trauma and anatomic causes of compression at the medial elbow.

Areas of Uncertainty

Specialty Training. The surgeons performing the surgery in these randomized trials are predominantly neurosurgeons. Does this reduce their generalizability to other specialty trained surgeons such as orthopedic, plastic, hand, and other peripheral nerve surgeons?

First, the reader should look to the description of the patient population. The reader will have to determine whether the patients treated are similar to those patients they might see. The results in these trials must be interpreted with caution because it is likely that the referral filter for a patient to see a neurosurgeon is different for a surgeon of a different specialty. It is known in other disciplines that patient populations referred to different specialty physicians who provide care for the "same condition" can be fundamentally different. Whether these differences exist in cubital tunnel syndrome and whether prognostically important variations persist to induce some difference in the efficacy of one surgical procedure or another is conjectural at this time.

Efficacy and Complication Rates of the Procedures. Do the results of these trials suggest these procedures, the efficacy, and the complication rates would be typical for other surgeons? Our attention is drawn to the cure rate that may be lower and the complication rate including infections that may be higher in these randomized trials than reported in large cohorts performed by other surgeons. For example, the importance of cutaneous nerves crossing the incision in cubital tunnel surgery has been pointed out in the literature.[15] The complications of subcutaneous transfer reported by Bartels and coworkers[9] could have been reduced by increased attention to this detail.

Similarly, the proportion of patients achieving complete relief of symptoms reported by Bartels and coworkers[9] seems low, and in contrast with the

systematic review of previous studies, the degree of compression did not appear to influence the results.

Carefully crafted large cohort studies should be a good method to identify the probability of events, such as complications, better than randomized trials, the size of which are planned to measure efficacy rather than complications. When the research design carefully seeks out complications and continuing symptoms, their prevalence will be greater than when they are evaluated in a later review of medical records or after general questioning. Differences in patient populations and ascertainment of results and complications can easily affect the reporting of results of surgery, which is one of the reasons randomized trials and cohort studies are preferred to case series especially when analyzed through review of medical records.

At this point, I believe it is not possible to determine whether the reported randomized trials by surgeons other than hand surgeons have a lower efficacy or a greater complication rate that would cause concern regarding the surgical technique or that would justify a belief that the results do not apply to fellowship trained hand surgeons, plastic surgeons, or orthopedic surgeons. Rather than take a xenophobic view, these randomized trials should be viewed as the best evidence available to guide surgical management.

Size of Studies

All studies reviewed were small trials, increasing the possibility that chance could play a role in the results. The largest study with Level I evidence[9] comparing simple release with subcutaneous transfer had enough power to detect a 25% or greater difference in the results. Those authors found a 13% difference in those patients "cured," favoring transposition. Biggs and Curtis's[11] study, when evaluating the more severe cases, found the reverse, favoring simple decompression, although the numbers are small. With small studies, the impact of methodologic problems or chance can sway the results of a trial. For example, in at least two of the trials, the measurement of the results was not blinded; in one trial, the allocation was not truly randomized; and in all the trials, the surgery was performed by a limited number of surgeons.

Nevertheless, these trials are the best evidence available to help a surgeon choose between the surgical alternatives for cubital tunnel syndrome. The direction of the results of these studies is consistent. No randomized trial has favored more involved surgery over lesser procedures.

CONCLUSIONS

Based on this review, I believe good to fair evidence exists (grade B, that is, consistent Level I and II evidence) to support simple decompression for cubital

Summary of Recommendations	
STATEMENT	LEVEL OF EVIDENCE/GRADE OF RECOMMENDATIONS
Simple decompression is as efficacious as transposition of the ulnar nerve in cubital tunnel syndrome	B

tunnel syndrome over transposition of the nerve. This evidence is limited to patients in whom the cubital tunnel syndrome is not secondary to trauma or an anatomic cause at the elbow. The evidence is strongest for use by neurosurgeons to guide their decision making. I believe evidence exists against transposition of the ulnar nerve, during cubital tunnel surgery. Also, I believe no evidence is available to differentiate between simple decompression and medial epicondylectomy in cubital tunnel surgery.

REFERENCES

1. Dellon AL: Review of treatment results for ulnar nerve entrapment at the elbow. J Hand Surg [Am] 14:688–700, 1989.
2. Kleinman WB, Bishop AT: Anterior intramuscular transposition of the ulnar nerve. J Hand Surg [Am] 14:972–979, 1989.
3. Dellon AL, Schlegel RW, Mackinnon SE: Validity of nerve conduction velocity studies after anterior transposition of the ulnar nerve. J Hand Surg [Am] 12:700–703, 1987.
4. Nathan PA, Keniston RC, Meadows KD: Outcome study of ulnar nerve compression at the elbow treated with simple decompression and an early programme of physical therapy. J Hand Surg [Br] 20;5:628–637.
5. Amako M, Nemoto K, Kawaguchi M, et al: Comparison between partial and minimal medial epicondylectomy combined with decompression for the treatment of cubital tunnel syndrome. J Hand Surg [Am] 25:1043–1050, 2000.
6. Dellon AL, Coert JH: Results of the musculofascial lengthening technique for submuscular transposition of the ulnar nerve at the elbow. J Bone Joint Surg Am 86-A(suppl 1):169–179, 2004.
7. Pasque CB, Rayan GM: Anterior submuscular transposition of the ulnar nerve for cubital tunnel syndrome. J Hand Surg [Br] 20:447–453, 1995.
8. Mowlavi A, Andrews K, Lille S, et al: The management of cubital tunnel syndrome: A meta-analysis of clinical studies. Plast Reconstr Surg 106:327–334, 2000.
9. Bartels RHMA, Verhagen WIM, van der Wilt GJ, et al: Prospective randomized controlled study comparing simple decompression versus anterior subcutaneous transposition for idiopathic neuropathy of the ulnar nerve at the elbow: Part 1. Neurosurgery 56:522–530, 2005.
10. Nabhan A, Ahlhelm F, Kelm J, et al: Simple decompression or subcutaneous anterior transposition of the ulnar nerve for cubital tunnel syndrome. J Hand Surg [Br] 30:521–524, 2005.
11. Biggs M, Curtis JA: Randomized, prospective study comparing ulnar neurolysis in situ with submuscular transposition. Neurosurgery 58:296–304, 2006.
12. Gervasio O, Gambardella G, Zaccone C, Branca D: Simple decompression versus anterior submuscular transposition of the ulnar nerve in severe cubital tunnel syndrome: A prospective randomized study. Neurosurgery 56:108–117, 2005.
13. Geutjens GG, Langstaff RJ, Smith NJ, et al: Medial epicondylectomy or ulnar-nerve transposition for ulnar neuropathy at the elbow? J Bone Joint Surg Br 78:777–779, 1996.
14. Baek GH, Kwon BC, Chung MS: Comparative study between minimal medial epicondylectomy and anterior subcutaneous transposition of the ulnar nerve for cubital tunnel syndrome. J Shoulder Elbow Surg 15:609–613, 2006.
15. Lowe JB 3rd, Maggi SP, Mackinnon SE: The position of crossing branches of the medial antebrachial cutaneous nerve during cubital tunnel surgery in humans. Plast Reconstr Surg 114:692–696, 2004.

What Is the Best Treatment for Displaced Fractures of the Distal Radius?

NEAL C. CHEN, MD AND JESSE B. JUPITER, MD

The optimal treatment for displaced distal radius fractures is unclear. Despite a literature filled with hundreds of studies examining biomechanics, treatment outcomes, and techniques, level I evidence is limited and does not provide an unambiguous answer. Many "prospective randomized" studies before 2000 have significant methodologic errors. Yet, more recent studies utilizing stringent blinding and more reproducible evaluation methods may offer some insight into choosing a treatment method.

OPTIONS

Numerous historical methods can be used to treat distal radius fractures; however, general categories are: (1) closed reduction and casting, (2) percutaneous pinning and casting, (3) external fixation, and (4) plate fixation. Subgroups exist within these general categories. External fixation may be bridging or nonbridging, uniplanar or multiplanar, and possibly augmented with percutaneous pins. Plate fixation may use an enormous variety of plate designs, approaches, and screw design and configurations. As one can imagine, this heterogeneity in treatment options is problematic when trying to design a study to evaluate treatment methods, as well as drawing conclusions from the various published studies.

Each treatment modality offers its own advantages and disadvantages. Closed reduction and casting avoids the general risks of surgery but requires routine follow-up and rehabilitation after bony healing. Percutaneous pinning offers treatment with minimal soft-tissue disruption but introduces risks for pin-tract infection. External fixation offers improved structural support than percutaneous pinning; however, problems of patient acceptance and pin-tract infection remain. Finally, open reduction and plate fixation allows direct manipulation and fixation of fracture fragments but requires soft-tissue disruption and risks late hardware problems.

It is unclear how each purported risk and benefit affects the overall outcome of each surgical technique. Prospective, randomized, controlled trials offer a global insight as to how much the cumulative risk and benefits differ between treatments.

EVIDENCE (LEVEL I AND II EVIDENCE)

Handoll and Madhok[1,2] performed a systematic review of the distal radius fracture literature before 2000. Significant methodologic deficiencies abounded: Most series had a small number of patients, allocation concealment was deficient in 42 of 44 studies, and a majority of outcomes were reported using a modified Gartland and Werley scheme, a nonvalidated surgeon-generated outcome measure. Despite these deficiencies, their systematic review suggests that external fixation and percutaneous pinning have better radiographic outcomes and may have improved functional outcomes compared with closed reduction and casting.

Studies after 2000 with improved methodology confirm results of previous studies. In a level I study, Kreder and colleagues[3] compared spanning external fixation to closed reduction and casting in distal radius fractures without joint incongruity and found trends toward improved 36-Item Short Form Health Survey (SF-36) bodily pain scores and Musculoskeletal Functional Assessment (MFA) scores at 2 years; however, these trends did not reach statistical significance. Radiologic outcomes also showed a trend that approached significance that favored external fixation. Comparisons of percutaneous pinning to closed reduction using validated outcomes also found that radiographic parameters were significantly improved with pinning; however, there was no difference in the SF-36 score.[4] Harley and colleagues'[5] level I study also examined outcomes of augmented external fixation versus percutaneous pinning at 1 year. Although validated and functional outcomes were similar, external fixation demonstrated better articular congruity on radiographic follow-up.

External fixation has also been compared with internal fixation. When comparing dorsal pi plating with external fixation in a level II study, Grewal and investigators[6] found no significant difference in Disabilities in Arm, Shoulder, and Hand (DASH) or SF-36 scores; however, the pi plate group had significantly weaker grip strengths and greater number of complications, especially tendonitis and the need for hardware removal. Kreder and colleagues[7] in a multicenter level I study found that although MFA and SF-36 scores were similar at 2 years between both external fixation with indirect reduction and percutaneous pinning and open reduction, internal fixation was statistically equivalent, internal fixation yielded a better SF-36 bodily pain subscore, but external fixation yielded better grip strengths at the 6-month period.

Although many studies have confirmed previous conclusions, some newer studies have brought these conclusions under question. In a 1998 level II study, McQueen[8] found that nonbridging external fixation yielded better radiographic results, grip strength, and flexion than bridging external fixation. However, Atroshi and colleagues[9] found that in a level I study, although radiographic outcomes were improved in patients treated with nonbridging fixators, DASH scores were statistically equivalent.

Trials have also examined adjunctive bone graft substitutes. In a level II randomized, controlled trial by Sanchez-Sotelo and coauthors,[10] Norian-treated wrists had better functional outcomes compared with wrists treated with closed reduction and casting. In the regression analysis, treatment without Norian increased the probability of a poor functional result by 12 and increased the probability of malunion by 11. Cassidy and colleagues[11] compared Norian SRS-treated wrists with external fixation in a level I study and found better subjective outcomes at 6 weeks; however, no significant clinical differences were observed at 1 year.

With regard to external fixation, Werber and researchers'[12] level II study demonstrated that use of a five-pin external fixator with one pin supporting the radial articular fragment yielded better radiographic and functional outcomes than a standard four-pin fixator. Egol and coworkers'[13] level I study demonstrated no significant difference in the incidence of pin-site infection regardless of pin-site care using dry dressings, peroxide pin-site care, or chlorhexidine impregnated discs.

Current level I and II evidence suggests that external fixation yields better radiographic results and trends toward improved validated outcomes than closed reduction and casting. Internal fixation and external fixation result in similar validated outcomes after 1 or 2 years. By induction, open reduction and internal fixation may lead to better outcomes than closed reduction and casting; however, a prospective, randomized, controlled study demonstrating this result is currently lacking.

AREAS OF UNCERTAINTY (LEVEL II AND III EVIDENCE)

Plating Techniques

A number of new plating techniques have become popular since the late 1990s. Volar fixed-angle plating was introduced with the pi plate in the late 1980s,[14] but now has undergone a renaissance. Orbay and Fernandez[15,16] have popularized this concept, and fixed-angle volar plating is now again in widespread use. Low-profile dorsal plating and dif-

ferent forms of fragment-specific fixation methods have been used successfully as documented in level IV case series.[17,18]

Despite this explosion of different types of plates and plating techniques, limited evidence has compared these different techniques. In Ruch and Papadonikolakis's[19] level III case–control series, no difference existed in the DASH between volar nonlocking plating versus dorsal nonlocking plating. In Koshimune and colleagues'[20] level II study, there was no clear advantage of volar locked versus volar nonlocked plating when evaluating radiographic parameters of palmar inclination, radial tilt, and radial length as final outcome.

Rehabilitation

Handoll and Madhok[21] also performed a systematic review of literature examining optimal methods for rehabilitation after surgical fixation of distal radius fracture. Despite the 15 trials that were able to be included in the review, the authors conclude that no specific guidelines can be made regarding rehabilitation after distal radius fracture.

Progression to Arthrosis

Previous studies have documented a statistical association with intra-articular step-off with radiographic arthrosis.[22] Kreder and investigators'[3] level I study from 2006 demonstrated that patients with a residual step-off were 10 times more likely to experience development of radiographic arthrosis. Patients with a step-off greater than 2 mm were eight times more likely to develop radiographic arthrosis than patients with a step-off less than 2 mm. Despite these dramatic numbers, the clinical impact of this radiographic arthrosis is unclear. A level II prospective, randomized trial by Young and coworkers'[23] with 7-year follow-up of 85 patients from the United Kingdom demonstrated radiographic arthrosis in 20 patients, but clinically significant arthrosis in only one patient. Goldfarb et al. demonstrated that radiographic arthrosis was present in 13 of 16 wrists at fifteen years after distal radius fracture, however clinical function was quite good despite the radiographic appearance.[24a] Long-term studies will be necessary to elucidate the incidence of clinically significant radiocarpal arthrosis after distal radius fracture, and it is likely that only a large cohort of patients will be able to distinguish whether one intervention is better than another in preventing clinical arthrosis.

CASE SERIES FOR FURTHER STUDY (LEVEL IV AND V EVIDENCE)

A number of authors have reported case series of different methods of plate fixation using various outcome measures ranging from Gartland and Werley functional scores to DASH and SF-36 scores.[15-17,24-26] This recent rash of case reports on plating reflect a growing worldwide trend favoring plate fixation; subsequently, they should be examined critically.

Case series involving volar-fixed angle plating demonstrated success in the potentially osteopenic elderly population[16] and also demonstrated DASH and Gartland and Werley scores comparable with previous series using other techniques.[26] Harness and colleagues[27] reported on a cohort of seven patients whose volar plating construct lost fixation. Careful review of this cohort found that the standard volar implants used did not adequately support the ulnar volar margin of the lunate facet. Dorsal plating series report minimal problems with extensor tendon irritation at 18 months with rare plate removal.[17,25] DASH and Gartland and Werley scores were also similar to other functional outcomes studies.

Recommendations

Application of Evidence

Grade A Recommendations, Good Evidence

High-quality evidence suggests that external fixation augmented with Kirschner wires and open reduction with plate fixation have similar validated outcomes at 1 to 2 years. It is reasonable to utilize either treatment modality for displaced distal radius fractures. Current evidence suggests better radiographic outcomes with open reduction, internal fixation, or augmented external fixation when compared with other less invasive measures. Utilization of closed reduction and casting or percutaneous pinning and casting are acceptable alternatives if the risks of surgery are prohibitive or patients are willing to accept a lesser radiographic result.

With regard to external fixation, the utilization of a fifth pin to support the articular surface of the radius has utility; however, it is unclear whether this is superior to external fixation with K-wire augmentation. Pin care using dry sterile dressing is sufficient, and peroxide or chlorhexidine augmentation does not confer a demonstrable benefit.

Grade B Recommendations, Fair Evidence

The type of fixation used in open-reduction, internal fixation does not yield a significant difference in outcome. It has been suggested that intra-articular step-off is associated with radiographic arthrosis; however, this finding is not as clearly defined in the current literature. Because of this association, it is reasonable to try to minimize articular step-off with treatment. No evidence exists demonstrating a superior method of rehabilitation after open-reduction, internal fixation at this time.

Grade C Recommendations, Poor Evidence

When compared with validated outcomes from level I studies, case series suggest new volar and dorsal plating techniques can provide comparable outcomes. No evidence currently exists to suggest superiority of newer fixed-angle plates or low-profile dorsal plating.

Loss of lunate facet fixation can compromise the overall result. As such, surgeons should be particularly wary of distal fractures of the intermediate column. Extensor tenosynovitis continues to be a complication with both volar and dorsal plating. No level I evidence shows that these complications occur at a lower rate than with other plating methods; however, in case series compared with historical controls, the incidence may be lower. It is reasonable to utilize newer plate technologies whereas paying close attention to noted potential complications. Table 11–1 provides a summary of recommendations for treatment of displaced fractures of the distal radius.

TABLE 11–1. Recommendations for Treatment of Displaced Distal Radius Fractures

STATEMENT	LEVEL OF EVIDENCE	GRADE OF RECOMMENDATION	REFERENCES
1. Augmented bridging external fixation yields better radiographic results than closed reduction and casting or percutaneous pinning; however, validated outcomes have not been demonstrated to be different.	I	A	3, 5
2. Augmented bridging external fixation and internal fixation yield similar validated outcomes.	I, II	A	6, 7
3. Pin care using dry sterile dressings are comparable with chlorhexidine or peroxide pin care.	I	A	13
4. Volar locked plating and nonlocked volar plating do not demonstrate differences in outcome.	II	B	20
5. Locked volar plating and dorsal plating have been used in small cohorts with acceptable validated outcomes.	IV	C	17, 25, 26
6. It is unclear whether bridging or nonbridging external fixation yields superior results in direct comparison.	I, II	I	8, 9

REFERENCES

1. Handoll HH, Madhok R: Surgical interventions for treating distal radial fractures in adults. Cochrane Database Syst Rev (3):CD003209, 2003.
2. Handoll HH, Madhok R: Surgical interventions for treating distal radial fractures in adults. Cochrane Database Syst Rev (3):CD003209, 2001.
3. Kreder HJ, Agel J, McKee MD, et al: A randomized, controlled trial of distal radius fractures with metaphyseal displacement but without joint incongruity: Closed reduction and casting versus closed reduction, spanning external fixation, and optional percutaneous K-wires. J Orthop Trauma 20:115–121, 2006.
4. Azzopardi T, Ehrendorfer S, Coulton T, et al: Unstable extra-articular fractures of the distal radius. J Bone Joint Surg Br 87:837–840, 2005.
5. Harley BJ, Scharfenberger A, Beaupre LA, et al: Augmented external fixation versus percutaneous pinning and casting for unstable fractures of the distal radius—A prospective randomized trial. J Hand Surg [Am] 29:815–824, 2004.
6. Grewal R, Perey B, Wilmink M et al: A randomized prospective study on the treatment of intra-articular distal radius fractures: Open reduction and internal fixation with dorsal plating versus mini open reduction, percutaneous fixation, and external fixation. J Hand Surg [Am] 30:764–772, 2005.
7. Kreder HJ, Hanel DP, Agel J, et al: Indirect reduction and percutaneous fixation versus open reduction and internal fixation for displaced intra-articular fractures of the radius. J Bone Joint Surg Br 87:829–836, 2005.
8. McQueen MM: Redisplaced unstable fractures of the distal radius: A randomized, prospective study of bridging versus non-bridging external fixation. J Bone Joint Surg Br 80:665–669, 1998.
9. Atroshi I, Brogren E, Larsson G-U, et al: Wrist-bridging versus non-bridging external fixation for displaced distal radius fractures: A randomized assessor-blind clinical trial of 38 patients followed for 1 year. Acta Orthop 77:445–453, 2006.
10. Sanchez-Sotelo J, Munuera L, Madero R: Treatment of fractures of the distal radius with a remodellable bone cement: A prospective randomized study using Norian SRS. J Bone Joint Surg Br 82:856–863, 2000.
11. Cassidy C, Jupiter JB, Cohen M, et al: Norian SRS cement compared with conventional fixation in distal radial fractures. J Bone Joint Surg Am 85:2127–2136, 2003.
12. Werber KD, Raeder F, Brauer RB, et al: External fixation of distal radial fractures: Four compared with five pins: A randomized prospective study. J Bone Joint Surg Am 85:660–666, 2003.
13. Egol KA, Paksima N, Puopolo S, et al: Treatment of external fixation pins about the wrist: A prospective, randomized trial. J Bone Joint Surg Am 88:349–354, 2006.
14. Ring D, Jupiter JB, Brennwald J, et al: Prospective multicenter trial of a plate for dorsal fixation of distal radius fractures. J Hand Surg [Am] 22:777–784, 1997.
15. Orbay, JL, Fernandez DL: Volar fixation for dorsally displaced fractures of the distal radius: A preliminary report. J Hand Surg [Am] 27:205–215, 2002.
16. Orbay JL, Fernandez DL: Volar fixed-angle plate fixation for unstable distal radius fractures in the elderly patient. J Hand Surg [Am] 29:96–102, 2004.
17. Simic PM, Robison J, Gardner MJ, et al: Treatment of distal radius fractures with a low-profile dorsal plating system: An outcomes assessment. J Hand Surg [Am] 31:382–386, 2006.
18. Benson LS, Minihane KP, Stern LD, et al: The outcome of intra-articular distal radius fractures treated with fragment-specific fixation. J Hand Surg [Am] 31:1333–1339, 2006.
19. Ruch DS, Papadonikolakis A: Volar versus dorsal plating in the management of intra-articular distal radius fractures. J Hand Surg [Am] 31:9–16, 2006.
20. Koshimune M, Kamano M, Takamatsu K, et al: A randomized comparison of locking and non-locking palmar plating for unstable Colles' fractures in the elderly. J Hand Surg [Br] 30:499–503, 2005.
21. Handoll HH, Madhok R, Howe TE: Rehabilitation for distal radial fractures in adults. Cochrane Database Syst Rev 3: CD003324, 2006.
22. Knirk, JL, Jupiter JB: Intra-articular fractures of the distal end of the radius in young adults. J Bone Joint Surg Am 68: 647–659, 1986.
23. Young CF, Nanu AM, Checketts RG: Seven-year outcome following Colles' type distal radial fracture. A comparison of two treatment methods. J Hand Surg [Br] 28:422–426, 2003.
24. Rozental TD, Beredjiklian PK, Bozentka DJ: Functional outcome and complications following two types of dorsal plating for unstable fractures of the distal part of the radius. J Bone Joint Surg Am 85:1956–1960, 2003.
24a. Goldfarb CA, Rudzki JR, Catalano LW, Hughes M, Borrelli J Jr. Fifteen-year outcome of displaced intra-articular fractures of the distal radius. J Hand Surg [Am]. 2006 Apr; 31(4):633–639.
25. Kamath AF, Zurakowski D, Day CS: Low-profile dorsal plating for dorsally angulated distal radius fractures: An outcomes study. J Hand Surg [Am] 31:1061–1067, 2006.
26. Rozental TD, Blazar PE: Functional outcome and complications after volar plating for dorsally displaced, unstable fractures of the distal radius. J Hand Surg [Am] 31:359–365, 2006.
27. Harness NG, Jupiter JB, Orbay JL, et al: Loss of fixation of the volar lunate facet fragment in fractures of the distal part of the radius. J Bone Joint Surg Am 86:1900–1908, 2004.

What Is the Best Surgical Treatment for Early Degenerative Osteoarthritis of the Wrist?

GREG A. MERRELL, MD AND ARNOLD-PETER C. WEISS, MD

SCAPHOTRAPEZIOTRAPEZOID JOINT ARTHRITIS

Although scaphotrapeziotrapezoid (STT) arthritis may be associated with chronic scapholunate injury and rotary subluxation of the scaphoid, it is also a relatively common site of focal arthritis, particularly in older women. The two most common surgical treatments for this problem are STT arthrodesis or distal scaphoid excision.

Evidence

No randomized trials have compared STT arthrodesis with distal scaphoid excision (Level I). No prospective comparative studies (Level II) or retrospective comparative studies (Level III) exist either. What is available to make a treatment decision is a collection of case series with few patients in each. Most of the reports on STT arthrodesis combine results from patients who had a fusion for scapholunate instability or other problems with patients who had the fusion for primary STT arthritis. This amalgamation of reported data also makes interpretation of outcome difficult.

In his monumental review of 800 triscaphe fusions, Dr. Watson[1] does identify 98 patients whose arthrodesis was for primary STT arthritis. The case series review states that 62% of the patients were examined in the office and the others had data pulled from chart reviews. The mean follow-up was 3.4 years. Patients were immobilized for 3 weeks in a long arm cast, followed by 3 weeks in a short arm cast. Pain was graded by the patients as mild, moderate, or severe. The flexion extension arc was 85% and 80%, respectively, of the contralateral side. Grip strength was 77% of the other side. The results with regard to pain were not broken out independently for STT arthritis versus other indications for STT fusion. The rate of nonunion across all indications for STT arthrodesis was only 4%.

In a review of eight patients with STT arthritis, Srinivasan and Matthews[2] found four were pain free, three had pain with certain activities, and one had constant pain. The flexion extension arc averaged 115 degrees compared with 124 degrees on the uninjured side. One of the eight had a nonunion. Follow-up averaged 4 years.

Only one case series describes results of distal scaphoid excision specifically for STT arthritis.[3]

Garcia-Elias and colleagues[3] reported on 21 patients with a mean follow-up of 29 months. Patients were immobilized for 2 to 3 weeks in a short arm splint. The preoperative visual analog scale (VAS) pain score was 7.5, and the postoperative score was 0.6, with 13 having no pain. Grip improved from 57% of the contralateral side preoperatively to 83% of the contralateral side after surgery. Wrist flexion averaged 57 degrees and wrist extension averaged 61 degrees. The radiolunate angle increased from 9 degrees before surgery to 17 degrees after surgery.

RECOMMENDATIONS

In conclusion, a paucity of clinical data exists with which to make informed treatment decisions for primary STT arthritis. There is some intuitive attraction to the simplicity, low complication rate, and early return to function of a distal scaphoid excision. However, cause for concern also exists with this procedure because the longer term impact of an increased dorsal intercalated segment instability carpal position that appears to develop after distal scaphoid excision is unknown. Therefore, for primary STT arthritis, we believe it is not appropriate to make a recommendation for treatment. Surgeons must take into account their experience base, the age of the patient, and other variables to decide on the best course of action.

SCAPHOLUNATE ADVANCED COLLAPSE AND SCAPHOID NON-UNION ADVANCED COLLAPSE

Scapholunate advanced collapse (SLAC) wrist is the most common post-traumatic form of arthritis in the wrist and follows a predictable progression of arthrosis. Scaphoid nonunion advanced collapse (SNAC) wrist follows the same pattern of arthrosis, although it is less common. As evidenced by the numerous treatments proposed for these forms of arthritis, the best surgical option remains a source of considerable debate.

The two most common surgical options for chronic SLAC and SNAC wrist are either a proximal row carpectomy (PRC) or a four-corner (Capitate–Lunate–Hamate–Triquetrum) fusion. Proponents of PRC point to its technical simplicity, decreased time for immobilization, and lack of nonunion risk. Proponents of four-corner fusion highlight the maintenance of physiologic carpal height and a congruent radiolunate joint, which may theoretically allow a more durable articulation.

Evidence

No randomized trials have compared PRC with a four-corner fusion (Level I). No prospective comparative studies exist (Level II). Four retrospective comparative studies (Level III) have been reported, only one of which has a methodology that would minimize patient selection bias and the results of which might therefore be valid.[4–7]

The highest quality study, by Cohen and Kozin[4] in 2001, retrospectively examined 2 cohorts of 19 patients at different institutions, which performed exclusively either PRC or four-corner fusions. Importantly, there were no preoperative differences with regard to age, sex, stage of arthritis, or preoperative pain or function. All patients were stage II, except one four-corner patient who was stage III. The most significant limitation is that the follow-up averaged 19 months for the PRC group and 28 months for the four-corner group. Typically, these procedures are performed on patients with the hope of decades of postoperative functionality, thus any conclusion based on 2 years of follow-up is limited. Nevertheless, it avoids the selection bias in other comparative studies where patients had one or the other procedure based on surgeon preference.

The authors found no statistical difference in range of motion, grip strength, pain relief, or patient satisfaction. A power analysis was not included in the study. The flexion-extension arc was 81 degrees in PRC and 80 degrees in four-corner fusion. Grip strength was 71% for PRC versus 79% for four-corner fusion. VAS pain scores at follow-up were 1.4 for PRC and 1.2 for four-corner fusion. Five of the PRC patients and four of the four-corner patients took nonsteroidal anti-inflammatory drugs or analgesics for wrist pain at final follow-up. Three patients in each group changed jobs or retired because of wrist pain and function.

One nonunion patient was in the arthrodesis cohort, which had a successful repeat arthrodesis. One patient with PRC had persistent pain and went on to a total wrist fusion. Radiographic analysis of the arthrodesis group demonstrated no evidence of progression of arthritic changes at the radiolunate articulation. Although three patients in the PRC group showed narrowing or sclerosis at the radiocapitate articulation, these findings did not correlate with pain or function.

Wyrick and coworkers'[5] retrospective review of 17 patients with four-corner and 10 patients with PRC treatment with a 27-month mean follow-up showed better grip strength, range of motion, and pain relief with a PRC.[5] There were three nonunions in the arthrodesis group, only one of which was symptomatic.

However, five of the patients with four-corner fusion required revision surgery, whereas none of the patients with PRC required revision.

Tomaino and researchers'[6] retrospective review examined 15 patients with PRC and 9 patients with arthrodesis at an average of 5.5 years. Mean postoperative pain and grip scores were comparable. PRC preserved a greater arc of motion, 77 versus 52 degrees for arthrodesis. Three patients with PRC treatment were unsatisfied, and one went on to a wrist fusion.

Krakauer and coauthors' retrospective review[7] compares results of mostly stage II PRC patients with mostly stage III four-corner patients and is therefore not believed to be helpful in providing a valid comparison of the two procedures.

RECOMMENDATIONS

Sufficient data are not available with which to make a recommendation of either a four-corner fusion or PRC for stage II SLAC or SNAC wrist. A multicenter, long-term, randomized trial would clearly be helpful and most likely achievable. The fact that four-corner fusion has been used since the 1980s and PRC for many years more, and that a Level III comparison is the best available in the orthopedic literature are perhaps characteristic of the overall quality of the orthopedic literature. This should be a wake-up call or a source of embarrassment for the orthopedic community, or both.

In the absence of better clinical trial data, there are some patient specific factors that may tip the scales one way or the other. The lack of long-term arthritic changes in a four-corner fusion and the presence of some arthritic progression in a PRC perhaps because of noncongruent articulations, even if asymptomatic, may suggest a four-corner fusion would be preferable for a young patient. That being said, the definition of what constitutes a "young" patient is up for debate and should really be based on the patient's physiologic rather than absolute chronologic age. On the other end of the spectrum, an older patient, lower demand patient, or smoker may be better suited for a PRC. In patients who have poor quality bone stock, a PRC may be favored because of the fixation requirements in a four-corner fusion.

OSTEOARTHRITIS OF THE DISTAL RADIOULNAR JOINT

Osteoarthritic changes at the distal radioulnar joint (DRUJ) are a challenging surgical dilemma. Our understanding of the anatomy and biomechanics of the joint and the related surgical options have increased substantially over the past two decades. In this analysis, we are focusing specifically on osteoarthritis of the DRUJ and not ulnocarpal impingement or other causes of ulnar-sided wrist pain and arthrosis. The most common surgical techniques have been complete distal resection (Darrach), hemiresection (with or without soft tissue interposition), Sauve–Kapandji (SK), or prosthetic replacement.

Evidence

No randomized trials have compared the surgical treatments for osteoarthritis of the DRUJ (Level I). No prospective comparative studies exist (Level II). One retrospective comparative study exists (Level III), which has serious methodologic flaws, as well as numerous case series (Level IV) with which to evaluate these procedures.

Minami and colleagues[8] retrospectively compare the results of 20 Darrach resections with 25 SK and 16 hemiresections for DRUJ osteoarthritis. The follow-up was impressively a minimum of 5 years and a mean of 8 of 11 years. The authors originally performed Darrach resections on all patients with symptomatic DRUJ osteoarthritis. Later, they performed SK procedures if the triangular fibrocartilage complex (TFCC) could not be reconstructed or there was positive ulnar variance of greater than 5 mm. If the TFCC was intact or reconstructible, a hemiresection with interposition (e.g., Bowers) was performed. Unfortunately, the Darrach resection group was older (68 versus 53 SK or 60 hemiresections), and 75% were arthritic changes caused by prior distal radius trauma, whereas only about 25% of the SK and hemiresection group conditions were due to secondary osteoarthritis and 75% were due to primary or idiopathic osteoarthritis. No ordinal preoperative pain scoring is available with which to compare postoperative pain results. These points make any comparison of postoperative pain, grip, or range of motion questionable. Of note, 40% of patients who had undergone Darrach resections had no postoperative pain, 20% had slight pain, 25% had moderate pain, and 15% had severe pain. Grip strength decreased in 65% of patients with a Darrach resection.

Watson and Gabuzda[9] reviewed results from 32 patients with matched hemiresection without interposition for post-traumatic osteoarthritis of the DRUJ. Two patients in the series had Madelung's deformity, and three had previously undergone a Darrach procedure. Twenty-one were examined personally and 11 by telephone. Follow-up averaged 51 months. Of the 21 patients examined, 6 experienced residual pain at the DRUJ. Of the 11 questioned by telephone, 5 had no pain, 3 had mild pain, 2 had moderate pain, and 1 had severe pain. Revisions for radioulnar impingement were performed on three patients.

Van Schoonhoven and coworkers[10] evaluated 36 patients with matched hemiresection with interposition for post-traumatic osteoarthritis of the DRUJ with an average follow-up of 34 months. Preoperative pain scores measured 7.8, whereas postoperative scores were 3.9. Grip strength improved from 40% to 64% of the uninjured side. In 21 patients, radioulnar impingement was observed and required revision in 5 patients.

Lamey and Fernandez[11] report on 18 patients with post-traumatic osteoarthritic changes of the DRUJ treated with a modified SK procedure. Follow-up averaged 4 years. Supination improved dramatically from 16 degrees before surgery to 76 degrees after surgery, and pronation improved from 42 to 81 degrees. Grip strength went from 36% of the unaffected side to 73% of the unaffected side. Fifteen patients reported no pain in the area of the DRUJ, and three reported mild pain with rotation. Eleven patients had repeat operations, primarily for removal of hardware. The ulnar stump was reported as stable in 16 patients.

The use of ulnar head prosthesis for salvage of failed distal ulnar resections has been reported. Results of ulnar head prosthetics for salvage or primary indications has been promising. For example, Schecker and Severo[12] reported on 23 patients, but with a mean follow-up of only 15 months. All 23 patients were reported to be free of pain with a normal pronation/supination arc. Eight of the 13 patients who were out of work because of DRUJ disability returned to work. Implant longevity, given the short follow-up of most of these case series on prosthetic options, continues to be a concern.

RECOMMENDATIONS

Persistent pain or stump instability continues to plague most proposed treatments for DRUJ arthritis. If the newer generation of ulnar head prosthetic replacements demonstrates durable results with time, they may be a preferred solution for some patients. The data to support any of these prosthetics in general or to support the preferential use of one prosthesis over another certainly does not exist yet. Table 12–1 provides a summary of recommendations.

TABLE 12–1. Summary of Recommendations

CONDITION	GRADE	RECOMMENDATION
STT arthritis	I	Insufficient evidence exists to allow a recommendation for or against STT arthrodesis versus distal scaphoid excision for the treatment of primary STT arthritis.
SLAC/SNAC	I	Insufficient evidence exist to suggest a PRC or a four-corner arthrodesis as the preferable treatment for stage II arthritic changes in a SLAC or SNAC wrist.
DRUJ arthritis	I	Insufficient evidence exists to suggest a preferred treatment for osteoarthritis of the DRUJ.

DRUJ, distal radioulnar joint; PRC, proximal row carpectomy; SLAC, scapholunate advanced collapse; SNAC, scaphoid nonunion advanced collapse; STT, scaphotrapeziotrapezoid.

REFERENCES

1. Watson KH, Wollstein R, Joseph E, et al: Scaphotrapeziotrapezoid arthrodesis: A follow-up study. J Hand Surg [Am] 28:397–404, 2003.
2. Srinivasan VB, Matthews JP: Results of scaphotrapeziotrapeziod fusion for isolated idiopathic arthritis. J Hand Surg [Br] 21:378–380, 1996.
3. Garcia-Elias M, Lluch AL, Farreres A, et al: Resection of the distal scaphoid for scaphotrapeziotrapezoid osteoarthritis. J Hand Surg [Br] 24:448–452, 1999.
4. Cohen MS, Kozin SH: Degenerative arthritis of the wrist: Proximal row carpectomy versus scaphoid excision and four-corner arthrodesis. J Hand Surg [Am] 26:94–104, 2001.
5. Wyrick JD, Stern PJ, Kiefhaber TR: Motion-preserving procedures in the treatment of scapholunate advanced collapse wrist: Proximal row carpectomy versus four-corner arthrodesis. J Hand Surg [Am] 20:965–970, 1995.
6. Tomaino MW, Miller RJ, Cole I, Burton R: Scapholunate advanced collapse wrist: Proximal row carpectomy or limited wrist arthrodesis with scaphoid excision. J Hand Surg [Am] 19:134–142, 199.
7. Krakauer JD, Bishop AT, Cooney WP: Surgical treatment of scapholunate advanced collapse. J Hand Surg [Am] 19:751–759, 1994.
8. Minami A, Iwasaki N, Ishikawa J, et al: Treatments of osteoarthritis of the distal radioulnar joint: Long-term results of three procedures. Hand Surg 10:243–248, 2005.
9. Watson KW, Gabuzda GM: Matched distal ulna resection for posttraumatic disorders of the distal radioulnar joint. J Hand Surg [Am] 17:724–730, 1992.
10. Van Schoonhoven J, Kall S, Schober F, et al: The Hemiresection-interposition arthroplasty as a salvage procedure for the arthrotically destroyed distal radioulnar joint. Handchir 35:175–180, 2003.
11. Lamey DM, Fernandez DL: Results of the modified Sauve-Kapandji procedure in the treatment of chronic posttraumatic derangement of the distal radioulnar joint. J Bone Joint Surg Am 80:1758–1769, 1998.
12. Schecker LR, Severo A: Ulnar shortening for the treatment of early post-traumatic osteoarthritis at the distal radioulnar joint. J Hand Surg 26:41–44, 2001.

Chapter 13

What Is the Best Treatment for Acute Injuries of the Scapholunate Ligament?

Paul Binhammer, MSc, MD, FRCS(C)

The scapholunate (SL) ligament is the fibrous structure that links the scaphoid and lunate bones of the wrist. It is composed of a thick and strong dorsal portion, a more pliable anterior portion, and finally an intervening membranous segment. It is the dorsal portion that plays the most important role for carpal stability.

Injury to the ligament usually occurs as a result of a fall on an outstretched hand resulting in wrist hyperextension, ulnar deviation, and midcarpal supination. Although the ligament can be injured in isolation, and the diagnosis missed, it can also be injured with fractures of the distal radius or scaphoid, which should raise clinical suspicion just as in perilunate dislocations.

Diagnosis of scapholunate dissociation (SLD) can usually be made on physical and radiologic examinations. Physical examination usually demonstrates localized tenderness and a positive scaphoid shift test. If there is a complete tear, radiologic findings may include an increased SL joint space and a "ring" sign where the scaphoid has an overlying ring or circle projection caused by its volar flexion deformity. Other tools that aid in the diagnosis are cineradiography, arthroscopy, and arthrography.

An acute injury to the SL ligament alters the linkage between the two bones resulting in a dissociative carpal instability, also known as an SLD. This can present clinically in a variety of stages depending on the severity of the original injury and the delay to clinical diagnosis. There is no consensus for the nomenclature for the various patterns of severity of SL injuries. Predynamic SLD is a partial injury where the ligament remains intact. Symptoms arise from the associated increase motion, but there is no instability. Dynamic SLD is a complete disruption of the ligament when it is still repairable. No cartilage damage exists, and secondary stabilizers are intact. No permanent malalignment and demonstration of the radiographic gap between the scaphoid exists, and the lunate may require special maneuvers. The third manifestation is static reducible SLD. Secondary stabilizers have become deficient. The radiographic appearance is quite apparent, but the deformity can still be reduced. Eventually, the insufficiency results in static fixed SLD where it cannot be reduced. Finally, there is progression to degenerative arthritis

with cartilage loss resulting in scapholunate advanced collapse (SLAC) wrist.[1] The rationale for treatment of acute SL injuries is to prevent the progression to a SLAC wrist.

SURGICAL TREATMENT OPTIONS

Acute injuries to the SL ligament are either predynamic or dynamic. Predynamic injuries may not always present acutely because the ligament is still intact and the time to diagnosis can be delayed. In acute predynamic cases, treatment is directed toward giving the stretched ligaments time to heal. The options indicated in the literature for management are either percutaneous fixation or arthroscopically guided fixation of the SL joint.

Dynamic SL injuries can present a spectrum of injury patterns to the ligament and have a variety of treatment. The ligament injury can be midsubstance, avulsed with or without bone. The quality of the ligament available for repair is also variable. The available options for treatment are closed reduction and cast immobilization, open reduction internal fixation and repair of the dorsal SL ligament, dorsal radioscaphoid capsulodesis, and other forms of acute reconstruction.

EVIDENCE

Predynamic Injuries

For acute predynamic SL injuries, this is primarily a diagnosis based on findings at the time of arthroscopy, and consistent symptoms and physical examination. No series in the literature have examined treatment of these patients conservatively either by observation alone or by casting. The evidence for percutaneous fixation for these injuries is limited to management review articles and book chapters.[2–4]

The evidence for arthroscopically guided fixation for acute incomplete injuries is also lacking. Studies for chronic symptoms and arthroscopic management of various types of wrist injuries have been reported; however, there are no acute injury case series.[5–8] Whipple[9] reported a non–peer-reviewed article on arthroscopically guided pin fixation in a series of 40 patients. In a subgroup of these 40 patients, with less than a 3-mm gap and less than 3 months of symptoms, 83% experienced symptom relief. However, the size of this subgroup and the severity of SL injury are not identified, and neither is the time from injury. Hirsh and colleagues[10] have reported on arthroscopic electrothermal shrinkage for SL laxity in 10 patients, of which there were 2 that were less than 6 weeks after injury. The outcomes for these two patients are unclear.

Dynamic Injuries

Cast Immobilization. Two case reports of successful management of an SLD associated with a distal radius fracture (DRF) managed by closed reduction and casting have been reported.[11,12] However, Tang and coworkers,[13] in a series of 20 patients with DRF and SLD, found at 1 year that 100% had clinical signs and positive radiographs. Eight patients underwent surgery at 1 year. Laulan and Bismuth,[14] in a radiographic study of DRF in 29 patients with an SL injury treated by casting alone, found at 1 year that progressive carpal collapse occurred in 61% of patients.

K-Wire Fixation. Treatment by temporary K-wire fixation alone has been reported by Peicha and coauthors[15] in 11 patients. These all had concomitant intra-articular DRF. The 11 patients had a spectrum of SL injuries including 2 cartilage injuries, 7 partial ligament tears, and 2 complete ligament tears. They had follow-up on 6 patients, but the results are not published in relation to the type of injury. The study was updated in 1999 with a total of 12 patients. The number of cartilage injuries had changed to one, and there were two complete and nine partial SL injuries. Seven patients were available for follow-up. Results are not provided for the injury groups except for three scales where the complete injuries score are worse.

K-wire fixation for SLD has been reported in a series of 27 cases.[16] In this series, the recurrence SL instability was found in 15 cases. The authors did not recommend this treatment for all cases but rather treatment to be tailored to severity of presentation.

Ligament Repair with or without Capsulodesis. Ligament repair in acute cases has been reported using a Mitek anchor.[17] There were 12 cases; however, only 2 were isolated SLDs, with the other being more complex perilunate injuries. It is not possible to determine the outcome of these two patients.

Ligament repair has been reported in children. Alt and coauthors[18] describe ligament repair in three children at approximately 10 weeks. Successful, pain-free, full-function outcomes were reported at about 28 months after surgery.

Many articles reference Lavernia and colleagues'[19] study. In this series of 24 cases, there were 24 patients treated with records for 21. The average time from injury to surgery was 17 months, so most of these records were not acute. Four had only a ligament repair, 14 repair and capsulodesis, and 3 a capsulodesis alone because the ligament was only attenuated. Patients did well at an average 33-month follow-up with regard to grip strength, pain, and satisfaction. It is not possible to determine the outcomes for the patients with acute injuries.

Wyrick and coworkers[20] have reported on their experience with 24 patients treated on average 3 months after injury (range, 3 days to 16 months). Follow-up was available for 17 patients at an average of 30 months; 13 had repair of the ligament and capsulodesis, and 4 had only a ligament repair. No patient was pain free, and four required further surgery. It is not possible to determine results in relation to time from injury.

In a study examining ligament repair and capsulodesis, Minami and coauthors[21] report on 17 patients with wrist ligament injuries; however, only 6 had an isolated SLD, and only 4 could be considered acute or subacute (15–45 days). These four patients did have reported good outcomes.

Other studies in the literature that examine outcomes of soft-tissue stabilization for chronic SLD, similar to Lavernia and colleagues'[19] study, have reported favorable results using similar surgical techniques.[22–25] However, these do not include acute management, and the spectrum of injury severity is variable. The different outcomes in the studies promote a favorable outcome for patients.

OTHER TYPES OF RECONSTRUCTION

Other forms of reconstruction have been described for the chronic state; however, their use in acute repair is quite limited.[26–28] A bone-retinaculum-bone flap taken from the dorsal distal radius has been reported in 19 cases, 2 of which were acute injuries.[23] For these two patients at a minimum follow-up at 24 months, one had no pain and the other had pain with heavy activity. Further specific results were unavailable.

A periosteal flap from the iliac crest has also been used acutely. Lutz and colleagues[28] describe its reconstruction in 11 cases at an average of 15 months after trauma, 3 of which they describe as subacute, less than 6 weeks.[24] It is not possible to determine the specific results for the acute group. Six of 11 were rated excellent to good results.

RECOMMENDATIONS

Predynamic

No strong evidence exists in the literature for the treatment of any kind in the predynamic injury subgroup of patients. There is also no clear understanding of the natural history of this condition if left untreated. Therefore, no specific recommendation for treatment of patients diagnosed with this specific injury currently can be offered.

Dynamic

For patients with dynamic injuries, it would appear from my understanding of the natural history of this condition that no treatment will lead to progressive collapse over time, and this is unacceptable. The available case series indicate that cast immobilization alone does not alter the natural history. K-wire fixation series are limited, and this treatment does not appear to be of benefit because recurrence is more than likely.

The case series of more aggressive forms of surgical intervention for acute SLD do not provide a clear picture of the outcomes. The time to treatment, severity of injury, and the form of intervention are all variable and make interpretation difficult. However, it would appear that, on average, patients who had some form of surgical reconstruction/repair, capsulodesis and ligament repair being most common, were more likely to have a better outcome than cast immobilization or K-wire fixation alone. No clear evidence supports one form of surgical repair/reconstruction. Therefore, for patients with acute dynamic injuries, the recommendation would be that they undergo repair/reconstruction. Table 13–1 provides a summary of recommendations for the treatment of SLD.

TABLE 13–1. Summary of Recommendations

STATEMENT	LEVEL OF EVIDENCE/GRADE OF RECOMMENDATION
Adults with acute dynamic scapholunate dissociation should have ligament repair/reconstruction. There is no evidence to support a specific technique of ligament repair/reconstruction.	C

REFERENCES

1. Garcia-Elias M, Geissler WB: Carpal instability. In Green DP, Pederson WC, Hotchkiss RN, Wolfe SW (eds): Green's Operative Hand Surgery. Philadelphia, Elsevier Churchill Livingstone, 2005, p 555.
2. Linscheid RL: Scapholunate ligamentous instabilities (dissociations, subdislocations, dislocations). Ann Chir Main 3:323–330, 1984.
3. O'Brien ET: Acute fractures and dislocations of the carpus. Orthop Clin North Am 15:237–258, 1984.
4. Taleisnik J: Scapholunate dissociation. In Strickland JW, Steichen JB (eds): Difficult Problems in Hand Surgery. St. Louis, CV Mosby, 1982, pp 341–348.
5. Ruch DS, Poehling GG: Arthroscopic management of partial scapholunate and lunotriquetral injuries of the wrist. J Hand Surg [Am] 21:412–417, 1996.
6. Westkaemper JG, Mitsianis G, Giannakopoulas PN: Wrist arthroscopy for the treatment of ligament and triangular fibrocartilage complex injuries. Arthroscopy 14:479–483, 1998.
7. Weiss AP, Sachar K, Glowacki KA: Arthroscopic debridement alone for intercarpal ligament tears. J Hand Surg [Am] 22: 344–349, 1997.
8. Earp BE, Waters PM, Wyzykowski RJ: Arthroscopic treatment of partial scapholunate ligament tears in children with chronic wrist pain. J Bone Joint Surg Am 88:2448–2455, 2006.
9. Whipple TL: The role of arthroscopy in the treatment of scapholunate instability. Hand Clin 11:37–40, 1995.
10. Hirsh L, Sodha S, Bozentka D, et al: Arthroscopic electrothermal collagen shrinkage for symptomatic laxity of the scapholunate interosseous ligament. J Hand Surg [Br] 30:643–647, 2005.
11. King RJ: Scapholunate diastasis associated with a Barton fracture treated by manipulation, or Terry-Thomas and the wine waiter. J R Soc Med 76:421–423, 1983.
12. Bell MJ: Perilunar dislocation of the carpus and an associated Colles' fracture. Hand 15:262–266, 1983.
13. Tang JB, Shi D, Gu YQ, Zhang QG: Can cast immobilization successfully treat scapholunate dissociation associated with distal radius fractures? J Hand Surg [Am] 21:583–590, 1996.
14. Laulan J, Bismuth JP: Intracarpal ligamentous lesions associated with fractures of the distal radius: Outcome at one year. A prospective study of 95 cases. Acta Orthop Belg 65: 418–423, 1999.
15. Peicha G, Seibert FJ, Fellinger M, et al: Lesions of the scapholunate ligaments in acute wrist trauma—arthroscopic diagnosis and minimally invasive treatment. Knee Surg Sports Traumatol Arthrosc 5:176–183, 1997.
16. Schadel-Hopfner M, Bohringer G, Gotzen L: Results after minimally invasive therapy of acute scapholunate dissociation. Handchir Mikrochir Plast Chir 32:333–338, 2000.
17. Bickert B, Sauerbier M, Germann G: Scapholunate ligament repair using the Mitek bone anchor. J Hand Surg [Br] 25: 188–192, 2000.
18. Alt V, Gasnier J, Sicre G: Injuries of the scapholunate ligament in children. J Ped Orthop 13:326–329, 2004.
19. Lavernia CJ, Cohen MS, Taleisnik J: Treatment of scapholunate dissociation by ligamentous repair and capsulodesis. J Hand Surg [Am] 17:354–359, 1992.
20. Wyrick JD, Youse BD, Kiefhaber TR: Scapholunate ligament repair and capsulodesis for the treatment of static scapholunate dissociation. J Hand Surg [Br] 23:776–780, 1998.
21. Minami A, Kato H, Iwasaki N: Treatment of scapholunate dissociation: Ligamentous repair associated with modified dorsal capsulodesis. Hand Surg 8:1–6, 2003.
22. Pomerance J: Outcome after repair of the scapholunate interosseous ligament and dorsal capsulodesis for dynamic scapholunate instability due to trauma. J Hand Surg [Am] 31:1380–1386, 2006.
23. Shih J-T, Lee H-M, Hou Y-T, et al: Dorsal capsulodesis and ligamentoplasty for chronic pre-dynamic and dynamic scapholunate dissociation. Hand Surg 8:173–178, 2003.
24. Muermans S, De Smet L, Van Ransbeeck H: Blatt dorsal capsulodesis for scapholunate instability. Acta Orthop Belg 65:434–439, 1999.
25. Saffar P, Sokolow C, Duclos L: Soft tissue stabilization in the management of chronic scapholunate instability without osteoarthritis. A 15-year series. Acta Orthop Belg 65:424–433, 1999.
26. Garcia-Elias M, Lluch AL, Stanley JK: Three-ligament tenodesis for the treatment of scapholunate dissociation: Indications and surgical technique. J Hand Surg [Am] 31:125–134, 2006.
27. Weiss AP: Scapholunate ligament reconstruction using a bone-retinaculum-bone autograft. J Hand Surg [Am] 23:205–215, 1998.
28. Lutz M, Kralinger F, Goldhahn J, et al: Dorsal scapholunate ligament reconstruction using a periosteal flap of the iliac crest. Arch Orthop Trauma Surg 124:197–202, 2004.

What Is the Best Method of Rehabilitation after Flexor Tendon Repair in Zone II: Passive Mobilization or Early Active Motion? What Is the Best Suture Configuration for Repair of Flexor Tendon Lacerations?

KYLE A. MITSUNAGA, MD AND ROBERT M. SZABO, MD, MPH

Restoration of satisfactory digital function after flexor tendon laceration and repair continues to be one of the most difficult problems in hand surgery. Early efforts to improve the performance of flexor tendon repairs are largely based on individual anecdotal experience, historical precedence, and clinical experimentation with little or no scientific support. Methods to repair flexor tendons have undergone a notable evolution since the 1950s. Early primary repair of flexor tendons in zone II, once called "no man's land," has replaced tendon grafting as the standard of care. Rehabilitation after repair of flexor tendon injuries has also evolved from complete immobilization to early passive motion and now early active motion. Nonetheless, the optimal treatment of a flexor tendon laceration in zone II remains an unresolved challenge for hand surgeons to define.[1] The basic tenet of current and historical investigative efforts has been to improve the strength of tendon repair to allow for earlier motion, thereby preventing adhesion formation. Recent studies have contributed to a better understanding of the biology of flexor tendon injuries, improved methods of tendon repair, a greater emphasis on flexor sheath and pulley management, and the development of early controlled motion rehabilitation protocols leading to better clinical results.[2] The purpose of this chapter is to provide a concise review of Level I and II studies on flexor tendon injury repair techniques and postoperative rehabilitation protocols.

TENDON REPAIR CONSIDERATIONS

During early phases of tendon healing, repair site strength is primarily dependent on the strength of the suture repair method. Strickland[2] describes six principles of an ideal repair: (1) easy placement of sutures in the tendon, (2) secure suture knots, (3) smooth juncture of tendon ends, (4) minimal gapping at the repair site, (5) minimal interference with tendon vascularity, and (6) sufficient strength throughout healing to permit the application of early motion stress to the tendon.[2] To satisfy these characteristics and therefore permit earlier active tendon mobilization, various suture techniques have been described that reportedly provide increased strength. Initial repair-site strength is roughly proportional to the intrinsic properties of the type of suture used, the number of suture strands traversing the repair site, and the number of grasping loops incorporated into the repair. Currently, hand surgeons agree that flexor tendon repairs should include a grasping or locking suture within the tendon, the "core" suture, and a continuous circumferential or "epitendinous" suture around the laceration site (Level IV). Addition of an epitendinous finishing suture has been shown to be of benefit in providing added tensile strength and gap resistance, as well as preventing triggering from uneven suture lines (Level IV).

CORE SUTURE CONFIGURATION

Early reports of active motion of tendons repaired with conventional two-strand repair documented rupture rates of up to 10%. Traditional two-strand suture methods are not sufficiently strong to consistently allow for early active digital motion. For this reason, several multistrand tendon suture techniques have been described. These techniques include the Kessler, Tajima, Savage, Lee, Tsuge, Tang, Sandow, and cruciate repair of Wolfe.[3–8] Recent in vitro studies have evaluated the biomechanical properties of various suture methods for flexor tendon repair in the canine model. Increased ultimate strength of repair was reported for the multistrand and multiple-grasping methods of Lee (38 N), Savage (53 N), and an eight-strand technique.[9] In vivo analysis demonstrated significant increases in strength for multistrand repair methods compared with traditional two-strand repairs at both 3 and 6 weeks in canine models. Reported ultimate strength values for an eight-strand repair was 52.6 and 70.9 N at 3 and 6 weeks, respectively.[10] Ex vivo and in vivo studies in human and canine models suggest that core suture configurations with the greatest tensile strength are those in which there are multiple sites of tendon suture interaction. The addition of a circumferential suture may increase the strength of core repairs by 10% to 50%, reduce gapping between tendon ends, and smooth the repair site.[11] Other variables shown to have a positive effect on the repair strength include a dorsovolar location of the core suture, adding locking or grasping stitches, and increasing the cross-sectional area of tendon that is grasped or locked by the redirecting loop of suture.[12] Ex vivo human model studies have demonstrated that greater strength is achieved with more dorsal rather than volar placement of the core suture within the tendon.[13-15] Positioning the redirecting loop of the core suture to "lock" rather than "grasp" the tendon stumps and increasing the number of suture locks or grasps further provides greater tensile strength of the repair site.[16,17]

Schuind and colleagues[18] report forces across flexor tendons of 0.9 kilogram force (kgf; 8.9 N) and 3.5 kgf (34.4 N) for passive and active digital motion, respectively, in an in vivo study of patients undergoing carpal tunnel surgery (Table 14–1). These values increased significantly to 12 kgf (117.5 N) with fingertip pinch.

TABLE 14–1. Forces That Occur in Finger Flexor Tendons

TYPE	KILOGRAMS FORCE	NEWTONS
Passive mobilization of wrist	0.6	5.9
Passive mobilization of fingers	0.9	8.9
Unresisted active mobilization of wrist	0.4	3.9
Unresisted active mobilization of fingers	3.5	34.4
Grasp (flexor digitorum profundus)	6.4	62.9
Tip pinch	12.0	117.5

Data from Schuind F, Garcia-Elias M, Cooney WP 3rd, An KN: Flexor tendon forces: In vivo measurements. J Hand Surg [Am] 17:291–298, 1992.

Urbaniak and coauthors[19] report an average tension in a human profundus tendon to be 14.7 N and found that tensile strength of tendon repairs decreases to approximately one fifth of its initial strength at 1 week. Taking into account increased resistance from edema after surgery and a decrease in suture strength during the initial weeks after repair, Urbaniak and coauthors[19] and Savage[20] therefore suggest that initial repair strength equal or exceed five times the average tension, 73.5 N, to withstand gentle or moderate active finger motion. To this end, numerous published investigations base treatment recommendations on Urbaniak[19] and Schuind's[18] reported in vivo force values.

Tang and coworkers[21] demonstrate in a human cadaver study that four newly developed suture methods (Fig. 14–1), the Tang, Silfverskiöld, Robertson, and cruciate, were biomechanically superior to the modified Kessler suture method when subjected to mechanical loads using the Instron tensile machine.

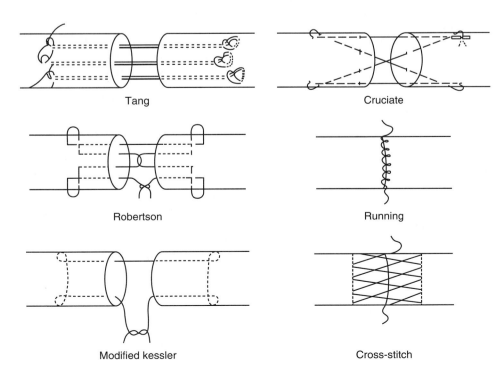

Tang

Cruciate

Robertson

Running

Modified kessler

Cross-stitch

FIGURE 14-1. Schematic illustration of tendon suture techniques. (Adapted from Tang JB, Gu YT, Rice K, et al: Evaluation of four methods of flexor tendon repair for postoperative active mobilization. Plast Reconstr Surg 107: 742–749, 2001, by permission.)

TABLE 14–2. Gap Formation Force, Ultimate Strength, and Energy to Failure of Repaired Tendons (Mean ± Standard Deviation)

| METHOD | SUTURE STRENGTH (N) | | ELASTIC MODULUS (N/mm) | ENERGY TO FAILURE (J) |
	2-mm GAP	ULTIMATE		
Tang	43.0 ± 3.5	53.6 ± 4.7	5.0 ± 0.4	0.30 ± 0.06
Cruciate	37.4 ± 3.8	46.3 ± 3.8	4.5 ± 0.3	0.26 ± 0.04
Robertson	25.0 ± 2.8	41.6 ± 3.9	3.1 ± 0.3	0.16 ± 0.03
Silfverskiöld	32.3 ± 4.7	41.0 ± 3.8	3.8 ± 0.3	0.19 ± 0.03
Kessler	21.2 ± 4.0	24.7 ± 3.0	3.1 ± 0.3	0.90 ± 0.02

Data from Tang JB, Gu YT, Rice K, et al: Evaluation of four methods of flexor tendon repair for postoperative active mobilization. Plast Reconstr Surg 107:742–749, 2001.

The Tang method possessed the greatest ultimate strength (53.6 N), 2-mm gap formation force (43.0 N), energy to failure, and capacity to resist tendon deformation among the five tested techniques. The cruciate method showed statistically higher tensile strength and energy to failure compared with the Robertson, Silfverskiöld, and modified Kessler methods. The gap formation force, ultimate strength, elastic modulus, and energy to failure were lowest for the modified Kessler method (Table 14–2).

Labana and investigators[22] similarly evaluated the biomechanical properties of three types of repairs—the standard Kessler–Tajima, double-loop (four-strand) modified Tsuge, and triple-loop (six-strand) modified Tsuge—in a human cadaver study. After subjecting the various repairs to mechanical testing using the Instron machine, the authors showed that the six-strand Tsuge suture was significantly stronger than both repairs, and that the four-strand Tsuge was significantly stronger than the Kessler–Tajima suture in terms of force to failure and initial gapping. Supramid 4–0 was used for core stitches in the modified Tsuge repairs and braided 4–0 nylon in the Kessler–Tajima repairs. 6–0 Prolene was used for epitenon repair in all cases. Labana and investigators[22] conclude that an ultimate tensile strength of 64 N for the six-strand modified Tsuge repair and 48 N for the four-strand modified Tsuge repair exceeds the forces measured by Schuind and colleagues[18] and, therefore, should withstand early range-of-motion rehabilitation protocols (Table 14–3).

Xie and researchers[23] compared the biomechanical properties of three six-strand tendon repair techniques with different configurations of core sutures: the modified Savage (Sandow's method), Tang, and Lim (Fig. 14–2; Table 14–4). 4–0 Ethilon was used in the modified Savage repairs and 4–0 Supramid in the Tang and Lim repairs in addition to a 6–0 Ethilon running peripheral suture in all cases. Statistically, ultimate strength of the modified Savage (57.8 N) and Tang (60.2 N) methods were similar and significantly higher than that of the Lim method (51.3 N). Gap formation force was also greater in the Tang method compared with the modified Savage and Lim methods. In addition, results indicate a significant difference between mode of failure between the modified

Savage and the Tang or Lim methods. Tendons repaired with the modified Savage method failed predominantly by suture breakage, which suggests that this repair may be strengthened by a larger caliber suture, whereas tendons repaired with the Tang and Lim methods failed mostly by suture pullout. The results of this study demonstrate that repair strength significantly varies with different configurations of six-strand repairs, and that location, number of locking junctions, and orientation of core sutures play an important role in repair strength despite an equal number of strands crossing the repair site.

Although in vitro studies can provide basic biomechanical data concerning specific repair techniques, it is impossible to reproduce in vitro the in vivo physiologic environment in which repaired human tendons heal. The weakness of in vitro studies is that actual healing does not take place, and mechanical testing in tendons without prior trauma may not accurately account for increases in work of flexion from postsurgical edema, stiffness, and adhesion formation. Until recently, most in vitro studies used a simple linear testing model to evaluate tensile strength in terms of extra-anatomic longitudinally applied loads. Komanduri and colleagues[14] propose using a dynamic "curvilinear" human cadaver model to test the strength of tendon repairs to more accurately simulate repair strength in vivo and account for biomechanical factors such as angulation at the repair site, differential loading, and frictional interference.

Komanduri and colleagues[14] show that dorsal tendon repairs using Kessler or Bunnell core suture

TABLE 14–3. Mean Force at Failure and Force to Initial Gapping for Three Repairs

REPAIR TYPE	MEAN ULTIMATE FORCE TO FAILURE (SD), N	MEAN INITIAL GAPPING (SD), N
Kessler–Tajima	31.8 (8.8)	29.6 (9.2)
Four-strand Tsuge	48.4 (10.7)	40.7 (12.3)
Six-strand Tsuge	64.2 (11.0)	56.1 (9.7)

SD, standard deviation.
Data from Labana N, Messer T, Lautenschlager E, et al: A biomechanical analysis of the modified Tsuge suture technique for repair of flexor tendon lacerations. J Hand Surg [Br] 26:297–300, 2001.

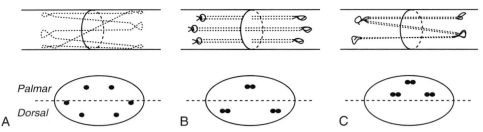

FIGURE 14–2. Schematic illustration of the configurations of tendon sutures and cross-sectional location of the strands in *(A)* modified Savage (Sandow), *(B)* Tang, and *(C)* Lim methods. (Adapted from Xie RG, Zhang S, Tang JB, Chen F: Biomechanical studies of 3 different 6-strand flexor tendon repair techniques. J Hand Surg [Am] 27:621–627, 2002, with permission of Elsevier.)

techniques were stronger than the standard volar repair.[14] Suture material was limited to 4–0 nylon core sutures and 6–0 nylon circumferential sutures. In all cases with and without epitenon repair, dorsally placed sutures provided significantly more tensile strength than palmarly placed sutures (Table 14–5).

Historically, concern has existed that crossing or cruciate sutures may not be as desirable as linear suture techniques because they may interfere with the blood supply of the tendon. In addition, the blood supply to the tendon is located in the dorsal portion of the tendon, which happens to be the stronger part of the tendon to anchor sutures. Because tendon nutrition is predominantly synovial, the effect compromising the blood supply by suture is theoretical and has not been evaluated experimentally or clinically. Expanding on Komanduri's work and using the same curvilinear model, Stein and colleagues[15] tested newer suture techniques: the Strickland, Robertson, and modified Becker. All core sutures were performed with 4–0 Ethibond and

6–0 nylon for epitenon repair. Stein and colleagues[15] demonstrate statistically significant increases in dorsal versus volar grasping strength with Kessler and Robertson repairs. No differences were found with the locking Strickland and modified Becker repairs. The four-strand techniques (Robertson and modified Becker) were also significantly stronger than the two-strand techniques (Kessler and Strickland). Wasserman and coworkers[24] further demonstrated the modified Becker repair to be significantly stronger and tougher than the modified Kessler repair whereas allowing equally efficient glide in a dynamic human cadaveric model (Table 14–6).

Based on in vivo clinical and experimental studies in canine and human models, four-strand (or higher) core suture techniques supplemented by a running epitendinous suture are recommended to achieve sufficient repair-site tensile strength to allow for postoperative passive motion rehabilitation without significant risk for gap formation at the repair site. Other variables shown that increase the tensile strength of the repair site include more dorsal placement of the core suture and increased number of locks or grasps.

SUTURE MATERIAL AND SIZE

Choice of suture material is an important factor in flexor tendon repair, which is reflected in efforts to determine the best tendon suture material. Few studies have investigated the range of suture materials available to the surgeon.[25] Monofilament stainless steel sutures have the greatest tensile strength but are difficult to use, tend to pull through the tendon, and may weaken by kinking.[26] The rate of material absorption and strength reduction of absorbable sutures in tendon repair often preclude their use in clinical settings.[27,28] Most surgeons use nonresorbable 3–0 or 4–0 braided polyester sutures because they have been found to be nearly as strong as stainless steel in comparable sizes and have much easier handling properties.[19]

Hatanaka and Manske[29] demonstrated a strength advantage of larger core sutures in a linear distraction model. Taras and investigators[30] similarly showed that larger caliber sutures significantly increase repair strength. In a cadaveric study using an

TABLE 14–4. Characteristics in Locking Junctions with the Tendon and Orientations of Core Sutures in Three Six-Strand Repair Techniques

CHARACTERISTICS	REPAIR TECHNIQUES			
	TANG	LIM	MODIFIED SAVAGE	SAVAGE*
Locking Junctions				
Total number of locking loops	6	4	6	12
Strands related to each loop	2	2 or 4	2	2
Locking loops in each strand[†]	1	1	1	2
Orientation of Strands[‡]				
Longitudinal	6	4	0	0
Oblique	0	2	6	6
Transverse	0	0	0	0
Relation of Strands to Tensile Loads				
Parallel to tension	6	4	0	0
Angular to tension	0	2	6	6

*Savage method is listed here for comparison.
[†]Indicates number of locking in each tendon stump.
[‡]Orientation listed is in respect to the longitudinal axis of the tendon.
Data from Xie RG, Zhang S, Tang JB, Chen F: Biomechanical studies of 3 different 6-strand flexor tendon repair techniques. J Hand Surg [Am] 27:621–627, 2002.

TABLE 14–5. Tensile Strength Data

TYPE OF REPAIR	PALMAR (N + SEM)	DORSAL (N + SEM)	LINEAR (N + SEM)
Bunnell	11.790 + 0.690	21.310 + 1.300*	21.280 + 3.740*
Kessler	15.090 + 0.850	23.940 + 1.380*	16.980 + 0.310
Kessler epitenon	17.860 + 1.980	30.120 + 1.510*	21.570 + 1.440*
Epitenon	Circumferential suture	5.790 + 1.760	Not done

*Statistically significant.
SEM, standard error of the mean.
Data from Komanduri M, Phillips CS, Mass DP: Tensile strength of flexor tendon repairs in a dynamic cadaver model. J Hand Surg [Am] 21:605–611, 1996.

TABLE 14–6. Mean Strength, Toughness, and Efficiency of Glide of Two Repairs

	TECHNIQUE		
	MODIFIED BECKER	MODIFIED KESSLER	P
Mean strength of repair (newtons ± SEM) as defined by peak load sustained before rupture	79 ± 3	64 ± 4	<0.01
Mean toughness of repairs (joules ± SEM) as defined by energy absorbed to rupture (integral of force displacement curve)	0.092 ± 0.002	0.078 ± 0.003	<0.01
Mean efficiency of glide (percentage ± SEM) as defined by intact tendon work to "full fist" divided by repaired tendon work to "full fist"	32 ± 6	33 ± 4	>0.9

SEM, standard error of the mean.
Data from Wassermann RJ, Howard R, Markee B, et al: Optimization of the MGH repair using an algorithm for tenorrhaphy evaluation. Plast Reconstr Surg 99:1688–1694, 1997.

anatomic curvilinear model, Alavanja and coauthors[31] compared the mechanical properties of a four-strand locked cruciate repair technique using 2–0, 3–0, and 4–0 braided polyester sutures. This study demonstrates that increasing suture caliber from 4–0 to 2–0 significantly increases maximum tensile strength but also results in an increased work of flexion and gliding resistance that may preclude its use in the clinical setting (Table 14–7). Gapping was not affected by suture caliber, and no significant difference between 3–0 or 4–0 braided polyester sutures was shown in terms of strength or gliding function. Repairs using 3–0 and 4–0 sutures in this study provided sufficient mechanical strength to withstand unrestricted finger flexion according to Schuind[18] and Urbaniak.[19]

Stainless-steel sutures have been shown to have increased tensile strength but are not widely used in flexor tendon surgery because of difficulty with handling and knot-tying. Su and coworkers[32] compared the biomechanical characteristics of the single-strand multifilament stainless-steel Teno Fix device (Ortheon Medical, Columbus, OH) designed for flexor tendon repair with a four-strand locked cruciate (3–0 or 4–0 braided polyester) suture repair using a linear model (Table 14–8). The Teno Fix is a knotless anchoring device composed of two intratendinous stainless steel anchors that adjoins transected tendon ends with a single multifilament 2–0 stainless-steel suture (Fig. 14–3).[33] The device was developed to take advantage of stainless-steel suture strength whereas avoiding difficulties with handling and knot-tying. The 2-mm gapping force was significantly greater for the Teno Fix and 3–0 repairs compared with 4–0 repairs. No statistically significant difference in peak force or energy absorbed at peak force

TABLE 14–7. Maximum Tensile Load and Mean Change of Work of Flexion

	2–0	3–0	4–0
Maximum tensile load	80 ± 12 N	74 ± 18 N	66 ± 12 N
Mean change of work of flexion	1.83	2.04	1.86

Data from Alavanja G, Dailey E, Mass DP: Repair of zone II flexor digitorum profundus lacerations using varying suture sizes: A comparative biomechanical study. J Hand Surg [Am] 30:448–454, 2005.

TABLE 14–8. Review of In Vitro Studies on Gapping and Ultimate Strength of Repair Techniques

REPAIR	STUDY	MATERIAL	ULTIMATE FORCE	GAPPING FORCE (GAP)
Modified Kessler (two-strand)	Stein et al.[15]	4–0 braided polyester, 6–0 nylon epitendinous	28.9 N	23.6 N (2 mm)
	McLarney et al.[6]	4–0 braided polyester, 6–0 polypropylene epitendinous	28 N	22 N (2 mm)
	Tang et al.[21]	3–0 nylon, 5–0 nylon epitendinous	28.2 N	23.4 N (2 mm)
Modified Becker (four-strand)	Stein et al.[15]	4–0 braided polyester, 6–0 nylon epitendinous	40.7 N	48.8 N (2 mm)
Cruciate (four-strand)	McLarney et al.[6]	4–0 braided polyester, 6–0 polypropylene epitendinous	56 N	44 N (2 mm)
	Tang et al.[21]	3–0 nylon, 5–0 nylon epitendinous	46.3 N	37.4 N (2 mm)
	Su et al.[32]	4–0 braided polyester, 5–0 polypropylene epitendinous	70 N	46.5 N (2 mm)
		3–0 braided polyester, 5–0 polypropylene epitendinous	73.8 N	53.8 N (2 mm)
	Alavanja et al.[31]	4–0 braided polyester, 6–0 Dermalon epitendinous	66 N	Not reported
		3–0 braided polyester, 6–0 Dermalon epitendinous	74 N	Not reported
		2–0 braided polyester, 6–0 Dermalon epitendinous	80 N	Not reported
Savage (six-strand)	Savage[20]	4–0 braided polyester, no epitendinous	67.2 N	58.9 N (2.7 mm)
Sandow (six-strand)	Xie et al.[23]	4–0 Ethilon, 6–0 Ethilon epitendinous	57.8 N	37.4 N (2 mm)
Tang (six-strand)	Tang et al.[21]	3 × 4–0 looped nylon, 6–0 nylon epitendinous	53.6 N	43 N (2 mm)
	Xie et al.[23]	4–0 Supramid, 6–0 Ethilon epitendinous	60.2 N	44.5 (2 mm)
Teno fix	Su et al.[34]	5–0 polypropylene epitendinous	66.7 N	54.5 N (2 mm)

Data from Su BW, Solomons M, Barrow A, et al: A device for zone-II flexor tendon repair. Surgical technique. J Bone Joint Surg Am 88(Suppl 1 pt 1):37–49, 2006.

was found among the three different repair techniques. This study also confirmed that addition of a circumferential epitendinous suture using 5–0 monofilament polypropylene to the Teno Fix repair increased the 2-mm gapping force by 40% and peak force by 48%. To further evaluate the clinical effectiveness of the Teno Fix, Su and coworkers[34] conducted a blinded, randomized clinical trial comparing its use with four-strand cruciate repairs using a single 4–0 or 3–0 polypropylene suture (depending on tendon size) with 6–0 nylon epitendinous repair.[34]

None of the Teno Fix repairs ruptured compared with 18% (9/51) of tendons repaired with the cruciate technique. Five of the nine ruptures were attributed to resistive motion against medical advice in noncompliant patients. No differences were reported between the two groups for range of motion, DASH (disability of the arm, shoulder, and hand) score, pinch and grip strength, pain, or swelling. The authors conclude that the Teno Fix is safe and effective for flexor tendon repair if tendon size and exposure are sufficient.

NEW DEVELOPMENTS

An adjunct to the mechanical approach of strong suture techniques is to minimize adhesion formation by various mechanical and pharmacologic agents including laser therapy, cytotoxics such as 5-fluorouracil, hyaluronidase (a lubricant), and most recently, Adcon-T/N (Gliatech Inc., Cleveland, OH). Adcon is a bioresorbable gel composed of porcine gelatin and proteoglycan ester in phosphate-buffered saline that is applied directly before wound closure. The effectiveness of Adcon as a physical barrier has been shown in animal studies for surgery on tendons and nerves. Several prospective, randomized, clinical trials have been published on the use of Adcon in flexor tendon repairs.

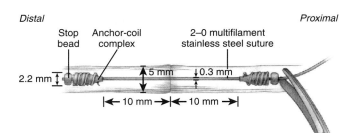

Distal   *Proximal*

FIGURE 14–3. Schematic diagram of the Teno Fix device. (From Su BW, Solomons M, Barrow A, et al: A device for zone-II flexor tendon repair. Surgical technique. J Bone Joint Surg Am 88(suppl 1 pt 1):37–49, 2006. Reprinted with permission from the Journal of Bone and Joint Surgery.)

Mentzel and researchers[35] compared the functional results 12 weeks after flexor tendon repair surgery with and without the use of Adcon-T/N. No significant difference was found with regard to total active motion and total extension lag between treated and untreated patients. Golash and investigators[36] also showed in a prospective, double-blinded, randomized, controlled, clinical trial that Adcon-T/N had no statistically significant effect on total active motion at 3, 6, and 12 months. However, the time taken to achieve final range of motion was significantly shorter in treated patients (10 vs. 14 weeks; $P = 0.02$). The authors suggest that Adcon-T/N may therefore limit adhesion formation in the early stages of healing. Greater rates of late rupture were observed in patients treated with Adcon-T/N (33% compared with 20% at a mean of 4 weeks compared with 2 weeks; $P = 0.016$), resulting in early conclusion of the study because of potential inhibitory effects of Adcon-T/N on tendon healing. In a similar double-blind, randomized, clinical study, Liew and coauthors[37] report a rupture rate of 25% in patients with tendon repairs treated with Adcon-T/N at an average of 33 days compared with a control group rupture rate of 26% at an average of 23 days. At 6-month follow-up examination, patients in the group treated with Adcon-T/N regained significantly more motion at the proximal interphalangeal joint (87% vs. 68%; $P = 0.005$), but not distal interphalangeal joint motion, hand grip, or pinch strength. Based on these results from early clinical studies, the benefit of using Adcon, as well as other mechanical barriers, in flexor tendon repairs remains unproven and, therefore, has not gained acceptance in clinical practice (grade B).

POSTOPERATIVE REHABILITATION

Postoperative rehabilitation protocols have evolved alongside advancement in flexor tendon repair techniques. Rehabilitation after flexor tendon repair must achieve a balance between protection of the repair from disrupting forces and prevention of adhesions. Studies have shown that early controlled forces applied to flexor tendon repairs are beneficial in providing more rapid recovery of tensile strength, fewer adhesions, improved tendon excursion, and minimal repair-site deformation in canine models.[38] Gelberman and coworkers[38] demonstrate an increase in tendon strength with passive motion at 12 weeks to within 50% of control, whereas a tendon completely immobilized had a strength equivalent to 20% of control. Tendon motion studies also show that immobilization results in 20% of normal excursion, whereas immediate mobilization produces up to 95% of normal tendon gliding. Motion clearly provides a stimulus for tendon healing.

Lister and colleagues[39] were among the first to report remarkable clinical results using active extension-passive flexion mobilization with the aid of a dynamic traction splint (Level IV). Two basic passive motion programs serve as the basis for other passive motion protocols: the Kleinert method and the Duran method[40] (Level IV). An effective postoperative program requires full range of passive flexion of both the distal and proximal interphalangeal joints. Both the Kleinert and Duran methods accomplish this goal when performed properly. Tables 14–9 and 14–10 outline the basic Kleinert and Duran protocols, respectively, that have been adapted and modified by hand surgeons.[41]

The timing, duration, and progression of rehabilitation, as well as optimal frequency of finger motion after flexor tendon repair, also have not been clearly established. Rehabilitation can begin anytime within 1 week after repair. Many surgeons report initiation of rehabilitation as immediate or starting the day after surgery. In a randomized clinical study, Adolfsson and researchers[42] investigated the effect of a shortened postoperative mobilization program after flexor tendon repair. All tendons were repaired with a modified 4–0 Maxon Kessler suture and running circumferential 6–0 Prolene suture. Patients were immobilized in a dorsal plaster splint with the wrist in 30 degrees and metacarpophalangeal (MCP) joints in 70 degrees of flexion. During the first 4 weeks, a passive flexion-active extension protocol described by Karlander[42a] was instituted followed by active flexion

TABLE 14–9. Kleinert Program

0–3 DAYS	0–4 WEEKS	4–6 WEEKS	6–8 WEEKS
• Dorsal protective splint applied with wrist and MCP joints in flexion and IP joints in full extension; elastic traction from fingernail, through palmar pulley, to volar forearm • Velcro strap to allow night release of elastic traction, splinting IPs in full extension	• Hourly active extension to limits of splints, followed by flexion with elastic traction only • Wound and scar management and education	• Dorsal protective splint discontinued, sometimes replaced with wrist cuff and elastic traction • Night protective splint to prevent flexion contracture • Active wrist and gentle active fisting initiated unless signs of minimal adhesions • At 6 weeks, blocking exercises begin	• Progressive resistive exercises begin

IP, proximal interphalangeal; MCP, metacarpophalangeal.
Data from Vucekovich K, Gallardo G, Fiala K: Rehabilitation after flexor tendon repair, reconstruction, and tenolysis. Hand Clin 21:257–265, 2005.

TABLE 14–10. Duran Program

0–3 DAYS	0–4.5 WEEKS	4.4–5.5 WEEKS	5.5 WEEKS	7.5 WEEKS
• Dorsal protective splint applied with wrist in 20-degree flexion, MCP joints in ~50-degree flexion, IP joints full extension	• Hourly exercises within the splint • 10 repetitions with PIP and MCP flexion • 10 repetitions passive PIP extension with MCP and DIP joint flexion	• Splint replaced by wrist cuff with elastic flexion traction from fingernail to cuff • Continue active extension/passive flexion	• Wrist cuff discontinued • Blocking and fisting exercises initiated	• Light resistive exercises with putty • Splinting to correct any joint or extrinsic flexor tightness

DIP, distal interphalangeal; IP, interphalangeal; MCP, metacarpophalangeal; PIP, proximal interphalangeal.

Data from Vucekovich K, Gallardo G, Fiala K: Rehabilitation after flexor tendon repair, reconstruction, and tenolysis. Hand Clin 21:257–265, 2005.

and extension without load for an additional 2 weeks. After the 6th week, patients were randomized to receive gradually increasing load and unrestricted activity at either 8 or 10 weeks. No significant differences were observed between the two groups in terms of functional results (Louisville, Tsuge, and Buck–Gramko), rupture rates, grip strength, or subjective assessments at 6 months. The authors conclude that a postoperative mobilization program after flexor tendon repair in zone II of the hand can be reduced to 8 weeks using the described regimen without significantly increasing risk for rupture or poorer functional results.

In a prospective, randomized, clinical study, Gelberman and coworkers[43] compared a traditional early passive motion protocol with a continuous passive motion protocol. All tendons were repaired with a Kessler 4–0 braided suture and 6–0 nylon epitenon suture. After surgery, dorsal plaster splints were applied with the wrist in 30-degree flexion, and MCP joints in 70-degree flexion. Patients were randomized into two treatments groups: (1) passive-motion rehabilitation using a continuous motion device for the first 4 weeks followed by combination active-motion rehabilitation alternating with continuous motion for a mean interval of 75 hours/week, and (2) controlled intermittent passive motion for the first 4 weeks followed by alternating active-motion and controlled-passive motion for a mean interval of controlled passive motion of 4 hours/week. Range of motion, both total active and mean active motion, as measured by the Strickland and Glogovac criteria showed a statistically significant difference between groups in favor of continuous motion.

More recently, early active motion protocols have been developed in response to experimental and clinical studies that demonstrate beneficial effects of early active motion. Early controlled active mobilization after flexor tendon repair may actually improve differential gliding between the flexor digitorum profundus (FDP) and flexor digitorum superficialis FDS tendons, and therefore reduce finger flexion contractures.[44] Strickland introduced an early active motion protocol for a four-strand repair with an epitendinous suture (Table 14–11).[45] Evans, Silfverskiöld,

RECOMMENDATIONS

Based on the summary recommendations of evidence (Table 14–12), we recommend a four-strand (or higher) core repair supplemented by a running epitendinous suture. We prefer a 3–0 (or 4–0 in smaller tendons) braided polyester core suture with Teflon coating and a 6–0 running Nylon epitendinous suture. We use a modified Savage technique as described by Sandow and McMahon[49] for repair of flexor tendons. The latest modification uses a four-strand, single cross core suture reinforced with a cross-stitch epitendinous suture (Fig. 14–4).[50,51] This repair method is technically easier and possesses gapping and strength characteristics as the original Savage technique strong enough to allow protected early active motion. After surgery, we recommend a modified Duran passive motion and place and hold rehabilitation protocol (Table 14–13).

May, and others have also introduced protocols that incorporate early active motion exercises (performed only under therapy supervision for the first few weeks) whereas using a Kleinert-type dorsal blocking splint.[46]

Despite the various active and passive motion protocols described in the literature, the optimal rehabilitation program after flexor tendon repair is yet to be determined. Kneafsey et al[47] reports no significant differences between controlled passive flexion with active extension (modified Kleinert) and controlled passive mobilization (modified Duran) in terms of active range of motion, power grip, pinch grip, and maximum finger pressure. In a Cochrane review, Thien and coworkers[48] conclude that there is insufficient evidence from randomized, controlled clinical trials to define the best mobilization strategy after flexor tendon repair.[48] The authors suggest that rehabilitation protocols using some early active mobilization should be used with multiple strand suture methods in compliant patients.

TABLE 14–11. Strickland (Indiana Hand Center) Early Active Motion Program

0–3 DAYS	0–4 WEEKS	4 WEEKS	5 WEEKS	6 WEEKS	8 WEEKS	14 WEEKS
• Dorsal blocking splint with wrist in 20-degree flexion, MCP joints in 50-degree flexion • Tenodesis splint allowing 30-degree wrist extension and full wrist flexion, maintaining MCP joints in 50-degree flexion (a single hinge splint with a detachable extension block can also be used)	• Duran passive motion performed 15 times every 2 hours • Tenodesis exercises within hinged splint 15 times every 2 hours	• Dorsal blocking splint removed during exercise but continued for protection • Tenodesis exercises continue • Instruction to avoid simultaneous wrist and finger extension	• Active IP flexion with MCP extension followed by full digital extension	• Blocking exercises begin if active tip to distal palmar crease is more than 3 cm • Passive extension can begin at 7 weeks	• Progressive resistive exercises initiated	• Unrestricted use of hand

IP, proximal interphalangeal; MCP, metacarpophalangeal.
Data from Vucekovich K, Gallardo G, Fiala K: Rehabilitation after flexor tendon repair, reconstruction, and tenolysis. Hand Clin 21:257–265, 2005.

TABLE 14–12. Summary of Recommendations

STATEMENT	LEVEL OF EVIDENCE/GRADE OF RECOMMENDATION	REFERENCES
1. Flexor tendon repairs should be performed using a 4-strand or greater core stitch technique.	Level III/Grade B	3-11, 14, 21, 22, 25
2. Flexor tendon repairs should include a horizontal mattress or running-lock peripheral circumferential epitendinous suture.	Level III/Grade B	11, 14
3. Flexor tendon repairs should be performed using a 4-0 or higher caliber nonresorbable suture.	Level III/Grade B	25-31
4. Postoperative rehabilitation protocols should employ early protected passive motion or active motion.	Level II/Grade B	39-48

Data from Hunter J, Macklin E, Callahan A: Rehabilitation of the Hand. St Louis, CV Mosby, 1995. Diagnosis & Treatment Manual for Physicians and Therapies, 4th ed. The Hand Rehabilitation Center of Indiana, Indianapolis, Indiana, 2001.

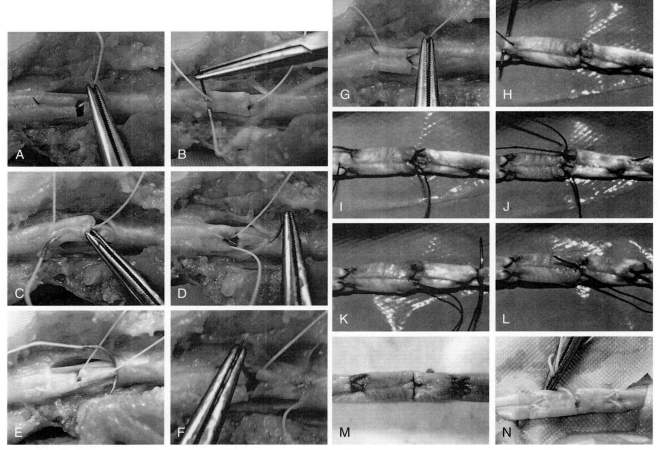

FIGURE 14–4. Four-strand modified Sandow technique. *A,* The first central core stitch exits the tendon centrally approximately 1 cm from the cut tendon end. *B,* The first cross-stitch exits in line with the first central core stitch approximately 1.1 to 1.2 cm from the cut tendon end. *C,* The first peripheral core stitch enters the tendon approximately 1 cm from the cut tendon end. *D,* The first opposite end peripheral core stitch. *E,* The first opposite end cross-stitch. Cross-stitches are always directed perpendicular to core sutures and exit 1 to 2 mm distal to the preceding throw. *F,* The first opposite end central core stitch. *G,* The second central core stitch. *H,* The second cross-stitch. *I,* The second peripheral core stitch. *J,* The second opposite end peripheral core stitch. *K,* The second opposite end cross-stitch. *L,* The second opposite end central core stitch. *M,* Repaired tendon. *N,* Repaired tendon. (Reproduced from Bernstein MA, Taras JS: Flexor tendon suture: A description of two core suture techniques and the Silfverskiold epitendinous suture. Tech Hand Up Extrem Surg 7:119–129, 2003, by permission.)

TABLE 14–13. University of California Davis Hand Flexor Tendon Zone II Protocol[52,53]

Treatment Protocol

I. Surgery to 10 days after surgery:
   - Patient is placed in a custom-fabricated dorsal extension block splint with the wrist in 0–30-degree flexion, the metacarpo-phalangeal joints (MPS) in 40–70 degrees of flexion, and the IP joints in neutral (full extension, with the exception of FDP in slight flexion at the DIP joint). The surgical dressing is removed, and a light compressive surgical dressing is used to redress the incision after it has been cleaned with sterile saline.
   - The splint is to be worn all the time until 4 to 6 weeks after surgery.
   - Digital nerve repairs may require positioning the PIP joint initially in 30 degrees of flexion and gradually increasing extension from 3 to 6 weeks.
   - On the first day after surgery, begin gentle passive flexion and active extension of each digit within the confines of the dressing and splint as follows:
     1. The DIP is flexed to at least 60-degree flexion and allowed to actively extend in the splint, 5–10 times/session.
     2. The PIP is flexed to at least 60 degrees flexion and allowed to actively extend in the splint, 5–10 times/session.
     3. Both IP joints are flexed together and allowed to actively extend in the splint, 5–10 times/session.
     4. These exercises are performed 5 times/day, or every 2 hours.
        - If patient is reliable, instructions are given to perform at home.
        - Edema control of digits from Coban or finger tube gauze can be started.
        - Active/passive range of motion A/PROM of uninvolved digits and joints can be started if there is not a direct effect on repaired structures, including the shoulder, elbows, and forearm.

II. 10 days to 3 weeks after surgery:
   - Patient continues on the same program of passive flexion and active extension in the splint.
   - Patient wears splint at all times.
   - 48 hours after suture removal, can begin scar massage and scar gel at night.
   - 2-week tenodesis to neutral only.

III. 3–6 weeks after surgery:
   - Splint can be changed to wrist neutral, if appropriate.
   - At 3 weeks, patient continues the passive flexion program as before, followed by place and hold in composite flexion.
   - Between 3 and 3½ weeks, pulsed ultrasound can be started.
   - At 3½ weeks after surgery, patient can begin blocking exercises within the confines of the splint. Patient is taught to actively flex the PIP and DIP joints as far as he/she can, hold, and repeat 10 times. Each joint is exercised individually. Patient performs these exercises at each involved joint 10 times every 1–2 hours.
   - Between 3½ and 4 weeks, active composite finger flexion with the wrist in neutral can be initiated.
   - At 4 weeks after surgery, protected tenodesis of simultaneous wrist flexion and finger extension, alternating with simultaneous wrist extension and finger flexion, can be started in therapy.
   - Neuromuscular electrostimulation can be added.
   - At 4½ weeks after surgery, exercises can include:
     1. Gentle active composite flexion with wrist flexion and gentle finger extension with wrist extension.
     2. Composite fist with wrist extension and flexion.
        - At 5 weeks after surgery, protected active differential tendon gliding exercises (hook fist, straight fist, and then full fist), with the wrist being blocked at 10 degrees of flexion, are performed by the patient 10 times in therapy. If appropriate, patient can begin weaning out of splint to do tenodesis, 4½-week exercises, and tendon gliding exercises.
        - Patient is seen two to three times per week in hand therapy.

IV. 6–8 weeks after surgery:
   - Splint can be discontinued.
   - Patient continues with the exercise program as before.
   - Blocking exercises may be initiated to the PIP joint and separately to the DIP joint, with the exception of the small finger.
   - Gentle passive extension exercises are initiated.
   - Can begin static volar extension pan splinting at night if needed.
   - Dynamic extension splinting may be initiated if PIP flexion contracture develops.
   - Patient is seen two to three times per week in hand therapy.

V. 8 weeks after surgery to discharge:
   - Resistive exercise can begin with putty for 5 minutes, three to four times a day, and with hand grippers or hand weights.
   - Patient continues to perform the same exercise program until normal range of motion is present.
   - Patient may need to wear static or dynamic splints to increase passive flexion or extension.
   - Patient is free for all daily activity except for sports or heavy work.
   - Patient is following monthly or as needed hand therapy.
   - At 12 weeks after surgery, there are no restrictions.

DIP, distal interphalangeal; FDP, flexor digitorum profundus; IP, interphalangeal; MCP, metacarpophalangeal; PIP, proximal interphalangeal.

REFERENCES

1. Strickland JW: Development of flexor tendon surgery: Twenty-five years of progress. J Hand Surg [Am] 25:214–235, 2000.
2. Strickland JW: Flexor tendon injuries: I. Foundations of treatment. J Am Acad Orthop Surg 3:44–54, 1995.
3. Lee H: Double loop locking suture: A technique of tendon repair for early active mobilization. Part I: Evolution of technique and experimental study. J Hand Surg [Am] 15:945–952, 1990.
4. Lee H: Double loop locking suture: A technique of tendon repair for early active mobilization. Part II: Clinical experience. J Hand Surg [Am] 15:953–958, 1990.
5. Tang JB, Shi D, Gu YQ, et al: Double and multiple looped suture tendon repair. J Hand Surg [Br] 19:699–703, 1994.
6. McLarney E, Hoffman H, Wolfe SW: Biomechanical analysis of the cruciate four-strand flexor tendon repair. J Hand Surg [Am] 24:295–301, 1999.
7. Tsuge K, Ikuta Y, Matsuishi Y: Intra-tendinous tendon suture in the hand—a new technique. Hand 7:250–255, 1975.
8. Kessler I, Nissim F: Primary repair without immobilization of flexor tendon division within the digital sheath. An experimental and clinical study. Acta Orthop Scand 40:587–601, 1969.
9. Noguchi M, Seiler JG 3rd, Gelberman RH, et al: In vitro biomechanical analysis of suture methods for flexor tendon repair. J Orthop Res 11:603–611, 1993.
10. Winters SC, Gelberman RH, Woo SL, et al: The effects of multiple-strand suture methods on the strength and excursion of repaired intrasynovial flexor tendons: A biomechanical study in dogs. J Hand Surg [Am] 23:97–104, 1998.
11. Wade PJ, Wetherell RG, Amis AA: Flexor tendon repair: Significant gain in strength from the Halsted peripheral suture technique. J Hand Surg [Br] 14:232–235, 1989.
12. Boyer MI, Strickland JW, Engles D, et al: Flexor tendon repair and rehabilitation: State of the art in 2002. Instr Course Lect 52:137–161, 2003.
13. Soejima O, Diao E, Lotz JC, Hariharan JS: Comparative mechanical analysis of dorsal versus palmar placement of core suture for flexor tendon repairs. J Hand Surg [Am] 20:801–807, 1995.
14. Komanduri M, Phillips CS, Mass DP: Tensile strength of flexor tendon repairs in a dynamic cadaver model. J Hand Surg 21:605–611, 1996.
15. Stein T, Ali A, Hamman J, Mass DP: A randomized biomechanical study of zone II human flexor tendon repairs analyzed in an in vitro model. J Hand Surg [Am] 23:1046–1051, 1998.
16. Hatanaka H, Zhang J, Manske PR: An in vivo study of locking and grasping techniques using a passive mobilization protocol in experimental animals. J Hand Surg [Am] 25:260–269, 2000.
17. Hatanaka H, Manske PR: Effect of the cross-sectional area of locking loops in flexor tendon repair. J Hand Surg [Am] 24:751–760, 1999.
18. Schuind F, Garcia-Elias M, Cooney WP 3rd, An KN: Flexor tendon forces: In vivo measurements. J Hand Surg [Am] 17:291–298, 1992.
19. Urbaniak JR, Cahill JD, Mortenson RA: Tendon suture methods: Analysis of tensile strength, in AAOS Symposium on Tendon Surgery in the Hand. St. Louis, Mosby, 1975, pp 70–80.
20. Savage R: In vitro studies of a new method of flexor tendon repair. J Hand Surg [Br] 10:135–141, 1985.
21. Tang JB, Gu YT, Rice K, et al: Evaluation of four methods of flexor tendon repair for postoperative active mobilization. Plast Reconstr Surg 107:742–749, 2001.
22. Labana N, Messer T, Lautenschlager E, et al: A biomechanical analysis of the modified Tsuge suture technique for repair of flexor tendon lacerations. J Hand Surg [Br] 26:297–300, 2001.
23. Xie RG, Zhang S, Tang JB, Chen F: Biomechanical studies of 3 different 6-strand flexor tendon repair techniques. J Hand Surg [Am] 27:621–627, 2002.
24. Wassermann RJ, Howard R, Markee B, et al: Optimization of the MGH repair using an algorithm for tenorrhaphy evaluation. Plast Reconstr Surg 99:1688–1694, 1997.

25. Lawrence TM, Davis TR: A biomechanical analysis of suture materials and their influence on a four-strand flexor tendon repair. J Hand Surg [Am] 30:836–841, 2005.
26. Nystrom B, Holmlund D: Separation of sutured tendon ends when different suture techniques and different suture materials are used. An experimental study in rabbits. Scand J Plast Reconstr Surg 17:19–23, 1983.
27. Mashadi ZB, Amis AA: Variation of holding strength of synthetic absorbable flexor tendon sutures with time. J Hand Surg [Br] 17:278–281, 1992.
28. O'Broin ES, Early MJ, Smyth H, Hooper AC: Absorbable sutures in tendon repair. A comparison of PDS with prolene in rabbit tendon repair. J Hand Surg [Br] 20:505–508, 1995.
29. Hatanaka H, Manske PR: Effect of suture size on locking and grasping flexor tendon repair techniques. Clin Orthop Relat Res (375):267–274, 2000.
30. Taras JS, Raphael JS, Marczyk SC, Bauerle WB: Evaluation of suture caliber in flexor tendon repair. J Hand Surg [Am] 26:1100–1104, 2001.
31. Alavanja G, Dailey E, Mass DP: Repair of zone II flexor digitorum profundus lacerations using varying suture sizes: A comparative biomechanical study. J Hand Surg [Am] 30:448–454, 2005.
32. Su BW, Protopsaltis TS, Koff MF, et al: The biomechanical analysis of a tendon fixation device for flexor tendon repair. J Hand Surg [Am] 30:237–245, 2005.
33. Su BW, Solomons M, Barrow A, et al: A device for zone-II flexor tendon repair. Surgical technique. J Bone Joint Surg Am 88(suppl 1 pt 1):37–49, 2006.
34. Su BW, Solomons M, Barrow A, et al: Device for zone-II flexor tendon repair. A multicenter, randomized, blinded, clinical trial. J Bone Joint Surg Am 87:923–935, 2005.
35. Mentzel M, Hoss H, Keppler P, et al: The effectiveness of ADCON-T/N, a new anti-adhesion barrier gel, in fresh divisions of the flexor tendons in Zone II. J Hand Surg [Br] 25:590–592, 2000.
36. Golash A, Kay A, Warner JG, et al: Efficacy of ADCON-T/N after primary flexor tendon repair in Zone II: A controlled clinical trial. J Hand Surg [Br] 28:113–115, 2003.
37. Liew SH, Potokar T, Bantick GL, et al: The use of ADCON-T/N after repair of zone II flexor tendons. Chir Main 20:384–387, 2001.
38. Gelberman RH, Woo SL, Lothringer K, et al: Effects of early intermittent passive mobilization on healing canine flexor tendons. J Hand Surg [Am] 7:170–175, 1982.
39. Lister GD, Kleinert HE, Kutz JE, Atasoy E: Primary flexor tendon repair followed by immediate controlled mobilization. J Hand Surg [Am] 2:441–451, 1977.
40. Vucekovich K, Gallardo G, Fiala K: Rehabilitation after flexor tendon repair, reconstruction, and tenolysis. Hand Clin 21:257–265, 2005.
41. Duran RJ, House RG: Controlled passive motion following flexor tendon repairs in zones 2 and 3. AAOS Symposium on Tendon Surgery in the Hand. St. Louis, Mosby, 1975.
42. Adolfsson L, Söderberg G, Larsson M, Karlander LE: The effects of a shortened postoperative mobilization programme after flexor tendon repair in zone 2. J Hand Surg [Br] 21:67–71, 1996.
42a. Karlander LE, Berggren M, Larsson M, Soderberg G, and Nylander G: Improved results in zone 2 flexor tendon injuries with a modified technique of immediate controlled mobilization. J Hand Surg [Br] 18(1): 26–30, 1993.
43. Gelberman RH, Nunley JA 2nd, Osterman AL, et al: Influences of the protected passive mobilization interval on flexor tendon healing. A prospective randomized clinical study. Clin Orthop Relat Res (264):189–196, 1991.
44. Tang JB: Indications, methods, postoperative motion and outcome evaluation of primary flexor tendon repairs in Zone 2. J Hand Surg [Br] 32:118–129, 2007.
45. Strickland JW, Cannon NM: Flexor tendon repair—Indiana method. Indiana Hand Center Newsletter 1–19, 1993.
46. Silfverskiold KL, May EJ: Flexor tendon repair in zone II with a new suture technique and an early mobilization program combining passive and active flexion. J Hand Surg [Am] 19:53–60, 1994.

47. Kneafsey B, O'Shaughnessy M, Vidal P, et al: Controlled mobilization after flexor tendon repair: A prospective comparison of two methods [abstract]. J Hand Surgery [Br] 19(suppl 1):37–38, 1994.

48. Thien TB, Becker JH, Theis JC: Rehabilitation after surgery for flexor tendon injuries in the hand. Cochrane Database Syst Rev (4):CD003979, 2004.

49. Sandow MJ, McMahon MM: Single cross-grasp six-strand repair for flexor tenorrhaphy modified Savage technique. Atlas Hand Clinics 1:41–64, 1996.

50. Bernstein MA, Taras JS: Flexor tendon suture: A description of two core suture techniques and the Silfverskiold epitendinous suture. Tech Hand Up Extrem Surg 7:119–129, 2003.

51. Wakefield Orthopedic Clinic: Upper limb research: Single-cross-grasp four strangd (Adelaide) tenorrhaphy. Available at: http://woc.com.au/content/14. Accessed December 2007.

52. Hunter J, Macklin E, Callahan A: Rehabilitation of the Hand. St. Louis, CV Mosby, 1995.

53. Diagnosis & Treatment Manual for Physicians and Therapists, 4th ed. The Hand Rehabilitation Center of Indiana, Indianapolis, Indiana, 2001.

Chapter 15

What Is the Best Management of Digital Triggering?

Christine J. Cheng, MD, MPH

Stenosing tenosynovitis, or trigger finger, was first described by Notta in 1850.[1] It is one of the most common hand conditions in adults treated by primary care providers, orthopedic and plastic surgeons, and hand surgeons, affecting a reported 2.6% of the general population.[2] The affected digit "triggers" or locks during active flexion, which is often associated with pain. In severe cases, the digit can become fixed in flexion or extension, leading to joint contracture. Despite its common occurrence, no clear consensus exists regarding the management of trigger fingers. Nonsurgical treatment has generally been advocated as the initial therapy, with either splinting of the affected digit or steroid injection into the flexor tendon sheath. Surgery traditionally has been reserved for those who do not respond to conservative therapy, with open division of the A1 pulley as the definitive treatment. In recent years, percutaneous release of the A1 pulley has gained popularity as an alternative surgical technique. Splinting and steroid injection are easily performed in the office, are relatively safe and inexpensive, and require no post-treatment activity restrictions for the patient. However, prolonged splinting regimens may be required, and persistent symptoms and recurrence are more likely to occur, especially if symptoms are long-standing.[3,4] Surgery usually provides permanent relief but is often more costly, involving potential time away from work and a risk for surgical complications. Systemic diseases such as amyloidosis, mucopolysaccharidoses, diabetes mellitus, and rheumatoid arthritis have been associated with digital triggering.[5] The most common of these is diabetes mellitus, in which the incidence rate of trigger finger is 4% to 10%.[6] Studies have suggested that conservative therapy is less effective in these patients, but complications such as infection and delayed wound healing may be special surgical concerns.

OPTIONS

Symptomatic patients may first present to primary care providers, who must decide which patients are unlikely to respond to conservative therapy and refer them to a surgeon. For the remaining patients, options include activity modifications, oral anti-inflammatory agents, splinting, and steroid injection.[5] For splinting regimens, the choice of joint for immobilization in the affected digit and length of treatment need to be

determined. For injection therapy, decisions include which steroid preparation to use, what volume and location to inject, how many injections to give, and at what time intervals repeat injections should be given. Although division of the A1 pulley is the widely accepted surgical procedure, the surgeon has a choice between open versus percutaneous technique. Ideally, systematic review of the published evidence should allow development of a treatment algorithm that can be followed reliably to achieve the safest, most effective results with the greatest level of patient satisfaction, whereas keeping costs at a minimum. In an effort toward reaching this goal, discussion in this chapter is limited to those comparative studies that provide the highest levels of evidence (Levels I-III) identified after systematic review of the published literature. Higher quality clinical studies are more likely to provide convincing evidence for influencing medical treatment decisions.

EVIDENCE

Few controlled studies comparing splinting with steroid injection have been published. In their prospective study, Patel and Bassini[4] compared 50 consecutive patients who were treated with metacarpophalangeal (MP) joint splinting with 50 patients who were treated with intrasheath injection of betamethasone (Level of Evidence II). Severity of triggering was graded, and patients with minimal pain, "uneven" movements that did not interfere with hand function, or who were symptom free at the end of the 1-year study period were considered successfully treated. One fourth of the injection group required a single repeat injection 2 weeks after the initial injection. Success was achieved in 66% of the splinted group and 84% of the injected group. Symptoms recurred in 12% of the splinted patients during the 1-year follow-up period; none recurred in the injection group. Patients with symptoms for longer than 6 months before treatment, multiple digital involvement, or triggering at time of presentation faired the worst. The authors comment that splinting was the least effective for trigger thumbs, and that more than 6 weeks of splinting was necessary to achieve success in one third of the patients.[4]

Although splinting is painless and noninvasive, it interferes with normal hand use, prolonged treatment may be necessary, and success relies directly on patient compliance. If a single steroid injection can provide comparable or better success rates, then it might be preferred over splinting, despite the discomfort associated with injection. Controlled prospective trials have compared a single injection of steroid into the flexor tendon sheath with placebo injection of local anesthetic.[7,8] In separate studies by Murphy and colleagues[7] and Lambert and co-workers[8] (Level II), a single intrasheath injection of betamethasone or methylprednisolone, respectively, cured 64% and 60% of the patients. Both studies were properly blinded, with the intervention and evaluations for each patient performed by different clinicians. Although the results were statistically significant, it is interesting to note that placebo injection was effective in 20% and 16% of patients in the two studies. No recurrences were reported within the relatively short (one[8] and four[7] months) follow-up periods.

Initial published results in the 1950s for corticosteroid injection in the treatment of trigger fingers demonstrated short-term efficacy,[9,10] with more lasting results achieved after the development of longer acting corticosteroid preparations.[10,11] Choice of steroid is usually based on physician preference, and no good comparison studies of steroid preparations have been done. Betamethasone, methylprednisolone, and triamcinolone are common choices. Injection volume and concentration of steroid have also varied widely among studies, with essentially all studies advocating injection into the flexor tendon sheath just distal to the A1 pulley. An interesting controlled prospective study by Taras and researchers[10] (Level II) explored this recommendation by comparing intrasheath with subcutaneous injection. The steroid was mixed with radio-opaque contrast dye. After their assigned injections, the actual location of each injection was verified radiographically. Symptom resolution was achieved in 71% of the subcutaneous group and 52% of the intrasheath group after 27-month average follow-up. Overall, 62% of the patients were treated successfully. Only 30% of the attempted injections into the tendon sheath were completely accurate. Recalculation of the results based on true location of steroid delivery had the following outcome: intrasheath, mixed, or subcutaneous showed no change in success rates. Although the results suggest that subcutaneous injection was as effective as intrasheath injection, the study lacked adequate power ($\beta = 0.92$). The study designs for these studies on efficacy of steroid injection are summarized in Table 15–1.

Although the physiologic explanation for greater incidence of trigger finger in patients with diabetes mellitus is unclear, it is usually reported as 4% to 10%, with some reports as high as 23%.[12] Steroid injections have been believed to be less effective in the treatment of diabetic trigger fingers. Stahl and investigators[13] prospectively compared the efficacy of steroid injections for trigger finger in 60 patients with diabetes with 60 nondiabetic control patients, matched for age, sex, digit involvement, occupation, and available follow-up (Level II). A maximum of three injections at 3-week intervals were allowed, with 12% of the patients with diabetes requiring three injections, whereas only 3% of the patients without diabetes did. Overall, 59% were treated successfully with steroid injection, but the response rate was significantly lower in patients with diabetes (49%) than in those without (76%). Insulin dependence and duration of symptoms before treatment did not affect the results. Long-term follow-up beyond 9 weeks was not provided. Likewise, retrospective review of 66 patients treated for trigger finger by Nimigan and coauthors[12] (Level III) showed 52% response rate to up to three steroid injections, with significantly lower response in patients with diabetes (26%) than in those without diabetes (57%).[12] Again, duration of symptoms and insulin dependence did not affect the results. Nearly all of the patients who underwent surgery either after did not respond to injection therapy or because of personal preference were successfully treated (97%), although 36% experienced complications. Patients with diabetes did not have greater complication rates, and stiffness was the most common postoperative problem. In contrast, Griggs and colleagues[14] (Level III) found patients with insulin-dependent diabetes less likely to respond to steroid injection (44%) compared with patients with non–insulin-dependent diabetes (71%) in their retrospective review. Steroid injection was successful in only 50% of 121 digits in the 54 patients in their study. The study designs for these studies on steroid injection in patients with diabetes are summarized in Table 15–2.

Reported efficacy for surgical release of the A1 pulley in the treatment of trigger finger has been generally excellent. However, complications resulting from steroid injection are rarely reported, whereas surgical complication rates in large controlled studies have ranged from 0%[15] to as high as 36%.[12] Kraemer and coworkers'[16] and Benson and Ptaszek's[15] retrospective reviews (Level III) showed comparable success rates for steroid injection and surgery, but power analysis was not mentioned. Treatment outcomes were 63% success after injection and 77% success after surgery in Kraemer and coworkers'[16] study.[16] In Benson and Ptaszek's[15] study, injection achieved 97% success, and all surgery patients responded well.[15] Sixty percent to 67% of the conservatively managed patients required only a single injection.[15,16] Seven percent of one surgery group experienced complications, which were usually persistent stiffness.[16] In the other study, none of the surgery patients had complications.[15] Despite excellent results from open surgical release, both authors discussed the "costs" to the patient associated with surgery, including operative charges, time spent for the procedure, subsequent time off work, and the potential additional cost with a complication. However, a calculation of costs must also take into account patient preferences. Interestingly, in Benson and Ptaszek's[15] study, 73% of the patients completed a follow-up satisfaction questionnaire, in which the majority of patients recalled the pain during injection to be equal to or more severe

TABLE 15–1. Study Designs: Comparative Studies of Steroid Injection

AUTHORS	JOURNAL	YEAR	GROUPS	PATIENTS (N)	DIGITS (N)	MEAN AGE (RANGE), YEARS	EXCLUSION CRITERIA	DESIGN	RANDOMIZED	BLINDED
Patel and Bassini[4]	*Journal of Hand Surgery (Am)*	1992	Splint	NR	50	60 (NR)	None	Prospective cohort	No	No
Lambert et al.[8]	*Journal of Hand Surgery (Br)*	1992	Steroid Steroid	20	50 20	61 (NR) 54 (22–56)	RA, IDDM, eczema, infection, injection within 3 months	Prospective cohort	NR	Yes
Murphy et al.[7]	*Journal of Hand Surgery (Am)*	1995	Placebo Steroid	21 14	21 14	54 (30–76) 54 (NR)	RA, IDDM, previous tendon laceration or trigger finger injection	Prospective cohort	Yes	Yes
Taras et al.[10]	*Journal of Hand Surgery (Am)*	1998	Placebo Subcutaneous injection Intrasheath injection	10 48 47	10 55 52	62 (NR) 60 (NR) 62 (NR)	Symptoms >6 months, DM, connective tissue disease	Prospective cohort	Yes	No

NR, not reported; RA, rheumatoid arthritis; IDDM, insulin-dependent diabetes mellitus; DM, diabetes mellitus.

TABLE 15–2. Study Designs: Comparative Studies of Steroid Injection in Patients with Diabetes

AUTHORS	JOURNAL	YEAR	GROUPS	PATIENTS (N)	DIGITS (N)	MEAN AGE (RANGE), YEARS	EXCLUSION CRITERIA	DESIGN	RANDOMIZED	BLINDED
Stahl et al.[13]	*Journal of Diabetes and its Complications*	1997	Diabetic	60	130	54 (19–70)	Lost to follow-up	Prospective cohort	No	No
			Nondiabetic (matched)	60	72	57 (24–81)				
Nimigan et al.[12]	*American Journal of Physical Medicine and Rehabilitation*	2006	Diabetic	26	26	61 (NR)	None	Retrospective cohort	No	No
			Nondiabetic	40	70					
Griggs et al.[14]	*Journal of Hand Surgery(Am)*	1995	IDDM	37	93	50 (20–70)	None	Retrospective cohort	No	No
			NIDDM	17	28					

NR = not reported; IDDM = insulin-dependent diabetes mellitus; NIDDM = non–insulin-dependent diabetes mellitus.

than pain with surgery, and planned to choose surgery sooner for future trigger digits.[15] None of the surveyed patients experienced surgical complications; their preferences might have differed if they had. Despite better results with surgery, both authors recommend that steroid injection remain the first-line treatment, with surgery reserved for nonresponders.[15,16]

Percutaneous release of the A1 pulley using a fine tenotome was first described in 1958 by Lorthioir.[17] In consideration of potential additional time and costs associated with open release for trigger fingers, Eastwood and colleagues[18] introduced percutaneous release using a large-gauge hypodermic needle as on office procedure. The complications most frequently reported after open release have been stiffness, scar sensitivity or pain, and wound infection or delayed healing. Presumably, needle percutaneous release would avoid painful scar and wound healing problems. However, cadaveric studies have raised the question of increased risks for incomplete pulley release, digital nerve injury, and flexor tendon injury. In 2001, Gilberts and researchers[19] (Level II) prospectively compared open and percutaneous needle release in the treatment of 100 trigger digits. Although the authors report random assignment to treatment groups, their methodology describes only the use of "sealed envelopes." Nearly all of the patients in both groups experienced symptom relief. A power analysis was not reported. No recurrences, nerve deficits, or tendon problems occurred in the 4-month follow-up period. Because both techniques were performed in an outpatient surgery facility, direct comparison of operating times was possible as an indirect measure of cost. Operating time, duration of postoperative pain, return to work, and time to regain full motion were significantly shorter in the percutaneous release group. One of the patients treated with open release required repeat surgery for "scar formation," and one patient in each group experienced development of a minor hematoma. Table 15–3 summarizes the study designs of the reviewed studies for open and percutaneous surgical treatment of trigger finger. Finally, Table 15–4 lists the results and levels of evidence for all of the comparative studies reviewed in this chapter.

AREAS OF UNCERTAINTY

Diagnosis

The diagnosis of trigger finger is believed to be straightforward by most clinicians. However, a spectrum of clinical presentations is recognized. In two of the reviewed articles, the authors use grading systems to describe the various symptoms in their patients, ranging from uneven motion only, painless triggering, to painful locked digits with palpable tendon nodules.[4,7] Whether these variations represent different levels of severity, different pathophysiology, or simply alternative presentations of a common disease process remains unclear. No standardized grading system is currently in use, making direct comparison of patient groups difficult. In their cost analysis of conservative and surgical treatments, Benson and Ptaszek[15] explore pain as a potential factor in their patients' personal preferences. If pain is, indeed, an influential factor, then studies that do not take it into account may not have homogeneous patient groups for risk-benefit analysis. These limitations of the diagnostic criteria also affect the measurement of treatment success. Fleisch and coauthors[20] address this in their systematic literature review of steroid injections for the treatment of trigger finger. They propose the use of a classification system for diagnosis, visual analog pain scale, and measured active digital motion to improve the assessment of treatment efficacy.

Treatment Protocols

No uniformity of treatment protocols exists, especially in the conservative management of stenosing tenosynovitis. Some authors advocate splinting of the MP joint alone,[4] but each of the interphalangeal joints have also been splinted in clinical practice, presumably with reasonable results. Similarly, the reviewed studies on steroid injection used various concentrations of a wide variety of long-acting agents (triamcinolone,[15] methylprednisolone,[8,13] betamethasone[4,7,10,12,14,15]). Some studies did not report the concentration or amount of drug injected, and the majority did not report the volume of injection administered, all of which may affect the result. No consensus exists regarding the duration of treatment for splinting or steroid injection, or the maximum number or intervals for injections, which makes the determination of treatment success or failure nearly impossible. Follow-up periods in the reviewed studies varied from 1 month[8] to 27 months.[14] Studies with shorter follow-up periods may have falsely increased success rates and vice versa, because the natural history of trigger finger after various treatment methods remains undefined.

Costs

In the two studies that directly compared steroid injection with surgery (open technique), the authors recommend that steroid injection remain the first line of treatment, despite achieving high rates of success in their surgical groups.[15,16] They based this recommendation on the "cost" associated with surgery. Cost is always difficult to estimate and generalize for analyses because charges may differ from actual costs, and time spent, as well as time lost (e.g., from work), need to be considered. In addition, the potential additional costs associated with a possible complication are often taken into account in the analysis. The costs of an intervention can vary based on the setting in which it is performed. Thus, the

TABLE 15–3. Study Designs: Comparative Studies of Surgery

AUTHORS	JOURNAL	YEAR	GROUPS	PATIENTS (N)	DIGITS (N)	MEAN AGE (RANGE), YEARS	EXCLUSION CRITERIA	DESIGN	RANDOMIZED	BLINDED
Kraemer et al.[16]	*Southern Medical Journal*	1990	Injection	129	164	60 (NR)	Previous hand injury or open tendon injury	Retrospective cohort	No	No
Benson and Ptaszek[15]	*Journal of Hand Surgery (Am)*	1997	Surgery	89	89	61 (NR)	None	Retrospective cohort	No	No
			Injection	102	75	61 (33–96)				
Gilberts et al.[19]	*Journal of Hand Surgery (Am)*	2001	Surgery		34		Inflammation or prior surgery of the digit	Prospective cohort	Yes	No
			Open release		46	60 (24–81)				
			Percutaneous release		54	62 (24–88)				

NR = not reported.

TABLE 15–4. Results and Levels of Evidence: Comparative Studies in the Treatment of Trigger Finger

AUTHORS	GROUPS	AVERAGE FOLLOW-UP (MONTHS)	FOLLOW-UP RATE	SUCCESS STUDY	CONTROL	% DIFFERENCE	*P*	SUFFICIENT POWER	LEVEL OF EVIDENCE
Patel and Bassini[4]	Splint vs. injection	>13	100%	66%	84%	18	NR	NR	2
Lambert et al.[8]	Steroid vs. placebo	1	95%	60%	15%	45	0.05*	NR	2
Murphy et al.[7]	Steroid vs. placebo	4	100%	64%	20%	44	0.05*		2
Taras et al.[10]	SQ injection vs. intrasheath injection	27	100%	71%	52%	19	Not significant	No	2
Stahl et al.[13]	DM vs. non-DM	>2.25	92%	49%	76%	27	0.0001*		2
Nimigan et al.[12]	DM vs. non-DM	23	NR	26%	57%	31	0.04†		3
Griggs et al.[14]	IDDM vs. NIDDM	27	100%	44%	71%	27	0.02‡		3
Kraemer et al.[16]	Injection vs. surgery	4	100%	63%	77%	14	0.42*	NR	3
Benson and Ptaszek[15]	Injection vs. surgery	18	73%	97%	100%	3	NR	NR	3
Gilberts et al.[19]	Open vs. percutaneous	3	100%	98%	100%	2	Not significant	NR	2

NR = not reported; SQ = subcutaneous; DM = diabetes mellitus; IDDM = insulin-dependent diabetes mellitus; NIDDM = non–insulin-dependent diabetes mellitus.
*Chi-square test.
†Forward exact test.
‡Fisher's exact test.

cost of a percutaneous A1 pulley release might change drastically if the procedure is performed in a hospital outpatient facility instead of a surgeon's office. For this reason, recommendations based on "cost" need to be considered in the context of the particular setting and may not translate outside of that setting.

Recommendations

Although activity modification and oral nonsteroidal anti-inflammatory medications are used for the treatment of trigger finger, this discussion remains limited to the more widely utilized treatments of splinting, steroid injection, and surgery. Published case series abound for each of these modalities, but only controlled studies were chosen for this chapter to try to present the strongest evidence available. Unfortunately, the resulting body of literature is quite small. The only controlled study on splinting prospectively compared it with steroid injection but failed to report any statistical analysis.[4] The method of assignment to the steroid injection group was not delineated, and clinical evaluations were not blinded. Thus, the body of evidence is insufficient to allow any recommendation for or against splinting as an effective treatment for trigger finger.

For steroid injection, the literature is stronger, with two prospective, triple-blinded, placebo-controlled studies available.[7,8] However, the randomization process was not reported in one[8] and was based on odd/even date for the other,[7] both of which may be sources of potential selection bias. The studies had relatively small groups, but steroid injection was significantly more effective than lidocaine placebo in both. Of note, both studies excluded patients with insulin-dependent diabetes mellitus. The study comparing subcutaneous with intrasheath steroid injection was novel, but unfortunately had insufficient power to support the alternative recommendation that subcutaneous injection is sufficient for treating trigger finger.[10] The authors report their β value as 0.08; recalculation shows the study power is actually 0.08 (8% power), with a β value of 0.92. Patients with diabetes mellitus had significantly poorer response to steroid injection than patients without diabetes, although follow-up evaluation was not blinded in any of the reviewed studies.[12,13] Longer duration of symptoms did not adversely affect response to steroid injection. Although neither study showed any difference between patients with insulin-dependent and non–insulin-dependent diabetes, a single small, retrospective study comparing these two populations showed that patients with insulin-dependent diabetes fared worse.[14] The evidence is fair in support of steroid injection in the treatment of trigger finger, with fair evidence that it is less effective in patients with diabetes mellitus, who may be more likely to require surgical management. No contraindication to its use in insulin-dependent patients has been found, but evidence regarding its efficacy is conflicted.

The two retrospective studies comparing steroid injection with open A1 pulley release showed no significant difference between the two treatments,[15,16] but power analyses were not performed

Continued

RECOMMENDATIONS—cont'd

to rule out the possibility of type II error. Lack of randomization and blinding make selection and ascertainment bias potential confounders as well. No complications were associated with steroid injection, but 7% of the open surgical release patients experienced minor complications.[16] A single prospective, randomized, controlled study comparing percutaneous needle release with open A1 pulley release showed equal efficacy with no major complications in either group.[19] However, the randomization process was not clearly defined and assessment was not blinded. Fair evidence exists to support the effectiveness of surgery in the treatment of trigger finger, but insufficient evidence to recommend it over steroid injection. The body of evidence is too small to make any recommendations regarding percutaneous versus open surgical techniques.

Based on currently published evidence, the following treatment algorithm is proposed by this author (Level V): splinting may be tried first for the treatment of stenosing tenosynovitis of the finger. Its effectiveness is dependent on the level of patient compliance. It is less likely to be effective for trigger thumb. Successful treatment is defined as pain-free resolution of symptoms with full active motion. If splinting fails, steroid injection is likely to be effective, regardless of the duration of symptoms prior to presentation. A maximum of three intrasheath injections of a long acting corticosteroid is given every 3 weeks as necessary. In patients with diabetes mellitus, only one steroid injection is recommended, followed by surgery if no response. If injection fails, open surgical release of the A1 pulley is recommended. Percutaneous needle release may be performed, based on surgeon experience, because a learning curve exists. The most common complication after surgery is stiffness. The major treatment recommendations are presented in summary form in Table 15–5, with their accompanying grades of recommendation.

Clearly, a great need exists for well-designed clinical trials even to improve the management of a common condition such as trigger finger. As a common condition that is treated by a wide variety of clinicians, the potential to conduct large, prospective, controlled studies with properly randomized treatment groups is good. Standardization of symptoms and clinical findings, possibly with a universal grading system, would improve validity. Long-term follow-up studies with each treatment modality would be useful to better define treatment successes or failures. Double or even triple blinding could be readily achieved, to minimize bias as a confounding factor. Careful attention to study design is the key to improving the body of available evidence.

TABLE 15–5. Summary of Recommendations for Treatment of Trigger Finger

RECOMMENDATIONS	ARTICLES AND LEVELS OF EVIDENCE	GRADE OF RECOMMENDATION
Splinting is effective in the treatment of trigger finger.	2	B
A single intrasheath steroid injection is effective in the treatment of trigger finger.	2, 2	B
Subcutaneous steroid injection at the A1 pulley is as effective as intrasheath injection.	2	B
Patients with diabetes with trigger finger are less likely to respond to steroid injection and should be treated surgically.	3, 3	B
Patients with insulin-dependent diabetes with trigger finger should not be treated with steroid injection.	3	B
A series of steroid injections is as effective as and less risky than surgery for trigger finger.	3, 3	B
Percutaneous A1 pulley release is as effective as and less morbid than open pulley release.	2	B

REFERENCES

1. Notta A: Recherches sur une affection particulier des gaines tendineuses de la main. Arch Gen Med 24:142, 1850.
2. Strom L: Trigger finger in diabetes. J Med Soc N J 74:951–954, 1977.
3. Rhoades CE, Gelberman RH, Manjarris JF: Stenosing tenosynovitis of the fingers and thumb. Clin Orthop 190:236–238, 1984.
4. Patel MR, Bassini L: Trigger fingers and thumb: When to splint, inject, or operate. J Hand Surg [Am] 17:110–113, 1992.
5. Ryzewicz M, Wolf JM: Trigger digits: Principles, management, and complications. J Hand Surg [Am] 31:135–146, 2006.
6. Lapidus PW, Guidotti EP: Stenosing tenovaginitis of the wrist and fingers. Clin Orthop 83:87–90, 1972.
7. Murphy D, Failla JM, Koniuch MP: Steroid versus placebo injection for trigger finger. J Hand Surg [Am] 628–631, 1995.
8. Lambert MA, Morton RJ, Sloan JP: Controlled study of the use of local steroid injection in the treatment of trigger finger and thumb. J Hand Surg [Br] 17:69–70, 1992.
9. Howard LD, Pratt DR, Bunnell S: The use of compound F (hydrocortisone) in operative and non-operative conditions of the hand. J Bone Joint Surg [Am] 35:994–1002, 1953.
10. Taras JS, Raphael JS, Pan WT, et al: Corticosteroid injections for trigger digits: Is intrasheath injection necessary? J Hand Surg [Am] 23:717–722, 1998.
11. Quinnell RC: Conservative management of trigger finger. Practitioner 244:187–190, 1980.
12. Nimigan AS, Ross DC, Gan BS, et al: Steroid injection in the management of trigger fingers. Am J Phys Med Rehabil 85: 36–43, 2006.
13. Stahl S, Kanter Y, Karnielli E: Outcome of trigger finger treatment in diabetes. J Diabetes Complications 11:287–290, 1997.

14. Griggs SM, Weiss APC, Lane LB, et al: Treatment of trigger finger in patients with diabetes mellitus. J Hand Surg [Am] 20:787–789, 1995.
15. Benson LS, Ptaszek AJ: Injection versus surgery in the treatment of trigger finger. J Hand Surg [Am] 22:138–144, 1997.
16. Kraemer BA, Young L, Arfken C: Stenosing flexor tenosynovitis. South Med J 83:806–811, 1990.
17. Lorthioir J: Surgical treatment of trigger finger by a subcutaneous method. J Bone Joint Surg [Am] 40:793–795, 1985.
18. Eastwood DM, Gupta KJ, Johnson DP: Percutaneous release of the trigger finger: An office procedure. J Hand Surg [Am] 17:114–117, 1992.
19. Gilberts ECAM, Beekman WH, Stevens HJPD, et al: Prospective randomized trial of open versus percutaneous surgery for trigger digits. J Hand Surg [Am] 26:497–500, 2001.
20. Fleisch SB, Spindler KP, Lee DH: Corticosteroid injections in the treatment of trigger finger: A level I and II systematic review. J Am Acad Orthop Surg 15:166–171, 2007.

What Is the Evidence for a Cause-and-Effect Linkage Between Occupational Hand Use and Symptoms of Carpal Tunnel Syndrome?

Isam Atroshi, MD, PhD

Because the cause of carpal tunnel syndrome (CTS) is in most cases still unknown, a number of explanatory theories have been proposed, one of which has been occupational hand use. The possible association between occupational hand use and CTS has been mainly based on the common belief that the pathophysiologic mechanism in CTS is increased pressure in the carpal tunnel. It has been suggested that certain hand or wrist activities or postures needed to perform occupational tasks may cause increased carpal tunnel pressure, which may lead to CTS. The hand and wrist activities and postures often linked to CTS have been mainly repetitive movements, force (or combinations of these two factors), and excessive flexion and extension.[1] The relationship between CTS and work has been argued for a long time[2]; an early review concludes that "exposure to physical work load factors, such as repetitive and forceful gripping, was probably a major risk factor for CTS in several types of worker populations."[3] The issue, however, has been debated intensely.[4,5]

Determining the possible association between certain occupations or occupational activities and CTS involves two essential aspects: measuring exposure and establishing the diagnosis (often called *CTS case definition*). These two aspects have not been managed in a standardized fashion in the literature. With regard to *exposure,* the methods of measuring occupational activities have mainly been self-report or expert judgment, with few studies using objective measures of hand posture or force (such as measuring number of cycles in a repetition, force exerted, or wrist angles). Other studies have used job titles to compare occupations, implying that they differ in their impact on the upper extremity. However, various work activities may differ even within the same categories, such as the amount of force or repetitiveness used in different activities classified as "low force" or "high repetitive," respectively. Besides, different types of work usually described as repetitive (e.g., computer work and packaging or assembling) are not similar. Hence, definition of high force versus low force and high repetition versus low repetition may not be consistent. In addition, no attempts have

been made to determine the length of exposure time for a given occupational stressor needed to cause disease. Regarding *case definition,* studies of CTS and occupational exposure have used different case definitions ranging from self-reported symptoms only to combination of symptoms, physical examination, and nerve conduction measurements. The use of different diagnostic criteria inevitably leads to different conclusions, and such studies cannot be considered to involve the same disease (i.e., numbness and tingling in the hand reported through a questionnaire is not the same entity as CTS diagnosed by a physician based on history and abnormal nerve conduction measurements). Demonstrating an association between occupation and symptoms cannot be interpreted as an association with CTS.

It is helpful to review the reported prevalence and incidence rates of CTS in the general population to interpret the results reported in the literature regarding the relationship between work and CTS. Using diagnostic criteria including nerve conduction measurements, researchers have reported the prevalence rates of CTS among women in general population studies to range from 3% to 6% and among men from 0.6% to 2.1%.[6–8] Based on symptoms and nerve conduction measurements, annual incidence rates of up to 0.5% among women and 0.1% among men have been reported.[9] If it is assumed that a certain occupation does not increase the risk for CTS, the prevalence of CTS in a random sample of workers from that occupation would likely be lower than that in an age- and sex-matched random general population sample because the latter would include former workers who are sick, disabled, or retired.

STUDY DESIGNS AND BIASES

To evaluate the strength of the evidence derived from the published studies that investigated the association between CTS and occupation, you must recognize the different types of study design and biases related to each study design.

Randomized Studies

Randomized studies investigating whether occupational hand use is associated with clinical CTS would probably be difficult to perform given the nature of the research question and the large samples needed; to my knowledge, no such studies have been performed.

Prospective Cohort Studies

Workers without CTS are enrolled and followed over a period during which occupational exposure is measured, and then the incidence of CTS is determined and compared between the exposed and the nonexposed persons (results usually shown as relative risks and their confidence intervals). The advantage of the prospective cohort study is that exposure is measured before the onset of disease, allowing determination of a causal relationship. A problem may be attrition of the sample during follow-up and the need for large samples that can generate an adequate number of CTS cases to allow firm conclusions.

Case–Control Studies

Workers who are CTS cases are identified through various methods and compared with control subjects (persons without CTS), ideally from the same population, regarding previous exposure (results usually shown as odds ratios and their confidence intervals). Problems associated with these studies include difficulties in obtaining representative samples of cases and controls, and accurate measurement of past occupational exposure.

Cross-sectional Studies

A sample from a general or occupational population is examined to identify CTS cases and measure occupational exposure at the same time, and the prevalence of CTS is compared between different occupations or between groups performing different occupational hand activities (results usually shown as odds or prevalence ratios and their confidence intervals). The problems with these studies include difficulties in obtaining a representative sample and in accurately measuring exposure. Moreover, cross-sectional studies cannot provide direct evidence for a causal relationship.

Reporting Bias

When exposure measurement and search for CTS cases are done at the same time, persons with hand symptoms, including those with CTS, may report exposure differently than persons without hand symptoms. The risk for reporting bias would be greater if the persons are asked specifically about hand symptoms and about activities that involve the hands at the same time. If workers with CTS report more exposure than workers without CTS because their reporting is influenced by the presence of disease and their belief that their symptoms are related to their occupation, this may result in a false-positive association. This type of bias should be considered in studies that show a positive association, especially when exposure is based on self-report. Case–control studies that rely on subjects' recollection of occupational exposure also are subject to reporting bias.

Misclassification

The magnitude of misclassification can be minimized with a more specific case definition that includes neurophysiologic examination and with objective measures of exposure.

Selection Bias

If there is a true causal relationship between a certain occupation and CTS that leads affected workers to leave that occupation, then a cross-sectional sample would mainly include persons without CTS (healthy worker effect). This bias may underestimate a true association between a certain occupation and CTS. Studies that use only healthy asymptomatic persons as control subjects carry the risk for overestimation of the association because control subjects should be as similar to the cases as possible except for the occupational exposure.

Confounders

It is well established that a number of factors such as age, sex, and body mass index are related to CTS.[6,8,10,11] If the exposed workers are older or have a greater proportion of overweight persons than the nonexposed workers, finding a greater prevalence of CTS may be related to these factors rather than to occupation. These factors need to be accounted for when comparing the prevalence of CTS in different occupational groups. Few studies have addressed nonoccupational hand use, but the importance of this factor is uncertain. Other medical conditions, such as inflammatory joint disease and diabetes, may also confound the association between CTS and occupation, but because of the relatively low prevalence of these conditions in occupational groups, their impact may not be large.

LITERATURE REVIEW

The evidence regarding the association between CTS and occupational hand use should be based on appropriate epidemiologic studies in which participants were selected from populations of exposed and nonexposed persons (different occupations or occupational activities), and the presence of CTS determined with reasonable accuracy. A review of the studies generated by the literature search showed several common problems that may affect the conclusions and subsequently the evidence derived from them. Inclusion and exclusion criteria were used to select appropriate studies for evaluation of the evidence.

Inclusion Criteria

Study Design. Although it is recognized that, in general, strong evidence would be based on Level I and II studies, the majority of the studies concerning the association between CTS and occupational hand use were Level III case–control or cross-sectional studies with few Level II prospective cohort studies and no Level I randomized studies. It was therefore believed appropriate to include Level III studies, but to take this fact into consideration when judging the strength of the overall evidence.

Selection of Participants

All studies that sampled participants from worker populations or general populations were considered. However, a number of studies selected participants from workers compensation or similar databases, a method subject to selection bias.

Carpal Tunnel Syndrome Case Definition

Many studies used self-reported symptoms, physical findings (usually Tinel's sign and Phalen's test), or both without nerve conduction measurement. Symptoms were usually self-reported either through questionnaire or interview often done by research assistants rather than by physicians experienced in the diagnosis of CTS. In addition, studies differed in their definition of symptoms required for the diagnosis with regard to location, severity, and frequency. The issue of CTS case definition was considered to be essential for the purpose of this report. A case definition based entirely on symptoms would probably lead to substantial misclassification. The prevalence of symptoms (numbness or tingling) in the hands is relatively high, and only a proportion of these symptomatic persons actually have CTS.[8,12] Although there may be some evidence supporting the common clinical practice that patients judged by the treating physician to have characteristic CTS symptoms may not need electrophysiologic confirmation, nerve conduction tests will increase the probability of a correct diagnosis in all types of settings. The severity of CTS in epidemiologic studies is expected to be lower than that in clinical settings, and because nerve conduction measurement results are more likely to be normal in mild than in severe CTS, this makes the diagnostic procedure in epidemiologic studies more difficult.

Questionnaires inquiring about symptoms would have low specificity, and although interviews can confirm the presence and location of the reported symptoms, an interview performed for the purpose of establishing a CTS diagnosis based on symptoms alone may need to be conducted by an examiner who can judge whether the symptoms are related to CTS or other disorder, or are nonspecific. Results based on reported symptoms alone are thus not appropriate as evidence of the association between work and CTS. However, the combination of symptoms and abnormal nerve conduction will substantially improve the specificity and would be reasonably reliable as a diagnostic procedure. In a general population study, the prevalence of symptoms was 14%, whereas with symptoms and abnormal nerve conduction, the prevalence rate was down to 5%.[8] A similar pattern has been reported in occupational populations.[13] This suggests that the degree of misclassification is substantially lower if a combination of symptoms and nerve conduction measurement is used in case definition for occupational studies than symptoms alone. The use of this case definition may still imply two problematic situations. First, a proportion of CTS cases with normal (i.e., false-negative) nerve conduction testing results would be excluded; this situation, which may occur in up to 20% of subjects,[8,14] is expected to affect both the exposed and nonexposed groups equally and, therefore, may affect the precision but not the size of the estimated association. Second, a proportion of persons with nonspecific numbness/tingling but with false-positive nerve conduction testing results would be included as CTS cases. In the presence of reporting bias (symptomatic persons reporting higher exposure), this situation may overestimate the association, but probably to a small degree. Although relatively high rates of abnormal nerve conduction testing results (15–20%) have been reported in general population samples[7,8] and among asymptomatic workers,[13,15] the combination of symptoms and nerve conduction measurements still constitutes the most accurate diagnostic method available in CTS. Any case definition will lead to misclassification of a proportion of cases, but in epidemiologic studies, the use of nerve conduction measurements combined with self-reported symptoms substantially reduces the degree of misclassification.[16] Similarly, studies that used a case definition based only on positive Tinel's sign and Phalen's test cannot be considered to provide adequate evidence because of the limitations of these tests in the diagnosis.[17]

Exclusion Criteria

Several studies that assessed the relationship between CTS and occupational hand use could not be considered in evaluating the evidence because of one or more of the following reasons:

1. Cases were identified through workers' compensation or other insurance claims databases. This

selection method is subject to high risk for bias that may substantially affect the conclusions.

2. No control/referent group was included.

3. CTS cases were diagnosed based on self-reported symptoms only, physical signs only, or nerve conduction measurements without symptoms. Studies with CTS case definition that did not include both symptoms and nerve conduction measurements were not considered in the evidence; however, studies with less specific case definitions but with large populations are described here.

4. CTS cases were workers with occupations that mainly involved use of handheld vibratory tools. In these workers, symptoms may have been related, at least in part, to vibration-induced neuropathy rather than compression neuropathy. Because of the difficulty in accurately differentiating CTS from hand-arm vibration syndrome, frequent use of vibratory tools is a significant confounder when other occupational factors are assessed.

5. Important confounders (age and sex) were not accounted for.

The studies retrieved through the literature search concerning occupational hand use and CTS (published through January 2007) were examined for relevance and whether they met the inclusion and exclusion criteria. Eligible studies were then classified according to the level of evidence and data regarding the populations studied, the exposure and the findings (prevalence, odds ratios, or relative risks) were recorded. The studies were grouped according to occupational activity and occupational title.

RESULTS

The review showed that most of the relevant studies had been included in two previous reviews, the most recent of which examined the literature published through 2004.[18,19] Several of the studies that have assessed the relationship between CTS and occupational activities (Table 16–1) or occupational title (Table 16–2), using an adequate case definition (symptoms and nerve conduction measurement),[8,20–31] have shown an association between CTS and either certain occupational activities (hand force, excessive wrist flexion/extension, or repetitive wrist motion) or certain occupations, with relative risks or odds ratios of up to 9.0 shown. However, some associations were inconsistent. In a number of "negative" studies that failed to show a statistically significant association, the lower limit of the 95% confidence interval for the odds ratio was just less than 1.0, suggesting a small sample size.

Studies with Less Specific Case Definitions

In a longitudinal cohort study from Denmark, Andersen and coworkers[32] investigated the relationship between computer work and CTS in a sample of 9480

technical assistants and machine technicians with a 1-year follow-up period; response rate was 73% at baseline and 82% at follow-up. Symptoms and exposure (mouse and keyboard use) were self-reported using a questionnaire and interview, but the case definition was based on symptoms only. The authors report an association between mouse use for more than 20 hours/week and risk for symptoms, but no statistically significant association with keyboard use, and conclude that "computer use does not pose a severe occupational hazard for developing symptoms of CTS."[32] The association between computer work and CTS has also been investigated in studies with adequate case definition. Gerr and colleagues[33] followed 582 persons newly hired into jobs requiring at least 15 hours per week of computer use for up to 3 years, finding a low incidence of electrophysiologically confirmed CTS (3 cases). Stevens and researchers[34] examined 256 employees described as frequent computer users at a medical facility, finding only 9 persons with electrophysiologically confirmed CTS and concluding that the prevalence was similar to that reported in general population studies. The overall evidence from a number of studies suggests that computer work is not associated with greater risk for CTS.

In a relatively large case–control study from France, Leclerc and coworkers[35] compared 1210 workers in repetitive work (assembly line, clothing and shoe industry, and food industry) from 53 different companies with a control group of 337 workers. Exposure was measured partly by self-report and partly assessed by occupational physicians, but the case definition demanded only positive Tinel's sign or Phalen's test (symptoms were not part of the criteria). The authors conclude that "CTS was associated with several factors including repetitive work, especially packaging."[35] Using the same case definition, the authors performed a longitudinal study of 598 workers (assembly, clothing, food, packaging, cashiers) who were re-examined after 3 years, and reported an association between CTS and forceful movements.[36] In a large cross-sectional study from France, Melchior and colleagues[37] examined a random sample of 2656 workers for a variety of upper limb musculoskeletal disorders including CTS, which was diagnosed based on symptoms and signs only. The authors report a greater risk for "CTS" in manual compared with nonmanual workers, which after adjusting for age, obesity, and medical conditions was statistically significant among women (prevalence ratio, 2.1; 95% confidence interval, 1.2–3.7) but not among men (prevalence ratio, 1.4; 95% confidence interval, 0.7–2.8).

In a longitudinal study, Nathan and investigators[38] examined a cohort of 471 workers from 4 industries in Oregon, at baseline and after 11 and 17 years; the case definition changed from only abnormal nerve conduction at baseline to what was described as "research-defined CTS" requiring symptoms (at least twice per month) and abnormal nerve conduction or previous

TABLE 16–1. Studies of Carpal Tunnel Syndrome and Occupational Activities Using a Carpal Tunnel Syndrome Case Definition of Symptoms and Abnormal Nerve Conduction Measurement Results (Unless Specified)

AUTHOR (YEAR OF PUBLICATION)	STUDY POPULATION	ACTIVITY	RR OR OR (95% CI)	CONFOUNDERS ACCOUNTED FOR	COMMENT
Atroshi et al. (1999)[8]	1422 active workers in random general population sample	Excessive force with hand (>1 hr/day) Excessively flexed or extended wrist (>1 hr/day)	3.2 (1.6–6.3) 2.6 (1.2–5.3)	Age, sex, BMI, medical conditions	Cross-sectional, population based; exposure, self-reported (general health questionnaire); CTS prevalence rate of 2.6%
de Krom et al. (1990)[20]	156 CTS cases (28 from random general population sample, 128 from hospital); 473 control subjects from general population	Flexed wrist, 20–40 hr/wk Extended wrist, 20–40 hr/wk	8.7 (3.1–24.1) 5.4 (1.1–27.4)	Age, sex, BMI, medical conditions	Mixture of cross-sectional and case–control study, cases drawn from two different populations; exposure, self-reported (interview)
Gell et al. (2005)[21]	432 industrial and clerical workers followed an average of 5.4 years	Threshold limit value for peak force–hand activity level = 3 (highest of 3 categories; derived from rating of force and repetition level, each 0–10 scale)	1.6 (0.9–2.9) (new-onset CTS)	Age, sex, BMI, symptoms, and nerve conduction at baseline	Longitudinal; participation rate 51% of original sample; exposure measured at baseline using job activity level rating; average annual incidence rate of 1.2%
Latko et al. (1999)[22]	336 workers from 3 manufacturing companies	Repetition: One-unit increase (0–10 scale) High vs. low repetition (3 levels)	1.2 (0.98–1.5) 3.1 (0.89–10.9)	Age, sex, wrist ratio	Cross-sectional; exposure measured with observational rating method; CTS prevalence rate of 5.6%
Roquelaure et al. (1997)[23]	65 CTS cases identified from occupational health records for plants manufacturing TV sets, shoes, and automobile breaks; 65 age-, sex-, and plant-matched referents	Hand force >1 kg (≥10 times/hr) Short elemental cycle (≤10 seconds) No job rotation	9.0 (2.4–33.4) 8.8 (1.8–44.4) 6.3 (2.1–19.3)	Age, sex	Small study; case definition was symptoms and nerve conduction or previous CTS surgery; exposure measured with direct observation
Thomsen et al. (2002)[24]	731 employees at a bank and 2 postal centers (389 repetitive nonforceful, 73 forceful nonrepetitive, 28 forceful repetitive, 219 nonforceful nonrepetitive)	Repetitive work (10-hour increase/wk of repetitive nonforceful work) Forceful work (10-hour increase/wk of forceful nonrepetitive work)	1.8 (1.1–3.2) 1.4 (0.9–2.3)	Age, sex, BMI	Cross-sectional and follow-up; detailed exposure measurement; no CTS cases among control subjects (nonrepetitive nonforceful work); follow-up part yielded few CTS cases
Werner et al. (2005)[25]	189 automobile assembly workers without CTS followed over 1 year	Elbow posture rating (1-point increase on 1–10 scale) Hand repetition level, peak hand force, and wrist flexion/extension	8.1 (1.5–44.2) Not significant (new-onset CTS)	Sex, BMI, baseline median neuropathy, diabetes	Longitudinal; only 279 of more than 1700 workers participated; exposure measured using job activity level rating; of the 20 new cases, only 10 had documented electrodiagnostic testing

Confidence interval (CI) for relative risk (RR) or odds ratio (OR) that does not include 1.0 indicates statistical significance.
BMI 5 body mass index; CTS 5 carpal tunnel syndrome.
Adapted from Palmer KT, Harris EC, Coggon D: Carpal tunnel syndrome and its relation to occupation: A systematic literature review. Occup Med (Lond) 57:57–66, 2007 by permission of Oxford University Press.

TABLE 16–2. Studies of Carpal Tunnel Syndrome and Job Title Using a Carpal Tunnel Syndrome Case Definition of Symptoms and Abnormal Nerve Conduction Measurement Results (Unless Specified)

AUTHOR (YEAR OF PUBLICATION)	EXPOSED/NONEXPOSED	RR OR OR (95% CI)	CONFOUNDERS ACCOUNTED FOR	COMMENT
Atroshi et al. (1999)[8]	710 active blue-collar workers/712 active white collar workers	2.1 (1.1–4.2)	Age, sex, BMI	Population-based employment data through general health questionnaire
Barnhart et al. (1991)[26]	106 ski-manufacturing workers in repetitive jobs/67 nonrepetitive jobs	1.6 (0.8–3.2)	Age, sex	Case definition: electrophysiology + positive Phalen's test or Tinel's sign and/or ever having had hand pain or tingling/numbness
Bonfiglioli et al. (2007)[27]	71 full-time cashiers, 155 part-time cashiers/98 office workers All female subjects from 4 big supermarket stores	Cashiers vs. office workers: Part-time: 1.06 (0.35–3.2) Full-time: 1.8 (0.52–6.3)	Age, BMI, other	High participation rate; significant association with symptoms but not with CTS (prevalence; full-time cashiers 9.9%, part-time cashiers 7.1%, office workers 8.2%)
Frost et al. (1998)[28]	743 slaughterhouse workers/398 control subjects (299 from chemical factory)	All: 4.0 (1.7–9.3) Nondeboning: 3.1 (1.3–8.0) Deboning: 4.9 (2.0–11.8)	Age, sex, BMI, smoking, medical conditions	Case definition: symptoms and nerve conduction or previous surgery for CTS; exposure described as high force/repetitive
Kutluhan et al. (2001)[29]	70 women carpet workers from 3 workshops in Turkey/30 healthy housewives	3.8 (1.05–14.1) (CTS in 30% of workers and 10% of control subjects)	Age, medical conditions	Small study with risk for bias in selection of cases (no data about participation rate) and control subjects (selection method not reported)
Osorio et al. (1994)[30]	56 supermarket workers (bakery icers, meat cutters, and cashiers) working ≥20 hr/wk/low-exposure group (others)	6.7 (0.8–52.9)	Age, sex	Small study
Rosecrance et al. (2002)[31]	Apprentice construction workers from a U.S. trades union (136 sheet metal workers, 486 operating engineers, 330 plumbers/pipe fitters)/163 apprentice electricians	Sheet metal workers: 2.0 (0.8–5.0) Engineers: 1.0 (0.5–2.2) Plumbers/pipe fitters: 1.2 (0.5–2.0)	Age, BMI	High participation rate; prevalence rate of CTS 8.3% among women and 8.2% among men

Confidence interval (CI) for relative risk (RR) or odds ratio (OR) that does not include 1.0 indicates statistical significance.
BMI = body mass index; CTS = carpal tunnel syndrome.
Adapted from Palmer KT, Harris EC, Coggon D: Carpal tunnel syndrome and its relation to occupation: A systematic literature review. Occup Med (Lond) 57:57–66, 2007 by permission of Oxford University Press.

CTS surgery at the final follow-up.[38-40] The baseline work exposure was used despite possible work change over time, and large attrition of the sample occurred with 54% and 35% participation rates at the two follow-up examinations, respectively. The authors consistently report no association between CTS and occupational repetition or force. The significant risk for bias limits the contribution of these studies to the overall evidence. In a case–control study Nordstrom and coauthors[41] identify 206 "newly diagnosed" CTS cases from clinic database in the Marshfield area in Wisconsin (physician-made diagnosis not requiring nerve conduction testing) and compare them with 211 randomly sampled residents with no CTS diagnosis; information on risk factors was obtained through telephone interviews and from medical records.[41] After adjustment for age, sex, body mass index, and other medical conditions, the occupational risk factors that showed statistically significant associations with "CTS" were frequent (>6 vs. 0 hours) use of power tools/machinery and bending/twisting of hands/wrists, with odds ratios (95% confidence interval) of 3.3 (1.1–9.8) and 2.1 (1.0–4.5), respectively.

In a case–control study from Canada, Rossignol and colleagues[42] used Montreal's surgery database of 1 year to identify 969 first-surgery CTS cases and conducted telephone interviews of a sample of 238 cases to obtain occupational history (94% reported having electrodiagnostic tests but no data on results). The authors conclude that among manual workers, "55% of surgical CTS in women and 76% in men was attributable to work," and that increased risk for surgical CTS was found in seven occupational groups. The study adjusted for age and sex but not for other confounders, and the use of surgery database and telephone interview of a sample to obtain occupational history may have introduced selection and reporting bias. In a frequently cited cross-sectional study, Silverstein and investigators[43] examined 652 workers in 39 jobs from 7 industries in the United States, using good exposure measurement (including observation and video analysis) to classify jobs into 4 groups (high/low force/repetition), but the case definition was based only on symptoms and physical signs. After adjustment for several potential confounders, the odds ratio of "CTS" in the high-force, high-repetition group compared with the low-force, low-repetition group was 15.5 (95% confidence interval, 1.7–142).

Experimental Studies

Several experimental studies have explored the hypothesis that working with certain wrist positions or force exertion may have potentially harmful effects on the median nerve in the carpal tunnel. A number of studies have measured carpal tunnel pressures in different wrist or hand positions or activities.[44-47] However, findings that wrist flexion and extension or certain finger positions or force levels lead to increased carpal canal pressure cannot be regarded as direct evidence that work with such positions will cause CTS. Similarly, studies have examined median nerve conduction or morphology in the carpal tunnel in certain occupational groups. The results of such experimental studies provide plausibility to the hypothesis, but not evidence, that specific work activities may lead to CTS.

CONCLUSIONS

To prove a causal relationship between occupational hand use and CTS, study investigators ideally would include an adequately large number of persons who have no symptoms of CTS at baseline, examine them clinically and neurophysiologically and follow them for an appropriate period, define and measure exposure with a reliable and valid method, and re-examine the persons at follow-up clinically and neurophysiologically to determine the incidence of CTS in the exposed and nonexposed groups. Most studies in the review were case–control or cross-sectional and had various limitations that affected the strength of the conclusions derived from them regarding the association between occupational hand use and CTS. The few longitudinal studies found typically were too small to yield adequate number of cases for strong conclusions regarding cause-and-effect relation. Dose–response associations have not been adequately demonstrated. Despite the limitations in the current literature, fairly consistent epidemiologic evidence has been reported of an association between certain work activities or certain occupations and CTS. However, the evidence does not permit firm conclusions about the exact nature of the cause, whether it is force, posture, repetitiveness, or a combination of these factors. A fair amount of evidence exists to support that occupations in which some or all of these factors are predominant (compared with other types of occupations) seem to be associated with a greater risk for CTS. Table 16–3 provides a summary of recommendations.

TABLE 16–3. Summary of Recommendations

ASSOCIATION BETWEEN OCCUPATIONAL ACTIVITY AND SYMPTOMS OF CARPAL TUNNEL SYNDROME	LEVEL OF EVIDENCE/GRADE OF RECOMMENDATION
Force (exertion of high force with the hand)	B
Repetitiveness (highly repetitive wrist motion)	B
Posture (prolonged extreme wrist flexion or extension)	B

Based on evidence from studies that involve one or more of these occupational activities, as well as studies that involve specific occupations in which one of these activities would be dominant.

REFERENCES

1. Keyserling WM, Stetson DS, Silverstein BA, et al: A checklist for evaluating ergonomic risk factors associated with upper extremity cumulative trauma disorders. Ergonomics 36:807–831, 1993.
2. Armstrong TJ, Chaffin DB: Carpal tunnel syndrome and selected personal attributes. J Occup Med 21:481–486, 1979.
3. Hagberg M, Morgenstern H, Kelsh M: Impact of occupations and job tasks on the prevalence of carpal tunnel syndrome. Scand J Work Environ Health 18:337–345, 1992.
4. Szabo RM, King KJ: Repetitive stress injury: Diagnosis or self-fulfilling prophecy? J Bone Joint Surg Am 82:1314–1322, 2000.
5. Amadio PC: Repetitive stress injury. J Bone Joint Surg Am 83:136–137, 2001.
6. de Krom MC, Knipschild PG, Kester AD, et al: Carpal tunnel syndrome: Prevalence in the general population. J Clin Epidemiol 45:373–376, 1992.
7. Ferry S, Pritchard T, Keenan J, et al: Estimating the prevalence of delayed median nerve conduction in the general population. Br J Rheumatol 37:630–635, 1998.
8. Atroshi I, Gummesson C, Johnsson R, et al: Prevalence of carpal tunnel syndrome in a general population. JAMA 282:153–158, 1999.
9. Mondelli M, Giannini F, Giacchi M: Carpal tunnel syndrome incidence in a general population. Neurology 58:289–294, 2002.
10. Werner RA, Albers JW, Franzblau A, et al: The relationship between body mass index and the diagnosis of carpal tunnel syndrome. Muscle Nerve 17:632–636, 1994.
11. Werner RA, Franzblau A, Albers JW, et al: Influence of body mass index and work activity on the prevalence of median mononeuropathy at the wrist. Occup Environ Med 54:268–271, 1997.
12. Anton D, Rosecrance J, Merlino L, et al: Prevalence of musculoskeletal symptoms and carpal tunnel syndrome among dental hygienists. Am J Ind Med 42:248–257, 2002.
13. Isolani L, Bonfiglioli R, Raffi GB, et al: Different case definitions to describe the prevalence of occupational carpal tunnel syndrome in meat industry workers. Int Arch Occup Environ Health 75:229–234, 2002.
14. Finsen V, Russwurm H: Neurophysiology not required before surgery for typical carpal tunnel syndrome. J Hand Surg [Br] 26:61–64, 2001.
15. Homan MM, Franzblau A, Werner RA, et al: Agreement between symptom surveys, physical examination procedures and electrodiagnostic findings for the carpal tunnel syndrome. Scand J Work Environ Health 25:115–124, 1999.
16. Rempel D, Evanoff B, Amadio PC, et al: Consensus criteria for the classification of carpal tunnel syndrome in epidemiologic studies. Am J Public Health 88:1447–1451, 1998.
17. Gerr F, Letz R: The sensitivity and specificity of tests for carpal tunnel syndrome vary with the comparison subjects. J Hand Surg [Br] 23:151–155, 1998.
18. National Institute for Occupational Health Safety: Musculoskeletal disorders and workplace factors: A critical review of epidemiologic evidence for work-related musculoskeletal disorders of the neck, upper extremity and low back. Cincinnati, OH: US Department of Health and Human Sciences/NIOSH, 1997.
19. Palmer KT, Harris EC, Coggon D: Carpal tunnel syndrome and its relation to occupation: A systematic literature review. Occup Med (Lond) 57:57–66, 2007.
20. de Krom MC, Kester AD, Knipschild PG, et al: Risk factors for carpal tunnel syndrome. Am J Epidemiol 132:1102–1110, 1990.
21. Gell N, Werner RA, Franzblau A, et al: A longitudinal study of industrial and clerical workers: Incidence of carpal tunnel syndrome and assessment of risk factors. J Occup Rehabil 15:47–55, 2005.
22. Latko WA, Armstrong TJ, Franzblau A, et al: Cross-sectional study of the relationship between repetitive work and the prevalence of upper limb musculoskeletal disorders. Am J Ind Med 36:248–259, 1999.
23. Roquelaure Y, Mechali S, Dano C, et al: Occupational and personal risk factors for carpal tunnel syndrome in industrial workers. Scand J Work Environ Health 23:364–369, 1997.
24. Thomsen JF, Hansson GA, Mikkelsen S, et al: Carpal tunnel syndrome in repetitive work: A follow-up study. Am J Ind Med 42:344–353, 2002.
25. Werner RA, Franzblau A, Gell N, et al: Incidence of carpal tunnel syndrome among automobile assembly workers and assessment of risk factors. J Occup Environ Med 47:1044–1050, 2005.
26. Barnhart S, Demers PA, Miller M, et al: Carpal tunnel syndrome among ski manufacturing workers. Scand J Work Environ Health 17:46–52, 1991.
27. Bonfiglioli R, Mattioli S, Fiorentini C, et al: Relationship between repetitive work and the prevalence of carpal tunnel syndrome in part-time and full-time female supermarket cashiers: A quasi-experimental study. Int Arch Occup Environ Health 80:248–253, 2007.
28. Frost P, Andersen JH, Nielsen VK: Occurrence of carpal tunnel syndrome among slaughterhouse workers. Scand J Work Environ Health 24:285–292, 1998.
29. Kutluhan S, Akhan G, Demirci S, et al: Carpal tunnel syndrome in carpet workers. Int Arch Occup Environ Health 74:454–457, 2001.
30. Osorio AM, Ames RG, Jones J, et al: Carpal tunnel syndrome among grocery store workers. Am J Ind Med 25:229–245, 1994.
31. Rosecrance JC, Cook TM, Anton DC, et al: Carpal tunnel syndrome among apprentice construction workers. Am J Ind Med 42:107–116, 2002.
32. Andersen JH, Thomsen JF, Overgaard E, et al: Computer use and carpal tunnel syndrome: A 1-year follow-up study. JAMA 289:2963–2969, 2003.
33. Gerr F, Marcus M, Ensor C, et al: A prospective study of computer users: I. Study design and incidence of musculoskeletal symptoms and disorders. Am J Ind Med 41:221–235, 2002.
34. Stevens JC, Witt JC, Smith BE, et al: The frequency of carpal tunnel syndrome in computer users at a medical facility. Neurology 56:1568–1570, 2001.
35. Leclerc A, Franchi P, Cristofari MF, et al: Carpal tunnel syndrome and work organisation in repetitive work: A cross sectional study in France. Study Group on Repetitive Work. Occup Environ Med 55:180–187, 1998.
36. Leclerc A, Landre MF, Chastang JF, et al: Upper-limb disorders in repetitive work. Scand J Work Environ Health 27:268–278, 2001.
37. Melchior M, Roquelaure Y, Evanoff B, et al: Why are manual workers at high risk of upper limb disorders? The role of physical work factors in a random sample of workers in France (the Pays de la Loire study). Occup Environ Med 63:754–761, 2006.
38. Nathan PA, Meadows KD, Doyle LS: Occupation as a risk factor for impaired sensory conduction of the median nerve at the carpal tunnel. J Hand Surg [Br] 13:167–170, 1988.
39. Nathan PA, Meadows KD, Istvan JA: Predictors of carpal tunnel syndrome: An 11-year study of industrial workers. J Hand Surg [Am] 27:644–651, 2002.
40. Nathan PA, Istvan JA, Meadows KD: A longitudinal study of predictors of research-defined carpal tunnel syndrome in industrial workers: Findings at 17 years. J Hand Surg [Br] 30:593–598, 2005.
41. Nordstrom DL, Vierkant RA, DeStefano F, et al: Risk factors for carpal tunnel syndrome in a general population. Occup Environ Med 54:734–740, 1997.
42. Rossignol M, Stock S, Patry L, et al: Carpal tunnel syndrome: What is attributable to work? The Montreal Study. Occup Environ Med 54:519–523, 1997.
43. Silverstein BA, Fine LJ, Armstrong TJ: Occupational factors and carpal tunnel syndrome. Am J Ind Med 11:343–358, 1987.
44. Szabo RM, Chidgey LK: Stress carpal tunnel pressures in patients with carpal tunnel syndrome and normal patients. J Hand Surg [Am] 14:624–627, 1989.
45. Werner R, Armstrong TJ, Bir C, et al: Intracarpal canal pressures: The role of finger, hand, wrist and forearm position. Clin Biomech (Bristol, Avon) 12:44–51, 1997.
46. Keir PJ, Bach JM, Rempel DM: Effects of finger posture on carpal tunnel pressure during wrist motion. J Hand Surg [Am] 23:1004–1009, 1998.
47. Keir PJ, Bach JM, Rempel DM: Fingertip loading and carpal tunnel pressure: Differences between a pinching and a pressing task. J Orthop Res 16:112–115, 1998.

What Are the Best Diagnostic Tests for Complex Regional Pain Syndrome?

Kevin C. Chung, MD, MS and Ahmer K. Ghori, BA

HISTORY

The French physician Claude Bernard (1813–1878) first described the condition now called *complex regional pain syndrome* (CRPS).[1] His student, Silas Weir Mitchell, attributed it to autonomic instability and proposed the term *causalgia* for this diagnosis.[2] Since then, a variety of other names has also been used to describe this condition, including algodystrophy, sympathalgia, post-traumatic spreading neuralgia, and reflex sympathetic dystrophy. Although *reflex sympathetic dystrophy* was the widely accepted diagnostic term for a long time, the role of the sympathetic nervous system in the pathophysiology of this syndrome has not been confirmed. Therefore, in a consensus workshop of the International Association for the Study of Pain (IASP) in 1995, it was recommended that the condition known as reflex sympathetic dystrophy be called *complex regional pain syndrome* (CRPS).

Complex Regional Pain Syndrome: Causative Factors and Natural Progression

CRPS is divided into two subtypes, I and II, on the basis of an association with peripheral nerve pathology.[3] CRPS I includes cases in whom no associated nerve pathology exists and in whom CRPS develops after a noxious event.[3] For example, the reported incidence of CRPS I after various fractures is 1% to 2% (7–35% after Colles' fractures).[4] CRPS II includes cases in which there are known nerve pathology, and it mostly affects large nerves such as the median or sciatic nerves.[3] For example, the reported incidence of CRPS II after peripheral nerve injuries is 2% to 5%; 10% to 26% of CRPS cases are idiopathic.[4]

CRPS may progress through three stages.[1] Stage 1 (acute) is a warm phase, and it is characterized by pain, sensory abnormalities, vasomotor dysfunction, edema, and sudomotor disturbances. Stage II (dystrophic) may be warm or cold, and it is characterized by worsening of stage I symptoms. In addition, motor and trophic (hair and nail growth) changes are first noted in stage II. Stage III (atrophic) is a cold phase in which pain and sensory disturbances decrease, but motor and trophic abnormalities worsen. In addition,

atrophy of affected muscles may be noted. In some cases, the specific stages of CRPS may be difficult to identify clinically because they may blend into one another in a more continuous spectrum of manifestations. In one study, 13% of patients with acute CRPS had cold affected areas.[2] In some patients, the warm phase has been noted to persist for as long as 8 to 12 years after the initial diagnosis of CRPS.[4] Overall, this staging system is widely accepted in literature.[1]

COMPLEX REGIONAL PAIN SYNDROME: CLINICAL DIAGNOSIS

The IASP has suggested diagnostic criteria on multiple occasions,[5] and these have been helpful in organizing the thought process in diagnosing CRPS. However, multiple studies have found that the IASP criteria have satisfactory sensitivity, but have poor specificity leading to a risk for overdiagnosis.[6–8] Because clinical symptoms can lead to overdiagnosis, in suspicious cases, more advanced tests that have better specificity may be administered to reduce false positives of clinical diagnosis. The clinical diagnosis criteria were revised in 2003, and the new standard that has better specificity[1] is described in Table 17–1. Clinical diagnosis has grade B level evidence (Table 17–2).

CLINICAL DIAGNOSIS: SPECIFIC SYMPTOMS AND DIAGNOSTIC METHODS

The clinical symptoms of CRPS fall into four broad categories: (1) sensory, (2) vasomotor, (3) sudomotor, (4) motor/trophic. The most common findings in each category and common techniques to diagnose these symptoms are presented in the following sections.

Sensory Changes

Pain is the most frequently encountered symptom in CRPS; 81% of CRPS patients suffer severe pain.[1] The nature of pain is often described as burning or stinging, which typically starts at the distal end of an extremity and propagates proximally.[9]

TABLE 17–1. Criteria for Clinical Diagnosis of Complex Regional Pain Syndrome

1. Continuing pain, which is disproportionate to any inciting event.
2. Patient must report at least three of the following symptoms:
   a. Sensory: reports of hyperesthesia
   b. Vasomotor: reports of temperature asymmetry and/or skin color changes and/or skin color asymmetry
   c. Sudomotor/Edema: reports of edema and/or sweating changes and/or sweating asymmetry
   d. Motor/Trophic: reports of decreased range of motion and/or motor dysfunction (weakness, tremor, dystonia) and/or trophic changes (hair, nail, skin)
3. Physician must verify at least two of the following signs:
   a. Sensory: evidence of hyperalgesia (to pinprick) and/or allodynia (to light touch)
   b. Vasomotor: evidence of temperature asymmetry and/or skin color changes and/or asymmetry
   c. Sudomotor/Edema: evidence of edema and/or sweating changes and/or sweating asymmetry
   d. Motor/Trophic: evidence of decreased range of motion and/or motor dysfunction (weakness, tremor, dystonia, neglect) and/or trophic changes (hair, nail, skin)

Adapted from Harden RN, Bruehl SP: Diagnosis of complex regional pain syndrome: Signs, symptoms, and new empirically derived diagnostic criteria. Clin J Pain 22:415–419, 2006.

Hyperesthesia and allodynia are reported in 65% of CRPS patients,[1] and they do not follow sensory nerve distribution patterns.[9] This can be used to distinguish CRPS from nerve pathologies, which are limited to the affected nerve's distribution. Mechanical allodynia can be tested by light touch or brushing over the affected area. Temperature allodynia may be assessed with warm and cold test tubes of water.

In addition, quantitative sensory testing, which is a computerized measure of temperature and vibrations sense,[10] can be used for objective assessment of allodynia.[11–13] Quantitative thermal testing may be done using a Marstock thermostimulator (Thermotest equipment; Somedic AB, Stockholm, Sweden).[12] This equipment has an electrode that is placed on the patient's skin. Patients have control over cooling or heating the electrode, and they are asked to raise/lower temperature until it induces pain. The thermal thresholds of the affected and unaffected region are measured and compared with each other to look for allodynia. Similarly, quantitative vibration testing can

TABLE 17–2. Grades of Recommendation for Diagnostic Tests

TEST	GRADE OF RECOMMENDATION*
Clinical diagnostic criteria	B
Radiograph	B
Magnetic resonance imaging	B
Bone scanning	B
Sympathetic skin response	B

*A = good evidence (Level I studies with consistent finding) for or against recommending intervention; B = fair evidence (Level II or III studies with consistent findings) for or against recommending intervention; C = poor-quality evidence (Level IV or V with consistent findings) for or against recommending intervention; I = there is insufficient or conflicting evidence not allowing a recommendation for or against intervention.

be done using a handheld vibrator (TVR model, HV-13 D; Heiwa Electronic Industrial, Osaka, Japan).[12]

Vasomotor Changes

Bilateral asymmetry in color, temperature, or both is a common symptom in CRPS; 87% of CRPS patients have asymmetry in color, and 79% have asymmetry in temperature.[1] Classically, the affected area is warmer, redder, and edematous (80% of patients) compared with the unaffected area in early-stage CRPS.[1] In 54% of patients, the affected area changes from hyperthermic to hypothermic presentation with progression of disease.[9]

In severe cases of CRPS, temperature asymmetry may be diagnosed by touching the affected and unaffected areas. In some cases, the temperature asymmetry is subtle and its diagnosis may require more sophisticated equipments. Simple infrared thermometers have been used for this purpose, and their sensitivity and specificity varies from 70% to 90% in literature.[14] In addition, more advanced computerized thermography devices are available.[13–15] For example, TIP 50 imaging unit (Bales Scientific, Walnut Creek, CA) can be used to measure the average temperature of the affected region and its contralateral normal region. The sensitivity, specificity, positive predictive value, and negative predictive value of computerized thermography depend on the cutoff asymmetry value (how different the temperature between affected and unaffected regions has to be before stating that the asymmetry is clinically significant). For example, if we choose a high cutoff value (e.g., difference of 1°C instead of 0.5°C), there would be fewer false positives, but we will not detect more patients with CRPS. One study reported that a temperature asymmetry of 0.6°C is most optimal to balance sensitivity and specificity, but if specificity is more important, then a higher cutoff (0.8°C) may be used.[15] Another study found thermography to have a sensitivity of 93%, specificity of 98%, positive predictive value (PPV) of 90%, and negative predictive value (NPV) of 94%.[16]

Sudomotor Changes

Sudomotor changes, most notably increased sweating on the affected side, is correlated with CRPS, and this sweating asymmetry is more pronounced on exertion.[9] In severe cases, asymmetry in sweating can be assessed with touch or sight. In moderate cases, dragging a smooth tool on skin can be used to approximate sweating. In addition, the following more advanced tests are available:

1. Resting Sweat Output test (RST): RST equipment quantitatively measures sweating. It has a capsule attached to patients' skin over the affected and contralateral unaffected regions. Nitrogen flows through the capsule, and an evaporative water-loss unit measures heat con-

ductance of the nitrogen flowing in and flowing out of the capsule. The difference in heat conductance gives a quantitative measure of sweating rate. This test has a high specificity (94%),[14] which serves to detect false positives that are prevalent in clinical diagnosis.

2. Quantitative Sudomotor Axon Reflex Test (QSART): In this test, acetylcholine is applied on the affected and contralateral unaffected skin, and it is forced into the skin by local application of a 2-mA current. The sweat response is then measured using equipment similar to that described for RST. The combination of RST and QSART achieves a specificity of 98%.[14]

Motor/Trophic Changes

Motor changes are common in CRPS patients; 80% of CRPS patients report decreased range of motion, 75% report muscle weakness in the involved area, and 20% of patients suffer tremors.[1] Trophic changes include brittle nails (24% of patients)[1] and increased hair growth (21% of patients).[1] Motor and trophic changes have to be assessed by clinical observation.

COMPLEX REGIONAL PAIN SYNDROME: ADDITIONAL TESTS

The current literature reports imaging, nuclear medicine, and sympathetic skin response (SSR) tests, which have grade B evidence (see Table 17–2) that can complement the clinical diagnosis of CRPS. The imaging techniques that may assist in the diagnosis of CRPS are plain x-ray films and magnetic resonance imaging (MRI). Radiographs are useful in the diagnosis of CRPS I after a fracture because the bone changes extend beyond the original fracture site in early stages,[17] and diffuse osteoporosis with severe patchy demineralization may appear in later stages.[18] In fact, the amount of bone loss in CRPS over a few months is tantamount to bone loss over 10 years of uncomplicated osteoporosis.[17] One study reported radiographs to have a sensitivity of 36%, specificity of 94%, NPV of 86%, and PPV of 58% in diagnosing CRPS.[18] The signs of CRPS observed on MRI are skin thickening/enhancement and joint effusion.[18–20] One study found MRI to have a specificity of 98% and sensitivity of 14% in diagnosing CPRS I, 16 weeks after initial trauma.[18] The literature recommends that because imaging studies have low sensitivity, they cannot be used as screening tests, but their high specificity makes them valuable as second-line tests in patients who are suspected of having CRPS after clinical observation.

In the bone scanning test, a tracer is administered to the patient, and bone imaging is done. CRPS extremities are correlated with increased uptake of tracer and accelerated blood flow to the affected limb.[18] The diagnostic parameters of this test in literature are as follows: sensitivity (54–100%), specificity (85–98%), PPV (67–95%), and NPV (61–100%).[21] The diagnostic accuracy is influenced by the following factors: stage of the disease, age of the patient, nature of inciting event, and location of the disease.

SSR test, which measures changes in skin conductance in response to electrical stimulation, may be useful to diagnose CRPS. The electrical stimulation is delivered using electrodes, and skin conductance is measured using electromyography. SSR is increased in the affected region of patients with early-stage CRPS.[22–25] One study found that SSR was less than normal in the affected region of patients with late-stage CRPS.[26] Therefore, it may be possible to differentiate stages of CRPS using SSR. No definitive data are available on the sensitivity, specificity, PPV, and NPV of SSR.

COMPLEX REGIONAL PAIN SYNDROME: A DIAGNOSTIC SCHEME

To understand the use of diagnostic acumen in CRPS, most clinicians, regardless of training background, will benefit from a refresher discussion on the use of diagnostic tests. In the uncertainties of medicine, diagnostic tests are used to establish the presence of a particular disease. These diagnostic tests vary in complexity, cost, and invasiveness. Typically, the best test is often referred to as the gold standard test, or more appropriately should be termed the *reference standard* test because gold is no longer used as a currency standard. However, the reference standard test cannot be used in all circumstances because it may be difficult to administer, time consuming, or prohibitively expensive. Therefore, more practical alternative tests are used first. The robustness of these alternative tests is judged against the reference standard. The problem with more practical alternative tests is that they have more false positives and false negatives. False-positive result is when the test identifies an individual as having the disease, but that individual does not have the disease according to the reference standard. False-negative result is when the test identifies an individual as not having the disease, but that individual actually has the disease according to the reference standard. The following concepts are important to critically evaluate diagnostic tests: (1) sensitivity, (2) specificity, (3) PPV, and (4) NPV.

1. Sensitivity
   - The percentage of true positive results that a diagnostic test identifies as positive.
   - High sensitivity reduces false-negative results.
2. Specificity
   - The percentage of true negative results that a diagnostic test identifies as negative.
   - High specificity reduces false-positive results.
3. PPV
   - The probability that a positive test result indicates a true positive result.
4. NPV
   - The probability that a negative test result indicates a true negative result.

The difficulty in diagnosing CRPS is, in part, because there is no widely accepted reference standard test for this condition. In its absence, clinical observation of symptoms serves as the standard. It has high sensitivity, as we described earlier, and is useful as a screening test when CRPS is suspected. Unfortunately, clinical diagnosis lacks in specificity, which results in a relatively high number of false-positive results. This is because the symptoms used to diagnose CRPS may be seen in a variety of other illnesses. Therefore, the first thing to do after a positive clinical diagnosis is to confirm that this is CRPS and not another disease.

The diagnosis of CRPS may, in many cases, be a diagnosis of exclusion. Rheumatologic, orthopedic, neurologic, and vascular disorders can resemble the clinical features of CRPS, and it is important to differentiate among these alternative diagnoses. Unlike most rheumatic disorders, CRPS is not usually associated with increased sedimentation rates or specific antigen-antibody complexes.[4] Orthopedic disorders such as osteoporosis, bone bruise, stress fracture, and delayed fracture healing may also resemble CRPS,[9] but they may be distinguished from it by radiography and bone scanning. Neurological disorders such as postherpetic neuralgia, plexopathy, and entrapment neuropathy may also resemble CRPS symptoms.[9] However, associated venous thrombosis seen in CRPS[4] does not occur in neurologic disorders. Vascular disorders, such as chronic arterial insufficiency and Raynaud's disease, may also resemble CRPS. The former can be differentiated from CRPS because in arterial insufficiency, pulses are absent, but they are present in CRPS. Raynaud's disease is exacerbated by cold, whereas CRPS symptoms are exacerbated by exercise.[4] Therefore, cold and exercise stress tests can be used to distinguish between Raynaud's disease and CRPS. CRPS symptoms may also be mistaken for infection. But with CRPS, there is no fever and no change in serology.[4] If CRPS is still suspected after the aforementioned differential diagnosis, then the probability that the positive result is a true positive can be further clarified by administering advanced tests that have better specificity.

We have discussed the advanced tests that can confirm the diagnosis of CRPS. For confirmation of sensory dysfunction, quantitative sensory testing may be used. For confirming temperature asymmetry, computerized thermography may be used because it has a high specificity (98%). For confirming sudomotor changes, the combination of RST and QSART may be used because it has a high specificity (98%). Furthermore, positive clinical diagnosis may be followed up with x-ray scanning, MRI, bone scanning, or SSR. These tests have high specificities and will reduce the number of false-positive results. If CRPS is confirmed after these advanced tests, then there is a relatively high probability that the diagnosis is correct.

COMPLEX REGIONAL PAIN SYNDROME: SUMMARY

Difficulties with the diagnosis of CRPS are partly due to the lack of a reference standard test and to our incomplete understanding of the exact patho-physiology of this disease. Given these limitations, clinical observation is the accepted standard and is used as a screening test when CRPS is suspected. It is important to differentiate CRPS from disorders that may resemble it, because in many cases, the diagnosis of CRPS may be based on exclusion. Other tests such as imaging, nuclear, and SSR tests may be useful as second-line tests to reduce over-diagnosis.

Table 17–3 provides a summary of recommendations for the treatment of CRPS.

TABLE 17–3. Summary of Recommendations

STATEMENT	LEVEL OF EVIDENCE/GRADE OF RECOMMENDATION	REFERENCES
Clinical diagnostic criteria	B	1,9
X-ray	B	17,18
MRI	B	18–20
Bone scanning	B	21
Sympathetic skin response	B	22–26

REFERENCES

1. Harden RN, Bruehl SP: Diagnosis of complex regional pain syndrome: Signs, symptoms, and new empirically derived diagnostic criteria. Clin J Pain 22:415–419, 2006.
2. Lau FH, Chung KC: Silas Weir Mitchell, MD: The physician who discovered causalgia. J Hand Surg [Am] 29:181–187, 2004.
3. Stanton-Hicks M, Janig W, Hassenbusch S, et al: Reflex sympathetic dystrophy: Changing concepts and taxonomy. Pain 63:127–133, 1995.
4. Veldman PH, Reynen HM, Arntz IE, Goris RJ: Signs and symptoms of reflex sympathetic dystrophy: Prospective study of 829 patients. Lancet 342:1012–1016, 1993.
5. IASP: Classification of chronic pain. Descriptions of chronic pain syndromes and definitions of pain terms. Prepared by the International Association for the Study of Pain, Subcommittee on Taxonomy. Pain Suppl 3:S1–S226, 1986.
6. Bruehl S, Harden RN, Galer BS, et al: External validation of IASP diagnostic criteria for Complex Regional Pain Syndrome and proposed research diagnostic criteria. International Association for the Study of Pain. Pain 81:147–154, 1999.
7. Galer BS, Bruehl S, Harden RN: IASP diagnostic criteria for complex regional pain syndrome: A preliminary empirical validation study. International Association for the Study of Pain. Clin J Pain 14:48–54, 1998.
8. Harden RN, Bruehl S, Galer BS, et al: Complex regional pain syndrome: Are the IASP diagnostic criteria valid and sufficiently comprehensive? Pain 83:211–219, 1999.
9. Vacariu G: Complex regional pain syndrome. Disabil Rehabil 24:435–442, 2002.
10. Chong PS, Cros DP: Technology literature review: Quantitative sensory testing. Muscle Nerve 29:734–747, 2004.
11. Fowler CJ, Carroll MB, Burns D, et al: A portable system for measuring cutaneous thresholds for warming and cooling. J Neurol Neurosurg Psychiatry 50:1211–1215, 1987.
12. Wahren LK, Torebjork E, Nystrom B: Quantitative sensory testing before and after regional guanethidine block in patients with neuralgia in the hand. Pain 46:23–30, 1991.
13. Gulevich SJ, Conwell TD, Lane J, et al: Stress infrared telethermography is useful in the diagnosis of complex regional pain syndrome, type I (formerly reflex sympathetic dystrophy). Clin J Pain 13:50–59, 1997.

14. Chelimsky TC, Low PA, Naessens JM, et al: Value of autonomic testing in reflex sympathetic dystrophy. Mayo Clin Proc 70:1029–1040, 1995.
15. Bruehl S, Lubenow TR, Nath H, Ivankovich O: Validation of thermography in the diagnosis of reflex sympathetic dystrophy. Clin J Pain 12:316–325, 1996.
16. Gulvich SJ, Conwell TD, Lane J, et al: Stress infrared telethermography is useful in the diagnosis of complex regional pain syndrome, Type I (formerly reflex sympathetic dystrophy). Conf Proc IEEE Eng Med Biol Soc 2:1178, 2004.
17. Masson C, Audran M, Pascaretti C, et al: Further vascular, bone and autonomic investigations in algodystrophy. Acta Orthop Belg 64:77–87, 1998.
18. Schurmann M, Zaspel J, Lohr P, et al: Imaging in early post-traumatic complex regional pain syndrome: A comparison of diagnostic methods. Clin J Pain 23:449–457, 2007.
19. Graif M, Schweitzer ME, Marks B, et al: Synovial effusion in reflex sympathetic dystrophy: An additional sign for diagnosis and staging. Skeletal Radiol 27:262–265, 1998.
20. Intenzo CM, Kim SM, Capuzzi DM: The role of nuclear medicine in the evaluation of complex regional pain syndrome type I. Clin Nucl Med 30:400–407, 2005.
21. Fournier RS, Holder LE: Reflex sympathetic dystrophy: Diagnostic controversies. Semin Nucl Med 28:116–123, 1998.
22. Cronin KD, Kirsner RL, Fitzroy VP: Diagnosis of reflex sympathetic dysfunction. Use of the skin potential response. Anaesthesia 37:848–852, 1982.
23. Aisen ML, Stallman J, Aisen PS: The sympathetic skin response in the shoulder-hand syndrome complicating tetraplegia. Paraplegia 33:602–605, 1995.
24. Clinchot DM, Lorch F: Sympathetic skin response in patients with reflex sympathetic dystrophy. Am J Phys Med Rehabil 75:252–256, 1996.
25. Bolel K, Hizmetli S, Akyuz A: Sympathetic skin responses in reflex sympathetic dystrophy. Rheumatol Int 26:788–791, 2006.
26. Rommel O, Tegenthoff M, Pern U, et al: Sympathetic skin response in patients with reflex sympathetic dystrophy. Clin Auton Res 5:205–210, 1995.

Chapter 18

What Is the Optimal Treatment of Displaced Midshaft Clavicle Fractures?

MICHAEL D. MCKEE, MD, FRCS(C)

Clavicle fractures most commonly occur in young active individuals as a result of a direct blow to the shoulder that produces axial compression of the bone. They account for approximately 2.6% of all fractures and are seen in most fracture clinics in large numbers. The most common type of injury is a fracture that occurs in the middle third (or midshaft) of the clavicle; this accounts for approximately 80% of all clavicle fractures and is the focus of this chapter. Proximal and distal third fractures are distinctly different entities with widely disparate mechanisms of injury, treatment methods, and prognoses; they are not discussed in this chapter. Even when significantly displaced, midshaft clavicle fractures traditionally have been treated without surgery. This treatment strategy was based on early reports suggesting that clavicular nonunion was extremely rare after nonoperative treatment, with an incidence rate of 0.1% to 1.0%.[1-3] Similarly, clavicular malunion was described as being of radiographic interest only with no clinical significance.[1-3]

However, recent studies that are restricted to completely displaced midshaft fractures in adults (the focus of this chapter), that use patient-oriented outcome measures, and that have improved follow-up dispute this generally accepted orthopedic dogma.[4-8] Nonunion rates between 11% and 21% have been reported, which are exponentially greater than described previously. Also, a significant proportion of patients with healed fractures but ongoing symptomatology have been described: It would appear that clavicular malunion is a distinct clinical entity with characteristic clinical and radiographic features.[9,10] A variety of potential explanations has been proposed to explain this change, including survival of critically injured trauma patients with more severe fracture patterns, increased patient expectations, more complete follow-up (including patient-oriented outcome measures), and eliminating children (with their inherently good prognosis) from studies.[4-11]

Sufficient evidence now exists to conclude that the results of closed treatment are much inferior to what has been reported previously. Because there are numerous recent studies that support the safety and efficacy of primary operative fixation for completely displaced midshaft clavicle fractures,[12-14] a discussion of the advantages and disadvantages of operative versus nonoperative treatment is warranted to augment what heretofore would have been a short chapter.

OPTIONS

Nonoperative Treatment

For centuries, attempts have been made to obtain and maintain "closed reduction" of displaced clavicular fractures, and literally hundreds of casts, splints, slings, and wraps have been described. Unfortunately, currently, no convincing evidence exists that any significant improvement can be made to the original position of the fracture. The "figure-of-eight" bandage has been popular in North America for many years, but no convincing clinical evidence is available that a closed reduction of a displaced clavicle fracture can be maintained by this device. The other popular nonoperative method is simple sling immobilization, followed by early motion. Andersen and colleagues[15] performed a randomized, clinical trial comparing a sling versus a figure-of-eight bandage for displaced clavicular shaft fractures. The study revealed no functional or radiographic difference between the two groups at final follow-up, and in general, patients favored the sling. Because no significant difference exists between the two groups, both forms of nonoperative treatment are amalgamated as "nonoperative treatment" for the purposes of this chapter.

Operative Treatment

Currently, two basic operative techniques exist for the fixation of displaced midshaft fractures of the clavicle. Arguably, the most popular method is open reduction and plate fixation. This technique has been well described, has a proven track record, and with modern implants, surgical techniques, and soft-tissue handling, has a high success rate and low complication rate.[12-14] For example, Smith and colleagues[16] report union in 30 of 30 cases treated in this manner in a prospective trial. The disadvantages of this technique include the prominence of the plate and potential wound complications from the soft-tissue dissection required. However, with newly available precontoured plates (as opposed to the straight plates used previously), this has become less of a problem. Some authors recommend the use of anterior-inferior placement of the plate as a means of decreasing local irritation (as well as avoiding neurovascular structures while drilling).[17] For the purposes of this chapter, open reduction and plating are considered as a single group (whether superior or anterior-inferior).

The second method that is discussed is intramedullary pinning of the clavicle. Although it is intrinsically difficult to perform intramedullary fixation of a curved bone with a straight intramedullary device, it is possible. The advantages of this technique include minimal soft-tissue dissection at the fracture site, less soft-tissue prominence of the hardware, and in some applications of this technique, the ability to remove the hardware relatively early through a small incision.[18–23] Chuang and coauthors[23] report success in 30 of 31 midshaft clavicle fractures treated with closed reduction and an intramedullary screw technique. Disadvantages of this technique, common to any unlocked intramedullary device, include difficulty in controlling shortening and rotation, especially in comminuted fractures. This led to a high rate of loss of reduction in one prospective, randomized study.[22]

EVIDENCE

Nonoperative Treatment

Whereas prior reports had described generally favorable results after nonoperative care of displaced midshaft fractures of the clavicle, Hill, McGuire, and Crosby's[7] landmark study published in 1997 reported a high degree of residual patient dissatisfaction. For the first time in this setting, they used a patient-based outcome tool and found that 31% of patients were dissatisfied with their outcomes, and noted a nonunion rate of 15%. Conversely, Nordqvist and coworkers[8] describe good results after long-term follow-up of 225 clavicle fractures, with 185 good, 39 fair, and only 1 poor result. However, in the sub-category of displaced, comminuted fractures (the topic of the article), 27% of patients rated their shoulder as "fair," which in the rating scale used, roughly corresponds to the dissatisfied group (31%) in Hill's study. Another Scandinavian study by Nowak and investigators[6] (the 2002 Neer Award article) found that 46% of 208 patients treated without surgery still had shoulder sequelae at 9- to 10-year follow-up. They found that comminution and displacement correlated with poor outcome. These and other nonoperative studies were summarized in a recent meta-analysis (see Comparative Studies section later in this chapter).

Operative Treatment

Initial reports regarding operative fixation of displaced clavicular fractures were plagued by selection bias (only the worst, comminuted, open fractures received surgery), poor soft-tissue handling, lack of antibiotic coverage (with correspondingly high infection rates), and especially inadequate or suboptimal fixation methods (i.e., cerclage wires or short, weak plates).[1–3] Thus, not surprisingly, operative failure rates were high and fixation was avoided. More recent articles with improved techniques have conclusively proved that properly performed, primary operative repair of displaced midshaft clavicle fractures is a safe, reliable technique with a low complication rate. Collinge and coworkers[17] report union in 39 of 42 cases treated with anterior/inferior plating, whereas Poigenfurst and coauthors[12] report similarly favorable results in 122 consecutive cases treated with superior plating. A summary of the results of operative fixation is given in the following section.

Comparative Studies

Despite the high numbers of clavicle fractures seen in clinical practice, a paucity of high-quality comparative studies is available for review. One of the few randomized clinical trials reported was recently completed by the Canadian Orthopaedic Trauma Society (COTS). They randomized 132 patients with completely displaced fractures of the midshaft clavicle to nonoperative (sling) versus operative (open-reduction and plate-fixation) treatment.[24] Follow-up of 111 patients at a year after injury revealed significantly improved Constant and DASH scores in the operative group (Figs. 18–1 and 18–2). Also, there were fewer nonunions (2/62 vs. 7/49; $P = 0.042$) and symptomatic malunions (0/62 vs. 9/49; $P = 0.001$) in the operative group. There were complications

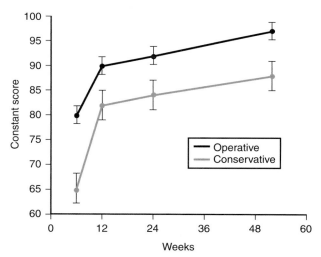

FIGURE 18–1. Acute displaced mid-shaft fractures of the clavicle. Graphical analysis of mean Constant Shoulder Scores in the operative plate fixation group versus non-operative group at 6 weeks, 12 weeks, 24 weeks, and 52 weeks follow-up. Values are statistically improved for the operative group at each time point (p<0.01 for all). (Adapted from Canadian Orthopaedic Trauma Soicety. Nonoperative Treatment compared with plate fixation of displaced midshaft clavicle fractures. A multicenter, randomized clinical trial. J Bone Joint Surg(A) 89:1–10, 2007. Reprinted with permission of the Journal of Bone and Joint Surgery.)

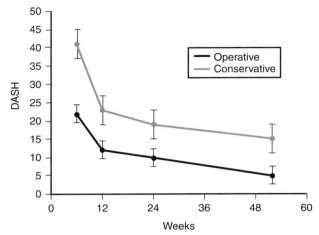

FIGURE 18–2. Acute displaced mid-shaft fractures of the clavicle. Graphical analysis of mean DASH scores in the operative plate fixation group versus non-operative groups at 6-, 12-, 24-, and 52-week follow-up. The DASH is a disability score where a "perfect" extremity would typically score 0 (mean values for a "normal" population are in the 4–8 range). Values are worse in the nonoperative group at each time point (6 week $P < 0.01$, 12 week $P = 0.04$, 24 week $P = 0.05$, 52 week $P < 0.01$). (Adapted from Canadian Orthopaedic Trauma Soiciety. Nonoperative Treatment compared with plate fixation of displaced mid-shaft clavicle fractures. A multicenter, randomized clinical trial. J Bone Joint Surg(A) 89:1–10, 2007. Reprinted with permission of the Journal of Bone and Joint Surgery.)

specific to the operative group (hardware removal, five cases; infection, three cases), but these usually responded to a single repeat operative procedure. Similar findings were reported by Smith and colleagues,[16] who, in a prospective randomized trial, found that open reduction and plate fixation resulted in union of 30 of 30 cases, whereas the nonoperative group had 12 nonunions in 35 cases ($P = 0.001$). These authors conclude that plate fixation was safe, effective, and superior to nonoperative care for preventing nonunion. However, they did note a 30% rate of hardware removal; this study took place before precontoured plates were readily available.

Only one randomized prospective trial compares nonoperative care with intramedullary fixation of displaced clavicle fractures. These data were presented in 2005 and noted that although shoulder outcome scores were similar at 1 year (93 for operative vs. 98 for nonoperative), complications were significantly greater in the operative group.[22] This included nonunion, refracture, infection, and pin prominence. However, almost half the patients in the operative group lost some of the original reduction, indicating fixation was suboptimal. A similar study, retrospective in nature, compared nonoperative (figure-of-eight bandage) versus operative (intramedullary pin fixation) treatment.[21] Again, although there were no significant differences in shoulder scores (85 for nonoperative vs. 83 for operative) at final follow-up, there were more complications in the operative group including 8 infections, 3 refractures, 2 hardware failures, and 2 nonunions (14/40 patients, 35%). It would appear that although this technique is

successful in expert hands, it is not as consistently reliable in general as compression plate fixation. This may relate to technique (it is a demanding procedure), patient selection (not ideal for comminuted fractures), or other unrecognized factors.

A recent meta-analysis was performed of available data from articles on midshaft clavicle fractures published between 1975 and 2005. Concentrating on data regarding displaced fractures, a nonunion rate of 15.1% was found after nonoperative care.[14] The nonunion rate for plating was 2.2% and for intramedullary pinning was 2%. Thus, for displaced midshaft clavicular fractures, plating provided a relative risk reduction of 86% (95% CI, 71–93%) for nonunion compared with nonoperative care.

AREAS OF CONTROVERSY

Sling versus Figure-of-Eight Bandage

Although traditionally favored as a means of obtaining and maintaining a closed reduction of a displaced clavicle fracture, the figure-of-eight bandage was found to be equivalent to a simple sling in terms of position of fracture healing in a randomized, prospective trial that Andersen and colleagues[15] conducted. In addition, patients preferred the sling (2/27 dissatisfied with sling vs. 9/34 dissatisfied with figure-of-eight bandage; $P = 0.09$).

Prediction of Unsatisfactory Outcome with Nonoperative Care

It is clear that many patients with displaced midshaft fractures of the clavicle will have good results with simple nonoperative care; however, it is clear that a substantial portion will not.[7–9] A goal of modern research in this field is to attempt to elicit prognostic factors that will identify individuals with an intrinsically poor outcome and then concentrate surgical resources on this group. Robinson and coauthors[4] report a prospective, observational cohort study of a consecutive series of 868 patients with clavicle fractures, 581 of whom had a midshaft diaphyseal fracture. They found a significantly greater nonunion rate (21%) in displaced comminuted midshaft fractures. A letter to the editor on this article by Brinker and coworkers[5] analyzing the data suggests a nonunion rate varying between 20% and 33% for displaced comminuted fractures in males. Hill and colleagues'[7] study of 52 displaced midshaft clavicle fractures revealed 8 nonunions and 16 patients who described dissatisfaction with their outcome based on patient-oriented measures: They conclude that displacement of the fracture fragments by greater than 2 cm was associated with an unsatisfactory result. Nowak and investigators[6] describe sequelae in 46% of patients treated without surgery 9 to 10 years after injury, and found that no bony contact (displacement), comminution, and increasing age were risk factors for a poor outcome.

Cosmesis

Although it has not traditionally been a focus of the orthopedic surgeon, it is well recognized that cosmesis is important to patients. An obvious and unsightly scar on the anterior aspect of the shoulder has been considered a deterrent to operative treatment of clavicular fractures. However, the significant shoulder asymmetry (with the typical depressed, medially translated, anteriorly rotated, "ptotic" position) that can result after a displaced fracture of the clavicle can be problematic for the modern body-image conscious patient. Several studies have addressed this question. The COTS study examined specifically the question of cosmesis, and patients were asked the question, "Are you satisfied with the appearance of your shoulder?" More patients in the operative group answered "yes" to this question than in the nonoperative group (52/62 vs. 26/49; $P = 0.001$).[24] Nowak and investigators'[6] study of long-term follow-up of nonoperative care revealed 27% of patients who were unhappy with the appearance of their shoulder. Smith's study[16] reports that 44% of the patients in the nonoperative group "had complaints about the cosmetic appearance of their shoulder at final follow-up." In this predominantly young population, nonoperative care can produce an unappeal-

RECOMMENDATIONS

It is important to remember that the following recommendations pertain to a specific subgroup of clavicle fractures: completely displaced fractures of the midshaft in healthy, active individuals between 16 and 60 years of age. This comprised 66 of 242 (27%) clavicle fractures in Hill's study.[7]

Sling versus Figure of Eight

Grade B evidence (single randomized trial) exists that a sling is as effective as a figure of eight in immobilizing fractures of the clavicle, and it is favored by patients.[15]

Position of Plate for Open Reduction with Internal Fixation

Grade C evidence (retrospective reviews and nonrandomized comparative study) exists that anterior-inferior plate placement is associated with a lower rate of symptomatic hardware compared with traditional straight plates used superiorly.[14,17] However, no comparison with superior precontoured plates has been reported in the literature, and the technique of anterior-inferior plating is one that has a significant learning curve.

Factors Associated with Poor Outcome after Nonoperative Care of Displaced Midshaft Clavicle Fractures

Grade A evidence has been reported from population-based, prospective, observational studies, randomized prospective trials, and retrospective reviews that increasing fracture displacement (especially greater than 2 cm of shortening), comminution/increasing number of fracture fragments, and advancing age are associated with poor outcome (nonunion, symptomatic malunion) after nonoperative care of displaced midshaft fractures of the clavicle.[4,7,9,10,14,16,24]

Plate Fixation versus Intramedullary Nailing

No specific recommendation can be made regarding plate fixation versus intramedullary nailing for displaced midshaft clavicle fractures. Currently, there is no direct comparative study published examining the outcome of plating versus intramedullary nailing of displaced clavicular fractures. However, although two separate randomized trials show clear advantages of open reduction with internal fixation with plating over nonoperative care,[16,24] similar studies examining the effect of intramedullary nailing provide contradictory results.[20–22] Currently, it is unclear whether the theoretic advantages of intramedullary nailing will outweigh the difficulties in maintaining length and rotation (critical elements of the reduction) of the fracture. One unpublished retrospective review with small numbers (17 patients per group) suggests some superiority of intramedullary pinning over plate fixation or nonoperative care in this setting.[20]

Plating versus Nonoperative Care of Displaced Midshaft Fractures of the Clavicle

Level B evidence (one published randomized, clinical trial; one presented randomized, clinical trial; one literature meta-analysis) exists that primary plate fixation results in a significant risk reduction for nonunion and symptomatic malunion compared with nonoperative treatment.[14,16,24] Also, as would be expected, patients return to their preoperative level of function more quickly. However, there is a significant reoperation rate, mainly for hardware removal.

ing "ptotic," droopy shoulder that can be of greater cosmetic concern than a scar.

SUMMARY

Completely displaced midshaft fractures in healthy, active individuals comprise approximately 25% of all clavicle fractures. A reasonable amount of evidence supports the use of a sling for those patients in whom nonoperative treatment is chosen. Sufficient evidence exists from high-quality prospective studies that certain risk factors (such as displacement or shortening of more than 2 cm or fracture comminution) portend a poor prognosis, and consideration should be given, in the appropriate patient, to operative treatment. Primary plate fixation of displaced clavicle fractures reduces the non-union and symptomatic malunion rate significantly and results in more rapid return of upper extremity function than nonoperative treatment. Optimal plate position (superior vs. anterior/inferior), or whether intramedullary pinning is as effective as plate fixation, remains unclear. Table 18–1 provides a summary of recommendations for the treatment of displaced midshaft clavicle fractures.

TABLE 18–1. A Meta-Analysis of Nonoperative Treatment, Intramedullary Pinning, and Plate Fixation for Displaced Midshaft Fractures of the Clavicle (Published 1975–2005)

TREATMENT METHOD	PERCENTAGE WITH NONUNION	INFECTIONS (TOTAL)	INFECTIONS (DEEP)	FIXATION FAILURES
Nonoperative (n = 159)	15.1	0	0	0
Plating (n = 460)	2.2	4.6	2.4	2.2
Intramedullary pinning (n = 152)	2.0	6.6	0	3.9

Data from Zlowodzki M, Zelle BA, Cole PA, et al: Treatment of mid-shaft clavicle fractures: Systemic review of 2144 fractures. J Orthop Trauma 19:504–508, 2005.

TABLE 18–2. Summary of Recommendations

STATEMENT	LEVEL OF EVIDENCE/GRADE OF RECOMMENDATION	REFERENCES
1. Young, active patients with completely displaced midshaft fractures of the clavicle will have superior results with primary fracture fixation.	B	14,16,24
2. Anterior-inferior plating may reduce the risk for symptomatic hardware compared with superior plating.	C	17
3. There is no difference in outcome between a regular sling and a figure-of-eight bandage when nonoperative treatment is selected.	B	15
4. There is no difference in outcome between plating and intramedullary nailing of displaced midshaft clavicle fractures.	I	10,12,14,18–21,23
5. Factors associated with poor outcome after nonoperative treatment of displaced midshaft clavicle fractures include shortening and increasing fracture comminution.	A	4–7,9,14,16

REFERENCES

1. Rowe CR: An atlas of anatomy and treatment of midclavicular fractures. Clin Orthop Relat Res 58:29–42, 1968.
2. Crenshaw AH: Fractures of the shoulder girdle, arm and forearm. Campbell's Operative Orthopaedics, 8th ed. St. Louis, Mosby-Yearbook, 1992, pp 989–995.
3. Neer C: Nonunion of the clavicle. JAMA 172:1006–1011, 1960.
4. Robinson CM, Court-Brown CM, McQueen MM, Wakefield AE: Estimating the risk of nonunion following non-operative treatment of a clavicle fracture. J Bone Joint Surg Am 86:1359–1365, 2004.
5. Brinker MR, Edwards TB, O'Connor DP: Letter to the editor. J Bone Joint Surg Am 87:677–678, 2005.
6. Nowak J, Holgersson M, Larsson S: Can we predict long-term sequelae after fractures of the clavicle based on initial findings? A prospective study with nine to ten years follow-up. J Shoulder Elbow Surg 13:479–486, 2004.
7. Hill JM, McGuire MH, Crosby LA: Closed treatment of displaced middle-third fractures of the clavicle gives poor results. J Bone Joint Surg Br 79:537–541, 1997.
8. Nordqvist A, Petersson CJ, Redlund-Johnell I: Mid-clavicle fractures in adults: End result study after conservative treatment. J Orthop Trauma 12:572–576, 1998.
9. McKee MD, Wild LM, Schemitsch EH: Midshaft malunions of the clavicle. J Bone Joint Surg Am 85:790–797, 2003.
10. Basamania CJ: Claviculoplasty. J Shoulder Elbow Surg 8:540, 1999. (Abstracts: Seventh International Conference on Surgery of the Shoulder, 1999.)
11. McKee MD, Stephen DJG, Kreder HJ, et al: Functional outcome following clavicle fractures in polytrauma patients. J Trauma 47:616, 2000.
12. Poigenfurst J, Rappold G, Fischer W: Plating of fresh clavicular fractures: Results of 122 operations. Injury 23:237–241, 1992.
13. McKee MD, Seiler JG, Jupiter JB: The application of the limited contact dynamic compression plate in the upper extremity: An analysis of 114 consecutive cases. Injury 26:661–666, 1995.
14. Zlowodzki M, Zelle BA, Cole PA, et al: Treatment of mid-shaft clavicle fractures: Systemic review of 2144 fractures. J Orthop Trauma 19:504–508, 2005.
15. Andersen K, Jensen PO, Lauritzen J: The treatment of clavicular fractures: Figure of eight bandage versus a simple sling. Acta Orthop Scand 58:71–74, 1987.
16. Smith CA, Rudd J, Crosby LA: Results of operative versus non-operative treatment for 100% displaced mid-shaft clavicle. Proceedings from the 16th Annual Open Meeting

of the American Shoulder and Elbow Surgeons, March 18, 2000, p 41.

17. Collinge C, Devinney S, Herscovici D, et al: Anterior-inferior plate fixation of middle-third fractures and nonunions of the clavicle. J Orthop Trauma 20:680–686, 2006.

18. Jubel A, Andermahr J, Schiffer G, et al: Elastic stable intra-medullary nailing of mid-clavicular fractures with a titanium nail. Clin Orthop Relat Res 408:279–285, 2003.

19. Boehme D, Curtis RJ, DeHaan JT, et al: Nonunion of fractures of the mid-shaft of the clavicle. Treatment with a modified Haigie intramedullary pin and autogenous bone-grafting. J Bone Joint Surg Am 73:1219–1226, 1991.

20. Sampath DS: Treatment of displaced midclavicle fractures with Rockwood pin: A comparative study. Proceedings of the 2005 AAOS Annual Meeting, p 566.

21. Grassi FA, Tajana MS, D'Angelo F: Management of midclavicu-lar fractures: Comparison between non-operative treatment and open intramedullary fixation in 80 patients. J Trauma 50:1096–1100, 2001.

22. Judd DB, Bottoni CR, Pallis MP, Smith E: Intramedullary fixa-tion versus non-operative treatment for mid-shaft clavicle fractures. Proceedings of the 2005 AAOS Annual Meeting, p 594.

23. Chuang TY, Ho WP, Hsieh PH, et al: Closed reduction and in-ternal fixation for acute midshaft clavicular fractures using cannulated screws. J Trauma 60:1315–1322, 2006.

24. Canadian Orthopaedic Trauma Society: Nonoperative treat-ment compared with plate fixation of displaced midshaft clavicle fractures. A multicenter, randomized clinical trial. J Bone Joint Surg Am 89:1–10, 2007.

What Is the Best Surgical Treatment for Cuff Tear Arthropathy?

Robert H. Hawkins, MD, FRCS(C)

HISTORICAL OVERVIEW

Cuff tear arthropathy (CTA) is the term Neer[1,2] originally proposed to describe a form of shoulder arthritis in association with long-standing rotator cuff deficiency. It is distinct clinically and radiographically from other forms of shoulder arthropathy in which joint destruction coexists with cuff deficiency such as rheumatoid arthritis or osteoarthritis with traumatically acquired cuff tear. The causative factor was first attributed to a crystal-mediated synovitis (the Milwaukee shoulder),[3,4] and it is still recognized that there is a correlation between large rotator cuff tears and high levels of calcium phosphate crystals in synovial fluid.[5] It is now generally agreed that this unique pattern of joint destruction occurs because of, not simply in association with, rotator cuff deficiency. Mechanical and nutritional factors associated with progressive upward humeral head migration from loss of cuff integrity are its causes. This combination of pain, glenohumeral joint destruction, and a nonfunctioning rotator cuff present treatment challenges that stand apart from other forms of shoulder arthropathy.

PATHOMECHANICS

An understanding of shoulder biomechanics is necessary to appreciate surgical treatment options. The fact that shoulder muscles function as force couples in the coronal plane was first appreciated by Inman and colleagues[6] and expanded subsequently by Burkhart,[7] who described a transverse force couple as well. Applying this theory to explain why full shoulder elevation is still possible in some shoulders with massive cuff tears and not in others, Burkhart[8] identified three groups of fulcrum kinematics. Despite major cuff tearing, transverse and coronal force couples may remain intact and the fulcrum is stable; the humeral head is contained within the glenoid socket, and full elevation is possible. When force couples are destroyed by cuff tearing, the humeral head rises out of the socket on attempted arm elevation; that is, the fulcrum is unstable, and so-called pseudoparalysis of elevation results. In some cases, the humeral head may restabilize in a superiorly subluxated position under an intact coracoacromial arch, the so-called captured fulcrum, again allowing arm elevation (Fig. 19–1).

The dynamic action of muscle forces including those of the rotator cuff, together with other capsuloligamentous restraints, stabilize the humeral head through the concavity compression mechanism. As explained by Matsen and coauthors[9] and in the biomechanical analysis of De Wilde and coworkers,[10] a loss of any of the normal osseous, capsuloligamentous, or muscular constraints leads to glenohumeral instability. Superior instability results from loss of the compression of the rotator cuff and spacer effect of the normal supraspinatus. Upward displacement of the humerus slackens the deltoid, making it less effective in humeral elevation and weakness, or even pseudoparalysis is the result. The coracoacromial arch is then the only remaining barrier to further upward migration. When this barrier has been compromised by frictional wear or aggressive surgical acromioplasty, anterosuperior escape of the humeral head occurs, further compounding pseudoparalysis.

CLINICAL PRESENTATION

CTA is the end stage of a continuum which begins with a simple cuff tear. The incidence of CTA is estimated to be anywhere from 4% to 20% of cuff tears.[11,12] Patients with CTA typically present with pain and weakness of the shoulder and glenohumeral joint destruction on radiographs. Jensen and investigators[13] collected clinical data on 104 cases from 10 different published reports and found the majority were elderly women (average age, 77.5 years), and almost 50% had bilateral involvement. Neer and researchers[2] describe the findings in 26 cases averaging 69 years of which 75% were women. No history of trauma was reported in 75%. The shoulders typically were swollen (Fig. 19–2), muscles were atrophic, and the long head of biceps ruptured. Passive motion was limited to an average of 90-degree elevation and 20-degree external rotation. Only 2 of 26 were able to actively elevate greater than 90 degrees. Positive lag signs for cuff deficiency[14] are frequently seen. These include the lift-off test for subscapularis,[15,16] the external rotation lag sign for supraspinatus and infraspinatus, and the drop sign for infraspinatus. In the presence of a normal deltoid, the drop-arm sign is indicative of a massive posterosuperior cuff tear with loss of the ability to create a stable fulcrum. The term *pseudoparalysis*[17] is also used when active

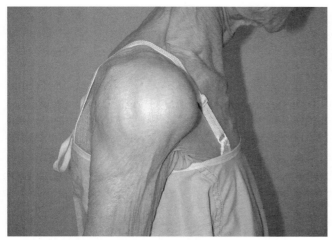

FIGURE 19–1. Swollen shoulder of an elderly woman with cuff tear arthropathy.

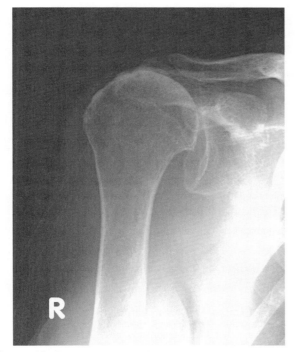

FIGURE 19–2. Radiograph of a shoulder with advanced cuff tear arthropathy.

shoulder elevation is less than 90 degrees in the presence of free anterior elevation with an intact deltoid.

RADIOGRAPHIC FEATURES

Radiographic indicators of major cuff deficiency such as acromiohumeral narrowing and superior migration of the humeral head represent the earliest

phases in a continuum that eventually leads to the joint destruction characteristic of true CTA.[18] Chronic wear of the superiorly displaced humeral head sculpts the undersurface of the coracoacromial arch and glenoid, termed *acetabularization*. Rounding off of the tuberosities leads to *femoralization* of the humerus (Fig. 19–3). In advanced cases, there may be collapse of the humeral head.[2]

Seebauer[19] has proposed a classification of CTA (Fig. 19–4) that combines radiographic features with an appreciation of the altered fulcrum mechanics that Burkhart[8] described. The four distinct groups are distinguished by the degree of superior migration from the center of rotation and the amount of instability at the center of rotation. In the most advanced category, IIB, the humeral head has escaped superiorly, removing any remaining fulcrum stability.

DIFFERENTIAL DIAGNOSIS

It is important to identify other forms of destructive arthopathy that resemble CTA but may require different treatment. Advanced rheumatoid arthritis of the shoulder often includes major cuff deficiency but typically is polyarticular in distribution. Osteoarthritis with incidental cuff tear lacks the characteristic component of vertical instability. Neuropathic arthropathy or Charcot shoulder presents radiographically with significant joint destruction but not of the coracoacromial arch.

TREATMENT

Medical management of CTA is based on specific needs and symptoms. When pain is minor and function remains good, mild analgesics and a gentle maintenance exercise program may be all that is necessary. Intra-articular steroid injections may give short-term relief, but repeated use is to be discouraged for fear of iatrogenic infection.

Quantifying Treatment Results in Cuff Tear Arthropathy

Many grading systems have become popular for clinical assessment of shoulder outcomes. Neer and researchers[20] recognized the need for a "limited goals" category in the case of patients with poorly functioning cuff musculature. This acknowledges that a result can still be considered successful if there is good pain relief and "useful" shoulder function even if the rigid criteria of success in those with intact cuff muscles are not met. Here, a result is considered successful if no significant pain is felt, the patient is pleased with the procedure, the patient remains independent for activities of daily living, and the patient has at least 90 degrees of arm elevation and 20-degree external rotation.

FORCE COUPLES OF THE SHOULDER

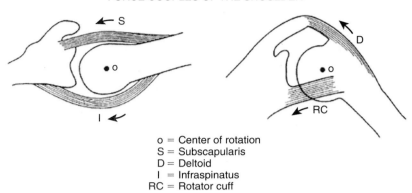

o = Center of rotation
S = Subscapularis
D = Deltoid
I = Infraspinatus
RC = Rotator cuff

FIGURE 19–3. Force couples of the shoulder.

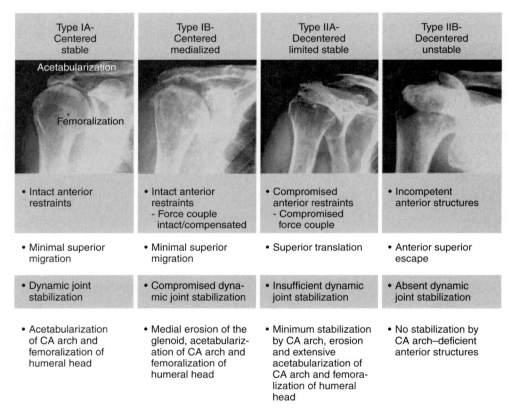

Type IA- Centered stable	Type IB- Centered medialized	Type IIA- Decentered limited stable	Type IIB- Decentered unstable
• Intact anterior restraints	• Intact anterior restraints - Force couple intact/compensated	• Compromised anterior restraints - Compromised force couple	• Incompetent anterior structures
• Minimal superior migration	• Minimal superior migration	• Superior translation	• Anterior superior escape
• Dynamic joint stabilization	• Compromised dynamic joint stabilization	• Insufficient dynamic joint stabilization	• Absent dynamic joint stabilization
• Acetabularization of CA arch and femoralization of humeral head	• Medial erosion of the glenoid, acetabularization of CA arch and femoralization of humeral head	• Minimum stabilization by CA arch, erosion and extensive acetabularization of CA arch and femoralization of humeral head	• No stabilization by CA arch–deficient anterior structures

FIGURE 19–4. Seebauer's radiographic and biomechanical classification of cuff tear arthropathy.

Surgical Management

Arthroscopic Debridement. Arthroscopic irrigation to remove activated enzymes and crystals offers only limited short-term relief[21] (Level IV). Any surgical violation of the coracoacromial arch, if still intact, is to be vigorously discouraged for fear of further destabilizing the humeral head.[13]

Arthrodesis. Glenohumeral arthrodesis has the potential to stabilize the glenohumeral joint and relieve pain but at the cost of reduced motion and function. However, most patients with CTA are unsuitable for arthrodesis because they are older, intolerant of prolonged immobilization, and frequently have bilateral disease.[2] Furthermore, osteoporosis in these typically elderly women presents problems with internal fixation. Arthrodesis is best reserved for younger high-demand patients disabled by an irreparable cuff tear, often with a nonfunctioning deltoid, and who require a strong stable shoulder girdle[22] (Level V). It may also have a place in other instances of massive irreparable cuff tear with deltoid dysfunction.

Unconstrained Shoulder Replacement. Shoulder prostheses with no built-in constraint rely on an intact and functioning rotator cuff to stabilize the humeral head within the socket. Although it is agreed that small cuff tears, regardless of whether they are repaired, have no effect on the outcome of total shoulder arthroplasty[23] (Level III); the same is not true for cases of major cuff deficiency. Franklin and coauthors[24] report a direct association between superior migration of the humeral component and a deficient rotator cuff (Level IV). They called the eccentric superior loading of the glenoid component the "rocking horse" phenomenon that leads to loosening and superior tilt. Therefore, unconstrained prostheses are not recommended for cuff tear arthroplasty.

Semiconstrained Shoulder Replacement. Semiconstrained glenoid components have also been used to give resistance to ascent of the humeral head in cuff deficient shoulders. Neer and researchers[2] experimented with 200% and 600% glenoid components for CTA in 11 cases followed for an average of 30 months, but they soon abandoned such designs because of the greater risk for failure and the difficulty of closing residual cuff defects[25] (Level IV). Amstutz and colleagues[26] and Gristina and investigators[27] have described the use of hooded glenoid components for use with nonconstrained systems but reported only short-term results (Level IV). It has been shown by finite element analysis[28] that the superior constraints of the component intending to prevent humeral head ascent increase stresses and may cause earlier loosening than with unconstrained designs.

Bipolar Shoulder Replacement. Bipolar hemiarthroplasty was introduced by Swanson and coworkers[29] for the treatment of advanced glenohumeral arthritis associated with superior migration of the humeral head and loss of rotator cuff function. It uses a larger diameter mobile shell around the head in an attempt to gain several advantages: increased mobility because of the lateralization of the center of rotation and the increase in the muscle lever arm; increased stability of the prosthetic shoulder; and reduced glenoid and acromial wear in contact with the prosthetic head.[30] Few published[31–33] and unpublished studies[34] exist that detail results but in general these indicate that even if pain relief is achieved, function remains low after the procedure (Level IV). Noting the better results reported with simple hemiarthroplasty particularly about mobility, Duranthon and investigators[33] conclude that the deltoid lever arm was being increased at the expense of overstretching capsular and residual cuff tissues, and that it was better to use a head size closer to normal anatomy. In addition to this overstuffing effect, concerns have been raised regarding rupture of the subscapularis tendon be-

cause of the vertical orientation of the component and the potential for excessive polyethylene wear.[35]

Hemiarthroplasty. The difficulties encountered with prosthetic designs that attempt to control the altered biomechanics of major cuff deficiency have led many to return to simple nonconstrained hemireplacement as the preferred procedure. Table 19–1 summarizes the published results. In the studies by Arntz and colleagues and Visotsky and coworkers,[19] close attention was paid to the issue of superior humeral escape (grade IIB in Seebauer's classification), and hemiarthroplasty was avoided in those cases. In Sanchez-Sotelo and coauthors'[51] study, postoperative anterosuperior instability occurred in seven of the eight cases that had had prior acromioplasty and resection of the coracoacromial arch. Although these studies show that symptoms can be improved by hemiarthroplasty, it is clear that these results fall far short of what can be achieved by replacement arthroplasty in other diagnoses, for example, total shoulder replacement for osteoarthritis, for both pain relief and arm elevation. The biomechanical computer analysis of De Wilde and coworkers[10] shows why simple hemiarthroplasty cannot be expected to solve the problem of weak arm elevation if the rotator cuff is not working and the humeral head is superiorly subluxated (Seebauer grade IIA), even if humeral escape had not yet occurred (Fig. 19–5). Simple hemiarthroplasty in these cases does not restore normal biomechanics, though it may relieve some pain.

Constrained Shoulder Replacement. Prosthetic arthroplasty with a constrained prosthesis has been used to treat all forms of shoulder arthropathy including cuff-deficient shoulders with arthritis. The fixed fulcrum mechanics of the Stanmore and Michael Reese prostheses used for many types of glenohumeral arthritis would appear to compensate for absence of functioning cuff but have resulted in high rates of mechanical failure and loosening of the glenoid component.[36–39] Table 19–2 summarizes the published results. Neer[40] abandoned his work in fixed fulcrum designs as early as 1974, concluding that the poor quality of scapular bone precludes adequate fixation of the glenoid component in a constrained prosthesis (Level IV).

Reverse Ball and Socket Replacement. A number of prostheses were introduced based on a reverse ball and socket concept to address the disappointing results reported earlier. Most remained essentially experimental. The Kessel (Fig. 19–6) and the early Grammont prosthesis featured a center of rotation well lateral to the glenoid surface, resulting in excessive torque or shear forces on the glenoid component and early loosening (Table 19–3). Recognizing this weakness, Grammont modified his original design with two important innovations (Fig. 19–7): The glenoid component diameter was enlarged, but the size of the sphere was reduced from two-thirds to half, thereby placing the center of rotation at the glenoid surface, and thus decreasing shear forces; the large diameter allows for a greater arc of motion before

TABLE 19–1. Reported Results of Hemiarthroplasty for Cuff Tear Arthropathy

STUDY	STUDY DESIGN	LEVEL OF EVIDENCE	N	AGE (RANGE), YR	DURATION OF FOLLOW-UP (RANGE), YR	PAIN SCORE (0 = NONE; 3 = SEVERE)		ACTIVE TOTAL ELEVATION (RANGE), DEGREES		SUCCESSFUL RESULTS (NEER LIMITED GOALS CRITERIA)	COMMENTS
						PREOPERATIVE	POSTOPERATIVE	PREOPERATIVE	POSTOPERATIVE		
Arntz et al. (1993)	Case series	IV	18	71 (54–84)	3 (2–10)	2.4	0.9	66 (44–90)	112 (70–160)	Not reported (all were at least "somewhat better")	Hemiarthroplasty done only if coracoacromial arch functionally intact
Williams and Rockwood (1996)	Case series	IV	21	72 (59–80)	4 (2–7)	2.8	0.7	70 (0–155)	120 (15–160)	76%	Postoperative radiographs not analyzed
Filed et al. (1997)	Case series	IV	16	74 (62–83)	3 (2–5)	2.4	0.8	60 (40–80)	100 (80–130)	63%	3 had humeral escape after surgery
Zuckerman et al. (2000)	Case series	IV	15	73 (65–81)	2 (1–5)	3	0.9	69 (20–140)	86 (45–140)	Not reported (86% were "satisfied")	Radiographs not analyzed for superior subluxation
Sanchez-Sotelo et al. (2001)	Case series	IV	33	69 (50–87)	5 (2–11)	2.5	1.3	72 (30–150)	91 (40–165)	67%	Superior subluxation after surgery was severe in 25/33
Visotsky et al. (2004)	Case series	IV	60	70 (5–89)	2.7 (minimum, 2 yr)	2.8	0.6	56	116	89%	Surgery not done if coracoacromial arch not intact (all were Seebauer grades IA, IB, and IIA)

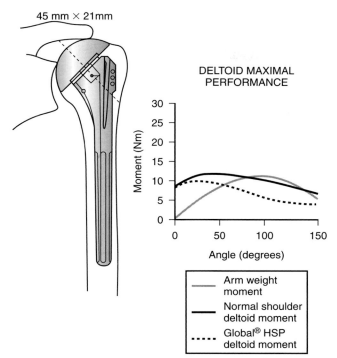

45 mm × 21mm

DELTOID MAXIMAL
PERFORMANCE

Arm weight
moment

Normal shoulder
deltoid moment

Global® HSP
deltoid moment

FIGURE 19–5. In a global hemiarthroplasty (DePuy Ortho-paedics Inc., Warsaw, IN) superiorly subluxated because of major cuff deficiency, the deltoid moment becomes less than the arm weight moment, resulting in no active abduction greater than 51 degrees.

impingement occurs. The humeral component has a small cup almost vertically oriented that covers less than half of the glenosphere, effectively lengthening or tensioning the deltoid (Fig. 19–8). This modified design offers several important biomechanical advantages[41] (Table 19–4). Although restoration of active elevation more than 90 degrees is achieved, active external rotation is often limited, particularly when the teres minor is not functioning. Internal rotation is also rarely restored because of the design limitations of the prosthesis.

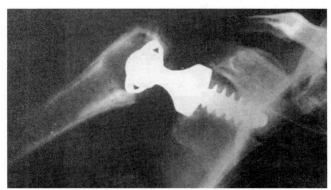

FIGURE 19–6. Radiograph of a Kessel prosthesis showing reverse ball and socket design with center of rotation well lateral to glenoid surface, creating high torque and shear forces at the glenoid component-bone interface.

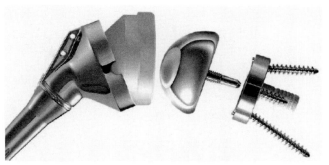

FIGURE 19–7. Photograph showing components of the Grammont reverse ball and socket prosthesis. From left to right: the humeral stem and metaphysic, the polyethylene humeral; concavity insert, the glenosphere and the meta-glene (Delta III; DePuy Orthopaedics Inc., Warsaw IN).

A feature unique to this prosthesis is bone loss believed to be caused by abutment of the adducted humeral prosthesis against the scapular neck. Termed *scapular notching,* it is seen in more than 50% of cases.[41] This contact is a direct consequence of the absence of a prosthetic neck to the glenosphere and the horizontal orientation of the humeral cup, which are the biomechanical solutions to avoid excessive forces on the glenoid component and improve the power of the deltoid. The degree of notching can be classified[42] as grade 1 if confined to the scapular pillar, grade 2 when it is in contact with the lower screw, grade 3 when it is over the lower screw, and grade 4 when it extends into the baseplate (Fig. 19–9). In a study using cadaveric shoulders, Nyffeler and investigators[43] showed that placing the glenoid component 2 to 4 mm lower than originally recommended significantly improves adduction and may reduce the risk for notching. Simovitch and colleagues[44] were able predict scapular notching by radiographic measurement of glenosphere placement and scapular neck angle. They correlated notching with significantly poorer outcomes in terms of Constant score, strength, and active flexion. Other causes for concern are polyethylene wear, prosthetic instability related to improper tensioning, and component disassociation.[23]

Clinical experience with the reverse ball and socket in the treatment of CTA has been impressive, with most patients achieving excellent pain relief and regaining elevation above horizontal. Some of the more recent reports are presented in Table 19–5. Sirveaux and researchers'[42] multicenter study does not specify inclusion criteria, so presumably the procedure was offered to all comers with painful CTA and none was offered hemiarthroplasty because of being younger, having a stabilized humeral head, or still being capable of active elevation of more than 90 degrees. The reoperation rate was 5.0% (glenoid loosening, infection, and component disassociation). Survivorship in this series (based on reoperation for component failure or significant pain) was 88% at 5 years and 29% at 7 years, which is a high rate of

TABLE 19–2. Published Series for Constrained Ball and Socket Prostheses for All Diagnoses

STUDY	STUDY DESIGN	LEVEL OF EVIDENCE	N	AGE (RANGE), YR	DURATION OF FOLLOW-UP (RANGE), YR	PAIN SCORE (0 = NONE; 3 = SEVERE)		ACTIVE TOTAL ELEVATION, DEGREES		SUCCESSFUL RESULTS (NEER LIMITED GOALS CRITERIA)	COMMENTS
						PREOPERATIVE	POSTOPERATIVE	PREOPERATIVE	POSTOPERATIVE		
Stanmore (Coughlin et al., 1979[36])	Case series	IV	16	57 (27–82)	3 (2–4)	2.6	0.3	57	104	N/A (most were very satisfied)	Reoperation in 3 cases (19%)
Michael Reese (Post et al., 1980[39])	Case series	IV	43	55 (27–75)	4–6	2.5	0.4	N/A	N/A	N/A	Reoperation in 15 cases (35%)
Stanmore (Lettin et al., 1982[27])	Case series	IV	50	57 (31–81)	N/A	N/A	N/A	N/A	N/A	N/A	Prosthesis removed in 9 cases (18%)
McNab-English (McElwain and English, 1987)	Case series	IV	13	62 (46–81)	3 (1–5)	N/A	N/A	57	84	N/A	Major complications in 7 cases (50%)

TABLE 19–3. Published Series for Reverse Ball and Socket Prostheses: Early Designs

STUDY	STUDY DESIGN	LEVEL OF EVIDENCE	N	AGE (RANGE), YR	DURATION OF FOLLOW-UP (RANGE)	PAIN SCORE (0 = NONE; 3 = SEVERE)		ACTIVE TOTAL ELEVATION, DEGREES		SUCCESSFUL RESULTS (NEER LIMITED GOALS CRITERIA)	COMMENTS
						PREOPERATIVE	POSTOPERATIVE	PREOPERATIVE	POSTOPERATIVE		
Kessel (Bayley and Kessel, 1982)	Case series	IV	31	64 (38–84)	3 yr (6 mo to 7 yr)	N/A	N/A	N/A	N/A	76% good or very good	Removed in 4 cases (12%)
Kessel (Brostrom et al., 1992) (results reported only for unrevised cases)	Case series	IV	22	54 (35–74)	7 (5–9) yr	3	No pain in 85% 1	90	105	N/A	6/22 cases (27%) had revision or removal of prosthesis
Grammont (Grammont et al., 1987) (initial design)	Case series	IV	8	70	6 mo	N/A	0	N/A	N/A <60 degrees in 3 cases	N/A	Large glenoid component (two thirds of a sphere) prone to loosening

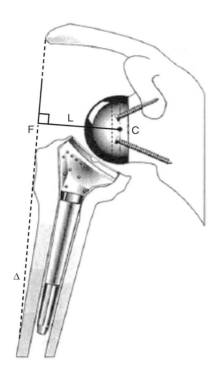

FIGURE 19–8. Diagram of a Grammont reverse prosthesis. The center of rotation *(C)* lies on the surface of the glenoid, protecting it from excessive shearing forces, and the humerus is lowered. L, lever arc of the force vector *(F)* and the deltoid (Δ).[23]

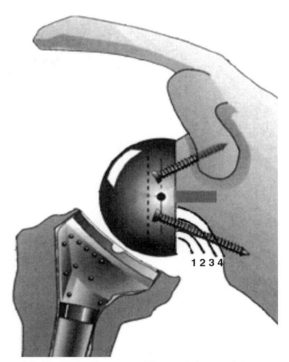

FIGURE 19–9. Classification of bone defects of the scapular neck.

failure. Those with an intact teres minor had better Constant scores. Scapular notching was noted in 64% of cases. In cases with more advanced notching, the Constant score was also adversely affected.

Boileau[45] presented the results of 45 Grammont prostheses, 21 of which were for CTA. In the whole group, the reoperation rate was 22% and the incidence rate of major complications was 31%. Results for CTA were better and were met with fewer complications. Again, the importance of an intact teres minor was stressed. Scapular notching was seen in 68% of cases.

Werner and coauthors[46] reviewed the results of 58 patients using the Grammont prosthesis. All had severe pain and pseudoparalysis (active elevation <90 degrees). In all cases, the rotator cuff was considered irreparable (chronic pseudoparalysis, acromiohumeral interval <7 mm, and fatty infiltration

of the surpaspinatus and infraspinatus at least Goutallier[47] grade 2). Substantial pain relief and improved function were achieved in all cases. Improvement was similar in all groups. Complications (including haematomas) occurred in 50% of cases but affected the outcome in only 10%. Component loosening or disassociation occurred in 9% of cases. Reoperation occurred in 33% overall but was 38% when there was a prior prosthesis and 40% when there was a prior nonprosthetic operation.

Frankle and colleagues[48] used a reverse ball and socket prosthesis of their own design (Reverse Shoulder Prosthesis; Encore Medical, Austin, TX) to treat 60 cases of CTA with good results. In their brief report, they note a 17% complication rate and a reoperation rate of 12%. They did not mention scapular notching possibly because the center of rotation is more lateralized.

Guery and researchers[49] studied survivorship of the Grammont prosthesis (Delta III) in 80 cases mostly for CTA. Using the end points of prosthetic revision and loosening, the survival rates were 91% and 84%, respectively, at 120 months for CTA, which they found significantly better than for other diagnoses. However, the survival rate was only 58% at 120 months using the end point of a Constant score less than 30.

In summary, several authors[9,49,50] have expressed caution regarding the use of a reverse ball and socket prosthesis in regard to complications and long-term survivorship. Currently, it should be reserved for the treatment of disabling CTA and exclusively in patients older than 70 years with low functional demands.

TABLE 19–4. Biomechanical Advantage of Reverse Ball and Socket Prosthesis

1. Large ball offers greater potential arc of motion and more stability than a small ball.
2. Small lateral offset (no neck) places center of rotation directly in contact with the glenoid surface and reduces torque at point of fixation of glenoid component.
3. Medializing center of rotation recruits more of deltoid fibers for elevation or abduction.
4. Lowering humerus increases tension on deltoid.

TABLE 19–5. Published Series for Reverse Ball and Socket Prostheses: Latest Design (Cuff Tear Arthropathy)

STUDY	STUDY DESIGN	LEVEL OF EVIDENCE	N	AGE (RANGE), YR	DURATION OF FOLLOW-UP (RANGE), YR	PAIN SCORE (0 = NONE; 3 = SEVERE)		ACTIVE TOTAL ELEVATION, DEGREES		CONSTANT MURLEY SCORE (MAXIMUM = 100)		REOPERATION RATE
						PREOPERATIVE	POSTOPERATIVE	PREOPERATIVE	POSTOPERATIVE	PREOPERATIVE	POSTOPERATIVE	
Sirveaux et al. (2004)[42]* (multicenter study)	Case series	IV	80	73 (60–86)	3.7 (2–8.1)	2.5	0.3	73	138	23	66	5%
Boileau et al. (2006)[45]*†	Case series	IV	21	77 (67–86)	3.3 (2–6)	N/A	0.5	53	123	18	66	5%
Werner et al. (2005)[44]*	Case series	IV	58	68 (44–84)	3.2 (minimum, 2)	2	0.9	42	100	29	64	33%
Frankle et al. (2006)[48]‡	Case series	IV	60	71	2.8 (minimum, 2)	1.9	0.7	55	105	N/A	N/A	12%

*Delta III prosthesis (DePuy Orthopaedics Inc., Warsaw, IN).
†RSP prosthesis (Encore Medical, Austin, TX).
‡Twenty-one cases of cuff tear arthropathy extracted from a total of 45.

RECOMMENDATIONS

To begin with, it must be recognized that most of the available evidence on which to base treatment decisions is only Level IV. With this in mind, however, rational and reasonable choices can still be made. The selection of the best surgical treatment for CTA begins with a thorough clinical assessment including history, physical, and imaging (plain radiographs and magnetic resonance imaging [MRI] in most cases). Not all cases of advanced cuff disease will have arthritis because the disease represents a continuum. Thorough assessment will establish the diagnosis and rule out other causes of joint destruction, particularly infection. The patient's fitness, age, and functional expectations (high or low demand) must be determined. Details of previous surgery are important. Physical examination should categorize the status of shoulder muscle force couples (active total elevation above or below 90 degrees). Up-to-date radiographs should be examined for the presence of acromiohumeral narrowing, superior humeral subluxation, and superior humeral head escape (deficient coracoacromial arch). An attempt to categorize the status of superior stability (stable or unstable fulcrum) should be made by assessing for pseudoparalysis and from inspection of plain radiographs (see Fig. 19–4). An MRI scan will reveal residual intact cuff, especially inferior subscapularis (which should be carefully preserved in any surgery) and teres minor (which will determine external rotation after surgery). The appropriate care can be selected with this information. The stage of the cuff disease may then be determined (Table 19–6).

The decision for surgery takes place after medical care has failed. Four options must be evaluated depending on circumstances:

1. *Rotator cuff repair:* should always be considered, especially in younger, more active patients for whom there is no arthropathy and the rotator cuff is judged to be reparable (grade C)
2. *Tendon transfer:* if there is no arthropathy and the cuff is deemed irreparable (acromiohumeral interval <7 mm; chronic pseudoparalysis; fat infiltration Goutallier grade 2 on MRI in surpaspinatus and infraspinatus). For antero-

superior deficiency, the pectoralis major is transferred, and for the more common posterosuperior deficiencies, the latissimus dorsi (grade C)
3. *Humeral head replacement:* in a painful shoulder when the force couple fulcrum is stable (Seebauer grades IA, IB, and IIA) (grade C)
4. *Reverse shoulder prosthesis:* in a painful shoulder when the patient is elderly (>70 years), has low functional demands, and there is chronic pseudoparalysis; if the teres minor in nonfunctional, latissimus dorsi transfer to restore external rotation may be considered (grade C)
5. *Glenohumeral arthrodesis:* in a younger high-demand patient who has a painful arthritic shoulder with pseudoparalysis and requires a stable shoulder girdle for function; in these instances, the deltoid will usually be nonfunctional (grade C)

Selection of the correct prosthesis is important. In hemiarthroplasty, overstuffing the joint with a large prosthesis must be avoided so that undue tension is not placed on soft tissues and residual cuff tendons. With the reverse arthroplasty, care should be taken to select a prosthesis that does not lateralize the center of rotation past the glenoid surface. The advantages of a lateralized center of rotation are greatly outweighed by real risk for early loosening.

In all cases of prosthetic replacement, patients must be followed at regular intervals afterward. With humeral head replacement, continued superior migration of the prosthesis has been observed.[51] With reverse shoulder replacement, there are serious concerns regarding late complications such as loosening and component disassociation. Table 19–7 provides a summary of recommendations for the surgical treatment of rotator cuff disease.

TABLE 19–6. Key Features in Cuff Tear Arthropathy Assessment

History	Degree of pain
	Functional expectations: ADL only vs. ADL plus sport and work
Physical	Active total elevation: >90 degrees (force couples into intact) vs. <90 degrees (force couples not intact)
Imaging	Head centered
	Head superiorly subluxated but CA arch intact
	Head superior escape, CA arch incompetent

ADL, activities of daily living; CA, coracoacromial.

TABLE 19–7. Summary of Recommendations

STAGE	RECOMMENDATION	LEVEL OF EVIDENCE/GRADE OF RECOMMENDATION
Reparable rotator cuff tear without arthropathy	Repair torn cuff	C
Irreparable cuff without arthropathy	Tendon transfer	C
Cuff tear arthropathy with stable fulcrum	Humeral head replacement	C
Cuff tear arthropathy with unstable fulcrum elderly, low demand	Reverse shoulder prosthesis	C
Cuff tear arthropathy with unstable fulcrum young, high demand	Glenohumeral arthrodesis	C

REFERENCES

1. Neer CSI, Cruess RL, Sledge CB, Wilde AH: Total glenohumeral replacement. A preliminary report. Orthop Trans 1:244–245, 1977.
2. Neer CS, Craig EV, Fukuda H: Cuff-tear arthropathy. J Bone Joint Surg Am 65:1232–1244, 1983.
3. Garancis JC, Cheung HS, Halverson PB, McCarty DJ: "Milwaukee shoulder"—association of microspheroids containing hydroxyapatite crystals, active collagenase, ad neutral protease with rotator cuff defects. III. Morphologic and biochemical studies of an excised synovium showing chondromatosis. Arthritis Rheum 24:484–491, 1981.
4. McCarty DJ: Milwaukee shoulder syndrome. X. Trans Am Clin Climatol Assoc 102:271–283, 1990.
5. Antoniou J, Tsai A, Baker D, et al: Milwaukee shoulder: Correlating possible etiologic variables. Clin Orthop Relat Res (407):79–85, 2003.
6. Inman VT, Saunders CM, Abbott LC: Observations on the function of the shoulder joint. J Bone Joint Surg 26:1–30, 1944.
7. Burkhart SS: Arthroscopic treatment of massive rotator cuff tears. Clinical results and biomechanical rationale. Clin Orthop 267:45–56, 1991.
8. Burkhart SS: Fluoroscopic comparison of kinematic patterns in massive rotator cuff tears. A suspension bridge model. Clin Orthop 284:144–152, 1992.
9. Matsen FA III, Boileau P, Walch G, et al: The reverse total shoulder arthroplasty. J Bone Joint Surg Am 89:660–667, 2007.
10. De Wilde LF, Audenaert EA, Berghs BM: Shoulder prostheses treating cuff tear arthropathy: A comparative biomechanical study. J Orthop Res 22:1222–1230, 2004.
11. Neer CS, Watson KC, Stanton FJ: Recent experience in total shoulder replacement. J Bone Joint Surg Am 64:319–337, 1982.
12. Worland RL, Jessup DE, Arredondo J, Warburton KJ: Bipolar shoulder arthroplasty for rotator cuff arthropathy. J Shoulder Elbow Surg 6:512–515, 1997.
13. Jensen KL, Williams GR, Russell IJ, Rockwood CA: Current concepts review—rotator cuff tear arthropathy. J Bone Joint Surg Am 81:1312–1324, 1999.
14. Hertel R, Ballmer FT, Lombert SM, Gerber C: Lag signs in the diagnosis of rotator cuff rupture. J Shoulder Elbow Surg 5:307–313, 1996.
15. Gerber C, Krushell R: Isolated ruptured of the tendon if the subscapularis muscle clinical features in 16 cases. J Bone Joint Surg Br 73:389–394, 1991.
16. Gerber C, Hersche O, Farron A: Isolated rupture of the subscapularis tendon. J Bone Joint Surg Am 78:1015–1023, 1996.
17. Werner CML, Steinmann PA, Gilbert M, Gerber C: Treatment of painful pseudoparesis due to irreparable rotator cuff dysfunction with the delta III reverse-ball-and-socket total shoulder prosthesis. J Bone Joint Surg Am 87:1476–1486, 2005.
18. Hamada K, Fukuda H, Mikasa M, Kobayashi Y: Roentgenographic findings in massive rotator cuff tears. A long-term observation. Clin Orthop Relat Res (254)92–96, 1990.
19. Visotsky JL, Basamania C, Seebauer L, et al: Cuff tear arthropathy: Pathogenesis, classification, and algorithm for treatment. J Bone Joint Surg Am 86(suppl 2):35–40, 2004.
20. Neer CS2, Watson KC, Stanton FJ: Recent experience in total shoulder replacement. J Bone Joint Surg Am 64:319–337, 1982.
21. Caporali R, Rossi S, Montecucco C: Tidal irrigation in Milwaukee shoulder syndrome. J Rheumatol 21:1781–1782, 1994.
22. Dines DM, Moynihan DP, Dines JS, McCann P: Irreparable rotator cuff tears: What to do and when to do it; the surgeon's dilemma. J Bone Joint Surg Am 88:2294–2302, 2006.
23. Boileau P, Sinnerton RJ, Chuinard C, Walch G: Arthroplasty of the shoulder. J Bone Joint Surg Br 88:562–575, 2006.
24. Franklin JL, Barrett WP, Jackins SE, Matsen FA: Glenoid loosening in total shoulder arthroplasty. Association with rotator cuff deficiency. J Arthroplasty 3:39–46, 1988.
25. Neer CSI: Glenohumeral arthroplasty. Shoulder reconstruction. Philadelphia, W.B. Saunders Company, 1990, p 153.
26. Amstutz HC, Thomas BJ, Kabo JM, et al: The Dana total shoulder arthroplasty. J Bone Joint Surg Am 70:1174–1182, 1988.
27. Gristina AG, Romano RL, Kammire GC, Webb LX: Total shoulder replacement. Orthop Clin North Am 18:445–453, 1987.
28. Orr TE, Carter DR, Schurman DJ: Stress analyses of glenoid component designs. Clin Orthop Relat Res (232):217–224, 1988.
29. Swanson AB, de Groot SG, Sattel AB, et al: Bipolar implant shoulder arthroplasty. Long-term results. Clin Orthop Relat Res (249):227–247, 1989.
30. Gregory T, Hansen U, Emery RJ, et al: Developments in shoulder arthroplasty. Proc Inst Mech Eng [H] 221:87–96, 2007.
31. Sarris IK, Papadimitriou NG, Sotereanos DG: Bipolar hemiarthroplasty for chronic rotator cuff tear arthropathy. J Arthroplasty 18:169–173, 2003.
32. Petroff E, Mestdagh H, Maynou C, Delobelle JM: [Arthroplasty with a mobile cup for shoulder arthrosis with irreparable rotator cuff rupture: Preliminary results and cineradiographic study]. [French]. Revue de Chirurgie Orthopedique et Reparatrice de l Appareil Moteur 85:245–256, 1999.
33. Duranthon LD, Augereau B, Thomazeau H, et al: [Bipolar arthroplasty in rotator cuff arthropathy: 13 cases]. [French]. Revue de Chirurgie Orthopedique et Reparatrice de l Appareil Moteur 88:28–34, 2002.
34. Worland RL, Jessup DE, Arredondo J, Warburton KJ: Bipolar shoulder arthroplasty for rotator cuff arthropathy. J Shoulder Elbow Surg 6:512–515, 1997.
35. Calton TF, Fehring TK, Griffin WL, McCoy TH: Failure of the polyethylene after bipolar hemiarthroplasty of the hip. A report of five cases. J Bone Joint Surg Am 80:420–423, 1998.
36. Coughlin MJ, Morris JM, West WF: The semiconstrained total shoulder arthroplasty. J Bone Joint Surg Am 61:574–581, 1979.
37. Lettin AW, Copeland SA, Scales JT: The Stanmore total shoulder replacement. J Bone Joint Surg Br 64:47–51, 1982.
38. Post M, Jablon M: Constrained total shoulder arthroplasty. Long-term follow-up observations. Clin Orthop Relat Res (173):109–116, 1983.
39. Post M, Haskell SS, Jablon M: Total shoulder replacement with a constrained prosthesis. J Bone Joint Surg Am 62:327–335, 1980.
40. Neer CSI: Glenohumeral arthroplasty. Shoulder reconstruction. Philadelphia, W.B. Saunders Company, 1990, pp 148–150.
41. Boileau P, Watkinson DJ, Hatzidakis AM, Balg F: Grammont reverse prosthesis: Design, rationale, and biomechanics. J Shoulder Elbow Surg 14(1 suppl S):147S–161S, 2005.
42. Sirveaux F, Favard L, Oudet D, et al: Grammont inverted total shoulder arthroplasty in the treatment of glenohumeral osteoarthritis with massive rupture of the cuff: Results of a multicentre study of 80 shoulders. J Bone Joint Surg Br 86:388–395, 2004.
43. Nyffeler RW, Sheikh R, Atkinson TS, et al: Effects of glenoid component version on humeral head displacement and joint reaction forces: An experimental study. J Shoulder Elbow Surg 15:625–629, 2006.
44. Simovitch RW, Zumstein MA, Lohri E, et al: Predictors of scapular notching in patients managed with the delta III reverse total shoulder replacement. J Bone Joint Surg Am 89:588–600, 2007.
45. Boileau P, Watkinson D, Hatzidakis AM, Hovorka I: Neer Award 2005. The Grammont reverse shoulder prosthesis: Results in cuff tear arthritis, fracture sequelae, and revision arthroplasty. J Shoulder Elbow Surg 15:527–540, 2006.
46. Werner CML, Steinmann PA, Gilbert M, Gerber C: Treatment of painful pseudoparesis due to irreparable rotator cuff dysfunction with the delta III reverse-ball-and-socket total shoulder prosthesis. J Bone Joint Surg Am 87:1476–1486, 2005.
47. Goutallier D, Postel JM, Gleyze P, et al: Influence of cuff muscle fatty degeneration on anatomic and functional outcomes after simple suture of full-thickness tears. J Shoulder Elbow Surg 12:550–554, 2003.
48. Frankle M, Levy JC, Pupello D, et al: The reverse shoulder prosthesis for glenohumeral arthritis associated with severe rotator cuff deficiency. A minimum two-year follow-up study

of sixty patients surgical technique. J Bone Joint Surg Am 88(1 suppl 2):178–190, 2006.

49. Guery J, Favard L, Sirveaux F, et al: Reverse total shoulder arthroplasty. Survivorship analysis of eighty replacements followed for five to ten years. J Bone Joint Surg Am 88: 1742–1747, 2006.

50. Wirth MA, Rockwood CA Jr: Complications of shoulder arthroplasty. Clin Orthop (307):47–69, 1994.

51. Sanchez-Sotelo J, Cofield RH, Rowland CM: Shoulder hemiarthroplasty for glenohumeral arthritis associated with severe rotator cuff deficiency. J Bone Joint Surg Am 83:1814–1822, 2001.

Chapter 20

What Is the Best Treatment for Complex Proximal Humerus Fractures? What Are the Main Determinants of Outcome after Arthroplasty?

Jason L. Hurd, MD and Joseph D. Zuckerman, MD

Proximal humerus fractures account for 4% to 5% of all fractures.[1] The majority of proximal humerus fractures (approximately 80%) are minimally displaced and can be treated with a sling and early mobilization.[2] Two-part fractures are most often treated with some form of osteosynthesis. Frequently, attempts to preserve the proximal humerus are also made in young, active patients with good bone quality who have three-part and valgus-impacted four-part fractures (level V). Osteosynthesis is usually considered preferable to hemiarthroplasty in young patients (level V) because of concerns about glenoid wear and implant longevity.[3-5]

Certain complex proximal humerus fractures, however, are either not amenable to fixation or are at significant risk for humeral head osteonecrosis, making osteosynthesis a less desirable option. These include widely displaced four-part fractures and fracture dislocations, head-splitting fractures with greater than 40% articular surface involvement, anatomic neck fractures, and selected three-part fractures in patients with osteopenia and nondisplaced comminution that precludes secure internal fixation.[6] In these cases where the risk for fixation failure is high, humeral head replacement is generally accepted as the best option. Support for this philosophy comes from the fact that primary hemiarthroplasties are technically easier and have been consistently shown in retrospective comparative series to have better outcomes than secondary hemiarthroplasties performed for failed internal fixation or nonoperative treatment.[7-11]

The literature on prosthetic treatment of complex proximal humerus fractures is sparse. Only three level I or II studies currently exist: one compares hemiarthroplasty with nonoperative treatment,[12] whereas the other two compare hemiarthroplasty with tension band wiring.[13,14]

In 1984, Stableforth[12] conducted a prospective, randomized, nonblinded comparison of uncemented hemiarthroplasty and nonoperative treatment. His study included 32 patients with an average age of 67 who had four-part proximal humerus fractures. The author found a significant reduction in pain, improved range of motion and strength, and greater ability to perform activities of daily living in patients treated with hemiarthroplasty. Criticisms of this limited study include its variable and relatively short follow-up period, unclear method of randomization, and poorly defined outcome measurements.[15]

In 1997, Hoellen and colleagues[13] compared hemiarthroplasty with open reduction and tension band wiring in a randomized, controlled trial of 30 patients, older than 65 years, with 4-part fractures. One-year follow-up was available for only 18 of the 30 patients. Results in the two groups were comparable with respect to pain, function, and ability to perform activities of daily living. The most significant difference between the two groups was that none of the patients in the arthroplasty group required reoperation, were five patients in the fixation group required further surgery for wire displacement (four patients) or failed fixation (one patient).

Two years after the study by Hoellen and colleagues,[13] Holbein and coworkers[14] published a follow-up report. This subsequent study included 39 patients with both 3- and 4-part fractures with up to 2-year follow-up. One-year data were available for 31 patients with 2-year follow-up for 24 patients. The results of this study were similar to those that Hoellen and colleagues[13] reported. The authors found no significant difference in patients with three- or four-part fractures treated with either tension band wiring or arthroplasty. At 2-year follow-up, however, nine patients in the fixation group required further surgery compared with none in the hemiarthroplasty group. It is difficult to make any sound conclusions from these studies because of the short follow-up period and significant dropout rate. The generalizability of these findings to younger patients is also unclear.

In 2003, Handoll and coworkers[15] conducted a Cochrane review on the treatment of proximal humerus fractures in adults. Based on their analysis, they were unable to provide any treatment recommendation. Both Bondi and coauthors[16] and Bhandari and investigators,[17] after systematic evidence-based reviews on proximal humerus fractures, also found insufficient evidence from randomized trials to determine optimal treatment. They conclude that until valid evidence exists, the management of proximal humerus fractures will be based on surgeon preference, ability, and experience. Although evidence-based support for arthroplasty in the treatment of complex proximal humerus fractures is lacking, some evidence exists that arthroplasty can optimize patient outcomes once the decision to treat has been made.

RESULTS AFTER HUMERAL HEAD REPLACEMENT

Reliable pain relief, patient satisfaction, and reasonable implant longevity have been consistently demonstrated in multiple retrospective reviews of patients who underwent hemiarthroplasty for complex proximal humerus fractures. Good-to-excellent pain relief has been reported in 73% to 97% of patients; overall, more than 80% of patients expressed satisfaction with their treatment, and prosthesis survival at 10 years ranges from 83% to 94%.[18]

Functional outcomes, however, have been much more unpredictable. Even within individual studies, outcomes vary widely from patient to patient. Less desirable functional outcomes are most often because of limited shoulder motion, decreased muscle power, and inability to perform activities of daily living. The challenge for surgeons is to identify methods of maximizing outcomes through meticulous patient selection, optimal surgical techniques, and appropriate postoperative treatment. With this in mind, several authors have explored the preoperative, surgical, and postoperative factors that appear to influence outcome.

PREOPERATIVE FACTORS

Robinson and investigators[19] performed a level II observational cohort study of 163 patients with complex humerus fractures treated with hemiarthroplasty. Of the 163 patients, 25 died or were lost to follow-up within the first postoperative year. The remaining 138 patients with an average age of 68.5 years were evaluated with Constant scores. Using a univariate linear regression model, the authors assessed the factors immediately after injury and at 6 weeks after surgery; these factors were predictive of the Constant score at 1 year.

Preoperative factors including advanced patient age, presence of a neurologic deficit, tobacco usage, and alcohol consumption were found to be significantly predictive of lower 1-year outcome scores. The age of the patient was the most significant of these factors, with the modified Constant score decreasing by eight points for every 10-year increase

in age. Neither fracture severity nor the presence of humeral head subluxation/dislocation affected 1-year outcomes.

OPERATIVE AND POSTOPERATIVE FACTORS

The most important operative factor that influences outcome after hemiarthroplasty for complex proximal humerus fractures is the ability to achieve anatomic reduction and union of the tuberosities, particularly the greater tuberosity. Achieving union of the tuberosities is dependent on proper positioning of the prosthesis and secure anatomic fixation of the tuberosities. These two factors are intimately related because it is virtually impossible to attain secure, anatomic tuberosity fixation if the prosthesis is not implanted in the correct position.

Robinson and investigators[19] also evaluated factors that affect outcome at 6 weeks after surgery. They found that the factors assessed at 6 weeks after surgery (which were mostly related to surgery) provided a more precise prediction of 1-year outcome than the patient-based factors assessed before surgery. The need for early reoperation, significant displacement of the prosthetic head from the central axis of the glenoid (radiographically), and radiographic evidence of retraction of one or more of the tuberosities were all predictive of worse outcomes. The authors emphasize the importance of an intact, functioning rotator cuff because many of the reoperations were due to displacement of the tuberosities, and subluxation was attributed to an incompetent rotator cuff. Advanced patient age and the presence of a persistent neurologic deficit were also shown to significantly predict poorer Constant scores at 1 year.

Boileau and colleagues,[20] in a prospective, multicenter, prognostic, level II study, attempted to determine the clinical and radiographic parameters that contribute to unsatisfactory results in some patients. Using regression tests for correlation, they demonstrate that final outcomes were directly related to tuberosity osteosynthesis. The factors associated with failure of tuberosity osteosynthesis were malpositioning of the greater tuberosity, poor initial position of the prosthesis, and age older than 75 in women.

Tuberosity malpositioning and/or migration, which was found in 50% of patients based on final follow-up radiographs or computed tomographic (CT) scans, was the most significant factor associated with poor outcomes. Malpositioning of the greater tuberosity was defined as greater than 5 mm superior or 10 mm inferior to the superior aspect of the humeral head, or as posterior placement such that the greater tuberosity was not visible on the postoperative anteroposterior radiograph in external or neutral rotation but could be seen on the internal rotation, axillary, scapular lateral, or CT views. Malpositioning of the prosthesis also significantly correlated with both tuberosity malpositioning and significantly worse functional results. Prosthesis malpositioning was defined as greater than 10 mm cephalad, 15 mm caudal, or retroversion of greater than 40 degrees. The negative influence of age on outcome was also confirmed. These authors found that women older than 75 years had a significantly greater failure rate of tuberosity osteosynthesis and subsequently worse outcomes than the other patients in their study. This was most likely due to a greater degree of osteopenia and, therefore, less secure fixation of the tuberosities.

SURGICAL RECOMMENDATIONS

Although patient-related factors are often out of the surgeon's control, the literature does provide some guidance on avoiding prosthesis malpositioning and attaining secure tuberosity fixation. Reestablishment of the patient's natural retroversion is difficult in the setting of a proximal humerus fracture. Some authors have suggested using the bicipital groove as a reference point.[21-23] By placing the lateral fin of the prosthesis a standard distance from the posterior edge of the bicipital groove, a predictable degree of retroversion can be attained. Several authors, however, have noted wide variations in the degree of humeral retroversion among different patients.[24-26] Use of a standard version may therefore result in significant malpositioning of the humeral stem.[24-26]

Kontakis and researchers,[26] in a study using 45 cadaveric specimens, showed that humeral head retroversion varies between −6.3 (i.e., anteversion) and 41.7 degrees. They found that placing the humeral prosthesis with the lateral fin at the posterior aspect of the bicipital groove, as commonly suggested, often resulted in excessive retroversion when compared with the patient's natural version. In some cases, this could lead to overtensioning of the greater tuberosity and ultimately failure of fixation when the arm is rotated internally. Using CT scans of cadaveric proximal humeri, they were able to estimate the natural version and measure the distance that the posterior fin of the prosthesis should be placed from the posterior aspect of the bicipital groove. They were able to use this method on six of their patients by obtaining CT scans of the opposite shoulder before surgery.

Murachovsky and coauthors[27] in another cadaveric study found that the pectoralis major tendon is a helpful landmark for restoring correct humeral height. After dissection of 40 shoulders, they found the distance from the upper border of the pectoralis major tendon insertion on the humerus to the top of the humeral head was 5.6 ± 0.5 cm with a confidence level of 95%. In addition, they found no correlation between the size of the patient and this measurement. In cases where severe comminution of the proximal humerus makes estimation of the appropriate humeral height difficult, this method may be useful. Other authors have suggested preoperative

templating of the opposite side, restoration of the medial calcar, reapproximation of the fracture fragments, or referencing based on the tension of the long head of the biceps to restore humeral height. All of these tools are at the surgeon's disposal and can be helpful when utilized.

Attaining secure, anatomic tuberosity fixation starts with anatomic positioning of the prosthesis using the tools just described. Correct positioning of the prosthesis makes anatomic positioning of the tuberosities much easier and reduces stress on the repair. Nonanatomic positioning of the greater tuberosity in a cadaveric model has been shown to significantly impair external rotation kinematics and increase torque requirements by eightfold.[28] When the tuberosities are anatomically placed, Frankel and coworkers[29] have shown that supplementation of the tuberosity repair with a circumferential medial cerclage incorporated into the prosthesis reduces strain on the greater tuberosity by more than 100%.

CONCLUSIONS

Currently, because of a lack of randomized, controlled trials, no recommendations can be made on the optimal treatment of three- and four-part proximal humerus fractures. However, recommendations can be made for optimizing outcomes once the decision to treat with arthroplasty has been made. Younger patients without neurologic deficits who do not smoke or consume alcohol tend to have better outcomes. Patients treated with early primary arthroplasty also have consistently better outcomes than patients who have secondary arthroplasty after failure of nonoperative or operative treatment. The most important factors for optimizing patient outcomes appear to be surgically related. Proper prosthesis positioning and secure anatomic tuberosity fixation lead to more reliable tuberosity osteosynthesis and improved outcome scores. Table 20–1 provides a summary of recommendations for the treatment of humerus fractures.

TABLE 20–1. Summary of Recommendations

STATEMENT	LEVEL OF EVIDENCE/GRADE OF RECOMMENDATION
1. No treatment recommendations can be made at this point.	I
2. Early treatment with hemiarthroplastyresults in better outcomes than delayed treatment.	C
3. Proper prosthesis positioning and anatomic, stable tuberosity fixation lead to better outcomes.	B

B = fair evidence (level II or III studies with consistent findings) for or against recommending intervention;
C = poor-quality evidence (level IV or V with consistent findings) for or against recommending intervention; I = insufficient or conflicting evidence not allowing a recommendation for or against intervention.

REFERENCES

1. Horak J, Nilsson BE: Epidemiology of fractures of the upper end of the humerus. Clin Orthop 112:250–253, 1975.
2. Shin SS, Zuckerman JD: One-part fractures. In Zuckerman JD, Koval KJ (eds): Shoulder Fractures: The Practical Guide to Management. New York: Thieme Medical Publishers, 2005, p 50.
3. Parsons IM 4th, Millett PJ, Warner JJ: Glenoid wear after shoulder hemiarthroplasty: Quantitative radiographic analysis. Clin Orthop Relat Res (421):120–125, 2004.
4. Sperling JW, Cofield RH: Revision total shoulder arthroplasty for the treatment of glenoid arthrosis. J Bone Joint Surg Am 80:860–867, 1998.
5. Sperling JW, Cofield RH, Rowland CM: Neer hemiarthroplasty and Neer total shoulder arthroplasty in patients fifty years old or less. Long-term results. J Bone Joint Surg Am 80:464–473, 1998.
6. Wirth MA: Late sequelae of proximal humerus fractures. Instr Course Lect 52:13–16, 2003.
7. Becker R, Pap G, Machner A, Neumann WH: Strength and motion after hemiarthroplasty in displaced four-fragment fracture of the proximal humerus: 27 patients followed for 1-6 years. Acta Orthop Scand 73:44–49, 2002.
8. Bosch U, Skutek M, Fremerey RW, Tscherne H: Outcome after primary and secondary hemiarthroplasty in elderly patients with fractures of the proximal humerus. J Shoulder Elbow Surg 7:479–484, 1998.
9. Demirhan M, Kilicoglu O, Altinel L, et al: Prognostic factors in prosthetic replacement for acute proximal humerus fractures. J Orthop Trauma 17:181–188, 2003.
10. Moeckel BH, Dines DM, Warren RF, Altchek DW: Modular hemiarthroplasty for fractures of the proximal part of the humerus. J Bone Joint Surg Am 74:884–889, 1992.
11. Frich LH, Sojbjerg JO, Sneppen O: Shoulder arthroplasty in complex acute and chronic proximal humeral fractures. Orthopedics 14:949–954, 1991.
12. Stableforth PG: Four-part fractures of the neck of the humerus. J Bone Joint Surg Br 66:104–108, 1984.
13. Hoellen IP, Bauer G, Holbein O: [Prosthetic humeral head replacement in dislocated humerus multi-fragment fracture in the elderly—an alternative to minimal osteosynthesis?] Zentralbl Chir 122:994–1001, 1997.
14. Holbein O, Bauer G, Hoellen I, et al: [Is primary endoprosthetic replacement of the humeral head an alternative treatment for comminuted fractures of the proximal humerus in elderly patients?] Osteosynthese Int 7(suppl 2):207–210, 1999.
15. Handoll HHG, Gibson JNA, Madhok R: Interventions for treating proximal humeral fractures in adults. Cochrane Database Syst Rev 4:CD000434, 2003.
16. Bondi R, Ceccarelli E, Campi S, Padua R: Shoulder arthroplasty for complex proximal humeral fractures. J Orthop Traumatol 6:57–60, 2005.
17. Bhandari M, Matthys G, McKee MD: Evidence-Based Orthopaedic Trauma Working Group: Four part fractures of the proximal humerus. J Orthop Trauma 18:126–127, 2004.
18. Kwon YW, Zuckerman JD: Outcome after treatment of proximal humeral fractures with humeral head replacement. Instr Course Lect 54:363–369, 2005.
19. Robinson CM, Page RS, Hill RM, et al: Primary hemiarthroplasty for treatment of proximal humeral fractures. J Bone Joint Surg Am 85:1215–1223, 2003.
20. Boileau P, Krishnan SG, Tinsi L, et al: Tuberosity malposition and migration: Reasons for poor outcomes after hemiarthroplasty for displaced fractures of the proximal humerus. J Shoulder Elbow Surg 11:401–412, 2002.
21. Tillett E, Smith M, Fulcher M, Shanklin J: Anatomic determination of humeral head retroversion: The relationship of the central axis of the humeral head to the bicipital groove. J Shoulder Elbow Surg 2:255–256, 1993.
22. Bigliani L: Proximal humeral arthroplasty for acute fractures. In: Craig EV (ed): The Shoulder. New York, Raven Press, 1995, pp 259–274.
23. Angibaud L, Zuckerman JD, Flurin PH, et al: Reconstructing proximal humeral fractures using the bicipital groove as a landmark. Clin Orthop 458:168–174, 2007.
24. Kummer FJ, Perkins R, Zuckerman JD: The use of the bicipital groove for alignment of the humeral stem in shoulder arthroplasty. J Shoulder Elbow Surg 7:144–146, 1998.
25. Edelson G: Variations in the retroversion of the humeral head. J Shoulder Elbow Surg 8:142–145, 1999.
26. Kontakis GM, Damilakis J, Christoforakis J, et al: The bicipital groove as a landmark for orientation of the humeral prosthesis in cases of fracture. J Shoulder Elbow Surg 10:136–139, 2001.
27. Murachovsky J, Ikemoto RY, Nascimento LG, et al: Pectoralis major tendon reference (PMT): A new method for accurate restoration of humeral length with hemiarthroplasty for fracture. J Shoulder Elbow Surg 15:675–678, 2006.
28. Frankle MA, Greenwald DP, Markee BA, et al: Biomechanical effects of malposition of tuberosity fragments on the humeral prosthetic reconstruction for four-part proximal humerus fractures. J Shoulder Elbow Surg 10:321–326, 2001.
29. Frankle MA, Ondrovic LE, Markee BA, et al: Stability of tuberosity reattachment in proximal humeral hemiarthroplasty. J Shoulder Elbow Surg 11:413–420, 2002.

Chapter 21

What Are the Best Diagnostic Criteria for Lateral Epicondylitis?

Constance M. LeBrun, MDCM, MPE, CCFP

Lateral epicondylitis is a common entity that affects up to 1% to 3% of the population. Historically, it has been termed *writer's cramp*,[1] *rider's sprain*,[2] and finally, the more familiar *tennis elbow*[3]; but in fact, only 5% to 10% of affected individuals actually play tennis. It is more frequent in sports and occupations that require repetitive actions of the hand and wrist, and can account for up to 50% of elbow injuries in athletes using overhead arm motions in their sport. The incidence is approximately 4 to 7 cases per 1000 patients, with a peak occurrence in patients aged 35 to 54 years. Similar symptoms can occur on the medial side of the elbow, but lateral elbow pain is more predominant with a 4:1 to 7:1 ratio. Symptoms last, on average, from 6 months to 2 years, with 89% of patients recovering within 1 year. Risk factors include overuse, repetitive movements, training errors, misalignments, flexibility problems, aging, poor circulation, strength deficits or muscle imbalance, and psychological factors.[4,5] More than 40 treatment options are described, with little scientific rationale for most of them.[6–8] Systematic literature reviews have identified substantive problems including the lack of proper randomized, controlled clinical trials, poor-quality studies, and vague inclusion criteria. No doubt contributing to the problem is the lack of evidence-based diagnostic criteria and outcome measures.

because *-itis* implies inflammation. Nirschl[11] rather described it as "tendinosis" or "angiofibroblastic hyperplasia," reflecting the degenerative changes based on histopathologic diagnosis. A review of histologic, immunohistochemical, and electron microscopy suggests that the condition is degenerative[12,13] with increased fibroblasts, vascular hyperplasia, proteoglycans and glycosaminoglycans, and disorganized and immature collagen. This is in keeping with current thinking about tendon pathology in general.[14,15]

Many names have been proposed for this condition—tennis elbow, radial or lateral epicondylalgia,[16] extensor tendinopathy, or epicondylitis lateralis humeri. The primary argument against lateral epicondylalgia (*algia* means "pain") is that lateral elbow pain can also result from PIN entrapment (radial tunnel syndrome) and from compression of the nerves of the cervical spine; therefore, this is probably too general a term for diagnosis. The term *extensor tendinopathy* is not inclusive enough because often more than the wrist extensor tendons are involved (ECRB and sometimes the supinator muscle). Some authors[17] have suggested that it is most appropriately termed *lateral elbow tendinopathy*, a painful overuse tendon condition in the area of lateral epicondyle. For purposes of consistency in the remainder of this review, however, the term *lateral epicondylitis* is used.

PATHOPHYSIOLOGY

Cyriax[9] in 1936 recognized that the origin of extensor carpi radialis brevis (ECRB) was the primary site of injury. Other muscles involved are the extensor carpi radialis longus, extensor carpi ulnaris extensor digitorum communis (in at least 50% of cases) and the supinator muscle (Fig. 21–1). The condition also requires detailed evaluation and consideration to exclude neuropathy, such as radial tunnel syndrome, posterior interosseous nerve (PIN) compression, or both.[10] The radial nerve can be entrapped at several sites (Fig. 21–2): by fibrous bands in front of the radial head, by the recurrent radial vessels (leash of Henry), at the arcade of Frohse (proximal thickened edge of superficial head of supinator muscle), and at the tendinous margin of the ECRB.

In chronic cases of lateral epicondylitis, it has been shown that there are little to no inflammatory cells, hence the term *tendonitis* is inappropriate

CLINICAL DIAGNOSTIC CRITERIA

Lateral epicondylitis is characterized by a corroborating history of injury and is a localized tenderness in the area where the common wrist extensors (especially ECRB) attach to the lateral epicondyle of the humerus.[18] Functional use, such as gripping or lifting heavy objects, exacerbates symptoms. Differential diagnoses include radial nerve entrapment (or rarely, lateral antebrachial cutaneous neuropathy), elbow joint disease (osteochondral desiccans, intra-articular loose bodies, osteoarthrosis), partial or complete tear of the tendon, and extrinsic causes (cervical dysfunction and nerve root compression).[19] Infrequently seen are degeneration or stenosis of the orbicular ligament, chronic impingement of the redundant synovial fold between the humerus and radial head, traumatic periostitis of the lateral epicondyle, and chondromalacia of the radial head and capitellum.

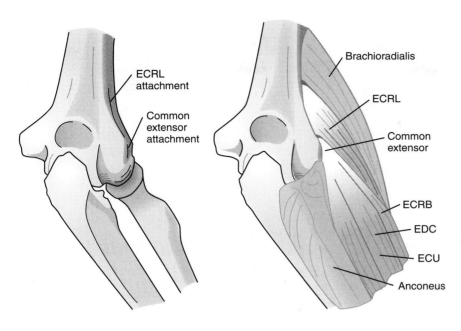

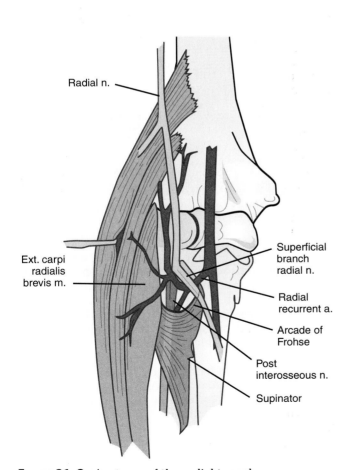

FIGURE 21-1. Anatomy of the lateral elbow. (Adapted with permission from Bishai SK, Plancher KD: The basic science of lateral epicondylosis: Update for the future. Tech Orthop 21:250–255, 2006.)

FIGURE 21-2. Anatomy of the radial tunnel.

Clinical examination should include visual inspection of the elbow for alignment (varus or valgus angulation), muscle bulk, and obvious bruising or swelling; however, none of these is diagnostic. Elbow range of motion is sometimes decreased; one study found a decrease of 10% in supination and 15% in pronation in 25 patients with chronic unilateral epicondylosis.[20] Previous cortisone injections may leave residual skin discoloration or lack of pigmentation. Neurovascular examination of the distal extremity is also necessary.

The diagnosis of lateral epicondylitis is substantiated by tenderness over the ECRB or common extensor origin. The therapist or physician should be able to reproduce the typical pain by the following methods: (1) digital palpation on the facet of the lateral epicondyle, (2) resisted wrist extension (Fig. 21–3) or resisted middle-finger extension with the elbow in extension (Fig. 21–4), or (3) having the patient grip an object. In addition to pain, patients almost always have decreased function. In radial tunnel syndrome[21] (which may coexist with lateral epicondylitis in up to 5% of cases), the pain is more diffuse and localized to the extensor mass, 3 to 4 cm distal to the lateral epicondyle. It may be provoked with supinator stress testing or resisted extension of the middle finger. Weakness of the distal muscle groups innervated by the PIN may also be present.

Other tests have been described,[22,23] including Cozen's test (with the elbow flexed and the forearm pronated, the patient is asked to make a fist and radially deviate and extend the wrist against resistance) (Fig. 21–5). Mill's test (Fig. 21–6) refers to pain (on resisted wrist extension) with the elbow extended and wrist flexed and pronated with radial deviation.[24] Coonrad and Hooper[24] have also described the "coffee cup test," where picking up a cup of coffee is painful. Another useful clinical tool is the "chair test"

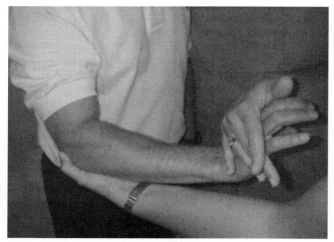

FIGURE 21–3. Resisted wrist extension.

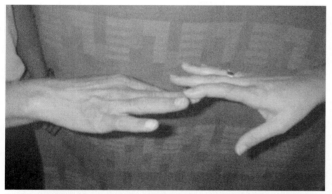

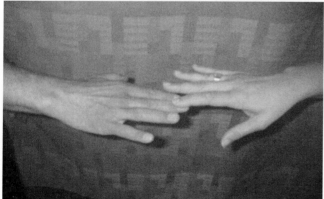

FIGURE 21–4. Resisted extension of the middle finger.

(Fig. 21–7), where the patient is asked to pick up a chair with the elbow extended and the wrist ulnarly deviated with the hand in palmar flexion.[25] One group studied a standardized and calibrated system to simulate the chair pick-up.[26] They demonstrated excellent reliability (inter-rater intraclass correlation coefficients [ICCs] ranging from 0.80–0.93 and intra-rater ICCs ranging from 0.9–0.97) and reproducibility of results. Measurements in a group of 16 patients with MRI-confirmed diagnosis suggested that this test could be valid for monitoring patients with lat-

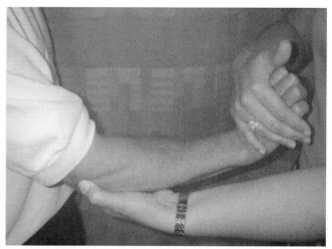

FIGURE 21–5. Cozen's test for lateral epicondylitis.

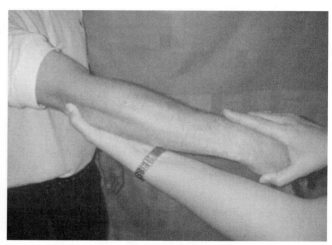

FIGURE 21–6. Mill's test for lateral epicondylitis.

eral epicondylosis. Other researchers[27] used an extensor grip test (where pain on resisted wrist extension was diminished by the examiner gripping the patients arm just below the elbow with an estimated 10–N pressure) to prospectively predict which patients would respond best to bracing. The validity (specifically the sensitivity and specificity) of the majority of these clinical tests has not yet been determined. This area is ripe for research, with a significant need for well-designed studies,[28] such as recently published for diagnosis of carpal tunnel syndrome.[29] Tests can also be validated against tissue observations of pathology or imaging studies.

OUTCOME MEASURES

A variety of specific outcome measures has been used to assess the effects of therapy. None is specifically diagnostic, and they are mainly used to quantify the severity of elbow injury and to monitor effectiveness of rehabilitation protocols. In some cases, they can

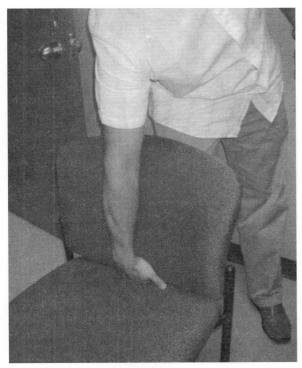

FIGURE 21–7. The "chair test."

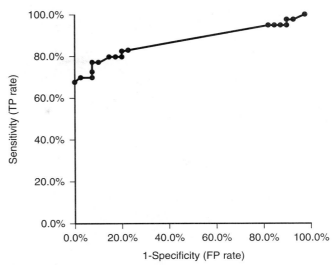

FIGURE 21–8. Sensitivity/specificity of a test of difference in grip strength to distinguish an extremity with lateral epicondylitis from a pain-free extremity. (Adapted from Dorf ER, Chhabra AB, Golish SR, et al: Effect of elbow position on grip strength in the evaluation of lateral epicondylitis. J Hand Surg [Am] 32A:882–886, 2007 with permission of Elsevier.)

help distinguish a patient population with the disease from healthy control subjects. Measures of pain include pain threshold test (dolorimeter), size of pain drawing, and visual analogue scales (VASs), but only pressure pain is associated with pain on palpation, grip strength, and manual tests.[30] Both maximal grip strength and pain free grip strength have been utilized,[31] and the latter has been shown to be moderately reliable.[32,33] Assessment of mean and maximal grip strength is done with an instrument such as a Jamar hydraulic hand dynamometer, with the elbow in 90 degrees of flexion and the elbow fully extended in front of patient. An average of multiple measurements is recommended, and from multiple sessions rather than from increasing the repetitions in a single test session. Dorf and colleagues[34] examined the sensitivity and specificity of grip strength in these positions in a population of 81 patients with lateral epicondylitis. In 41 patients, the affected side only was tested, whereas 40 had bilateral measurements done. The affected extremity was 29% stronger in flexion than in extension. The authors suggest that loss of grip strength between flexion and extension in a single extremity should be considered as a test to distinguish an extremity with lateral epicondylitis from a pain-free extremity. With a 5% decrease in grip strength between flexion and extension, the sensitivity was 83% and specificity 80%; with a 10% decrease, sensitivity was 78% and specificity 90% (Fig. 21–8). DeSmet and colleagues[35,36] had similar findings: a statistically significant mean grip strength loss of 43% from flexion to extension for the pathologic side in 55 consecutive patients with lateral epicondylitis compared with a less than 2% difference for the control side. In their studies, grip strength in both elbow extension and flexion significantly improved after surgery and correlated with a good clinical outcome.

Forearm muscle imbalance or shoulder muscle pathology may also be important in the development of tennis elbow. It has been suggested that there is a greater fatigability of wrist extensors compared with wrist flexors.[37] Alizadehkhaiyat and coworkers[38] actually developed an extension/flexion dynamometer type instrument to measure this (Fig. 21–9), but no other systematic studies have been done on this wrist-forearm-shoulder segment. Isokinetic dynamometer measurements have shown peak torque at a radial velocity of 90 degrees/sec, and work in wrist flexion reduced by 17% in lateral epicondylitis and 13% in medial epicondylitis.

Another study looked at strength with a device called the *Marcy Wedge-Pro (MWP)*, commonly used by tennis players for training,[39] to quantitatively assess ability to perform wrist extension exercises. The MWP results were compared with clinical measures and found to accurately identify patients who responded to treatment ($P < 0.05$). Another group[40] explored the clinical utility of a middle digit isokinetic eccentric strength dynamometer for evaluating the effects of lateral epicondylitis therapy. Eccentric isokinetic torque, work power, and angle at peak torque of the third finger were tested in 2 groups of patients: one without physician-diagnosed lateral epicondylitis (13 male and 14 female patients) and the other with lateral epicondylitis (13 male and 14 female patients). Test-retest correlation values ranged from 0.83 to 0.45, and analysis of variance showed a significant difference in all variables between the two subject groups.

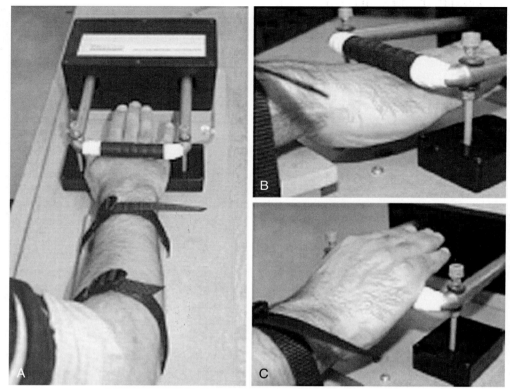

FIGURE 21–9. Wrist-hand dynamometer. (Reprinted from Alizadehkhaiyat O, Fisher AC, Kemp GJ, Frostick SP: Strength and fatiguability of selected muscles in upper limb: Assessing muscle imbalance relevant to tennis elbow. J Electromyogr Kinesiol 17:428–436, 2007, with permission of Elsevier.)

ELECTROMYOGRAPHY

Electromyography is used mainly for diagnosis of radial tunnel syndrome, but it is not often positive. Roles and Maudsley[10] note a delay in motor conduction velocity in "some cases," but normal electrophysiologic findings do not exclude the entrapment diagnosis. Bauer and Murray[41] used surface electromyography and demonstrated significantly earlier, longer, and greater activation of the wrist extensor muscles in a group suffering from lateral tennis elbow versus healthy control subjects. This type of work may lead to some insight into the pathogenesis of this chronic condition and suggest therapies.

PATIENT-RATED QUESTIONNAIRES

Traditional pain and disability questionnaires, such as the Disabilities of the Arm, Shoulder and Hand (DASH) questionnaire, and VAS are used in outcome studies, but they are nonspecific. A Patient-Rated Forearm Evaluation Questionnaire has been developed, using 5 items to assess pain and 10 items to assess function during the previous week.[42] This has been shown to have high reliability, but only fair correlation with pain-free grip strength. Further refinements have confirmed the reliability and reproducibility, and have validated that it is at least as sensitive to change as other commonly used outcome scales.[43]

It has subsequently been renamed the Patient-Rated Tennis Elbow Evaluation (PRTEE).[44] Recently, it has been utilized concurrently with an outcome therapy study in 78 patients who play tennis and have MRI-confirmed lateral elbow tendinopathy.[45] Detailed and favorable assessment of internal consistency, construct validity, reproducibility, and sensitivity to change led these authors to suggest that the PRTEE should become the standard primary outcome measure in research on tennis elbow.

DIAGNOSTIC IMAGING

Diagnostic imaging of the elbow may include radiographic evaluation, diagnostic ultrasound, computed tomography (CT) arthrogram, MRI, and/or bone scan. The cost benefit of such studies should be considered in the diagnosis of lateral epicondylitis.

PLAIN RADIOGRAPHS

Although sometimes useful to exclude other pathology, plain radiographs are not diagnostic for this condition, and thus are not necessary as an initial step in evaluation. In a consecutive series of 294 radiographs (standard anteroposterior, lateral, and radiocapitellar views in patients with lateral epicondylitis), 16% had findings present, most commonly faint calcification along the lateral epicondyle in 20 patients (7%) (Fig. 21–10). However, management was altered by only 2 of the sets of films.[46]

DIAGNOSTIC ULTRASOUND

Diagnostic ultrasound is a noninvasive imaging modality that uses sound waves in the frequency range of more than 20,000 Hz. Better resolutions are attained with higher frequencies of scanning, but at the expense of less depth of field. This technique is best for assessment of tendon integrity. Additional passive or resisted dynamic imaging can further evaluate function and continuity of the tendon, as well as visualize any gaps.[47] Disadvantages of diagnostic ultrasound include the fact that it is very much operator dependent, and it is also limited by the resolution of the equipment. Printed images are only a snapshot of the dynamic process of evaluation, and thus cannot be used in isolation.[48]

On ultrasound, tendon degeneration is visualized as irregularities of fibrillar appearance, with thickening, focal hypoechoic areas, calcification, and sometimes cortical irregularity or spur formation of the epicondyle (Fig. 21–11). In tendons with a synovial sheath, widening of the sheath can be seen, as well as increased fluid within it. Tendon ruptures appear as fragmented contiguous fibrils. It has been suggested that intrinsic changes in the tendon can be

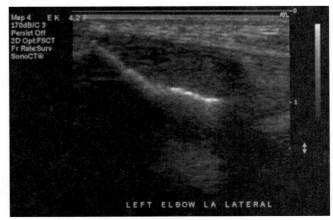

Figure 21–11. Ultrasound images of patient with lateral epicondylitis. Note focal thickening and hypoechoic region at the common extensor origin (CEO) onto the lateral epicondyle. Lateral: long axis view. CEO, and lateral epicondyle.

detected earlier with ultrasound than with MRI. Calcification is also noted earlier with ultrasound than with MRI. The addition of color Doppler permits visualization of neovascularization (Fig. 21–12), which is thought to be a source of the pain in such tendinopathies (growth factors, pain fibers, etc.). It also provides a method by which these pathologic neovessels can be treated with various sclerosing agents such as polidocanal or glycerol.

Some studies of clinical correlation have been performed. Maffulli and investigators[49] were able to identify six different entities: enthesopathy, tendonitis, peritendinitis, bursitis, intramuscular lesions, and mixed lesions, and suggested a possible prognostic value in patients with tennis elbow. They were able to confirm the clinical diagnosis of lateral epicondylitis by sonographic abnormalities in 93% of their patients. Connell and coworkers[50] studied

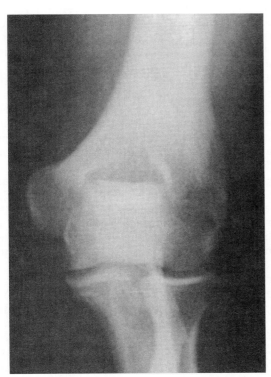

Figure 21–10. "Gun-sight oblique view" radiograph showing punctuate calcifications by lateral epicondyle. (Courtesy DeLee and Drez.)

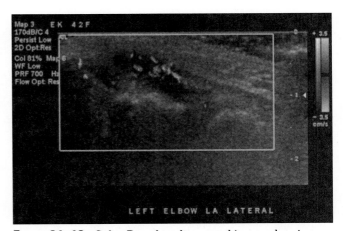

Figure 21–12. Color Doppler ultrasound image showing inflammation and increased blood flow at the common extensor origin (CEO). Lateral: long axis view.

75 patients, with a 95% confirmation rate (4 tendons were normal). The most common finding was a hypoechoic area in 64% of these images. Another group,[51] in a well-designed study, documented hyperechogenicity, swelling, calcification, bursitis, enthesopathy, and tendinosis in 75% of patients with an injured extremity. Positive and negative predictive values are shown in Tables 21–1 and 21–2. However, no significant predictive values of sonographic abnormalities were found for either success rate of treatment or mean decrease in pain.

The most thorough study so far[52] retrospectively reviewed images of 20 elbows in 10 asymptomatic volunteers (6 men, 4 women; age range, 22–38 years; mean, 29.6 years) compared with 37 elbows in 22 patients with symptoms of lateral epicondylitis (10 men, 12 women; age range, 30–59 years; mean, 46 years). A total of 57 images were randomly selected and interpreted by 3 individual readers for 1 or more of 8 ultrasound findings. Intrareader variability was assessed at two separate sessions. Sensitivity varied from 72% to 88%, and specificity from 36% to 48.5%. The odds ratio was significant ($P < 0.05\%$) for calcification of common extensor tendon, tendon thickening, adjacent bone irregularity, focal hyoechoic regions, and diffuse heterogeneity, but not significant for linear intrasubstance tears and peritendinous fluid.

Using another method called *spatial compound-sonography,* sonographic information is obtained from several different angles and combined to produce a single image. In one study of 34 patients,[53] real-time spatial compound sonography (with a 12-5-MHz multifrequency linear array transducer) significantly improved definition of soft-tissue planes, reduced speckle and other noise, and improved image detail when compared with conventional high-resolution sonography ($P < 0.0001$ for all evaluated parameters). Nevertheless, this technique is not routinely used.

Finally, Miller and coworkers[54] used ultrasound to examine 11 patients with tennis elbow and a normal contralateral elbow. In 10 of these patients, as well as in 6 asymptomatic volunteers, they were able to compare MRIs. Sonographic features of epicondylitis

included outward bowing of the common tendon, presence of hypoechoic fluid subadjacent to the common tendon, thickening, decreased echogenicity, and ill-defined margins of the common tendon. Sensitivity for detecting epicondylitis ranged from 64% to 82% for sonography and from 90% to 100% for MRI. Specificity ranged from 67% to 100% for sonography and from 83% to 100% for MRI. The authors conclude that sonography is as specific but not as sensitive as MRI for evaluating epicondylitis. Used as an initial imaging tool, sonography may be adequate for diagnosing this condition in many patients, thus allowing MRI to be reserved for patients with symptoms whose sonographic findings are normal.

MAGNETIC RESONANCE IMAGING

MRI gives excellent detail and soft-tissue contrast. Coronal and axial fast short-T1 inversion recovery and fat-suppressed T2-weighted images are good for interstitial fluid and edema in and around tendon and bone, whereas T1-weighted or proton density–weighted images illustrate anatomic structures and fat planes.[55,56] Tendinosis can be seen with or without superimposed partial- or full-thickness tearing, as well as chondromalacia, synovitis, osteophytic spurring, or loose bodies. Pathologic features suggesting lateral epicondylitis include thickening and high-intensity signal in tendon, as well as dystrophic calcification on gradient-echo techniques (Figs. 21–13 through 21–15). Bone marrow edema of the lateral epicondyle, anconeus muscle edema, and fluid within the radial head bursa may also be visualized.[57] MRI is also useful in differential diagnosis of the less common radial tunnel syndrome, through demonstration of denervation edema or atrophy within muscles innervated by the PIN, and mass effects along the course of the nerve.[58] A reasonable correlation of MRI findings with the stages of tendinosis also exists[59] (Table 21–3). Although most imaging is currently performed on high-field whole-body scanners (>1.0 Tesla), there is also increasing interest in low (<0.5 Tesla) and medium (0.5–1.0 Tesla) field strengths, available with smaller, less expensive scanners, which can be installed in physicians' offices.[60] Patients can then be scanned in sitting or recumbent positions, making this test much more practical and accessible.

TABLE 21–2. Diagnostic Values per Entity, Injured Arm

FINDING	SENSITIVITY	SPECIFICITY	PPV	NPV	LIKELIHOOD RATIO
Hypoechoic area	0.67	0.81	0.78	0.71	3.52
Swelling	0.61	0.84	0.80	0.69	3.81
Enthesopathy	0.65	0.86	0.82	0.71	4.64
Tendinosis	0.19	0.95	0.79	0.46	3.80
Any entity	0.75	0.81	0.80	0.23	3.95

NPV, negative predictive value; PPV, positive predictive value.
Data from Levin D, Nazarian LN, Miller TT, et al: Lateral epicondylitis of the elbow: US findings. Radiology 237:230–234, 2005.

TABLE 21–1. Diagnostic Values of Sonographic Findings in Lateral Epicondylitis

FINDING	INJURED SIDE (N = 57)		NONINJURED SIDE (N = 57)	
	N	%	N	%
Hypoechoic area	38	67	11	19
Hyperechoic area	3	5	0	0
Swelling	35	61	16	16
Calcifications	3	5	0	0
Bursitis	1	2	0	0
Enthesopathy	37	65	14	14
Tendinosis	11	19	5	5
Any entity	43	75	19	19
No entity	14	25	81	91

Data from Levin D, Nazarian LN, Miller TT, et al: Lateral epicondylitis of the elbow: US findings. Radiology 237:230–234, 2005.

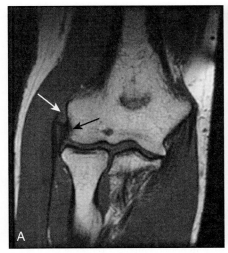
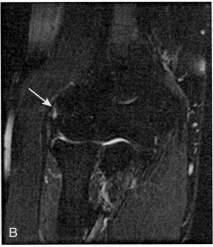

FIGURE 21–13. Magnetic resonance imaging findings in lateral epicondylitis. (From Saliman JD, Beaulieu CF, McAdas TR: Ligament and tendon injury to the elbow: Clinical surgical and imaging features. Top Magn Reson Imaging 17:327–336, 2006, 2006, reprinted with permission.)

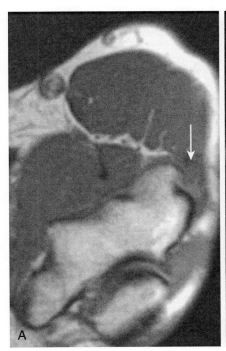
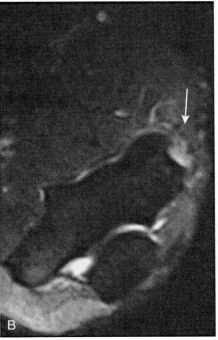

FIGURE 21–14. Magnetic resonance imaging findings in lateral epicondylitis. (Reprinted from Banks KP, Ly JZ, Beall DP, et al: Overuse injuries of the upper extremity in the competitive athlete: Magnetic resonance imaging findings associated with repetitive trauma. Curr Probl Diagn Radiol 34:127–142, 2005, with permission of Elsevier.)

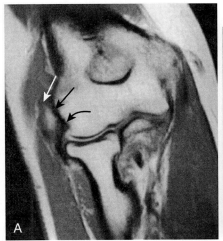
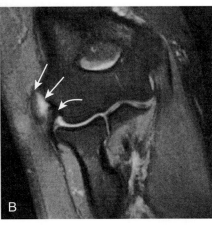

FIGURE 21–15. Magnetic resonance imaging findings in lateral epicondylitis. (Reprinted with permission From Fritz RC, Breidahl WH: Radiographic and special studies: Recent advances in imaging of the elbow. Clin Sports Med 23:567–580, 2004 .)

TABLE 21–3. Correlation of Magnetic Resonance Imaging Findings with Pathologic Stages of Lateral Epicondylitis

	PATHOLOGIC STAGES OF TENDINOSIS	MAGNETIC RESONANCE IMAGING	FINDINGS
Stage 1	Temporary irritation (possible chemical inflammation)	T1 and T2 increased signal	Usually the origin of the extensor carpi radialis brevis
Stage 2	Permanent tendinosis—less than 50% of tendon cross section	T2—increased signal	Corresponds with area of mucoid degeneration and neovascularization
Stage 3	Permanent tendinosis—greater than 50% of tendon cross section	T2—increased signal	Corresponds with area of significant disruption of collagen fibers and tear of tendon
Stage 4	Partial or total rupture of tendon	T2—increased signal	Disruption of the tendon and edema

Data from Bishai SK, Plancher KD: The basic science of lateral epicondylosis: Update for the future. Tech Orthop 21:250–255, 2006.

RECOMMENDATIONS

In conclusion, little to no evidence (grade C) exists to support the validity of the various clinical findings and special examination techniques for the diagnosis of lateral epicondylitis. Some nonspecific strength and pain measures are useful in predicting response to therapy but are less helpful for diagnosis. Fair evidence (grade B recommendation) has been reported for utilization of some specialized outcome scales (such as the PRTEE), especially for longitudinal therapeutic studies. Imaging modalities for this common entity, in particular, diagnostic ultrasound and MRI, continue to become more detailed and refined in confirming the diagnosis, as well as more easily available to the clinician. Despite the fact that they are not the first step in evaluation of this condition, fair evidence (grade B) exists for their diagnostic utility and precision. It would seem important, therefore, to establish a "gold standard" for diagnosis of lateral epicondylitis, comparing anatomic and/or radiologic findings with clinical diagnostic criteria. This will reduce inconsistencies and improve the accuracy of diagnosis, as well as enable larger-scale epidemiologic studies and establishment of evidence-based conservative or surgical treatment guidelines. Table 21–4 provides a summary of recommendations.

TABLE 21–4. Summary of Recommendations

	LEVEL OF EVIDENCE / GRADE OF RECOMMENDATION	RATIONALE
Clinical evaluation	C	Little or no evidence exists to support the validity of the various clinical findings and special examination techniques.
Outcome measurement	B	Fair evidence has been reported for utilization of some specialized outcome scales (e.g., Patient-Rated Tennis Elbow Evaluation).
Imaging modalities	B	Fair evidence exists for the diagnostic utility and precision of diagnostic ultrasound and magnetic resonance imaging.

REFERENCES

1. Runge F: Zur genese und behandlung des schreibe kranfes. Bed Kin Worchenschr 10:245–248, 1873.
2. Morris H: The rider's sprain. Lancet 2:133–134, 1882.
3. Major HP: Lawn tennis elbow. J Br Med 2:557, 1883.
4. Allander E: Prevalence, incidence and remission rates of some common rheumatic diseases and syndromes. Scand J Rheum 3:145–153, 1974.
5. Almekinders LC, Temple JD: Etiology, diagnosis, and treatment of tendonitis: An analysis of the literature. Med Sci Sports Exerc 30:1183–1190, 1998.
6. Labelle H, Guibert R, Joncas J, et al: Lack of scientific evidence for the treatment of lateral epicondylitis of the elbow. An attempted meta-analysis. J Bone Joint Surg 74:646–651, 1992.
7. Hudak P, Cole D, Haines A: Understanding prognosis to improve rehabilitation: The example of lateral elbow pain. Arch Phys Med 77:586–592, 1996.
8. Assendelft W, Green S, Buchbinder R, et al: Tennis elbow (lateral epicondylitis). Clin Evid 9:1388–1398, 2003.
9. Cyriax JH: The pathology and treatment of tennis elbow. J Bone Joint Surg Am 18:921–938, 1936.
10. Roles NC, Maudsley RH: Radial tunnel syndrome: Resistant tennis elbow as nerve entrapment. J Bone Joint Surg Br 54:499–508, 1972.
11. Nirschl RP: Tennis elbow. Orthop Clin North Am 4:787–800, 1973.
12. Nirschl RP: Elbow tendinosis/tennis elbow. Clin Sports Med 11:851–870, 1992.
13. Kraushaar BS, Nirschl RP: Tendinosis of the elbow (tennis elbow). Clinical features and findings of histological, immunohistochemical and electron microscopy studies. J Bone Joint Surg Am 81:259–278, 1999.
14. Khan K, Cook J, Taunton J, et al: Overuse tendinosis, not tendonitis: A new paradigm for a difficult clinical problem. Phys Sport Med 28:38–48, 2000.
15. Khan KM, Cook JL, Kannus P, et al: Time to abandon the "tendinitis" myth. Br Med J 324:626–627, 2002.
16. Waugh E: Lateral epicondylalgia or epicondylitis: What's in a name? J Orthop Sport Phys Ther 35:200–202, 2005.
17. Stansinopoulos D, Johnson MI: 'Lateral elbow tendinopathy' is the most appropriate diagnostic term for the condition commonly referred to as lateral epicondylitis. Med Hypotheses 67:1399–1401, 2006.
18. Nirschl R, Ashman E: Elbow tendinopathy: Tennis elbow. Clin J Sport Med 22:813–836, 2003.
19. Hume PA, Reid D, Edwards T: Epicondylar injury in sport: Epidemiology, type, mechanisms, assessment, management and prevention. Sports Med 36:151–170, 2006.
20. Pienimäki TT, Siira PT, Vanharanta H: Chronic medial and lateral epicondylitis: A comparison of pain, disability and function. Arch Phys Med Rehabil 83:317–321, 2002.
21. Lister GD, Belsole RB, Keinert HE: The radial tunnel syndrome. J Hand Surg 4:52–59, 1979.
22. Dutton M: Orthopedic Examination, Evaluation and Intervention. New York, McGraw-Hill Companies, 2004, pp 543–544.
23. Wadsworth TG: Tennis elbow: Conservative, surgical and manipulative treatment. BMJ 294:621–624, 1987.

24. Coonrad RW, Hooper WR: Tennis elbow: Its course, natural history, conservative and surgical management. J Bone Joint Surg 55A:1117–1182, 1973.
25. Gardner RC: Tennis elbow: Diagnosis, pathology and treatment. Clin Orthop 72:248–253, 1970.
26. Paoloni JA, Appleyard RC, Murrell GAC: The Orthopedic Research Institute-Tennis Elbow Testing System: A modified chair pick-u test—Interrrater and intrarater reliability testing and validity for monitoring lateral epicondylosis. J Shoulder Elbow Surg 13:72–77, 2004.
27. Struijs PAA, Assendelft WJJ, Kerkhoffs GMM, et al: The predictive value of the extensor grip test for the effectiveness of bracing for tennis elbow. Am J Sports Med 33:1905–1909, 2005.
28. Boyer MI, Hastings H: Lateral tennis elbow: "Is there any science out there?" J Shoulder Elbow Surg 8:481–491, 1999.
29. Graham B, Regehr G, Naglie G, Wrist JG: Development and validation of diagnostic criteria for carpal tunnel syndrome. J Hand Surg [Am] 31A:919e1–919e7, 2006.
30. Pienimäki T, Tarvainen T, Siira P, et al: Associations between pain, grip strength and manual tests in the treatment evaluation of chronic tennis elbow. Clin J Pain 18:164–170, 2002.
31. Smidt N, van der Windt DA, Assendelft WJ, et al: Interobserver reproducibility of the assessment of severity of complaints, grip strength, and pressure pain threshold in patients with lateral epicondylitis. Arch Phys Med Rehabil 83:1145–1150, 2002.
32. Stratford PW, Norman GR, McIntosh JM: Generalizability of grip strength measurements in patients with tennis elbow. Phys Ther 68:276–281, 1989.
33. Hamilton A, Balnave R, Adams R: Grip strength testing reliability. J Hand Ther 7:163–170, 1994.
34. Dorf ER, Chhabra AB, Golish SR, et al: Effect of elbow position on grip strength in the evaluation of lateral epicondylitis. J Hand Surg [Am] 32A:882–886, 2007.
35. DeSmet L, Fabry G: Grip strength in patients with tennis elbow. Influence of elbow position. Acta Orthop Belg 62:26–29, 1996.
36. DeSmet L, Van Ransbeeck H, Fabry G: Grip strength in tennis elbow: Long-term results of operative treatment. Acta Orthop Belg 64:167–169, 1998.
37. Hagg GM, Milerad E: Forearm extensor and flexor muscle exertion during simulated gripping work—an electromyographic study. Clin Biomech 12:39–43, 1997.
38. Alizadehkhaiyat O, Fisher AC, Kemp GJ, Frostick SP: Strength and fatiguability of selected muscles in upper limb: Assessing muscle imbalance relevant to tennis elbow. J Electromyogr Kinesiol 17:428–436, 2007.
39. Smith RW, Mani R, Cawley MID, et al: Assessment of tennis elbow using the Marcy Wedge-Pro. Br J Sports Med 27:233–235, 1993.
40. Pearson D, Gehlsen GM, Wilson JK, et al: An objective measure of lateral epicondylitis. Isokinet Exerc Sci 7:27–31, 1998.
41. Bauer JA, Murray RD: Electromyographic patterns of individuals suffering from lateral tennis elbow. J Electromyogr Kinesiol 9:245–252, 1999.
42. Overend TJ, Wuori-Fearn JL, Kramer JF, MacDermid JC: Reliability of a patient-rated forearm evaluation questionnaire for patients with lateral epicondylitis. J Hand Ther 12:31–37, 1999.
43. Newcomer KL, Martinez-Silvestrini JA, Schaefer MR, et al: Sensitivity of the Patient-rated Forearm Evaluation Questionnaire in lateral epicondylitis. J Hand Ther 18:400–406, 2005.
44. MacDermid J: Update: The Patient-rated Forearm Evaluation Questionnaire is now the Patient-rated Tennis Elbow Evaluation. J Hand Ther 18:407–410, 2005.
45. Rompe JD, Overend TJ, MacDermid JC: Validation of the Patient-rated Tennis Elbow Evaluation Questionnaire. J Hand Ther 20:3–11, 2007.
46. Pomerance J: Radiographic analysis of lateral epicondylitis. J Shoulder Elbow Surg 11:156–157, 2002.
47. Lew HL, Chen CPC, Wang T-G, Chew KTL: Introduction to musculoskeletal diagnostic ultrasound: Examination of the upper limbs. Am J Phys Med Rehabil 86:310–321, 2007.
48. Allen GM, Wilson DJ: Ultrasound in sports medicine—a critical evaluation. Eur J Radiol 62:79–85, 2007.
49. Maffulli N, Regine R, Carrillo F, et al: Tennis elbow: An ultrasonographic study in tennis players. Br J Sports Med 24:151–155, 1990.
50. Connell D, Burke P, Coombes P, et al: Sonographic examination of lateral epicondylitis. AJR Am J Roentgenol 176:777–782, 2001.
51. Struijs PAAA, Spruyt M, Assendelft WJJ, van Dijk CN: The predictive value of diagnostic sonography for the effectiveness of conservative treatment of tennis elbow. AJR Am J Roentgenol 185:1113–1118, 2005.
52. Levin D, Nazarian LN, Miller TT, et al: Lateral epicondylitis of the elbow: US findings. Radiology 237:230–234, 2005.
53. Lin DC, Nazarian LN, O'Kane PL, et al: Advantages of real-time spatial compound sonography of the musculoskeletal system versus conventional sonography. AJR Am J Roentgenol 179:1629–1631, 2002.
54. Miller TT, Shapiro MA, Schultz E, Kalish PE: Comparison of sonography and MRI for diagnosing epicondylitis. J Clin Ultrasound 30:193–202, 2002.
55. Saliman JD, Beaulieu CF, McAdas TR: Ligament and tendon injury to the elbow: Clinical surgical and imaging features. Top Magn Reson Imaging 17:327–336, 2006.
56. Kijowski R, Tuite M, Sanford M: Magnetic resonance imaging of the elbow. Part II: Abnormalities of the ligaments, tendons, and nerves. Skelet Radiol 34:1–18, 2004.
57. Tuitje MJ, Kijowski R: Sport-related injuries of the elbow: An approach to MRI interpretation. Clin Sports Med 25:387–408, 2006.
58. Ferdinand BD, Rosenberg ZS, Schweitzer ME: MR imaging features of radial tunnel syndrome: Initial experience. Radiology 240:161–168, 2006.
59. Nirschl RP, Pettrone FA: Tennis elbow. The surgical treatment of lateral epicondylitis. J Bone Joint Surg Am 61:832–839, 1979.
60. Ghazinoor S, Crues JV III: Low field MRI: A review of the literature and our experience in upper extremity imaging. Clin Sports Med 25:591–606, 2005.

Chapter 22

What Are the Indications for Surgery, and What Is the Best Surgical Treatment for Chronic Lateral Epicondylitis?

BILL REGAN, MD, FRCSC AND PHILIPPE GRONDIN, MD

Lateral epicondylitis (LE), or tennis elbow, was first described in the 1880s[1] by Major as a condition causing elbow pain in lawn tennis players. Clinically, this entity is characterized by lateral-sided elbow pain with activities of daily living, such as turning knobs and opening jars. Sufferers of LE may also notice a weakness in their grip strength or difficulty carrying objects in their hands.

Differential diagnoses of LE include C5-6 radiculopathy, posterolateral instability, posterior interosseus nerve (PIN) entrapment, osteochondritis dissecans, and radiocapitellar osteoarthritis. Proper history taking must include inquiry into previous acute trauma such as a dislocation, paresthesia and neck pain, and catching and locking, in addition to standard questions on symptom chronology, alleviating and aggravating factors, previous treatments, and review of systems.

On physical examination, LE causes pain on palpation 5 to 10 mm anterior to the lateral epicondyle. Pain is elicited with resisted wrist dorsiflexion, resisted supination, and resisted middle finger extension.

Physical examination must distinguish between LE and the main differential diagnoses. A cervical examination including nerve root examinations must be done especially if the history is suggestive of cervical pathology. Palpation must be thorough, systematic, and include palpating the radiocapitellar joint for osteoarthritis and the capitellum for osteochondritis dissecans. PIN entrapment tenderness is typically more distal than in LE. Range of motion and stability of the elbow must be tested, including the lateral pivot shift test for posterolateral rotatory instability.[2-4]

A thorough history and physical examination are usually all that is required for the diagnosis, but radiographs may help to rule out other abnormalities when the diagnosis is doubtful or when history and physical examination suggest coexisting pathologies. In a review of 294 radiographs of patients diagnosed with LE, Pomerance[5] found only 16% of patients had positive findings, with the most common abnormality, being faint calcific deposits along the extensor carpi radialis brevis (ECRB) occurring in 7% . In only two cases (0.7%) did radiographs change management plans.

Although ultrasonography and magnetic resonance imaging have reported sensitivities of 64% to 82% and 90% to 100%, respectively, and specificities of 67% to 100% and 83% to 100%, respectively, they are not traditionally ordered.[6]

Although up to 40% of tennis players will experience tennis elbow at some point,[7] LE is more often seen in workplaces that involve repetitive or forceful activities of the forearm, wrist, or hand.[8] In a 31-month study, Kurppa[9] found the annual incidence rate in a meat-processing factory housing 377 employees to be 1% for those working in nonstrenuous jobs and 7% to 11% for those working in strenuous jobs. In the general population, Shiri and colleagues[8] found the incidence rate of LE to be 1.3% in people aged 30 to 64 years, with a peak incidence in the 45- to 54-year age group in a Finnish study involving 4,783 subjects. Men and women were affected equally.

The precise pathophysiology of LE remains incompletely understood, but the most commonly accepted mechanism appears to be microscopic tearing of the ECRB muscle caused by repetitive trauma.[10,11] In up to one third of patients, the extensor digitorum communis (EDC) is also involved. This trauma causes growth of reparative tissue known as *angiofibroblastic hyperplasia* or *angiofibroblastic tendinosis*.[11,12] Histologic studies confirm that LE is a misnomer because no inflammatory cells are seen at the time of surgical intervention. A more representative term would be *lateral epicondylar tendinosis*.

OPTIONS

Many conservative treatments have been advocated for LE, including acupuncture, topical and oral nonsteroidal anti-inflammatory drugs (NSAIDs), corticosteroid injections, physiotherapy, bracing, extracorporeal shock wave therapy (ESWT), and more recently, botulinum toxin injections. Level I and II evidence found on MEDLINE and EMBASE searches on each modality are presented in this chapter, and where possible, conclusions are drawn.

Although conservative treatment is said to be successful in more than 90% of cases,[14] various operations have been described to treat recalcitrant LE. These operations fall into three broad categories: open release, percutaneous release, and arthroscopic release. The best data available on these interventions based on MEDLINE and EMBASE searches are also presented.

EVIDENCE

Acupuncture

Three studies reviewed acupuncture therapy. In a randomized, controlled, double-blind study involving 45 patients, Fink and coauthors[15] noticed a significant improvement in maximum grip strength, pain, and function based on the disability of the arm, shoulder, and hand (DASH) form at 2 weeks in the true acupuncture versus sham acupuncture. At 2 months, however, this benefit was no longer seen. In a single blinded, randomized, controlled trial involving 48 patients, Molsberger and Hille[16] found acupuncture pain relief superior and longer lasting (20.2 vs. 1.4 hours average) than sham acupuncture. Davidson and coworkers[17] compared acupuncture with ultrasound in a study enrolling 16 patients and found significant improvement in both treatments over baseline in DASH scores, pain, and pain-free grip strength but found no significant difference between the two modalities at 1 month. In conclusion, not enough evidence exists to support acupuncture definitively, but studies suggest (grade B) it may have a role in the short term (<6 weeks) only.

Nonsteroidal Anti-Inflammatory Medication

Three randomized, controlled trials on topical NSAIDs versus placebo were done, and meta-analyses were conducted by Green and researchers.[18] The trials (Burnham et al., 1998,[19] Burton 1988,[20] and Jenoure et al., 1997[21]) had a combined population of 130 subjects and assessed the effect of topical NSAIDs (2 trials used diclofenac, 1 trial used difflam) on pain. The pooled weighted mean difference (WMD) was -1.88 (95% confidence interval [CI], -2.54 to -1.21) in the short term (1–3 weeks). That is, those in the topical NSAID group had 1.88 of 10 points less pain on a visual analogue scale (VAS) at the end of the trial than those using placebo.[18]

No clinically significant differences were found between topical NSAIDs and placebo in the effect on strength, tenderness, range of motion, or physician's opinion regarding effect. Side effects were reviewed in two of the three trials, and no significant differences were found.

Two trials examined oral NSAIDs versus placebo with contradictory results. Labelle and Guibert,[22] examining diclofenac daily use for 1 month plus cast immobilization versus immobilization and placebo in a double-blinded, randomized study involving 129 patients, found a significant difference in pain reduction (1.4/10 less pain) but not in grip strength or function in the diclofenac group. The diclofenac group, however, had a greater incidence rate of abdominal pain (30% vs. 9%) and diarrhea (39% vs. 20%) than the placebo group. Hay and investigators,[23] examining naproxen use in a study involving 111 randomized patients, however, found no significant difference in improvement in pain after 1 month and 1 year. Side effects were not mentioned in the study.

In conclusion, good evidence (grade A) exists that topical NSAIDs have a role in short-term pain relief. Oral NSAIDs have conflicting (grade I) evidence supporting their use and are associated with more side effects. Further studies are needed.

Corticosteroid Injections

Three randomized studies were found on corticosteroid injections. Two of these studies involve a control group in which avoidance of aggravating activities is the only treatment, and they give us the best available data on the natural history of LE.

Altay and coauthors,[24] in a prospective, randomized trial involving 120 patients, compared injecting triamcinolone with lidocaine to lidocaine alone using the peppering technique (injecting 40–50 times through the same skin entry point) and found no differences in the two groups at 2 months in the number of excellent results defined as complete pain relief, completely satisfied and devoid of pain on resisted wrist dorsiflexion (93% in the triamcinolone arm vs. 95% in the control group). Results were not changed at 6 months or 1 year.

Smidt and researchers[25] compared physiotherapy with corticosteroid injection with a wait-and-see approach in a randomized, controlled trial involving 185 patients. Exclusion criteria included physiotherapy treatment or injections for the elbow complaint in the last 6 months. Corticosteroid injections consisted of 1 mL triamcinolone (10 mg/mL) and 1 mL 2% lidocaine injected into all painful areas until resisted dorsiflexion was no longer painful. A maximum of 3 injections over a 6-week period were allowed. Fifty-eight percent (58%) used one injection, 27% used two, and 15% used three. The physiotherapy consisted of nine treatments of pulsed ultrasound, deep friction massage, and a home exercise program over 6 weeks. The wait-and-see group was educated on the disease and how to avoid provoking pain. All groups were told to avoid aggravating activities, discouraged from using other forms of treatment but allowed pain medication (naproxen [Naprosyn] and paracetamol). Patients kept a diary of other forms of treatments used, but activity level was not recorded. Success was defined as pain completely resolved or much improved. The researchers also reviewed patient self-rated general improvement, severity of the main complaint, pain, elbow disability, and patient satisfaction. Severity of elbow complaint, grip strength, and pressure pain threshold were assessed by a research physiotherapist.

As shown in Figure 22–1, at 6 weeks, corticosteroids had significantly greater success rate (92%) than both physiotherapy (47%) and wait-and-see (32%) approaches, but this was no longer true at 3 months. The corticosteroid injection group had a greater relapse rate (defined as no longer completely resolved or much improved) at 72% than the physiotherapy and wait-and- see groups (at 8% and 9%, respectively). At 1 year, the injection group had a lower success rate (69%) than both the physiotherapy (91%) and the wait-and-see (83%) groups.

In the follow-up period (week 7 to 1 year), 76% of the wait-and-see group used no other forms of treatment compared with 57% in the corticosteroids group and 19% in the physiotherapy group. In the wait-and-see group, 20% used pain medication. In the corticosteroids group, 21% used physiotherapy, 34% used more injections, and 27% used pain medication. In the physiotherapy group, 66% used more physiotherapy. In 38 of the 42 patients who used more physiotherapy, the duration of the extra physiotherapy was less than 6 weeks.

Bisset and colleagues[26] also compared corticosteroid injections to physiotherapy to a wait-and-see approach in a single-blinded, randomized, controlled trial involving 198 participants with follow-up of 1 year. Participants had symptoms of LE for more than 6 weeks. Exclusion criteria included any treatment for LE by any health practitioner in the last 6 months. The corticosteroid injection group received 1 mL triamcinolone (10 mg/mL) and 1 mL of 1% lidocaine to painful elbow points. A second injection was allowed at 2 weeks if needed. Eighty-six percent received one injection, whereas 12% received two and 1.5% (one patient) received three. Physiotherapy

consisted of eight sessions of elbow manipulations and exercises over a 6-week period. All patients were given an information booklet outlining the disease process and providing practical advice on self-management and ergonomics. A diary recording any other forms of treatment was kept. Analgesics were allowed, but other treatment modalities were discouraged. Primary end points were global improvement scale where completely resolved or much improved were deemed successful, pain-free grip strength as a percentage of normal side, and assessor's rating of severity. As shown in Figure 22–2, at 6 weeks, corticosteroid injections were significantly better in all 3 end points, having 78% success rate compared with 65% in the physiotherapy group and 27% in the wait-and-see group. At 3 months, however, this was reversed, with the injection group having only 45% success as opposed to 76% success with physiotherapy or 59% with the wait-and-see approach. This relation was maintained at 1 year, with the corticosteroid group having less success (68%) compared with the physiotherapy group at 94% success and the wait-and-see group at 90% success.

Area under the curve analysis demonstrated a significant advantage in favor of physiotherapy over injection for all primary outcome measures and over wait and see for pain-free grip (mean difference [MD], 534; 99% CI, 3–1065) and assessor-rated severity (MD, 447; 99% CI, 137–758). It also demonstrated a significant advantage for wait and see over injection for global improvement (MD, −8.3; 99% CI, −15.0 to −1.5) and assessor-rated severity (−337; 99% CI, −642 to −32).[26]

The physiotherapy group had the most patients who used no other forms of treatment (79%), followed by the corticosteroid group (51%) and the wait-and-see group (45%).

In conclusion, although there is good evidence (grade A) supporting corticosteroid injection in the short term, there is also good evidence that corticosteroid injections are less successful than wait and see in the long term (grade A).

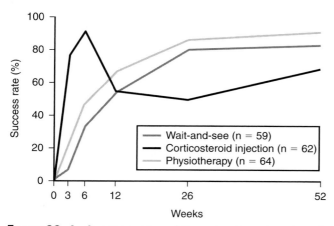

Figure 22–1. Success rates of three treatment regiment. (Adapted from Smidt N, van der Windt DA, Assendelft WJ, Deville WL, Korthals-de Bos IB, Bouter LM. Corticosteroid injections, physiotherapy, or a wait-and-see policy for lateral epicondylitis: a randomised controlled trial. Lancet 23;359[9307]:657-662, 2002 with permission of Elsevier.)

Physiotherapy

Two studies (see Corticosteroid Injections earlier in chapter) reviewed physiotherapy versus a wait-and-see approach[25,26] and had conflicting results. Smidt and researchers[25] found nine treatments of pulsed ultrasound, deep friction massage, and a home exercise program over 6 weeks to be better than wait and see over the short and long term but not by a significant amount. Wait and see also had more patients not use any other forms of treatment (79%) than the physiotherapy group (19%). If one excludes physiotherapy done within 6 weeks of the end of the treatment period, however, both groups have similar percentages of patients not using any other forms of treatments (85% in the physiotherapy group and 83% in the wait-and-see group).

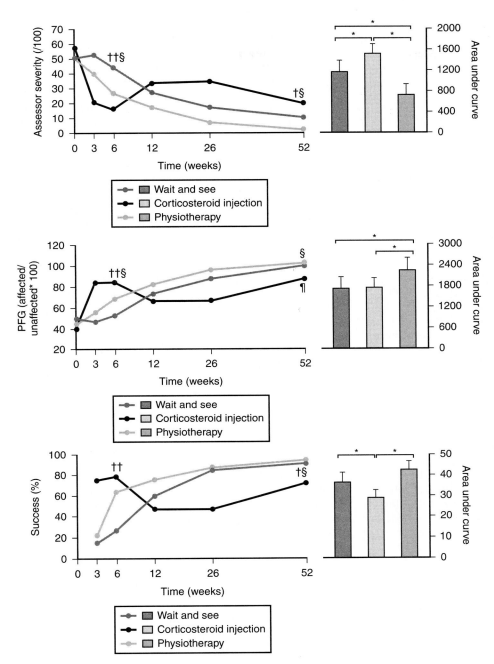

FIGURE 22–2. Primary outcome measure: mean assessor's rating of severity (visual analog scale), mean pain-free grip (PFG—affected/unaffected expressed as a percentage), and percentage success. Significant differences between study arms at 6 and 12 weeks: [†]corticosteroid injection versus wait-and-see approach; [‡]physiotherapy versus wait-and-see approach; [§]corticosteroid injection versus physiotherapy; [¶]significant difference between corticosteroid and wait-and-see approach on per protocol analysis. Bar graphs represent mean (99% confidence interval) area under curve (trapezium method[24]) analysis of assessor severity, PFG, and global improvement. *Significant differences between groups ($P < 0.01$). Adapted from Bisset L, Beller E, Jull G, Brooks P, Darnell R, Vicenzino B. Mobilisation with movement and exercise, corticosteroid injection, or wait and see for tennis elbow: randomised trial. BMJ 333(7575):939, 2006 with permission of the BMJ Publishing Group.

Bisset and colleagues[26] found eight sessions of elbow manipulations combined with an exercise program for 6 weeks was favorable over wait and see at 6 weeks in terms of the number of patients with complaints completely resolved or much improved, pain-free grip strength and assessor-rated severity but no longer at 1 year. Furthermore, more of the patients in the physiotherapy group used no other forms of treatment (79%) versus 45% in the wait-and-see group.

Evidence is contradictory on the benefits of physiotherapy in LE preventing a clear conclusion. Physiotherapy may help but benefits when found are modest at best (grade I).

Smidt and researchers'[25] and Bisset and colleagues'[26] studies give the closest approximation of the natural history of LE to date. In both studies, more than 80% of patients had symptoms that were much improved or completely resolved by 6 months with little or no treatment beyond activity modification and patient education.

Brace

Studies on braces are limited by small numbers, short follow-up, and heterogeneity of the braces studied. Conclusions on the role braces play are hard to make based on these data.

Faes and investigators[27] compared a dynamic extensor brace (Carp-x; Somas, St-Anthonis, Netherlands) with no brace in a randomized, controlled trial involving 63 patients and found significant differences favoring the brace group in pain, pain-free maximum grip strength, and function of the arm at 12 and 24 weeks. In that article, graphs are presented but no numbers are given.

Jensen and coworkers[28] compared an off-the-shelf orthotic (Rehband) with corticosteroid injections in 30 randomized patients over a period of 6 weeks and found no significant differences between the groups in pain, maximum grip strength, dumbbell test, function VAS, or global improvement.[29] Similarly, Erturk and colleagues[30] compared an epicondylitis bandage with a steroid injection in 36 randomized patients and found no significant difference at 3 weeks in pain on resisted wrist extension and no difference in maximum grip strength. Haker and Lundeberg,[31] in a study involving 61 patients, compared an elbow strap and a wrist splint with corticosteroid injections looking at global function and pain-free grip strength, and found improved global function with the injection group at 2 weeks but no difference in pain-free grip strength. No differences were found between the groups at 6 months or at 1 year.

Dwars and researchers[32] compared the Epitrain orthosis with physiotherapy (unspecified) looking at pain and global function in a randomized study involving 84 patients, and found no significant differences. Struijs and colleagues[33] compared an elbow strap brace (Epipoint) to physiotherapy (pulsed ultrasound, friction massage, and strengthening and stretching exercises) to the Epipoint brace plus physiotherapy in a randomized trial involving 180 patients looking at 9 outcomes (global function, severity of the patient's complaints, severity of the patient's main complaint, modified pain-free function questionnaire [PFFQ], inconvenience during daily activities, pain-free grip strength, maximal grip strength, pressure pain, and satisfaction). Over the short term (6 weeks), combination therapy was superior over bracing alone in severity of complaints (MD, 11/100; 95% CI, 6–18), PFFQ (MD, 9; 95% CI, 2–15), and satisfaction (MD, 11; 95% CI, 3–19), but not in the other 6 outcomes measured. Combination treatment offered little or no benefit over physical therapy alone. Physical therapy and bracing also fared similarly. Over the mid term (26 weeks) and long term (1 year), all three groups scored similarly with no significant differences in any of the 9 outcomes measured.

Bracing may help in LE but there is insufficient data to promote or refute it's use.

Extracorporeal Shock Wave Therapy

Nine randomized, controlled trials were found comparing ESWT against placebo with conflicting results. Three studies[34–36] favored ESWT over placebo, whereas four trials[38–41] showed no advantage to ESWT. When available data from the trials were pooled by Buchbinder and coauthors,[37] however, most benefits observed in the positive trials were no longer statistically significant.

Data from 6 trials could be pooled, and based on these data, most of the evidence supports the conclusion that ESWT is no more effective than placebo for lateral elbow pain. For example, pooled analysis of 3 trials (446 participants)[34,38,39] showed that ESWT is no more effective than placebo with respect to pain at rest at 4 to 6 weeks after the final treatment (WMD pain out of 100 = −9.42 [95% CI, −20.70 to 1.86]); pooled analysis of three trials (455 participants)[35–38] (Pettrone, 2005) showed that ESWT is no more effective than placebo at 12 weeks after the final treatment with respect to pain provoked by resisted wrist extension (Thomsen test) (WMD pain out of 100 = −9.04 [95% CI, −19.37 to 1.28]) and grip strength (SMD [standardized mean difference], 0.05 [95% CI, −0.13 to 0.24]).

Pooled analyses combining results of other trials failed to demonstrate statistically significant benefits for ESWT over placebo across a range of outcomes including mean pain with resisted middle-finger extension or resisted wrist extension at 6 weeks after completion of treatment, night pain at 3 to 4 weeks after completion of treatment, or failure of treatment defined by a Roles and Maudsley score of 4 at 6 weeks and 12 months after completion of treatment.[38,39,41] Based on these studies and their pooling,[37] good evidence (grade A) exists to refute the use of ESWT for treating LE.

Botulinum (Botox) Injection

Four randomized, controlled trials were found on botulinum (Botox) injections. Three studies compared Botox with saline injection and one compared Botox with surgical release. Two of the three studies comparing Botox with placebo support Botox, whereas the third refutes it. In all three studies, Botox injection results in significant weakness in a significant amount.

Wong and colleagues[42] compared Botox A injection (1 cm distal to the epicondyle) with normal saline injection in a randomized, double-blinded, controlled study involving 60 patients with symptoms of LE for at least 3 months looking at pain VAS and grip strength. Exclusion criteria included having received any corticosteroid injection. Significant differences in improvement in pain between the groups of 24.4 mm at 4 weeks and 19.3 mm at 12 weeks favoring Botox were found. Significant grip strength improvement was present in both groups but not significantly different between the groups. Mild paresis of the fingers occurred in 4 (13%) patients in the botulinum group at 4 weeks. One patient's (3%) symptoms persisted until week 12, whereas none of the patients receiving placebo had the same complaint. At 4 weeks, 10 patients (33%) in the botulinum group and 6 patients (20%) in the placebo group experienced weak finger extension on the same side as the injection site. At 12 weeks, 2 patients in the Botox group (7%) and 1 patient (3%) in the placebo group still reported weak finger extension.

Placzek and coauthors[43] studied Botox injection (0.6 mL 3–4cm distal to epicondyle tender region) versus placebo (normal saline injection) in a randomized, controlled, double-blinded clinical trial involving 130 patients with follow-up at 2, 6, 12, and 18 weeks, and found modest improvements with the Botox group. Continuous pain VAS in the last 48 hours was significantly better for Botox than for placebo at 6 and 18 weeks, but not at 2 and 12 weeks. The MD was 1.14 (out of 10) at 6 weeks and 0.86 at 18 weeks. Maximum pain VAS in the last 48 hours, however, was not significantly better between the groups at any time point. Global assessment rated by the physician and global assessment as rated by the patient, where 4 was substantially better, 3 was slightly better, 2 was unchanged, 1 was slightly worse, and 0 was substantially worse, were significantly better from 6 weeks onward for the Botox group. The MDs in patient global assessment are 0.56, 0.31, and 0.55 at 6, 12, and 18 weeks, respectively. At 18 weeks, the greatest mean scores for both groups were 3.31 for the Botox group and 2.76 for the placebo group. As a side effect, the Botox group experienced significant decrease in third finger extension strength compared with the control group starting at 2 weeks. By 12 weeks, the strength was back to preinjection levels, and by 18 weeks, the difference between the groups was no longer significant. Wrist extension and grip strength was not significantly different between the groups.

Keizer and coworkers[44] compared Botox injection into ECRB muscle with surgical extensor release as described by Hohmann in a randomized prospective study involving 40 patients and follow-up at 3, 6, 12, and 24 months. At 1 year, the number of patients with good to excellent results were similar; namely, 65% in the Botox group and 75% in the operative group.

Hayton and coauthors[45] had different results, however, comparing Botox A injections (2 mL 5 cm distal to tender region of epicondyle) with normal saline injections in 40 patients in a double-blinded study. Inclusion criteria included symptoms for at least 6 months and having received at least one corticosteroid injection. At 3 months, there were no significant differences found in pain VAS, Short Form 12 (SF-12) scores, or grip strength. Two of 18 patients in the Botox group experienced third finger extension weakness that interfered with their quality of life.

Several reasons may explain the different results obtained in Hayton and coauthors'[45] study from Wong and colleagues'[42] and Placzek and coauthors'[43] studies. First, at 40 patients (vs. 60 and 130), perhaps Hayton and coauthors'[45] study lacks the necessary power to detect a significant benefit to the Botox injection. Second, all patients in Hayton and coauthors'[45] study had received corticosteroid injections, whereas only some in Placzek and coauthors'[43] and none in Wong and colleagues'[42] study had received any. Perhaps the tendon degeneration that may occur with corticosteroid injection blunts the beneficial effect that the Botox-induced rest provides.

Overall, it appears that Botox injection has better results than placebo (grade B) but at the cost of sometimes bothersome weakness that can last up to 3 months.

Surgery

Open Surgery. Table 22–1 outlines the results of various studies on surgical lateral release for LE.

Nirschl and Pettrone[46] described a technique in 1979 where the interval between ECRL and EDC is utilized through a 2.5-cm skin incision to expose and resect the diseased ECRB tendon. In this technique, the joint is not routinely inspected, any diseased EDC is also resected, and one to two holes are drilled in the exposed lateral humeral condyle to enhance bleeding and healing. With this technique, Nirschl and Pettrone[46] achieved 75% excellent results and 10% good results in 88 elbows. There was an improvement rate of 97.7% and 85% returned to full activities.

Verhaar and researchers[47] in a prospective study reported somewhat worse results, with 76% of their 63 cases having no or slight pain at 1 year after surgery. At 1 year, there were 32% excellent results, 37% good results, 19% fair results, and 11% poor results. At 5 years, there were 32 excellent results (56%), 19 good results (33%), 4 fair results (7%), and 2 poor results (4%).

Rosenberg and Henderson[48] reported on open lateral releases in 19 patients, with 95% achieving pain relief and strength gain, on average, 3 and 4 months after surgery, respectively.

Khashaba[49] questioned the need for drilling the lateral condyle in a randomized, single-blinded trial involving 23 elbows where the lateral epicondyle was drilled in half of the cases and no drilling was performed in the other half looking at subjective pain and objective wrist extension strength at 3 and 6 months. Despite this article's results being cited in many other publications[50,51] and the article being a single-blinded randomized trial, the article's presentation makes it difficult to know whether the findings are backed by rigorous method. Inclusion and exclusion criteria are not clearly defined. No mention is made of the comparability of the two arms before surgery (age, duration of symptoms, number of corticosteroid injection, etc.). No *P* values, no standard deviations, and no confidence intervals are indicated. Postoperative pain is compared with remembered preoperative pain at 3 and 6 months instead of pain documented before surgery. The only numbers mentioned are the average increase in power at 6 months (3 months not indicated), and these are 5.2 kg in the drilled group versus 6.5 kg in the nondrilled group. Average decrease in pain (3 and 6 months combined and averaged) was 4.6 of 10 in the drilled group versus 6.8 of 10 in the nondrilled group.

TABLE 22–1. Outcomes of Open, Percutaneous and Arthroscopic Lateral Release Surgeries

AUTHORS	NUMBER OF PATIENTS	PROCEDURE	STUDY TYPE/LEVEL	RESULTS/TIME	BACK TO WORK
Nirschl and Pettrone[46]	88	Open release	Case series (Level 4)	75% excellent 10% good	
Verhaar et al.[47]	63	Open release	Case series (Level 4)	32% excellent 37% good at 1 year	
Rosenberg and Henderson[48]	19	Open release	Case series (Level 4)	95% pain relief/strength at 3, 4 months	
Grundberg and Dobson[53]	32	Percutaneous release	Case series (Level 4)	90% good or excellent at 9 weeks	
Kaleli et al.[54]	26	Percutaneous release	Case series (Level 4)	92% excellent results at 8 weeks	
Savoie[55]	21	Percutaneous release	Case series (Level 4)	Andrews–Carson score 166 → 198/200	
Dunkow et al.[56]	47	Open vs. percutaneous release	Randomized prospective comparative (Level 2)	Open: 25% pleased 67% satisfied Percutaneous: 61% pleased 39% satisfied Percutaneous significantly better DASH than open	Open: 5 weeks Percutaneous: 2 weeks
Baker et al.[61]	42	Arthroscopic release	Case series (Level 4)	100% better/much better	
Owens et al.[62]	16	Arthroscopic release	Case series (Level 4)	83% much better	6 days (0–28)
Rubenthaler et al.[64]	10 open vs. 20 arthroscopic	Open vs. arthroscopic	Retrospective comparative (Level 3)	Morrey score not significantly different between groups	
Peart et al.[65]	54 open vs. 33 arthroscopic	Open vs. arthroscopic	Retrospective comparison (Level 3)	Open: 69% good/excellent Arthroscopic: 72% good excellent	Arthroscopic earlier at work
Szabo et al.[66]	38 open vs. 41 arthroscopic vs. 23 percutaneous	Open vs. arthroscopic vs. percutaneous	Retrospective comparison (Level 3)	Pain visual analogue scale, Andrews–Carson score, complications, recurrence no different	

Data from Smidt N, van der Windt DA, Assendelft WJ, Deville WL, Korthals-de Bos IB, Bouter LM. Corticosteroid injections, physiotherapy, or a wait-and-see policy for lateral epicondylitis: a randomised controlled trial. Lancet 23;359(9307):657-662, 2002.

Percutaneous Lateral Release. In 1933, Hohmann[52] described epicondylar stripping done percutaneously for LE with good success. More recently, Grundberg and Dobson[53] reported on results from percutaneous common extensor release in 32 elbows that had been having symptoms for, on average, 18 months. Ninety percent (90%) had excellent or good results, with the pain relieved, on average, 9 weeks after operation. Grip strength improved from an average of 60% of the opposite side to 90% after operation. Kaleli and investigators[54] investigated 26 patients with symptoms of LE for an average of 8.9 months before having a percutaneous extensor release and found excellent results in 92% of cases, with pain relief coming, on average, 8 weeks after surgery.

In the percutaneous release described by Savoie,[55] a #11 blade knife is introduced 2 to 3 mm anterior to the epicondyle with the elbow flexed at 90 degrees. The blade inserted parallel to the long axis of the humerus is then pivoted so that its tip reaches the more superior aspect of the ECRB proximally. Distally, the blade tip stops short of the articular margin of the humerus. The surgeon's thumb is kept on the posterolateral aspect of the radiocapitellar joint to protect the radial collateral ligament. A small rasp is then used to excoriate the epicondyle in the area to stimulate a healing response. Using this technique, Savoie[55] had an average increase of 32 in Andrews–Carson scores in 21 percutaneous releases after surgery, obtaining an average score of 198 out of 200. A high Andrews–Carson score indicates good function.

One advantage of a percutaneous release over the open release is lower morbidity. Dunkow and colleagues[56] conducted a randomized trial comparing an open release with a percutaneous release in 47 elbows of patients with unsuccessful results after 1 year of conservative treatment and found the percutaneous release group returned to work at an average of 2 weeks after surgery, 3 weeks earlier than the open group ($P = 0.001$). Furthermore, the decrease in DASH score after surgery showing improved function was significantly larger in the percutaneous release group. In addition, 50% of patients were pleased with procedure in the percutaneous group versus 25% in the open group.

One disadvantage of the percutaneous release compared with the open release may be inability to resect all the degenerative pathology. Organ and coworkers[57] reviewed 35 cases of failed lateral releases with the distribution of the most recent techniques as follows: 19 slide and release procedures, 6 slide and release procedures with partial resection of the annular ligament (Bosworth), 7 unknown surgical interventions, 2 primary radial nerve decompressions, and 1 Nirschl procedure. In 27 elbows, the pathologic changes in the ECRB tendon had not been previously addressed at all, and in 7 elbows, the damaged tissue had not been completely excised. Salvage surgery included excision of pathologic tissue in the ECRB tendon origin combined with excision of excessive scar tissue and repair of the extensor aponeurosis when necessary. Based on a 40-point functional rating scale proposed here, 83% of the elbows (29/35) had good or excellent results at an average follow-up of 64 months (range, 17 months to 17 years).

Arthroscopic Lateral Release. In 1995, Grifka and colleagues[58] described an arthroscopic method of doing a Hohman lateral release for recalcitrant tennis elbow. Kuklo and researchers[59] conducted a cadaveric study using 10 specimens to study the safety of the lateral arthroscopic release. He found the radial nerve to be in close proximity to the proximal lateral portal (average, 5.4 mm), but failed to find instability in the elbow after intervention. Smith and investigators[60] confirmed the efficacy of the arthroscopic procedure using seven cadavers. They note that the ECRB and EDC origin was resected a mean of 100% and 90%, respectively. Elbow stability was maintained when resection did not extend posteriorly to an intra-articular line bisecting the radial head. Arthroscopy also allows for a faster recovery than open releases in theory. Furthermore, intra-articular pathology can be addressed concomitantly.

Baker and coauthors[61] published their results in 42 arthroscopic releases. Patients had, on average, 14 months of symptoms prior to the release and were followed for an average of 2.8 years after the procedure. The average pain at rest after surgery was 0.9 out of 10, pain with daily activity was 1.4, and pain with sport was 1.9. Of the 39 elbows in the 37 patients who were available for follow-up, 37 were rated "better" or "much better." Patients returned to work in an average of 2.2 weeks. Grip strength averaged 96% of the strength of the unaffected limb. Notably, there was a 69% rate of associated intra-articular pathologies found at the time of arthroscopy. Owens and colleagues,[62] in a case series of 16 arthroscopic ECRB releases in patients with symptoms lasting for an average of 31.7 months, found 83% of cases to be much better, with an average pain with activities of daily living of 1.58 out of 10 and an average return to unrestricted work in 6 days (range, 0–28 days).

Cohen et al. (unpublished data; however, work is incorrectly cited as published in Cohen and colleagues[63]) compared open with arthroscopic releases in a study involving 30 patients. They conclude that there were no differences between the two procedures regarding outcomes, return of strength, and postoperative symptoms. However, the arthroscopic group returned to sports and work much sooner, at 35 versus 66 days after the open surgery. Rubenthaler and investigators[64] compared retrospectively open lateral Hohmann releases (10 cases) with arthroscopic (20 cases) Hohmann lateral releases and found similar results in the 2 groups. The score of Morrey showed an average scoring of 93.2 for the endoscopic group and 87.5 for the open group ($P > 0.05$). Peart and cowork-

ers[65] retrospectively compared 54 open lateral releases with 33 arthroscopic ones and found no significant differences in outcomes. Sixty-nine (69%) of open cases and 72% of arthroscopic cases had good or excellent outcomes. Notably, patients treated with arthroscopic release returned to work earlier than patients treated with open release, and required less postoperative therapy.

Szabo and coauthors[66] retrospectively reviewed 38 open lateral release cases, 41 arthroscopic cases, and 23 percutaneous cases. The groups were matched for age, sex, dominance, conservative measures used, cortisone injections, and preoperative pain VAS scores, but the percutaneous cases had a better preoperative Andrews–Carson score at 164.6 (vs. 160.2 for open and 158.9 for arthroscopic) and a shorter duration of conservative care (6.6 months for percutaneous vs. 15.3 for open cases and 12.9 for arthroscopic cases). Possibly confounding the interpretation of the data, however, more than one procedure was performed in many cases. In the arthroscopic release group, 44% had intra-articular pathology addressed at the time of arthroscopy, consisting of 14 plicae, 2 loose bodies, and 2 posterolateral ligamentous repairs. Twenty-two (22%) arthroscopic cases also had extra-articular procedures performed, consisting of 5 posterior interosseous nerve releases, 2 carpal tunnel releases, and 2 open posterolateral ligamentous reconstructions. Approximately 21.1% of the open group had other procedures performed consisting of three shoulder arthroscopies, two ulnohumeral arthroplasties, two posterior interosseous nerve releases, and one carpal tunnel release. It is noted that when these procedures and their possible influence on the postoperative Andrews–Carson score were examined, no difference was found, but no data is given. Nevertheless, Szabo and coauthors[66] found that postoperative pain VASs, Andrews–Carson scores, number of complications, failures, and recurrences were not significantly different for the 3 groups. The Andrews–Carson score was 195.3, 195.4, and 193 for open, arthroscopic, and percutaneous groups, respectively.

A need exists for better studies on surgical interventions. Only the study by Keizer and coworkers,[44] which prospectively compared Botox injections with a Hohmann open release, has prospectively compared surgery with a conservative measure. Only one study conducted by Dunkow and colleagues[56] has compared one surgical technique with another in a randomized prospective manner. It is thus difficult to make conclusive statements about the value of surgical interventions over certain less invasive conservative measures or the value of one technique over another. The evidence suggests, however, that all three techniques—open, percutaneous, and arthroscopic releases—are effective in treating recalcitrant LE. It would also seem percutaneous and arthroscopic releases lead to a quicker return to activities after surgery than do open surgeries.

RECOMMENDATIONS

LE is usually a self-limiting disease. More than 80% of patients have symptoms that are completely resolved or much better by 6 months with little treatment when aggravating activities are avoided for 6 weeks and the patient is educated.

We disfavor the use of corticosteroid injections because patients appear to benefit short term only to relapse and have a worse outcome than wait and see in the medium to long term. ESWT is also not recommended because no beneficial effect has been shown. Physiotherapy, bracing, and nonsteroidal anti-inflammatory medication may be useful, but the evidence is contradictory, incomplete, or both. Topical NSAIDs and acupuncture have evidence for their use in the short term.

Botox injections have evidence supporting their use for the short to long term but at the cost of sometimes bothersome weakness that may last up to 3 months.

Failure of conservative treatment for more than 6 months warrants surgical intervention. Earlier surgical intervention may be warranted if symptoms are incapacitating. Although open, percutaneous, and arthroscopic lateral releases are acceptable options, we favor arthroscopic release. Arthroscopic release allows inspection and treatment of joint pathology, leads to good pain relief and strength gain, and returns the patients quicker to work. Table 22–2 provides a summary of recommendations for the treatment of LE.

TABLE 22–2. Summary of Recommendations

STATEMENT	LEVEL OF EVIDENCE/GRADE OF RECOMMENDATION	REFERENCES
1. LE responds well to education and avoidance of aggravating activities with 80% of patients having symptoms completely resolved or much better by 6 months.	A	25,26
2. Corticosteroid injections may be useful diagnostically but are disfavored as a therapeutic intervention.	A	24-26
3. ESWT is not recommended.	A	34-41
4. Acupuncture is not recommended.	A	15-18
5. Though perhaps useful, no conclusions can be made on bracing.	I	27-33
6. No conclusions can be made on oral NSAIDs.	I	22,23
7. Topical NSAIDs have benefit in the short term. (1-3wks). Further studies are need for beyond 3wks.	A	19-21
8. Physiotherapy may be modestly beneficial but evidence is contradictory.	I	25,26
9. Botox injection is recommended only if the patient accepts possibly acquiring significant weakness for modest symptom relief.	I	42-45
10. Lateral release done open, percutaneously, or arthroscopically is indicated in symptomatic LE persisting beyond 6 months.	C	46-48, 53-56, 61,62,64-66
11. Results of all 3 techniques are similar but percutaneous[56] and arthroscopic release[65] may return patients to work earlier than open.	B	56,64,65,66

REFERENCES

1. Major HP: Lawn-tennis elbow. Br Med J 2:557, 1883.
2. Murphy KP, Giuliani JR, Freedman BA: Management of lateral epicondylitis in the athlete. Oper Tech Sports Med 14:67–74, 2006.
3. Mehta JA, Bain GI: Posterolateral rotatory instability of the elbow. J Am Acad Orthop Surg 12:405–415, 2004.
4. O'Driscoll SW, Bell DF, Morrey BF: Posterolateral rotatory instability of the elbow. J Bone Joint Surg Am 73:440–446, 1991.
5. Pomerance J: Radiographic analysis of lateral epicondylitis. J Shoulder Elbow Surg 11:156–157, 2002.
6. Miller TT, Shapiro MA, Schultz E, Kalish PE: Comparison of sonography and MRI for diagnosing epicondylitis. J Clin Ultrasound 30:193–202, 2002.
7. Bisset L, Paungmali A, Vicenzino B, Beller E: A systematic review and meta-analysis of clinical trials on physical interventions for lateral epicondylalgia. Br J Sports Med 39: 411–422, 2005.
8. Shiri R, Viikari-Juntura E, Varonen H, Heliovaara M: Prevalence and determinants of lateral and medial epicondylitis: A population study. Am J Epidemiol 164:1065–1074, 2006.
9. Kurppa K, Viikari-Juntura E, Kuosma E, et al: Incidence of tenosynovitis or peritendinitis and epicondylitis in a meat-processing factory. Scand J Work Environ Health 17:32–37, 1991.
10. Cyriax JH: The pathology and treatment of tennis elbow. J Bone Joint Surg 18:921–940, 1936.
11. Kraushaar BS, Nirschl RP: Tendinosis of the elbow (tennis elbow). Clinical features and findings of histological, immunohistochemical, and electron microscopy studies. J Bone Joint Surg Am 81:259–278, 1999.
12. Regan W, Wold LE, Coonrad R, Morrey BF: Microscopic histopathology of chronic refractory lateral epicondylitis. Am J Sports Med 20:746–749, 1992.
13. Deleted in proof.
14. Coonrad RW, Hopper WR: Tennis elbow: It's course, natural history, conservative and surgical management. J Bone Joint Surg Am 55:1177–1182, 1973.
15. Fink M, Wolkenstein E, Karst M, Gehrke A: Acupuncture in chronic epicondylitis: A randomized controlled trial. Rheumatology (Oxford) 41:205–209, 2002.

16. Molsberger A, Hille E: The analgesic effect of acupuncture in chronic tennis elbow pain. Br J Rheumatol 33:1162–1165, 1994.
17. Davidson J, Vandervoort A, Lessard L, et al: The effect of acupuncture versus ultrasound on pain level, grip strength and disability in individuals with lateral epicondylitis: A pilot study. Physiother Can 53:195–202, 211, 2001.
18. Green S, Buchbinder R, Barnsley L, et al: Non-steroidal anti-inflammatory drugs (NSAIDs) for treating lateral elbow pain in adults. Cochrane Database Syst Rev (2):CD003686, 2002.
19. Burnham R, Gregg R, Healy P, Steadward RL: The effectiveness of topical diclofenac for lateral epicondylitis. Clin J Sports Med 8:78–81, 1998.
20. Burton A: A comparative trial of forearm strap and topical anti-inflammatory as adjuncts to manual therapy in tennis elbow. Man Med 3:141–143, 1988.
21. Jenoure P, Rostan A, Gremion G, et al: Multi-centre, double-blind, controlled clinical study on the efficacy of diclofenac epolamine tissugel plaster in patients with epicondylitis. Medicina Dello Sport 50:285–292, 1997.
22. Labelle H, Guibert R: Efficacy of diclofenac in lateral epicondylitis of the elbow also treated with immobilization. Arch Fam Med 6:257–262, 1997.
23. Hay E, Paterson S, Lewis M, et al: Pragmatic randomised controlled trial of local corticosteroid injection and naproxen for treatment of lateral epicondylitis of elbow in primary care. BMJ 319:964–968, 1999.
24. Altay T, Gunal I, Ozturk H: Local injection treatment for lateral epicondylitis. Clin Orthop Relat Res (398):127–130, 2002.
25. Smidt N, van der Windt DA, Assendelft WJ, et al: Corticosteroid injections, physiotherapy, or a wait-and-see policy for lateral epicondylitis: A randomised controlled trial. Lancet 359:657–662, 2002.
26. Bisset L, Beller E, Jull G, et al: Mobilisation with movement and exercise, corticosteroid injection, or wait and see for tennis elbow: Randomised trial. BMJ 333:939, 2006.
27. Faes M, van den Akker B, de Lint JA, et al: Dynamic extensor brace for lateral epicondylitis. Clin Orthop Relat Res 442: 149–157, 2006.
28. Jensen B, Bliddal H, Danneskiold-Samsore B: Comparison of two different treatments of lateral humral epicondylitis—"tennis elbow." A randomized controlled trial (in Danish). Ugeskr Laeger 163:1427–1431, 2001.
29. Struijs PA, Smidt N, Arola H, et al; Orthotic devices for tennis elbow. Cochrane Database Syst Rev (2):CD001821, 2001.
30. Erturk H, Celiker R, Sivri A, et al: The efficacy of different treatment regiments that are commonly used in tennis elbow [Tenisci dirseginde sik kullanilan farkli tedavi yaklasimlarinin etkinligi]. J Rheum Med Rehab 8:298–301, 1997.
31. Haker E, Lundeberg T: Elbow-band, splintage and steroids in lateral epicondylalgia (tennis elbow). Pain Clinic 6:103–112, 1993.
32. Dwars BJ, de Feiter P, Patka P, Haarman HJThM. Functional treatment of tennis elbow. In: Hermans G, ed. Proceedings of the 24th world congress of Sports Medicine, 1990. Amsterdam: Elsevier Science Publishers (Biomedical Division) pp. 237-41, 1990.
33. Struijs PA, Kerkhoffs GM, Assendelft WJ, Van Dijk CN: Conservative treatment of lateral epicondylitis: Brace versus physical therapy or a combination of both—a randomized clinical trial. Am J Sports Med 32:462–469, 2004.
34. Rompe J, Hopf C, Kullmer K, et al: Low-energy extracorporeal shock-wave therapy for persistent tennis elbow. Int Orthop 20:23–27, 1996.
35. Rompe JD, Decking J, Schoellner C, Theis C: Repetitive low-energy shock wave treatment for chronic lateral epicondylitis in tennis players. Am J Sports Med 32:734–743, 2004.
36. Petronne FA, McCall BR. Extracorporeal shock wave therapy without local anesthesia for chronic lateral epicondylitis. J Bone Joint Surg (Am) 87(6):1297-1304, 2005.
37. Buchbinder R, Green SE, Youd JM, et al: Shock wave therapy for lateral elbow pain. Cochrane Database Syst Rev (4): CD003524, 2005.
38. Haake M, Boddeker IR, Decker T, et al: Side effects of extracorporeal shock wave therapy (ESWT) in the treatment of tennis elbow. Arch Orthop Trauma Surg 122:222–228, 2002.
39. Speed C, Nichols D, Richards C, et al: Extracorporeal shock wave therapy for lateral epicondylitis—a double blind randomized controlled trial. J Orthop Res 20:895–898, 2002.
40. Melikyan EY, Shahin E, Miles J, Bainbridge LC: Extracorporeal shock-wave treatment for tennis elbow. A randomised double-blind study. J Bone Joint Surg Br 85:852–855, 2003.
41. Chung B, Wiley JP: Effectiveness of extracorporeal shock wave therapy in the treatment of previously untreated lateral epicondylitis: A randomised controlled trial. Am J Sports Med 32:1660–1667, 2004.
42. Wong SM, Hui AC, Tong PY, et al: Treatment of lateral epicondylitis with botulinum toxin: A randomized, double-blind, placebo-controlled trial. Ann Intern Med 143:793–797, 2005.
43. Placzek R, Drescher W, Deuretzbacher G, et al: Treatment of chronic radial epicondylitis with botulinum toxin A. A double-blind, placebo-controlled, randomized multicenter study. J Bone Joint Surg Am 89:255–260, 2007.
44. Keizer SB, Rutten HP, Pilot P, et al: Botulinum toxin injection versus surgical treatment for tennis elbow: A randomized pilot study. Clin Orthop Relat Res (401):125–131, 2002.
45. Hayton MJ, Santini AJ, Hughes PJ, et al: Botulinum toxin injection in the treatment of tennis elbow. A double-blind, randomized, controlled, pilot study. J Bone Joint Surg Am 87:503–507, 2005.
46. Nirschl RP, Pettrone FA: Tennis elbow. The surgical treatment of lateral epicondylitis. J Bone Joint Surg Am 61:832–839, 1979.
47. Verhaar J, Walenkamp G, Kester A, et al: Lateral extensor release for tennis elbow. A prospective long-term follow-up study. J Bone Joint Surg Am 75:1034–1043, 1993.
48. Rosenberg N, Henderson I: Surgical treatment of resistant lateral epicondylitis. Follow-up study of 19 patients after excision, release and repair of proximal common extensor tendon origin. Arch Orthop Trauma Surg 122:514–517, 2002.
49. Khashaba A: Nirschl tennis elbow release with or without drilling. Br J Sports Med 35:200–201, 2001.
50. Whaley AL, Baker CL: Lateral epicondylitis. Clin Sports Med 23:677–691, x, 2004.
51. Murphy KP, Giuliani JR, Freedman BA: Management of lateral epicondylitis in the athlete. Oper Tech Sports Med 14:67–74.
52. Hohmann G: Das wesen und die behandlung des sogenannten tennisellenbogens (the nature and treatment of so-called tennis elbow). Much Med Wochnschr 80:250–252, 1999.
53. Grundberg AB, Dobson JF: Percutaneous release of the common extensor origin for tennis elbow. Clin Orthop Relat Res (376):137–144, 2000.
54. Kaleli T, Ozturk C, Temiz A, Tirelioglu O: Surgical treatment of tennis elbow: Percutaneous release of the common extensor origin. Acta Orthop Belg 70:131–133, 2004.
55. Savoie FH: Management of lateral epicondylitis with percutaneous release. Tech Shoulder Elbow Surg 2:243–246, 2001.
56. Dunkow PD, Jatti M, Muddu BN: A comparison of open and percutaneous techniques in the surgical treatment of tennis elbow. J Bone Joint Surg Br 86:701–704, 2004.
57. Organ SW, Nirschl RP, Kraushaar BS, Guidi EJ: Salvage surgery for lateral tennis elbow. Am J Sports Med 25:746–750, 1997.
58. Grifka J, Boenke S, Kramer J: Endoscopic therapy in epicondylitis radialis humeri. Arthroscopy 11:743–748, 1995.
59. Kuklo TR, Taylor KF, Murphy KP, et al: Arthroscopic release for lateral epicondylitis: A cadaveric model. Arthroscopy 15:259–264, 1999.
60. Smith AM, Castle JA, Ruch DS: Arthroscopic resection of the common extensor origin: Anatomic considerations. J Shoulder Elbow Surg 12:375–379, 2003.
61. Baker CL Jr, Murphy KP, Gottlob CA, Curd DT: Arthroscopic classification and treatment of lateral epicondylitis: Two-year clinical results. J Shoulder Elbow Surg 9:475–482, 2000.
62. Owens BD, Murphy KP, Kuklo TR: Arthroscopic release for lateral epicondylitis. Arthroscopy 17:582–587, 2001.
63. Cohen M, Romeo A: Lateral epicondylitis: Open and arthroscopic treatment. J Am Soc Surg Hand 1:172–176, 2001.
64. Rubenthaler F, Wiese M, Senge A, et al: Long-term follow-up of open and endoscopic Hohmann procedures for lateral epicondylitis. Arthroscopy 21:684–690, 2005.
65. Peart RE, Strickler SS, Schweitzer KM Jr: Lateral epicondylitis: A comparative study of open and arthroscopic lateral release. Am J Orthop 33:565–567, 2004.
66. Szabo SJ, Savoie FH 3rd, Field LD, et al: Tendinosis of the extensor carpi radialis brevis: An evaluation of three methods of operative treatment. J Shoulder Elbow Surg 15:721–727, 2006.

Chapter 23

What Is the Optimal Rehabilitative Approach to Post-Traumatic Elbow Stiffness?

Joy C. MacDermid, PT, PhD

CHALLENGES IN IMPLEMENTING EVIDENCE-BASED PRACTICE IN THIS CASE

Evidence-based practice dictates that we use best available evidence when making clinical decisions. In this regard, the question posed in this chapter presents a number of challenges:

1. Rehabilitation is an area of clinical practice, not a specific intervention. Studies are designed to answer whether specific approaches within rehabilitation are effective, and not to answer the broad question posed above.
2. Rehabilitation programs are multimodal. Studies that evaluate isolated components of rehabilitation must necessarily detect the isolated smaller effect sizes that contribute to the overall rehabilitation program, and thus would require extremely large sample sizes to be fully powered. Ideally, studies should be designed to compare the treatment of interest with one that is substantially different in philosophy or intensity (ideally a placebo), but standards of practice, ethics, and professional beliefs often restrict this approach.
3. Unlike surgery, which happens at a single point in time, recovery and rehabilitation occurs over time. Goals, interventions, and effectiveness of rehabilitation can vary at different time points, complicating the comparison across different studies. For example, in the acute rehabilitation phase, the focus of rehabilitation for a stiff elbow would be restoration of joint mobility, whereas later the focus might be strengthening, functional endurance, retraining, and work accommodation. (Joint mobility is the focus of this clinical question, with interventions subgrouped into joint mobility interventions, adjunctive interventions, and functional interventions.)
4. Classification and definition of the various techniques/options involved in rehabilitation have not been agreed on.
5. Description of the various techniques involved in rehabilitation in most studies is insufficient to fully understand what has been done. (I have attempted to deal with item 4 by creating specific definitions but was limited by item 5.)

6. Like orthopedic surgery research, the majority of studies are of low quality (see the following paragraph).

The net result of these problems is that there is difficulty locating sufficient high-quality evidence to make comprehensive specific recommendations for rehabilitation of post-traumatic elbow stiffness. This became evident in the first attempts at searching the literature, where few relevant studies could be identified using the classic approaches to searching the literature.

Despite these challenges, evidence-based practice does provide guidance on how to proceed when specific high-quality evidence is lacking. One approach is to include lower levels of evidence; thus, this chapter includes any studies that addressed rehabilitation of the stiff elbow (Levels I–IV) and then separately lists peer-reviewed published expert opinions. A second approach used was the extrapolation of results from studies that were similar to the specific problem of interest. For this reason, this chapter includes a systematic review that addressed rehabilitation of stiffness after trauma to other upper extremity joints. In this case an ESB approach required multiple literature searches and an understanding of the clinical issues to find appropriate and useful evidence.

OPTIONS

To be clear about what is being administered in any joint mobility intervention, one has to be able to describe the active ingredient of the intervention (in a way that others could replicate it). This is not characteristic of how interventions are described in the literature. I proposed a classification system by which the nature of specific rehabilitative interventions designed for joint mobility may be understood. It is important to define the composition and intensity of the intervention using consistent terminology to understand or replicate any given intervention. The composition of the intervention is defined by who delivers the active ingredient (patient, therapist, mobilization device, constraint device) and what type of mobilization is performed (defined by activation mode, arc of movement, and end range time). Intensity is defined by the force applied, the number of repetitions per session, and the number of sessions per day.

DEFINING THE COMPOSITION AND INTENSITY OF JOINT MOBILITY INTERVENTIONS (FIGURE 1)

A. Composition of Intervention

1. <u>Control</u>
a. *Patient*: patient delivers the stimulus
b. *Therapist*: the therapist delivers the stimulus
c. *Device*:
- Mobilization device: A device whose purpose is to directly mobilize specific impaired joints. It is applied to patient, usually under direction of the health professional (includes dynamic and static splints, as well as CPM).
- Constraint device: A device whose purpose is to immobilize specific unimpaired joints, and thereby indirectly mobilize impaired joints; supplied to the patient usually under direction of health professional (includes blocking splints and casting of unaffected joints).

2. <u>Type of movement</u> (activation mode, arc of movement, end range time)
a. *Activation mode*
- Active: active muscle contraction is used to produce movement
- Passive: passive force is used to produce movement
- Combined activation: combination of active and passive movement
b. *Arc of movement*
- Physiologic: The body segment is moved throughout a defined range that is consistent with the normal movement of the joint; this is sometimes referred to as *range of motion (ROM) exercise* because patients or through a ROM (can be active or passive); but to avoid confusion, this chapter uses the more specific term *physiologic motion;* note blocking of motion refers to a restriction on the full physiologic arc of motion.
- Accessory: The body segment is moved to produce the accessory joint "play" movement that occurs during normal physiologic motion; this is sometimes referred to a "joint mobilization," but as the latter terms encompass other techniques, the more specific term *accessory motion* is used here.
- End range: The body segment is maintained at the end of the available range of the joint.
- Manipulation: The body segment is thrust beyond is available end range of the joint.
c. *End range time*
- Intermittent: The joint is maintained at its end range time for a variable amount of time and then released and returned in cyclic fashion.
- Sustained: The joint is maintained at its end range time for a sustained amount of time (often based/progressed according to tolerance).

B. Intensity of intervention

1. <u>Force applied</u>
Ideally, force applied and specific end range time should be described, particularly for splinting

Conversely, these can be described as:
- low load where the joint is held at the end of range with minimal mobilizing force (intended to grow tissue extensibility)
- moderate deforming load where a tolerable load is applied to move the segment and lengthen tissue to improve extensibility
- thrust where force is intended to disrupt tissue adhesions/blocks.

Number of repetitions per application or set
Number of sets or applications per day

Figure 1 describes some common mobilization interventions using their common names and categories: active, passive, and manipulation. These fall on a continuum of increasingly intense mobility interventions. The common names are associated with the more specific terminology defined below to define the different delivery/control methods (patient, therapist, mobilization device).

ADJUNCTIVE INTERVENTIONS

The second group of rehabilitation intervention used to manage joint mobility must be considered adjunctive. These are interventions that support the main goal—that is, joint mobility by facilitating the mobilization intervention. Interventions that are designed to control pain or promote tissue extensibility as a prerequisite to improving joint mobility are the most common that would fit in this category.

The final groups of interventions are considered to be functional. These are interventions designed to restore function. They may or may not improve joint stiffness but are implemented with the goal of restoring the patient to maximum function and quality of life. Examples include strengthening programs, work hardening, adaptive devices, education, or functional splinting. Given our question, these issues are not addressed in this chapter.

DEFINING AN ANSWERABLE QUESTION

Given the earlier discussion, our specific evidence-based practice question is: What evidence exists to support or refute the use of mobilization or adjunctive interventions to mitigate elbow stiffness in patients after joint trauma or surgery?

Finding the Evidence

We used several typical database searches (Table 23–1). The classic PICO approach had to be modified due to paucity of evidence.

Appraising and Extracting the Evidence

Systematic Reviews. Michlovitz and colleagues[1] conducted an SR on conservative interventions to improve mobility after upper extremity musculoskeletal trauma.

AGENT OF DELIVERY

	Movement	Patient	Therapist	Mobilization device*
Beyond end range motion	*Beyond end range motion*	N/a (except by accident)	Joint manipulation Under anesthesia Joint manipulation	*N/a* *device is monitored by a person*
	Passive end range mobilization	Self-assisted Accessory joint mobilization (self-mobilization) Self-assisted Physiological end-range hold (stretch)	Joint mobilization with movement Accessory joint Mobilization (joint mobilization) Physiological stretch (stretch)	**Passive end-range mobilizing device-static progressive force (static progressive splints)** **Passive end-range mobilizing device-dynamic force (dynamic splints)**
	Passive physiological mobilization	Self-assisted physiological (passive ROM)	Passive physiological (passive ROM)	**Passive physiologic movement device (continuous passive ROM = CPM)**
	Active (ROM) mobilization	Active physiological (ROM)	Muscle activation training (includes PNF, muscle energy and others)	**Constrained adjacent joint motion devices (constrained movement therapy, casting motion to mobilize stiffness; blocking splints)**

Intensity of intervention →

FIGURE 23–1. Physiological movement: the body segment is moved throughout a defined range that is consistent with the normal movement of the joint. Accessory movement: the body segment is moved to produce the accessory joint "play" movement that occurs during normal physiologic motion; End range: the body segment is maintained at the end of the available range of the joint. The intensity of intervention should be defined by the Force applied, and duration (including the number of repetitions or time/application or set and the number of sets or applications/day).
* Device is monitored by a person.

Medline, CINAHL, PEDRO, PubMed, and Cochrane were searched. Two reviewers performed abstract selection and critical appraisal (n = 26 studies; 24-item critical appraisal and level of evidence). The primary outcome considered was ROM measurement. Overall, the quantity and quality of evidence were moderate to low. Level IIb, III, and IV evidence supported the use of joint mobilization, a supervised exercise program, and splinting. No studies found examined techniques of physical agent or electrotherapeutic modalities. The authors conclude that future studies are needed to delineate selection of appropriate candidates for these techniques and effective dosage.

Evidence of Mobilizations

Active Mobilization

1. Level III evidence exists that active motion alone is effective after closed reduction of elbow dislocation. Twenty consecutive patients from a naval academy with closed posterior elbow dislocations were treated prospectively on a rapid motion, functional regimen. Final ROM averaged 24 to 139 degrees. All patients attained final extension within 5 degrees of the contralateral side; within an average of 19 days after reduction of the dislocation. Arm circumference returned to normal at an average of 6.5 days.[2]

2. Two Level II evidence reports indicate that early active ROM is more effective than late ROM after cubital tunnel decompression and medial epicondylectomy. Warwick compared early versus ROM exercises after cubital tunnel release and medial epicondylectomy. Fifty-seven consecutive cases

were studied and divided into 2 groups. Physical therapy consisting of active and passive ROM exercises was started 14 days after surgery for the first group and 3 days after surgery for the second group. Fifty-two percent of the patients in the delayed motion group sustained flexion contractures of more than 5 degrees compared with only 4% of the patients in the early motion group. Patient starting exercise earlier returned to work in half the time. A second smaller trial in 45 consecutive procedures patients were randomized to rehabilitation at an average of 3 days after surgery *or* an average of 14 days after surgery. Flexion contracture of more than 5 degrees was observed in 5% of the early mobilization group compared with 52% of the late mobilization group ($P < 0.001$). On average, patients in the early mobilization group returned to work twice as early as those in the late mobilization group and did not experience any adverse effects on their grip strength or other hand functions.[3]

3. Level II evidence exists that splinting for more than 3 weeks is detrimental to achieving ROM after elbow dislocation. In 45 patients with a simple elbow dislocation/closed reduction (61 months after injury), the overall results were good or excellent with regard to pain and function. The most common finding was a loss of terminal extension (9% had a lack of extension up to 30 degrees). Better results were observed in those immobilized either less than 2 weeks or for 2 to 3 weeks as compared with those who were immobilized more than 3 weeks.[4]

TABLE 23–1. Search Strategies were Modified to Find Evidence on Elbow Rehabilitation

APPROACH	SEARCH TERMS	Results		
		NUMBER RETRIEVED	ON TOPIC	FIT*
Expert search strategy	MEDLINE: clinical trials/ or clinical trials, phase i/ or clinical trials, phase ii/ or clinical trials, phase iii/ or clinical trials, phase iv/ or controlled clinical trials/ or randomized controlled trials/ or multicenter studies/ or cross-over studies/ or double-blind method/ or meta-analysis/ or random allocation/ or single-blind method/ or systematic review$.ti,ab. or ((singl$ or doubl$ or tripl$) adj (mask$ or blind$)).ti,ab. or (blind$ or random$).ti,ab.	97	0	0
	EMBASE: randomized controlled trial/ or (controlled study/ or comparative study/) and (clinical trial/ or phase 1 clinical trial/ or phase 2 clinical trial/ or phase 3 clinical trial/ or phase 4 clinical trial/ or major clinical study/ or prospective study/)) or "systematic review"/ or randomization/ or double blind procedure/ or single blind procedure/ or triple blind procedure/ or ((singl$ or doubl$ or tripl$) adj (mask$ or blind$)).ti,ab. or (blind$ or random$).ti,ab.			
	To identify the Level III and beyond evidence, again the same terms were used except they were paired with the following methodology-related terms to weed out the appropriate types of studies:			
	MEDLINE: case-control studies/ or retrospective studies/ or comparative study/ or case series.tw. or exp treatment outcome/ or exp Cohort Studies/			
	EMBASE: case control study/ or retrospective study/ or comparative study/ or case series.tw. or treatment outcome/ or exp treatment failure/ or cohort analysis/			
	All of the above searches were restricted to human and English language articles only. The number of results from the Level I and Level II evidence search are below:			
	MEDLINE: 13 identified			
	EMBASE: 6 identified			
PICO specific	Elbow AND stiffness AND rehabilitation	42	6	4
PICO broad	MEDLINE: (elbow/ or elbow joint/ or (elbow$ adj3 stiff$).ti,ab.) and (physical therapy modalities/ or rehabilitation/ or rehab$.ti,ab.)	97	0	0
	EMBASE: Joint Stiffness/ and (ELBOW/ or ELBOW INJURY/)			
Expanded population				
Expanded database	CINAHL Elbow/ or elbow injuries/ or elbow fracture and physical therapy	45	0	0
	CINAHL			
Personal database and files search	Searched hard files and personal database using elbow and (stiffness OR range of motion)	108	12	4

*With evidence-based medicine approach (Levels I–IV specific or Level 1 extrapolated).

Mobilization Splinting

1. Level 3 evidence has been found that static progressive stretch splinting for 1 to 3 months is effective in patients who had limited success with other treatment modalities including serial casting, dynamic splinting, physical therapy, and/or surgery; results were an average of 31 degrees or 69% improvement. All patients expressed satisfaction, with no complications and no deterioration in ROM at the 1-year follow-up evaluation.[5]

2. Multiple Level III or IV studies support that low-load prolonged stretch orthoses can reduce elbow joint contractures. In one study (17 patients; 12 with elbow contracture), secondary neurologic and orthopedic pathologies improved; elbow results were not summarized separately[6] in another[7].

3. Level IV evidence has been reported that a dynamic supination splint that does not cross the humeroulnar and humeroradial joints is effective in increasing ROM. Eleven subjects treated for various elbow and/or wrist fractures leading to losses of forearm supination significantly increased their passive ROM from 34.0 degrees at the initial visit to 82.3 degrees at discharge, and active range of motion from 27.0 to 72.3 degrees. Surface electromyography (EMG) confirmed the passive nature of the splint: Average supinator EMG activity was 7.9 mV at rest, 7.8 mV in the splint, and 68.0 mV with maximal isometric contraction.[8]

4. Level II evidence exists that CPM is an effective adjunct to surgery in treating elbow stiffness secondary to heterotopic periarticular ossifications. Heterotopic ossificans was surgically excised in 16 elbows of 14 patients with traumatic brain injury, an average of 18.9 months after the end of coma. During the follow-up period, all the elbows showed improvement in ROM, and the arc of flexion averaged 95 degrees in the surgery group, versus 116 degrees in the surgery/CPM group. Authors attribute their better outcomes compared

with those obtained by previous investigators to be due to the prolonged application of continuous passive motion after surgery.[9]

Evidence of Adjunctive Interventions. Level II evidence exists that cryotherapy is effective in managing muscle stiffness and pain related to a bout of damage-inducing eccentric exercise (8 sets of 5 maximal reciprocal contractions at 0.58 rad $\times$ sec^{-1}) of the elbow flexors on an isokinetic dynamometer (n = 15 female subjects). Subjects in the cryotherapy group immersed their exercised arm in cold water ($15°C$) for 15 minutes immediately after eccentric exercise and then every 12 hours for 15 minutes for a total of seven sessions. Relaxed elbow angle was greater and creatine kinase activity lower for the cryotherapy group than the control group on days 2 and 3 after the eccentric exercise.[10]

Level V (Expert Recommendations)

A variety of Level V recommendations were extracted from review articles.

- Nonoperative management of stiffness should be considered for up to 6 months (after contracture).[11–13] Note: Evidence has been found that even prolonged contractures benefit from splinting.
- More recent contractures are more likely to respond to nonoperative management.[12]
- Ice and inflammatory medication are useful adjuncts.[12,13]
- Overly aggressive physical therapy may increase pain, stiffness, and swelling, and possibly lead to HO.[13]
- Night splinting should be used in the direction of greatest limitation.[12]
- Splinting for 20 hours of wear alternating directions with intermittent exercise is effective.[12]
- Staging of intervention should include cryotherapy, gentle passive and active ROM exercise during inflammatory stage; thermal modalities and activities of daily living are added during fibroblastic stage; in the remodeling stage, all modalities and strengthening exercises are indicated.[14]
- Low-load passive exercise progressed to active, then end-range exercise/stretch.[14]
- Exercise of 5 to 10 repetitions every 2 to 3 hours is progressed to 15 to 20 repetitions every hour based on tissue response.[14]
- Forearm/pronation exercise should be performed at 90 degrees of elbow flexion to protect ligaments.[14]
- Joint mobilization (increased from lesser grades to end range mobilizations) are effective when combined with splinting.[14]
- Splinting for mobilization should be avoided for 3 to 6 weeks after injury.[14]
- The static progressive flexion cuff, serial static extension splint, static progressive turnbuckle splints for flexion/extension, and either a static progressive or dynamic splint for pronation/supination are affective mobilizing splint choices.[14]
- Splinting can start with 1–2 hours, 3–4 times/day in the fibroblastic phase combined with night and splinting.[14]

- Splinting is more effective when combined with intensive therapy.[11,14]
- Traditional treatment during the day and night and use of CPM is effective.[14]
- CPM is used when fractures/ligament repairs are stable.[14]
- Ultrasound is less useful for improving tissue extensibility at the elbow (vs. hot packs or whirlpool) because of the size and depth of tissue.[14]
- EMG biofeedback is useful for re-educating agonist muscles or to reduce antagonist activity that contributes to joint stiffness.[14]
- Injury-specific guidelines (Level V)[14]

Fracture distal humerus
- Early ROM begins on day 1 (if triceps sparing extension is allowed).
- Home programs should consist of elevation/ice, active-assisted flexion, gravity-assisted extension, active pronation/supination, maintained exercise shoulder/wrist and hand.
- Once callus forms, passive ROM and mobilization splinting are added.

Radial head fractures
- elbow extension and flexion should be performed in pronation (supination increases the radiocapitellar load).
- Forearm rotation should be performed with elbow flexed to 90 degrees.
- Fractures with open reduction with internal fixation without ligament injury are positioned in a collar and cuff for day use and an elbow extension splint at night.
- If the lateral collateral ligament is deficient, the elbow is splinted in 90-degree flexion and forearm pronation during the day.
- Early active flexion/extension with the elbow greater than 90 degrees is started on day 1.
- Strengthening can start at 8 weeks, progressing from pronation to supination.

Coronoid fractures
- Early active ROM within a stable arc is indicated.
- Extension should be blocked by a splints for last 40 to 60 degrees (block reduced 10 degrees/week); for total use of 4 to 6 weeks.
- Passive extension/mobilizations delayed until fracture is healed.
- Pronation/supinations performed at 90 degrees out of splint.
- Early contracture control is needed—serial extension splinting starts at 4 weeks.
- Strengthening delayed until 8 to 10 weeks.

Elbow dislocations
- Initially, patients are splinted in a posterior elbow splint holding the joint at 90 degrees for 5 to 7 days.
- If stable, elbow ROM in an unrestricted range is initiated; if stability is a concern, extension protection is indicated.
- Passive elbow flexion stretches are avoided for 6 weeks.

AREAS OF UNCERTAINTY

The following issues have not been resolved in relation to optimal rehabilitation of post-trauma elbow stiffness:
- The optimal choice and timing for physical agent or electrotherapeutic modalities
- Factors that indicate prognosis or need for specific interventions
- Optimal type or dosage of active exercise (and condition specific restrictions)
- Optimal type or dosage of splinting
- Optimal type or dosage of joint mobilization

SUMMARY OF RECOMMENDATIONS

Fair evidence exists to suggest the following conclusions:
- Supervised active exercise is effective in reducing elbow joint stiffness.
- Early motion is more effective than later motion.
- Joint mobilization is effective in reducing joint contractures.

- Dynamic and progressive static splinting are effective in reducing joint contracture.
- CPM may assist in resolving selected types of joint stiffness.
- Cold can reduce acute symptoms of exercise-induced swelling and pain.
- Multiple interventions are more effective than isolated interventions.
- Specific injuries and surgical approaches will impose specific challenges, restrictions, and indications.

The preponderance of evidence supports a role for a progressive rehabilitation program, although the specifics of an optimal rehabilitation program cannot be defined on the basis of current exercise. Further research and consensus exercise around condition-specific restrictions and more consistent use of outcome measures would benefit the field. Table 23–2 provides a summary or recommendations for the treatment of post-traumatic elbow stiffness.

ACKNOWLEDGMENT

J.C.M. was funded by a New Investigator Award, Canadian Institutes of Health Research.

TABLE 23–2. Summary of Recommendations

STATEMENT	LEVEL OF EVIDENCE	REFERENCES
1. Joint mobilization, supervised exercise and splinting are effective in improving mobility of upper extremity joints.	A	1
2. Earlier active motion is effective in reducing joint contracture and work lost time in patients with elbow dislocation or cubital tunnel surgery	B	2,3
3. Immobilization for longer than three weeks following simple elbow dislocation results in loss of extension range of motion	B	4
4. Static progressive end range mobilization splinting improves motion in resistant elbow contracture	B	5
5. Prolonged low load end range splinting can reduce elbow joint contracture in a spectrum elbow pathologies.	C	6,7
6. Continuous passive motion is effective in improving the arc of motion attained following surgery for heterotopic ossification	B	9
7. Cryotherapy immediately following maximal eccentric elbow flexion exercise reduces delayed (2-3 day) muscle stiffness and pain experience	B	10

REFERENCES

1. Michlovitz SL, Harris BA, Watkins MP: Therapy interventions for improving joint range of motion: A systematic review. J Hand Ther 17:118–131, 2004.
2. Ross G, McDevitt ER, Chronister R, Ove PN: Treatment of simple elbow dislocation using an immediate motion protocol. Am J Sports Med 27:308–311, 1999.
3. Seradge H: Cubital tunnel release and medial epicondylectomy: Effect of timing of mobilization. J Hand Surg [Am] 22:863–866, 1997.
4. Schippinger G, Seibert FJ, Steinbock J, Kucharczyk M: Management of simple elbow dislocations. Does the period of immobilization affect the eventual results? Langenbecks Arch Surg 384:294–297, 1999.
5. Bonutti PM, Windau JE, Ables BA, Miller BG: Static progressive stretch to reestablish elbow range of motion. Clin Orthop Relat Res (303):128–134, 1994.
6. Nuismer BA, Ekes AM, Holm MB: The use of low-load prolonged stretch devices in rehabilitation programs in the Pacific northwest. Am J Occup Ther 51:538–543, 1997.
7. Green DP, McCoy H: Turnbuckle orthotic correction of elbow flexion contractures after acute injuires. J Bone Joint Surg Am 61:1092–1095, 2007.
8. Lee MJ, LaStayo PC, von Kersburg AE: A supination splint worn distal to the elbow: A radiographic, electromyographic, and retrospective report. J Hand Ther 16:190–198, 2003.
9. Ippolito E, Formisano R, Caterini R, et al: Resection of elbow ossification and continuous passive motion in postcomatose patients. J Hand Surg [Am] 24:546–553, 1999.

10. Eston R, Peters D: Effects of cold water immersion on the symptoms of exercise-induced muscle damage. J Sports Sci 17:231–238, 1999.
11. Issack PS, Egol KA: Posttraumatic contracture of the elbow: Current management issues. Bull Hosp Jt Dis 63(3-4):129–136, 2006.
12. King GJ, Faber KJ: Posttraumatic elbow stiffness. Orthop Clin North Am 31:129–143, 2000.
13. Morrey BF: The posttraumatic stiff elbow. Clin Orthop Relat Res (431):26–35, 2005.
14. Chinchalkar SJ, Szekeres M: Rehabilitation of elbow trauma. Hand Clin 20:363–374, 2004.

PEDIATRIC TOPICS

Can We Prevent Children's Fractures?

Andrew Howard, MD, MSc, FRCSC

Injury is currently one of the leading causes of burden of disease, accounting for 9% of worldwide morbidity and mortality combined in 1998. Injury is expected to account for a much greater share—14% of global morbidity and mortality by 2020.[1,2] The expected increase is attributable both to increased motorization leading to a greater burden of road traffic crashes, and to the demographic and epidemiologic transition whereby diseases of poverty (malnutrition, infections) become replaced by those of affluence (trauma, diabetes, heart disease, cancer) as global wealth increases and population growth rates slow.[3]

Many fields of medicine (e.g., cardiology) consider the scientific understanding of prevention of disease as implicit in clinical practice. The prevention of fractures, both at the individual and at the population level, is an important aim toward which orthopedic surgeons have much to contribute. Injury prevention is in itself a broad scientific field as exemplified by the scope and depth of articles presented in a leading journal, *Injury Prevention*. Fractures are a common feature of many injury events from the high- (e.g., road traffic) to the low-energy (sports, falls) mechanisms. It is not the purpose of this chapter to review the general evidence supporting the statement that most injury events among children are, in fact, preventable. Rather, this chapter focuses on clinical aspects of the prevention of fractures in the population pediatric orthopedists treat as patients specifically. The relationship between bone health and fractures among healthy children and among children with medical comorbidities is considered. Evidence about the prevention of refractures in clinical practice is examined.

BONE HEALTH AND FRACTURES AMONG HEALTHY CHILDREN

Increasing longevity puts more of the population at risk for osteoporotic fractures in old age. Ensuring attainment of the greatest possible peak bone mass in childhood and adolescence is an obvious but difficult to implement step at a societal level. Attainment and maintenance of bone mass relies on adequate dietary calcium, availability of vitamin D, weightbearing exercise, and hormonal milieu. Peak bone mass is attained by early adulthood and declines thereafter; therefore improving bone health

for a lifetime requires interventions in childhood and adolescence.[4] Whether these same interventions will reduce childhood or adolescent fractures is unclear. A transient osteoporosis of adolescence coinciding with peak height growth velocity has been hypothesized, and it may increase fracture incidence at this time.

Randomized, controlled trial (level I) evidence demonstrates that oral calcium supplementation increases the bone mineral density (BMD) of female children during the pubertal growth spurt; however, at 7 years of follow-up, there was no difference in total body BMD and distal radius BMD.[5] A randomized, controlled trial combining exercise intervention and calcium supplementation in 16- and 18-year-old girls found a significant increase in BMD (at 1 year) with calcium supplementation, but no additional effect from a weightbearing exercise program prescribed to individuals.[6] A prospective, nonrandomized study from Sweden (level II evidence) used a school-based exercise program and showed that classes of girls given daily physical exercises had improved BMD and bone width compared with classes doing physical exercise once per week.[7]

An increased risk for forearm fractures from reduced BMD has been established prospectively for girls using a cohort design (level II evidence)[8] and retrospectively for boys using a case–control design (level III evidence).[9] In both of these studies, an increased body mass index was also found to be an independent predictor of increased fracture risk.

In summary, among healthy children, it is possible to increase the BMD over the short term by adding calcium to the diet and perhaps by implementing group exercise programs. Children with lower BMD are at increased risk for forearm fractures. Intervention trials with fracture outcomes (rather than bone density outcomes) have not yet been done among children.

BONE HEALTH AND FRACTURES AMONG CHILDREN WITH COMORBIDITIES

Osteogenesis Imperfecta

Osteogenesis imperfecta is a group of related conditions in which defects in collagen production lead to bony fragility and fractures. Bone turnover is high, particularly during the growing years. Bisphosphonates decrease osteoclastic resorption of bone, leading to increased bone mass and bone strength. Two randomized, controlled trials (level I evidence) support treating patients with osteogenesis imperfecta with oral bisphosphonates. One trial randomized 34 children to either oral olpadronate (10 mg/m^2 daily) or placebo, in addition to calcium and vitamin D for all patients. A 2-year parallel arm design was used. Olpadronate-treated patients had a 31% reduction in long-bone fracture risk. Increases in BMD and bone mineral content were statistically significantly greater among olpadronate-treated patients. No difference was found in overall quality of life.[10] A second trial randomized 17 children to oral alendronate or placebo in a blinded crossover study and showed increases in BMD, increases in quality of life in the domains of pain, analgesic use, and well-being, as well as decreases in the number of fractures during the time of alendronate treatment.[11]

Earlier studies regarding bisphosphonates for Osteogenesis imperfecta were case series (level IV evidence) that documented increased bone mineral densities, decreased serum markers of bone turnover, and decreased numbers of fractures after treatment with intravenous pamidronate.[12–15]

Cerebral Palsy/Neuromuscular Conditions

Patients with cerebral palsy are at risk for osteoporosis and fractures. Decreased weightbearing stimulus and altered vitamin D metabolism, related to lack of sun exposure and to anticonvulsant medication, have been postulated as mechanisms. A randomized, controlled trial (level I evidence) of increasing the time of the standing program for nonambulant children with cerebral palsy demonstrated an increase in vertebral but not tibial BMD with increased standing. Only 26 patients were randomized, no effect on fractures was noted (perhaps because of small numbers), and the clinical significance of the vertebral BMD differences was unclear.[16] A causative study using a case–control design (level III evidence) compared 20 patients with fractures with 20 age-matched control subjects from a population of children and young adults with spastic quadriplegia in residential care.[17] Anticonvulsant therapy was strongly associated with both the occurrence of fractures and abnormally high serum alkaline phosphatase, indicating high bone turnover. Radiographic signs of rickets were present in many of the fracture patients. After administration of vitamin D and calcium, the radiographic findings and the high serum alkaline phosphatase normalized (level IV evidence, case series), although there was not adequate follow-up to determine subsequent fracture risk. Two level IV studies support the use of oral[18] or intravenous[19] bisphosphonate in nonambulant patients with cerebral palsy by documenting increased BMD and decreased fracture incidence during treatment.

Steroid Treatment

Steroid-induced osteoporosis is a well-described consequence of chronic steroid use, which is indicated in many pediatric medical conditions. A retrospective cohort study (level III evidence) found that inhaled steroid use (for asthma) of 800 μg/day or more significantly decreased lumbar spine BMD. The effect was more pronounced if oral steroids were also used. Only 76 patients were analyzed, and fracture outcomes were not reported.[20]

Among patients with renal transplant taking chronic oral steroid, one randomized trial (level I evidence) has shown significant increase in BMD with oral vitamin D treatment or with nasal calcitonin treatment, but no significant effect of alendronate alone.[21] Using alendronate without supplementing calcium and vitamin D is an unusual choice, and the negative result regarding alendronate from this trial is therefore suspect.

Another study grouped children receiving chronic oral steroids who had suffered fractures and compared them with those receiving steroids who did not have fractures. Those who had had fractures were treated with intravenous pamidronate plus steroid, and those who had not continued on steroid alone. All children in both groups were prescribed calcium and vitamin D. After pamidronate treatment, there was significant improvement in lumbar spine BMD, compared with significant loss among the steroid alone group. This comparative cohort study can be considered level of evidence III because only one of the arms was gathered prospectively.[22]

PREVENTION OF REFRACTURES IN CLINICAL PRACTICE

Forearm Fractures

A case series (level IV evidence) published in 1996 described 28 forearm refractures of which 25 had known causes. Twenty-one (84%) of them were related to incomplete consolidation of the tensile side of a diaphyseal greenstick fracture.[23] The article did not include data on patients without refractures, so no firm conclusions can be drawn about preventing this event.

A subsequent article published in 1999 used a retrospective case–control design to analyze 768 primary forearm fractures in children of which 38 (4.9%) had refractures.[24] All primary fractures included were treated under general anesthesia by closed or open means. The strongest predictor of refracture risk was the location of the fracture, with 14.7% of diaphyseal fractures suffering a refracture, compared with 2.7% of metaphyseal radius fractures, 1.5% of metaphyseal both bones fractures, and 0% of physeal fractures ($P < 0.001$). The second most important predictor was the duration of cast immobilization, with a refracture rate of 6% among fractures immobilized 6 weeks or less, 4% among fractures immobilized 4 to 6 weeks, and 1% among those immobilized over 6 weeks. The median time to fracture after cast removal was 8 weeks, with most refractures happening within 16 weeks of cast removal. Based on this level III evidence, one can recommend 6 weeks of cast immobilization for diaphyseal fractures and activity restriction for 16 weeks after cast removal.[24]

Femur Fractures

External fixation of femur fractures may present a greater risk for refracture than other treatment methods because the stiff frame may delay consolidation and then is removed abruptly. The true risk for refracture is not known and may be no greater with external fixation than with other means. The only randomized trial comparing external fixators to casts found a 4% refracture rate with external fixators and 0% with casts, a difference that was not statistically significant given the numbers involved (level of evidence I).[25]

A retrospective comparative study of 66 femoral fractures treated with external fixation found 8 refractures (12%) and found that the risk for refracture was 33% if fewer than 3 cortices had bridging callus at the time of fixator removal compared with 4% if 3 or 4 cortices demonstrated bridging callus.[26] According to this level III evidence, the recommendation would be to leave external fixators in place until three or four cortices show bridging callus, to minimize the risk for refracture with this technique. Table 24–1 provides a summary of recommendations.

TABLE 24–1. Summary of Recommendations

STATEMENT	LEVEL OF EVIDENCE/GRADE OF RECOMMENDATION	REFERENCES
Weightbearing exercise and dietary calcium supplementation improve bone mass in female adolescents.	A	5, 6
Forearm fracture risk is greater during childhood among girls and boys with lower bone mineral density.	B	8, 9
Oral bisphosphonates reduce fracture risk and increase quality of life in patients with severe osteogenesis imperfecta.	A	10, 11
Intravenous bisphosphonates increase bone mineral density and decrease fractures in patients with severe osteogenesis imperfecta.	C	12–15
Inhaled steroids of more than 800 μg/day decrease bone mineral density in growing children.	B	20
Bisphosphonate plus calcium and vitamin D substantially improves bone mineral density among patients taking chronic oral steroids.	B	22
Forearm refractures in children are strongly associated with cast removal before 6 weeks.	B	24
Femoral refractures after external fixator removal are uncommon if three or four cortices have bridging callus at the time of fixator removal and more common if two or fewer cortices have bridging callus.	A,B	25, 26

REFERENCES

1. Murray C, Lopez A: Alternative projections of mortality and disability by cause 1990-2020: Global Burden of Disease Study. Lancet 349:1498–1504, 1997.
2. Krug EG, Sharma GK, Lozano R: The global burden of injuries. Am J Public Health 90:523–526, 2000.
3. Beveridge M, Howard A: The burden of orthopaedic disease in developing countries. J Bone Joint Surg Am 86-A:1819–1822, 2004.
4. Osteoporosis prevention, diagnosis, and therapy. NIH Consensus Statement. 17:1–45, 2000 consensus.nih.gov.
5. Matkovic V, Goel PK, Badenhop-Stevens NE, et al: Calcium supplementation and bone mineral density in females from childhood to young adulthood: A randomized controlled trial. Am J Clin Nutr 81:175–188, 2005.
6. Stear SJ, Prentice A, Jones SC, Cole TJ: Effect of a calcium and exercise intervention on the bone mineral status of 16–18-y-old adolescent girls. Am J Clin Nutr 77:985–992, 2003.
7. Valdimarsson O, Linden C, Johnell O, et al: Daily physical education in the school curriculum in prepubertal girls during 1 year is followed by an increase in bone mineral accrual and bone width—data from the prospective controlled Malmo pediatric osteoporosis prevention study. Calcif Tissue Int 78:65–71, 2006.
8. Goulding A, Jones IE, Taylor RW, et al: More broken bones: A 4-year double cohort study of young girls with and without distal forearm fractures. J Bone Miner Res 15:2011–2018, 2000.
9. Goulding A, Jones IE, Taylor RW, et al: Bone mineral density and body composition in boys with distal forearm fractures: A dual-energy x-ray absorptiometry study. J Pediatr 139:509–515, 2001.
10. Sakkers R, Kok D, Engelbert R, et al: Skeletal effects and functional outcome with olpadronate in children with osteogenesis imperfecta: A 2-year randomised placebo-controlled study. Lancet 363:1427–1431, 2004.
11. Seikaly MG, Kopanati S, Salhab N, et al: Impact of alendronate on quality of life in children with osteogenesis imperfecta. J Pediatr Orthop 25:786–791, 2005.
12. Grissom LE, Kecskemethy HH, Bachrach SJ, et al: Bone densitometry in pediatric patients treated with pamidronate. Pediatr Radiol 35:511–517, 2005.
13. DiMeglio LA, Ford L, McClintock C, Peacock M: Intravenous pamidronate treatment of children under 36 months of age with osteogenesis imperfecta. Bone 35:1038–1045, 2004.
14. Lee YS, Low SL, Lim LA, Loke KY: Cyclic pamidronate infusion improves bone mineralisation and reduces fracture incidence in osteogenesis imperfecta. Eur J Pediatr 160:641–644, 2001.
15. Glorieux FH, Bishop NJ, Plotkin H, et al: Cyclic administration of pamidronate in children with severe osteogenesis imperfecta. N Engl J Med 339:947, 1998.
16. Caulton JM, Ward KA, Alsop CW, et al: A randomised controlled trial of standing programme on bone mineral density in non-ambulant children with cerebral palsy. Arch Dis Child 89:131–135, 2004.

17. Bischof F, Basu D, Pettifor JM: Pathological long-bone fractures in residents with cerebral palsy in a long-term care facility in South Africa. Dev Med Child Neurol 44:119–122, 2002.

18. Sholas MG, Tann B, Gaebler-Spira D: Oral bisphosphonates to treat disuse osteopenia in children with disabilities: A case series. J Pediatr Orthop 25:326–331, 2005.

19. Plotkin H, Coughlin S, Kreikemeier R, et al: Low doses of pamidronate to treat osteopenia in children with severe cerebral palsy: A pilot study. Dev Med Child Neurol 48:709–712, 2006.

20. Harris M, Hauser S, Nguyen TV, et al: Bone mineral density in prepubertal asthmatics receiving corticosteroid treatment. J Paediatr Child Health 37:67–71, 2001.

21. El-Husseini AA, El-Agroudy AE, El-Sayed MF, et al: Treatment of osteopenia and osteoporosis in renal transplant children and adolescents. Pediatr Transplant 8:357–361, 2004.

22. Acott PD, Wong JA, Lang BA, Crocker JFS: Pamidronate treatment of pediatric fracture patients on chronic steroid therapy. Pediatr Nephrol 20:368–373, 2005.

23. Schwarz N, Pienaar S, Schwarz AF, et al: Refracture of the forearm in children. J Bone Joint Surg Br 78:740–744, 1996.

24. Bould M, Bannister GC: Refractures of the radius and ulna in children. Injury 30:583–586, 1999.

25. Wright JG, Wang EE, Owen JL, et al: Treatments for paediatric femoral fractures: A randomised trial. Lancet 365:1153–1158, 2005.

26. Skaggs DL, Leet AI, Money MD, et al: Secondary fractures associated with external fixation in pediatric femur fractures. J Pediatr Orthop 19:582–586, 1999.

Chapter 25

What Is the Best Treatment for Wrist Fractures?

ROBERT D. GALPIN, MD, FRCSC

Pediatric wrist fractures may be classified based on the level of injury and the degree of soft-tissue damage (Table 25–1). The level of injury may be physeal or metaphyseal. Physeal injuries may be further subdivided into Salter–Harris type I and II injuries. The literature demonstrates that the majority of physeal injuries at the wrist are Salter–Harris type II.[1] Metaphyseal fractures may be subdivided into torus (buckle fractures), greenstick, and complete fractures. Complete fractures may be angulated, translated, or completely displaced with shortening. Most wrist fractures in the pediatric age group are closed injuries. Open fractures, which indicate a greater degree of soft-tissue damage, may increase the risk for complications including loss of reduction, infection, and growth arrest.

An extensive review of recent English-speaking orthopedic literature from 1997–2007 was undertaken to identify areas of uncertainty and to determine the best evidence available to justify the current treatment of wrist fractures in the pediatric age group. This search identified five articles that reach evidence level I or II (*Journal of Bone and Joint Surgery* combined volumes [JBJS] Levels of Evidence for Primary Research Question).[2,3] Three of these five articles concern management of torus fractures of the distal radius.[4–6] Eleven more articles reached levels of evidence III and IV.

Torus Fractures

By definition, torus fractures are incomplete fractures with a failure of the cortex on the compression side of the bone. The convex (or tension side) cortex remains intact. These are stable injuries, and five articles support a minimalist approach to management of these injuries.[4–9]

Three randomized clinical trials addressed the subject of torus fractures. Davidson and colleagues[4] randomized 201 patients to treatment with a cast versus a removable "Futura-type" wrist splint for 3 weeks with no difference in outcome as measured by a mail-in questionnaire. Plint and coauthors[5] found similar results using a validated outcome tool—the Activities Scales for Kids performance version (ASKp). This study reported better functioning in the splint group, with less interference with bathing. Symons and coworkers[6] reviewed 87 patients

treated with splints to assess home management versus standard hospital follow-up. Forty patients who had their splints removed at home were compared with 47 patients treated by removal of the cast in the orthopedic clinic. Results were similar between the groups, but both groups, if given the choice, would prefer removal of the splint at home. Several authors believe there is no evidence that further follow-up is needed after splint removal.[4,6]

Several articles report cost savings with these minor injuries, because of fewer clinic and physician visits, fewer radiographs, and a reduction in family's time lost from school and work.[4,6–8]

In summary, this evidence-based literature demonstrates that buckle fractures of the distal radius can be managed with application of a splint in the emergency ward, followed by one orthopedic clinic visit to confirm the diagnosis. Support of the injured limb with a removable splint should continue for approximately 3 weeks, followed by removal of the splint in the home setting and initiation of self-administered range-of-motion exercises. Parental education in the emergency department and clinic, with a written description of expected course of management, results in uniformly good outcomes and high levels of patient satisfaction.

Displaced Fractures

After achievement of adequate analgesia, a closed reduction and immobilization of the wrist and forearm in a well-molded, short-arm plaster of Paris or fiberglass cast is the accepted treatment and standard of care for displaced fractures.[10,11] Analgesia in the emergency department may be in the form of intravenous regional anesthesia (Bier block) or intravenous sedation with narcotics and benzodiazepines. Numerous case report studies in the orthopaedic literature (levels of evidence IV and V) confirm the safety and efficacy of various techniques for regional or general pain control during fracture manipulation.[12]

Displacement Limits Postreduction

Limits on what is considered an acceptable reduction vary with the bone involved, the direction of displacement, and patient age. Remodeling after

TABLE 25–1. Classification of Pediatric Wrist Fractures

Physeal fractures
    Salter–Harris type 1
    Salter–Harris type 2
Metaphyseal fractures
    Torus
    Greenstick
    Complete
        Partial displacement
        Complete displacement
Open fractures

malunited wrist and distal forearm fractures in children is common and often dramatic. Price and researchers[10] have previously demonstrated the remodeling potential in malunited forearm fractures in childhood. Only six of their patients had distal third fractures, but they believed that "distal fractures have a more favorable prognosis" than diaphyseal injuries.[13] Do and colleagues[14] demonstrated in 34 pediatric metaphyseal wrist fractures that all healed within an average of 6 weeks and completely remodeled within an average of 7.5 months. They recommend that angulation in either plane (coronal or sagittal) of less than 15 degrees, and shortening of less than 1 cm, are acceptable limits and consistent with a normal functional outcome. They also demonstrated a significant cost saving (50%) compared with the patients who were managed with formal reduction and casting. Zimmermann and coauthors[15] have shown equal remodeling potential for dorsal and volar displaced wrist fractures.

The literature defining acceptable limits for displacement after reduction is, in the majority, level III (case–control study)[14-16] or IV (case series).[17,18] No randomized clinical trials (levels of evidence I and II) address this question, although most practicing pediatric orthopedic surgeons are inclined to accept up to 15 degrees of angulation in the sagittal plane and slightly less deformity in the coronal plane. Translation, especially in the coronal plane, with encroachment on the interosseus space is less likely to be accepted. Age of the patient is also an important parameter in determining limits of malreduction, recognizing the greater remodeling potential of the younger child. A randomized clinical trial

would be required to more definitively address the limits of acceptable displacement (amount and plane of deformity) that are consistent with good clinical outcomes, and how these limits are modified by the age of the patient.

Cast Treatment after Fracture Reduction

Immobilization in a short-arm cast will prevent loss of reduction as long as cast molding is adequate. Three articles confirm the cast index (the ratio of the cast dimension, at the level of the fracture, on the anteroposterior vs. lateral radiograph) as a predictor of loss of reduction.[10,11,15] Webb and investigators[10] demonstrate a direct correlation between higher cast indices (indicative of poor cast molding) and loss of reduction. This study also demonstrates that a well-molded short-arm cast is just as effective at maintaining reduction as long-arm casts for fractures in the wrist and distal third of the forearm. Short-arm casting also resulted in fewer lost school days and reduced need for assistance with activities of daily living.[10] Bhatia and researchers[1] demonstrated a further reduction in redisplacement rates by improvement in casting technique.

Indications for Open Reduction or Internal Fixation

Indications for open reduction of pediatric wrist fractures include failure to achieve or maintain an adequate closed reduction. For fractures with significant instability, which may not be held reduced with external cast immobilization, smooth pin fixation is indicated.[19] Although these principles are generally accepted in the orthopedic texts and literature, the levels of supporting evidence in the literature are generally no higher than level III or IV. One randomized clinical trial (level of evidence I) compared cast immobilization with percutaneous pin fixation for pediatric distal radius fractures. This was a small study (34 patients) that found a similar short-term complication rate with both methods of treatment, but the complications were different: patients with casts had a high rate of loss of reduction (39%), whereas the pinned patients developed pin tract problems (38%). At long-term follow-up, there were no differences in results between the treatment groups.[20]

TABLE 25–2. Summary of Recommendations

STATEMENT	LEVEL OF EVIDENCE/GRADE OF RECOMMENDATION	REFERENCES
1. There is *good* evidence supporting a minimalist approach to the management of torus fractures.	I, A II	3
2. There is *good* evidence that short-arm casts are adequate after closed reduction of distal third radius fractures providing the cast index is less than 0.8.	I, A	4, 5
3. There is *poor* evidence concerning how much displacement may be compatible with adequate radiographic and functional outcome.	IV, C	8, 9 1, 14, 15

Open Fractures

Grade 1 open wrist fractures are managed with conscious sedation, slight enlargement of the wound with adequate irrigation in the emergency department, followed by closed reduction and casting. A short course of antibiotics and early inspection of the wound result in low complication rates. Grade 2 and 3 open injuries with a greater degree of soft-tissue injury should be débrided in the operating room, with consideration given to delayed closure to reduce the risk for deep infection. Again, levels of supporting evidence in the literature, for management of open fractures, are levels III to IV.[16] Many years of clinical experience, and low complication rates in the level IV series, which do exist, support continuation of these management protocols. Table 25–2 provides a summary of recommendations for the treatment of wrist fractures.

REFERENCES

1. Bhatia M, Housden PH: Re-displacement of paediatric forearm fractures: Role of plaster moulding and padding [erratum appears in Injury. 2006 Aug;37(8):801]. Injury 37:259–268, 2006.
2. Bhandari M, Swiontkowski MF, Einhorn TA, et al: Interobserver agreement in the application of levels of evidence to scientific papers. J Bone Joint Surg Am 86:1717–1720, 2004.
3. Wright JG, Swiontkowski MF, Heckman JD: Introducing levels of evidence to the journal. J Bone Joint Surg Am 85:1–3, 2003.
4. Davidson JS, Brown DJ, Barnes SN, Bruce CE: Simple treatment for torus fractures of the distal radius. J Bone Joint Surg Br 83:1173–1175, 2001.
5. Plint AC, Perry JJ, Correll R, et al: A randomized, controlled trial of removable splinting versus casting for wrist buckle fractures in children. Pediatrics 117:691–697, 2006.
6. Symons S, Rowsell M, Bhowal B, Dias JJ: Hospital versus home management of children with buckle fractures of the distal radius. A prospective, randomised trial. J Bone Joint Surg Br 83:556–560, 2001.
7. Meier R, Prommersberger K-J, van Griensven M, Lanz U: Surgical correction of deformities of the distal radius due to fractures in pediatric patients. Arch Orthop Trauma Surg 124:1–9, 2004.
8. Solan MC, Rees R, Daly K: Current management of torus fractures of the distal radius. Injury 33:503–505, 2002.
9. Van Bosse HJP, Patel RJ, Thacker M, Sala DA: Minimalistic approach to treating wrist torus fractures. J Pediatr Orthop 25:495–500, 2005.
10. Webb GR, Galpin RD, Armstrong DG: Comparison of short and long arm plaster casts for displaced fractures in the distal third of the forearm in children. J Bone Joint Surg Am 88:9–17, 2006.
11. Bohm ER, Bubbar V, Yong Hing KY, Dzus A: Above and below-the-elbow plaster casts for distal forearm fractures in children. A randomized clinical trial. J Bone Joint Surg Am 88:1–8, 2006.
12. Colizza WA, Said E: Intravenous regional anesthesia in the treatment of forearm and wrist fractures and dislocations in children. Can J Surg 36:225–228, 1993.
13. Price CT, Scott DS, Kurzner ME, Flynn JC: Malunited forearm fractures in children. J Paediatr Orthop 10:705–712, 1990.
14. Do TT, Strub WM, Foad SL, et al: Reduction versus remodeling in pediatric distal forearm fractures: A preliminary cost analysis. J Pediatr Orthop Part B 12:109–115, 2003.
15. Zimmermann R, Gschwentner M, Pechlaner S, Gabl M: Remodeling capacity and functional outcome of palmarly versus dorsally displaced pediatric radius fractures in the distal one-third. Arch Orthop Trauma Surg 124:42–48, 2004.
16. Luhmann SJ, Schootman M, Schoenecker PL, et al: Complications and outcomes of open pediatric forearm fractures. J Pediatr Orthop 24:1–6, 2004.
17. Cannata G, De Maio F, Mancini F, Ippolito E: Physeal fractures of the distal radius and ulna: Long-term prognosis. J Orthop Trauma 17:172–180, 2003.
18. Kiely PD, Kiely PJ, Stephens MM, Dowling FE: Atypical distal radial fractures in children. J Pediatr Orthop B 13:202–205, 2004.
19. Choi KY, Chan WS, Lam TP, Cheng JC: Percutaneous Kirschner-wire pinning for severely displaced distal radial fractures in children. A report of 157 cases. J Bone Joint Surg Br 77:797–801, 1995.
20. Miller B, Taylor B, Widmann R, et al: Cast immobilization versus percutaneous pin fixation of displaced distal radius fractures in children: A prospective, randomized study. J Pediatr Orthop 25:490–494, 2005.

What Is the Best Treatment for Forearm Fractures?

Keith Noonan, MD and Rebecca Carl, MD

Fractures of the radius and ulna account for more than 40% of fractures treated in the United States. Forearm fractures are most common in the pediatric age group.[1] Because radius and ulna fractures are so common, orthopedic practitioners are comfortable managing this type of injury. Skeletally immature patients have the potential to remodel bone; therefore, children generally have good outcomes after forearm fractures. Even when bony remodeling is incomplete, children rarely have functional limitations as a result of these injuries. Price and colleagues[2] managed patients with malunion after forearm fractures and showed that 92% had an excellent or good result and none had a poor result. Although most orthopedists are well-versed in conventional algorithms for managing forearm fractures in children, recent studies have addressed some outstanding clinical questions regarding the subtleties of caring for these injuries.

TREATMENT OF BUCKLE FRACTURES

Buckle fractures of the distal radius are common in children. Traditionally, this type of fracture has been treated with a period of immobilization in a short-arm cast. True buckle fractures are not at risk for displacement, and many practitioners choose to put patients in a removable splint rather than in a cast. Several recent studies have compared casting and splinting in terms of patient comfort and satisfaction, risk for complications, and cost. These studies all illustrate that children with buckle fractures have excellent outcomes regardless of whether they are treated with a splint or with a cast.

Davidson and coworkers[3] surveyed specialists in England and found that 78% of emergency department doctors treated patients with distal radius buckle fractures with molded plaster splints. Orthopedic consultants/specialists tended to use casts. In addition, they randomized 201 patients with buckle fractures to treatment with a premade wrist splint or a short-arm plaster cast. All fractures were well-healed 3 weeks after injury without radiographic evidence of deformity. The follow-up rate was lower for patients who were splinted. A cost-benefit analysis showed that splint treatment was approximately half as expensive as cast treatment (assuming the splinted patients are not seen in follow-up).[3] In a randomized, controlled study by Plint and coworkers,[4] patients with distal

radius or ulna buckle fractures were treated with either a short-arm plaster cast or a molded plaster backslab/splint. Parents and patients were asked to fill out an activities questionnaire at weekly intervals for 4 weeks and to attend a follow-up visit at 3 weeks. Children who were treated with splints had an easier time with writing and bathing, and had an earlier return to activities. No complications occurred in either group; however, five children in the cast group required replacement of their casts.[4] West and investigators[5] performed a similar study in children with distal radius buckle fractures. They randomized 39 patients to treatment with a soft bandage or a cast. Investigators instructed patients in the former group to wean out of the bandage when they felt comfortable doing so. Bandaged patients regained wrist flexion and extension more quickly. No complications were reported in either treatment group.[5]

Conclusions

For many types of forearm fractures, casts offer the best protection from refracture and malunion. When treating patients with a buckle fracture, a physician's primary goal must be to protect the child from further injury. However, casts are not without risk and inconvenience. Risks of casting include skin breakdown and loss of motion. The studies presented earlier indicate that patients with buckle fractures may have improved comfort and ability to perform activities of daily living when treated with a splint. In addition, it may be possible to save time and costs and avoid radiation exposure by forgoing the follow-up visits in patients with forearm buckle fractures.

CAST TYPE AND POSITION

Many casting methods have been used to maintain the position of pediatric forearm fractures. Investigators have attempted to determine whether factors such as cast molding, forearm and elbow position, and extension of cast above the elbow influence the rate of fracture reangulation and thus outcome.

Cast index is the ratio of cast width on lateral radiograph to the width on anteroposterior (AP) radiograph. Chess and researchers[6] have identified 0.7 as the optimal cast index based on measurements of the pediatric forearm. This group performed a retrospective analysis of 558 distal third forearm fractures requiring closed reduction; patients were immobilized in short-arm casts. All of the patients with significant angulation had "poor cast molding"; unfortunately, this phrase was not clearly defined, nor did the examiners describe the criteria for remanipulation.[6] Bhatia and Housden[7] reviewed 144 charts retrospectively and followed 34 children prospectively. All patients had forearm fractures requiring closed reduction. They measured cast index and defined a padding index (ratio of padding diameter on lateral radiograph to interosseous space on AP radiograph). The authors looked for redisplacement 1 to 2 weeks after injury and defined this as angulation of greater than 20 degrees and/or translation greater than 50%. The mean padding index for the group with redisplacement was 0.42 compared with 0.11 for the group without redisplacement. The redisplacement group mean cast index was 0.87; the mean cast index for patients without redisplacement was 0.71. Both sets of findings were statistically significant with *P* values less than 0.005.[7]

Boyer and researchers[8] conducted a prospective trial randomizing 100 patients with distal third forearm fractures to be casted with the forearm in pronation, supination, or neutral position. One patient casted in supination and one casted in pronation had significant loss of reduction. In their study, cast index did not correlate with residual angulation at follow-up. Bochang and coworkers[9] managed one group of children with forearm fractures treated with the elbow in extension and compared them with a group at another center treated with flexed-elbow casting. In the flexed-elbow group, the rate of redisplacement was 17.6%. None of the children in the extended-elbow group had significant angulation on repeat radiographic examination. Other investigators who had looked at extended elbow casting in small retrospective studies also found low rates of redisplacement.[10,11]

Two prospective, controlled trials have compared long- and short-arm plaster casts for the treatment of distal forearm fractures. Bohm and investigators[12] randomized 102 skeletally immature children with displaced distal third forearm fractures randomized to be placed in a long- or a short-arm cast. Casts were well molded with an average cast index of 0.71. There was actually a greater rate of need for remanipulation in patients treated with long-arm cast; this difference was not statistically significant. Webb and researchers[13] had similar finding when they randomized 127 children with displaced distal third forearm fractures to be placed in short- versus long-arm casts. They found no difference in angulation or displacement at follow-up. Patients with long arm casts reported more difficulty in performing activities of daily living.

Conclusions

Proper molding of a plaster cast appears to decrease the need for future fracture manipulation, and it does not appear that casting in supination or pronation affords any advantage in distal fractures. Two well-constructed studies show that a below-the-elbow cast may be sufficient to prevent recurrence of angulation in children with displaced *distal* forearm fractures. In both of these studies, cast molding was optimal with cast indices averaging close to 0.7. This information may not apply to midshaft or proximal forearm fractures where little data exist to prove that short-arm casts are equivalent to the time-tested results from standard long-arm casting in these injuries. Casting with the elbow in extension may increase fracture stability. A well-randomized, prospective study is needed to examine this further.

SEDATION

Physicians have used many different techniques and medications to provide anesthesia for reducing forearm fractures in children. In the emergency department setting, anesthetic regimens must provide safe and effective analgesia and anxiolysis without a prolonged recovery time. Parents and patients often prefer deep sedation to local anesthesia because they feel more comfortable with the idea that they will be completely unaware of the fracture reduction or will have amnesia for the event. However, recent studies have shown that regional anesthesia methods such as hematoma and nerve blocks can be effective in children. These methods offer the advantage of quicker recovery times and decreased monitoring.

Luhmann and researchers[14] randomly assigned 102 children who required closed reduction of forearm fractures to receive either nitrous oxide (NO) and hematoma block or intravenous ketamine and midazolam. Videotapes of the fracture reduction were reviewed by an investigator and scored using a behavioral checklist. Both groups had low scores indicating good pain control, but pain scores were significantly lower for the group that received NO and a hematoma block ($P = 0.02$). Recovery time was less for children in the NO group. Children who received ketamine and midazolam had a greater rate of nightmares, hallucinations, and ataxia; otherwise, complication rates and side effects were similar.[14] In Evans and colleagues'[15] randomized, prospective study, children treated with NO had similar pain scores during fracture reduction as children who were given an intramuscular injection of meperidine and promethazine; the patients treated with NO were significantly more likely to report they would choose the same agent again for anesthesia. Gregory and Sullivan[16] compared NO sedation with Bier block and found no significant difference in pain scores. In their study, one Bier block failed because of accidental deflation of the blood pressure cuff.

Axillary nerve block is another alternative to deep sedation. Kriwanek and coauthors'[17] compared pain control in children receiving an axillary block and those treated with intravenous ketamine for forearm fracture reduction. Both groups of patients were given midazolam in this study. Examiners did not detect a significant difference in behavior scores between the two groups. However, two patients in the axillary block required supplemental anesthesia, and patient satisfaction was lower for this method.

Davidson and coworkers[18] compared prilocaine and lidocaine as intravenous agents for Bier block in 279 patients undergoing forearm fracture reduction. They found that 90% of patients who received lidocaine had no or minimal pain as opposed to 78% in the prilocaine group.

Conclusions

Many safe and effective protocols have been developed for delivering anesthesia to children undergoing fracture reduction. The availability of different types of specialists and individual hospital policies regarding sedation techniques often influence how analgesia is provided to children. The various studies presented highlight advantages and disadvantages of several types of anesthetic agents. Comparing anesthetic regimens is problematic because pain is subjective, and thus difficult to measure. Nonetheless, these studies demonstrate that regional anesthesia is a viable alternative to deep sedation. One major advantage to regional blocks is that they can be used in children who have recently eaten, obviating the need to wait until a patient has been nil per os (nothing by mouth) for a sufficient length of time.

FIXATION OF FRACTURES

Most pediatric forearm fractures are treated with casting with or without prior closed manipulation. Skeletally immature patients have the capacity to significantly remodel bone at the site of fractures. A certain degree of angular deformity and displacement are acceptable because of the known potential for bony remodeling. Jones and Weiner[19] retrospectively evaluated 730 children with forearm fractures and found that only 12 patients required fixation, indicating that the treatment of this type of fracture is usually nonsurgical. However, a subset of pediatric forearm fractures exists that are either irreducible or susceptible to redisplacement after reduction. These fractures will require some type of fixation. Because children rarely require intervention beyond closed reduction of their forearm fractures, there are no large, randomized trials comparing the various methods of fixation.

Several authors have published case series that illustrate that intramedullary fixation of forearm fractures generally yields excellent results. In these studies, complication rates, including neuropraxias, superficial and deep infections, refracture, lost reduction, and persistent angulation, range from 8% to 28%.[20-26] In two recent articles, authors have reported compartment syndrome as a complication of intramedullary fixation. Yuan and investigators[27] retrospectively analyzed data from 285 patients with forearm fractures. None of the 205 patients treated with closed reduction and casting experienced development of compartment syndrome. However, 6 of the 80 patients (7.5%) treated with intramedullary fixation experienced development of compartment syndrome; none of these patients had a high-velocity mechanism of injury. The increase in compartment syndrome rates for patients managed surgically was significant with a P value less than 0.001. Increased time in the operating room for fracture fixation was associated with a greater rate of compartment syndrome ($P = 0.01$).[27] Kapoor and colleagues[28] looked retrospectively at 50 children who underwent flexible intramedullary nailing of forearm fractures. Two patients in their series developed compartment syndrome; both of these patients had a high-energy mechanism of injury.

In two retrospective comparative studies, investigators compared elastic stable intramedullary nailing with Kirschner wire fixation in children with diaphyseal forearm fractures. No significant differences in complication rates were found, as would be expected in both of these intramedullary methods of fixation. In Majed and Bacos' study,[29] all patients had excellent functional outcomes. Calder and coauthors[30] found a clinically evident limitation in forearm rotation in 11% of their patients; however, they did not quantify range-of-motion measurements in their records.

Retrospective comparative studies have also been used to examine the difference in outcomes between patients who undergo intramedullary fixation versus plate fixation of their forearm fractures. Fernandez and researchers[31] reviewed records of 45 patients who underwent elastic stable intramedullary nailing of their middle-third and transitional zone forearm fractures, and compared the results with those of 19 patients who had plate fixation of their fractures. No significant difference in complication rates was found between the two groups. However, patients with plate fixation had longer hospital stays, longer time under anesthesia, and worse cosmetic results. Similarly, Van der Reis and colleagues[32] compared results from the charts of 23 patients who had Rush rod fixation of their diaphyseal both-bone forearm fractures with those of 18 patients whose fractures were fixed with plates. No significant difference was found in complication rates or functional outcomes. The authors did note that two patients in the intramuscular fixation group had mild rotational deformities; this type of deformity did not occur in any patients in the plate fixation group.[32]

Conclusions

Closed reduction and casting continues to be the mainstay of treatment for pediatric forearm fractures. In cases where closed manipulation fails to maintain fracture fragments in an adequate alignment, internal fixation must be considered. Both

TABLE 26–1. Summary of Recommendations

STATEMENT	LEVEL OF EVIDENCE/GRADE OF RECOMMENDATION	REFERENCES
1. Buckle fractures can be safely treated with either removable splints or short-arm casts.	A	3–5
2. Well-molded casts decrease rate of fracture reangulation in displaced forearm fractures.	B	7
3. Well-molded short-arm casts are equivalent to long-arm casts in maintaining reduction of displaced distal forearm fractures.	A	12, 13
4. Casting with the elbow in extension is superior to casting in flexion for maintaining reduction in patients with displaced forearm fractures.	B	9–11
5. Intramedullary fixation and plate fixation have similar acceptable complication rates. Anesthesia times and scarring are minimized with intramedullary fixation.	B	31, 32
6. Regional anesthesia offers comparable analgesia with systemic, deep sedation.	B	14–16

intramedullary and plate fixation can be performed safely. Intramedullary fixation offers the advantages of shorter time under anesthesia and better cosmetic results. Currently, a large prospective study comparing the two methods has not been conducted. Table 26–1 provides a summary of recommendations for the treatment of forearm fractures.

REFERENCES

1. Chung KC, Spilson SV: The frequency and epidemiology of hand and forearm fractures in the United States. J Hand Surg [Am] 26:908–915, 2001.
2. Price CT, Scott DS, Kurzner ME, Flynn JC: Malunited forearm fractures in children. J Pediatr Orthop 10:705–712, 1990.
3. Davidson JS, et al: Simple treatment for torus fractures of the distal radius. J Bone Joint Surg Br 83:1173–1175, 2001.
4. Plint AC, et al: A randomized, controlled trial of removable splinting versus casting for wrist buckle fractures in children. Pediatrics 117:691–697, 2006.
5. West S, et al: Buckle fractures of the distal radius are safely treated in a soft bandage: A randomized prospective trial of bandage versus plaster cast. J Pediatr Orthop 25:322–325, 2005.
6. Chess DG, et al: Short arm plaster cast for distal pediatric forearm fractures. J Pediatr Orthop 14:211–213, 1994.
7. Bhatia M, Housden PH: Re-displacement of paediatric forearm fractures: Role of plaster moulding and padding. Injury 37:259–268, 2006.
8. Boyer BA, et al: Position of immobilization for pediatric forearm fractures. J Pediatr Orthop 22:185–187, 2002.
9. Bochang C, Jie Y, Zhigang W, et al: Immobilisation of forearm fractures in children. Extended versus flexed elbow. J Bone Joint Surg Br 87:994–996, 2005.
10. Shaer JA, Smith B, Turco VJ: Mid-third forearm fractures in children: An unorthodox treatment. Am J Orthop 28:60–63, 1999.
11. Walker JL, Rang M: Forearm fractures in children. Cast treatment with the elbow extended. J Bone Joint Surg Br 73:299–301, 1991.
12. Bohm ER, Bubbar V, Yong Hing K, Dzus A: Above and below-the-elbow plaster casts for distal forearm fractures in children. A randomized controlled trial. J Bone Joint Surg Am 88:1–8, 2006.
13. Webb GR, Galpin RD, Armstrong DG: Comparison of short and long arm plaster casts for displaced fractures in the distal third of the forearm in children. J Bone Joint Surg Am 88:9–17, 2006.
14. Luhmann JD, et al: A randomized comparison of nitrous oxide plus hematoma block versus ketamine plus midazolam for emergency department forearm fracture reduction in children. Pediatrics 118:e1078–e1086, 2006.
15. Evans JK, et al: Analgesia for the reduction of fractures in children: A comparison of nitrous oxide with intramuscular sedation. J Pediatr Orthop 15:73–77, 1995.
16. Gregory PR, Sullivan JA: Nitrous oxide compared with intravenous regional anesthesia in pediatric forearm fracture manipulation. 16:187–191, 1996.
17. Kriwanek KL, Wan J, Beaty JH, Pershad J: Axillary block for analgesia during manipulation of forearm fractures in the pediatric emergency department: A prospective randomized comparative trial. J Pediatr Orthop 26:737–740, 2006.
18. Davidson AJ, Eyres RL, Cole WG: A comparison of prilocaine and lidocaine for intravenous regional anaesthesia for forearm fracture reduction in children. Paediatr Anaesth 12:1 46–150, 2002.
19. Jones K, Weiner DS: The management of forearm fractures in children: A plea for conservatism. J Pediatr Orthop 19:811–815, 1999.
20. Flynn JM, Waters PM: Single-bone fixation of both-bone forearm fractures. J Pediatr Orthop 16:655–659, 1996.
21. Qidwai SA: Treatment of diaphyseal forearm fractures in children by intramedullary Kirschner wires. J Trauma 50:303–307, 2001.
22. Shoemaker SD, et al: Intramedullary Kirschner wire fixation of open or unstable forearm fractures in children. J Pediatr Orthop 19:329–337, 1999.
23. Yung PS, et al: Percutaneous transphyseal intramedullary Kirschner wire pinning: A safe and effective procedure for treatment of displaced diaphyseal forearm fracture in children. J Pediatr Orthop 24:7–12, 2004.
24. Cullen MC, et al: Complications of intramedullary fixation of pediatric forearm fractures. J Pediatr Orthop 18:14–21, 1998.
25. Kucukkaya M, et al: The application of open intramedullary fixation in the treatment of pediatric radial and ulnar shaft fractures. J Orthop Trauma 16:340–344, 2002.
26. Lascombes P, et al: Elastic stable intramedullary nailing in forearm shaft fractures in children: 85 cases. J Pediatr Orthop 10:167–171, 1990.
27. Yuan PS, Pring ME, Gaynor TP, et al: Compartment syndrome following intramedullary fixation of pediatric forearm fractures. J Pediatr Orthop 24:370–375, 2004.
28. Kapoor V, Theruvil B, Edwards SE, et al: Flexible intramedullary nailing of displaced diaphyseal forearm fractures in children. Injury 36:1221–1225, 2005.
29. Majed A, Baco AM: Nancy nail versus intramedullary-wire fixation of paediatric forearm fractures. J Pediatr Orthop B 16:129–132, 2007.
30. Calder PR, Achan P, Barry M: Diaphyseal forearm fractures in children treated with intramedullary fixation: Outcome of K-wire versus elastic stable intramedullary nail. Injury 34:278–282, 2003.
31. Fernandez FF, et al: Unstable diaphyseal fractures of both bones of the forearm in children: Plate fixation versus intramedullary nailing. Injury 36:1210–1216, 2005.
32. Van der Reis WL, et al: Intramedullary nailing versus plate fixation for unstable forearm fractures in children. J Pediatr Orthop 18:9–13, 1998.

How Should We Treat Elbow Fractures in Children?

Andrew Howard, MD, MSc, FRCSC

Fractures of the child's elbow are a touchstone of pediatric orthopedics, and often the heaviest contributor to operative emergency lists. The relatively low level of evidence in the literature belies a relatively large clinical load, a high level of comfort, and confidence among pediatric orthopedic surgeons, and fulfilled high expectations of good results from patients. Many principles and tenets of pediatric orthopedic practice have not been tested or proved scientifically, and many never will be. For example, the common practice of closed reduction and pinning for displaced supracondylar fractures is based on Level III evidence[1]; yet, there is little expectation that Level I or II evidence comparing pinning with flexion strapping or casting is desirable or forthcoming, the latter treatment methods having been largely abandoned. Is there a problem with this? Perhaps there is.

Pediatric orthopedic surgeons view the world from their own perspective. In urban centers in North America, a high likelihood exists that many children will have access to a pediatric orthopedic surgeon for the primary care of selected fractures, including many operative elbow traumas. Outside this setting, primary fracture care is undertaken by general orthopedic surgeons. Childhood fractures are so common that appropriate care of the injured child, globally speaking, must not rely on the pediatric orthopedic surgeon. The decisions to be made in the care of children's fractures should be able to be made by any trained surgeon with access to the literature.

This chapter considers the English language literature describing management of fractures around the child's elbow. It does not adhere strictly to a "level of evidence" hierarchy because I believe that a large, carefully done, retrospective study can be deservedly more influential in practice than a small randomized trial with methodologic problems—not that either represents the ideal. Specifically, I have intended to comment on all randomized or prospective (Level I or II) evidence related to the topic, have selectively included retrospective comparative (Level III) or case series (Level IV) evidence where I believe it makes an important contribution, and have ignored large volumes of Level III zand IV evidence, which I do not use in my practice.

SUPRACONDYLAR FRACTURES: ACUTE TREATMENT

Closed Reduction and Percutaneous Pinning

Level III evidence has been instrumental in defining closed reduction and percutaneous pinning as the current treatment for displaced supracondylar fractures. The first such comparative study, in 1979 by Prietto,[2] retrospectively compared 27 patients treated with Dunlop's traction (at one hospital) with 20 patients treated with closed reduction and percutaneous pin fixation. Clinical "gunstock" varus malunion occurred in 9 of 27 patients treated with traction (33%) and 1 of 20 patients with percutaneous pinning (5%). Mean hospital stay was 17 days for the traction group and 3 for the pinned group. Complications were low, and functional results were good in each group.

A much larger retrospective comparative study (Level III evidence) was published in 1988.[1] A total of 325 patients with displaced extension supracondylar fractures were treated by 1 of 4 methods, and 230 returned for late review. Treatments compared were closed reduction and casting (130), closed reduction and percutaneous K-wire fixation (78), traction (15), or open reduction and internal fixation (7). Among 130 patients initially treated with a flexion cast, 29 had the treatment discontinued because of problems with forearm circulation; 14 had varus malunion, of whom 8 had osteotomies, 6 had loss of motion, and 1 experienced development of a Volkmann's ischemic contracture. Among 78 patients treated with K wires primarily plus 18 converted from casting to K-wire fixation, there were 3 varus malunions, of whom 1 had an osteotomy, 2 had loss of motion, and no patients had ischemia of muscle, although several had an initially absent radial pulse with an otherwise well-perfused hand. Pin placement was crossed medial and lateral pins in 47, and 2 lateral pins in 49 patients. No pin-related nerve complications with either placement were reported, and there were two superficial pin infections. About 78% of patients in the pinning group had both the carrying angle and range of motion within five degrees of the contralateral side at final follow-up; this was true of only 51% of the patients in the group treated with casts. The series was neither randomized nor prospective, and only 230 of 325 potential patients returned for a late review. Among those reviewed, the outcomes were much better and the complication rates lower in the closed reduction and percutaneous pinning group, and this remains the best available evidence supporting this practice. In summary, a large, well-done, retrospective cohort study (Level III evidence) supports closed reduction and percutaneous pinning of all displaced supracondylar fractures over closed reduction and plaster immobilization.

Crossed Pins or Lateral Entry Pins

A large retrospective series (Level III evidence) was published in 2001[3] comparing the results of lateral pins versus crossed pins in 345 displaced extension-type supracondylar fractures. The configuration of the pins did not affect the maintenance of reduction. Fracture displacement was noted on 4% (4/103) of radiographs where lateral pins were used, 3% (4/120) where crossed pins were applied without hyperflexion, and 2% (1/58) where crossed pins were applied with hyperflexion. Ulnar nerve injury was not seen in the 125 patients in whom only lateral pins were used. The use of a medial pin was associated with ulnar nerve injury in 4% (6) of 149 patients in whom the pin was applied without hyperflexion of the elbow and in 15% (11) of 71 in whom the medial pin was applied with the elbow hyperflexed. Because the maintenance of reduction was equal with lateral or crossed pins, but the ulnar nerve injury rate was greater with crossed pins, the authors conclude that lateral pins alone provide adequate fixation. Two smaller Level III comparative studies had reached this conclusion previously.[4,5] A subsequent prospective Level IV study[6] reports on 124 consecutive unselected displaced supracondylar fractures with no loss of reduction and no nerve injuries using lateral entry pins only, 2 pins for more stable, and 3 pins for less stable fracture patterns.

Two Level I studies (prospective, randomized trials) have since been performed addressing the question of lateral pins versus crossed pins.[7,8] Both trials were small. The first trial, with good methodologic quality, found no differences in minor loss of reduction (1/24 crossed, 6/28 lateral), ulnar nerve injury (none), or major loss of reduction (none).[7] The second trial, with less complete description of the methodologic issues, had 5 ulnar nerve injuries among 34 patients with crossed pins, and 2 ulnar nerve and 1 radial nerve injuries among 32 patients with lateral entry pins.[8] Although these are Level I studies, which remove selection bias, the small number of patients does not allow a precise estimation of the rate of rare events such as nerve injuries or loss of reduction. A systematic review pooling all data from previously published case and comparative series reports an iatrogenic nerve injury rate of 1.9% for lateral entry pins and 3.5% for crossed pins (among 1909 patients), and a loss of reduction rate of 0.7% for lateral entry pins and 0% for crossed pins (among 1455 patients).[9] Evidence from the Level I studies alone is insufficient to decide about treatment because the series are

small relative to the expected outcome rate, and because one of the studies had a high complication rate inconsistent with the rest of the literature.

One Level III retrospective study used a case–control design to analyze anatomic details of the medial pin placement comparing 18 patients with ulnar nerve injury with 72 patients without injury.[10] The medial pin was inserted with much more anterior to posterior angulation (12.1 ± 11.7 degrees) in the group with ulnar nerve injuries compared with the group without (1.6 ± 11.0 degrees). Although this article gives some guidance on how to place a medial pin, the authors mention in the discussion that they have abandoned routine use of the medial pin in favor of lateral entry pinning, which was not discussed.

A final Level III retrospective study used a case–control design comparing 8 fractures that lost fixation with 271 that remained well reduced.[11] In each case with lost fixation, a technical error of initial pin placement was (retrospectively) identified: single pins in the distal fragment, lack of bicortical purchase, and lack of 2 mm separation of pins at the fracture site.

Although a larger Level I study could be suggested, a practical interpretation of the current literature is that lateral pinning is preferred (based on Level III and IV evidence and one good but small Level I study) because the loss of reduction is low in large, prospective, consecutive and retrospective, comparative series, and because we may value prevention of iatrogenic nerve injuries more highly than reduction of a low malunion rate.

Open Reduction versus Closed Reduction

Open reduction has been used selectively for closed supracondylar fractures that are "irreducible" and are mentioned in many series, but with no standard definition of "irreducible" or indeed of an acceptable reduction, it is difficult to judge what is being compared. One article[12] compares a policy of primary open reduction of 44 consecutive patients with a policy of closed reduction and pinning in 55 subsequent patients treated at the same institution (Level III evidence). Although the open reduction group was observed longer (35 vs. 21 months), more patients in the open reduction group were stiff at final follow-up examination (38%) than in the closed reduction group (20%), defining stiffness as 10 degrees or more loss of motion compared with the other side. No differences were reported in infections (three open, two closed) or ulnar nerve lesions (two open, two closed). The authors conclude that closed reduction with percutaneous pinning is preferable to a routine policy of open reduction.

Flexion Supracondylar Fractures

Flexion supracondylar fractures are much less common than extension-type injuries and have been thought to be less stable and more difficult to reduce because the posterior periosteum is torn at the fracture site with a flexion injury. A retrospective comparative cohort (Level III) from a single center found the rate of flexion injuries to be 3%, and reported 31% open reductions for flexion injuries compared with 10% for extension injuries and 19% preoperative ulnar nerve symptoms for flexion injuries compared with 3% for extension injuries.[13]

Pulseless Hand

Two case series from 1996 drew opposite conclusions from similar clinical material regarding the pulseless pink hand. The first was a case series of seven patients with a pulseless arm, all of whom had a "seemingly viable" hand after closed reduction and pinning, were treated by arterial exploration with vein grafting[3] or microdissection vessel mobilization,[4] and did well at follow-up.[14] The authors of this first study recommend routine arterial exploration and repair for a pulseless but viable hand.

A larger case series of 22 children with a supracondylar fracture and an absent radial pulse on admission included 15 with a well-perfused hand after closed reduction and K-wire fixation, of whom 5 had no radial pulse. All patients with a well-perfused hand were treated with observation, including the five without a pulse, and none had any clinical circulatory problems at follow-up examination. Seven patients who had a cold white hand after closed reduction of the fracture underwent arterial exploration with or without repair. The authors conclude that routine exploration of the brachial artery is unnecessary in the circumstance of a pink, perfused hand with an absent radial pulse after closed treatment of a supracondylar fracture.[15]

One year later, a case series of 13 patients with pulseless, pink hands treated by closed with or without open[10] reductions and various vascular treatments including vein patch angioplasty[4] was published and included more information on the fate of the vessel using follow-up magnetic resonance angiography. Late magnetic resonance angiograms obtained on 10 patients showed occlusion or restenosis at the brachial artery in 5 patients, including 2 of 3 who had had a successful vein patch. Collateral flow was excellent in all arms with brachial artery compromise on magnetic resonance angiography, all patients had a palpable radial pulse on follow-up examination, and no patient had claudication or cold intolerance. Based on this experience, the authors recommend close observation instead of immediate invasive treatment for pink, viable hands without a radial pulse after reduction because regardless of repairing the vessel in the short term, arms were reliant on collateral circulation over the long term anyway, and none had poor clinically results.[16]

The pulseless, pink hand is rare enough that case series (Level IV) evidence is all that is present in the literature. Although routine exploration had a good outcome in one series, observation had an equally good outcome in another, and the fate of repaired vessels (restenosis) described in the third series, on balance, allows a conclusion that currently the pulseless, pink hand should be treated by observation, with vascular interventions reserved for cold, white hands. This conclusion is based on Level IV evidence.

Timing of Treatment

Several retrospective cohort studies (Level III evidence) have compared early (<8 hours after presentation) versus late (>8 hours after presentation) treatment of closed supracondylar fractures without vascular compromise. The first of these was published in 2001[17] and showed no difference in complications, no compartment syndromes in either group, and equal low rates of conversion to open reduction, pin infections, and iatrogenic nerve injuries among 52 patients treated at less than 8 hours compared with 146 patients treated at more than 8 hours. The recommendation from the article was that treatment of closed supracondylar fractures without vascular compromise could be delayed beyond 8 hours without compromising patient outcome. Similar findings and conclusions came from subsequent Level III studies[18,19] showing no differences in position at healing either. A single Level III study drew the opposite conclusion comparing 126 patients treated less than 8 hours after presentation who had an 11.2% open reduction rate, with 45 patients treated more than 8 hours after presentation who had a 33% open reduction rate.[20] The overall open reduction rate in the latter article is much greater than that suggested in the general literature; without well-defined criteria for performing an open reduction, it is an imperfect measure of outcome. In summary, the balance of the Level III evidence suggests that patients with closed fractures without vascular compromise have equivalent outcomes whether the surgery is performed immediately or is delayed beyond 8 hours after presentation.

Physical Therapy

A randomized study with blinded outcome assessment (Level I) compared 22 patients treated with physiotherapy (30 minutes 3 times per week, passive stretching plus active exercises) with 21 patients not receiving physiotherapy. There was about 10 degrees more flexion-extension range at 12 and 18 weeks in the physiotherapy group, but no difference at 1 year. The authors conclude that postoperative physical therapy is unnecessary for routine care.[21]

VARUS MALUNIONS OF SUPRACONDYLAR FRACTURES

The most common late complication of supracondylar fractures treated surgically is varus malunion, also known as "gunstock" deformity for its characteristic appearance. The deformity occurs readily in untreated fractures because the narrow fracture surface seen on the lateral means instability with any rotation, and the tendency is for the distal fragment to internally rotate, then tip into varus. A variety of osteotomies has been described to treat the cosmetic deformity of a supracondylar fracture healed in varus, and two comparative studies describe the results of these osteotomies.

The first study describes itself as a randomized trial,[22] but patients were treated with one of two osteotomies in alternation, so true randomization did not occur and the study is best categorized as Level II evidence. Treatments compared were the French technique and a dome osteotomy. The French technique used a lateral closing wedge osteotomy with an intact medial hinge that was closed by tightening a wire around unicortical screws above and below the osteotomy. The dome osteotomy was complete and was stabilized temporarily with an external fixator, then definitively with crossed Kirschner wires. Both osteotomies adequately corrected the carrying angle and had similar cosmetic results. Complications were greater in the dome group. Elbow stiffness was seen in 2 of 13 patients with the French osteotomy and 5 of 12 with the dome. Correction was reported as inadequate in 2 of 13 patients with the French osteotomy and 1 of 12 with the dome. The dome group also had one infection, one nerve palsy, and one vascular complication. The authors report that the dome osteotomy was more technically difficult and had a greater complication rate, and recommended use of the French technique.

A prior Level III study had compared the French technique with fixation with Kirschner wires or a plaster cast and had reported better cosmetic results and fewer complications with the French technique,[23] although numbers were small in all groups. In summary, Level II and III evidence supports the use of the French technique of supracondylar osteotomy to treat varus malunion.

LATERAL CONDYLE FRACTURES: ACUTE TREATMENT

Acute treatment of lateral condyle fractures is based on the fact that this fracture can go on to nonunion if left untreated; however, this is rare for children's fractures. A chronic nonunion of the lateral humeral epicondyle can lead to progressive valgus deformity of the elbow and a delayed-onset (many years) ulnar nerve palsy.

Diagnosis of Displacement

The degree of fracture displacement is considered important in the treatment of lateral condyle fractures but can be difficult to judge on plain radiographs. A prospective cohort (Level II evidence) showed that the internal oblique radiograph was more sensitive than a plain anteroposterior radiograph at detecting displacement in 30 of 54 patients.[24] Both sonography and magnetic resonance imaging (MRI) have been suggested as adjuncts to plain radiographs, particularly where plain radiographs show minimal or no displacement. In this circumstance, a fracture with an intact articular cartilage hinge might be treated with immobilization, whereas a complete fracture might be treated with percutaneous pinning. High-resolution sonography showed intact cartilage hinge in four of six patients, none of whom had subsequent displacement on plain radiographs after nonoperative management, and showed fracture through the joint cartilage in two of six children with confirmation by MRI or intraoperative findings.[25] A larger study used MRI on 16 patients, 12 of whom had plain radiograph displacement of less than 3 mm. Of those 12 patients, 10 had intact joint cartilage on MRI, and none displaced; 2 had broken joint cartilage, and 1 displaced. The authors conclude that MRI was useful in identifying stable fracture patterns with intact joint cartilage.[26] Similar use of the MRI had been reported previously.[27] In conclusion, Level II evidence exists that internal oblique radiographs are more sensitive at detecting displacement than anteroposterior radiographs. For undisplaced fractures, Level IV evidence has been reported that MRI is useful in confirming an intact joint cartilage, in which case the fracture would not be expected to displace with immobilization alone.

Undisplaced or Minimally Displaced Fractures

A retrospective, comparative series (Level III evidence) describes 30 fractures with initial displacement of less than 2 mm, of which 17 were treated in a long arm cast and 13 were treated with closed or open K-wire stabilization.[28] Of 17 treated in a cast, 5 displaced, 4 of these required later surgery, and at final follow-up, there were 2 nonunions and 2 malunions. Of the 13 patients treated operatively, 2 lost reduction and had malunions; there were no nonunions.

A larger case series (Level IV) reported on 95 fractures treated without surgery for initial displacements less than 2 mm; 93 healed with plaster immobilization, and 2 displaced and were treated with open K-wires and healed.[29]

It is difficult to reconcile a larger case series with almost uniformly good outcome from immobilization of minimally displaced fractures and a smaller retrospective comparative study with better results after operative stabilization of minimally displaced fractures. The treatment articles did not use MRI to diagnose the potentially stable fractures as suggested in the diagnostic literature; perhaps subsequent articles that base treatment decisions on more sophisticated diagnostic techniques will allow differentiation of the potentially unstable fracture and will resolve the controversy.

Displaced Fractures

The retrospective comparative series described earlier (Level III evidence)[28] included 67 displaced fractures, of which 10 were treated without surgery despite an initial displacement of 2 mm or more. These 10 fractures had been initially deemed undisplaced or minimally displaced by the treating surgeons but were reclassified as displaced more than 2 mm on review. Of these 10, 4 displaced farther and 2 were treated with surgery; at healing, 5 healed adequately, 3 were nonunions, and 2 were malunited. By comparison, among the other 57 displaced fractures initially treated with surgery, 4 displaced, 1 was revised, and 5 malunions and no nonunions occurred.

A retrospective comparison of the clinical and radiographic outcomes after open reduction compared 12 displaced fractures with anatomic position after treatment with 10 with 2 to 6 mm of residual displacement.[30] Among 10 patients with residual displacement, 9 experienced development of a radiographic "fishtail" deformity indicating growth disturbance in the central physis, and 2 had marked restriction of flexion/extension. Among 12 with anatomic reduction, there were no radiographic deformities seen and none had stiff elbows.

A larger case series (Level IV evidence) showed 1 nonunion among 104 displaced lateral condyle fractures treated with open reduction and 3 weeks of K-wire immobilization,[31] suggesting that this time period is adequate for healing of operatively stabilized fractures. Although the evidence is of lower quality, a consistent recommendation for accurate reduction and K-wire immobilization of displaced lateral condyle fractures can be made.

MEDIAL EPICONDYLE FRACTURES: ACUTE TREATMENT

Controversy exists regarding whether medial epicondyle fractures require operative reduction and stabilization, or whether they can be treated closed. Most authors consider a medial epicondyle irreducibly trapped within the joint as a definite indication for open reduction. Beyond that, disagreement exists regarding what degree of displacement (if any) warrants open reduction and internal fixation.

A long-term comparative series (level III evidence) compared three treatments: closed treatment, open reduction and internal fixation, and primary excision of the epicondyle. Follow-up periods averaged 33 years (30–61 years). Among 19 patients treated with long arm casting, 17 had a nonunion radiographically. All had stable elbows to valgus stress testing, and two had minor symptoms related to the elbow. Among 17 patients treated with open reduction and internal fixation, all had radiographic union, all were stable, and three had minor symptoms. Among six patients treated with excision of the epicondylar fragment, four had constant pain, ulnar paraesthesias, and an unstable elbow. The authors conclude that despite a high rate of radiographic

nonunion, the functional results suggest that nonoperative management was recommended for medial epicondyle fractures displaced 5 to 15 mm. Excision of the fragment should be avoided because results are poor.[32]

A second retrospective comparative study (Level III evidence) reviewed 43 children 2 to 5 years after open[23] or closed[20] management of displaced medial epicondyle fractures and also concluded that closed management was preferred. Bony union was seen in 87% of those treated surgically and 55% of those treated closed, but 39% of those treated surgically had ongoing symptoms (pain, stiffness) at the elbow at medium-term follow-up compared with 5% of those treated without surgery.[33]

In summary, the comparative series show better results for those patients treated without surgery, but the evidence is only Level III (retrospective), and given the strong possibility of selection bias (i.e., operations performed more often for patients in a poorer prognostic group to begin with), it is entirely possible, though unproven, that there is a group of patients who may benefit from open management.

RADIAL NECK FRACTURES: ACUTE TREATMENT

Radial neck fractures best exemplify the pervasive selection bias in operative versus nonoperative retrospective cohorts. In 1978, a retrospective cohort (Level III evidence) observed 43 children with radial neck fractures for 8 years (range, 1–18 years).[34] Among 23 patients treated without surgery, 19 had a "good" outcome, and among 14 treated with surgery, only 5 had a "good" outcome. However, among those treated without surgery, only 1 had an initial displacement greater than 60 degrees, whereas among 14 treated with surgery, 7 had an initial displacement greater than 60 degrees.[34] Such a cohort allows us to recommend nonoperative treatment for less severe fractures but does not help with treatment decisions on more severe fractures because we do not know whether to ascribe the bad outcomes to the severity of the fracture or to the operative intervention.

A later retrospective cohort study (Level III evidence) reported on 100 patients treated by immobilization, closed reduction, or open reduction, and again found a disappointingly large number of painful, stiff elbows among those treated with open reductions compared with better results with closed reduction or no reduction.[35] Again, this cohort can only suggest how to treat the less severe fractures because the poor results in the more severe fractures may be related to the severity of the injury or to the operation itself.

Avoiding open dissection of this fracture avoids both capsular stiffness and potential damage to the blood supply of the radial head; thus, recent literature has focused on operative reduction and fixation techniques for severely displaced fractures that avoid incisions and capsular dissections where possible.

TABLE 27–1. Summary of Recommendations

STATEMENT	LEVEL OF EVIDENCE/GRADE OF RECOMMENDATION	REFERENCES
Supracondylar Fractures		
Closed reduction and lateral entry percutaneous pinning is acceptable initial treatment for displaced supracondylar fractures.	A	7
Closed reduction and lateral entry percutaneous pinning is the preferred initial treatment for displaced supracondylar fractures.	B, C	1, 3–6
A viable, pulseless hand after closed reduction and percutaneous pinning can be treated by observation rather than routine arterial exploration.	C	15, 16
Surgical treatment of closed supracondylar fractures without vascular compromise may be delayed 8 hours or more after presentation without increasing complications.	B	17–19
Varus malunion after supracondylar fracture is best treated with the French osteotomy.	B	22, 23
Lateral Condyle Fractures		
Cast treatment or percutaneous pinning can be used for undisplaced lateral condyle fractures.	B, C	28, 29
Accurate open reduction and pinning is the preferred treatment for displaced lateral condyle fractures.	B, C	28, 30, 31
Medial Epicondyle Fractures		
Displaced medial epicondyle fractures treated operatively have a greater rate of fracture union and a greater rate of pain, stiffness, or other symptoms compared with those treated without surgery.	B (probable selection bias)	32, 33
Radial Neck Fractures		
Radial neck fractures treated by no reduction or closed reduction have less pain, stiffness, and complications than those treated by open reductions.	B (probable selection bias)	34, 35
Most displaced radial neck fractures can be successfully reduced by percutaneous K-wire manipulation.	C	36
Displaced radial neck fractures that can be reduced by closed or percutaneous techniques can be stabilized by intramedullary titanium nails with good outcomes.	C	37, 38

In 1992, a case series (Level IV evidence) of 36 consecutive fractures displaced more than 30 degrees reported 33 successful reductions using a percutaneous K-wire technique, of which 31 had full motion at follow-up examination.[36] No internal fixation was used to maintain the reduction. Subsequent case series combining closed or percutaneous reduction with stabilization by a flexible intramedullary nail introduced through the distal radial metaphysic have reported similarly good results.[37,38] The consensus in the recent literature indicates that closed or percutaneous reduction techniques, perhaps supplemented by intramedullary fixation, generally gives good results *where it is possible*. The bias in the recent literature is that the cases are selected and reported based on the success of the technique; therefore, although we may be whittling away at the group of potential bad outcomes with perhaps a more sophisticated set of tools, we still have little information about the results of all badly displaced fractures, including those (if any) that cannot be reduced by the means described. Furthermore, the case series described earlier cannot inform us when, if ever, intramedullary fixation is required to supplement closed or percutaneous reduction.

SUMMARY

Table 27–1 summarizes the literature on elbow fractures around common clinical presentations or questions. Little controversy exists surrounding closed reduction and pinning as the main treatment for supracondylar fractures, or open reduction and pinning as the main treatment for displaced lateral condyle fractures. The current state of the literature, however, does not allow us to confidently assert whether pinning or cast treatment is better for undisplaced lateral condyle fractures, which are common. In addition, displaced medial epicondyle fractures may be treated open or closed depending on the trade-off between radiographic union and residual symptoms. The literature regarding treatment of radial neck fractures is fraught with bias. However, it is fairly clear that avoiding open operations is likely to lead to better patient outcomes. More recent literature arms us with percutaneous reduction and fixation techniques that have good results when they can be applied successfully. Little in the literature addresses the preferred treatment of pediatric elbow trauma in settings devoid of c-arms and Kirschner wires, even though such settings are the reality of most of the children in the world.

REFERENCES

1. Pirone AM, Graham HK, Krajbich JI: Management of displaced extension-type supracondylar fractures of the humerus in children. J Bone Joint Surg Am 70:641–650, 1988.
2. Prietto CA: Supracondylar fractures of the humerus. A comparative study of Dunlop's traction versus percutaneous pinning. J Bone Joint Surg Am 61:425–428, 1979.
3. Skaggs DL, Hale JM, Bassett J, et al: Operative treatment of supracondylar fractures of the humerus in children.

The consequences of pin placement. J Bone Joint Surg Am 83-A:735–740, 2001.

4. France J, Strong M: Deformity and function in supracondylar fractures of the humerus in children variously treated by closed reduction and splinting, traction, and percutaneous pinning. J Pediatr Orthop 12:494–498, 1992.

5. Topping RE, Blanco JS, Davis TJ: Clinical evaluation of crossed-pin versus lateral-pin fixation in displaced supracondylar humerus fractures. J Pediatr Orthop 15:435–439, 1995.

6. Skaggs DL, Cluck MW, Mostofi A, et al: Lateral-entry pin fixation in the management of supracondylar fractures in children. J Bone Joint Surg Am 86-A:702–707, 2004.

7. Kocher MS, Kasser JR, Waters PM, et al: Lateral entry compared with medial and lateral entry pin fixation for completely displaced supracondylar humeral fractures in children. A randomized clinical trial. J Bone Joint Surg Am 89:706–712, 2007.

8. Foead A, Penafort R, Saw A, Sengupta S: Comparison of two methods of percutaneous pin fixation in displaced supracondylar fractures of the humerus in children. J 12:76–82, 2004.

9. Brauer CA, Lee BM, Bae DS, et al: A systematic review of medial and lateral entry pinning versus lateral entry pinning for supracondylar fractures of the humerus. J Pediatr Orthop 27:181–186, 2007.

10. Ozcelik A, Tekcan A, Omeroglu H: Correlation between iatrogenic ulnar nerve injury and angular insertion of the medial pin in supracondylar humerus fractures. J Pediatr Orthop B 15:58–61, 2006.

11. Sankar WN, Hebela NM, Skaggs DL, Flynn JM: Loss of pin fixation in displaced supracondylar humeral fractures in children: Causes and prevention. J Bone Joint Surg Am 89:713–717, 2007.

12. Ozkoc G, Gonc U, Kayaalp A, et al: Displaced supracondylar humeral fractures in children: Open reduction vs. closed reduction and pinning. Arch Orthop Trauma Surg 124:547–551, 2004.

13. Mahan ST, May CD, Kocher MS: Operative management of displaced flexion supracondylar humerus fractures in children. J Pediatr Orthop 27:551–556, 2007.

14. Schoenecker PL, Delgado E, Rotman M, et al: Pulseless arm in association with totally displaced supracondylar fracture. J Orthop Trauma 10:410–415, 1996.

15. Garbuz DS, Leitch K, Wright JG: The treatment of supracondylar fractures in children with an absent radial pulse. J Pediatr Orthop 16:594–596, 1996.

16. Sabharwal S, Tredwell SJ, Beauchamp RD, et al: Management of pulseless pink hand in pediatric supracondylar fractures of humerus. J Pediatr Orthop 17:303–310, 1997.

17. Mehlman CT, Strub WM, Roy DR, et al: The effect of surgical timing on the perioperative complications of treatment of supracondylar humeral fractures in children. J Bone Joint Surg Am 83-A:323–327, 2001.

18. Carmichael KD, Joyner K: Quality of reduction versus timing of surgical intervention for pediatric supracondylar humerus fractures. Orthopedics 29:628–632, 2006.

19. Sibinski M, Sharma H, Bennet GC: Early versus delayed treatment of extension type-3 supracondylar fractures of the humerus in children. J Bone Joint Surg Br 88:380–381, 2006.

20. Walmsley PJ, Kelly MB, Robb JE, et al: Delay increases the need for open reduction of type-III supracondylar fractures of the humerus. J Bone Joint Surg Br 88:528–530, 2006.

21. Keppler P, Salem K, Schwarting B, Kinzl L: The effectiveness of physiotherapy after operative treatment of supracondylar humeral fractures in children. J Pediatr Orthop 25:314–316, 2005.

22. Kumar K, Sharma R, Maffulli N: Correction of cubitus varus by French or dome osteotomy: A comparative study. J Trauma 49:717–721, 2000.

23. Bellemore MC, Barrett IR, Middleton RW, et al: Supracondylar osteotomy of the humerus for correction of cubitus varus. J Bone Joint Surg Br 66:566–572, 1984.

24. Song KS, Kang CH, Min BW, et al: Internal oblique radiographs for diagnosis of nondisplaced or minimally displaced lateral condylar fractures of the humerus in children. J Bone Joint Surg Am 89:58–63, 2007.

25. Vocke-Hell AK, Schmid A: Sonographic differentiation of stable and unstable lateral condyle fractures of the humerus in children. J Pediatr Orthop B 10:138–141, 2001.

26. Horn BD, Herman MJ, Crisci K, et al: Fractures of the lateral humeral condyle: Role of the cartilage hinge in fracture stability. J Pediatr Orthop 22:8–11, 2002.

27. Kamegaya M, Shinohara Y, Kurokawa M, Ogata S: Assessment of stability in children's minimally displaced lateral humeral condyle fracture by magnetic resonance imaging. J Pediatr Orthop 19:570–572, 1999.

28. Launay F, Leet AI, Jacopin S, et al: Lateral humeral condyle fractures in children: A comparison of two approaches to treatment. J Pediatr Orthop 24:385–391, 2004.

29. Bast SC, Hoffer MM, Aval S: Nonoperative treatment for minimally and nondisplaced lateral humeral condyle fractures in children. J Pediatr Orthop 18:448–450, 1998.

30. Rutherford A: Fractures of the lateral humeral condyle in children. J Bone Joint Surg Am 67:851–856, 1985.

31. Thomas DP, Howard AW, Cole WG, Hedden DM: Three weeks of Kirschner wire fixation for displaced lateral condylar fractures of the humerus in children. J Pediatr Orthop 21:565–569, 2001.

32. Farsetti P, Potenza V, Caterini R, Ippolito E: Long-term results of treatment of fractures of the medial humeral epicondyle in children. J Bone Joint Surg Am 83-A:1299–1305, 2001.

33. Wilson NI, Ingram R, Rymaszewski L, Miller JH: Treatment of fractures of the medial epicondyle of the humerus. Injury 19:342–344, 1988.

34. Vahvanen V, Gripenberg L: Fracture of the radial neck in children. A long-term follow-up study of 43 cases. Acta Orthop Scand 49:32–38, 1978.

35. D'souza S, Vaishya R, Klenerman L: Management of radial neck fractures in children: A retrospective analysis of one hundred patients. J Pediatr Orthop 13:232–238, 1993.

36. Steele JA, Graham HK: Angulated radial neck fractures in children. A prospective study of percutaneous reduction. J Bone Joint Surg Br 74:760–764, 1992.

37. Stiefel D, Meuli M, Altermatt S: Fractures of the neck of the radius in children. J Bone Joint Surg Br 83:536–541, 2001.

38. Schmittenbecher PP, Haevernick B, Herold A, et al: Treatment decision, method of osteosynthesis, and outcome in radial neck fractures in children: A multicenter study. J Pediatr Orthop 25:45–50, 2005.

What Is the Best Treatment for Femoral Fractures?

JENNIFER GOEBEL, BA AND JOHN M. FLYNN, MD

Pediatric femoral shaft fractures are among the most common injuries treated by the orthopedic surgeon. These fractures represent 1.6% of all bony injuries in children,[1–3] with the majority healing without any long-term sequelae. A review of recent literature illustrates that abuse and falls represent the most common mechanisms of injury for femoral fractures in children 4 years of age and younger. In children older than 11 years, the femoral shaft is much stronger, so fracture is more often caused by high-energy injuries, such as motor vehicle accidents or gunshot wounds.[2,4–6]

Initial evaluation includes a comprehensive history and physical examination evaluating for the presence of swelling, instability, and/or tenderness. Imaging begins with anteroposterior and lateral radiographs of the entire femur, as well as views of the hip and knee. Rarely, a bone scan or magnetic resonance imaging is valuable, such as in the diagnosis of stress fractures.[7]

OVERVIEW

Femoral fractures are often separated into three broad categories according to the geographic location of the fracture, which include proximal femur fractures, femoral shaft fractures, and supracondylar femur fractures. The character of the fracture can also be classified based on its appearance: (1) transverse, spiral, or oblique; (2) comminuted or noncomminuted; and (3) open or closed.[7] The nature of the injury, the character of the fracture, the child's age, and the amount of soft-tissue involvement are important factors that ultimately influence treatment options.

Treatment options may be divided into traction/casting versus operative fixation management with the decision ultimately based on the child's age, weight, and fracture stability. Closed reduction and casting is the treatment of choice in younger children, whereas fixation is used for older patients (Table 28–1).

In infants (birth to 6 months old), a stable proximal or midshaft femoral fracture can be treated with a simple splint or Pavlik harness. An infant with an unstable femoral fracture may need a Pavlik harness with a splint around the thigh to provide extra support. Immediate spica casting may be required in infants who present with femoral fractures of excessive shortening or angulation.[7] A Pavlik harness facilitates skin care but does not offer the pain relief of full immobilization in a spica cast.

For children 6 months to 4 years of age, immediate (or early) spica casting is the method of choice for femoral fractures with less than 2 cm of initial shortening. Children in this age group with greater than 2 cm of initial shortening may require 3 to 10 days of skeletal traction followed by spica casting.[7] In rare cases, external fixation and flexible intramedullary nailing (FIN) are used in this age group.

For children 4 to 11 years old, many treatment methods can be used, based on the surgeons' preference, fracture type, and family's wishes. Treatment options include early spica casting, skeletal traction followed by spica casting, FIN, plate fixation, solid antegrade nailing, and external fixation.[7] The optimal treatment for femur fractures in this 4- to 11-year-old age group is based on the nature of the injury, the character of the fracture, the skeletal maturity, the patient's weight, and the experience and skill of the surgeon with a given treatment method.

Children 11 years of age to skeletal maturity require maximum fixation strength whereas avoiding avascular necrosis or growth arrest. Treatment options include FIN, plating, locked intramedullary nails, and external fixation.[7] Rigid, locked intramedullary nailing utilizes a trochanteric starting point and is popular particularly in those children who are closer to skeletal maturity. Submuscular plating is becoming increasingly popular for this age group. Traction followed by spica casting, which was a standard treatment in the 1990s, is rarely used for this age group today (Fig. 28–1).[8]

EVIDENCE

Six Months to 4 Years

Several studies have shown that both the Pavlik harness (younger than 6 months) and spica casting (6 months to 4 years of age) are acceptable treatment options (Table 28–2). A retrospective study (Level III evidence) of 40 patients by Podeszwa and colleagues[9] compared application of the Pavlik harness versus spica casting for the treatment of children younger than 1 year. No difference was found in radiographic outcomes, but approximately one third of all spica

TABLE 28–1. Treatment Options for Pediatric Femoral Shaft Fractures

AGE	TREATMENT
Younger than 6 months	Pavlik harness
	Immediate spica casting
6 months to 4 years	Immediate spica casting
	Skeletal traction followed by spica casting
4–11 years	Skeletal traction followed by spica casting
11 years to maturity	Flexible intramedullary nailing
	Plating
	External fixation
	Flexible intramedullary nailing
	Plating
	Locked intramedullary nailing
	External fixation

TABLE 28–2. Table of Recommendations

STUDY	LEVEL OF EVIDENCE	GRADE OF RECOMMENDATION
Podeszwa et al.[9]	III	B
Buckley[10]	III	B
Allen et al.[11]	IV	C
Wright[12]	II	B
Bar-On et al.[13]	II	B
Barlas et al.[14]	III	B
Caird et al.[15]	IV	C
Ward et al.[16]	IV	C
Caglar et al.[17]	III	B
Sink et al.[18]	IV	B
Kanlic et al.[19]	III	B
Buechsenschuetz et al.[20]	II	B
Flynn et al.[21]	II	B
Wright et al.[22]	I	A
Coyte et al.[23]	III	B
Carey et al.[24]	III	B
Aronson et al.[25]	IV	C
Davis et al.[26]	IV	C
Domb et al.[27]	II	B
Leet et al.[28]	III	B
Moroz et al.[29]	III	B

patients experienced development of a skin complication. The authors conclude that all children younger than 1 year with a femoral shaft fracture should be considered for treatment with a Pavlik harness.[9] Buckley[10] reports the current trends in the treatment of femoral shaft fractures in children and adolescents. By analyzing healthcare costs and the desire for early discharge, he concludes that immediate hip spica casting remains the optimum method of treatment for most children 4 years and younger (Level III evidence). Allen and colleagues[11] likewise recommend immediate spica casting for femoral shaft fractures in infants and children. They reviewed 55 femoral shaft fractures in children treated by closed reduction and immediate application of a double hip spica cast, and showed satisfactory results in all cases

(level IV evidence case series, but with uniform outcome).[11] In a study comparing spica casting and skeletal traction, Wright[12] shows that early application of a hip spica cast had lower costs and malunion rates than traction (Level II evidence).

Four to 11 Years

Femur fracture treatment for the 4- to 11-year-old age group has been the most frequently studied cohort. Bar-On and researchers[13] prospectively reviewed ex-

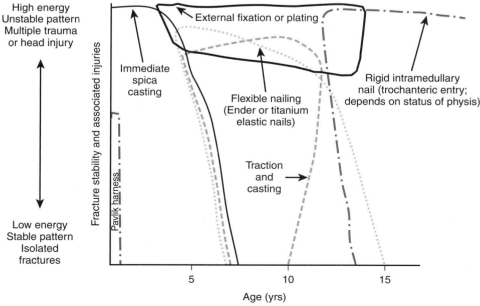

FIGURE 28–1. Treatment options for pediatric femoral fractures based on type of injury and patient age. (Adapted from Flynn JM, Schwend RM: Management of pediatric femoral shaft fractures. J Am Acad Orthop Surg 12:347–359, 2004 with permission of the American Academy of Orthopedic Surgeons.)

ternal fixation versus FIN for the femoral shaft in 19 children aged 5.2 to 13.2 years with 20 fractures of the femoral shaft (Level II evidence). The FIN group showed much more callous formation, and the time to full weight bearing, full range of movement, and return to school were all shorter. Bar-On and researchers[13] conclude, "External fixation should be reserved for open or severely comminuted fractures." Barlas and Beg[14] similarly reviewed external fixation and FIN in 40 children between 5.4 and 14.1 years of age. They also found an earlier return to function in the FIN group with minimal complications (Level III evidence). Their recommendations further support the efficacy of FIN over external fixation for patients in this age group.[14]

Other techniques in the 4- to 11-year-old age group including plating have also been evaluated. Caird and coauthors[15] reviewed open compression plating and found 100% union rate in 60 children younger than 16 years with minimal complications (Level IV). Ward and coauthors[16] likewise reviewed 25 children 6 to 16 years old treated with plate fixation, and found 23 of 25 fractures to heal in 11 weeks, on average, with leg length discrepancy not being a clinical problem (Level IV). Their indications for using this technique include a severe head injury or associated polytrauma. Caglar and colleagues[17] compare compression plating and FIN in pediatric femoral shaft fractures. Their results illustrate that FIN provided a high union rate with a shorter operation time when compared with the patients treated with compression plating (Level III).

Sink and coworkers[18] report the results of 27 patients treated with submuscular bridge plating for unstable femoral fractures (Level IV). No intraoperative or postoperative complications resulted. No instrumentation failure or loss of reduction was seen, whereas early callus was seen by 6 to 8 weeks and stable bony union by 12 weeks in all patients. Sink and coworkers[18] conclude, "Submuscular plating is a reasonable option for operative stabilization of communited and unstable pediatric femoral fractures." Kanlic and researchers[19] similarly reported the advantages of submuscular bridge plating. All 51 patients with an average age of 10 years had fractures united with excellent clinical results (Level IV). Kanlic and researchers[19] conclude, "This technique offers the advantage of adequate stability for early functional treatment and predictable healing with maintenance of length and alignment for all pediatric femoral shaft fractures."

Other groups have compared nonoperative versus operative management techniques. Buechsenschuetz and coworkers[20] have examined traction and casting versus elastic stable intramedullary nailing. Cost analyses and a comparison of clinical/functional parameters were done. No difference existed between the two groups for standard clinical/functional criteria. Elastic stable intramedullary nailing was associated with a lower overall cost than traction and casting. The authors found that a lower cost and comparable clinical outcome make elastic stable intramedullary nailing a better option than the traditional traction and casting for patients with femoral fractures (Level II).[20] Flynn and investigators[21] have compared titanium elastic nailing with traction and a spica cast. By prospectively following 83 patients, the results illustrate that children treated with titanium elastic nailing had shorter hospitalization, walked with support sooner, walked independently sooner, and returned to school earlier. These differences were significant ($P < 0.0001$) (Level II).

External fixation has also been compared with casting. Wright and coauthors[22] performed a multicenter prospective study comparing malunion rates after external fixation and after early hip spica cast application. Their results illustrated that the rate of malunion was significantly greater in the spica group than in the external fixator group 2 years after fracture (Level I). Coyte and investigators,[23] however, saw a greater expected total cost for patients and their families treated with external fixation as compared with those who were treated with an early hip spica cast (Level III). Fifty percent of this difference was attributable to the longer inpatient stays for patients treated with an external fixation device.

Other studies have focused on a single technique separately. Carey and Galpin[24] conclude that FIN seems to be a safe and effective method of treatment of femoral fractures for patients between 6 and 12 years of age (Level IV). Aronson and Tursky,[25] however, examined external fixation and found promising results with this technique. Most patients returned to school by 4 weeks, and all had full knee motion 6 weeks after fixator removal (Level IV). Davis and colleagues[26] also conclude in their small cohort (n = 14) that external fixation is an effective means of treating isolated femoral fractures in the pediatric population (Level IV). A major disadvantage of external fixation is stress-shielding and refracture. Domb and researchers[27] hypothesize that the use of axial dynamization may improve the speed and strength of callus formation. Looking at dynamization versus static external fixation in 52 patients, the author provide results that there was no difference in healing or frequency of complications for dynamic versus static external fixation techniques (Level II) (Tables 28–3 and 28–4).

Areas of Uncertainty

Age Group: 4 to 11 Years of Age. When treating a patient in the 4 to 11 year age group, it is important to consider the many available treatment options. FIN offers predictably excellent results in stable fractures with ease and safety of implantation and removal. Trochanteric entry locked nailing and submuscular plating has gained some popularity, especially for length-unstable fractures. External fixation, and rarely traction and casting, still have their place in this age group.

Larger and Older Children. Leet and coauthors[28] illustrate that obese children have an increased rate of

TABLE 28–3. Review of the Literature

STUDY	LEVEL OF EVIDENCE	NO. OF FRACTURES	AGE	TYPE OF TREATMENT	RECOMMENDATION
Podeszwa et al.[9]	III	39	<1 year	Pavlik harness vs. spica cast	Pavlik harness > Spica Cast for all children < 1 year of age
Buckley[10]	III	N/A	N/A	Traction, spica cast, traction and spica casting, cast brace, ex fix, plate fix, flexible IM rod, rigid IM rod	Each child must be individualized regarding treatment
Allen et al.[11]	IV	55	3 weeks to 14 years	Immediate spica cast	Immediate spica cast > traction
Wright[12]	II	N/A	*	All treatment methods were reviewed	Spica cast > traction
Bar-On et al.[13]	II	20	5.2–13.2	Ex fix vs. FIN	FIN: fractures of femoral shaft that require surgery Ex fix: open or severely comminuted fractures
Barlas et al.[14]	III	40	5.4–14.1	FIN vs. ex fix	FIN: fractures of femoral shaft which require surgery Ex fix: open or severely comminuted fractures
Caird et al.[15]	IV	60	<16 years	Compression plating	Compression plating
Ward et al.[16]	IV	25	6–16	Compression plating	Plate fix
Caglar et al.[17]	III	40	6–12	Compression plating vs. FIN	FIN > plate fix
Sink et al.[18]	IV	27	4–15	Submuscular bridge plating	Submuscular bridge plating for unstable pediatric femoral fractures
Kanlic et al.[19]	III	51	3.8–15.5	Submuscular bridge plating	Submuscular bridge plating
Buechsenschuetz et al.[20]	II	71	*	Traction and spica casting vs. ESIN	ESIN > traction and spica casting
Flynn et al.[21]	II	84	6–16	TEN vs. traction and spica cast	TEN
Wright et al.[22]	I	108	4–10	Ex fix vs. spica cast	Higher rates of malunion in Spica Cast > Ex Fix
Coyte et al.[23]	III		*	Ex fix vs. spica treatment	Ex fix: greater costs > spica treatment
Carey et al.[24]	III	27	6–12	FIN	FIN
Aronson et al.[25]	IV	44	2.5–17.8	Ex fix	Ex fix
Davis et al.[26]	IV	15	3–13	Ex fix	Ex fix
Domb et al.[27]	II	53	6–11	Dynamic vs. static ex fix	Static ex fix Dynamic ex fix: no significant effect on time to healing
Leet et al.[28]	III	104	6–14	Ex fix, IM rodding	Parents of obese children need to be aware of potentially greater risk for complications
Moroz et al.[29]	III	234	3–18	TEN	TEN Weight of child = important factor in treatment choice

*All children with femur fractures.
ESIN, elastic stable IM nailing; ex fix, external fixation; FIN, flexible intramedullary nailing; IM, intramedullary; plate fix, plate fixation; TEN, titanium elastic nailing.

TABLE 28–4. Summary of Recommendations

STATEMENT	LEVEL OF EVIDENCE/GRADE OF RECOMMENDATION	REFERENCES
1. Children younger than 1 year with a femoral shaft fracture should be considered for treatment with a Pavlik harness.	III/B	9
2. Immediate hip spica casting remains the optimum method of treatment for most children 4 years and younger.	III/B	10
3. Immediate spica casting for femoral shaft fractures is recommended in infants and children.	IV/C	11
4. Early application of a hip spica cast has lower costs and malunion rates than traction.	II/B	12
5. External fixation should be reserved for open or severely comminuted fractures.	II/B	13
6. Flexible intramedullary nailing is recommended over external fixation for pediatric patients.	III/B	14
7. Open compression plating is recommended for children younger than 16 years.	IV/C	15
8. Plate fixation is recommended for children between 6 and 16 years old.	IV/C	16
9. Flexible intramedullary nailing may have a high union rate with a shorter operation time when compared with compression plating.	III/B	17
10. Submuscular plating is a reasonable option for operative stabilization of communited and unstable pediatric femoral fractures.	IV/C	18
11. Submuscular plating offers the advantage of adequate stability for early functional treatment.	III/B	19
12. Lower cost and comparable clinical outcome makes elastic stable intramedullary nailing a better option than the traditional traction and casting for patients with femoral fractures.	II/B	20
13. Children treated with titanium elastic nailing have shorter hospitalization, walk with support sooner, walk independently sooner, and return to school earlier.	II/B	21
14. Early application of hip spica results in significantly greater rates of malunion 2 years after the fracture as compared with external fixation for patients between 4 and 10 years of age.	I/A	22
15. There is a greater expected total cost for patients and their families treated with external fixation as compared with those who were treated with an early hip spica cast.	III/B	23
16. Flexible intramedullary nailing seems to be a safe and effective method of treatment of femoral fractures for patients between 6 and 12 years of age.	III/B	24
17. External fixation is recommended to treat pediatric patients with femoral fractures.	IV/C	25
18. External fixation is an effective means of treating isolated femoral fractures in the pediatric population.	IV/C	26
19. No difference exists in healing or frequency of complications for dynamic vs. static external fixation techniques.	II/B	27
20. Obese children have an increased rate of complications after surgical treatment of femoral shaft fractures as compared with children of normal body weight.	III/B	28
21. In patients treated with titanium elastic nailing, heavier children have a poorer outcome.	III/B	29

complications after surgical treatment of femoral shaft fractures as compared with children of normal body weight. Moroz and colleagues[29] have conducted a multicenter study between 1996 and 2003 of 234 femur fractures treated by titanium elastic nailing. Although the outcome was excellent in the majority of the patients, 150 of 234 (65%) heavier children were more likely to have a poor outcome. In fact, a poor outcome was five times more likely in children who weighed more than 49 kg (Level II). Both studies illustrate that the child's weight is an important criteria in choosing an appropriate treatment option.

Removing Surgical Implants. Much debate remains about whether it is necessary to remove elastic nails, solid nails, or plates after the fracture has healed. No strong evidence exists on either side; therefore, this decision is currently based on the patient's and family's wishes, as well as the surgeon's preference.

Guidelines

Currently, no guidelines from the American Academy of Orthopaedic Surgeons (AAOS), Pediatric Orthopaedic Society of North America (POSNA), or Orthopaedic Trauma Association (OTA) for treatment of pediatric femur fractures have been published.

RECOMMENDATIONS

In children 4 years or younger, early spica casting yields satisfactory results, with low rates of malunion, shortening, and skin problems. There are no surgical incisions, no risk for infection, and no implants to remove. For this reason, spica casting remains the standard of care for this age group. The Pavlik harness remains an option for infants.

Continued

For children 4 to 11 years old, length-stable fractures are best managed with elastic nailing in most cases. Some surgeons prefer submuscular plating for this group. Submuscular plates offer more stability, but the implants are harder to remove. For length-unstable fractures, submuscular plating and external fixation (depending on the surgeon's preference and experience) are probably the best options in most cases. Elastic nailing can be used for length unstable fractures, especially in smaller, younger patients, but supplementary cast immobilization may be necessary for a short period, and the risk for malunion is somewhat greater. Solid antegrade nailing can also be used in this group and is usually reserved for the older, heavier children.

For children and adolescents in the 11-year-old to skeletal maturity age group, solid antegrade nailing through the greater trochanteric and submuscular plating may be the best option for most cases. Elastic nailing can be used in this age group with caution, particularly if the fracture is a length stable transverse fracture in a relatively small patient in this age group. External fixation is rarely used, except in some fractures at the junction of the distal diaphysis and metaphysis.

Skeletally mature adolescents are treated with solid antegrade or retrograde interlocking nails.

REFERENCES

1. Fry K, Hoffer MM, Brink J: Femoral shaft fractures in brain-injured children. J Trauma 16:371–373, 1976.
2. Hedlund R, Lindgren U: The incidence of femoral shaft fractures in children and adolescents. J Pediatr Orthop 6:47–50, 1986.
3. Landin LA: Fracture patterns in children. Analysis of 8,682 fractures with special reference to incidence, etiology and secular changes in a Swedish urban population 1950–1979. Acta Orthop Scand Suppl 202:1–109, 1983.
4. Blakemore LC, Loder RT, Hensinger RN: Role of intentional abuse in children 1 to 5 years old with isolated femoral shaft fractures. J Pediatr Orthop 16:585–588, 1996.
5. Daly KE, Calvert PT: Accidental femoral fracture in infants. Injury 22:337–338, 1991.
6. Loder RT: Pediatric polytrauma: Orthopaedic care and hospital course. J Orthop Trauma 1:48–54, 1987.
7. Beaty J, Kasser J: Rockwood and Wllkins' Fractures in Children, 6th ed. Philadelphia, Lippincott Williams & Wilkins, 2006.
8. Flynn JM, Schwend RM: Management of pediatric femoral shaft fractures. J Am Acad Orthop Surg 12:347–359, 2004.
9. Podeszwa DA, Mooney JF 3rd, Cramer KE, Mendelow MJ: Comparison of Pavlik harness application and immediate spica casting for femur fractures in infants. J Pediatr Orthop 24:460–462, 2004.
10. Buckley SL: Current trends in the treatment of femoral shaft fractures in children and adolescents. Clin Orthop Relat Res (338):60–73, 1997.
11. Allen BL Jr, Schoch EP 3rd, Emery FE: Immediate spica cast system for femoral shaft fractures in infants and children. South Med J 71:18–22, 1978.
12. Wright JG: The treatment of femoral shaft fractures in children: A systematic overview and critical appraisal of the literature. Can J Surg 43:180–189, 2000.
13. Bar-On E, Sagiv S, Porat S: External fixation or flexible intramedullary nailing for femoral shaft fractures in children. A prospective, randomised study. J Bone Joint Surg Br 79:975–978, 1997.
14. Barlas K, Beg H: Flexible intramedullary nailing versus external fixation of paediatric femoral fractures. Acta Orthop Belg 72:159–163, 2006.
15. Caird MS, Mueller KA, Puryear A, Farley FA: Compression plating of pediatric femoral shaft fractures. J Pediatr Orthop 23:448–452, 2003.
16. Ward WT, Levy J, Kaye A: Compression plating for child and adolescent femur fractures. J Pediatr Orthop 12:626–632, 1992.
17. Caglar O, Aksoy MC, Yazici M, Surat A: Comparison of compression plate and flexible intramedullary nail fixation in pediatric femoral shaft fractures. J Pediatr Orthop B 15:210–214, 2006.
18. Sink EL, Hedequist D, Morgan SJ, Hresko T: Results and technique of unstable pediatric femoral fractures treated with submuscular bridge plating. J Pediatr Orthop 26:177–181, 2006.
19. Kanlic EM, Anglen JO, Smith DG, et al: Advantages of submuscular bridge plating for complex pediatric femur fractures. Clin Orthop Relat Res 426:244–251, 2004.
20. Buechsenschuetz KE, Mehlman CT, Shaw KJ, et al: Femoral shaft fractures in children: Traction and casting versus elastic stable intramedullary nailing. J Trauma 53:914–921, 2002.
21. Flynn JM, Luedtke LM, Ganley TJ, et al: Comparison of titanium elastic nails with traction and a spica cast to treat femoral fractures in children. J Bone Joint Surg Am 86-A:770–777, 2004.
22. Wright JG, Wang EE, Owen JL, et al: Treatments for paediatric femoral fractures: A randomised trial. Lancet 365:1153–1158, 2005.
23. Coyte PC, Bronskill SE, Hirji ZZ, et al: Economic evaluation of 2 treatments for pediatric femoral shaft fractures. Clin Orthop Relat Res (336):205–215, 1997.
24. Carey TP, Galpin RD: Flexible intramedullary nail fixation of pediatric femoral fractures. Clin Orthop Relat Res 332:110–118, 1996.
25. Aronson J, Tursky EA: External fixation of femur fractures in children. J Pediatr Orthop 12:157–163, 1992.
26. Davis TJ, Topping RE, Blanco JS: External fixation of pediatric femoral fractures. Clin Orthop Relat Res (318):191–198, 1995.
27. Domb BG, Sponseller PD, Ain M, Miller NH: Comparison of dynamic versus static external fixation for pediatric femur fractures. J Pediatr Orthop 22:428–430, 2002.
28. Leet AI, Pichard CP, Ain MC: Surgical treatment of femoral fractures in obese children: Does excessive body weight increase the rate of complications? J Bone Joint Surg Am 87:2609–2613, 2005.
29. Moroz LA, Launay F, Kocher MS, et al: Titanium elastic nailing of fractures of the femur in children. Predictors of complications and poor outcome. J Bone Joint Surg Br 88:1361–1366, 2006.

What Is the Best Treatment for Growth Plate Injuries?

Andrew Wainwright, BSc (Hons), MB, ChB, FRSC (Tr and Orth) and
Tim Theologis, MD, MSc, PhD, FRCS

A growth plate is a disc of cartilage that is organized into a physiologic pattern that, as it matures, is responsible for longitudinal growth of long bones. The cause of growth plate injuries may be acute or chronic. An injury is most commonly caused by trauma. Less frequent causes include infection, thermal injury, effects of metabolic abnormalities, tumors, or neuromuscular conditions, and there are iatrogenic causes such as exposure to irradiation or LASER.[1]

Treatment of growth plate injuries may be considered in the following situations: (1) the treatment of an acute fracture involving a growth plate, (2) the treatment of a chronic growth plate injury, and (3) the treatment of the injured growth plate.

WHAT IS THE BEST TREATMENT OF A GROWTH PLATE INJURY CAUSED BY A FRACTURE?

Epidemiologic Studies

In a study of 2650 long-bone fractures in children younger than 16 years, 30% involved the growth plate.[2] A population-based study was performed assessing 951 physeal fractures over a 10-year period in Minnesota.[3] The following bones were involved in decreasing frequency: finger phalanges (37%), distal radius (18%), distal tibia (11%), distal fibula (7%), metacarpals, toe phalanges, distal humerus, distal ulna, proximal humerus, distal femur, metatarsals proximal tibia, and proximal radius fibula. In these and other studies, male individuals were affected twice as often as female individuals. Female individuals were most commonly injured at a younger age (11–12 years compared with 12–14 years in boys). When all types of growth plate fractures are considered, the rate of growth disturbance is approximately 30%. Some sites are more prone than others; however, only 2% of such fractures result in a significant functional disturbance.

How Should These Injuries Be Followed Up?

For all of these fractures, it is generally agreed that they should be re-examined with radiographs in the short term to ensure reduction has been maintained, and in the longer term to ensure that growth arrest has not occurred. No evidence is available to indicate how long review should continue; most experts are of the opinion (Level V evidence) that a parallel Harris line[4] at some distance from the growth plate at 6 to 12 months is a sign that normal growth has resumed.

Factors That Affect Treatment.

Experts agree that the most important factors that affect decisions for treatment of growth plate fractures include: (1) the age of the child (and the growth potential of the bone), (2) the fracture pattern (i.e., the direction of fracture relative to the growth plate), and (3) the site of the growth plate affected.

Age of the Child. It is self-evident that a child's age has a correlation with the amount of growth remaining and, therefore, the amount of potential growth disturbance that may be caused by a partial or complete growth arrest.

Pattern of the Fracture. There have been many classification systems proposed based on the pattern of the fracture. These include the systems of Salter and Harris, Ogden, and Peterson. The most widely known is that of Salter and Harris.[5] Evidence for the best treatment of each type of fracture is summarized in the following sections. In general, this evidence is not based on comparative studies but on received wisdom (Level V evidence) and case series (Level IV).

Best Treatment for a Salter–Harris Type I or II Growth Plate Fracture. With a transverse fracture through the hypertrophic zone (Type I), the germinal layer usually is not primarily involved, although there may be some microfracture that extends into the germinal zone,[6] and significant growth disturbance is uncommon, unless there is associated injury to the blood supply.[5] In the more common, type II fracture, which runs through the growth plate with a triangular fragment of metaphysis (Thurston–Holland fragment), there is usually an intact periosteal hinge[5] that can aid closed reduction.

In laboratory rats after a type I or II fracture, a brief growth arrest is noted. However, the growth plate appears normal after 25 days other than a thickened hypertrophic zone.[7]

Specific treatment depends on the site of the fractures. There are no high-level studies that compare open with closed treatment or use of fixation. The accepted wisdom is that reduction should be gentle to avoid scraping the growth plate on bone fragment or damaging the germinal layers during manipulation.[1,5,8] It is generally agreed that closed reduction and casting is successful; however, that it may be necessary to use internal fixation after open or closed reduction if it is unstable.[8] In some circumstances, the periosteum may become interposed into the fracture and block satisfactory or anatomic reduction requiring exploration.[9]

Best Treatment for Salter–Harris Type III or IV Growth Plate Fractures. In both type III and IV fractures, the fracture includes a growth plate injury with a disruption in the articular surface of the joint. Although a type III fracture runs through the epiphysis and a type IV runs through the metaphysis and epiphysis, they may both result in malalignment of the layer zones of the growth plate and lead to development of a bony bridge.

No randomized studies have compared open with closed treatment or use of fixation. According to Bright,[9] anatomic alignment of the growth plate and articular surface is important and requires anatomic reduction and internal fixation. There are case reports of nondisplaced fragments becoming displaced if fixation is not used.

No studies have compared methods of fixation. It is generally accepted that nonthreaded wires should be used in the epiphysis or metaphysis that run parallel to the growth plate.[8] Alternatively, screw fixation parallel to the growth plate can be used. If stable anatomic fixation cannot be attained with transverse pins, it is also accepted that oblique nonthreaded wires across the growth plate may be used.[8] There have been case-series reports (Level IV evidence) of the use of biodegradable rods, Polylactide-glycolide polymer,[10] across the growth plates without disturbance of growth.

Best Treatment of Salter–Harris Type V and "VI" Fractures. Compression or crush injuries to the growth plate (type V) are rarely diagnosed acutely. Some debate exists in the literature whether this mechanism exists. Although several reports have demonstrated that growth plate compression injuries occur, they usually result in a complete arrest (rather than partial growth arrest that is indicated in the Salter–Harris article).[1] The average time until diagnosis of this type of injury is 17 months.

Although not included in the original Salter–Harris classification, a type "VI" fracture is included in Rang's book.[11] He reports that Kessel suggested an additional type of growth plate injury, that is, an injury to the periosteum or perichondrial ring resulting in a bony bridge. It is suggested that this may lead to angular deformity from a bone bridge. Few cases series have reported this injury type.

Because these fractures are not usually diagnosed acutely, there is no specific treatment recommendation at the time of injury. If a Salter–Harris type V or "VI" growth plate injury does result, further treatment may be necessary to prevent or correct deformity.

Site of Growth Plate Injury. Some growth plates are more susceptible to injury than others. Some particular sites warrant separate discussion.

Acetabular Triradiate Cartilage Fractures. Injury to the acetabular triradiate growth plate cartilage is rare, but it may be associated with progressive acetabular dysplasia and subluxation of the hip. Bucholz and colleagues[12] found nine patients with triradiate growth plate injury (Level IV evidence). Shearing (SH type I or II) injury seems to have a favorable prognosis. However, a crushing SH type V growth plate injury has a poor prognosis, with premature closure. Prognosis is dependent on the age of the patient at the time of injury and on the extent of chondro-osseous disruption.

DISTAL FEMUR FRACTURES. Fractures of the distal femoral growth plate account for approximately 5% of growth plate injuries. From case reports, it is apparent that damage to the neurovascular structures in the popliteal fossa may occur when displacement occurs in the saggital plane and should be sought for and treated.

Approximately 50% of distal femur growth plate fractures are associated with growth disturbance, even the type I or II fractures (Level IV evidence, case series).[13,14]

Expert advice is that closed reduction should also be attempted for all minimally to moderately displaced Salter–Harris type I and II fractures.[15] However, a study of 10 distal femoral physeal fractures found that 7 displaced, and the authors suggest that internal fixation should be used.[16] Fractures with greater displacement, especially those with a hyperextension pattern, are associated with an increased risk for redisplacement; therefore, percutaneous fixation is recommended.[17]

Salter–Harris type II fractures can be stabilized by fixation across the Thurston Holland metaphyseal spike if it is large. Percutaneous screws are preferred for fixation if they can be inserted without crossing the physis. If metaphyseal stability cannot be obtained, Salter–Harris type I and II fractures can be fixed with one or two smooth Steinmann pins from the epiphysis to the metaphysis. If the pins are left outside of the skin, they can cause irritation and may even lead to infection septic arthritis.[15] Salter–Harris type III and IV fractures can be fixed with intraepiphyseal screws.[14]

Proximal Tibia Fractures. Fractures of the proximal tibia growth plate are among the most uncommon but have the greatest rate of serious complications. Displacement of the fracture can result in significant problems related to popliteal artery disruption in 5% to 7% of cases[18,19] or common peroneal nerve injury, and these should be looked for. In these retrospective series (Level IV evidence), it is also noted that there may be a growth arrest that does not correlate well with fracture pattern, and close follow-up should be made to detect angular or leg-length deformity.

Expert advice is that fractures that can be reduced by closed methods can usually be held in alignment with a long leg cast. If the fracture is displaced, the cast should be bivalved and the patient should be observed overnight for vascular complications. The circulation should be carefully assessed, and an intraoperative arteriogram should be made when the vascular supply is compromised, and compartment syndrome should be ruled out clinically.[15]

Salter–Harris type III pattern of injury is rare in the proximal part of the tibia (except as a pattern of tibial tubercle avulsion), which has been attributed to the shape of the epiphysis. Unstable fractures of any pattern and all displaced type IV fractures should be reduced and stabilized with internal fixation such as smooth Steinmann pins.

Distal Tibia Fractures. Fractures of the distal end of the tibia in children often involve the growth plate. They may result in partial growth arrest, angulation, leg-length difference, or joint incongruity.[20]

Salter–Harris I and II fractures can usually be treated with closed reduction. A series of 56 type II fractures treated in casts resulted in no deformity or premature physeal closure[21] (Level IV evidence). Acceptable alignment of displaced fractures in children with at least 2 years of growth remaining consists of no more than 15 degrees of plantar tilt, 10 degrees of valgus, and no varus. In children with less than 2 years of growth remaining, the amount of acceptable angulation is reduced to 5 degrees in all planes (Level V evidence, expert opinion).[22]

General agreement exists that type III and IV fractures require surgical intervention.[15,23] In a retrospective series, it was concluded that major deformity can be avoided with aggressive follow-up and early corrective treatment.[20] Open or arthroscopic visualization of the joint surface has been recommended to confirm reduction, and stabilization with 3.5- or 4.0-mm cannulated screws assessing the screw placement carefully in two planes.[15]

Treatment recommendation for Tillaux fractures (SH III of the anterolateral portion of the distal tibial epiphysis) is directed to reducing and holding the fragment with less than 2 mm displacement, and this is best judged with computed tomography.[15] Closed reduction, open reduction, and a percutaneous method have been described.[24]

Treatment recommendations for Triplane fractures (complex Salter–Harris type IV fractures in three planes) include radiographic and computed tomographic evaluation initially. An articular step-off of more than 2 mm or a fracture gap of more than 2 to 4 mm is an indication for open reduction.[15] This is based on a study that showed that more than 2 mm articular displacement leads to poorer long-term results according to a follow-up study by Ertl et al.[25] An open exploration and fixation is usually necessary to achieve reduction.[15]

Distal Radius and Ulna. The growth plate of the distal radius is the most frequently injured, usually with a SH type I or II pattern. Three quarters of the growth of the forearm occurs at the distal growth plates, with good potential for remodeling, but also potential for a significant mismatch if one of these paired bones has an arrest. Significant growth disturbance occurs in 7% of distal radius fractures.[26] This is important as a study of 30 patients who had surgical management of distal radial growth arrest that was found to improve pain and range of motion in symptomatic patients and prevent symptoms in asymptomatic patients.[27]

BEST TREATMENT OF A CHRONIC GROWTH PLATE INJURY

In addition to the acute physeal injuries sustained through sports,[28] there is an increasing body of evidence demonstrating that growth plate injuries can occur by repetitive physical loading required in sports. A recent systematic review found that most reports were case reports or case series.[29]

This injury appears to be related to mineralization of the hypertrophic zone because of altered metaphyseal perfusion.[30] The hypertrophic zone continues to get wider, as shown experimentally by Jaramillo et al[31] in rabbits with similar magnetic resonance imaging findings seen in competitive gymnasts. This is usually temporary,[30] but it may lead to permanent changes, with either a partial or complete growth plate disturbance.

This is best known in conditions such as "little league shoulder"; there are many reports of stress changes in the proximal humeral physis of baseball pitchers' throwing arms.[29] Although this tends to improve with rest, there is one report of premature physeal closure.[32] Similar reports of physeal widening in association with other sports, and even piano playing, in the upper and lower limbs of growing athletes can be found in the literature.[29]

Recommendations for managing these problems primarily relate to prevention. These include the education of coaches, altering the training regimens for children, especially during rapid growth, and referral to a physician in the case of significant pain around a joint. If rested, there is evidence that the process is reversible.

BEST TREATMENT FOR AN INJURED GROWTH PLATE

An injured or disrupted growth plate may lead to premature fusion of part or all of the growth plate, with a bone "bar" across the area that should be made of the specialized arrangement of growth cartilage. There is consequent tethering that may lead to partial (angular) or complete (longitudinal) growth disturbance at the growth plate.[33] This bar may be visible on a conventional radiograph, but multiplanar imaging such as computed tomography or magnetic resonance can be helpful in localizing the lesion.

Different forms of treatment have been described for growth plate arrest. The best treatment depends on the following factors: the location of the growth plate; the amount of growth remaining at that growth plate; whether complete arrest has been maintained; or if partial, the proportion of the growth plate that is involved and the circumstances of the child.[1] No high-level evidence has compared outcomes of different treatments for these relatively rare events, and management recommendations are based on Level V evidence (expert opinion).

For complete arrest, treatment is directed to the management of length inequality. Management options include no intervention, compensatory orthoses (shoe lift), epiphyseodesis or shortening of the

TABLE 29–1. Summary of Recommendations

STATEMENT	LEVEL OF EVIDENCE/GRADE OF RECOMMENDATION	REFERENCES
Most Salter–Harris type I and II fractures may be adequately treated by closed manipulation and stabilization in a cast.	IV	21
Open reduction and fixation is better than closed manipulation for most Salter–Harris type III and IV fractures.	IV	15, 20, 25
Salter–Harris type V fractures exist.	V	5
Chronic repetitive injury can result in physeal arrest that can be prevented by rest.	IV	29
Growth plate fractures with higher Salter–Harris grades have a greater risk for partial or complete growth arrest.	IV, V	1, 5
Approximately 50% of distal femur growth plate fractures are associated with growth disturbance, even the type I or II fractures.	IV	13, 14
Physeal bridge resection with interposition material is an effective way of treating partial growth arrest.	IV	9, 33–42

contralateral or companion bone, ipsilateral bone lengthening, or a combination.[1]

For partial growth arrest, treatment is directed to managing the length inequality and angulation. Treatment options include a combination of the following: no intervention; compensatory orthoses (shoe lift); epiphyseodesis of the remaining bone, or contralateral or companion bone; correction of the angulation by acute (osteotomy) or gradual correction (distraction osteogenesis); excision of the bar and interposition of an inert material; and distraction of the growth plate and bar (in children nearing maturity).[1]

Resection of a Bone Bridge

To prevent arrest of growth after physeal injury, investigators have performed bone bar resection and used various interposition materials: fat,[33,34] muscle,[35] polymeric silicone,[36–39] bone wax,[40] and bone cement.[41] These studies are Level IV evidence (case series); regarding the results of treatment, no study shows the superiority of one material over the others.

Experts agree that resection is indicated if less than 30% to 50% of growth plate is involved[1] (Level of Evidence V). Younger children tend to have a better prognosis. Less than 2 years of remaining growth is a relative contraindication for bone bridge resection. It has also been noted that central bars are more amenable to resection than peripheral, which is probably related to the adjacent periosteal stripping in peripheral lesions. Ischemic or septic-related bone bars have a poorer prognosis (Level of Evidence V).

In one study, 28 skeletally immature patients underwent 29 primary physeal bridge resections. Of 22 resections followed for 2 years, there were 11 excellent, 5 good, 2 fair, and 4 poor results. Overall mean growth was 83%, with 98% in the excellent group and 96% in the good group. The authors conclude that physeal bridge resection is an effective method of treating partial physeal growth arrest (Level IV evidence). Results with fat compare favorably with results of other interposition materials without the disadvantages of local reaction and implant removal.[42]

Physeal Distraction

Hemichondrodiastasis, closed gradual distraction of the growth plate, to correct angular deformity has been described.[43,44] This technique in a group of 35 patients worked best in post-traumatic deformities when the bony bridge occupied less than 30% of the plate. It was used toward the end of growth (or earlier in the case of progressive deformity of more than 20 degrees).

Recent experimental studies have explored the use of autogenous chondrocytes to fill the defect.[45,46] However there are still some problems to overcome. Principally, it is difficult to find suitable donor sites other than apophyses, and apophyseal cartilage may lack the growth potential of epiphyseal cartilage. These experimental studies are preclinical and do not receive level of evidence grades.

SUMMARY

The evidence for the best treatment of growth plate injuries is based mainly on epidemiologic studies, retrospective reviews, animal model experiments, and expert opinion. Table 29–1 provides a summary of recommendations for the treatment of growth plate injuries.

REFERENCES

1. Peterson HA: Physeal injuries and growth arrest. In Beaty JH, Kasser JR (eds): Rockwood and Wilkins' Fractures in Children, 5th ed. Philadelphia: Lippincott Williams & Wilkins, 2001, pp 91–138.
2. Mann DC, Rajmaira S: Distribution of physeal and nonphyseal fractures in 2,650 long-bone fractures in children aged 0-16 years. J Pediatr Orthop 10:713–716, 1990.
3. Peterson HA, Madhok R, Benson JT, et al: Physeal fractures part 1 epidemiology in Olmsted county Minnesota, 1979-88. J Pediatr Orthop 41:423–430, 1994.
4. Harris HA: Lines of arrested growth in the long bones in childhood: The correlation of histological and radiographic appearance in clinical and experimental conditions. Br J Radiol 4:561–588, 1931.
5. Salter RB, Harris WR: Injuries involving the epiphyseal plate. J Bone Joint Surg Am 45-A:587–622, 1963.

6. Ogden JA: Injury to the growth mechanism of the immature skeleton. Skeletal Radiol 6:237–253, 1981.
7. Gomes LS, Valpon JB, Gonclaves RP: Traumatic separation of epiphyses; an experimental study in rats. Clin Orthop Relat Res (236):286–295, 1988.
8. Canale ST: Physeal injuries. In: Green NE, Swiontowski MF (eds): Skeletal Trauma in Children, 2nd ed. Philadelphia: WB Saunders Company, 1997, pp 17–58.
9. Bright RW: Physeal injuries. Fractures: Fractures in Children, 3rd ed. Philadelphia: Lippincott-Raven, 1991, pp 87–186.
10. Makela EA, Bostman O, Kekomaki M, et al: Biodegradable fixation of distal humeral fractures. Clin Orthop Relat Res 283:237–243, 1992.
11. Rang M (ed): The Growth Plate and Its Disorders. Edinburgh and London: E&S Livingstone, 1969.
12. Bucholz RW, Ezaki M, Ogden JA: Injury to the acetabular triradiate physeal cartilage. J Bone Joint Surg Am 64:600–609, 1982.
13. Eid AM, Hafez MA: Traumatic injury of the distal femoral physis. Retrospective study on 150 cases. Injury 33:251–255, 2002.
14. Riseborough EJ, Barrett IR, Shapiro F: Growth disturbances following distal femoral physeal fracture separations. J Bone Joint Surg Am 65:885–893, 1983.
15. Flynn J, et al: The operative management of pediatric fractures of the lower extremity. J Bone Joint Surg Am 84: 2288–2300, 2002.
16. Graham JM, Gross RH: Distal femoral physeal problem fractures. Clin Orthop Relat Res (255):51–53, 1990.
17. Thomson JD, Stricker SJ, Williams MM: Fractures of the distal femoral epiphyseal plate. J Pediatr Orthop 15:474–478, 1995.
18. Shelton WR, Canale ST: Fractures of the tibia through the proximal tibial epiphyseal cartilage. J Bone Joint Surg Am 61:167–173, 1979.
19. Burkhart SS, Peterson HA: Fractures of the proximal tibial epiphysis. J Bone Joint Surg Am 61:996–1002, 1979.
20. Lalonde K-A, Letts M: Traumatic growth arrest of the distal tibia: a clinical and radiographic review. Can J Surg 48: 143–147, 2004.
21. Dugan G, Herndon WA, McGuire R: Distal tibial injuries in children: a different treatment concept. J Orthop Trauma 1:63–67, 1987.
22. Cummings RJ: Distal tibial and fibular fractures. In: Rockwood CA Jr, Wilkins KE, Beaty JH (eds): Fractures in Children, 4th ed. Philadelphia: Lippincott-Raven, 1996, pp 1377–1428.
23. deSanctis N, Della Corte S, Pempinello C: Distal tibial and fibular epiphyseal fractures in children: Prognostic criteria and long term results in 158 patients. J Pediatr Orthop B 9:40–44, 2000.
24. Schlesinger L, Wedge JH: Percutaneous reduction and fixation of displaced juvenile Tillaux fractures: A new surgical technique. J Pediatr Orthop 13:389–391, 1993.
25. Ertl JP, Barrack RL, Alexander AH, VanBuecken K: Triplane fracture of the distal tibial epiphysis. Long-term follow-up. J Bone Joint Surg Am 70:967–976, 1988.
26. Lee BS, Esterhai JL Jr, Das M: Fracture of the distal radial epiphysis. Characteristics and surgical treatment of premature, post-traumatic epiphyseal closure. Clin Orthop (185):90–96, 1984.
27. Waters PM, Bae DS, Montgomery KD: Surgical management of post traumatic distal radial growth arrest in adolescents. J Pediatr Orthop 22:717–724, 2002.
28. Krueger-Franke M, Siebert CH, Pfoerringer W: Sports related epiphyseal injuries of the lower extremity. An epidemiological study. J Sports Med Phys Fitness 32:106–111, 1992.
29. Caine D, DiFiori J, Maffulli N: Physeal injuries in children's and youth sports: Reason for concern? Br J Sports Med 40:749–760, 2006.
30. Ogden JA: Skeletal Injury in the Child. New York: Springer-Verlag, 2000.
31. Jaramillo D, Laor T, Zaleske DJ: Indirect trauma to the growth plate. Radiology 187:171–178, 1993.
32. Carson WG, Gasser SI: Little leaguer's shoulder: A report of 23 cases. Am J Sports Med 26:575–580, 1998.
33. Langenskiöld A: The possibilities of eliminating premature partial closure of an epiphyseal plate caused by trauma or disease. Acta Orthop Scand 38:267–279, 1967.
34. Österman K: Operative elimination of partial premature epiphyseal closure. An experimental study. Acta Orthop Scand Suppl (147):3–79, 1972.
35. Martiana K, Low CK, Tan SK, Pang MWY: Comparison of various interpositional materials in the prevention of transphyseal bone bridge formation. Clin Orthop 325:218–224, 1996.
36. Campbell CJ, Grisolia A, Zanconato G: The effects produced in the cartilaginous epiphyseal plate of immature dogs by experimental surgical trauma. J Bone Joint Surg Am 41: 1221–1242, 1959.
37. Bright RW: Operative correction of partial epiphyseal plate closure by osseous bridge resection and silicone rubber implant. An experimental study in dogs. J Bone Joint Surg Am 56:655–664, 1974.
38. Macksoud WS, Bright R: Bar resection and silastic interposition in distal radial physeal arrest. Orthop Trans 13:1–2, 1989.
39. Lee EH, Gao GX, Bose K: Management of partial growth arrest: Physis, fat, or silastic? J Pediatr Orthop 13:368–372, 1993.
40. Broughton NS, Dickens DRV, Cole WG, Menelaus MB: Epiphysiolysis for partial growth plate arrest. J Bone joint Surg Br 71:13–16, 1989.
41. Klassen RA, Peterson MA: Excision of physeal bars: The Mayo Clinic experience 1968–1978. Orthop Trans 2:65, 1982.
42. Williamson RV, Staheli LT: Partial physeal growth arrest: Treatment by bridge resection and fat interposition. J Pediatr Orthop 10:769–776, 1990.
43. Aldegheri R, Trivella G, Lavini F: Epiphyseal distraction hemichondrodisatasis. Clin Orthop Relat Res (241):128–136, 1989.
44. Canadell J, de Pablos J: Correction of angular deformities by physeal distraction. Clin Orthop Relat Res 98–105, 1992.
45. Olin A, Creasman C, Shapiro F: Free physeal transplantation in the rabbit. J Bone Joint Surg Am 66:7–20, 1984.
46. Lee EH, Chen F, Chan J, Bose K: Treatment of growth arrest by transfer of cultured chondrocytes into physeal defects. J Pediatr Orthop 18:155–160, 1998.

Chapter 30

How Do You Best Diagnose Septic Arthritis of the Hip?

MININDER S. KOCHER, MD, MPH

The initial presentation of a child with an acutely irritable hip can pose a diagnostic challenge to the orthopedic surgeon, pediatrician, emergency department physician, or primary care physician. After ruling out the more apparent radiographic abnormalities of Legg–Perthes disease, slipped capital femoral epiphysis, and fracture, the differential diagnosis commonly involves septic arthritis versus transient synovitis.

The differentiation between septic arthritis and transient synovitis of the hip in children is essential because the two clinical entities have quite different treatments and potential for negative sequelae. Septic arthritis is treated with operative drainage and antibiotics, whereas transient synovitis is usually self-limited and treated symptomatically.[1–7] Complications of septic arthritis include osteonecrosis, growth arrest, and sepsis, whereas transient synovitis usually has a benign clinical course.[8–15] In addition, the early, accurate diagnosis of septic arthritis is essential because poor outcomes after septic hip in children have been associated with delay in diagnosis.[16–20]

The differentiation of septic arthritis and transient synovitis of the hip in children can be difficult because both often have similar presentations: an atraumatic, acutely irritable hip in a child with progressive symptoms and signs of fever, limp or refusal to bear weight, limited motion, joint effusion, and abnormal laboratory evaluation. Empirically, clinicians have used various clinical, laboratory, and radiographic variables to distinguish between septic arthritis and transient synovitis.

This chapter overviews the diagnostic accuracy of clinical, laboratory, and radiographic variables in the diagnosis of septic arthritis of the hip in children, and provides recommendations based on best available evidence.

OVERVIEW

Septic Arthritis

Septic arthritis of the hip in a child constitutes a surgical emergency. Prompt recognition, diagnosis, and treatment of this entity are essential. Bacterial infection of the joint space results in an inflammatory effusion consisting of up to 90% polymorphonuclear cells (PMNs).[21] The release of proteolytic enzymes by PMNs and bacteria, in conjunction with increased intra-articular pressure, can result in rapid and irreversible hyaline cartilage degradation in as little as 6 hours. If unrecognized or left untreated, this process can result in joint destruction with subsequent severe deformity and devastating lifelong disability. Joint infections can ultimately lead to disseminated infection, systemic bacterial sepsis, multiorgan failure, and death. However, if recognized and treated in a timely fashion with surgical drainage and appropriate antimicrobial therapy, a good outcome with minimal sequelae can be expected. Poor outcomes are most closely associated with delay in diagnosis. Other factors related to poor outcome include patient age younger than 6 months, prematurity, *Staphylococcus* species infection, and concomitant osteomyelitis.

Septic arthritis may occur as a result of hematogenous seeding, local spread from a contiguous infection, or primary seeding of a joint secondary to surgery or trauma. In the hip, shoulder, ankle, and elbow (90% of cases), septic arthritis often develops after metaphyseal osteomyelitis with subperiosteal erosion, abscess formation, and subsequent joint communication (because of the intra-articular location of the metaphyses in these joints). Premature and immunocompromised children are at greater risk. The most commonly identified causative organisms are *Staphylococcus aureus*, group A streptococci, *Streptococcus pneumococcus,* other gram-negative organisms (may be seen in special hosts or after trauma-klebsiellae, salmonellae, kingellae), and *Neisseria gonorrhea.*[22] Before the advent of an effective vaccine, *Haemophilus influenzae* type B was responsible for up to 40% of cases but has largely disappeared because of successful immunization programs.[23,24] In the neonate, group B β-hemolytic streptococcus and gram-negative bacilli are common causative agents in addition to *S. aureus.* Gram-negative infections are common among intravenous (IV) drug abusers. Mycobacteria and fungi must be considered in patients with chronic infection.

Diagnosis

Children with septic arthritis will often have a history of recent upper respiratory or local soft-tissue infection, as well a recent course of antibiotics. A high level of suspicion is important when evaluating premature and immunocompromised infants. Septic arthritis is more commonly seen in boys and is most common in children younger than 2 years. Patients may report pain, stiffness, and malaise, but such a history is often impossible to ascertain from small children or infants. Fever, limp, inability or refusal to weight bear, limited and painful range of motion (secondary to capsular stretching), erythema, warmth, tenderness, and swelling are common physical findings. The child may complain of anterior hip, groin, thigh, or knee pain. The child may lie with the hip in external rotation, adduction, and mild flexion to maximize joint volume and decrease capsular stretch. Physical examination of the infant can be challenging and may only demonstrate limited or a lack of active motion in the affected extremity (pseudoparalysis).

Laboratory tests that are frequently ordered in cases of suspected septic arthritis of the hip include C-reactive protein (CRP) level, erythrocyte sedimentation rate (ESR), complete blood cell count (CBC) with differential, blood cultures, and throat culture/rapid strep test. Lyme titers are often added in endemic areas. Plain radiographs of the hip or pelvis are routinely ordered. Ultrasound may be useful to detect joint effusion. Magnetic resonance imaging (MRI) may be useful to detect associated osteomyelitis. The definitive diagnosis of septic arthritis is made by joint aspiration and analysis of joint fluid. Joint fluid white blood cell (WBC) count and cultures establish the diagnosis. Organisms can be detected on joint fluid Gram stain or culture. Cases with negative cultures but increased joint fluid WBC counts ($>50,000/mm^3$) are considered to be presumed septic arthritis or culture-negative septic arthritis.

Treatment

Poor outcome is most closely associated with delay in diagnosis with subsequent delay in treatment. Once septic arthritis is diagnosed, prompt treatment with adequate surgical drainage and empiric IV antimicrobial therapy is cardinal. Ideally, synovial and blood cultures are obtained before treatment to increase the likelihood of identifying an organism. Open surgical irrigation and debridement to remove the microorganisms, host and bacterial enzymes, and particulate debris is indicated for most patients. However, arthroscopy has been used successfully in the shoulder, elbow, knee, and ankle, but it has not been widely utilized in the hip. Empiric IV antimicrobial therapy should be initiated as soon as cultures are obtained. Empiric coverage must include an anti-staphylococcal agent, either a β-lactamase–resistant penicillin or a first-generation cephalosporin. Cefazolin is chosen as the drug for initial empiric therapy because it is effective against *S. aureus,* group A streptococcus, and *S. pneumococcus,* which should account for nearly all of the organisms among normal hosts with acute hematogenous osteomyelitis. Gram-negative coverage is indicated in the neonate (causative organisms may also include

group B streptococci and gram-negative bacilli) and adolescents (to cover gonococcus). In children who are allergic to penicillin, clindamycin can be used. Ceftriaxone should be considered for coverage of gonococcal or Lyme arthritis. The antimicrobial regimen is adjusted according to culture speciation; if another organism is identified as the causative agent, an infectious disease consultation should be sought. IV antibiotics are continued for 72 hours. If the child shows evidence of clinical improvement (afebrile, decreased localized swelling, decreased/no pain, increased range of motion) and lyme titers are negative, conversion to oral antibiotics can be considered. The criteria for oral antibiotics include diagnosis within 4 days of the onset of symptoms, no concurrent osteomyelitis, and an ability to tolerate and be rigorously compliant with taking oral antibiotics. Patients treated with cefazolin may be given cephalexin 100 mg/kg/day divided in 4 daily doses (maximum dose, 4 g/day), and those treated with ceftriaxone can receive cefixime 8 mg/kg/day every 12 to 24 hours (maximum dose, 400 mg/day) for 21 days. The median duration of IV antibiotics is 5 to 15 days, and the total duration of antibiotics has been 4 to 6 weeks in uncomplicated cases.

EVIDENCE

Imaging

Ultrasonography has been demonstrated good accuracy in detecting an effusion associated with septic arthritis of the hip in children. Zamzam[25] retrospectively studied 81 children with septic arthritis and 73 children with transient synovitis, finding sensitivity of 86.4% and specificity of 89.7%. Dörr and colleagues[26] also found ultrasound to be useful in detecting effusion in 204 acutely irritable hips. In addition, they found certain characteristics, such as synovial hypertrophy and capsular thickening, to be helpful in differentiation between septic arthritis and transient synovitis. In a prospective analysis of 500 children with a painful hip or limp, Miralles and researchers[27] found ultrasonography to be useful in the detection of effusion. In addition, these authors showed that transient synovitis had resolution of the effusion at repeat ultrasound 2 weeks later.

MRI has been shown to be useful in detecting associated osteomyelitis but may also be useful in differentiating septic arthritis from transient synovitis. In a retrospective case series of 49 children with transient synovitis and 18 children with septic arthritis, Yang and investigators[28] found that patients with transient synovitis were more likely to have contralateral effusion and absence of signal intensity in the surrounding soft tissue and bone marrow.

Laboratory Tests

Clinicians have empirically utilized different laboratory variables to help distinguish between septic arthritis and transient synovitis. Bennett and Namnyak[29] emphasize leukocyte count in children older than 3 years. Morrey and coauthors[20] and Klein and researchers[21] accent increased ESR. Chen and colleagues[30] found both leukocytosis and increased ESR to be common. However, because these retrospective case series of children with septic arthritis did not have a comparison group of children with transient synovitis, they were unable to identify differences between the groups and were unable to determine the diagnostic performance of assorted variables.

On comparing children with septic arthritis and transient synovitis in retrospective case series, poor diagnostic utility has been found for various screening clinical, laboratory, and radiographic data because of substantial overlap between the two groups. Molteni[22] retrospectively reviewed 97 patients with so-called nonspecific arthritis and 37 patients with septic arthritis of various joints including the hip, knee, ankle elbow, and wrist. Diagnoses were established presumptively, with joint fluid analysis of 12 of 97 patients with nonspecific arthritis and of 32 of 37 patients with septic arthritis. Fifty percent of the patients with septic arthritis had negative cultures and joint fluid WBC count varied from 5 to 385 × 1000/mm^3. Without statistically comparing the two groups, Molteni[22] describes the clinical and laboratory findings in each (septic arthritis vs. nonspecific arthritis): age (5.8 vs. 6.0 years), male sex (22/37 vs. 49/97), temperature >101°F (82% vs. 38%), serum WBC count (7.23 vs. 6.3 × 1000/mm^3), and ESR (50 vs. 35 mm/hr). Because of the similarities in values and the extent of overlap, he concludes that reliable data were not found to distinguish the two different joint processes. Del Beccaro and colleagues[31] also found that overlap between screening variables impeded the differentiation of septic arthritis and transient synovitis of the hip in children. They compare 94 children with transient synovitis (defined retrospectively via clinical course) with 38 patients with septic arthritis (defined as pyarthrosis). In the transient synovitis group, 21 of 94 patients had joint fluid analysis, and in the septic arthritis group, 28 of 38 patients had joint fluid cell counts. They found significant ($P < 0.05$) univariate differences between the two groups with respect to the following factors (septic arthritis vs. transient synovitis): temperature (38.1°C vs. 37.2°C), ESR (44 vs. 19 mm/hr), PMN (7.8 vs. 6.3 × 1000/mm^3), and bands (903 vs. 295/mm^3). Of note, with the numbers available for study, serum WBC count could not be shown to differ significantly ($P > 0.05$) (13.2 vs 11.2 × 1000/mm^3). Although ESR was significantly ($P < 0.05$) different between the two groups, the substantial amount of overlap made it a poor discriminator. The range of ESR for the septic hip group was 6 to 90 mm/hr (with 24% of patients with ESR <20 mm/hr), and the range for the synovitis group was 1 to 125 mm/hr (with 28% of patients with ESR >20 mm/hr). By combining ESR >20 mm/hr with temperature >37.5°C, they were able to identify 97% of the septic arthritis cases; however, those parameters also included 47% of the transient syno-

vitis cases. Kunnamo and coworkers[32] reviewed 278 children younger than 16 years with various arthritides, including transient synovitis, juvenile arthritis, septic arthritis, serum sickness, enteroarthritis, and Schonlein–Henoch purpura. They found the patients with septic arthritis ($n = 18$) to differ significantly ($P < 0.05$) from the other patients with respect to CRP level, temperature >38.5°C, and serum WBC count >12 (×1000/mm^3).[20] Levine and colleagues[33] emphasize the value of CRP in the diagnosis of septic arthritis of the hip. In a retrospective review of 133 children with an irritable joint, CRP level had better predictive ability than ESR. In particular, if the CRP level was less than 1.0 mg/dL, the probability that the patient did not have septic arthritis was 87%.

Prediction Rules

Prediction rules based on presenting variables have been developed to differentiate septic arthritis from transient synovitis of the hip. Kocher and reviewers[34] retrospectively analyzed 82 children with septic arthritis and 86 children with transient synovitis of the hip treated at Children's Hospital Boston from 1979 to 1996. Diagnoses of true septic arthritis, presumed septic arthritis, and transient synovitis were made based on joint fluid WBC, blood and joint fluid cultures, and clinical course. Using multivariate analysis, they identified four independent predictors of septic arthritis (history of fever, non–weight bearing, ESR ≥40 mm/hr, and serum WBC >12,000/mm^3). The predicted probability of septic arthritis was calculated for all 16 combinations of these 4 predictors (Table 30–1) and was summarized as 0.2% for 0 predictor, 3.0% for 1 predictor, 40.0% for 2 predictors, 93.1% for 3 predictors, and 99.6% for 4 predictors (Table 30–2). This prediction rule demonstrated excellent diagnostic performance with an area under the receiver operating characteristic (ROC) curve of 0.96 (Fig. 30–1).

These authors then validated this prediction rule in a new series of patients.[35] They prospectively analyzed 51 children with septic arthritis of the hip and 103 children with transient synovitis of the hip treated at Children's Hospital Boston from 1997 to 2002. Using the same diagnostic parameters and similar analysis, they identified the same four multivariate predictors of septic arthritis (history of fever, non–weight bearing, ESR ≥40mm/hr, and serum WBC >12,000/mm^3). The predicted probability of septic arthritis demonstrated similar but not identical values (see Table 30–1) and was summarized as 2.0% for one predictor, 9.5% for one predictor, 35.0% for 2 predictors, 72.8% for 3 predictors, and 93.0% for 4 predictors (see Table 30–2). The diagnostic accuracy showed diminished but still good performance with an area under the ROC curve of 0.86.

Jung and colleagues[36] performed a similar study to establish a prediction rule for the differentiation of septic arthritis and transient synovitis of the hip

TABLE 30–1. Probability of Septic Arthritis Algorithm

HISTORY OF FEVER	NON–WEIGHT BEARING	ESR ≥ 40 mm/hr	SERUM WBC COUNT > 12,000/mm³	PREDICTED PROBABILITY OF SEPTIC ARTHRITIS	DISTRIBUTION OF SEPTIC ARTHRITIS (NEW POPULATION)
Yes	Yes	Yes	Yes	99.8%	91.8%
Yes	Yes	Yes	No	97.3%	83.3%
Yes	Yes	No	Yes	95.2%	71.7%
Yes	Yes	No	No	57.8%	38.0%
Yes	No	Yes	Yes	95.5%	65.7%
Yes	No	Yes	No	62.2%	31.7%
Yes	No	No	Yes	44.8%	30.0%
Yes	No	No	No	5.3%	9.4%
No	Yes	Yes	Yes	93.0%	72.2%
No	Yes	Yes	No	48.0%	38.6%
No	Yes	No	Yes	33.8%	36.8%
No	Yes	No	No	3.4%	12.3%
No	No	Yes	Yes	35.3%	30.5%
No	No	Yes	No	3.7%	9.6%
No	No	No	Yes	2.1%	9.0%
No	No	No	No	1 in 700	2.3%

ESR, erythrocyte sedimentation rate; WBC, white blood cell.
Data from Kocher MS, Zurakowski D, Kasser JR: Differentiating between septic arthritis and transient synovitis of the hip in children: An evidence-based clinical prediction algorithm. J Bone Joint Surg Am 81-A:1662–1670, 1999; and Kocher MS, Mandiga R, Zurakowski D, et al: Validation of a clinical prediction rule for the differentiation of septic arthritis and transient synovitis of the hip in children. J Bone Joint Surg Am 86-A:1629–1635, 2004.

TABLE 30–2. Probability of Septic Arthritis

NO. OF PREDICTORS*	TRANSIENT SYNOVITIS (N = 86)	SEPTIC ARTHRITIS (N = 82)	PREDICTED PROBABILITY OF SEPTIC ARTHRITIS	DISTRIBUTION OF SEPTIC ARTHRITIS (NEW POPULATION)
0	19 (22.1%)	0 (0%)	<0.2%	2.0%
1	47 (54.7%)	1 (1.2%)	3.0%	9.5%
2	16 (18.6%)	12 (14.6%)	40.0%	35.0%
3	4 (4.7%)	44 (53.7%)	93.1%	72.8%
4	0 (0%)	25 (30.5%)	99.6%	93.0%

*Predictors are history of fever, non–weight bearing, erythrocyte sedimentation rate ≥40 (mm/hr), and serum white blood cell count >12 (×1000/mm³).
Data from Kocher MS, Zurakowski D, Kasser JR: Differentiating between septic arthritis and transient synovitis of the hip in children: An evidence-based clinical prediction algorithm. J Bone Joint Surg Am 81-A:1662–1670, 1999; and Kocher MS, Mandiga R, Zurakowski D, et al: Validation of a clinical prediction rule for the differentiation of septic arthritis and transient synovitis of the hip in children. J Bone Joint Surg Am 86-A:1629–1635, 2004.

(Fig. 30–2). In a retrospective series of 97 children with transient synovitis of the hip and 27 children with septic arthritis of the hip, they identified five independent multivariate predictors of septic arthritis: temperature >37°C, ESR >20 mm/hr, CRP level >1.0 mg/dL, serum WBC count >11,000/mm³, and >2 mm joint space difference on radiographs. Four of these five predictors were similar to those of Kocher and reviewers.[34] They developed an algorithm based on the 32 combinations of the 5 predictors. The area under the ROC curve for their prediction rule was 0.986 (Table 30–3). This prediction rule has not been validated in a new patient population.

Luhmann and coworkers[37] developed a new clinical prediction rule and analyzed the performance of the prediction rule of Kocher and reviewers[34] in a retrospective series of 47 septic hips and 118 transient synovitis hips at St. Louis Children's Hospital from 1992 to 2000. Their multivariate model identified three predictors of septic arthritis: history of fever, serum WBC >12,000/mm³, and prior healthcare visit. Two of the four predictors from the algorithm of Kocher and reviewers[34] were not predictive in their model: ESR and non–weight bearing. The area under the ROC curve for their model was 77.1%, and the area under the ROC curve for the algorithm of Kocher and reviewers[34] in their population was 79.9%.

Caird and researchers[38] also developed a prediction rule for the differentiation of children with septic arthritis versus transient synovitis of the hip. In a prospective study of 53 children who underwent aspiration for an acutely irritable hip over a 4-year period at Children's Hospital of Philadelphia, they identified 5 predictors of septic arthritis: fever >38.5°C, CRP level >2.0 mg/L, ESR >40 mm/hr, refusal to bear weight, and serum WBC >12,000/mm³. The four predictors from the algorithm of Kocher and reviewers[34] were predictive in this model, and CRP level showed enhanced diagnostic performance over ESR. The

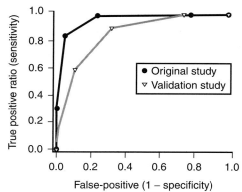

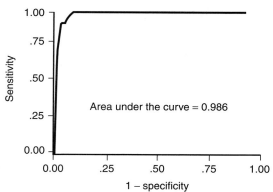

FIGURE 30–1. Receiver-operating characteristic curves for the clinical prediction rule of Kocher and coworkers[34,35] in the original patient population (area under curve = 0.96) and the new patient population (area under curve = 0.86). (Data from Kocher MS, Zurakowski D, Kasser JR: Differentiating between septic arthritis and transient synovitis of the hip in children: An evidence-based clinical prediction algorithm. J Bone Joint Surg Am 81-A:1662–1670, 1999; and Kocher MS, Mandiga R, Zurakowski D, et al: Validation of a clinical prediction rule for the differentiation of septic arthritis and transient synovitis of the hip in children. J Bone Joint Surg Am 86-A:1629–1635, 2004.)

FIGURE 30–2. Receiver-operating characteristic curve for clinical prediction rule of Jung and colleagues.[36] (Data from Jung ST, Rowe SM, Moon ES, et al: Significance of laboratory and radiologic findings for differentiating between septic arthritis and transient synovitis of the hip. J Pediatr Orthop 23:368–372, 2003.)

TABLE 30–3. Probability of Septic Arthritis

TEMPERATURE >37°C	ESR >20 mm/hr	CRP LEVEL >1.0 mg/dL	WBC COUNT >11,000 cells/mL	DIFFERENCE OF JOINT SPACE DISTANCE >2 mm	PREDICTIVE PROBABILITY OF SEPTIC ARTHRITIS (%)
Yes	Yes	Yes	Yes	Yes	99.1
Yes	Yes	Yes	Yes	No	97.3
Yes	Yes	Yes	No	Yes	84.8
Yes	Yes	Yes	No	No	65.5
Yes	Yes	No	Yes	Yes	90.9
Yes	Yes	No	Yes	No	77.2
Yes	Yes	No	No	Yes	34.5
Yes	Yes	No	No	No	15.2
Yes	No	Yes	Yes	Yes	85.9
Yes	No	Yes	Yes	No	67.4
Yes	No	Yes	No	Yes	24.3
Yes	No	Yes	No	No	9.9
Yes	No	No	Yes	Yes	36.5
Yes	No	No	Yes	No	16.4
Yes	No	No	No	Yes	2.9
Yes	No	No	No	No	1.0
No	Yes	Yes	Yes	Yes	90.1
No	Yes	Yes	Yes	No	75.6
No	Yes	Yes	No	Yes	32.5
No	Yes	Yes	No	No	14.1
No	Yes	No	Yes	Yes	46.2
No	Yes	No	Yes	No	22.7
No	Yes	No	No	Yes	4.3
No	Yes	No	No	No	1.5
No	No	Yes	Yes	Yes	34.4
No	No	Yes	Yes	No	15.2
No	No	Yes	No	Yes	2.7
No	No	Yes	No	No	0.9
No	No	No	Yes	Yes	4.7
No	No	No	Yes	No	1.7
No	No	No	No	Yes	0.3
No	No	No	No	No	0.1

ESR, erythrocyte sedimentation rate; CRP, C-reactive protein; WBC, white blood cell.
Data from Jung ST, Rowe SM, Moon ES, et al: Significance of laboratory and radiologic findings for differentiating between septic arthritis and transient synovitis of the hip. J Pediatr Orthop 23:368–372, 2003.

TABLE 30–4. Probability of Septic Arthritis

			Predicted Probability of Septic Arthritis (%)	
NO. OF FACTORS	SEPTIC ARTHRITIS (*N* = 34), *n* (%)	TRANSIENT SYNOVITIS (*N* = 14), *n* (%)	CURRENTSTUDY	KOCHER ET AL.'S STUDY[34]
0	1 (3)	3 (21)	16.9	0.2
1	3 (9)	6 (43)	36.7	3
2	3 (9)	2 (14)	62.4	40
3	9 (26)	2 (14)	82.6	93.1
4	15 (44)	1 (7)	93.1	99.6
5	3 (9)	0	97.5	

Data from Caird MS, Flynn JM, Leung YL, et al: Factors distinguishing septic arthritis from transient synovitis of the hip in children. A prospective study. J Bone Joint Surg Am 88:1251–1257, 2006.

probability of septic arthritis was 16.9% for 0 predictors, 36.7% for 1 predictor, 62.4% for 2 predictors, 82.6% for 3 predictors, 93.1% for 4 predictors, and 97.5% for 5 predictors (Table 30–4).

Clinical Practice Guidelines

Kocher and coworkers[39] developed a clinical practice guideline (CPG) for the diagnosis and management of patients with septic arthritis of the hip (Fig. 30–3). The diagnostic arm of the algorithm included laboratory analysis of CRP level, ESR, CBC count with differential, Lyme titer, blood culture, throat culture, and antistreptolysin O titer (ALSO). The imaging arm of the algorithm included radiographs and ultrasound. In a case–control study of the performance of this algorithm, the authors found that CPG patients had significantly greater rates of obtaining initial and follow-up CRP tests (93% vs. 13% and 70% vs. 7%), lower use of initial bone scan (13% vs. 40%), lower rates of presumptive drainage (13% vs. 47%), greater compliance with recommended antibiotic therapy (93% vs. 7%), faster change to oral antibiotics (3.9 vs. 6.9 days), and shorter hospital course (4.8 vs. 8.3 days). No significant differences were found for outcome variables of readmission, recurrent infection, recurrent drainage, development of osteomyelitis, septic osteonecrosis, or limitation of motion. They conclude that patients on the septic arthritis CPG had less variation of process and improved efficiency of care, without a significant difference in outcome.

RECOMMENDATIONS

The diagnosis of septic arthritis of the hip can be vexing. The differentiation between septic arthritis and transient synovitis is important because the clinical entities have vastly different treatment and prognosis. Furthermore, delay in diagnosis of septic arthritis is a risk factor for poor outcome.

Certain presenting variables can be useful in the diagnosis of septic arthritis. Based on history, a history of fever and of non–weight bearing have been identified as predictors of septic arthritis. Based on laboratory tests, increased serum WBC count, ESR, and CRP level are predictive of septic arthritis. In particular, CRP level has greater diagnostic value than ESR. Based on imaging, ultrasonography can identify an effusion and can help guide arthrocentesis (Table 30–5).

Clinical prediction rules can be useful for stratifying the risk for septic arthritis. This may guide further management. For example, patients with extremely high risk for septic arthritis may be best managed with aspiration in the operating room given the high probability of needing surgical drainage. Patients with extremely low risk for septic arthritis may be managed with observation in the correct clinical context. Patients with intermediate risk should undergo arthrocentesis to establish the diagnosis.

Ultimately, there are no laboratory tests, imaging modalities, or prediction rules that are pathognomonic for the diagnosis of septic arthritis. Clinical prediction rules are not designed to replace clinical judgment. Because the risks of missing the diagnosis of septic arthritis of the hip are so consequential, there should be a low threshold for joint aspiration to establish the diagnosis and surgical drainage for definitive treatment.

SEPTIC ARTHRITIS CPG ALGORITHM

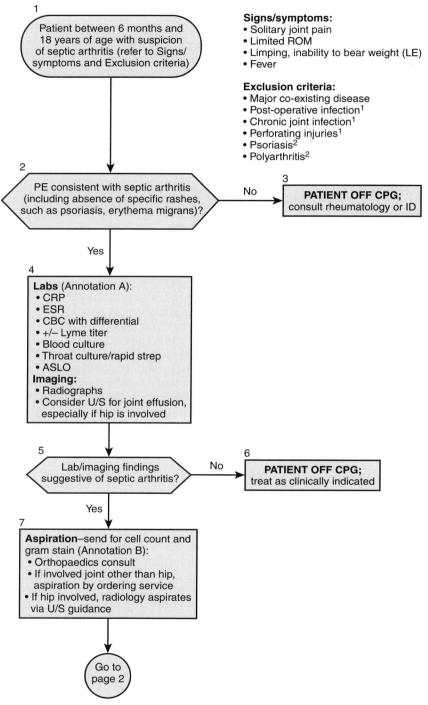

¹Consult ID
²Consult rheumatology

FIGURE 30–3. Clinical practice guideline for septic arthritis. (Adapted from Kocher MS, Mandiga R, Murphy J, et al: A clinical practice guideline for septic arthritis in children: Efficacy on process and outcome for septic arthritis of the hip. J Bone Joint Surg Am 85-A:994–999, 2003, with permission of the Journal of Bone and Joint Surgery.)

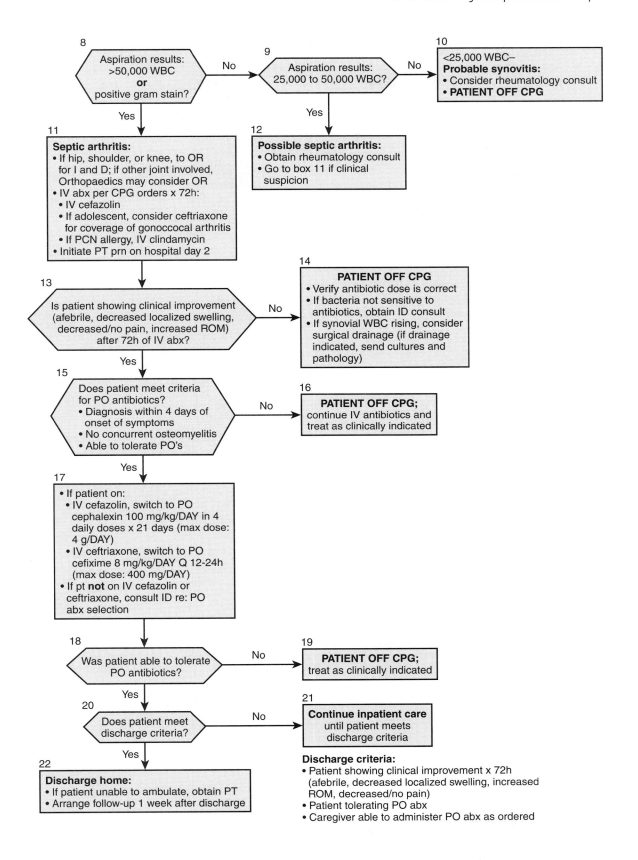

8 Aspiration results: >50,000 WBC **or** positive gram stain? — No → **9** Aspiration results: 25,000 to 50,000 WBC? — No → **10** <25,000 WBC– **Probable synovitis:** • Consider rheumatology consult • **PATIENT OFF CPG**

8 Yes ↓

9 Yes ↓ **12** **Possible septic arthritis:** • Obtain rheumatology consult • Go to box 11 if clinical suspicion

11 **Septic arthritis:**
• If hip, shoulder, or knee, to OR for I and D; if other joint involved, Orthopaedics may consider OR
• IV abx per CPG orders x 72h:
  • IV cefazolin
  • If adolescent, consider ceftriaxone for coverage of gonoccocal arthritis
  • If PCN allergy, IV clindamycin
• Initiate PT prn on hospital day 2

13 Is patient showing clinical improvement (afebrile, decreased localized swelling, decreased/no pain, increased ROM) after 72h of IV abx? — No → **14** **PATIENT OFF CPG**
• Verify antibiotic dose is correct
• If bacteria not sensitive to antibiotics, obtain ID consult
• If synovial WBC rising, consider surgical drainage (if drainage indicated, send cultures and pathology)

13 Yes ↓

15 Does patient meet criteria for PO antibiotics?
• Diagnosis within 4 days of onset of symptoms
• No concurrent osteomyelitis
• Able to tolerate PO's — No → **16** **PATIENT OFF CPG;** continue IV antibiotics and treat as clinically indicated

15 Yes ↓

17 • If patient on:
  • IV cefazolin, switch to PO cephalexin 100 mg/kg/DAY in 4 daily doses x 21 days (max dose: 4 g/DAY)
  • IV ceftriaxone, switch to PO cefixime 8 mg/kg/DAY Q 12-24h (max dose: 400 mg/DAY)
• If pt **not** on IV cefazolin or ceftriaxone, consult ID re: PO abx selection

18 Was patient able to tolerate PO antibiotics? — No → **19** **PATIENT OFF CPG;** treat as clinically indicated

18 Yes ↓

20 Does patient meet discharge criteria? — No → **21** **Continue inpatient care** until patient meets discharge criteria

20 Yes ↓

22 **Discharge home:**
• If patient unable to ambulate, obtain PT
• Arrange follow-up 1 week after discharge

Discharge criteria:
• Patient showing clinical improvement x 72h (afebrile, decreased localized swelling, increased ROM, decreased/no pain)
• Patient tolerating PO abx
• Caregiver able to administer PO abx as ordered

TABLE 30–5. Review of the Literature: Clinical Prediction Rules

STUDY	LEVEL OF EVIDENCE	PROSPECTIVE VS. RETROSPECTIVE	PATIENTS WITH SEPTIC ARTHRITIS, *n*	PATIENTS WITH TRANSIENT SYNOVITIS, *n*	PREDICTORS	SUMMARY STATISTICS
Kocher et al. (1999)[34]	IV	Retrospective	82	86	1. History of fever 2. Non–weight bearing 3. ESR ≥40 mm/hr 4. WBC >12,000/mm³	Area under ROC curve: 0.96
Kocher et al. (2004)[35]	II	Prospective	51	103	1. History of fever 2. Non–weight bearing 3. ESR ≥40 mm/hr 4. WBC >12,000/mm³	Area under ROC curve: 0.86
Jung et al. (2003)[36]	IV	Retrospective	27	97	1. Temperature >37°C 2. ESR >20 mm/hr 3. CRP level >1.0 mg/dL 4. WBC >11,000/mm³ 5. >2 mm joint space widening on radiographs	Area under ROC curve: 0.986
Luhmann et al. (2004)[37]	IV	Retrospective	47	118	1. History of fever 2. WBC count >12,000/mm³ 3. Prior healthcare visit	Area under ROC curve: 0.771
Caird et al. (2006)[38]	II	Prospective	34	14	1. Temperature >38.5°C 2. CRP level >2.0 mg/L 3. ESR >40 mm/hr 4. Refusal to bear weight 5. Serum WBC count >12,000/mm³.	

ESR, erythrocyte sedimentation rate; WBC, white blood cell; ROC, receiver operating characteristic; CRP, C-reactive protein.

TABLE 30–6. Summary of Recommendations

STATEMENT	LEVEL OF EVIDENCE/GRADE OF RECOMMENDATION	REFERENCES
1. Poor outcomes have been associated with delay in diagnosis of septic arthritis of the hip in children.	B	16-20
2. Widespread use of the vaccine for Haemophilus influenza type B has substantially reduced the incidence of septic arthritis from this pathogen.	B	23, 24
3. Ultrasonography accurately identifies hip effusion in children.	B	27
4. MRI can differentiate septic arthritis from transient synovitis of the hip in children.	B	28
5. CRP level <1.0 mg/dL is suggestive of transient synovitis.	B	33
6. Predictors that differentiate septic arthritis from transient synovitis include history of fever, non–weight bearing, ESR >40 mm/hr, and serum WBC >12,000/mm3.	B	34, 35
7. Predictors that differentiate septic arthritis from transient synovitis include temperature >37°C, ESR >20 mm/hr, CRP level >1.0 mg/dL, serum WBC count >11,000/mm3, and >2 mm joint space difference on radiographs.	B	36
8. Predictors that differentiate septic arthritis from transient synovitis include history of fever, serum WBC >12,000/mm3, and prior healthcare visit.	B	37
9. Predictors that differentiate septic arthritis from transient synovitis include fever >38.5°C, CRP level >2.0 mg/L, ESR >40 mm/hr, refusal to bear weight, and serum WBC >12,000/mm3.	B	38
10. A clinical practice guideline (CPG) for management of children with septic arthritis of the hip can result in less variation of process and improved efficiency of care, without a significant difference in outcome.	B	39

REFERENCES

1. Adams JA: Transient synovitis of the hip in children. J Bone Joint Surg 45B:471–476, 1963.
2. Dan M: Septic arthritis in young infants: Clinical and microbiologic correlations and therapeutic implications. Rev Infect Dis 6:147–155, 1984.
3. Edwards EG: Transient synovitis of the hip joint in children. JAMA 148:30–36, 1952.
4. Haueisen DC, Weiner DS, Weiner SD: The characterization of transient synovitis of the hip in children. J Pediatr Orthop 6:11–17, 1986.
5. Petersen S, Knudsen FU, Andersen EA, Egeblad M: Acute haematogenous osteomyelitis and septic arthritis in childhood: A 10-year review and follow-up. Acta Orthop Scand 51:451–457, 1980.
6. Sharwood PF: The irritable hip syndrome in children. Acta Orthop Scand 52:633–638, 1981.
7. Wingstrand H: Transient synovitis of the hip in the child. Acta Orthop Scand 57(supp):1–61, 1986.
8. Betz RR, Cooperman DR, Wopperer JM, et al: Late sequelae of septic arthritis of the hip in infancy and childhood. J Pediatr Orthop 10:365–372, 1990.
9. De Valderrama JAF: The "observation hip" and its late sequelae. J Bone Joint Surg Br 45:462–470, 1963.
10. Hermel MB, Albert SM: Transient synovitis of the hip. Clin Orthop 22:21–26, 1962.
11. Hunka L, Said SE, MacKenzie DA, et al: Classification and surgical management of the severe sequelae of septic hips in children. Clin Orthop 171:30–36, 1982.
12. Jacobs BW: Synovitis of the hip in children and its significance. Pediatrics 47:558–566, 1971.
13. Nachemson A, Scheller S: A clinical and radiological follow-up study of transient synovitis of the hip. Acta Orthop Scand 40:479–500, 1969.
14. Spock A: Transient synovitis of the hip in children. Pediatrics 24:1042–1048, 1959.
15. Wopperer JM, White JJ, Gillespie R, Obletz BE: Long-term follow-up of infantile hip sepsis. J Pediatr Orthop 8:322–325, 1988.
16. Fabry G, Meire E: Septic arthritis of the hip in children: Poor results after late and inadequate treatment. J Pediatr Orthop 3:461–466, 1983.
17. Gillespie R: Septic arthritis of childhood. Clin Orthop 96:152–159, 1973.
18. Jackson MA, Nelson JD: Etiology and medical management of acute suppurative bone and joint infections in pediatric patients. J Pediatr Orthop 2:313–323, 1982.
19. Lunseth PA, Heiple KG: Prognosis in septic arthritis of the hip in children. Clin Orthop 139:81–85, 1979.
20. Morrey BF, Bianco AJ Jr, Rhodes KH: Septic arthritis in children. Orthop Clin North Am 6:923–934, 1975.
21. Klein DM, Barbera C, Gray ST, et al: Sensitivity of objective parameters in the diagnosis of pediatric septic hips. Clin Orthop 338:153–159, 1997.
22. Molteni RA: The differential diagnosis of benign and septic joint disease in children. Clin Pediatr 17:19–23, 1978.
23. Howard AW, Viskontas D, Sabbagh C: Reduction in osteomyelitis and septic arthritis related to Haemophilus influenzae type B vaccination. J Pediatr Orthop 19:705–709, 1999.
24. Peltola H, Kallio MJ, Unkila-Kallio L: Reduced incidence of septic arthritis in children by Haemophilus influenzae type-b vaccination. Implications for treatment. J Bone Joint Surg Br 80:471–473, 1998.
25. Zamzam MM: The role of ultrasound in differentiating septic arthritis from transient synovitis of the hip in children. J Pediatr Orthop 15:418–422, 2006.
26. Dörr U, Zieger M, Hauke H: Ultrasonography of the painful hip. Prospective studies in 204 patients. Pediatr Radiol 19:36–40, 1988.
27. Miralles M, Gonzalez G, Pulpeiro JR, et al: Sonography of the painful hip in children: 500 consecutive cases. Am J Roentgenol 152:579–582, 1989.
28. Yang WJ, Im SA, Lim GY, et al: MR imaging of transient synovitis: Differentiation from septic arthritis. Pediatr Radiol 36:1154–1158, 2006.
29. Bennett OM, Namnyak SS: Acute septic arthritis of the hip joint in infancy and childhood. Clin Orthop 281:123–132, 1992.
30. Chen CH, Lee ZL, Yang WE, et al: Acute septic arthritis of the hip in children: Clinical analysis of 31 cases. Changgeng Yi Xue Za Zhi 16:239–245, 1993.
31. Del Beccaro MA, Champoux AN, Bockers T, Mendelman PM: Septic arthritis versus transient synovitis of the hip: The value of screening laboratory tests. Ann Emerg Med 21:1418–1422, 1992.
32. Kunnamo I, Kallio P, Pelkonen P, Hovi T: Clinical signs and laboratory tests in the differential diagnosis of arthritis in children. Am J Dis Child 141:34–40, 1987.
33. Levine MJ, McGuire KJ, McGowan KL, et al: Assessment of the test characteristics of C-reactive protein for septic arthritis in children. J Pediatr Orthop 23:373–377, 2003.
34. Kocher MS, Zurakowski D, Kasser JR: Differentiating between septic arthritis and transient synovitis of the hip in children: An evidence-based clinical prediction algorithm. J Bone Joint Surg Am 81-A:1662–1670, 1999.
35. Kocher MS, Mandiga R, Zurakowski D, et al: Validation of a clinical prediction rule for the differentiation of septic arthritis and transient synovitis of the hip in children. J Bone Joint Surg Am 86-A:1629–1635, 2004.
36. Jung ST, Rowe SM, Moon ES, et al: Significance of laboratory and radiologic findings for differentiating between septic arthritis and transient synovitis of the hip. J Pediatr Orthop 23:368–372, 2003.
37. Luhmann SJ, Jones A, Schootman M, et al: Differentiation between septic arthritis and transient synovitis of the hip in children with clinical prediction algorithms. J Bone Joint Surg Am 86-A:956–962, 2004.
38. Caird MS, Flynn JM, Leung YL, et al: Factors distinguishing septic arthritis from transient synovitis of the hip in children. A prospective study. J Bone Joint Surg Am 88:1251–1257, 2006.
39. Kocher MS, Mandiga R, Murphy J, et al: A clinical practice guideline for septic arthritis in children: Efficacy on process and outcome for septic arthritis of the hip. J Bone Joint Surg Am 85-A:994–999, 2003.

What Is the Best Treatment for Anterior Cruciate Ligament Injuries in Skeletally Immature Individuals?

R. Baxter Willis, MD, FRCSC

Anterior cruciate ligament (ACL) injury in a growing child is being diagnosed with some degree of frequency, probably because of increased skill in diagnostic ability including specialized imaging studies such as magnetic resonance imaging.[1-7] The true incidence of ACL injury in the skeletally immature athlete is unknown. In a series of 1000 consecutive ACL injuries treated at the Cleveland Clinic, 5 patients were younger than 12 years.[8]

From insurance claim data in the United States for youth soccer leagues, the overall incidence rate is about 0.01% with 550 claims for ACL injury out of 6 million children and youths who were insured during the time period.[9] Girls have been noted to be 2 to 9 times more likely to sustain this injury than boys.[10]

NATURAL HISTORY OF ANTERIOR CRUCIATE LIGAMENT INJURY IN CHILDREN

In adults, chronic ACL insufficiency leads to intra-articular damage. Meniscal tears and chondral damage occur in individuals who continue to participate in sports and recreational activities without the benefit of a stable knee.[11-13] What is the evidence? A number of Level II and III studies confirm the same dismal prognosis in children with open physes; namely, if the ACL is left untreated, the patient has a markedly increased risk for development of meniscal tears and chondral damage leading to eventual osteoarthritis.[4,5,14-18]

Level III studies by Graf and colleagues,[4] McCarroll and coworkers,[5] and Angel and Hall[1] all report on the high incidence of meniscal tears and the inability to resume preinjury activity levels. Level II studies by Aichroth and investigators,[14] Pressman and researchers,[18] and Kannus and Jarvinen[19] have confirmed the results of these earlier studies.

MAKING THE DIAGNOSIS

Since the early 1990s, the orthopedic literature has discussed in depth the possibility of an ACL disruption in the growing child. Before these detailed descriptions, it was generally believed that children did not tear the ACL with the exception of the pediatric equivalent, namely, the tibial eminence fracture.[20-23] With that background, it is important for the physician to have a high index of suspicion in a child presenting with a presumed hemarthrosis (swollen knee) after a knee injury.

In a number of series of knee injuries in the pediatric population, the incidence rate of ACL disruption has been reported to be as low as 10% and as high as 65% in series with the number of patients ranging from 35 to 138 patients.[24-28]

A physical examination in this clinical setting should include a careful examination for ACL insufficiency. The examination should consist of a careful and gentle Lachman test for anteroposterior instability with the knee at 20 to 30 degrees of flexion, an anterior drawer test at 90 degrees if the patient's pain and tense effusion will allow, and finally, a gentle examination for a positive pivot shift.

Again, a high index of suspicion is necessary. Except in the incidence of tibial or femoral bony avulsion, there is no need for urgent surgical reconstruction (Level of Evidence V). The patient can be instructed to ice the knee, start active range-of-motion exercises and strengthening, and be re-evaluated in 2 to 3 weeks when the physical examination will be more reliable and easier to perform because the patient will be more comfortable and the majority of the hemarthrosis will be resorbed.

DIAGNOSTIC IMAGING

All patients with a significant knee injury and presenting with an effusion (hemarthrosis) should have plain radiographs of the knee to rule out tibial eminence fracture or other bony avulsions and osteochondral fractures.

The decision to order magnetic resonance imaging still remains somewhat controversial. However, in 2007, it is recommended for patients with suspected ACL tears to be evaluated for meniscal tear and osteochondral lesions (such as a fracture or a "bone bruise") (Fig. 32–1) (Level of Evidence V).

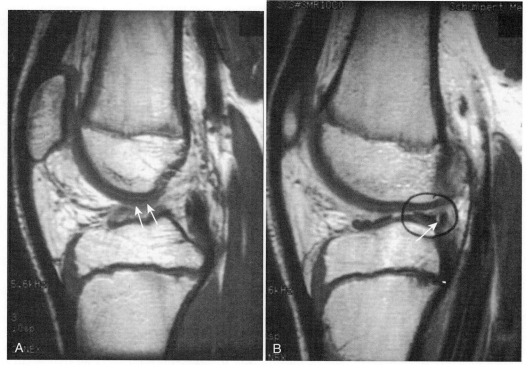

FIGURE 31–1. *A,* Magnetic resonance imaging (MRI) of a skeletally immature adolescent with disruption of anterior cruciate ligament (ACL) tear. Note disruption of anterior cruciate ligament *(white arrows)* and open physes. *B,* Same patient. Note peripheral separation of lateral meniscus, an injury commonly seen in patients with ACL disruption.

TREATMENT

Special Considerations in the Growing Child

Children with open growth plates may present challenges to the treating orthopedic surgeon familiar with reconstruction techniques used in adults. Most ACL reconstructions in adults use autograft tendon (hamstring or patellar tendon) to replace the torn ACL. The surgical technique involves a central drill hole in the proximal tibia and another in the distal femur to place the tendon graft to closely resemble the anatomic location of the normal ACL. Utilizing this surgical technique in a growing child may result in a growth arrest or altered growth in either the proximal tibia or the distal femur. Growth disturbances using conventional surgical techniques have been reported in both animal models[29-31] and clinical series of reconstructions in pediatric patients.[32-34]

Is There a Place for Nonoperative Treatment?

A number of commercially available knee orthoses are available that theoretically prevent the knee instability seen in patients with chronic ACL insufficiency. Unfortunately, no evidence has been presented to show they prevent the dreaded consequences of further meniscal damage and chondral change despite the claims of rendering the knee more stable[16-18] (Level of Evidence IV). Also, few growing children are willing to alter their active lifestyle and give up change-of-direction sports.

Operative Treatment

Given the unique anatomic aspects of the growing child, nontraditional surgical methods have been used in an attempt to prevent knee instability whereas at the same time preventing or reducing the risk for growth disturbance.

These surgical methods can be divided into the following categories:

1. Extra-articular surgical reconstructions
2. Physis-sparing surgical reconstructions including graft fixation in the epiphysis
3. Partial physeal-sparing reconstructions
4. Transphyseal reconstructions

Extra-articular Surgical Reconstruction. Extra-articular surgical reconstruction was popular in adults in the 1970s. Unfortunately, the location of the graft in a nonanatomic location was unsuccessful in controlling anterior translation of the tibia on the femur. Nevertheless, these extra-articular reconstructions have been proposed as a "temporizing" procedure in the skeletally immature patient[2,4,5] (Level of Evidence IV). No evidence suggests that they will act any more efficiently than reported previously.

Physis-Sparing Reconstructions. In an attempt to avoid crossing the physis with the graft, a number of grafts have been used with variations on a theme. The graft

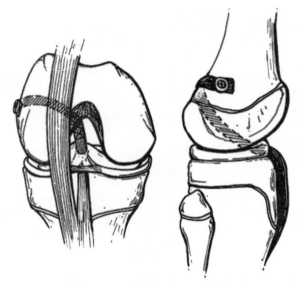

FIGURE 31–2. Physis-sparing technique of anterior cruciate ligament reconstruction utilizing autogenous patellar tendon as the graft. The graft remains attached distally to the tibia and is passed through a notch in the proximal tibial epiphysis beneath the intermeniscal ligament to an intra-articular position, and subsequently is passed through the posterior capsule to an "over-the-top" position on the distal femur above the distal femoral physis.

avoids the proximal tibial physis by using a drill hole in the proximal epiphysis only.[35–37] In addition, the distal femoral physis is avoided by placing the graft in an "over-the-top" position through the posterior capsule[35,37] or by a drill hole into the epiphysis only[36] (Fig. 31–2). Only Level III and IV studies have documented the efficacy of these surgical treatments, with the longest follow-up being 5 years.[35,36,38–43]

A variation of the combined intra-articular and extra-articular reconstruction popularized by McIntosh and Darby has been proposed by Kocher[37] in prepubescent skeletally immature children and adolescents to provide knee stability whereas at the same time avoiding the dreaded iatrogenic complication of growth disturbance seen with drill holes through either the proximal tibial or the distal femoral physis, or both (Level of Evidence IV) (Fig. 31–3).

In their Level IV study, 44 skeletally immature children (Tanner stage I or II) underwent the combined intra-articular and extra-articular reconstruction using iliotibial band. The factors evaluated were functional outcome, graft survival, and radiographic outcome with special emphasis on any growth disturbance. Follow-up period ranged from 2.0 to 15.1 years with a mean of 5.3 years. No growth disturbances were noted after the surgery as measured clinically and radiographically. Functional

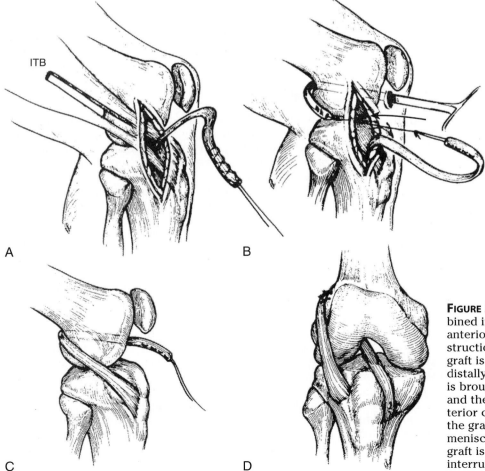

FIGURE 31–3. Physeal-sparing, combined intra-articular and extra-articular anterior cruciate ligament (ACL) reconstruction. *A,* Autogenous iliotibial band graft is harvested keeping it attached distally to Gerdy's tubercle. *B,* The graft is brought to an "over-the-top" position and then into the joint through the posterior capsule. *C,* From the knee joint, the graft is brought under the intermeniscal ligament anteriorly. *D,* The graft is sutured to the periosteum using interrupted mattress sutures.

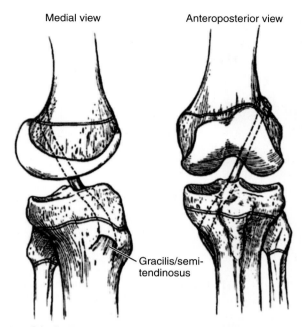

Medial view   Anteroposterior view

Gracilis/semi-tendinosus

FIGURE 31–4. Partial physeal-sparing anterior cruciate ligament (ACL) reconstruction. Hamstring tendons (semitendinosus and gracilis) are harvested and fed through a 6- to 8-mm vertical drill hole in the proximal tibia, then out through the posterior capsule to an "over-the-top" position on the distal femur. The graft is fixed to the distal femur with staples or sutures.

outcome was excellent with subjective knee scores of 96.7 ± 6.7 (range, 74–100) using the Lysholm knee score. Examination for stability of the knee revealed normal Lachman test results in 23 patients and near-normal results in 18 patients, whereas pivot shift examination was normal in 31 patients and near normal in 11 patients. Four patients who had undergone concurrent meniscal repair at the time of the ligamentous reconstruction (out of a total of 24 patients) underwent repeat meniscal surgery, either repair or partial resection.

Partial Physeal-Sparing Techniques. Partial physeal-sparing techniques use a small, central, and vertical drill hole through the proximal tibial physis and placement of the graft through the posterior capsule to an "over-the-top" position on the distal femur. Level IV studies indicate this technique renders the knee stable with little or no further meniscal damage, and no alteration of growth in either the distal femur or proximal tibia[42,44,45] (Fig. 31–4).

Transphyseal Reconstructions. Transphyseal reconstructions use a 6- to 8-mm drill hole in the proximal tibia and distal femur. The drill holes are placed in as vertical orientation as possible to minimize the cross-sectional damage to the physes. The graft is placed in the same anatomic location as the native ACL (Figs. 31–5 and 31–6). A number of authors have concluded that transphyseal reconstructions are safe with no disruption of longitudinal growth (Fig. 31–7).

However, there are reports of growth disturbance utilizing a transphyseal reconstruction in children with open physes.[34] Level II and III studies have documented that this reconstruction offers the benefits of long-term knee stability.[5,46] In most cases, it should be reserved for the adolescent at or near the end of growth. Figure 31–8 presents an algorithm for treatment of ACL tears in children.

POSTOPERATIVE REHABILITATION

Postoperative therapy is important to the success of the surgery and is recommended for all patients. Patients are kept toe touch weight bearing for up to 6 weeks in the prepubescent patients and up to 2 to 3 weeks in older adolescents.

Therapy consists of the use of a removable brace, although there is no evidence to suggest the outcome is any better, but it tends to restrict overzealous

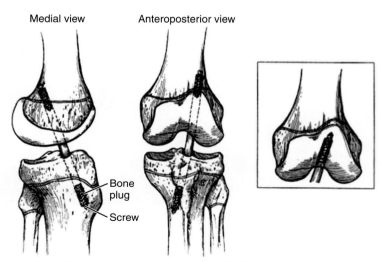

Medial view   Anteroposterior view

Bone plug

Screw

FIGURE 31–5. Diagram of transphyseal anterior cruciate ligament (ACL) reconstruction used in older adolescents and adults. Free hamstring tendons are used, and the fixation devices should not encroach on either physis if the physis is still open.

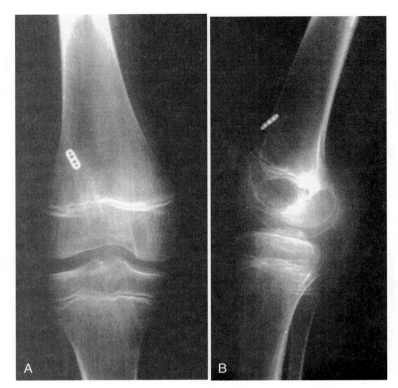

FIGURE 31–6. *A,* Anteroposterior radiograph of skeletally immature child after transphyseal anterior cruciate ligament (ACL) reconstruction using autogenous hamstring tendons. Note vertical orientation of drill holes in proximal tibia and distal femur. *B,* Lateral radiograph of same patient.

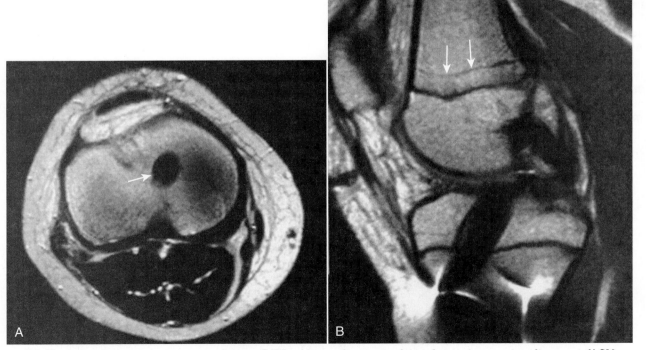

FIGURE 31–7. *A,* Axial magnetic resonance image (MRI) of knee after transphyseal anterior cruciate ligament (ACL) reconstruction. Note small, centrally placed drill hole in proximal tibia *(white arrow). B,* Lateral MRI of same patient showing graft filling tibial tunnel. Note Park–Harris growth arrest lines *(white arrows)* on distal femur proximal to physis indicating continued growth.

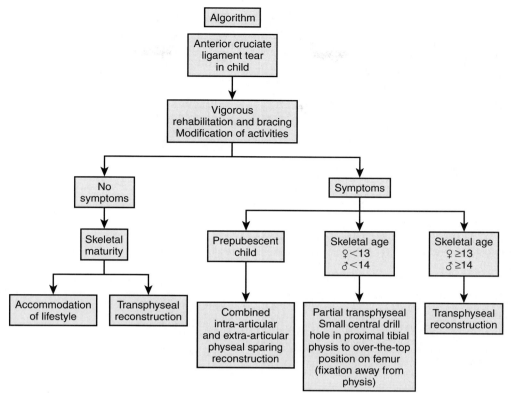

FIGURE 31–8. Algorithm for treatment of anterior cruciate ligament tears in children.

patients from too much activity (Level of Evidence V). The therapist works with the patient to decrease swelling, increase range of motion, and increase strength with closed chain exercises followed by pro-prioceptive training. At 3 months, jogging and sports-specific exercises are permitted with change of direction, cutting activities, and expected return to sports 6 months after the surgery.

RECOMMENDATIONS

Based on a number of Level III and IV studies, the following recommendations can be made. For the young child with an ACL disruption and 3 to 4 years or more of growth remaining, a trial of bracing and activity modification is warranted until the child is older or until such time as the treatment is deemed a failure.

In younger children with 3 or more years of growth remaining, there are 2 options. In prepubescent patients, a physeal-sparing technique should be used. Although not exactly replicating the anatomic location of the native ACL, studies suggest the efficacy of this treatment in controlling instability and preventing further intra-articular damage whereas at the same time not disrupting growth at either the distal femur or proximal tibia[35–43] (grade C).

A strip of iliotibial band about 2 to 3 cm wide and 15 cm long is harvested, keeping the strip attached distally to Gerdy's tubercle and detaching it proximally. Arthroscopy is performed, and the graft is passed in a retrograde fashion from an "over-the-top" position through the posterior capsule and intercondylar notch, underneath the intermeniscal ligament to a second incision on the proximal tibia. It is sutured to the periosteum distally to the proximal tibial physis after a small notch is placed in the proximal tibial epiphysis.[37] The graft is first fixed on the femoral side at the insertion of the lateral intermuscular septum to the lateral femoral condyle with the knee flexed 90 degrees. It is then fixed under tension to the periosteum of the proximal tibia with the knee flexed 20 degrees.

In adolescent patients with approximately 2 years of growth remaining, partial transphyseal reconstructions are recommended. A small (6–8-mm) drill hole is placed in the proximal tibia in a more vertical orientation than is performed in skeletally mature individuals. Hamstring tendons (semitendinosus and gracilis) are used and

Continued

are passed through the tibial tunnel and through the intercondylar notch and posterior capsule of the knee joint to an "over-the-top" position on the distal femur. A number of different fixation techniques have been used including staples and screws and washers for the distal femur fixation.[42,44,45]

The fixation devices should be used at a distance of 1.5 to 2.0 cm from the physis. The hamstring tendons can be left attached on the proximal tibia and fed up the tunnel or detached and fixed in the tibial tunnel with a bioabsorbable screw. The drill hole needs to be placed in a more vertical orientation than is used in adults to allow the insertion of the interference screw without damaging the proximal tibial physis.

In the adolescent near skeletal maturity, the transphyseal method of reconstruction is safe and provides a stable knee. If the adolescent has 1 year or less of growth remaining, it is recommended to perform a transphyseal reconstruction of the ACL using autograft hamstring tendon, autograft bone-patellar tendon-bone, or allograft tendon (Achilles).[5,46] The recommendations are summarized in the algorithm in Figure 31–8 and in Table 31–1.

TABLE 31–1. Levels of Evidence for Anterior Cruciate Ligament Injuries in Skeletally Immature Individuals

STATEMENT	LEVEL OF EVIDENCE/GRADE OF RECOMMENDATION	REFERENCES
1. Untreated anterior cruciate ligament injuries in children lead to meniscal tears and chondral damage.	B B	1, 4, 5 14, 18, 19
2. Knee braces do not alter the long-term natural history.	B B	16, 18 17
3. Extra-articular anterior cruciate ligament reconstruction does not correct the clinical problem of knee instability.	B	2, 4, 5
4. Physis-sparing reconstructions can offer the advantage of stabilizing the knee without the risk for growth arrest at the proximal tibia or distal femur.	C	35–43
5. Partial physeal-sparing techniques appear to offer knee stability without the risk for growth arrest.	C	42, 44, 45
6. Transphyseal ligamentous reconstructions offer long-term stability but some risk for growth disturbance. They should be reserved for the adolescent near the end of growth.	B B	5, 46 34

REFERENCES

1. Angel KR, Hall DJ: Anterior cruciate ligament injury in children and adolescents. Arthroscopy 5:197–200, 1989.
2. Delee JC, Curtis R: Anterior cruciate ligament insufficiency in children. Clin Orthop 172:112–118, 1983.
3. Eskjaer S, Larsen ST: Arthroscopy of the knee in children. Acta Orthop Scand 58:273–276, 1987.
4. Graf BK, Lange RH, Frijisaki CK, et al: Anterior cruciate ligament tears in skeletally immature patients: Meniscal pathology at presentation and after attempted conservative treatment. Arthroscopy 8:229–233, 1992.
5. McCarroll JR, Rettig AC, Shelbourne KD: Anterior cruciate ligament injuries in the young athlete with open physes. Am J Sports Med 16:44–47, 1988.
6. Stanitski CL, Harvell JC, Fu F: Observations on acute knee hemarthrosis in children and adolescents. J Pediatr Orthop 13:506–510, 1993.
7. Steiner ME, Grana WA: The young athlete's knee: Recent advances. Clin Sports Med 7:527–546, 1988.
8. Andrish JT: Anterior cruciate ligament injuries in the skeletally immature patient. Am J Orthop 30:103–110, 2001.
9. Shea K, Pfeiffer R, Wang J, et al: ACL injury in pediatric and adolescent athletes: Differences between males and females. Presented at the Annual Meeting of Pediatric Orthopaedic Society of North America; Amelia Island, FL; May 2003.
10. Ireland ML: The female ACL: Why is it more prone to injury? Orthop Clin North Am 33:637–651, 2002.
11. Daniel DM, Stone ML, Dobson BE, et al: Fate of the ACL injured patient. A prospective outcome study. Am J Sports Med 22:632–644, 1994.
12. Hawkins RJ, Misamore GW, Merritt TR: Follow-up of the acute nonoperated isolated anterior cruciate ligament tear. Am J Sports Med 14:205–210, 1986.
13. Buckley SL, Barrack RL, Alexander AH: The natural history of conservatively treated partial anterior cruciate tears. Am J Sports Med 17:221–225, 1989.
14. Aichroth PM, Patel DV, Zorrilla P: The natural history and treatment of rupture of the anterior cruciate ligament in children and adolescents. A prospective review. J Bone Joint Surg Br 84:618–619, 2002.
15. Janarv PM, Nystrom A, Werner S, et al: Anterior cruciate ligament injuries in skeletally immature patients. J Pediatr Orthop 16:673–677, 1996.
16. Millett PJ, Willis AA, Warren RF: Associated injuries in pediatric and adolescent anterior cruciate ligament tears: Does a delay in treatment increase the risk of meniscal tear? Arthroscopy 18:955–999, 2002.
17. Mizuta H, Kubota K, Shiraishi M, et al: The conservative treatment of complete tears of the anterior cruciate ligament in skeletally immature patients. J Bone Joint Surg Br 77:890–894, 1995.
18. Pressman AE, Letts RM, Jarvis JG: Anterior cruciate ligament tears in children: An analysis of operative versus non-operative treatment. J Pediatr Orthop 17:505–511, 1997.
19. Kannus P, Jarvinen M: Knee ligament injuries in adolescents. Eight year follow-up of conservative management. J Bone Joint Surg Br 70:772–776, 1988.
20. Rang M: Children's Fractures, 2nd ed. Philadelphia, Lippincott, 1983.
21. Kocher MS, Micheli LJ, Gerbino P, et al: Tibial eminence fractures in children: Prevalence of meniscal entrapment. Am J Sports Med 31:404–407, 2003.
22. Kocher MS, Foreman ES, Micheli LJ: Laxity and functional outcome after arthroscopic reduction and internal fixation of displaced tibial spine fractures in children. Arthroscopy 19:1085–1090, 2003.
23. Kocher MS, Mandiga R, Klingele KE, et al: Anterior cruciate ligament injury versus tibial spine fracture in the skeletally

immature knee: A comparison of skeletal maturation and notch width index. J Pediatr Orthop 24:185–188, 2004.

24. Eiskjaer S, Larsen ST, Schmidt MB: The significance of hemarthrosis of the knee in children. Arch Orthop Trauma Surg 107:96–98, 1988.
25. Kloeppel-Wirth S, Koltai JL, Dittmer H: Significance of arthroscopy in children with knee joint injuries. Eur J Pediatr Surg 2:169–172, 1992.
26. Vahasarja V, Kinnuen P, Serlo W: Arthroscopy of the acute traumatic knee in children. Prospective study of 138 cases. Acta Orthop Scand 64:580–582, 1993.
27. Kocher MS, DiCanzio J, Zurakowski D, et al: Diagnostic performance of clinical examination and selective magnetic resonance imaging in the evaluation of intraarticular knee disorders in children and adolescents. Am J Sports Med 29:292–296, 2001.
28. Luhmann SJ: Acute traumatic knee effusions in children and adolescents. J Pediatr Orthop 23:199–202, 2003.
29. Guzzanti V, Falciglia F, Gigante A, et al: The effects of intraarticular ACL reconstruction on the growth plate of rabbits. J Bone Joint Surg Br 76:960–963, 1994.
30. Houle JB, Letts M, Yang J: Effects of tensioned tendon graft in a bone tunnel across the rabbit physis. Clin Orthop 391:275–281, 2001.
31. Edwards TB, Greene CC, Baratta RV, et al: The effect of placing a tensioned graft across open growth plates. A gross and histologic analysis. J Bone Joint Surg Am 83A:725–734, 2001.
32. Lipscomb AB, Anderson AF: Tears of the anterior cruciate ligament in adolescents. J Bone Joint Surg Am 68:19–28, 1986.
33. Koman JD, Sanders JO: Valgus deformity after reconstruction of the anterior cruciate ligament in a skeletally immature patient. A case report. J Bone Joint Surg Am 81:711–715, 1999.
34. Kocher MS, Saxon HS, Hovis WD, et al: Management and complications of anterior cruciate ligament injuries in skeletally immature patients: Survey of the Herodicus Society and The ACL Study Group. J Pediatr Orthop 22:452–457, 2002.
35. Parker AW, Drez D, Cooper JL: Anterior cruciate ligament injuries in patients with open physes. Am J Sports Med 22:44–47, 1994.
36. Anderson AF: Transepiphyseal replacement of the anterior cruciate ligament in skeletally immature patients. A preliminary report. J Bone Joint Surg Am 85-A:1255–1263, 2003.
37. Kocher MS: Anterior cruciate ligament reconstruction in the skeletally immature patient. Oper Tech Sports Med 14:124–134, 2006.
38. Vahasarja V, Kinnuen P, Serlo W: Arthroscopy of the acute traumatic knee in children. Prospective study of 138 cases. Acta Orthop Scand 64:580–582, 1993.
39. Brief LB: Anterior cruciate ligament reconstruction without drill holes. Arthroscopy 7:350–357, 1991.
40. DeLee J, Curtis R: Anterior cruciate ligament insufficiency in children. Clin Orthop 172:112–118, 1983.
41. Kim SH, Ha KI, Ahn JH, et al: Anterior cruciate ligament reconstruction in the young patient without violation of the epiphyseal plate. Arthroscopy 15:792–795, 1999.
42. Guzzanti V, Falciglia F, Stanitski CL: Physeal-sparing intraarticular anterior cruciate ligament reconstruction in preadolescents. Am J Sports Med 31:949–953, 2003.
43. Micheli LJ, Rask B, Gerberg L: Anterior cruciate ligament reconstruction in patients who are prepubescent. Clin Orthop 364:40–47, 1999.
44. Lo IK, Kirkley A, Fowler PJ, et al: The outcome of operatively treated anterior cruciate ligament disruptions in the skeletally immature child. Arthroscopy 13:627–634, 1997.
45. Bisson LJ, Wickiewicz T, Levinson M, Warren R: ACL reconstruction in children with open physes. Orthopedics 21:659–663, 1998.
46. Aronowitz ER, Ganley TJ, Goode JR, et al: Anterior cruciate ligament reconstruction in adolescents with open physes. Am J Sports Med 28:168–175, 2000.

Chapter 32

What Is the Optimal Treatment for Slipped Capital Femoral Epiphysis?

Randall T. Loder, MD

Slipped capital femoral epiphysis (SCFE) is an adolescent hip disorder in which there is a displacement of the capital femoral epiphysis from the metaphysis through the physis. Most cases are "idiopathic," although they may also occur from a known endocrine disorder,[1-3] renal failure osteodystrophy,[4] or previous radiation therapy.[3,5,6] This chapter is limited to the idiopathic SCFE. SCFEs are classified both by their clinical nature and magnitude. The traditional clinical classification was acute, chronic, and acute on chronic,[7-11] and it was based on the patient's history, physical examination, and roentgenograms. An acute SCFE case is defined as those with symptoms for less than 3 weeks with an abrupt displacement through the proximal physis in which there was a preexisting epiphyseolysis.[7] Chronic SCFE cases account for 85% of all slips[12] and present with more than 3 weeks of groin, thigh, and knee pain, often for months to years. These patients often have a history of exacerbations and remissions of the pain and limp. Acute-on-chronic SCFEs are those with chronic symptoms initially and the subsequent development of acute symptoms. A newer, more clinically useful classification is dependent on physeal stability, which imparts a prognosis to the hip regarding subsequent avascular necrosis (AVN).[13] A stable SCFE is defined as one where the child is able to ambulate, with or without crutches. An unstable SCFE is defined as one where the child cannot ambulate, with or without crutches. Unstable SCFE cases have a much greater incidence rate of AVN, up to 50% in some series, compared with stable SCFEs (nearly 0%).[13]

OPTIONS

Once a diagnosis of SCFE is made, treatment is indicated to prevent slip progression[14-16] and to avoid complications, especially AVN and chondrolysis. Multiple treatment options are available, each having specific advantages and disadvantages. These options are divided into those for patients with stable SCFE and those for patients with unstable SCFE.

Treatment options for a stable SCFE include: (1) in situ stabilization with a single screw[8,9,17-21] or multiple pins[17,22-25]; (2) epiphyseodesis[25-30]; (3) open reduction with corrective osteotomy through the physis and internal fixation[18,22,30-39]; (4) basilar neck osteotomy[40-42]; (5) intertrochanteric osteotomy[24,42-46]; and (6) surgical

dislocation of the hip with transphyseal callus removal, reduction, and fixation.[47-51]

The treatment of a patient with unstable SCFE is quite controversial. Treatment options include internal fixation with or without reduction and joint decompression, epiphysiodesis, and open reduction with corrective osteotomy through the physis and internal fixation. Considerable discussion has occurred regarding the timing (emergent or urgent reduction vs. elective) of the reduction, the magnitude of reduction (incidental reduction [improvement in the SCFE that occurs with positioning the patient on the operating table] vs. a complete reduction), the role of joint decompression, and the number of internal fixation devices.

LEVELS OF EVIDENCE

The treatment of SCFE has been one of gradual evolution over time. The available studies (Table 32-1) are, at best, Level III; no randomized, controlled studies and few prospective comparative studies involve SCFE. For this reason, I review the few Level III and the most appropriate Level IV series, compare and contrast them regarding long-term outcomes and complications, synthesize the data, and propose as best as possible the optimal treatment of SCFE.

As a background to considering the various different treatments for SCFE, it is first necessary to understand the long-term natural history of the untreated SCFE and the long-term outcomes from SCFEs treated many years ago. The two major concerns in the untreated individual with SCFE are the risk for further progression and the risk for degenerative joint disease in adult life. Few long-term studies of patients with SCFE and even fewer untreated individual are included in these series.[11,22,52-56] Ordeberg and researchers[57] studied a series of patients with SCFE without primary treatment 20 to 40 years after diagnosis. Few patients had restrictions in working capacity or social life. However, there was a risk for slip progression as long as the physis remained open.[58] Carney and coauthors[22] reported on 35 patients with SCFE who were initially observed; in 6 hips (17%), gradual progression occurred, with 5 becoming severe. An additional 11 patients had an acute episode superimposed on the chronic SCFE;

TABLE 32–1. Levels of Evidence in Studies of Idiopathic Slipped Capital Femoral Epiphysis

STUDY	DESIGN	LEVEL OF EVIDENCE	GRADE
Stable SCFE			
Multiple Treatment Methods			
Aronson and Loder (1992)[94]	RR	III	B
Carlioz et al. (1984)[18]	RR	III	B
Carney et al. (1991)[22]	RR	III	B
Diab et al. (2004)[35]	RR	III	B
Dreghorn et al. (1987)[23]	RR	III	B
El-Mowafi et al. (2005)[42]	RR	III	B
Jerre et al. (1996)[38]	RR	III	B
Parsch et al. (1999)[24]	RR	III	B
Szypryt et al. (1987)[30]	RR	III	B
Zahrawi et al. (1983)[25]	RR	III	B
Single Central Screw Fixation			
Aronson and Carlson (1992)[8]	PS with RR	IV	C
Herman et al. (1996)[19]	RR	IV	C
Kenny et al. (2003)[20]	RR	IV	C
Koval et al. (1989)[21]	RR	IV	C
Ward et al. (1992)[9]	PS with RR	IV	C
Multipin Fixation			
Aronson et al. (1992)[17]	RR	IV	C
Physeal/Cuneiform Osteotomy			
Barros et al. (2000)[34]	RR	IV	C
Broughton et al. (1988)[95]	RR	IV	C
DeRosa et al. (1996)[31]	RR	IV	C
Dunn et al. (1978)[36]	RR	IV	C
Fish (1994)[33]	RR	IV	C
Fron et al. (2000)[37]	RR	IV	C
Nishiyama et al. (1989)[39]	RR	IV	C
Velasco et al. (1998)[32]	RR	IV	C
Basilar Neck Osteotomy			
Abraham et al. (1993)[96]	RR	IV	C
Kramer et al. (1976)[41]	RR	IV	C
Intertrochanteric Osteotomy			
Ireland and Newman (1978)[97]	RR	IV	C
Kartenbender et al. (2000)[46]	RR	IV	C
Parsch et al. (1999)[24]	RR	IV	C
Rao et al. (1984)[98]	RR	IV	C
Salvati et al. (1980)[99]	RR	IV	C
Schai et al. (1996)[44]	RR	IV	C
Southwick (1967)[43]	RR	IV	C
Spica Cast Treatment			
Betz et al. (1990)[100]	RR	IV	C
Meier et al. (1992)[101]	RR	IV	C
Epiphysiodesis			
Adamczyk et al. (2003)[29]	RR	IV	C
Rao et al. (1996)[27]	RR	IV	C
Schmidt et al. (1996)[28]	RR	IV	C

PS, prospective series; RR, retrospective review; SCFE, slipped capital femoral epiphysis.

all progressed to severe displacement and required surgical stabilization.

Howorth[59] (Level V evidence) states that SCFE is likely the most frequent cause of degenerative joint disease of the hip in middle life, and a common source of pain and disability. This is not necessarily supported by other studies. The number of patients with known SCFE is low (average 5%) in reviewing large series of patients with degenerative joint disease.[60–62] The severity of deformity in the untreated SCFE is known to correlate with the long-term prognosis regarding degenerative joint disease.[22,52,54,56,63,64] Oram[54] reports on 22 patients with untreated SCFEs; patients with moderate SCFEs retained good function for years, whereas patients with severe SCFEs experienced development of degenerative joint disease within 15 years. Jerre[63,64] and Ross and colleagues[56] report increasingly poor results with longer follow-up periods; many patients responded well early on but experienced development of increasing symptoms and decreasing function with increasing age. Carney and Weinstein[52] studied the natural history of the untreated, chronic SCFE in 31 hips at an average follow-up period of 41 years. The average Iowa Hip Rating was 92 in the 17 patients with mild SCFE, 87 in the 11 patients with moderate SCFE, and 75 in the 3 patients with severe SCFE. Although a patient with a mild SCFE appears to have a favorable prognosis, patients with moderate and severe SCFE have a high incidence of degenerative joint disease. Poor results, however, can occasionally be seen even with minimal SCFEs.[11,22,52,56] In summary, the natural history of chronic (stable) SCFE is favorable provided that displacement is mild and remains so. Thus, all treatments should stabilize the SCFE and prevent complications.

What are the long-term historical results of treatment? Wilson and coworkers[65] reviewed 300 hips treated between 1936 and 1960. Good results were seen in 81% of those treated with in situ fixation and in 60% of those with deformity correction. Hall[53] reviewed 138 patients; excellent results were seen in 80% of those treated with multiple pin fixation; realignment with osteotomy of the femoral neck resulted in a 38% AVN rate with 36% poor results. Ordeberg and researchers[66] reviewed 44 patients with untreated SCFE followed for more than 30 years. Symptomatic treatment or fixation in situ gave excellent results, with only 2% needing a secondary reconstructive procedure. Closed reduction or spica cast treatment had a combined rate of AVN and chondrolysis of 13%, with 35% needing a reconstructive procedure; femoral neck osteotomy resulted in a combined rate of AVN and chondrolysis of 30%, with 15% needing a reconstructive procedure.[57] Carney and coauthors[22] report on 155 hips at a mean follow-up of 41 years. Poorer results were associated with more severe slips and realignment; chondrolysis (16%) and AVN (12%) were more common with increasing slip severity. All these long-term studies support the use of in situ fixation as the treatment of choice for SCFE regardless of slip severity. Realignment was associated with significant complications and poorer results. It must be remembered, however, that the surgical fixation techniques and imaging modalities used in these historical series are much different from those currently used.

Stable Slipped Capital Femoral Epiphysis

The incidence rates of AVN range from 0% to 10%, of chondrolysis from 0.8% to 16%, and slip progression from 0.5% to 5.7% (Tables 32–2, 32–3, and 32–4). The lowest rates of AVN, chondrolysis, and slip progression in aggregate are those treated with a single central screw (see Table 32–4). The advantages of single-screw fixation for a patient with a stable SCFE include a high success rate, a low incidence rate of further slippage, and a low incidence rate of complications.[8,67,68]

Epiphysiodesis attempted to avoid the complications associated with internal fixation (unrecognized pin protrusion, damage to the lateral epiphyseal vessels, and hardware failure); however, the fixation provided by the bone graft was less secure than that with internal fixation, having a 5.7% incidence rate of slip progression. As a result of this higher slip progression rate and other disadvantages (blood loss, large scar, long anesthesia time, neck and subtrochanteric fracture), epiphysiodesis is no longer the first choice of treatment for an SCFE.

Osteotomies are used in an attempt to correct the deformity associated with SCFE. The overall incidence rate of both chondrolysis and AVN in 350 cases of physeal/cuneiform osteotomy compiled from the literature was 10%. Because of this high risk for AVN and subsequent poor results in most series, a physeal cuneiform osteotomy is not recommended in the treatment of SCFE. A compensating base-of-neck osteotomy is an attempt to maintain the advantages of a physeal osteotomy (deformity correction) but with a lower risk for AVN. Indeed, the incidence rate of AVN is less with basilar neck osteotomies compared with the cuneiform osteotomy (10% vs. 1%). The intertrochanteric osteotomy is an attempt to improve hip motion, obtain some correction of the deformity (albeit a compensatory correction), and completely avoid AVN. The compiled results demonstrate that AVN still occurs with a 2.2% incidence rate and also carries a significant risk for chondrolysis (11.9%). The results of intertrochanteric osteotomy using the Southwick technique are much poorer than those of in situ single-screw fixation.[43,44,69] The simpler Imhäuser flexion intertrochanteric osteotomy[24,45,46] has replaced the Southwick osteotomy. Because it is not a valgus, limb-lengthening osteotomy, the increase in joint pressure created by the traditional Southwick osteotomy, a likely cause of chondrolysis, is avoided. When comparing the results (Table 32–5) between the flexion and South-

wick types of osteotomies, the rate of AVN and chondrolysis is 2.5% (5/198) and 4.9% (7/142) for the flexion osteotomy and 0% (0/112) and 15.2% (17/112) for the Southwick osteotomy. Although the rate of chondrolysis is lower for the flexion osteotomy, there is an increase in the rate of AVN with the flexion osteotomy.

In conclusion, when reviewing all the evidence and published series to date, it is clear that the optimal treatment for the stable, idiopathic SCFE is single central screw fixation (Figs. 32–1 and 32–2).

Unstable Slipped Capital Femoral Epiphysis

The treatment for the unstable SCFE is controversial as shown by survey studies of both North American[70] and European[71] pediatric orthopedic surgeons. An urgent/emergent treatment was favored by 88% of North American and European surgeons; a manipulative reduction was favored by 32% of European and 12% of North American surgeons, whereas more North American surgeons (84%) favored an incidental reduction. Single-screw fixation was recommended by 57% of North American surgeons and 79% of European surgeons, with double-screw fixation being recommended by 40% of North American and only 18% of European surgeons. Capsular decompression was recommended by 29% of the European and 35% of the North American surgeons. This Level V evidence clearly indicates that the best treatment for an unstable SCFE is not yet known.

In the initial study that described the unstable SCFE, the risk for AVN was 47%.[13] It was 88% in those when operative stabilization occurred less than 48 hours after the onset of symptoms versus 32% in those more than 48 hours. However, the cause-and-effect relation between the timing of operative stabilization and the development of AVN could not be determined.

Several authors have attempted to answer these questions (Table 32–6). Some[72–74] believe that reduction reduces the incidence of AVN, others[75,76] believe that reduction has no influence on the development of AVN, and a few[77] believe that reduction increases the incidence of AVN. Peterson and colleagues,[73] in 91 patients with unstable SCFEs at an average follow-up period of 44 months, note that the incidence rate of AVN was 7% when a closed reduction was performed less than 24 hours from presentation and 20% when performed more than 24 hours from presentation. The authors believe that the acute displacement of the femoral epiphysis compromises the blood flow, which may be restored by a timely reduction of the SCFE. Gordon and coworkers[72] support this concept, with no cases of AVN in 10 patients with unstable SCFE treated within 24 hours by reduction, arthrotomy, and double-screw fixation. Maeda and researchers,[78] using angiography, demonstrated restoration of blood supply to the epiphysis after reduction of an unstable SCFE. Phillips and coauthors[74] reviewed

14 patients with unstable SCFE, and noted no complication in those who were treated with early reduction and stabilization. By contrast, Tokmakova and coworkers[77] reviewed 36 patients with unstable SCFEs and noted a 58% AVN incidence rate. Their multiple logistic regression analysis showed that a complete or partial reduction of an unstable SCFE increased the chances of AVN; they thus recommend in situ fixation with a single central screw as the treatment for the unstable SCFE. Kalogrianitis and investigators[79] recommend that the reduction be performed within 24 hours, and that after that the epiphysis is much more susceptible to AVN and thus to defer definitive treatment until at least 1 week has passed.

Several studies address the number of screws that should be used in the patient with unstable SCFE, but nearly all are in vitro animal models and different than the clinical situation. Karol and researchers[80] and Kibiloski and colleagues[81] compared single- and double-screw fixation in a calf model, testing in both a single load to failure and the effects of physiologic shear loading. Double-screw fixation did not double the strength compared with single-screw fixation for either a single load to failure or simulated walking. Both articles recommend protected weight bearing in the postoperative period for the unstable SCFE regardless of whether 1 or 2 screws are used. Again, in an immature bovine model, Kishan and coworkers[82] evaluated one and two screws in varying degrees of configuration at physiologically relevant loads, and they found no significant differences among three different screw configurations, but that double-screw constructs were 66% stiffer and 66% stronger than single-screw constructs. In an immature porcine model, Snyder and coauthors[83] studied torsional strength after removal of the perichondrium at the physeal level (analogous to the situation, the unstable SCFE where the perichondrium at the physeal level has been compromised). Two-screw fixation after removal of the perichondrium provided 43% of the stiffness and 74% of the strength of the intact physis in torsion.

Thus, any recommendation for the treatment of the unstable SCFE is at best Level IV evidence and mostly Level V. Keeping this in mind, this author's current management strategy for the unstable SCFE is immediate admission, urgent gentle repositioning under a general anesthetic and fluoroscopic guidance, double-screw fixation, joint decompression, and protected weight bearing for 6 to 12 weeks. Because of the rarity of the unstable SCFE, a prospective study of different treatment methods is needed.

Prophylactic Treatment of the Opposite Hip

The risk for a contralateral SCFE developing in a patient with unilateral SCFE is reported to be 2335 times greater than the risk for an initial SCFE,[84] yet even if the bilaterality incidence rate is 60%, then 40% of children with SCFE will have unnecessary surgery if prophylactic fixation is performed on all children with idiopathic SCFE. Prophylactic fixation is recommended by some researchers,[85–87] whereas close observation is recommended by others.[88,89] Therefore, what is the level of evidence regarding prophylactic fixation?

First, is prophylactic fixation safe? Few series report the results of prophylactic fixation[86,87,90–92] (Table 32–7). The combined number of hips treated prophylactically in these 5 studies is 305. No AVN or chondrolysis was found, although in some cases, the epiphysis grew off the fixation (7.3% in the 3 series in which it was recorded accurately[87,90,91]). Thus, it seems relatively clear that with today's methods of single central screw fixation, prophylactic fixation can be performed with a low incidence of complications.

Considering this relative safety, it then becomes necessary to determine when prophylactic fixation should be performed in child with a unilateral stable, idiopathic SCFE. A POSNA membership survey (Level V evidence) recommends prophylactic fixation of the opposite hip[70] in only 12.2% of cases. Two recent studies using decision analysis models have been performed to assist in this dilemma, but they have come to differing conclusions. Schultz and investigators[84] developed a model with probabilities for the occurrence of a contralateral SCFE. They conclude that prophylactic fixation of the contralateral hip was beneficial to the long-term outcome of the hip, but cautioned that the clinician use sound clinical judgment with respect to the age, sex, and endocrine status of the patient, including the preferences of the patient and family, before recommending prophylactic fixation of the contralateral hip. Kocher and coworkers[93] similarly used a decision analysis model with probabilities for the occurrence of a contralateral SCFE and reached the conclusion that when the probability of a contralateral SCFE is greater than 27% or in cases where reliable follow-up is not feasible, then prophylactic fixation of the contralateral hip is favored. The difference between these studies is how the probabilities of a contralateral SCFE were determined. Schultz and investigators[84] used values from the literature for various incidences and probabilities of events (e.g., AVN, chondrolysis, severity of SCFE, etc.). Kocher and coworkers[93] used a questionnaire to determine patient preferences in a group of children without SCFE; the questionnaire posed scenarios for different outcomes and asked the patients to rate preferences regarding prophylactic fixation in that framework. Unfortunately, these decision analysis models have not yet answered this controversial question: What are the exact indications for prophylactic treatment? Table 32–8 provides a summary of recommendations for the treatment of SCFE.

TABLE 32–2. Treatment Outcomes in Stable, Idiopathic Slipped Capital Femoral Epiphysis

STUDY	LEVEL OF EVIDENCE	STABLE SCFEs, N	SEVERITY OF SCFE (M/M/S)	TREATMENT	AVERAGE FOLLOW-UP (YR)	OUTCOME % SATISFACTORY*	AVN, N (%)	CHONDROLYSIS, N (%)	PROGRESSION OF SCFE	GROWING OFF THE FIXATION
Multiple Treatment Methods										
Aronson and Loder (1992)[94]	III	MPF—54, SCS—43	—	MPF—54, SCS—43	MPF—4.0, SCS—3.3	MPF—74, SCS—91	MPF—2 (4), SCS—0	MPF—3(6), SCS—0	0 (0), 2 (5)	NA
Carlioz et al. (1984)[18]	III	59, SCS—33, PO—26	20/18/21	SCS—33, PO—26	4.4	85, SCS—91, PO—77	0	PO—3 (8), SCS—0	NA	NA
Carney et al. (1991)[22]	III	37	Moderate/severe, Moderate/severe, Moderate/severe	MPF—11, PO—12, ITO—14	41	NA	1 (9), 3 (25), 1 (7)	1 (9), 6 (50), 5 (36)	0, 0, 0	0, 0, 0
Diab et al. (2004)[35]	III	26, ITOF—15, PO—11	0/0/26	ITOF—15, PO—11	ITOF—6.33, PO—4.17	NA	PO—2 (18), ITOF—1 (7)	PO—0, ITOF—1 (7)	NA	NA
Dreghorn et al. (1987)[23]	III	97 cases, number stable not known	—	MPF—66, CRIF—32, PO/ITO—8	2.1	NA	0, 2 (10), 2 (18)	2 (3), 0, 0	0, 0, 0	1 (1.5), 0, —
El-Mowafi et al. (2005)[42]	III	35, BNO—15, ITOS—20	0/5/10, 0/12/8	BNO—15, ITOS—20	3.5	BNO—87, ITOS—90	BNO—1 (7), ITOS—0	BNO—1 (7), ITOS—5 (25)	NA	NA
Jerre et al. (1996)[38]	III	33, 22 PO, 11 ITO	All moderate or severe	ITO, PO	PO—33.5, ITO—36.1	PO—41, ITO—36	PO—5 (23), ITO—1 (9)	1 (5), 1 (9)	NA	NA
Parsch et al. (1999)[24]	III	84	34/0/0	MPF	All > 8	97%	0	0	NA	NA
Szypryt et al. (1987)[30]	III	51, PO—22, EPI—29	PO—all severe, EPI—0/12/18	PO—22, EPI—29	5	PO—77, EPI—59	PO—4 (18), EPI—2 (7)	PO—0, EPI—3 (10)	NA	NA
Zahrawi et al. (1983)[25]	III	94	Average 22-degree slip, Average 30-degree slip	MPF—61, EPI—33	MPF—7.3, EPI—6.6	MPF—92, EPI—72	0, 0	MPF—2 (3), EPI—1 (3)	MPF—2 (3), EPI—0	NA, NA
Single Central Screw Fixation										
Aronson and Carlson (1992)[8]	IV	50	38/7/5	SCS	3.0	94	0	0	1 (2)	0
Herman et al. (1996)[19]	IV	10	0/0/10	SCS	2.6	—	0	1 (10)	NA	NA
Kenny et al. (2003)[20]	IV	35		SCS	2	94	0	1 (3)	0	0
Koval et al. (1989)[21]	IV	67	—	SCS	2.9	—	0	0	0	1 (1.5)
Ward et al. (1992)[9]	IV	51	16/26/9	SCS	2.7	NA	0	0	0	3 (5.8)

Study										
Multiple Pin Fixation										
Aronson et al. (1992)[17]	IV	80	49/20/11	MPF	3.3	70	3	4	0	0
Physeal/Cuneiform Osteotomy										
Barros et al. (2000)[34]	IV	20	0/0/20	PO	5.8	75	3 (15)	2 (10)	1 (5)	NA
Broughton et al. (1988)[95]	IV	70		PO	12.92	71	3 (5)	6 (9)	NA	NA
DeRosa et al. (1996)[31]	IV	27	0/0/27	PO	8.5	70	4 (15)	8 (30)	2 (7)	0
Dunn et al. (1978)[36]	IV	40	0/0/40	PO	8.83	75	1 (3)	3 (8)	NA	NA
Fish (1994)[33]	IV	50	0/23/27	PO	12.8	98	0	1 (2)	NA	NA
Fron et al. (2000)[37]	IV	50	0/0/50	PO	4.5	82	6 (12)	3 (6)	NA	NA
Nishiyama et al. (1989)[39]	IV	18	0/0/18	PO	10.25	78	1 (6)	1 (6)	NA	NA
Velasco et al. (1998)[32]	IV	22	2/4/14	PO	22.4	41	4 (18)	5 (23)	NA	NA
Basilar Neck Osteotomy										
Abraham et al. (1993)[96]	IV	36	0/14/22	BNO	9	90	0	3 (8)	NA	NA
Kramer et al. (1976)[41]	IV	56	All >40 degrees	BN	2–11	79	0	1 (2)	NA	NA
Intertrochanteric Osteotomy										
Ireland and Newman (1978)[97]	IV	35	0/0/35	ITOS	7.5	60	0	4 (11)	†	†
Kartenbender et al. (2000)[46]	IV	39	0/0/39	ITOF	23.4	67	2 (5)	3 (8)	†	†
Parsch et al. (1999)[24]	IV	47 + 49 = 96	0/80/16	ITOF	All >8	70	1 (1)	3 (3)	†	†
Rao et al. (1984)[98]	IV	29	0/12/17	ITOS	7.5	79	0	2 (6)	†	†
Salvati et al. (1980)[99]	IV	24	0/7/17	ITO	4.3	67	1 (4)	7 (29)	†	†
Schai et al. (1996)[44]	IV	51	0/67/0	ITOF	24.1	55	1 (2)	NA	†	†
Southwick (1967)[43]	IV	28	0/14/14	ITOS	8	75	0	6 (21)	†	†
Spica Cast Treatment										
Betz et al. (1990)[100]	IV	32	23/5/4	SC	4.1	—	0	4 (13)	1 (3)	†
Meier et al. (1992)[101]	IV	13	6/5/2	SC	4.1	—	—	6 (46)	3 (23)	†
Epiphysiodesis										
Adamczyk et al. (2003)[29]	IV	273	NA	EPI	All >1 year	NA	4 (1.5)	0	17 (6%)	†
Rao et al. (1996)[27]	IV	46	18/20/8	EPI	2.9	NA	3 (7)	2 (4)	0	†
Schmidt et al. (1996)[28]	IV	33	29/4/0	EPI	3.6	91%	0	0	3 (9)	†

In several of the studies, the data were extracted from the original manuscript and analyzed as best as possible allowing for insufficient data or data not given.

*Satisfactory is defined as excellent/very good and good; fair and poor are considered unsatisfactory.

†Does not apply to this particular treatment method.

AVN, avascular necrosis; BNO, basilar neck osteotomy; CRIF, closed reduction internal fixation; EPI, epiphysiodesis; ITOS, intertrochanteric osteotomy (Southwick type); ITOF, intertrochanteric osteotomy (flexion Imhaüser type); M/M/S, mild, moderate, severe; MPF, multipin fixation; NA, data not available in the study; PO, physeal osteotomy; PS, prospective series; RR, retrospective review; SC, spica cast; SCFE, slipped capital femoral epiphysis; SCS, single central screw.

TABLE 32–3. Compiled Results of Outcomes for Different Methods of Treatment in Stable Idiopathic Slipped Capital Femoral Epiphysis

STUDY	N	AVN, n	CHONDROLYSIS, n	SLIP PROGRESSION, n	EPIPHYSIS GROWING OFF FIXATION, n
Multipin Fixation					
Aronson et al. (1992)[17]	80	3	4	0	0
Carney et al. (1991)[22]	11	1	1	0	0
Dreghorn et al. (1987)[23]	66	0	2	0	1
Parsch et al. (1999)[24]	84	0	0	NA	NA
Zahrawi et al. (1983)[25]	61	0	2	2	NA
Total (%)	302	4/302 (1.3)	9/302 (3)	2/218 (0.9)	1/157 (0.6)
Single Central Screw					
Aronson and Carlson (1992)[8]	50	0	0	1	0
Carlioz et al. (1984)[18]	33	0	0	NA	NA
Herman et al. (1996)[19]	10	0	1	NA	NA
Kenny et al. (2003)[20]	35	0	1	0	0
Koval et al. (1989)[21]	67	0	0	0	1
Ward et al. (1992)[9]	51	0	0	0	3
Total (%)	246	0/246 (0)	2/246 (0.8)	1/203 (0.5)	4/203 (2)
Intertrochanteric Osteotomy					
Carney et al. (1991)[22]	14	1	5	*	*
Diab et al. (2004)[35]	15	1	1	*	*
El-Mowafi et al. (2005)[42]	20	0	5	*	*
Ireland and Newman (1978)[97]	35	0	4	*	*
Jerre et al. (1996)[38]	11	1	1	*	*
Kartenbender et al. (2000)[46]	39	2	3	*	*
Parsch et al. (1999)[24]	96	1	3	*	*
Rao et al. (1984)[98]	29	0	2	*	*
Salvati et al. (1980)[99]	24	1	7	*	*
Schai et al. (1996)[44]	51	1	NA	*	*
Southwick (1967)[43]	28	0	6	*	*
Total (%)	362	8/362 (2.2)	37/311 (11.9)		
Physeal/Cuneiform/Dunn					
Barros et al. (2000)[34]	20	3	2	*	*
Carlioz et al. (1984)[18]	26	0	3	*	*
Carney et al. (1991)[22]	12	3	6	*	*
DeRosa et al. (1996)[31]	27	4	8	*	*
Diab et al. (2004)[35]	11	2	0	*	*
Dunn et al. (1978)[36]	70	3	6	*	*
Fish (1994)[33]	50	0	1	*	*
Fron et al. (2000)[37]	50	6	3	*	*
Jerre et al. (1996)[38]	22	5	1	*	*
Nishiyama et al. (1989)[39]	18	1	1	*	*
Szypryt et al. (1987)[30]	22	4	0	*	*
Velasco et al. (1998)[32]	22	4	5	*	*
Total (%)	350	35/350 (10.0)	36/350 (10.3)		
Basilar Neck					
Abraham et al. (1993)[96]	36	0	3	*	*
El-Mowafi et al. (2005)[42]	15	1	1	*	*
Kramer et al. (1976)[41]	56	0	1	*	*
Total (%)	107	1/107 (1.0)	5/107 (4.7)		
Spica Cast					
Betz et al. (1990)[100]	32	0	4	1	*
Meier et al. (1992)[101]	13	6	3	NA	*
Total (%)	45	6/45 (13)	7/45 (16)	1/32 (3)	

TABLE 32–3. Compiled Results of Outcomes for Different Methods of Treatment in Stable Idiopathic Slipped Capital Femoral Epiphysis—cont'd

STUDY	N	AVN, n	CHONDROLYSIS, n	SLIP PROGRESSION, n	EPIPHYSIS GROWING OFF FIXATION, n
Epiphysiodesis					
Adamczyk et al. (2003)[29]	273	4	0	17	*
Rao et al. (1996)[27]	46	3	2	0	*
Schmidt et al. (1996)[28]	33	0	0	3	*
Szypryt et al. (1987)[30]	29	2	3	NA	*
Zahrawi et al. (1983)[25]	33	0	1	NA	*
Total	414	7/414 (1.7)	6/414 (1.5)	20/352 (5.7)	

*Does not apply to this particular treatment method.
AVN, avascular necrosis; NA, data not available in the study.

TABLE 32–4. Summary of Literature Results in the Treatment of Stable, Idiopathic Slipped Capital Femoral Epiphysis

TREATMENT	N	AVN (%)	CHONDROLYSIS (%)	SLIP PROGRESSION (%)	EPIPHYSIS GROWING OFF FIXATION (%)
Single central screw	246	0	0.8	0.5	1.0
Multipin fixation	302	1.3	3	0.9	0.6
Physeal/Cuneiform osteotomy	350	10.0	10.3	*	*
Basilar neck osteotomy	107	1.0	4.7	*	*
Intertrochanteric osteotomy	362	2.2	11.9	*	*
Spica cast	45	13	16	3	*
Epiphysiodesis	414	1.5	1.5	5.7	*

*Does not apply to this particular treatment method.
AVN, avascular necrosis.

TABLE 32–5. Comparisons between the Flexion and Southwick Types of Intertrochanteric Osteotomies in the Treatment of Stable, Idiopathic Slipped Capital Femoral Epiphysis

SERIES	N	AVN	CHONDROLYSIS
Flexion Osteotomy			
Diab et al. (2004)[35]	7	1	1
Kartenbender et al. (2000)[46]	39	2	3
Parsch et al. (1999)[24]	96	1	3
Schai et al. (1996)[44]	56	1	NA
Total (%)	198	5/198 (2.5)	7/142 (4.9)
Southwick Osteotomy			
El-Mowafi et al. (2005)[42]	20	0	5
Ireland and Newman (1978)[97]	35	0	4
Rao et al. (1984)[98]	29	0	2
Southwick (1967)[43]	28	0	6
Total	112	0	17/112 (15.2)

AVN, avascular necrosis; NA, data not available in the study.

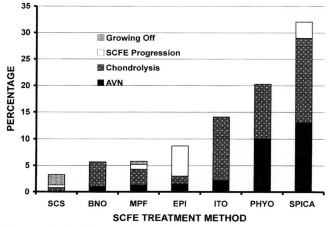

FIGURE 32–1. The incidence of cumulative complications for various treatment methods in idiopathic, stable slipped capital femoral epiphysis (SCFE), as derived from multiple series in the literature. BNO, basilar neck osteotomy; EPI, epiphysiodesis; ITO, intertrochanteric osteotomy; MPF, in situ multipin fixation; PHYO, physeal/cuneiform osteotomy; SCS, in situ single central screw fixation; SPICA, spica cast.

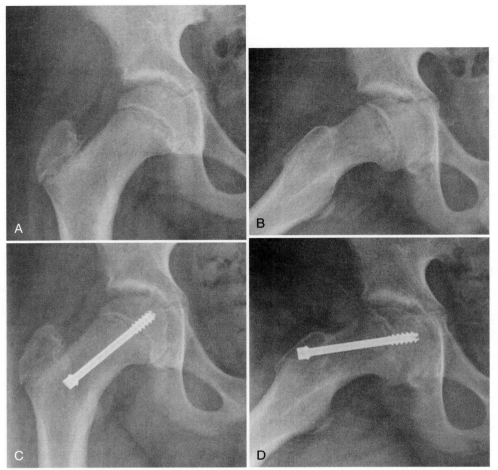

FIGURE 32–2. The anteroposterior (AP) *(A)* and frog-lateral *(B)* radiographs of a child with a right slipped capital femoral epiphysis (SCFE). Treatment was provided by a single central screw in the center of the epiphysis and perpendicular to the physis in both the AP *(C)* and frog-lateral *(D)* positions.

TABLE 32–6. Treatment Outcomes for Prophylactic Fixation of the Opposite Hip in Children with Slipped Capital Femoral Epiphysis

STUDY	LEVEL OF EVIDENCE	GRADE	NO. OF HIPS	AVERAGE FOLLOW-UP (YR)	AVN, *n*	CHONDROLYSIS, *n*	GROWING OFF THE FIXATION
Single Central Screw Fixation							
Dewnany and Radford (2005)[90]	IV	C	65	6.5	0	0	0
Kumm et al. (1996)[91]	IV	C	34	5.4	0	0	10 (29)
MacLean and Reddy (2006)[86]	IV	C	17	NA	0	0	NA
Multipin Fixation							
Emery et al. (1990)[92]	IV	C	95	NA	0	0	29% of pins
Multiple Kirschner-Wire Fixation							
Seller et al. (2001)[87]	IV	C	94	All >1 year	0	0	4 (4)

AVN, avascular necrosis; NA, data not available in the study.

TABLE 32–7. Treatment Outcomes for Prophylactic Fixation of the Opposite Hip in Children with Slipped Capital Femoral Epiphysis

STUDY	LEVEL OF EVIDENCE	GRADE	NO. OF HIPS	AVERAGE FOLLOW-UP (YR)	AVN, *n*	CHONDROLYSIS, *n*	GROWING OFF THE FIXATION
Single Central Screw Fixation							
Dewnany and Radford (2005)[90]	IV	C	65	6.5	0	0	0
Kumm et al. (1996)[91]	IV	C	34	5.4	0	0	10 (29)
MacLean and Reddy (2006)[86]	IV	C	17	NA	0	0	NA
Multipin Fixation							
Emery et al. (1990)[92]	IV	C	95	NA	0	0	29% of pins
Multiple Kirschner-Wire Fixation							
Seller et al. (2001)[87]	IV	C	94	All >1 yr	0	0	4 (4)

AVN, avascular necrosis; NA, data not available in the study.

TABLE 32–8. Summary of Recommendations

STATEMENT	LEVEL OF EVIDENCE/GRADE OF RECOMMENDATION	REFERENCES
1. Stable SCFEs are initially best treated with single central screw fixation.	B, C	8, 9, 17-25, 27-34, 36-39, 41-44, 46, 97-101
2. If an intertrochaneric osteotomy is selected for secondary reorientation of a SCFE, the flexion type rather than the Southwick type should be used.	C	24, 34, 43-44, 97-98
3. The ideal type of treatment for an unstable SCFE is very controversial, but the treatment strategy recommended for the average orthopaedic surgeon is urgent gentle repositioning, double screw fixation, joint decompression, and protected weightbearing.	C, I	70-83

REFERENCES

1. Loder RT, Wittenberg B, DeSilva G: Slipped capital femoral epiphysis associated with endocrine disorders. J Pediatr Orthop 15:349–356, 1995.
2. Wells D, King JD, Roe TF, et al: Review of slipped capital femoral epiphysis associated with endocrine disease. J Pediatr Orthop 13:610–614, 1993.
3. McAffee PC, Cady RB: Endocrinologic and metabolic factors in atypical presentations of slipped capital femoral epiphysis. Report of four cases and review of the literature. Clin Orthop 180:188–196, 1983.
4. Loder RT, Hensinger RN: Slipped capital femoral epiphysis associated with renal failure osteodystrophy. J Pediatr Orthop 17:205–211, 1997.
5. Loder RT, Hensinger RN, Alburger PD, et al: Slipped capital femoral epiphysis associated with radiation therapy. J Pediatr Orthop 18:630–636, 1998.
6. Liu S-C, Tsai C-C, Huang C-H: Atypical slipped capital femoral epiphysis after radiotherapy and chemotherapy. Clin Orthop 426:212–218, 2004.
7. Fahey JJ, O'Brien ET: Acute slipped capital femoral epiphysis. J Bone Joint Surg Am 47-A:1105–1127, 1965.
8. Aronson DD, Carlson WE: Slipped capital femoral epiphysis: A prospective study of fixation with a single screw. J Bone Joint Surg Am 74-A:810–819, 1992.
9. Ward WT, Stefko J, Wood KB, et al: Fixation with a single screw for slipped capital femoral epiphysis. J Bone Joint Surg Am 74-A:799–809, 1992.
10. Aadalen RJ, Weiner DS, Hoyt W, et al: Acute slipped capital femoral epiphysis. J Bone Joint Surg Am 56-A:1473–1487, 1974.
11. Boyer DW, Mickelson MR, Ponseti IV: Slipped capital femoral epiphysis. Long-term follow-up of one hundred and twenty-one patients. J Bone Joint Surg Am 63-A:85–95, 1981.
12. Loder RT, Aronson DD, Greenfield ML: The epidemiology of bilateral slipped capital femoral epiphysis. A study of children in Michigan. J Bone Joint Surg Am 75-A:1141–1147, 1993.
13. Loder RT, Richards BS, Shapiro PS, et al: Acute slipped capital femoral epiphysis: The importance of physeal stability. J Bone Joint Surg Am 75-A:1134–1140, 1993.
14. Kocher MS, Bishop JA, Weed B, et al: Delay in diagnosis of slipped capital femoral epiphysis. Pediatrics 113:e322–e325, 2004.
15. Loder RT, Starnes T, Dikos G, et al: Demographic predictors of severity of stable slipped capital femoral epiphyses. J Bone Joint Surg Am 88-A:97–105, 2006.
16. Rahme D, Comley A, Foster B, et al: Consequences of diagnostic delays in slipped capital femoral epiphyhsis. J Pediatr Orthop B 15:93–97, 2006.
17. Aronson DD, Peterson DA, Miller DV: Slipped capital femoral epiphysis: The case for internal fixation in situ. Clin Orthop 281:115–122, 1992.
18. Carlioz H, Vogt JC, Barba L, et al: Treatment of slipped upper femoral epiphysis: 80 cases operated on over 10 years (1968–1978). J Pediatr Orthop 4:153–161, 1984.
19. Herman MJ, Dormans JP, Davidson RS, et al: Screw fixation of grade III slipped capital femoral epiphysis. Clin Orthop 322:77–85, 1996.
20. Kenny P, Higgisn T, Sedhom M, et al: Slipped upper femoral epiphysis. A retrospective, clinical and radiological study of fixation with a single screw. J Pediatr Orthop B 12:97–99, 2003.
21. Koval KJ, Lehman WB, Rose D, et al: Treatment of slipped capital femoral epiphysis with a cannulated-screw technique. J Bone Joint Surg Am 71-A:1370–1377, 1989.
22. Carney BT, Weinstein SW, Noble J: Long-term follow-up of slipped capital femoral epiphysis. J Bone Joint Surg Am 73-A:667–674, 1991.

23. Dreghorn CR, Knight D, Mainds CC, et al: Slipped upper femoral epiphysis-a review of 12 years of experience in Glasgow (1972–1983). J Pediatr Orthop 7:283–287, 1987.

24. Parsch K, Bühl T, Weller S: Intertrochanteric corrective osteotomy for moderate and severe chronic slipped capital femoral epiphysis. J Pediatr Orthop B 8:223–230, 1999.

25. Zahrawi FB, Stephens TL, Spencer Jr GE, et al: Comparitive study of pinning in situ and open epiphysiodesis in 105 patients with slipped capital femoral epiphysis. Clin Orthop 177:160–168, 1983.

26. Weiner DS, Weiner S, Melby A, et al: A 30-year experience with bone graft epiphysiodesis in the treatment of slipped capital femoral epiphysis. J Pediatr Orthop 4:145–152, 1984.

27. Rao SB, Crawford AH, Burger RR, et al: Open bone peg epiphysiodesis for slipped capital femoral epiphysis. J Pediatr Orthop 16:37–48, 1996.

28. Schmidt TL, Cimino WG, Seidel FG: Allograft epiphysiodesis for slipped capital femoral epiphysis. Clin Orthop 322:61–76, 1996.

29. Adamczyk MJ, Weiner DS, Hawk D: A 50-year experience with bone graft epiphysiodesis in the treatment of slipped capital femoral epiphysis. J Pediatr Orthop 23:578–583, 2003.

30. Szypryt EP, Clement DA, Colton CL: Open reduction or epiphysiodesis for slipped upper femoral epiphysis. J Bone Joint Surg Br 69-B:737–742, 1987.

31. DeRosa GP, Mullins RC, Kling TF Jr: Cuneiform osteotomy of the femoral neck in severe slipped capital femoral epiphysis. Clin Orthop 322:48–60, 1996.

32. Velasco R, Schai PA, Exner GU: Slipped capital femoral epiphysis: A long-term follow-up study after open reduction of the femoral head combined with subcapital wedge resection. J Pediatr Orthop B 7:43–52, 1998.

33. Fish JB: Cuneiform osteotomy of the femoral neck in the treatment of slipped capital femoral epiphysis. J Bone Joint Surg Am 76-A:46–59, 1994.

34. Barros JW, Tukiama G, Fontoura C, et al: Trapezoid osteotomy for slipped capital femoral epiphysis. Int Orthop 24: 83–87, 2000.

35. Diab M, Hresko MT, Millis MB: Intertrochanteric versus subcapital osteotomy in slipped capital femoral epiphysis. Clin Orthop 427:204–212, 2004.

36. Dunn DM, Angel JC: Replacement of the femoral head by open operation in severe adolescent slipping of the upper femoral epiphysis. J Bone Joint Surg Br 60-B:394–403, 1978.

37. Fron D, Forgues D, Mayrargue E, et al: Follow-up study of severe slipped capital femoral epiphysis treated with Dunn's osteotomy. J Pediatr Orthop 20:320–325, 2000.

38. Jerre R, Billing L, Karlsson J: Long-term results after realignment operations for slipped upper femoral epiphysis. J Bone Joint Surg Br 78-B:745–750, 1996.

39. Nishiyama K, Sakamaki T, Ishii Y: Follow-up of the subcapital wedge osteotomy for severe chronic slipped capital femoral epiphysis. J Pediatr Orthop 9:412–416, 1989.

40. Barmada R, Bruch RF, Gimbel JS, et al: Base of the neck extracapsular osteotomy for correction of deformity in slipped capital femoral epiphysis. Clin Orthop 132:98–101, 1978.

41. Kramer WG, Craig WA, Noel S: Compensating osteotomy at the base of the femoral neck for slipped capital femoral epiphysis. J Bone Joint Surg Am 58-A:796–800, 1976.

42. El-Mowafi H, El-Adl G, El-Lakkany MR: Extracapsular base of neck osteotomy versus Southwick oseotomy in treatment of moderate to severe chronic slipped capital femoral epiphysis. J Pediatr Orthop 25:171–177, 2005.

43. Southwick WO: Osteotomy through the lesser trochanter for slipped capital femoral epiphysis. J Bone Joint Surg Am 49-A: 807–835, 1967.

44. Schai PA, Exner GU, Hansch O: Prevention of secondary coxarthrosis in slipped capital femoral epiphysis: A long-term follow-up study after corrective intertrochanteric osteotomy. J Pediatr Orthop B 5:135–143, 1996.

45. Kamegaya M, Saisu T, Ochiai N, et al: Preopertive assessment for intertrochanteric femoral osteotomies in severe chronic slipped capital femoral epiphysis using computed tomography. J Pediatr Orthop B 14:71–78, 2005.

46. Kartenbender K, Cordier W, Katthagen B-D: Long-term follow-up study after corrective Imhäuser osteotomy for severe slipped capital femoral epiphysis. J Pediatr Orthop 20: 749–756, 2000.

47. Leunig M, Casillas MM, Hamlet M, et al: Slipped capital femoral epiphysis. Early mechanical damage to the acetabular cartilage by a prominent femoral metaphysis. Acta Orthop Scand 71:370–375, 2000.

48. Ganz R, Gill TJ, Gautier E, et al: Surgical dislocation of the adult hip. A technique with full access to the femoral head and acetabulum without the risk of avascular necrosis. J Bone Joint Surg Br 83-B:1119–1124, 2001.

49. Spencer S, Millis MB, Kim Y-J: Early results of treatment for hip impingement syndrome in slipped capital femoral epiphysis and pistol grip deformity of the femoral head-neck junction using the surgical dislocation technique. J Pediatr Orthop 26:281–285, 2006.

50. Beck M, Leunig M, Parvizi J, et al: Anterior femoroacetabular impingement. Part II. Midterm results of surgical treatment. Clin Orthop 418:67–73, 2004.

51. Lavigne M, Parvizi J, Beck M, et al: Anterior femoroacetabular impingement. Part 1. Techniques of joint preserving surgery. Clin Orthop 418:61–66, 2004.

52. Carney BT, Weinstein SL: Natural history of untreated chronic slipped capital femoral epiphysis. Clin Orthop 322:43–47, 1996.

53. Hall JE: The results of treatment of slipped upper femoral epiphysis. J Bone Joint Surg Br 39-B:659–673, 1957.

54. Oram V: Epiphysiolysis of the head of the femur. A follow-up examination with special reference to end results and the social prognosis. Acta Orthop Scand 23:100–120, 1953.

55. Ponseti I, Barta CK: Evaluation of treatment of slipping of the capital femoral epiphysis. Surg Gynecol Obstet 86:87–97, 1948.

56. Ross PM, Lyne ED, Morawa LG: Slipped capital femoral epiphysis. Long term results after 10–38 years. Clin Orthop 141:176–180, 1979.

57. Ordeberg G, Hansson LI, Sandström S: Slipped capital femoral epiphysis in southern Sweden. Clin Orthop 220: 148–154, 1987.

58. Jerre R, Hansson G, Wallin J, et al: Does a single device prevent further slipping of the epiphysis in children with slipped capital femoral epiphysis? Arch Orthop Trauma Surg 116:348–351, 1997.

59. Howorth B: History. Slipping of the capital femoral epiphysis. Clin Orthop 48:12–32, 1966.

60. Johnston RC, Larson CB: Results of treatment of hip disorders with cup arthroplasty. J Bone Joint Surg Am 51-A:1461, 1969.

61. Murray RO: The etiology of primary osteoarthritis of the hip. Br J Radiol 38:810–824, 1965.

62. Solomon L: Patterns of osteoarthritis of the hip. J Bone Joint Surg Br 58-B:176–183, 1976.

63. Jerre T: A study in slipped upper femoral epiphysis with special reference to late functional and reontgenological results and the value of closed reduction. Acta Orthop Scand 6(suppl), 1950.

64. Jerre T: Early complications of osteosynthesis with a three flanged nail in situ for slipped epiphysis. Acta Orthop Scand 27:126, 1958.

65. Wilson PD, Jacobs B, Schecter L: Slipped capital femoral epiphysis. An end-result study. J Bone Joint Surg Am 47-A: 1128–1145, 1965.

66. Ordeberg G, Hansson LI, Sandström S: Slipped capital femoral epiphysis in southern Sweden. Long-term results with no treatment or symptomatic primary treatment. Clin Orthop Relat Res (191):95–104, 1984.

67. Goodman WW, Johnson JT, Robertson Jr WW: Single screw fixation for acute and acute-on-chronic slipped capital femoral epiphysis. Clin Orthop 322:86–90, 1996.

68. Stevens DB, Short BA, Burch JM: In situ fixation of the slipped capital femoral epiphysis with a single screw. J Pediatr Orthop B 5:85–89, 1996.

69. Southwick WO: Compression fixation after biplane intertrochanteric osteotomy for slipped capital femoral epiphysis. J Bone Joint Surg Am 55-A:1218–1224, 1973.

70. Mooney III JF, Sanders JO, Browne RH, et al: Management of unstable/acute slipped capital femoral epiphysis. Results of a survey of the POSNA membership. J Pediatr Orthop 25:162–166, 2005.

71. Witbreuk M, Besselaar P, Eastwood D: Current practice in the management of the acute/unstable slipped capital femoral epiphysis in the United Kingdom and the Netherlands: Results of a survey of the membership of the British Society of Children's Orthopaedic Surgery and the Wekrgroep Kinder Orthopaedie. J Pediatr Orthop B 16:79–83, 2007.

72. Gordon JE, Abrahams MS, Dobbs MB, et al: Early reduction, arthrotomy, and cannulated screw fixation in unstable slipped capital femoral epiphysis treatment. J Pediatr Orthop 22:352–358, 2002.

73. Peterson MD, Weiner DS, Green NE, et al: Acute slipped capital femoral epiphysis: The value and safety of urgent manipulative reduction. J Pediatr Orthop 17:648–654, 1997.

74. Phillips SA, Griffiths WEG, Clarke NMP: The timing and reduction and stabilisation of the acute, unstable slipped upper femoral epiphysis. J Bone Joint Surg Br 83-B:1046–1049, 2001.

75. Fallath S, Letts M: Slipped capital femoral epiphysis: An analysis of treatment outcome according to physeal stability. Can J Surg 47:284–289, 2004.

76. Rattey T, Piehl F, Wright JG: Acute slipped capital femoral epiphysis. Review of outcomes and rates of avascular necrosis. J Bone Joint Surg Am 78-A:398–402, 1996.

77. Tokmakova KP, Stanton RP, Mason DE: Factors influencing the development of osteonecrosis in patients treated for slipped capital femoral epiphysis. J Bone Joint Surg Am 85-A:798–801, 2003.

78. Maeda S, Kita A, Funayama K, et al: Vascular supply to slipped capital femoral epiphysis. J Pediatr Orthop 21:664–667, 2001.

79. Kalogrianitis S, Tan CK, Kemp GJ, et al: Does unstable slipped capital femoral epiphysis require urgent stabilization? J Pediatr Orthop B 16:6–9, 2007.

80. Karol LA, Doane RM, Cornicelli SF, et al: Single versus double screw fixation for treatment of slipped capital femoral epiphysis: A biomechanical analysis. J Pediatr Orthop 12:741–745, 1992.

81. Kibiloski LJ, Doane RM, Karol LA, et al: Biomechanical analysis of single- versus double-screw fixation in slipped capital femoral epiphysis at physiological load levels. J Pediatr Orthop 14:627–630, 1994.

82. Kishan S, Upasani V, Mahar A, et al: Biomechanical stability of single-screw versus two-screw fixation of an unstable slipped capital femoral epiphysis model: Effect of screw position in the femoral neck. J Pediatr Orthop 26:601–605, 2006.

83. Snyder RR, Williams JL, Schmidt TL, et al: Torsional strength of double- versus single-screw fixation in a pig model of unstable slipped capital femoral epiphysis. J Pediatr Orthop 26:295–299, 2006.

84. Schultz WR, Weinstein JN, Weinstein SL, et al: Prophylactic pinning of the contralateral hip in slipped capital femoral epiphysis. Evaluation of long-term outcome for the contralateral hip with use of decision analysis. J Bone Joint Surg Am 84-A:1305–1314, 2002.

85. Hägglund G: The contralateral hip in slipped capital femoral epiphysis. J Pediatr Orthop B 5:158–161, 1996.

86. MacLean JGB, Reddy SK: The contralateral slip. An avoidable complication and indication for prophylactic pinning in slipped upper femoral epiphysis. J Bone Joint Surg Br 88-B:1497–1501, 2006.

87. Seller K, Raab P, Wild A, et al: Risk-benefit analysis of prophylactic pinning in slipped capital femoral epiphysis. J Pediatr Orthop B 10-B:192–196, 2001.

88. Castro Jr. FP, Bennett JT, Doulens K: Epidemiological perspective on prophylactic pinning in patients with unilateral slipped capital femoral epiphysis. J Pediatr Orthop 20:745–748, 2000.

89. Jerre R, Billing L, Hansson G, et al: The contralateral hip in patients primarily treated for unilateral slipped upper femoral epiphysis. J Bone Joint Surg Br 76-B:563–567, 1994.

90. Dewnany G, Radford P: Prophylactic contralateral fixation in slipped upper epiphysis: Is it safe? J Pediatr Orthop B 14:429–433, 2005.

91. Kumm DA, Schmidt J, Eisenburger S-H, et al: Prophylactic dynamic screw fixation of the asymptomatic hip in slipped capital femoral epiphysis. J Pediatr Orthop 16:249–253, 1996.

92. Emery RJH, Todd RC, Dunn DM: Prophylactic pinning slipped upper femoral epiphysis. Prevention of complications. J Bone Joint Surg Br 72-B:217–219, 1990.

93. Kocher MS, Bishop JA, Hresko MT, et al: Prophylactic pinning of the contralateral hip after unilateral slipped capital femoral epiphysis. J Bone Joint Surg Am 86-A:2658–2665, 2004.

94. Aronson DD, Loder RT: Slipped capital femoral epiphysis in Black children. J Pediatr Orthop 12:74–79, 1992.

95. Broughton NS, Todd RC, Dunn DM, et al: Open reduction of the severely slipped upper femoral epiphysis. J Bone Joint Surg Br 70-B:435–439, 1988.

96. Abraham E, Garst J, Barmada R: Treatment of moderate to severe slipped capital femoral epiphysis with extracapsular base of neck osteotomy. J Pediatr Orthop 13:294–302, 1993.

97. Ireland J, Newman PH: Triplane osteotomy for severely slipped upper femoral epiphysis. J Bone Joint Surg Br 60-B:390–393, 1978.

98. Rao JP, Francis AM, Siwek CW: The treatment of chronic slipped capital femoral epiphysis by biplane osteotomy. J Bone Joint Surg Am 66-A:1169–1175, 1984.

99. Salvati EA, Robinson Jr HJ, O'Dowd TJ: Southwick osteotomy for severe chronic slipped capital femoral epiphysis: Results and complications. J Bone Joint Surg Am 62-A:561–570, 1980.

100. Betz RR, Steel HH, Emper WD, et al: Treatment of slipped capital femoral epiphysis. Spica cast immobilization. J Bone Joint Surg Am 72-A:587–600, 1990.

101. Meier MC, Meyer LC, Ferguson RL: Treatment of slipped capital femoral epiphysis with a spica cast. J Bone Joint Surg Am 74-A:1522–1529, 1992.

Best Treatment for Adolescent Idiopathic Scoliosis: What Do Current Systematic Reviews Tell Us?

Lori A. Dolan, PhD and Stuart L. Weinstein, MD

Adolescent idiopathic scoliosis (AIS) is a structural, lateral, rotated curvature of the spine of at least 10 degrees (using the Cobb measurement method) arising in otherwise normal children at or around puberty. The diagnosis is one of exclusion, made only when other causes of scoliosis, such as vertebral malformation, neuromuscular disorder, and syndromic conditions have been ruled out. Curvatures less than 10 degrees are viewed as a variation of normal because they have little potential for progression.

When defined as at least a 10-degree angle, epidemiologic studies estimate that 1% to 3% of the at-risk population (children aged 10–16 years) will have some degree of curvature, with most curves requiring no intervention.[1,2]

Treatment of any condition is an attempt to alleviate current problematic signs and symptoms, and to ultimately alter long-term natural history. Most patients with AIS do not initially seek treatment because of symptoms, but rather because of the finding of trunk asymmetry noted during screening or incidentally during well-child examinations. Most subjects have no complaints and will continue to do well throughout their lives. Therefore, the treatment of AIS during adolescence is mainly an attempt to prevent future problems.

Despite the fact that idiopathic scoliosis has been studied and treated for many centuries, the lack of knowledge concerning the etiopathogenesis of the condition has limited clinicians' ability to prevent the disease. They are therefore left to interventions aimed at secondary prevention, where the goal is to avoid the negative side effects of the established disease. And although operative interventions have become safer and more effective at restoring normal anatomy since the 1950s, one could argue that few, if any, advances have been made in nonoperative treatment. Roach[3] reports that as early as 400 BC, Hippocrates recognized the condition and used a system of intermittently applied forces to apply distraction and lateral pressure to reduce the deformity (Fig. 33–1, *A*). The Milwaukee brace and, more recently, thoracolumbosacral orthosis (TLSO) use these same principles to effect curve reduction (see Figs. 33–1, *B* and *C*). This lack of advancement would be acceptable if clinicians were certain that the interventions actually demonstrated the ability to achieve anatomic and quality-of-life goals of the

patient. However, this is not necessarily the case. Curves continue to progress to the point where only surgery can correct the deformity, and prevent future progression and possible pulmonary compromise; patients continue to report dissatisfaction with daily bracing and exercise regimens, and as adults, many face back pain, alterations in body image, and pulmonary impairment. Therefore, in light of these shortcomings, it is imperative that clinicians and patients have access to evidence concerning the effectiveness and side effects of these treatments, so they can knowledgeably make decisions based on their own personal risk/benefit ratios. Systematic reviews, the explicit combination of findings from multiple studies, can provide the reliable and accurate conclusions about effectiveness that patients should receive to make informed decisions. This chapter summarizes the existing systematic reviews of nonoperative treatments for AIS and discusses the practical implications of the findings.

SUMMARY OF REVIEWS

We conducted a search of the Cochrane, Medline, DARE (Database of Abstracts of Reviews of Effects), and ACP Journal Club databases for meta-analyses and systematic reviews of AIS treatment. After excluding articles concerning operative treatments, the search yielded six studies. The major objectives of these studies included effectiveness of mass screening, exercises, bracing, observation, and electrical stimulation. All but one were quantitative reviews that attempted to combine outcome rates across studies. Table 33–1 summarizes the studies that were included in each of the reviews.

Effectiveness of Nonsurgical Treatment for Idiopathic Scoliosis

The first systematic review of nonoperative treatment for AIS was conducted by an Italian group and published in 1991.[4] This study was conducted to gather evidence for or against routine screening for AIS, assuming that early detection must be justified by early, effective treatment. Thus, the question: Are available nonoperative treatments effective in changing the natural history of the condition?

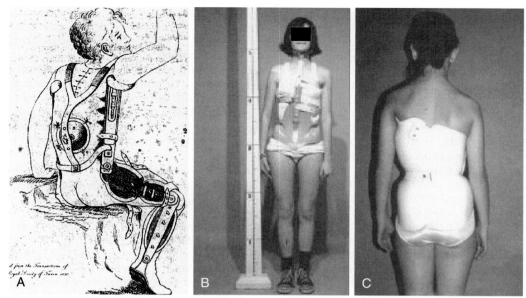

FIGURE 33–1. Orthoses to treat scoliosis. *A*, An early scoliosis orthosis case. *B*, A Milwaukee orthosis case. *C*, A Rosenberger thoracolumbosacral orthosis case. (*A*: From Roach JW: Adolescent idiopathic scoliosis. Nonsurgical treatment. In Weinstein SL (ed): The Pediatric Spine. New York, Raven Press, 1994, pp 498, 503, by permission; *B, C*: Courtesy Stuart L. Weinstein, MD.)

TABLE 33–1. Characteristics of Primary Studies Included in the Reviews

REVIEW	CLINICAL QUESTION	INTERVENTIONS	NO. OF STUDIES	AGE AT TREATMENT INITIATION	COBB AT TREATMENT INITIATION	FOLLOW-UP	STUDY DESIGNS
Focarile et al.[4]	Difference in outcome between treated and untreated patients, between mild and severe curves, and between different therapies	Observation Bracing and LESS	7 17	7–16 years	>5, <50 <50	Not specified	Prognostic: II, III, IV Therapeutic: III, IV
U.S. Preventive Services Task Force[5,6]	Link between screening and treatment and health outcomes	Observation Bracing, LESS, and surgery	Unknown	Unknown	Unknown	Unknown	Unknown
Rowe et al.[10]	Effect of treatment, maturity, and criterion for failure on effectiveness of nonoperative treatments	Observation Bracing and LESS	20	Juvenile, immature, mature	?	Until treatment completion	Therapeutic: II, III, IV
Negrini et al.[14]	Effectiveness of physical exercises	Physical exercises	11	4–49 years	4–114	4 weeks to 7 years	Therapeutic: II, III, IV
Lenssinck et al.[15]	Effectiveness of brace and other nonoperative therapies	Observation Bracing and LESS	13	<18	<60	0–24 months	Therapeutic: II, III
Dolan and Weinstein[16]	Surgery rates after bracing and observation	Observation and bracing	18	8–15	20–45	Until skeletal maturity	Therapeutic: III, IV

LESS, lateral electrical surface stimulation.

The authors conducted a literature search of the Medline database, searching for English-language articles published between 1975 and 1987. Keywords included "therapy," "scoliosis," "random allocation," "natural history," "prevention," "control," "occurrence," "mass screening," "child," "adolescent," and "follow-up studies." The search yielded 111 articles that were reviewed by 2 of the authors. Studies were combined into natural history and therapy studies. Criteria for including natural history studies were few; they required a radiograph at the beginning and end of treatment, criteria for progression, and the number of patients who progressed. Thus, seven studies were included in the final review. The therapy studies included those with patients whose curves were less than 50 degrees at treatment initiation, and 17 articles were included in the final review. The authors calculated the percentage of patients who progressed more than 5 degrees or did not respond favorably (finished treatment with a curve greater than 45 degrees or went on to surgery) and then derived a 95% confidence interval (CI) around the proportion for the individual natural history and treatment studies. In addition, pooled rates were developed by calculating the direct standardized ratio and 95% CI.

The seven natural history studies included curves greater than 5 degrees in patients between the ages of 7 and 16, with Risser signs ranging from 0 to 5. The authors note that the studies were heterogeneous in terms of the rates and note that study design was a factor: The percentage of patients with progressive curves was lower in the prospective studies (7%) than in the retrospective studies (25%). Overall, the range of progression was from 5% to 56%, with a pooled proportion of 15% (95% CI, 3–27%). The 17 therapy studies included 11 studies of bracing; the rest concerned lateral electrical surface stimulation (LESS), posture training, and exercise. They found an overlap in the CIs for LESS (17.5–39.5%) and bracing (13.3–45.5%), although they note these studies were heterogenous in terms of the study end points, and that they also differed according to study design. When failure was the outcome, the failure rate of treatment among curves less than 30 degrees at initiation of bracing was lower (4%) than for those curves greater than 30 degrees (24%).

Overall, this review makes 2 conclusions. First, curves less than 30 degrees had a better prognosis, regardless of whether they were treated, than those greater than 30 degrees, indicating the usefulness of early detection and treatment. Second, unlike the case of failure, the proportion of progressive curves was not different between the treated and untreated groups. To explain this second finding, the authors postulate that 3 conditions may exist: (1) available treatments do not work; (2) treatments cannot stop progression, but they can slow it until maturity; or (3) treatments do work, but they could not demonstrate their effectiveness because of the heterogeneity of the treated and untreated groups. For the clinician, this review indicates that bracing of small-to-moderate-sized curves can decrease the risk for failure relative to observation or LESS. However, when considering curve progression itself, this systematic review draws a range of conclusions, including that treatments to prevent curve progression (bracing and LESS) do not work, and the essentially opposite conclusion that treatments do work, but the literature cannot prove their effectiveness. This review alone, therefore, could not provide evidence to make any decision in practice.

Screening for Idiopathic Scoliosis in Adolescents: U.S. Preventive Services Task Force

The U.S. Preventive Services Task Force (USPSTF) released their recommendations for screening in 1996[5] and updated them in 2004.[6] In 1996, they stated, "There is insufficient evidence to recommend for or against routine screening of asymptomatic adolescents for idiopathic scoliosis"[6] partly because of the lack of convincing evidence that nonoperative treatment of curves detected early results in better health outcomes. In 2004, the USPSTF re-examined their recommendation in light of research published between 1994 and 2002, and attempted to answer several questions including: Is there new evidence that early treatments lead to better health outcomes if applied at an early stage?

The USPSTF used a search of electronic databases for a wide variety of studies, including randomized controlled trials (RCTs), meta-analyses, systematic reviews, well-designed observational studies, editorials, and commentaries. They used the search terms "scoliosis," "idiopathic scoliosis," "treatment," and "population-based screening." The search was limited to adolescents and the English language. Their search found 120 studies, of which 16 were pertinent to the study questions. Of these 16, only 1 study was an RCT. They provided no description of the methods they used to analyze the evidence, although balance sheets and expert consensus were used to form the recommendations.

The RCT compared studies of the effects of exercise alone, exercise and bracing combined, and exercise and electrical stimulation combined.[7] The subjects were between 6 and 16 years old, with curves ranging from 15 to 45 degrees. After 12 weeks of treatment, overall improvement was found for all three groups, and no significant difference was found between the different combinations of treatments. The USPSTF also evaluated the results of two cohort studies. One was a long-term retrospective study of patients treated with bracing or surgery, or both, compared with an age-matched, population-based control group.[8] The follow-up occurred an average of 22 to 23 years after completion of treatment. Both patient groups responded well in terms of curve progression, and no difference in degenerative spine changes was found between the braced and surgical group, although both groups had more degenerative disc changes than the control group. The USPSTF also considered a multinational, controlled study of bracing, observation, and electrical stimulation.[9] Treatment was considered successful if the curve progressed less than 6 degrees by the time the subjects were 16 years of age. A highly significant effect favored bracing over the other 2 treatments. One meta-analysis was available to the USPSTF.[10] The analysis (more fully described later in this chapter) included only observational studies, of which only 1 included a control group. The definition of failure was 3 to 10 degrees of progression. Overall, the primary authors conclude that bracing for 23 or more hours per day is the superior treatment for AIS to prevent curve progression.

Given these new studies, the 2004 USPSTF summary[5] states they could find no new evidence concerning the effectiveness of screening. They also report that conclusions about treatments are limited by the mixed quality of treatment outcomes studies, including inadequate adjustment for confounding factors, and the lack of health outcomes data. The evidence was rated as fair, defined as "sufficient to determine effects on health outcomes, but the strength of the evidence is limited by the number, quality or consistency of the individual studies, generalizability to routine practice or indirect nature of the evidence on health outcomes."[5] Their recommendation carries a grade of D, recommending against routine screening of asymptomatic patients because of at least fair evidence that screening is ineffective or that harms outweigh the benefits. This conclusion represents the current (U.S.) consensus not to screen routinely for scoliosis in schools, and thus informs public health practice. The question regarding the effectiveness of brace treatment in clinical practice is secondary, although crucial, because screening cannot be justified unless early, effective treatment is available. Recent evidence suggesting that bracing might be effective[9,10] was incorporated into the review. Evidence for the clinical effectiveness of brace treatment was not compelling enough to support screening to brace early. Again, insufficient evidence is provided in this review to inform the clinical decision on whether to brace.

Meta-analysis of the Efficacy of Nonoperative Treatments for Idiopathic Scoliosis

Rowe and coworkers,[10] as charged by the Prevalence and Natural History Committee of the Scoliosis Research Association, used meta-analysis to determine whether bracing substantially reduces the number of curves that progress to the degree where surgical intervention is warranted. They were interested in the nonoperative options of observation, bracing, and LESS.

The authors began not with a search of electronic databases, but with the bibliography of a major textbook of operative pediatric orthopedics. Three reviewers identified and included 20 studies, including an unpublished prospective, controlled series and an unpublished doctoral dissertation.

These were 13 studies of bracing, 6 of LESS, and only 1 of observation. Juvenile (age, <9 years), immature (age, 10–13 years), and mature patients (age, >13 years) were included. Braces included the Charleston, Milwaukee, and generic TLSOs. All study designs were included. Nineteen articles were rejected because they included only nonradiographic outcomes, or the data were insufficient regarding treatment, follow-up, or completion rates. They performed a traditional meta-analysis, including categoric and regression analyses of the study findings, which were weighted according to sample size to give more impact to findings from larger numbers of patients.

Three variables were sufficiently described in all studies and were included in the meta-analysis as predictor and outcome variables: level of maturity, definition of progression, and type of treatment. The authors note that the quality scores of the studies increased over time, but that there was no correlation between the year of publication and the effect size found in each study. They did not report the correlation between quality score and effect size. Several problems were found within the individual studies. In some studies, the criteria for failure were unspecified. In others, failure ranged from an increase of 3 to 10 degrees in curve severity. They note that if the typical measurement error is 5 degrees, there is a high likelihood that patients were misclassified as failed. In addition, there was insufficient information concerning the curve type (location of the apex) in the studies.

Rowe and coworkers[10] found that the unweighted rate of success in the bracing studies ranged from 57%[11] to 100%,[12,13] and the weighted mean rate of success was 92%. For the LESS studies, unweighted success rates ranged from 22% to 64%, and the weighted mean rate was 39%. In the one study of observation, the rate of success was 49%. The definition of outcome was found to influence the results: When defined as less than 6 degrees, the success rate was 68%, almost identical as the success rate when defined as progression of less than 10 degrees (67%). However, in the 5 bracing studies where success/failure was undefined, the success rate was 97%. This indicates that the results of the studies where the outcome was not defined inflated the success rate when weighted and averaged over studies.

The authors also found curves were less likely to progress the more mature the patient was at the beginning of treatment, and that wearing the brace for 23 hours/day was significantly more successful than 16- or 8-hour (Charleston brace) regimens. Overall, they conclude that the results of this meta-analysis support the efficacy of bracing compared with LESS and observation only. This review was an attempt to answer a direct clinical question about whether to brace and comes to a conclusion supporting bracing. Strengths of the review include the quantitative pooling of data from different studies. Limitations include the search methodology (beginning with a textbook) being nonstandard, the source articles being of low and variable quality, and hence more difficult to pool, and the failure to account for publication bias. In addition, the pooling of natural history data from one source of patients with treatment data from other cities at other times is inextricably biased. Applying this review to clinical practice would mean bracing immature patients with small curves, but on evidence with sufficient documented limitations and potential biases that it would not meet methodologic standards for prescribing a drug treatment, for example.

Physical Exercises as a Treatment for Adolescent Idiopathic Scoliosis: A Systematic Review[13]

The objective of a review by an Italian group was to assess the effectiveness of physical exercises for AIS in terms of delaying or preventing the need for bracing and in keeping the curve less than 30 degrees (mild scoliosis).[13] Figure 33–2 shows a patient with scoliosis performing a postural exercise to avoid compression in the concave side of the curve.

Articles were found via a search of multiple electronic databases and via hand-searching of multiple non–English-language journals. No language restrictions were set. The group searched for articles including patients with AIS, treated solely by physical exercises, with a control group. The Cobb angle was designated as the outcome of interest. All study designs were included. The full text of 27 articles was reviewed, and the final analysis included 11 articles. The authors rated the internal validity of each study, noting that overall the quality was poor. Five of the studies were uncontrolled (had no control group, or no pretherapy and post-therapy comparisons). Of the six controlled studies, three were prospective, but of these, two included only historical control. Of the four with a concurrent control group, only one specified how patients were allocated to

treatment. None included a blinded outcomes assessment, and only one study attempted to control for important sources of confounding. The articles included several methods of exercise to control curve progression via mobilization, posture control, strengthening, balance, and autocorrection.

The authors found that the poor quality of the studies made it impossible to draw any valid conclusions on the effectiveness of physical exercises in AIS, but that overall, the results of the studies tend to favor physical exercises: The degree of curvature in the PE groups seems to reduce or remain stable regardless of the baseline Cobb angle, whereas the results in the various control groups (who started with smaller Cobb angles) were worse. In terms of practice, the authors believe that the option of PE should be presented to patients so they can make a decision in light of their own preferences, but that further research is required before any definitive conclusions can be made. Applying this review to clinical practice, we found that any support for physical therapy modalities is currently based on studies of low quality.

Effect of Bracing and Other Conservative Interventions in the Treatment of Idiopathic Scoliosis in Adolescents: A Systematic Review of Clinical Trials

Lenssinck and coauthors'[15] review from a group of physical therapists in the Netherlands begins by stating that there is a consensus about surgical treatment for the small group of patients with curves exceeding 45 degrees, but that there is currently no systematic review of the effectiveness of conservative (i.e., nonoperative) care for AIS. They also deemed Rowe and coworkers'[10] study as invalid because it does not meet the criteria for reviews set down by the

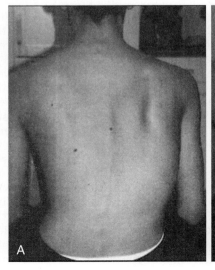
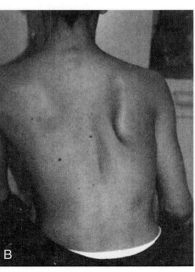

Figure 33–2. Physical exercises. *A,* Sitting as usual. *B,* Sitting in a relaxed but straightened position or prevent compression on the concave side of the curve. (From Weiss HR, Weiss G, Petermann F: Incidence of curvature progression in idiopathic scoliosis patients treated with scoliosis in-patient rehabilitation (SIR): An age- and sex-matched controlled study. Pediatr Rehabil 6:23–30, 2003, reprinted with permission of the publisher (Taylor & Francis Ltd, http://www.tandf.co.uk/journals).

Cochrane Collaboration. Therefore, the aim of their study was to evaluate the effectiveness of nonoperative care using the Cochrane criteria.

The authors used the Cochrane, PubMed, CINAHL, and PEDro databases from inception to 2003 to search for randomized trials and controlled clinical trials, using the keywords pertaining to bracing, exercises, AIS, and treatment. Three authors independently conducted the search and examined all abstracts. The following criteria were used to select studies: (1) RCT or CCT (controlled clinical trial) (including an intervention and 1 or more nonrandomized control groups), (2) AIS, (3) age younger than 18 years, and (4) conservative intervention (no drug or surgery studies). No language restrictions were set. Two reviewers rated the quality of the studies and extracted the data. A total of 437 articles were found, and 13 studies were included (3 RCTs and 10 CCTs).

Quality scores (theoretically ranging from 0–9 points) varied between 0 and 5. The studies covered a wide range of interventions, including bracing, LESS, exercises, and behavioral treatment; many studies included a combination of most frequently bracing and another intervention. Different braces were compared in 5 studies. Treatment duration ranged from 8 days to 8 years, but was often not specified. Follow-up period ranged from none to 24 months. The effect of therapy was most often measured using the Cobb angle, but other studies evaluated pulmonary function, torso overhang, curve rotation, and loads on instrumented pads in the brace. Six studies reported surgery rates. Low power was an issue for the majority of studies; in 9 studies, 1 or more of the groups included less than 25 patients.

No statistical pooling was done because of the heterogeneity of the studies with regard to interventions, populations, and treatment duration. Overall, no statistical differences between groups within studies were found, but using a brace tended to result in the most frequent reduction of the curve. Lenssinck and coauthors'[15] cite only 1 study with a statistically significant difference, Nachemson and Peterson,[9] but conclude that this study was of low quality, and that the treatment assignment was not random. They also found no differences among braces or between bracing and LESS. They then conclude that the effectiveness of bracing and exercises is promising but not yet established. This review may again frustrate the practitioner by concluding that insufficient evidence has been reported in the literature to guide selection of either bracing or physical therapy treatment. The review attempted to uphold higher methodologic review standards rather than to draw a "pragmatic" conclusion. It underlines the current seeming paradox in systematic reviews—the higher the quality of the review itself, the lower the grade of recommendation it tends to make. This paradox exists in fields such as children's orthopedics where RCTs are the exception rather than the norm in assessing the results of treatment.

Surgical Rates after Observation and Bracing for Adolescent Idiopathic Scoliosis: An Evidence-Based Review

Dolan and Weinstein's[16] review derived a pooled rate of the prevalence of surgery in untreated and braced patients, and attempted to evaluate the effect of certain known risk factors for curve progression on surgical rates. The authors attempted to mimic current indications for bracing by limiting the study to patients with curves between 20 and 45 degrees, and age between 8 and 15, and a Risser sign of 0, 1, or 2. Follow-up to skeletal maturity was also mandatory. Interventions included observation, TLSOs, and bending (nighttime) braces. Studies were limited to those reporting rates of surgery, recommended surgery or curves progressing to greater than 50 degrees.

The authors used electronic databases (Medline, Cochrane, Web of Science, Clinical Evidence) and the bibliography of all reviewed articles, and limited the search to English language and children 0 to 18 years of age. Search terms included "AIS," "natural history," "bracing," "observation," and "orthotics." Only one reviewer selected the studies and extracted the data, although the extraction was repeated to improve reliability. Analysis consisted of pooling the number of surgeries across all studies and dividing by the number of subjects across all studies; therefore, the unit of analysis was the individual patient and not the study. Ninety-five percent CIs were calculated for all rates.

Of 152 studies reviewed, only 18 met the inclusion criteria. In total, 15 studies reviewed bracing and 3 reviewed observation. Minor exceptions were made to the criteria to include 2 observation and five bracing studies. All studies were Level III comparison studies or Level IV case series. The sample size of the individual studies ranges from 15 to 319 (median sample size, 78). Surgical indications included progression, a curve greater than 45 degrees, or a curve greater than 50 degrees. Some studies took other characteristics into consideration, such as complaints of pain, deformity, and the wishes of the patient and family. The surgical rates in the observation studies ranged from 13%[17,18] to 38%[19] (pooled estimate, 22%; 95% CI, 16–29%). This rate was comparable with that found for the bracing studies, where rates ranged from 1%[13] to 43%,[20] for a pooled rate of 23% (95% CI, 20–24%). The authors state that comparing the surgery rates for observation and bracing shows no clear advantage to either approach, and that the practice of bracing patients with these characteristics to avoid surgery is supported by inconsistent or inconclusive studies. This review asks a clearly defined question: Does bracing decrease the surgical rate? Selecting only articles that contribute directly to that question (and therefore excluding many studies using radiographic progression as an end point), the answer to the question is that bracing does not decrease the rate of surgery among patients with AIS with Risser signs of 0 to 2. Pooling Level III and IV studies gives a larger sample but does not increase the level of evidence. Therefore, this study could be interpreted as weak evidence supporting not using a brace in clinical practice or as additional evidence that the realistic conclusion to be drawn from the current literature is one of equipoise—that is, we simply do not know enough or have enough evidence to decide whether to use a brace.

METHODOLOGIC CONSIDERATIONS

Just as individual studies can be biased or otherwise flawed, so can systematic reviews. First, the question asked by a review needs to be defined precisely so that only the appropriate primary studies will be included. Of the systematic reviews summarized here, all were designed to answer questions of effectiveness, but the USPSTF[5,6] searched broadly to collect information about screening and subsequent treatment, whereas Dolan and Weinstein's[16] review specifically examined two treatment approaches and one outcome. The quality of a systematic review should be assessed as stringently as primary studies. Table 33–2 summarizes the reviews in terms of the Oxman and Guyatt Overview Quality Assessment Questionnaire (OQAQ) to access the scientific quality of the materials and methods leading up to the conclusions.[21] First, the search methods used to find the primary studies should be stated explicitly and be comprehensive. The sources should be named (e.g., Medline, Embase), and the years covered by the search should be specified. In addition, the search must be comprehensive, demonstrated by a listing of keywords used in the search (OQAQ items 1 and 2). All the reviews in this chapter searched electronic databases, except for Rowe and coworkers,[10] which included only articles from a textbook bibliography. Rowe and coworkers[10] also included Nachemson and Peterson's[9] manuscript (before its peer review and publication) and an unpublished doctoral thesis,[22] but it did not explicitly give the authors' reasons for doing so. Notably, both of these articles had a relatively high rate of success and large sample size. The criteria for including and excluding primary studies should be explicit; in addition, more than one reviewer should decide independently which papers meet these criteria, and a consensus should be reached, to eliminate bias in selecting the materials (OQAQ items 3 and 4). In addition to finding all pertinent articles, reviewers should also make an effort to assess the validity of the primary articles. The criteria for validity (i.e., scoring system or level of evidence based on research design) should be mentioned and incorporated into decisions either concerning which papers to include or when analyzing the studies that are cited (OQAQ items 5 and 6). All authors note methodologic problems with the articles they include;

TABLE 33–2. Characteristics of the Reviews Using the Oxman and Guyatt Overview Quality Assessment Questionnaire System[21]

QUESTIONS	SYSTEMATIC REVIEWS					
	FOCARILE ET AL.[4]	U.S. PREVENTIVE SERVICES TASK FORCE[5,6]	ROWE ET AL.[10]	NEGRINI ET AL.[14]	LENSSINCK ET AL.[15]	DOLAN AND WEINSTEIN[16]
1. Were the search methods used to find evidence stated?	+	+	+	+	+	+
2. Was the search for evidence reasonably comprehensive?	+	+	–	+	+	+
3. Were the criteria for deciding which studies to include in the overview reported?	+	+	O	+	+	+
4. Was bias in the selection of studies avoided?	+	+	–	o	+	–
5. Were the criteria used for assessing the validity of the included studies reported?	+	O	o	+	+	+
6. Was the validity of all studies referred to in the text assessed using appropriate criteria?	+	O	o	+	+	+
7. Were the methods used to combine the findings of the relevant studies reported?	+	+	+	NA	+	+
8. Were the findings of the relevant studies combined appropriately relative to the primary question the overview addresses?	+	+	+	NA	+	+
9. Were the conclusions made by the authors(s) supported by the data and/or analysis reported in the overview?	+	+	+	+	+	+
Oxman and Guyatt Index	7	5	3	5	7	5

+, yes; ‾, no; O, can't tell from review.

only Lenssinck and coauthors[15] limited their review to controlled studies. Rowe and coworkers[10] rated each study according to a list of quality indicators. The methods used to combine the findings of the study should be stated and appropriate relative to the primary question (OQAQ items 7 and 8). None of the pooled results was weighted according to quality scores. Rowe and coworkers[10] weighted their success rates according to sample size. The point estimate from a larger study is more precise than that from a smaller study; however, weighting by sample size does not ensure that studies with the most evidence for internal validity are given more impact than others. In addition, sensitivity analysis or some other method of evaluating the sensitivity of the pooled results to certain characteristics of the studies should be included. For example, Focarile and researchers[4] found that retrospective studies (or those where the patients were selected for study) had greater rates of progression than prospective studies. Dolan and Weinstein[16] note that including results of one study almost doubled the pooled surgical rate from the observational studies. Lastly, the numeric result and the conclusions must be interpreted with common sense and the context of the question being asked (OQAQ item 9). The reviewer must decide how the result should influence the care of an individual patient.[21] All of the reviews except for the USPSTF[5,6] and Rowe and coworkers[10] acknowledge that their results do not support or deny the effectiveness of the treatments they reviewed. The USPSTF[5,6] recommends against screening after they balanced the potential benefits and potential harms of both screening and early treatment. Rowe and coworkers[10] recommend full-time bracing relative to part-time bracing, LESS, or observation, on the basis of statistical pooling of the data. And although, statistically, bracing does appear to be relatively effective, the authors did not take the poor quality of the studies into account, and they did not acknowledge the questionable reliability of the success and failure rates in the sole study reflecting the outcomes of observation. They additionally included multiple studies of bracing where the criteria for success were not explicitly defined, despite the fact that these rates were acknowledged to be among the greatest reviewed. The criteria for failure were based on Cobb angle progression rather than on surgical rate. Based on the OQAQ criteria and Oxman and Guyatt's suggested scoring and interpretation of overall scientific quality[21] (OQAQ item 10), scores for these reviews ranged from 3[10] to 7.[4,15] A score of 1 to 4 points indicates extensive flaws, 5 or 6 points indicates minor flaws, and 7 points indicates minimal flaws. Based on this system, Rowe and coworkers'[10] review is extensively flawed, and its recommendations should be questioned. Focarile and researchers'[4] and Lenssinck and coauthors'[15] reviews were the highest quality in this series, and as such, their recommendations should be considered the most valid and informative concerning treatment decisions.

IMPLICATIONS FOR PRACTICE

Clinicians looking to these studies for an answer to the question, "What is the best treatment for scoliosis?" could be rightfully frustrated. After many years of treating this condition, the research literature, both primary studies and systematic reviews, still lacks a clear consensus concerning the effectiveness of bracing, LESS, and exercises. In making a decision about treatment, the first step should be to clarify the goals of the patient, convey the pertinent findings together with the quality of the evidence behind the findings, discuss the possible side effects, and then to let the patient make the decision based on a personal risk/benefit ratio. Table 33–3 provides a guide to clinicians who wish to impart information from these reviews to their patients.

Preventing curve progression is a different goal from preventing surgery. Curve progression can occur without reaching the threshold (generally, 45–50 degrees) where there is a high risk for continued progression and of developing an unacceptable deformity that can be treated only by instrumentation and fusion. Therefore, if the patient's goal is to prevent even a few degrees of progression, the clinician could relate the following information: No high-quality evidence has demonstrated an advantage of bracing over observation or any other nonoperative treatment to prevent progression. However, one low-quality systematic review[10] suggests that bracing may be advantageous, but only if the brace is worn for 23 hours/day. The adverse effects of bracing include skin irritation and some risk for psychosocial problems such as self-consciousness; however, these problems are extremely variable, and some patients have no problems with the treatment at all.

If the patient is comfortable with the risk for some curve progression but is more concerned with preventing progression to the point of surgery, then the following information could be given: Only two systematic reviews in the literature examine the rate of surgery after bracing and observation. One was of high quality,[4] and the other was of adequate quality.[16] The higher quality study suggests that bracing significantly decreases the risk for surgery when started early, that is, when the curve is less than 30 degrees, compared with starting for a more severe curve. The study of lesser quality found the same advantage to bracing early, but overall did not find any difference in surgical rates, for any curve size, between bracing and observation. Bracing has been associated with some adverse effects. Observation is a difficult choice, especially when the impulse is to seek active treatment. Patients who watch and wait may feel remorse if surgery is advised, because of their decision not to treat.

DISCUSSION

Systematic reviews represent the best sources of quantitative information for making evidence-based choices in medicine. Also, they are especially needed

TABLE 33–3. Major Findings of Reviews

FINDINGS	FOCARILE ET AL.[4]	U.S. PREVENTIVE SERVICES TASK FORCE[5,6]	ROWE ET AL. [10]	NEGRINI E AL. [14]	LENSSINCK ET AL.[15]	DOLAN AND WEINSTEIN[16]
Overview Quality Assessment Questionnaire score	7	5	3	5	7	5
Finding with curve progression as outcome	No advantage to bracing over LESS or observation	Inconclusive effect of bracing Not specified	Bracing more effective than LESS or observation Bracing 23 hours is more effective than <23 hours No difference between <23 hour bracing, LESS, and observation	Inconclusive effect of exercises	Inconclusive effect of bracing, LESS, and exercises	Not studied
Finding with surgery (or proxy) as outcome	Bracing when curve is <30 results in fewer surgeries than in curves >30 degrees	Not specified	Not studied	Not studied	Not studied	No difference between bracing and observation for any curve size Bracing when curve is <30 results in fewer surgeries than in curves >30 degrees

LESS, lateral electrical surface stimulation.

in an area such as AIS for several reasons. The sample size available to any one researcher is generally too small to make a definitive statement about effectiveness, especially when subgroup analysis is necessary to evaluate outcomes according to risk factors such as curve size, maturity, and curve location. The practice of bracing around the world is anything but standardized; multiple types of braces are used in North America alone, as well as the different types used in Europe. In addition, some countries such as Germany, Spain, and Italy[23,24] tend to begin treatment with exercises, followed by a combination of exercises and bracing if the curve progresses. This variability in practice requires large, multinational efforts with clearly specified treatment regimens to discern the relative merits of each treatment program. The reviews in this chapter illustrate the disparate findings in the primary literature. For example, the range of surgical rates after bracing in the Dolan and Weinstein[16] review was 1% to 43%; not included in their review were two recent articles, one with a surgical rate of 0%[25] to 76%.[26] But perhaps the most compelling reason for systematic reviews in this population is the costs to the healthcare system and to families.

Mass screening for AIS diverts resources from other public health programs at the same time that it creates unnecessary costs through referral of children with "schooliosis." Observation can be difficult for families who want to actively treat the condition, even if the risk of surgery is not definitely decreased. Braces are expensive, both in terms of money and psychosocial costs to the family. In some cases, patients perceive the brace to be more deforming than the anatomy they are trying to correct. Currently, the USPSTF review[5,6] continues to find insufficient evidence that early diagnosis produces net benefit, and thus does not recommend routine school screening for scoliosis, in part because the lack of evidence for the effectiveness of early clinical treatment.

Regarding clinical treatment, insufficient evidence exists to support physical therapy as an effective modality when curve progression is the desired outcome.[14,15] Bracing is more complicated. One meta-analysis[10] concludes that bracing is effective (92% "success" rate with bracing, 49% "success" rate with control) by pooling patient data from Level II, III, and IV studies of varying quality. This conclusion was based on either Cobb angle progression or unspecified criteria for failure. The review itself was done in a manner quite differently from that currently accepted. Two additional meta-analyses[5,16] with strict search and inclusion criteria have failed to support bracing. In the case of the Dolan and Weinstein[16] review, the question was, What is the surgical rate with (23%) and without (22%) bracing? This well-defined outcome was addressed only in level III and IV studies. In the case of the Lennsinck and coauthors'[15] review, the application of quality criteria to the included studies limited the ability of the reviewers to draw any firm conclusions about the effectiveness of bracing. For the clinician, the lesson is that a single meta-analysis does not conclusively answer a clinical question. Meta-analyses differ in quality and detail, and all are limited by the availability and quality of published clinical evidence. Where level III and IV studies predominate, systematic reviews may produce results that contradict each other or that are inconclusive, or both. Such is the state of knowledge regarding bracing: The balance of published evidence neither supports nor prohibits using a brace to treat scoliosis in the growing child. Table 33–4 provides a summary of recommendations.

TABLE 33–4. Summary of Recommendations

STATEMENT	LEVEL OF EVIDENCE/GRADE OF RECOMMENATION	REFERENCES
1. Bracing *does not* reduce the incidence of surgery among growing adolescents with curves 25 to 40 degrees relative to observation.	I	4, 16
2. Bracing when the curve is <30 degrees *may* result in fewer surgeries than when the curve is >30 degrees.	I	4, 16
3. Bracing *may* reduce the incidence of curve progression among adolescents.	I	10
4. Conservative treatment (bracing, LESS and/or exercise) *may not* reduce the incidence of curve progression among adolescents.	I	4-6, 15
5. Physical exercises *may* stop or reduce curve progression among adolescents.	I	13

REFERENCES

1. Parent S, Newton PO, Wenger DR: Adolescent idiopathic scoliosis: Etiology, anatomy, natural history, and bracing. Instr Course Lect 54:529–536, 2005.
2. Shindle MK, Khanna AJ, Bhatnagar R, et al: Adolescent idiopathic scoliosis: Modern management guidelines. J Surg Orthop Adv 15:43–52, 2006.
3. Roach JW: Adolescent idiopathic scoliosis. Nonsurgical treatment. In Weinstein SL (ed): The Pediatric Spine. New York: Raven Press, 1994, pp 497–510.
4. Focarile FA, Bonaldi A, Giarolo MA, et al: Effectiveness of nonsurgical treatment for idiopathic scoliosis. Overview of available evidence. Spine 16:395–401, 1991.
5. U.S. Preventive Services Task Force: Screening for Idiopathic Scoliosis in Adolescents: Recommendation Statement [Agency for Healthcare Research and Quality], June 2004. Available at: http://www.ahrq.gov/clinic/3rduspstf/scoliosis/scoliors.htm. Accessed July 3, 2008.
6. U.S. Preventive Services Task Force: Screening for adolescent idiopathic scoliosis. Review article. JAMA 269:2667-2672, 1993.
7. el-Sayyad M, Conine TA: Effect of exercise, bracing and electrical surface stimulation on idiopathic scoliosis: A preliminary study. Int J Rehab Res 17:70–74, 1994.
8. Danielsson AJ, Nachemson AL: Radiologic findings and curve progression 22 years after treatment for adolescent idiopathic scoliosis: Comparison of brace and surgical treatment with matching control group of straight individuals. Spine 26:515–525, 2001.
9. Nachemson AL, Peterson LE: Effectiveness of treatment with a brace in girls who have adolescent idiopathic scoliosis. A prospective, controlled study based on data from the Brace Study of the Scoliosis Research Society. J Bone Joint Surg Am 77:815–822, 1995.
10. Rowe DE, Bernstein SM, Riddick MF, et al: A meta-analysis of the efficacy of non-operative treatments for idiopathic scoliosis. J Bone Joint Surg Am 79:664–674, 1997.
11. Green NE: Part-time bracing of adolescent idiopathic scoliosis. J Bone Joint Surg Am 68:738–742, 1986.
12. Edmonsson AS, Morris JT: Follow-up study of Milwaukee brace treatment in patients with idiopathic scoliosis. Clin Orthop Relat Res 58–61, 1977.
13. Ylikoski M, Peltonen J, Poussa M: Biological factors and predictability of bracing in adolescent idiopathic scoliosis. J Pediatr Orthop 9:680–683, 1989.
14. Negrini S, Antonini G, Carabalona R, et al: Physical exercises as a treatment for adolescent idiopathic scoliosis. A systematic review. Pediatr Rehabil 6:227–235, 2003.
15. Lenssinck ML, Frijlink AC, Berger MY, et al: Effect of bracing and other conservative interventions in the treatment of idiopathic scoliosis in adolescents: A systematic review of clinical trials. Phys Ther 85:1329–1339, 2005.
16. Dolan LA, Weinstein SL: Surgical rates after observation and bracing for adolescent idiopathic scoliosis: An evidence-based review. Spine 32:S91–S100, 2007.
17. Goldberg CJ, Dowling FE, Hall JE, et al: A statistical comparison between natural history of idiopathic scoliosis and brace treatment in skeletally immature adolescent girls. Spine 18:902–908, 1993.
18. Goldberg CJ, Moore DP, Fogarty EE, et al: Adolescent idiopathic scoliosis: The effect of brace treatment on the incidence of surgery. Spine 26:42–47, 2001.
19. Fernandez-Feliberti R, Flynn J, Ramirez N, et al: Effectiveness of TLSO bracing in the conservative treatment of idiopathic scoliosis. J Pediatr Orthop 15:176–181, 1995.
20. Little DG, Song KM, Katz D, et al: Relationship of peak height velocity to other maturity indicators in idiopathic scoliosis in girls. J Bone Joint Surg Am 82:685–693, 2000.
21. Bhandari M, Morrow F, Kulkarni A, Tornetta P: Meta-analysee in orthopaedic surgery. A systematic review of their methodologies. J Bone Joint Surg Am 83:15–24, 2001.
22. Styblo K: Conservative Treatment of Juvenile and Adolescent Idiopathic Scoliosis. Leiden, The Netherlands, Rijksuniversiteit te Leiden, 1991.

23. Negrini S, Aulisa L, Ferraro C, et al: Italian guidelines on rehabilitation treatment of adolescents with scoliosis or other spinal deformities. Eura Medicophys 41:183–201, 2005.
24. Weiss HR, Negrini S, Rigo M, et al: Indications for conservative management of scoliosis (guidelines). Scoliosis 1:5, 2006.
25. Danielsson AJ, Hasserius R, Ohlin A, et al: A prospective study of brace treatment versus observation alone in adolescent idiopathic scoliosis: A follow-up mean of 16 years after maturity. Spine 32:2198–2207, 2007.
26. Janicki JA, Poe-Kochert C, Armstrong DG, et al: A comparison of the thoracolumbosacral orthoses and providence orthosis in the treatment of adolescent idiopathic scoliosis: Results using the new SRS inclusion and assessment criteria for bracing studies. J Pediatr Orthop 27:369–374, 2007.

Chapter 34

What Is the Best Treatment for Ambulatory Cerebral Palsy?

Unni G. Narayanan, MBBS, MSc, FRCSC

WHAT IS CEREBRAL PALSY? NEW DEFINITION AND CLASSIFICATION

Cerebral palsy (CP) constitutes one of the most common causes of chronic childhood disability, with rates estimated between 2 and 2.5 per 1000 live births.[1] This chapter discusses the evidence for interventions for ambulant children with CP. Any discussion about the effectiveness of interventions in CP must first consider what CP and its associated pathophysiology are, and take into account the heterogeneity and natural history of CP to put definitions of "effectiveness" into perspective.

An international multidisciplinary collaborative effort to arrive at a consensus definition and classification system for CP was begun in 2004.[2] This culminated in the Report on the Definition and Classification of Cerebral Palsy, which states that the term "CP describes a group of permanent disorders of the development of movement and posture, causing activity limitation, that are attributed to non-progressive disturbances that occurred in the developing fetal or infant brain. The motor disorders are often accompanied by disturbances of sensation, perception, cognition, communication and behaviour, by epilepsy, and by secondary musculoskeletal problems."[3] The robustness (reliability and validity) of this definition is yet to be established, and it is not the only one in current use, but this report based on collective expert opinion, represents the best effort to date to standardize the definition, inclusion/exclusion criteria, and the characteristics used currently for describing children with CP.

In this report, the international group also proposed a new classification system[3] because the traditional classifications of CP based on the movement disorder (spastic, ataxic, or dyskinetic) and/or topographic distribution (hemiplegia, diplegia, and quadriplegia) alone were not reproducible, not reliably prognostic, or adequately descriptive of the heterogeneous population of children with CP. The new classification is based on 4 dimensions:

1a. *Nature and typology of the motor disorder:* They are based on the dominant type of tone and movement abnormality (spastic, ataxic, dystonic, athetoid).

1b. *Functional motor abilities:* The Gross Motor Functional Classification System (GMFCS) is a five-level ordinal system that has become the international standard for categorizing individuals based on the severity of their motor disability.[4] The GMFCS has been shown to be reliable and valid,[5] and its prognostic utility has been established in a prospective, longitudinal, population-based cohort study of 657 children (Level I evidence).[6] Children in GMFCSS level I can perform all the activities of their age-matched peers, albeit with some difficulties with their speed, balance, and coordination. In level II, children have similar functional abilities on flat and familiar surfaces, but they require support on uneven surfaces or when climbing stairs. Children in level III are also independent walkers but require an assist device such as a crutch or a walker, and they may use wheelchairs for longer distances. Children in levels IV and V are nonambulatory. In level IV, they may bear weight for transfers and use a walker for exercise purposes, whereas in level V, children cannot achieve any functional weight bearing and are usually totally dependent on caregivers. The GMFCS provides an excellent basis for stratification of patients in outcome evaluations.

2. *Accompanying impairments:* Accompanying impairments may have a greater impact on the functional abilities of the individual than the primary motor abnormality (e.g., seizure disorders, hearing and visual problems, cognitive and attention deficits, emotional and behavioral issues, and secondary musculoskeletal problems).

3. *Anatomic distribution* (limb, truncal, and bulbar involvement) and *neuroimaging findings.*

4. *Cause and timing,* to the extent that this is determinable, since these are likely to influence the presentation and natural history.

The new classification was developed by international expert opinion, and its overall reliability and validity is yet to be established.

PATHOPHYSIOLOGY

The hallmark of CP is abnormal muscle tone, of which spasticity is the most common type, accompanied by loss of selective motor control, muscle weakness, and impaired balance.[7] Muscles grow in response to the stimulus of stretch derived from normal physical activity. Hypertonia and limited use of muscles because of developmental delay result in dynamic (velocity-dependent) muscle contractures, which become static joint contractures over time as the tight muscles fail to grow proportionately with their skeletal attachments (Level V evidence from animal studies).[8] These abnormal forces on the growing skeleton lead to secondary bony deformities and joint instability, and related lever arm dysfunction.[9] In children with ambulatory potential, the interaction of joint contractures, muscle weakness, bony deformities, and joint instability at multiple levels affect the quality and efficiency of gait and other aspects of their physical function. This understanding of the pathophysiology of CP is based on Level IV and V evidence.

IMPLICATIONS OF NATURAL HISTORY OF CEREBRAL PALSY ON OUTCOMES EVALUATION

Based on a prospective longitudinal cohort study of 657 children, Level I evidence has been reported that shows that gross motor function improves in children up to the age of 6 or 7 years, albeit with different trajectories for each GMFCS level, but it remains stable after motor development is complete.[6] "Improvements" after any interventions in younger children must therefore be placed in the context of expected improvements in gross motor function before the age of 7 years. In contrast, although the primary central nervous system pathology is static, the secondary musculoskeletal pathology and its consequences are known to deteriorate over time in older children. Bell and colleagues[10] report deterioration in passive range of motion, and spatiotemporal and kinematic parameters on gait analyses an average of 4.5 years apart in a group of 28 ambulatory children with CP who had not undergone any surgery during this interval.[10] Johnson and coworkers[11] found similar rates of deterioration in gait over a 32-month period in 18 ambulatory children (4–18 years old) regardless of age or history of prior surgery. Despite their small sample sizes, both these longitudinal case series (Level IV evidence) suggest that effectiveness of surgical interventions for this population must be interpreted in the context of natural deterioration of gait with growth. Consequently, preintervention versus postintervention comparisons in uncontrolled case series may underestimate the outcomes of these interventions in the short term.[12] However, short-term outcomes are also less meaningful because the growing child is at risk for recurrent deformity and gradual loss of mobility over the long term, because the primary central nervous system pathology remains unaffected by the intervention. Mobility in adulthood may also deteriorate over time (Level IV evidence).[13–15] These issues have implications both on the optimal age at which the surgical interventions should be performed and the timing of outcome assessments.

GOALS OF TREATMENT AND OUTCOMES TO CONSIDER

The goals of treatment of ambulatory children with CP are to preserve or improve present and future gait efficiency and physical function, and secondarily to improve the appearance of gait.[16] The treatment principles to accomplish these goals are: (1) *prevention* of joint contractures and skeletal deformities by muscle stretching, spasticity reduction, and muscle strengthening; and (2) *correction* of significant contractures and bony deformities when these have already occurred. Evaluating the effectiveness of interventions to achieve these goals requires defining the outcomes of interest and the longevity of these outcomes.[17,18]

The American Academy for Cerebral Palsy and Developmental Medicine (AACPDM) advocates the use of a two-part conceptual framework to evaluate the effectiveness of interventions.[19,20] The framework analyzes and categorizes treatment outcomes according to the components of the International Classification of Functioning, Disability and Health (ICF),[21] and judges the strength of the evidence according to the study design and rigor in the conduct of the study. The ICF model has two parts, each with two components (Table 34–1).

A common, but often untested assumption is that treatment at one level (e.g., body structure and function: knee flexion contracture) may positively affect another level (e.g., activity and participation: by permitting independent walking over longer distances). Similarly, interventions do not always have simple effects on a single dimension. For example, powered mobility may increase activities by providing an alternative means of efficient locomotion, which may also increase participation by allowing a student to be independent and move around the school faster and with less effort, but may have negative effects in the body structure and function such as increased knee flexion contractures.[22] A multicenter cross-sectional study found at best a fair correlation between measures of spasticity or range of motion (body structure and function) and measures of gross motor function or physical function.[23]

INTERVENTION STRATEGIES FOR AMBULATORY CEREBRAL PALSY

A number of complementary strategies are used sequentially or in combination, including physical therapy, orthotics (braces), and serial casting to simulate the stretch that would normally be derived from usual physical activity, to stimulate muscle growth. These strategies are often accompanied by measures to reduce muscle tone by pharmacologic (botulinum toxin type A [BTX-A], phenol) or neurosurgical methods (selective dorsal rhizotomy [SDR], intrathecal baclofen). These are believed to facilitate the stretch from therapy and serial casting, and to improve tolerance of brace wear, which, in turn, may prevent or delay

TABLE 34–1. International Classification of Functioning, Disability, and Health Model

COMPONENTS	DEFINITION AND EXAMPLES
Part I: Functioning & Disability	
1. Body Structure & Body Function (negative term = impairment)	Body structure: anatomic parts of the body such as organs, limbs, and their components (e.g., periventricular leukomalacia in premature infant's brain, torsional deformity)
	Body function: physiologic functions of body systems including psychological functions (e.g., range of motion, muscle strength)
2. Activity & Participation (negative terms = activity limitation; participation restriction)	Activity: execution of a task or action by an individual (e.g., walking difficulties such as balance, endurance or fatigue, climbing stairs)
	Participation: involvement in a life situation (e.g., limited sports participation, interference with social interaction)
Part II: Contextual Factors	
1. Environmental Factors (facilitators or barriers)	Make up the physical, social, and attitudinal environment in which people live and conduct their lives; factors are external to the affected individuals, and facilitate or restrict full participation in society
	Facilitator: examples include ramp for wheelchair access and assisted-living units
	Barriers: examples include exclusion from employment, limited access to medical equipment/health insurance, and limited wheelchair access to public facilities
2. Personal Factors	Background of an individual's life and living and comprise features of the individual that are not part of a health condition (e.g., sex, race, age, and other health conditions)

the onset of static contractures and bony deformities.[24,25] The musculoskeletal changes, collectively referred to as "lever arm disease" are best addressed with orthopedic surgery.[9]

The remainder of this chapter reviews the evidence for the effectiveness of these strategies in the management of ambulant children with CP.

EVIDENCE FOR EFFECTIVENESS OF SPASTICITY REDUCTION METHODS

Botulinum Toxin A

A systematic review published in the Cochrane database in 2000 could not find sufficient evidence to support or refute the use of BTX-A in the treatment of lower-limb spasticity in children with CP.[26] Systematic reviews of more recent randomized trials (Level 1 evidence) confirm that injection of BTX-A compared with placebo[27–30] does reduce calf (equinus) spasticity, increase ankle dorsiflexion, and improve gait pattern in the short term.[31,32] When compared with serial casting, two small randomized clinical trials (RCTs) with only 10 patients in each arm (Level II evidence) showed that BTX-A injections were as efficacious as serial casting in the management of dynamic equinus.[33,34] The BTX-A group had a more sustained response than casting, although median time to reintervention was similar in both groups.[33] This evidence was contradicted by a subsequent small RCT of 23 patients randomized to receive either serial casting alone or serial casting with BTX-A, which showed equivalent reduction in spasticity and increased dorsiflexion at 3 months in both groups, but more sustained benefits in the cast alone group at 12 months.[35] However, in an-

other small double-blind RCT, 39 patients were randomized to receive BTX-A alone, placebo injection plus casting, or BTX-A plus casting. The BTX-A injection group did not show any significant change, whereas the two groups that were casted with placebo injection or BTX-A showed significant but equivalent improvements in spasticity reduction, passive range of motion, and ankle kinematics at 12 months.[36]

In summary, BTX-A injections are superior to placebo injections in reducing calf muscle spasticity and increasing ankle dorsiflexion in the short term, but show only equivalent efficacy in the short term when compared with serial casting, with mixed evidence regarding the combination of serial casting plus BTX-A. Limited evidence exists in the literature to support the widely held belief that the reduction in spasticity brought on by BTX-A potentiates the effect of therapy interventions to reduce the mechanical aspects of the hypertonicity,[24] and even less evidence that these effects translate into measurable functional benefits in terms of activities and participation.

In a systematic review to evaluate the evidence for the effectiveness of therapy (including serial casting) after BTX-A injections, Lannin and colleagues[37] found only two studies with control groups that compared BTX-A alone with botulinum toxin plus some form of therapy. In a small prospective series of 25 children (Level IV evidence), Boyd and coworkers[38] found that a short period of casting improves passive range of motion and ankle kinetics, whereas Desloovere and coauthors[39] found that it makes no difference if such casting is provided immediately before or after BTX-A injections in a small randomized trial of 34 children (Level II evidence). In a multicenter clinical trial in the Netherlands, 46 children were randomized to receive multilevel BTX-A followed by comprehensive rehabilitation or just usual physiotherapy (PT). The BTX-A plus comprehensive rehabilitation group experienced significantly greater improvements in the gross motor function measure (GMFM) outcome measure at 24 weeks (3.5 points better than usual physical therapy group). This effect, although clinically significant, is modest at best, and this study cannot separate the relative contributions of BTX-A from those of the cointervention of comprehensive rehabilitation to the improved outcome.[40]

Although a retrospective cohort study of 424 patients (Level III evidence) concluded that a program of serial multilevel Botox injections might delay the need for, and reduce the frequency of, orthopedic surgery,[41] this evidence is undermined by the unknown comparability of the treatment cohorts at baseline, the different periods that the cohorts were treated, and the possibility of bias by indication. Furthermore, the long-term effects or benefits of BTX-A in terms of improved muscle growth, mobility, and function remain unknown.[42]

Selective Dorsal Rhizotomy

Three published randomized trials have evaluated the efficacy of selective dorsal rhizotomy followed by physiotherapy (SDR + PT) compared with PT alone.[43–45] All 3 trials showed that SDR + PT consistently reduced spasticity, but only in the Toronto ($n = 24$) and Vancouver ($n = 30$) trials was there a significantly greater improvement in function as measured by the GMFM in the SDR + PT groups at 1 year. In the Seattle trial ($n = 38$), there was no demonstrable difference in functional outcomes (GMFM) between the 2 groups either at 12 or 24 months, with both groups demonstrating equivalent functional gains. A possible explanation may be that patients in the PT group in the Seattle trial received an intensive and prolonged course of PT, far more than their counterparts in the other two trials, and the rhizotomies performed in Seattle involved transaction of significantly fewer rootlets than at the other 2 locations, which could also explain the smaller gains demonstrated by the SDR + PT groups in the Seattle trial. A meta-analysis of these 3 randomized trials (Level 1 evidence) confirmed that for children between 4 and 8 years of age with spastic CP, SDR + PT does produce a clinically significant reduction in spasticity at 12 months and a statistically significant but relatively small functional advantage of 4 percentage points on the GMFM when compared with PT alone.[46] In the multivariate analysis, a positive association was found between the percentage of rootlets transected and the magnitude of functional improvement. Despite the effectiveness of SDR in the short term, the question remains whether these small benefits are worth the time, effort, and expense involved. Only limited evidence (Levels III and IV) exists that SDR reduces the

need for or amount of subsequent orthopedic surgery,[47–49] and the long-term effects and benefits of SDR have yet to be elucidated.

EVIDENCE FOR MULTILEVEL ORTHOPEDIC SURGERY

Established musculoskeletal problems are thought to be best addressed with simultaneous (single-event) multilevel orthopedic surgery (SEMLS) including tendon lengthening or transfers and corrective osteotomies based on small uncontrolled case series[50,51] and expert opinion (Level IV and V evidence). Addressing all deformities simultaneously avoids the "birthday syndrome" of staged isolated procedures[16] and limits the interventions to one hospitalization and one period of rehabilitation (Level V evidence). However, to date, no comparative studies have tested the superiority of this approach, leaving room for some debate. Some surgeons recommend (Level V evidence) early surgical interventions during childhood development with the expectation that this will enhance function and allow further improvement of motor skills, with further surgery as needed when the child is older.[52] This approach also uses multilevel procedures as needed and has been referred to as Staged Multilevel Interventions in the Lower Extremity (SMILE). There is some weak Level IV evidence from small case series that children with spastic diplegia who underwent staged orthopedic procedures had unpredictable results.[53] In contrast, there is little evidence that the single-event multilevel surgery performed at the optimal (older) age eliminates the need for additional surgery in the future.

Outcomes of Multilevel Orthopedic Surgery Compared with Natural History

Only 1 retrospective cohort study (Level III evidence) compares the short-term outcomes in a small group of ambulatory children with spastic diplegia treated with multilevel surgery ($n = 12$) with those of a control group of comparable children ($n = 12$) who were recommended but did not undergo similar types of multilevel surgery.[12] Effects of treatment were derived from change in gait analyses between the baseline assessment and 12 months later. Gait of children in the control group deteriorated between analyses, whereas for the treatment group, parents' perceived walking distance and reliance on assist devices improved. Whether these benefits were a consequence of the multilevel surgery or the intensive postoperative PT (or both) that the operated patients received is unknowable from this study, and whether these benefits will last over the long term remains a concern in light of some Level IV evidence from longitudinal case series that mobility will deteriorate in growing children even after surgery.[11] Few published studies evaluate the long-term effects of multilevel orthopedic surgery at skeletal maturity, let alone into adulthood.[18]

Outcomes of Multilevel Orthopedic Surgery Compared with Other Interventions

In a prospective cohort study of ambulant children with spastic diplegia who underwent either SDR or multilevel orthopedic surgery as their initial surgical procedure, children who underwent SDR ($n = 16$) demonstrated improvements in 3 of 5 dimensions, as well as the total score of the GMFM, but more than 60% of these patients experienced a reduction in gait velocity. Those who underwent orthopedic surgery ($n = 14$) had more predictable improvements in spatiotemporal gait parameters, although their improvements in the GMFM was limited to only 1 dimension (walking, running, and jumping) and the total score.[54] This study comprised 2 separate treatment cohorts studied prospectively that had the same preoperative and postoperative measures, allowing for the comparison at about 12 months after surgery, rather than a randomized (or nonrandomized trial) of similar patients (Level II evidence). In another prospective cohort study of children with spastic diplegia with a mean age of 73 months, 18 children who underwent SDR were compared with 7 who underwent orthopedic surgery (Level II evidence). Significant improvements were seen in passive range of motion, muscle tone, gait kinematics, and oxygen cost in both groups 2 years after surgery.[48] In both of these studies, the unknown comparability of the groups at baseline and the different indications for choosing SDR or orthopedic surgery bias any inferences. Furthermore, the 2 interventions should be seen as complementary because they address different facets of the problem (spasticity in the case of SDR and fixed contractures, and/or bony deformities in the case of multilevel orthopedic surgery), rather than as competing alternatives to manage the ambulant child with spastic CP.

Evidence for Specific Orthopedic Procedures and Techniques

The most common soft-tissue procedures include intramuscular lengthening of the psoas over the pelvic brim,[55–57] fractional lengthening of the medial hamstrings,[50,55,58–61] transfer of the rectus femoris for a stiff knee gait,[62–66] and recession of the gastrocnemius.[67,68] Open lengthening of the hip adductors, iliopsoas tenotomy, lengthening of the lateral hamstrings,[61] and tendo-Achilles lengthening[69] are rarely required and may lead to overcorrection and weakness, especially in bilateral involvement.[70] Significant equinovalgus/planovalgus deformities of the feet can be corrected with calcaneal lengthening,[71] sometimes combined with subtalar arthrodesis to prevent recurrence. Equinovarus deformities can be managed with split tibialis posterior tendon transfers for flexible deformities[72] and split tibialis anterior tendon transfer combined with intramuscular lengthening of the tibialis posterior and tendo-Achilles for stiffer deformities in older children.[73,74] Severe torsional deformities can be addressed with derotational osteotomies of the femur either distally or proximally,[75–77] and supramalleolar derotational osteotomies of the tibia and fibula.[78]

The quality of evidence in support of these specific interventions to improve gait in ambulatory children with CP is weak and based almost entirely on uncontrolled case series (Level IV evidence). This is equally true of studies evaluating the efficacy of multilevel orthopedic surgery as a whole. These studies are typically small, retrospective, uncontrolled case series looking at preintervention and postintervention comparisons that demonstrate some improvements in the short term in outcomes limited to the level of body structures and body functions, such as range of motion, spatiotemporal gait parameters, and kinematic or kinetic improvements on gait analysis.[18,59,79–81] The clinical significance of these findings is less clear, with only a few case series (Level IV evidence) reporting benefits in some functional outcomes at the level of activities and participation.[80–84]

A few retrospective, case–control or cohort studies (Level III evidence) compare different surgical techniques, but few prospective clinical trials compare the effectiveness of these procedures. In a case–control study, rectus femoris transfer ($n = 98$) has been reported to be superior to distal rectus release ($n = 31$), especially for children with less than 80% knee range of motion.[63] One case–control study showed little difference in functional outcomes or complication rates between proximal ($n = 27$) and distal femoral ($n = 51$) derotational osteotomies.[77] In a prospective cohort study of 28 patients with spastic diplegia and intoed gait, there was no difference in the gait outcomes between the proximal and distal femoral derotational osteotomies, but the distal osteotomies were reportedly faster with significantly lower blood loss (Level II evidence).[76]

In a systematic review of different interventions to improve gait, these interventions did have a statistically significant effect on the spatiotemporal parameters of gait.[85] This was true for specific orthopedic procedures as well, when the analysis was stratified based on the type of intervention. However, the authors were unable to make any clinical recommendations about relative efficacy of different interventions. The majority of the individual studies included were Level III or IV studies with sample sizes smaller than necessary to detect the effect sizes they found from the meta-analysis. Nearly every study failed to categorize patients by (and therefore adjust for) severity, age, or type of CP, and did not take into account the effect of cointerventions that are inevitable in multilevel surgery and are likely to have an impact on the outcomes.

EVIDENCE FOR USE OF GAIT ANALYSIS FOR SURGICAL DECISION MAKING BEFORE MULTILEVEL ORTHOPEDIC SURGERY

Little consensus exists about the indications or choice of which procedures to perform during multilevel surgery.[86,87] For ambulatory patients, gait analysis has been recommended to guide surgical decision making, but it remains an area of much controversy among pediatric orthopedic surgeons.[88–90] The basic premise of gait analysis is that gait data generated in a motion laboratory provide insight beyond what is derivable from observational analysis alone, and that it has the potential to influence or alter treatment decisions for at least some patients whose outcomes presumably would have been worse had they had surgery based on decisions made by observational analysis alone.

Does Gait Analysis Alter Decision Making?

Level IV evidence has been reported that gait analysis alters surgical decision making for patients with CP. In 3 separate case series, treatment recommendations based on observation of gait changed with the addition of gait analysis data in 52%, 93%, and 40% of the cases.[91–93] However, in all 3 studies, the investigators were not blinded to their decisions based on observation alone. We also do not know whether these decisions would have been consistent if retested at a later time (reproducibility). In the Hartford study, all patients reportedly underwent treatment based on the gait analysis recommendations; therefore, in the absence of control subjects, we do not know whether implementing these recommendations did, indeed, result in different, let alone better, outcomes.[91] The authors conclude that because in their series gait analysis data led to an overall reduction in the number of procedures recommended, this would be associated with a reduction in cost of surgery. However, we do not know whether the treatment decisions based on gait analysis were the ones that were, in fact, carried out. Furthermore, conclusions regarding potential cost reductions are somewhat speculative because a valid health economic evaluation was not performed. The 2 other studies also demonstrated that decisions were altered by the addition of gait analysis data, but once again with little evidence that these altered decisions were either reproducible or better than the original decisions made by observation alone.[92,93]

Does the Use of Gait Analysis for Surgical Decision Making Result in Better Functional Outcomes after Multilevel Orthopedic Surgery?

A systematic review of the literature on the use of gait analysis in children with walking disorders reported that there was little published evidence that outcomes of surgery based on gait analysis are any better than outcomes of surgery based on observational analysis alone.[94] One case–control study (Level III evidence) attempts to answer this question. Lee and colleagues[95] retrospectively selected 23 patients with ambulatory CP who had complete preoperative and postoperative gait analysis available out of 100 patients who had been evaluated in their gait laboratory

over a 5-year period.[95] Eight of these 23 children underwent surgery based on the visual analysis alone rather than the recommendations based on gait analysis. The authors provide no information as to why these 8 patients underwent operations different from what was recommended or whether their surgeons had had access to the gait studies. The outcomes of these 8 children were compared with those of the 15 children who were treated according to the recommendations based on preoperative gait analysis. Of the 7 children who reportedly did not improve based on the postoperative gait analysis data as the outcome measure, 5 of these 7 children belonged to the control group that received treatment based on clinical (visual) analysis alone. Thirteen of 15 children showed improved gait outcomes in the gait analysis group compared with only 3 of 8 in the control group. The authors conclude that gait analysis was responsible for the difference in outcomes between the 2 groups. However, the small numbers of patients, the absence of information on the comparability of the 2 groups at baseline, the short follow-up, and the absence of any functional outcomes undermine any conclusions regarding the necessity for, or the benefits of, preoperative gait analysis.

Other retrospective case series (Level IV studies) of children with ambulatory CP undergoing multilevel orthopedic surgery, in which patients underwent preoperative and postoperative gait analyses, have documented postoperative improvement in outcomes.[59,82,96] However, in the absence of any control subjects, it is not possible to conclude with any confidence that these improvements are attributable to the use of gait analysis either.

Molenaers and coauthors[41] suggest that gait analysis delays the first orthopedic procedures in children with CP based on a retrospective review of 424 children with ambulatory CP treated at one center from 1985 to 2001. Three historical cohorts were compared (Level III evidence): group 1 (1985–1989), group 2 (1996–1997), and group 3 (2000–2001). These groups were separated by the introduction of gait analysis in 1990 and the addition of BTX-A in the early treatment of these children in 1996. Children in group 1 who did not have the benefit of gait analysis or botulinum toxin underwent surgery significantly earlier than those in group 2 who had the benefit of gait analysis. There was also a significant decrease in the frequency of surgery for groups 3 and 2 compared with group 1. The authors acknowledge the limitations of such a study and are careful to qualify their conclusions. The association between the introduction of gait analysis and the delay of surgery could be attributable to change in philosophy with the times rather than the introduction of gait analysis. Furthermore, delay of surgery is at best a proxy for, and not necessarily representative of, improved outcomes.

Chang and researchers[97] evaluated retrospectively 20 children with ambulatory CP who were recommended orthopedic surgery treatment after undergoing gait analysis. For reasons not explained,

10 children did not follow through with these recommendations and underwent unspecified alternative nonoperative treatments, whereas the other 10 completed the surgical procedures recommended. The surgical group experienced "a higher percentage" of positive (44%) gait outcomes compared with the group who did not follow the gait analysis-based surgical recommendations (26%). The authors conclude that "gait performance can be significantly improved when gait analysis is used to determine the appropriate surgical intervention."[97] However, little information is available about the comparability of the 2 groups at baseline other than the similarity of the surgical recommendations based on gait analysis. The "outcomes" are based on desired or expected changes in the gait kinematics. This definition is unsatisfactory because all changes are arbitrarily treated as equal. We also have no knowledge of how these changes relate to the outcome of real interest, which is physical function. The only conclusion is that, in this series, patients treated with surgery responded better based on the authors' definition of gait outcomes than patients treated by nonoperative methods (Level III). The actual contribution of gait analysis to these outcomes is speculative. For gait analysis to be effective in this role, it needs to be shown to alter decision making in a reproducible or consistent way.[90]

Effect of Variability in Gait Analysis

Many sources of variability stem from gait analysis, including patients themselves,[98,99] and between gait laboratories[100] because of variation in equipment, marker placement, and lack of standardization. After implementation of a standardized protocol in gait laboratories in the Shriner's system in North America, there was only a moderate decrease in the variability across the 12 sites, which the authors conclude must be improved on before the data between laboratories can be considered comparable.[101] These technical problems are likely to be solved with technical solutions, which will not, however, address the issue of variability of interpretation and treatment recommendations.[90]

Reproducibility of Gait Analysis Interpretation and Surgical Recommendations

When the same gait analysis data were examined by gait analysis experts from 6 different institutions in the United States, there was only slight-to-moderate agreement in the list of problems (Kappa values: 0.14–0.46) generated by the experts.[102] Agreement about specific surgical recommendations was similarly poor, except for hamstring lengthening (Kappa value: 0.64). The authors conclude that, although gait analysis data are themselves objective, there is subjectivity in interpretation even among recognized experts, with diagnoses and treatment recommendations seemingly influenced

by the institution at which the interpretation was performed.[102] However, the authors did not report the inter-rater reliability at the institutional level, which would have provided some support to the latter conclusion.

Variability was present in the kinematic data generated in 4 different motion laboratories that tested the same 11 patients.[100] Although the clinical significance of some of this variability has been challenged, the treatment recommendations generated from these data were widely different across the 4 centers for 9 of the 11 patients. Perhaps such variability might not have been demonstrated had the patients been tested in other gait centers, as was implied in the accompanying editorial,[103] but evidence to support this contention remains elusive.

In the presence of significant variability, the data cannot be used with confidence to influence decision making. Variability in the interpretation of gait data reflects the prevailing uncertainty (or controversies) about the causes and/or significance of specific findings, and will be resolved only with ongoing clinical research and experience using gait analysis.[104] Similarly, variability in treatment recommendations based on the same gait data also reflects differences of opinion about best strategies to deal with specific problems, which, in turn, can be definitively resolved only with comparative clinical trials. Neither the variability in interpretation nor the variability in surgical recommendations is the fault of gait analysis per se, but as long as such significant variability exists, the recommendation that gait analysis is essential for preoperative decision making before multilevel orthopedic surgery is currently not supported by the literature.[90] Consequently, there is wide variation across North America in the rates of utilization of gait analysis for surgical decision making in the management of children with ambulatory CP.[105] It is not clear whether there is corresponding variation in functional outcomes of children receiving multilevel orthopedic surgery in different centers in North America, and if so, whether these differences are attributable to the use of gait analysis or other factors, such as surgical skill and experience, or the quality of the postoperative rehabilitation.

CONCLUSION

A paucity of high-level evidence exists of the efficacy of orthopedic procedures used for children with CP. Moreover, the methodologic rigor of these studies even within their level of study design is low. A lack of consensus has been shown on the indications for these specific procedures. Although there is some evidence (mostly Level IV) that multilevel orthopedic surgery may benefit the gait of ambulatory children with CP in the short term, especially when compared with the natural history (Level III evidence), there is less evidence that these short-term benefits translate into any meaningful improvements in the dimensions of activities and participation, or that these benefits

TABLE 34–2. Summary of Recommendations

STATEMENT	LEVEL OF EVIDENCE/GRADE OF RECOMMENDATION	REFERENCES
1. BTX-A is superior to placebo in reducing calf spasticity and improving ankle dorsiflexion in the short term.	A	27–32
2. BTX-A is equivalent to serial casting in reducing calf spasticity and improving ankle dorsiflexion in the short term.	A, B	32–34
3. Botox injection plus serial casting increases passive range of motion more than serial casting alone.	I	35, 36, 38
4. Serial multilevel BTX-A delays the need for and reduces the frequency or orthopedic surgery.	B	41
5. SDR plus PT is more effective than PT alone in reducing lower extremity spasticity in children with spastic diplegia between 4 and 8 years of age.	A	46 43–45
6. SDR plus PT has a significant but small functional benefit over PT alone in children with spastic diplegia between 4 and 8 years of age.	A	46 43–45
7. SEMLS preserves (or improves) gait outcomes when compared with natural history and SDR.	B	12
8. SEMLS is superior to staged orthopedic procedures.	I	
9. Orthopedic surgery in children with ambulatory CP results in short-term functional gains in the domains of activities and participation.	C	80, 82–84
10. Orthopedic procedures result in benefits at the body structure and body function domains in the short term.	C	18, 59, 79–81
11. Gait analysis alters decision making.	C	91–93
12. Gait analysis for surgical decision improves functional outcomes after multilevel orthopedic surgery.	I	94, 95, 97

BTX-A, botulinum toxin type A; CP, cerebral palsy; PT, physiotherapy; SDR, selective dorsal rhizotomy; SEMLS, single-event multilevel orthopedic surgery.

are long lasting, let alone permanent. A growing recognition exists for the need to improve and expand the evidence base for the orthopedic management of children with chronic developmental disabilities.[104,106] Further studies are needed to define the long-term outcomes in these children to improve our understanding of the indications for and the effects of multilevel surgery for this population.[12] Although RCTs are desirable, these are not immediately forthcoming because of the high cost, multiplicity of interventions, need for long-term outcomes, and problems of recruitment and retention associated with the large numbers of patients from multiple centers needed to participate, which make such trials difficult to conduct.[106] Alternatives to RCTs are beginning to emerge including pragmatic or practical clinical trials[107] and Clinical Practice Improvement, which uses a large-scale, prospective, observational design incorporating comprehensive review of key patient characteristics, all treatment and care processes and outcomes,[108] and multivariate analyses to account for heterogeneity of patient populations. Even the quality of lower-level study designs can be greatly improved by following established guidelines.[109] Table 34–2 provides a summary of recommendations.

REFERENCES

1. Stanley F, Alberman ED, Blair E: Cerebral Palsies: Epidemiology and Causal Pathways. London: Mac Keith, 2000.
2. Bax M, Goldstein M, Rosenbaum P, et al: Proposed definition and classification of cerebral palsy, April 2005. Dev Med Child Neurol 47:571–576, 2005.
3. Rosenbaum P, Paneth N, Leviton A, et al: A report: The definition and classification of cerebral palsy April 2006. Dev Med Child Neurol Suppl 109:8–14, 2007.
4. Palisano R, Rosenbaum P, Walter S, et al: Development and reliability of a system to classify gross motor function in children with cerebral palsy. Dev Med Child Neurol 39:214–223, 1997.
5. Wood E, Rosenbaum P: The gross motor function classification system for cerebral palsy: A study of reliability and stability over time. Dev Med Child Neurol 42:292–296, 2000.
6. Rosenbaum PL, Walter SD, Hanna SE, et al: Prognosis for gross motor function in cerebral palsy: Creation of motor development curves. Jama 288:1357–1363, 2002.
7. Gage JR; Spastics Society: The neurological control system for normal gait. In Gage JR (ed): Gait Analysis in Cerebral Palsy. London, MacKeith Press, 1991, pp 37–60.
8. Ziv I, Blackburn N, Rang M, Koreska J: Muscle growth in normal and spastic mice. Dev Med Child Neurol 26:94–99, 1984.
9. Gage JR, Schwartz M: Pathologic gait and lever arm dysfunction. In Gage JR (ed): The Treatment of Gait Problems in Cerebral Palsy. London, Mac Keith, distributed by Cambridge University Press, 2004, pp 180–204.
10. Bell KJ, Ounpuu S, DeLuca PA, Romness MJ: Natural progression of gait in children with cerebral palsy. J Pediatr Orthop 22:677–682, 2002.
11. Johnson DC, Damiano DL, Abel MF: The evolution of gait in childhood and adolescent cerebral palsy. J Pediatr Orthop 17:392–396, 1997.
12. Gough M, Eve LC, Robinson RO, Shortland AP: Short-term outcome of multilevel surgical intervention in spastic diplegic cerebral palsy compared with the natural history. Dev Med Child Neurol 46:91–97, 2004.
13. Murphy KP, Molnar GE, Lankasky K: Medical and functional status of adults with cerebral palsy. Dev Med Child Neurol 37:1075–1084, 1995.
14. Andersson C, Mattsson E: Adults with cerebral palsy: A survey describing problems, needs, and resources, with special emphasis on locomotion. Dev Med Child Neurol 43:76–82, 2001.
15. Bottos M, Feliciangeli A, Sciuto L, et al: Functional status of adults with cerebral palsy and implications for treatment of children. Dev Med Child Neurol 43:516–528, 2001.

16. Rang M: Cerebral palsy. In Lovell WW, Morrissy RT, Winter RB (eds): Lovell and Winter's Pediatric Orthopaedics, 3rd ed. Philadelphia, Lippincott, 1990, pp 465–506.
17. Goldberg MJ: Measuring outcomes in cerebral palsy. J Pediatr Orthop 11:682–685, 1991.
18. Saraph V, Zwick EB, Auner C, et al: Gait improvement surgery in diplegic children: How long do the improvements last? J Pediatr Orthop 25:263–267, 2005.
19. Butler C, Chambers H, Goldstein M, et al: Evaluating research in developmental disabilities: A conceptual framework for reviewing treatment outcomes. Dev Med Child Neurol 41:55–59, 1999.
20. O'Donnell M, Darrah J, Adams R, et al: AACPDM methodology to develop systematic reviews of treatment interventions. 2004. Available from http://www.aacpdm.org/resources/systematicReviewsMethodology.pdf
21. World Health Organization: International Classification of Functioning, Disability and Health. Geneva, WHO, 2001. Available from http://www.who.int/classifications/icf/en/
22. Butler C, Chambers H, Goldstein M, et al: Evaluating research in developmental disabilities: A conceptual framework for reviewing treatment outcomes. AACPDM Treatment Outcomes Committee Report 1998–1999. Available from http://www.aacpdm.org/index?service=page/treatmentOutcomesReport
23. Abel MF, Damiano DL, Blanco JS, et al: Relationships among musculoskeletal impairments and functional health status in ambulatory cerebral palsy. J Pediatr Orthop 23:535–541, 2003.
24. Dumas HM, O'Neil ME, Fragala MA: Expert Consensus on Physical Therapist Intervention after Botulinum Toxin A Injection for Children with Cerebral Palsy. Pediatr Phys Ther 13:122–132, 2001.
25. Graham HK, Aoki KR, Autti-Ramo I, et al: Recommendations for the use of botulinum toxin type A in the management of cerebral palsy. Gait Posture 11:67–79, 2000.
26. Ade-Hall RA, Moore AP: Botulinum toxin type A in the treatment of lower limb spasticity in cerebral palsy. Cochrane Database Syst Rev (2):CD001408, 2000.
27. Bjornson K, Hays R, Graubert C, et al: Botulinum toxin for spasticity in children with cerebral palsy: A comprehensive evaluation. Pediatrics 120:49–58, 2007.
28. Ubhi T, Bhakta BB, Ives HL, et al: Randomised double blind placebo controlled trial of the effect of botulinum toxin on walking in cerebral palsy. Arch Dis Child 83:481–487, 2000.
29. Koman LA, Mooney JFr, Smith BP, et al: Botulinum toxin type A neuromuscular blockade in the treatment of lower extremity spasticity in cerebral palsy: A randomized, double-blind, placebo-controlled trial. BOTOX Study Group. J Pediatr Orthop 20:108–115, 2000.
30. Sutherland DH, Kaufman KR, Wyatt MP, et al: Double-blind study of botulinum A toxin injections into the gastrocnemius muscle in patients with cerebral palsy. Gait Posture 10:1–9, 1999.
31. Cardoso ES, Rodrigues BM, Barroso M, et al: Botulinum toxin type A for the treatment of the spastic equinus foot in cerebral palsy. Pediatr Neurol 34:106–109, 2006.
32. Boyd RN, Hays RM: Current evidence for the use of botulinum toxin type A in the management of children with cerebral palsy: A systematic review. Eur J Neurol 8(suppl 5):1–20, 2001.
33. Corry IS, Cosgrove AP, Duffy CM, et al: Botulinum toxin A compared with stretching casts in the treatment of spastic equinus: A randomised prospective trial. J Pediatr Orthop 18:304–311, 1998.
34. Flett PJ, Stern LM, Waddy H, et al: Botulinum toxin A versus fixed cast stretching for dynamic calf tightness in cerebral palsy. J Paediatr Child Health 35:71–77, 1999.
35. Kay RM, Rethlefsen SA, Fern-Buneo A, et al: Botulinum toxin as an adjunct to serial casting treatment in children with cerebral palsy. J Bone Joint Surg Am 86:2377–2384, 2004.
36. Ackman JD, Russman BS, Thomas SS, et al: Comparing botulinum toxin A with casting for treatment of dynamic equinus in children with cerebral palsy. Dev Med Child Neurol 47:620–627, 2005.
37. Lannin N, Scheinberg A, Clark K: AACPDM systematic review of the effectiveness of therapy for children with cerebral palsy after botulinum toxin A injections. Dev Med Child Neurol 48:533–539, 2006.
38. Boyd RN, Pliatsios V, Starr R, et al: Biomechanical transformation of the gastroc-soleus muscle with botulinum toxin A in children with cerebral palsy. Dev Med Child Neurol 42:32–41, 2000.
39. Desloovere K, Molenaers G, Jonkers I, et al: A randomized study of combined botulinum toxin type A and casting in the ambulant child with cerebral palsy using objective outcome measures. Eur J Neurol 8(suppl 5):75–87, 2001.
40. Scholtes VA, Dallmeijer AJ, Knol DL, et al: The combined effect of lower-limb multilevel botulinum toxin type A and comprehensive rehabilitation on mobility in children with cerebral palsy: A randomized clinical trial. Arch Phys Med Rehabil 87:1551–1558, 2006.
41. Molenaers G, Desloovere K, Fabry G, De Cock P: The effects of quantitative gait assessment and botulinum toxin A on musculoskeletal surgery in children with cerebral palsy. J Bone Joint Surg Am 88:161–170, 2006.
42. Gough M, Fairhurst C, Shortland AP: Botulinum toxin and cerebral palsy: Time for reflection? Dev Med Child Neurol 47:709–712, 2005.
43. Steinbok P, Reiner AM, Beauchamp R, et al: A randomized clinical trial to compare selective posterior rhizotomy plus physiotherapy with physiotherapy alone in children with spastic diplegic cerebral palsy. Dev Med Child Neurol 39:178–184, 1997.
44. McLaughlin JF, Bjornson KF, Astley SJ, et al: Selective dorsal rhizotomy: Efficacy and safety in an investigator-masked randomized clinical trial. Dev Med Child Neurol 40:220–232, 1998.
45. Wright FV, Sheil EM, Drake JM, et al: Evaluation of selective dorsal rhizotomy for the reduction of spasticity in cerebral palsy: A randomized controlled trial. Dev Med Child Neurol 40:239–247, 1998.
46. McLaughlin J, Bjornson K, Temkin N, et al: Selective dorsal rhizotomy: Meta-analysis of three randomized controlled trials. Dev Med Child Neurol 44:17–25, 2002.
47. Hagglund G, Andersson S, Duppe H, et al: Prevention of severe contractures might replace multilevel surgery in cerebral palsy: Results of a population-based health care programme and new techniques to reduce spasticity. J Pediatr Orthop B 14:269–273, 2005.
48. Thomas SS, Buckon CE, Piatt JH, et al: A 2-year follow-up of outcomes following orthopedic surgery or selective dorsal rhizotomy in children with spastic diplegia. J Pediatr Orthop B 13:358–366, 2004.
49. Steinbok P: Outcomes after selective dorsal rhizotomy for spastic cerebral palsy. Childs Nerv Syst 17:1–18, 2001.
50. Nene AV, Evans GA, Patrick JH: Simultaneous multiple operations for spastic diplegia. Outcome and functional assessment of walking in 18 patients. J Bone Joint Surg Br 75:488–494, 1993.
51. Norlin R, Tkaczuk H: One session surgery on the lower limb in children with cerebral palsy. A five year follow-up. Int Orthop 16:291–293, 1992.
52. Sussman MD, Aiona MD: Treatment of spastic diplegia in patients with cerebral palsy. J Pediatr Orthop B 13:S1–S12, 2004.
53. Fabry G, Liu XC, Molenaers G: Gait pattern in patients with spastic diplegic cerebral palsy who underwent staged operations. J Pediatr Orthop B 8:33–38, 1999.
54. Abel MF, Damiano DL, McLaughlin JF, et al: Comparison of functional outcomes from orthopedic and neurosurgical interventions in spastic diplegia. Neurosurg Focus 4:e2, 1998.
55. DeLuca PA, Ounpuu S, Davis RB, Walsh JH: Effect of hamstring and psoas lengthening on pelvic tilt in patients with spastic diplegic cerebral palsy. J Pediatr Orthop 18:712–718, 1998.
56. Sutherland DH, Zilberfarb JL, Kaufman KR, et al: Psoas release at the pelvic brim in ambulatory patients with cerebral palsy: Operative technique and functional outcome. J Pediatr Orthop 17:563–570, 1997.
57. Novacheck TF, Trost JP, Schwartz MH: Intramuscular psoas lengthening improves dynamic hip function in children with cerebral palsy. J Pediatr Orthop 22:158–164, 2002.
58. Hoffinger SA, Rab GT, Abou-Ghaida H: Hamstrings in cerebral palsy crouch gait. J Pediatr Orthop 13:722–726, 1993.
59. Saraph V, Zwick EB, Zwick G, et al: Multilevel surgery in spastic diplegia: Evaluation by physical examination and gait analysis in 25 children. J Pediatr Orthop 22:150–157, 2002.

60. Thometz J, Simon S, Rosenthal R: The effect on gait of lengthening of the medial hamstrings in cerebral palsy. J Bone Joint Surg Am 71:345–353, 1989.

61. Kay RM, Rethlefsen SA, Skaggs D, Leet A: Outcome of medial versus combined medial and lateral hamstring lengthening surgery in cerebral palsy. J Pediatr Orthop 22:169–172, 2002.

62. Gage JR, Perry J, Hicks RR, et al: Rectus femoris transfer to improve knee function of children with cerebral palsy. Dev Med Child Neurol 29:159–166, 1987.

63. Ounpuu S, Muik E, Davis RB 3rd, et al: Rectus femoris surgery in children with cerebral palsy. Part II: A comparison between the effect of transfer and release of the distal rectus femoris on knee motion. J Pediatr Orthop 13:331–335, 1993.

64. Chambers H, Lauer A, Kaufman K, et al: Prediction of outcome after rectus femoris surgery in cerebral palsy: The role of cocontraction of the rectus femoris and vastus lateralis. J Pediatr Orthop 18:703–711, 1998.

65. Rethlefsen S, Tolo VT, Reynolds RA, Kay R: Outcome of hamstring lengthening and distal rectus femoris transfer surgery. J Pediatr Orthop B 8:75–79, 1999.

66. Saw A, Smith PA, Sirirungruangsarn Y, et al: Rectus femoris transfer for children with cerebral palsy: Long-term outcome. J Pediatr Orthop 23:672–678, 2003.

67. Rose SA, DeLuca PA, Davis RB 3rd, et al: Kinematic and kinetic evaluation of the ankle after lengthening of the gastrocnemius fascia in children with cerebral palsy. J Pediatr Orthop 13:727–732, 1993.

68. Steinwender G, Saraph V, Zwick EB, et al: Fixed and dynamic equinus in cerebral palsy: Evaluation of ankle function after multilevel surgery. J Pediatr Orthop 21:102–107, 2001.

69. Dietz FR, Albright JC, Dolan L: Medium-term follow-up of Achilles tendon lengthening in the treatment of ankle equinus in cerebral palsy. Iowa Orthop J 26:27–32, 2006.

70. Graham HK, Selber P: Musculoskeltal aspects of cerebral palsy. J Bone Joint Surg Br 85:157–166, 2003.

71. Mosca VS: Calcaneal lengthening for valgus deformity of the hindfoot. Results in children who had severe, symptomatic flatfoot and skewfoot. J Bone Joint Surg Am 77:500–512, 1995.

72. Green NE, Griffin PP, Shiavi R: Split posterior tibial-tendon transfer in spastic cerebral palsy. J Bone Joint Surg Am 65:748–754, 1983.

73. Hoffer MM, Barakat G, Koffman M: 10-year follow-up of split anterior tibial tendon transfer in cerebral palsied patients with spastic equinovarus deformity. J Pediatr Orthop 5:432–434, 1985.

74. Barnes MJ, Herring JA: Combined split anterior tibial-tendon transfer and intramuscular lengthening of the posterior tibial tendon. Results in patients who have a varus deformity of the foot due to spastic cerebral palsy. J Bone Joint Surg Am 73:734–738, 1991.

75. Ounpuu S, DeLuca P, Davis R, Romness M: Long-term effects of femoral derotation osteotomies: An evaluation using three-dimensional gait analysis. J Pediatr Orthop 22:139–145, 2002.

76. Pirpiris M, Trivett A, Baker R, et al: Femoral derotation osteotomy in spastic diplegia. Proximal or distal? J Bone Joint Surg Br 85:265–272, 2003.

77. Kay RM, Rethlefsen SA, Hale JM, et al: Comparison of proximal and distal rotational femoral osteotomy in children with cerebral palsy. J Pediatr Orthop 23:150–154, 2003.

78. Dodgin DA, De Swart RJ, Stefko RM, et al: Distal tibial/fibular derotation osteotomy for correction of tibial torsion: Review of technique and results in 63 cases. J Pediatr Orthop 18:95–101, 1998.

79. Gannotti ME, Gorton GE 3rd, Nahorniak MT, et al: Postoperative gait velocity and mean knee flexion in stance of ambulatory children with spastic diplegia four years or more after multilevel surgery. J Pediatr Orthop 27:451–456, 2007.

80. Rodda JM, Graham HK, Nattrass GR, et al: Correction of severe crouch gait in patients with spastic diplegia with use of multilevel orthopaedic surgery. J Bone Joint Surg Am 88:2653–2664, 2006.

81. Yngve DA, Scarborough N, Goode B, Haynes R: Rectus and hamstring surgery in cerebral palsy: A gait analysis study of results by functional ambulation level. J Pediatr Orthop 22:672–676, 2002.

82. Schwartz MH, Viehweger E, Stout J, et al: Comprehensive treatment of ambulatory children with cerebral palsy: An outcome assessment. J Pediatr Orthop 24:45–53, 2004.

83. Damiano DL, Gilgannon MD, Abel MF: Responsiveness and uniqueness of the pediatric outcomes data collection instrument compared to the gross motor function measure for measuring orthopaedic and neurosurgical outcomes in cerebral palsy. J Pediatr Orthop 25:641–645, 2005.

84. Abel MF, Damiano DL, Pannunzio M, Bush J: Muscle-tendon surgery in diplegic cerebral palsy: Functional and mechanical changes. J Pediatr Orthop 19:366–375, 1999.

85. Paul SM, Siegel KL, Malley J, Jaeger RJ: Evaluating interventions to improve gait in cerebral palsy: A meta-analysis of spatiotemporal measures. Dev Med Child Neurol 49:542–549, 2007.

86. Patrick JH, Roberts AP, Cole GF: Therapeutic choices in the locomotor management of the child with cerebral palsy—more luck than judgement? Arch Dis Child 85:275–279, 2001.

87. Sussman MD: Pediatric Orthopaedic Society of North America., Shriners Hospitals for Crippled Children. Surgical decision making—consensus statement. In Sussman MD (ed): The Diplegic Child: Evaluation and Management. Rosemont, IL, American Academy of Orthopaedic Surgeons, 1992, pp 203–206.

88. Gage JR: The role of gait analysis in the treatment of cerebral palsy. J Pediatr Orthop 14:701–702, 1994.

89. Watts HG: Gait laboratory analysis for preoperative decision making in spastic cerebral palsy: Is it all it's cracked up to be? J Pediatr Orthop 14:703–704, 1994.

90. Narayanan UG: The role of gait analysis in the orthopaedic management of ambulatory cerebral palsy. Curr Opin Pediatr 19:38–43, 2007.

91. DeLuca PA, Davis RB 3rd, Ounpuu S, et al: Alterations in surgical decision making in patients with cerebral palsy based on three-dimensional gait analysis. J Pediatr Orthop 17:608–614, 1997.

92. Kay RM, Dennis S, Rethlefsen S, et al: The effect of preoperative gait analysis on orthopaedic decision making. Clin Orthop Relat Res (372):217–222, 2000.

93. Cook RE, Schneider I, Hazlewood ME, et al: Gait analysis alters decision-making in cerebral palsy. J Pediatr Orthop 23:292–295, 2003.

94. Hailey D, Tomie JA: An assessment of gait analysis in the rehabilitation of children with walking difficulties. Disabil Rehabil 22:275–280, 2000.

95. Lee EH, Goh JC, Bose K: Value of gait analysis in the assessment of surgery in cerebral palsy. Arch Phys Med Rehabil 73:642–646, 1992.

96. Gage JR, Fabian D, Hicks R, Tashman S: Pre- and postoperative gait analysis in patients with spastic diplegia: A preliminary report. J Pediatr Orthop 4:715–725, 1984.

97. Chang FM, Seidl AJ, Muthusamy K, et al: Effectiveness of instrumented gait analysis in children with cerebral palsy—comparison of outcomes. J Pediatr Orthop 26:612–616, 2006.

98. Kirkpatrick M, Wytch R, Cole G, Helms P: Is the objective assessment of cerebral palsy gait reproducible? J Pediatr Orthop 14:705–708, 1994.

99. Steinwender G, Saraph V, Scheiber S, et al: Intrasubject repeatability of gait analysis data in normal and spastic children. Clin Biomech (Bristol, Avon) 15:134–139, 2000.

100. Noonan KJ, Halliday S, Browne R, et al: Interobserver variability of gait analysis in patients with cerebral palsy. J Pediatr Orthop 23:279–291, 2003.

101. Gorton G, Hebert D, Goode B: Assessment of the kinematic variability between 12 Shriner's motion analysis laboratories (SMALnet) following implementation of the minimum standardized gait analysis protocol (MSGAP) [abstract]. Gait Posture 13:247, 2001.

102. Skaggs DL, Rethlefsen SA, Kay RM, et al: Variability in gait analysis interpretation. J Pediatr Orthop 20:759–764, 2000.

103. Gage J. Con: Interobserver variability of gait analysis. Editorial. J Pediatr Orthop. 2003 May-Jun;23(3):290–1.

104. Davids JR, Ounpuu S, DeLuca PA, Davis RB 3rd: Optimization of walking ability of children with cerebral palsy. Instr Course Lect 53:511–522, 2004.

105. Narayanan UG, Weir S, Morris A, Redekop S: Rates of utilization of gait analysis for surgical decision making for ambulatory cerebral palsy in North America [abstract]. Dev Med Child Neurol 49(S111):11–16, 2007.
106. Graham HK: The trials of trials. Dev Med Child Neurol 49:163–163, 2007.
107. Tunis SR, Stryer DB, Clancy CM: Practical clinical trials: Increasing the value of clinical research for decision making in clinical and health policy. Jama 290:1624–1632, 2003.
108. Horn SD, DeJong G, Ryser DK, et al: Another look at observational studies in rehabilitation research: Going beyond the holy grail of the randomized controlled trial. Arch Phys Med Rehabil 86(12 suppl 2):S8–S15, 2005.
109. Slim K, Nini E, Forestier D, et al: Methodological index for non-randomized studies (minors): Development and validation of a new instrument. ANZ J Surg 73:712–716, 2003.

Chapter 35

What Is the Best Treatment for Developmental Dysplasia of the Hip?

Andreas Roposch, MD, MSc, FRCS

The majority of high-quality research into developmental dysplasia of the hip (DDH) has focused on the neonatal period and early infancy. It was the introduction of hip ultrasound in the early 1980s that led to a paradigm shift in the diagnosis and management of DDH in this age group. Ultrasound allowed visualization of hip morphology in newborns and added further information to the physical examination of the hip. The main question posed by the introduction of ultrasound was whether better outcomes can be achieved by utilizing ultrasound as opposed to relying on clinical tests alone. Many questions followed: If ultrasound is utilized, at what age should it be done? Should all infants receive the test or only those with remarkable findings on physical examination? Which abnormal sonographic findings warrant immediate treatment, which warrant repeat scanning, and which hips can be discharged from any further follow-up?

Although hip ultrasound has the potential to contribute valuable information in hips with unclear findings on physical examination, its accuracy has never been well established from basic principles and remains unclear.[1] As a result, not only physical examination but also ultrasound testing leaves much room for debate and uncertainty in the diagnosis and management of DDH.[2,3]

Uncertainty exists as to which forms of neonatal DDH warrant treatment and which will improve spontaneously; how long can we wait for a hip to improve on its own, and when is it justified to initiate costly treatment that includes serious risks, as well as burden to affected families. Randomized, controlled trials have been performed to answer some of these questions (Table 35–1). They were mainly driven by a desire to determine whether ultrasound can improve health outcomes in neonates with DDH. This chapter focuses on those areas of DDH studied by randomized, controlled trials.

DIAGNOSIS

The neonate with DDH may reveal remarkable findings on clinical examination. Although the majority of the hips with a positive Barlow or Ortolani test reveal some form of DDH (high sensitivity), these tests are not positive in all patients with DDH (imperfect specificity). Clearly, factors such as the age of the patient and the experience of the examiner influence test performance. Therefore, the accuracy of these tests cannot be quantified by one single number. Limited hip abduction is another potential but unreliable clinical sign for DDH. In a sample of Dutch infants aged 3 to 10 months, the finding of unilateral limitation of abduction had an overall sensitivity for the diagnosis of DDH of 69%, a specificity of 54%, a positive predictive value of 43%, and a negative predictive value of 78%; 46% of infants without DDH exhibited definite limited abduction.[4]

In addition to the clinical examination, ultrasound can be used to evaluate the neonatal hip. The result of the ultrasound test may be consistent with the clinical findings, or it may be inconsistent and provide additional information. For instance, an Ortolani-positive hip will show dislocation on ultrasound (findings are consistent). However, a clinically stable and unremarkable hip may reveal a shallow acetabulum and reduced femoral head coverage on ultrasound, which is an abnormal sonographic finding. The management of such hips remains highly controversial because the significance of some sonographic findings is unclear.

Abnormalities of the neonatal hip can be grouped into clinical abnormalities (instability of the hip, dislocatability of the hip, limited unilateral abduction of the hip) and by sonographic abnormalities (sonographic instability, reduced femoral head coverage, shallow acetabulum). No standardized diagnostic criteria have been established, however, with which these abnormalities can be distinguished from forms of DDH that will not resolve spontaneously.[3]

Because abnormalities of the hip present at birth are modulated by ongoing growth and because resolution of less severe abnormalities (Barlow-positive hips) was reported in up to 95% of patients,[5,6] a relevant question is up to which age treatment can be delayed without altering outcomes.

NEONATAL HIP INSTABILITY

Gardiner and Dunn[6] performed a randomized clinical trial to address this question.[6] Abduction splinting was delayed until the age of 10 to 14 days, or

TABLE 35-1. Research Questions of Randomized Clinical Trials on Developmental Dysplasia of the Hip in the Neonate

STUDY	LOE	RESEARCH QUESTION	ANSWER	CONCLUSIONS
Rosendahl et al. (1994)[5]	II	Does general (all newborns) or selective (with risk factors for DDH or hips showing positive findings on clinical examination) ultrasound screening provide more appropriate criteria for treatment of DDH, hence reducing the prevalence of late DDH compared with clinical screening alone?	No. The absolute number of late DDH was greatest in those not offered ultrasound and lowest in those who had general ultrasound screening, but these differences were not statistically significant.	General ultrasound screening increased the number of ultrasound follow-ups for hips that were clinically unremarkable. Of these, 97% showed spontaneous resolution, but because of clinicians' uncertainty, scanning was performed repeatedly until resolution was documented.
Gardiner and Dunn (1990)[6]	II	In neonates with clinical hip instability (positive Barlow test), does delaying abduction splinting for 2 weeks allow for spontaneous resolution of neonatal hip instability?	Yes. Sonographic and radiographic outcomes and clinical findings at 1 year were similar between those treated immediately and those who were observed for 2 weeks and splinted when necessary thereafter (29%).	Dislocatable hips at birth may be safely monitored sonographically for 2 weeks before determining the need for treatment without altering the outcome at 1 year.
Elbourne et al. (2002)[7]	II	In neonates with clinical hip instability, can an ultrasound examination (in addition to the clinical examination) reduce the likelihood of babies to be splinted without doubling of the risk for late treatment compared with clinical examination alone?	Yes. Ultrasound testing reduced rates of abduction splinting in newborns with neonatal hip instability significantly and is not associated with an increase in abnormal hip development by 2 years.	Ultrasound should be used in the management of those neonates with clinical hip instability.
Wood et al. (2000)[8]	II	Do 0- to 6-week-old newborns who present with clinically and sonographically stable hips but show sonographic dysplasia benefit from abduction splinting compared with no treatment?	No. Acetabular morphology improved regardless of abduction treatment and was not different between groups at 4 to 6 or 12 months, respectively.	Do not recommend splintage for stable but dysplastic hips within the first 6 weeks. Recommend follow-up at 3 months and beyond by both ultrasound and radiography to avoid treating nonsignificant acetabular dysplasia.
Holen et al. (2002)[10]	II	Is ultrasound screening of all neonates superior to ultrasound screening of those with risk factors (family history, instability of hip, foot deformities, breech position) for DDH?	No. The rates of late-presenting cases of DDH were similar in both groups.	Universal ultrasound screening is not superior over selected screening if clinical screening is of high quality.

DDH, developmental dysplasia of the hip; LOE, level of evidence.

commenced immediately in neonates (≤2 days old) with dislocatable hips (positive Barlow test). All infants in the "delay group" were monitored by means of ultrasound at the age of 2 weeks and were treated thereafter if hips had not improved. Treatment became necessary in 29% of all infants. The trial revealed similar outcomes for those who received immediate treatment at the age of 2 days or younger, and for those who received delayed treatment (if it was still indicated because the hip did not resolve spontaneously) at the age of 2 weeks.

Outcomes included sonographic and radiographic parameters at 6 and 12 months of age. The findings of this trial suggest that ultrasound can reduce the number of neonates with unstable hips treated with splinting by as much as 70%. The authors conclude that dislocatable hips at birth may be safely watched sonographically for 2 weeks before determining the need for treatment without altering the outcome.

Of interest, the authors distinguished between hips that were dislocatable (positive Barlow test) and those dislocated at birth (positive Ortolani test). The latter was not part of their trial because common practice is that such hips warrant immediate treatment.

Based on the findings of this trial,[6] the U.K. Collaborative Hip Trial group[7] wanted to establish whether it was safe not to splint hips that were clinically suspect but seemed normal on ultrasound surveillance. Their concern was that such a regimen might increase the numbers of children requiring late treatment for DDH. The primary outcome of the trial was radiographic hip appearance at the age of 2 years. Eligible were infants 0 to 6 weeks old who had been diagnosed with neonatal hip instability by a senior physician.

The experimental intervention was ultrasound of the hip at the age of 2 weeks or older; if ultrasound showed significant displacement or instability, splinting was initiated. The nonexperimental intervention was treatment based on clinical examination alone. In the latter group, it was at the treating clinicians' discretion to splint hips early (as soon as they were seen for assessment at 0–6 weeks of life), or to monitor hips clinically up to 8 weeks of age. If by the age of 8 weeks the hip was still of concern on clinical evaluation, splinting was initiated.

This randomized trial clearly showed that the use of ultrasound for the diagnosis and treatment of DDH significantly reduced the number of abduction splinting. Fewer children in the ultrasound group received treatment in the first 2 years of life. In contrast, splinting was done much earlier when the diagnosis was based on clinical examination alone—81% had splints fitted within the first 2 weeks. This trial also demonstrated that the total mean costs per used resources were similar in both groups.

How can these results be compared with those of Gardiner and Dunn's trial?[6] Gardiner and Dunn studied babies with dislocatable hips on clinical examination (positive Barlow test) and randomized them into early treatment or ultrasound and observation for 2 weeks. Also, the U.K. Collaborative Hip Trial group[7] included such patients—that is, infants who presented with the same remarkable findings on clinical examination warranting immediate treatment. If this particular stratum is considered for comparison, the relative risk (i.e., the risk of an outcome among patients receiving an intervention, in comparison with patients not receiving the intervention of interest) to receive any form of treatment during the trial period was 30% for the ultrasound group. That is, the rate of receiving any form of treatment in the ultrasound group was one third of that in the nonultrasound group. This effect was similar to Gardiner and Dunn's trial.[6]

SONOGRAPHIC DYSPLASIA IN CLINICALLY STABLE HIPS

Another controversial issue is the sonographically "shallow" acetabulum. This hip is unremarkable on clinical examination, stable on dynamic ultrasound, but reveals reduced femoral head coverage and/or a shallow acetabulum (alpha angle <50 degrees in neonates).

Wood and colleagues[8] investigated whether sonographically shallow hips that were stable on clinical

and ultrasound examination should be treated. Infants who had either remarkable hips on physical examination or who were considered at risk for DDH received ultrasound scanning at the age of 2 to 6 weeks. Approximately 13.6% were found to have stable (<2 mm displacement of the femoral head from the floor of the acetabulum) but sonographically dysplastic (<40% femoral head cover) hips. These infants were randomly allocated to either splinting or observation alone. All patients were managed 6 and 12 weeks later by ultrasound. Radiographic outcomes were determined at the age of 3 to 4 months, and in some at the age of 12 months. Neither sonographic nor radiographic outcome parameters were significantly different between groups. The sample size of this study was small with a statistical power of less than 80%.

Based on results of retrospective studies, Graf and coauthors[9] believe that treatment of sonographic dysplastic hips (Graf types IIc and D) must be initiated within the first 4 to 6 weeks of life; however, results from prospective studies suggest that such hips do well without treatment as long as they are stable.[5] Because the outcome of untreated Graf types IIc and D hips has never been established in well-designed comparative studies, the significance of such sonographic findings remains unclear, especially in the long term. Sonographic monitoring of such hips seems to be sensible.

SCREENING

There is agreement that the hips of all newborns should be screened for DDH by physical examination performed by a trained healthcare professional. Recognizing that a proportion of newborns with an unremarkable physical examination still might be affected by DDH, research has been performed to determine whether the addition of ultrasound as a screening tool can lead to better outcomes. Two large studies were performed about hip ultrasound screening.

Rosendahl and coworkers[5] managed 11,925 Norwegian newborns who underwent physical examination within the first 2 days of life. Newborns were assigned to one of three groups by convenience: general ultrasound screening, selective ultrasound screening of newborns found to be at high risk for DDH, and no ultrasound screening (allocation to the no-screening group if the sonographer was absent). The high-risk group included infants with hip dislocation, dislocatable hip, breech position, or family history of DDH (first- or second-degree relatives). Serial clinical examinations were performed in the first 2 years of life, supplemented by ultrasound tests for those in the ultrasound groups. All high-risk infants were referred for radiographs of the hips at 4 to 5 months of age. Ultrasound screening was performed within the first 2 days of delivery; modified Graf criteria (including hip morphology and hip stability) were applied.

Ortolani- or Barlow-positive hips were treated immediately with abduction splints, as were hips that were dislocated on ultrasound (Graf type III). The primary outcome of the trial was DDH discovered after the first month of life. There were 24 such cases, and they were classified by means of radiography in dysplasia, subluxation, and dislocation. The median age of late-presenting cases was 4.5 months. The total number was almost similar in the nonultrasound ($n = 10$) and selective ultrasound groups ($n = 9$), but lower in the universal ultrasound group ($n = 5$). The rates of late dislocations or subluxation were 0.3, 0.7, and 1.3 per 1000 live births, respectively. These differences were not significant, however. Three infants (nonscreening and selective screening groups) required surgery for dislocated hips.

Treatment in general was significantly more often conducted in the universal ultrasound group than in the other 2 groups (3.4% vs. 2.0% and 1.8%). Universal ultrasound screening identified 130 cases per 1000 clinically healthy infants as having abnormalities requiring sonographic monitoring. Of these, 97% showed spontaneous resolution by 3 months of age, but each infant had 3 to 5 ultrasound tests before being declared to have normal hips.

Although no late presentations of DDH were observed after universal ultrasound screening, statistically, there was no difference among the 3 screening regimens, and ultrasound, therefore, was not superior to physical examination by well-trained personnel. However, like others studies,[6,8] the results of this study suggest that the need for clinical follow-up can be minimized by the reassuring findings of a normal ultrasound test.

Holen and researchers[10] investigated whether universal ultrasound screening is superior to selective ultrasound screening. After a physical examination by an experienced single pediatrician, a newborn's risk factors for DDH were established. These included any form of instability of the hip (positive or uncertain Barlow test), positive family history, breech position, and foot deformities. Infants were randomized into 2 groups. One group received both physical and ultrasound examinations. Infants in the second group received ultrasound only if they had a risk factor. DDH detected after the first month of life was the primary outcome, and it was measured by sonographic and radiographic criteria, respectively. In the universal ultrasound group, 1 case (0.13/1000 live births) was found, and 5 were found in the selected ultrasound group (0.65/1000 live births). The relative risk for late detected DDH in the universal screening group was 0.21 (95% confidence interval, 0.03–1.45). This study clearly showed that universal ultrasound screening is not superior over selected screening if clinical screening is of high quality.

The authors raised the question whether ultrasound could have the potential to eradicate late-presenting cases of DDH because there was only 1 such case in their universal ultrasound screening group. Universal ultrasound screening was established in 1996 in Germany, and all newborns have been screened by means of ultrasound before the sixth week of life. Despite a population screening rate of more than 95%,

13% of infants required an operative procedure later on to treat DDH. Of interest, 13% of these hips were judged to be normal on ultrasound screening.[11] These findings show that ultrasound screening may have the potential to reduce the number of late-presenting cases of DDH or the need for surgical treatment but will not eliminate them.

EXISTING GUIDELINES

The American Academy of Pediatrics[12] recommend, based on a model-driven approach with a comprehensive synthesis of the evidence base, clinical screening for DDH by a trained health professional for all newborns. Ultrasound is not recommended except for girls born in the breech position. These infants should undergo either hip ultrasound at the age of 6 weeks or radiographs at 4 months because of the significantly high risk for DDH (absolute risk, 70–120/1000). Hips remarkable in the postnatal examination can be watched for 2 weeks or should be referred to an orthopedic specialist, but no abduction splinting is recommended at that stage.

The U.S. Preventative Services Task Force[13] recommends against routine screening for DDH. The task force argues that the natural history of DDH is poorly defined, and there is lack of evidence that screening would improve health outcomes, although there is evidence that interventions have the potential to cause harm such as avascular necrosis of the hip.

The Canadian Task Force for Preventative Health Care[14] recommend serial physical examination by a trained clinician in the periodic health examinations. Also, this guideline does not recommend ultrasound as a screening tool, not even in infants at high risk such as girls born in the breech position. The author argues that selective screening is ineffective in reducing the operating rates because most newborns have no risk factors.

The U.K. National Screening Committee recommends ultrasound to be used in the management of infants with clinical hip instability.[15] Population screening programmes using ultrasound in all newborns have been implemented in some Mid-European countries where ultrasound is performed within the first 6 weeks of life.

RECOMMENDATIONS

The treatment of late-presenting DDH (>6 month of age) in general is more complex and prolonged compared with treatment initiated earlier on. Clinicians therefore should aim for an early diagnosis of DDH, ideally within the first 6 weeks.

Good evidence exists for the management of the dislocatable hip of the neonate. Treatment of such hips can be safely delayed until the age of 2 to 3 weeks without altering the final outcome. In fact, a large proportion of such hips will stabilize

Continued

RECOMMENDATIONS—CONT'D

spontaneously within this period. Based on current evidence, treatment should be initiated if the hip is not improving beyond the age of 2 weeks.

If a hip is dislocated but reducible (Ortolani positive) in the neonatal period, abduction splinting by means of a reduction device such the Pavlik harness should be commenced at any age. Although never proved to be effective in a randomized trial, this strategy was part of all randomized trials in DDH; early reduction of a dislocated hip seems sensible. It is generally accepted that such treatment must be monitored by means of ultrasound every other week to ensure that femoral head position and acetabular dysplasia are improving. In the child beyond the neonatal period, the process of reduction will take longer, and documentation of sonographic improvement is even more important. Various harnesses are available, but none has proven its relative efficacy in well-designed comparative studies. Avascular necrosis of the proximal femoral epiphysis is a potential but rare complication of harness treatment (<1% in observational studies), and the benefits of a reduced hip outweigh this risk.

The best management of hips that are Ortolani and Barlow negative but sonographically abnormal remains obscure. Because of the variety of definitions used to define sonographic dysplasia in previous studies, and because of the inconsistency with which these criteria were applied, no general recommendations can be made on how to treat this particular subgroup. However, the way these abnormalities are detected seems to influence the likelihood for abduction splinting. If these abnormalities were detected by means of screening, treatment was significantly more likely to be initiated. However, if they were detected because of an unclear physical examination, ultrasound monitoring reduced the number splinted at the expense of repeat ultrasound scanning.

Sufficient evidence does not exist to support general ultrasound screening. Two trials demonstrated that general ultrasound is not superior to selective ultrasound. If the physical examination is performed by well-trained and experienced personnel, ultrasound should be utilized for hips that show unclear findings on clinical examination because it will reduce the number of splinting. Girls born in the breech position have a significantly greater absolute risk (up to 12 times greater) for severe forms of DDH. Ultrasound screening of this subgroup within the first 6 weeks seems plausible. Table 35–2 provides a summary of recommendations for the treatment of DDH.

TABLE 35–2. Summary of Recommendations

STATEMENT	LEVEL OF EVIDENCE /GRADE OF RECOMMENDATION
1. Treatment of dislocatable hips in neonates can be delayed until the age of 2 weeks under ultrasound surveillance without altering outcomes.	B
2. Treatment of dislocated hips in neonates (positive Ortolani test) should be initiated immediately and not be delayed.	C
3. Sonographically stable (<2 mm displacement of the femoral head from the floor of the acetabulum) but sonographically dysplastic (<40% femoral head cover) hips do not warrant abduction treatment when diagnosed at the age of 2 to 6 weeks.	B
4. Hips that are stable on clinical examination (negative Ortolani and Barlow tests) but sonographically dysplastic with Graf alpha angles of 43 to 50 degrees should receive immediate abduction splinting to avoid residual acetabular dysplasia.	I
5. Hips that are unremarkable on clinical examination but reveal sonographic dysplasia of the acetabulum without sonographic instability do not warrant abduction splinting because they will improve within the first 3 months of life in up to 97% of infants.	B

REFERENCES

1. Roposch A, Moreau NM, Uleryk E, et al: Developmental dysplasia of the hip: Quality of reporting of diagnostic accuracy for US. Radiology 241:854, 2006.
2. Woolacott NF, Puhan MA, Steurer J, et al: Ultrasonography in screening for developmental dysplasia of the hip in newborns: Systematic review. BMJ 330:1413, 2005.
3. Roposch A, Wright JG: Increased diagnostic information and understanding disease: Uncertainty in the diagnosis of developmental hip dysplasia. Radiology 242:355, 2007.
4. Castelein RM, Korte J: Limited hip abduction in the infant. J Pediatr Orthop 21:668, 2001.
5. Rosendahl K, Markestad T, Lie RT: Ultrasound screening for developmental dysplasia of the hip in the neonate: The effect on treatment rate and prevalence of late cases. Pediatrics 94:47, 1994.
6. Gardiner HM, Dunn PM: Controlled trial of immediate splinting versus ultrasonographic surveillance in congenitally dislocatable hips. Lancet 336:1553, 1990.
7. Elbourne D, Dezateux C, Arthur R, et al: Ultrasonography in the diagnosis and management of developmental hip dysplasia (UK Hip Trial): Clinical and economic results of a multicentre randomised controlled trial. Lancet 360:2009, 2002.
8. Wood MK, Conboy V, Benson MK: Does early treatment by abduction splintage improve the development of dysplastic but stable neonatal hips? J Pediatr Orthop 20:302, 2000.
9. Graf R. Ultrasound measurements of the newborn hip—comparison of two methods in 657 newborns. Acta Orthop Scand 69:550, 1998.

10. Holen KJ, Tegnander A, Bredland T, et al: Universal or selective screening of the neonatal hip using ultrasound? A prospective, randomised trial of 15,529 newborn infants. J Bone Joint Surg Br 84:886, 2002.
11. von Kries R, Ihme N, Oberle D, et al: Effect of ultrasound screening on the rate of first operative procedures for developmental hip dysplasia in Germany. Lancet 362:1883, 2003.
12. Lehmann HP, Hinton R, Morello P, et al: Developmental dysplasia of the hip practice guideline: Technical report. Committee on Quality Improvement, and Subcommittee on Developmental Dysplasia of the Hip. Pediatrics 105:E57, 2000.
13. Screening for developmental dysplasia of the hip: Recommendation statement. US Preventative Services Task Force. Paediatrics 117:898, 2006.
14. Patel H: Preventive health care, 2001 update: Screening and management of developmental dysplasia of the hip in newborns. CMAJ 164:1669, 2001.
15. Elliman DA, Dezateux C, Bedford HE: Newborn and childhood screening programmes: Criteria, evidence, and current policy. Arch Dis Child 87:6, 2002.

Chapter 36

What Is the Best Treatment for Idiopathic Clubfoot?

Frederick R. Dietz, MD

The best treatment for idiopathic clubfoot is the simplest, safest, least expensive, and most rapid method to correct the clubfoot deformity, maintain correction, and allow lifelong normal foot function. Clearly, several potential questions need to be addressed. For example, the treatment that most rapidly corrects deformity may result in painful feet long term. The safest technique for initial correction may be less effective than other techniques. Clarifying the questions to be answered is critical to evaluating the quality of evidence available.

This chapter addresses the following questions: (1) What treatment best obtains initial correction in idiopathic clubfoot? (2) What treatment best maintains correction? (3) What treatment gives the best long-term foot function? Treatment techniques for severe recurrent deformities from failed treatment such a triple arthrodesis and Ilizarov approaches are not addressed.

Few investigations of "high-level" evidence address these questions. There are several reasons for this. First, true randomized studies of very different treatment methods have not been performed and will not be performed for ethical reasons. No orthopedic surgeons are agnostic with respect to the best treatment for clubfoot. Minor variations within a treatment approach are much more likely to be randomized. Second, the severity of clubfeet appears to vary in ways that are difficult to quantitate. This inability to classify feet results in stratification of individuals within a cohort of clubfoot patients who are treated in different ways based on nonquantifiable distinctions of their treating physicians, resulting in selection bias for a particular treatment. One practitioner's "mild" deformity may be another practitioner's "moderate" deformity. If these practitioners choose treatment with manipulation or posteromedial release (PMR) based on the "severity" of deformity, the results of their treatment regimens will not be comparable. Rating scales of severity at birth have not been shown to identify difficulty with initial correction, maintenance of correction, or long-term function for different treatment techniques. That a particular scale can predict success with a particular treatment technique has been shown, but this result cannot be generalized a priori to other techniques.[1] When a technique, such as the Ponseti method, results in near-universal early correction, there is no value of rating scales for predicting the likelihood of initial

deformity correction. A useful rating scale would need to predict recurrence risk or long-term outcome. No such rating scale exists. Therefore, we do not have a common starting point for comparing treatment techniques that is validated, and there may never be one. This is particularly important because many case series are a mixture of techniques based on the treating physician's view of the severity of the deformity. Thus, many case series describe a treatment given to a selected group of patients with clubfoot from a cohort that is not defined. Third, recurrence of deformity, as opposed to failure of complete correction, is ill-defined. Generally, recurrence is in the eye of the beholding physician. Proxy measures, such as repeat surgery or need for further casting, are crude measures of recurrence. Fourth, outcome studies of sufficient length and quality to answer the question "What treatment method gives the best lifelong foot function?" are rare. A true comparative study of different methods that met Level I or II standards would require funding and commitment at a level that such studies have not and may never be performed. One confounding factor that occurs commonly in all surgical fields is that the surgical procedure is constantly "tweaked" so that long-term studies are rarely strictly comparable with the present "best" surgical treatment.

Despite these problems, data do exist that suggest best treatments. Case series studies of similar patients treated by different treatments because of a change in practice of a single or group of practitioners can be compared. Outcome studies utilizing validated outcome instruments of case series are beginning to be performed, and such studies can be compared. Multiple case series of a specific technique can be compared with multiple case series using a different technique.

The data used to attempt to answer the questions come from an Embase and Medline search for Level I and II evidence studies written in the English language from 1950 to 2007. Almost no relevant studies were found. Using the same research strategy from 2000 to 2007, a few Level III evidence studies and several Level II studies, not initially identified, were found. Because of the paucity of information, the same databases were searched for Level IV evidence studies from 2000 to 2007, of which there were 77 identified. These case series studies were supplemented with earlier case series studies that the author believes were most informative. The analysis does not meet the standard of a systematic review. The quantity of case series studies before 2000 and in non–English language publications that would need to be surveyed for a systematic review was beyond the scope of this project but may be a worthwhile undertaking. I will attempt to give an accurate appraisal of the quality of evidence, but it should be noted that the quality of evidence is not what would be desired or expected for such a relatively common disorder.

WHAT TREATMENT BEST OBTAINS INITIAL CORRECTION IN IDIOPATHIC CLUBFOOT?

The question of what treatment best obtains initial correction in idiopathic clubfoot asks what nonoperative (or largely nonoperative technique if percutaneous tendo Achilles lengthening [TAL] is included) treatment is most effective is correcting clubfoot deformities. Neonatal surgical correction by major ligament release has not succeeded in giving lasting correction and has been abandoned. Many idiosyncratic techniques for manipulating and immobilizing clubfeet exist. In much of the literature, the question is not addressed because the studies are of surgical treatments. The authors simply state that feet uncorrected conservatively had their surgical treatment. When stated, the number of feet that were conservatively corrected varies from 5% to 60% in most studies, but specific treatment techniques are rarely specified. The most prominent published techniques are those of Kite and Denis Browne from the 1930s, Ponseti from the 1960s, and Dimeglio and Bensahel from the 1990s. The Kite method was by far the most common technique used in the United States until the recent popularity of the Ponseti method.

Sud and colleagues[2] compared rates of initial correction and relapse comparing the Ponseti and Kite methods in a prospective, randomized study with outcome assessment by a surgeon who was blinded to the treatment. The clinic in which the children were treated had used the Kite method for 15 years and the Ponseti method for 1 year before beginning the study. Fifty-three patients with 81 feet were enrolled, and 8 were lost to follow-up and excluded from analysis. Thirty-six feet treated by the Ponseti method and 31 feet treated by the Kite method were followed for an average of 26 months. The Ponseti method had a 91.7% initial correction rate compared with 66.7% by the Kite technique. Ponseti method feet had a 21.1% relapse rate over the course of the study compared with a 38.1% relapse rate for the Kite method. The mean number of casts was statistically significantly less for the Ponseti method (6.2, Ponseti method; 10.7, Kite method), and the mean time to correction was significantly shorter for the Ponseti method (49.2 days, Ponseti method; 91.2 days, Kite method).

Three other studies address the question of early correction by comparing different methods. Herzenberg, Radler, and Bor[3] in Maryland and Israel compared their first 27 patients treated by the Ponseti method with 27 patients matched from their database who had been treated by a variety of manipulative techniques by the authors or referring physicians. Their major outcome variable was need for PMR in the first year of life because of failure to correct the deformity. Only 1 foot required PMR (97%) correction with the Ponseti technique compared with only 2 feet corrected without PMR in the historical control group, which had a 6% success rate. Segev and coworkers[4] compared 61 clubfeet treated by a modification of the Kite and Lovell method and managed an average of 55 months with their initial 48 feet treated with the Ponseti method that were managed for an average of 29 months with a 16-month minimum. The feet treated by the Kite and Lovell method required surgical correction in 56% of the feet. Of the feet treated by the Ponseti method, 3 (6%) required surgical correction.

Aurell and researchers[5] in Sweden report a center randomized study of clubfeet treated by 2 different techniques. A consecutive series of children with clubfoot was treated by the Ponseti method at 1 hospital (9 feet) and by the Copenhagen method at another hospital (19 feet). The Copenhagen method involves manipulation by a physiotherapist 4 to 5 times per week with correction maintained by a plexidur splint for 1 month, followed by 1 or 2 times per week manipulation in the second week. At 2 months of age, a pediatric orthopedic surgeon decided whether further treatment was needed. All 9 feet treated by the Ponseti technique required only a percutaneous TAL. Of the 19 feet treated by the Copenhagen method, 12 required PMR (63%) and 1 required a posterior release (5%).

Many case series studies address the effectiveness of the Ponseti method for early correction. Changulani and researchers[6] report their initial experience in the United Kingdom using the Ponseti method in 100 feet in 66 children. Ninety-six of 100 feet were fully corrected with 85 requiring percutaneous tenotomy. Colburn and Williams[7] report complete initial correction of 54 of 57 feet (95%) of the first babies they treated by Ponseti method in San Francisco. Goksan and coauthors[8] report on 134 feet with 97% follow-up to mean age of 46 months with a minimum of 2 years after initial casting in Turkey. Only 4 patients required PMR. Lehman and colleagues[9] in New York reported successful correction in 92% of the first 45 feet treated by the Ponseti method. Tindall and coworkers[10] report initial correction of 98 of 100 in Malawi by nonphysician orthopedic paraprofessionals. Shack and Eastwood[11] report initial correction of 39 of 40 children in a physiotherapist-delivered Ponseti program in the United Kingdom. Morcuende and colleagues[12] report initial correction in 98% of 256 feet treated by Dr. Ponseti and others at the University of Iowa.

A number of case series reports have been published of the French or Montpellier method of physiotherapy correction of clubfoot. Physiotherapy was developed and refined by Masse, Bensehal, Dimeglio, Metaizeau, and others. The technique has been published in English, but several case series in French are not included here. Dimeglio reported on three groups of feet during the evolution of the treatment in 1996. The best group consisted of 52 clubfeet. Forty percent were corrected without surgery; 35% required PMR or PMRL; and 25% required posterior release. Van Campenhout and investigators[13] evaluated their results of physiotherapy and continuous passive motion machine in 64 babies with 100 feet. The authors included only infants presenting at younger than 3 months whose family strictly adhered to the protocol. With a minimum follow-up of 18 months and a mean follow-up of 3.2 years, 75 (75%) of the feet required surgery. Richards and coauthors[14] report on 142 feet in 98 babies treated by the French method.[14] With an average follow-up of 35 months, 20% required PMR and 29% required posterior release. Souchet and colleagues[15] report what appears to be a largely personal series of Bensahel of 350 clubfeet followed to skeletal maturity. Twenty-three percent required surgical treatment at a mean age of 1 year. Stromqvist and coworkers[16] report on 75 feet treated by a strict physiotherapy and bracing regimen, and managed for an average of 8 years. Sixty-seven (89%) of the feet underwent posterior release (PR) (two thirds) or PMR (one third) between 2 and 5 months of age.[16] Twenty-five feet (33%) required a second operation at a mean of 4 years, and 4 feet had a third operation.

Summary

Reasonably strong evidence exists that the Ponseti method is the best treatment to obtain initial correction in idiopathic clubfoot. Although high-level evidence studies are few, they are entirely consistent in supporting the Ponseti method as the most effective and rapid technique. Case series are persuasive because all show a more than 90% initial correction rate, which is greater than that reported in *any* report for other methods. Furthermore, most series report the authors' early experience, and results would be expected to improve with experience. That the results have been replicated in many parts of the world by medical practitioners of varying levels of training, all support the conclusion that the Ponseti method is the "best" method for initial correction of idiopathic clubfoot.

WHAT TREATMENT BEST MAINTAINS CORRECTION?

Relapse of deformity that requires treatment in clubfoot is in the "eye of the beholder." No technical cutoff exists to say when a correction is inadequate versus when a recurrence of deformity has developed. Therefore, relapse rates are likely to vary between different investigators. Nonoperatively treated clubfeet that lose correction will relapse into a clubfoot deformity with varying amounts of recurrent equinus, varus, adductus, and cavus. Operatively treated feet may relapse in a similar way but may also lose correction into foot positions such as severe planovalgus, severe cavus from dorsal dislocation of the navicular, dorsal bunion development, and any combination of relapse and overcorrection of the initial deformities. In general, recurrent deformity requiring further treatment is reported to compromise results. One long-term report of the Ponseti method suggests that relapse of a certain type, at a certain age, can be managed in a way (anterior tibial tendon transfer to the third cuneiform) that does not compromise long-term foot function.[17] Nonetheless, most relapses in corrected clubfoot treated nonoperatively occur in the first 5 years of life. The surgical literature, which is largely short- to medium-term follow-up studies (2–8 years), also suggests that recurrent deformity or overcorrection tends to occur during the rapid growing period of the foot.

For the purposes of this section, I define "need for further surgery after initial correction" as a surrogate for relapse in reports of surgically treated feet. Investigations of feet treated surgically in infancy almost never report using manipulation and casting to treat recurrent deformity. Therefore, only further surgery indicates a change in foot morphology that the investigator thought required treatment. Adherents of the Ponseti method will treat relapse at an early stage with repeat casting, and at a later age with an anterior tibial transfer under most circumstances. This is not considered a failure based on current long-term follow-up data and, therefore, is discussed somewhat differently than a recurrence requiring further surgery. Note that some feet may require further treatment because of symptoms, without incurring new deformity. Therefore, need for further surgery is not a distinct end point but is the best available surrogate.

The literature I use to address this question is largely case series studies with follow-up periods shorter than skeletal maturity for most patients. Most of these studies purport to be "outcome" studies. Most of these studies use unvalidated, idiosyncratic rating scales that mix symptoms, physical finding, and radiographic findings in arbitrary ways to develop "excellent/good/fair/and poor" ratings. The only value of these studies is for assessing early complication rates such as relapse. These are not considered in the last section on long-term outcome. Bad results can be identified at any age, but I will not consider a study to address long-term foot function until the cohort studied is at least mostly skeletally mature. Another weakness of many of these studies is that comparisons of different treatment methods were done based on a change in practice so that the follow-up lengths are markedly different between the treatment groups. Finally, the reporting of basic data such as age at operation, length of follow-up, rate of follow-up, and rate of reoperation are often absent or unclear in the published manuscripts. Some interpretation is occasionally necessary, which certainly reduces accurate assessment of the data reported.

A number of Level III evidence studies comparing different surgical treatment techniques demonstrate the problem of markedly different follow-up periods between different techniques that were utilized at various times at single institutions.

Tschopp and colleagues reported on 18 feet treated by PMR managed for an average of 98 months and compared them with 17 feet undergoing complete subtalar release with an average follow-up of 39 months.[18] Four feet needed further surgery in the PMR group, and one foot needed further surgery in the subtalar release group.

Centel and investigators[19] compared 17 feet treated by PMR and managed for 5 years with 46 feet treated by subtalar release and managed for 2 years. The PMR group had a 19% reoperation rate, and the subtalar release group had an 11% reoperation rate. Centel and investigators[19] also reported on 20 patients who presented with only residual equinus who were treated by posterior release alone and who were managed for 4 years and had a 29% reoperation rate.

Nimityongskul and researchers[20] compared 16 feet treated by Turco PMR and managed for an average of 8.5 years with 12 feet treated by McKay/Simons circumferential release managed for less than 4 years on average. Six of 16 PMR feet (37.5%) required further surgery, whereas no complete subtalar release feet needed further surgery during this short follow-up. The authors' anticipated 55% of the PMR group and 17% of the complete subtalar release group would require further surgery.

Pavlovcic and Pecak[21] compared the results of posterior release in 96 feet (chosen for this treatment because of mild deformity) with PMR in 75 feet (chosen for this treatment because of severe deformity). Both groups were managed for slightly more than 12 years on average. Sixty-eight percent of the PR feet required further surgery, and 42% of the PMR feet underwent further surgery.

A single study compared 30 feet treated by PMR with 30 feet treated by PMR and an anterior tibial tendon lengthening.[22] Follow-up was 11 and 9 years for the respective groups. Eight of 30 (27%) of the PMR-treated feet, and 2 of 30 (7%) of the feet with PMR plus anterior tibial tendon lengthening required further surgery. Seventeen percent of all feet required further surgery.

Simons[23] report on 21 feet treated by PMR and lateral release with 25 feet treated with a complete subtalar release. A short follow-up of 3 years revealed that 4 feet (9% of the entire group) required further surgery. Two feet had PMR and 2 had complete subtalar release. Furthermore, Simons[23] describe, major complications that may require further surgery in an additional 24 patients (52%).

Otremski and coworkers[24] compared 30 feet treated by PMR with an 8- to 14-year follow-up with 22 feet treated by a modified PMR with a 5-year average follow-up period. Five patients treated by PMR and 1 patient treated by modified PMR had further surgery at last follow-up examination (12% of the entire group).

Thompson and colleagues[24a] fashioned three groups from a population of 244 clubfeet of which 73% were managed for less than 10 years and 27% had longer than a 10-year follow-up period. The group treated with a limited or *à la carte* release (112 feet) required further surgery in 74% of feet and recasting in 8%. A second group was defined as having had a failed incomplete release and had undergone a complete PMR (39 feet). Ten percent of this group had subsequent surgery, and 28% were recasted. A group of 93 feet treated primarily by PMR had a 9% reoperation rate and an 11% recasting rate.

Case series studies with short-term results that shed light on recurrence rates are common but are subject to all the biases inherent in such studies. Fourteen representative studies are summarized with respect to recurrence of deformity requiring surgical treatment. Surgical treatment in these 14 reports were variously described as "Turco procedure," "modified Turco," "soft tissue release," "selected soft tissue release," "a la carte," "complete subtalar release," "Simon release," "McKay release," "early posterior release," "Goldner release," and "staged plantar medial followed by postero lateral release." Follow-up ranged from 2 to 16 years with an average follow-up period of 8 years. Number of feet reported ranged from 16 to 271 with an average of 91 feet. Further surgery rates ranged from 0% to 68% with an average of 24%. These articles are by no means exhaustive of the case series published on short-term results of clubfoot, but they are representative of the English language articles including the work of Turco and McKay.[25–38]

The method of physiotherapy is difficult to assess in this section because of the high rate of failed initial correction. However, the percentage of feet requiring extensive release surgery using this method is between 25% and 89% as reported earlier (see What Treatment Best Obtains Initial Correction in Idiopathic Clubfoot? section).

Relapse in the Ponseti method requires a somewhat different assessment. Few Ponseti method–treated feet undergo surgery at an early age (excluding percutaneous tenotomy), and relapses are treated by repeat manipulation and casting until the child is mature enough for an anterior tibial tendon transfer to the third cuneiform to be performed. Morcuende and colleagues[12] reviewed 256 feet treated at the University of Iowa between 1991 and 2001 with an average follow-up of 26 months (6–96 months). Seventeen patients suffered a relapse (11% of feet). Four feet (2.5%) required PR or PMR, and four feet required anterior tibial transfer to the third cuneiform. The authors found that 2 of 140 patients (~1%) whose parents reported compliance with the bracing regimen relapsed, whereas 15 of 17 patients whose parents were not compliant relapsed (89%).

Dobbs and researchers[39] evaluated recurrence risk in 51 consecutive infants with 86 idiopathic clubfeet managed for an average of 27 months (24–35 months). They report complete initial correction. Twenty-seven feet relapsed, and all relapses were treated successfully by manipulation and recasting. All of the relapsed feet occurred in families who were noncompliant with brace wear. Compliance was related to relapse with an odds ratio of 183 ($P < 0.00001$).

Haft and coworkers[40] report on 73 feet in 51 infants treated in New Zealand with a mean follow-up period of 35 months (24–65 months). They report a 41% relapse rate with only 51% brace compliance. Relapses were minor in 18% of patients and required only TAL or anterior tibial tendon transfer, or both. Relapses were major in 24% of patients and required PR or PMR. Noncompliance with brace treatment conferred a five times increased risk for relapse.

Summary

What can be concluded with regard to the question, What treatment best maintains clubfoot correction? Very little from an evidence basis. The studies are generally of poor design, and confounding factors are multiple and often invisible in the articles. Virtually all studies that compare a less with a more aggressive surgical procedure (PR vs. PMR; à la carte vs. PMR, PMR vs. complete subtalar release) found a lower reoperation rate with the more aggressive procedure. The more aggressive procedure was due to a change in practice and, therefore, had a shorter follow-up period. The wide range of recurrence requiring treatment in the early PR, PMR, and complete subtalar release series may depend on details of surgical technique, follow-up protocol, variability in defining a recurrence length of follow-up period, and a host of other factors. Relapse after Ponseti method correction appears to be dependent on compliance with the postcorrection brace protocol. Compliance with bracing could reasonably be expected to vary by population, physician, culture, among other factors. Comparison of relapse rate between Ponseti method and joint invasive surgical techniques is not possible given the available data.

WHAT TREATMENT GIVES BEST LONG-TERM FOOT FUNCTION?

Multiple reports of "long-term" follow-up of clubfoot exist. Few of these studies report on a cohort whose members are all skeletally mature much less middle aged or elderly and, therefore, can scarcely be called long term. The mean life span in most of the developed world is the late 70s. These studies are only long term from the perspective of an orthopedic surgeon's career, which is not an appropriate determinant of length of follow-up. Data from long-term follow-up studies of Legg–Calve–Perthes disease should be cautionary. Most patients responded well until the middle of the sixth decade of life, at which time disabling arthritis requiring THR became common. "Good" functional results in the teens, 20s, 30s,

and so on cannot be extrapolated without data. For example, Krauspe and colleagues[41] used the McKay rating system (a nonvalidated, multidomain, idiosyncratic measuring scheme) to assess the outcomes of 104 feet in 64 patients treated by the Scheel technique (a PR with PMR as needed with a traction suture on the calcaneus). The results deteriorated markedly from less than 10 to 10 to 20 years to greater than 20 years (Table 36–1).

Long-term results of clubfoot treatment are generally a confused mix of ages, procedures, and evaluations. A classic and typical report is the 1964 report by Wynne-Davies.[42] She reports on 84 patients with 121 feet (88% follow up) who had completed treatment. Completion of treatment was arbitrarily defined as older than 10 years. Ninety-three feet belonged to patients 10 to 21 years of age, and 28 feet belonged to patients 22 to 35 years of age. Twenty-eight feet had closed treatment only; 51 feet had PMR, anterior tendon transfer laterally, or both; and 24 feet had arthrodesis, of which 10 had had a prior soft-tissue procedure. Patient-centered outcomes consisted of the following copied directly from the article:

Occupation—Few of the patients limited their activities on account of deformed feet [Table 36–2].[42]
Symptoms—These were few. The commonest complaint, only elicited by direct questioning, was of callosities on the lateral border of the foot (in one-quarter of the patients). Occasional pain and "tiring easily" was noted in only fifteen out of eighty-four patients. Although there were many stiff feet, only seven patients had noticed any difficulty in walking on rough ground.

Unfortunately, much of the literature of the ensuing 40 years is no more informative than this early attempt at an outcome study.

Only one investigation has been published that reports outcomes in skeletally mature clubfoot patients

TABLE 36–1. Deterioration of Surgical Clubfoot Results with Advancing Age

AGE (years)	GRADE (%)				
	2 EXCELLENT	3 GOOD	4 SATISFACTORY	5 POOR	6 FAILURE
<10	23	38	49		
10–20	8	13	42	12	25
>20		5	34	28	33

TABLE 36–2. Activities ($N = 84$)

ACTIVITIES	PATIENTS (N)		
	MALE	FEMALE	TOTAL
Still at school	26	13	39
Sedentary occupation	2	7	9
Standing or heavy work	31	3	34
Mental defectives	2	—	2
Total	61	23	84
Played active games	54	24	75

evaluated by a validated outcomes instrument. Dobbs and coworkers[43] report on 73 feet in 45 patients treated by posterior and plantar release in 13 feet (average follow-up, 31 years; range, 30–32 years) and Turco-type PMR in 60 feet (average follow-up, 28 years; range, 25–29 years). They were able to find 73% of eligible patients. Using the health survey Short Form-36 (SF-36) for evaluation of health-related quality of life, this cohort scored nearly 2 standard deviations less than the average on the physical functioning scale and average on the mental functioning scale. No study has been reported with which to compare this validated outcome result, but the physical functioning level was similar to cohorts of patients with chronic heart failure, awaiting coronary bypass surgery, and suffering cervical radiculopathy. The authors of this study used other outcome measures as well that, although not validated, have been used in other long-term follow-up studies of patients with clubfoot.

Cooper and Dietz[17] reviewed 45 patients with 71 clubfeet who were treated under the supervision of Dr. Ponseti at an average age of 34 years (range, 25–42 years). Only 36% of the eligible cohort was evaluated. The authors of this study administered a questionnaire to a control group of 97 patients of similar age (21–50 years old) and sex to the clubfoot cohort who were screened only for the absence of a congenital foot abnormality. The questionnaire began as follows:

1. My foot (feet)
   a. is never painful
   b. occasionally causes mild pain
   c. is painful after strenuous activities only
   d. is painful in routine day to day activities
   e. is painful in routine walking
   f. is painful at rest or at night
2. In my daily living, my foot (feet)
   a. does not limit my activities
   b. occasionally limits my activities
   c. limits me in strenuous activities
   d. limits me in routine day to day activities
   e. limits me in routine walking

After reviewing the responses of the first 34 control participants' responses to these questions, the authors defined the following groups:

Excellent = a foot that does not limit activities of daily living and is never painful or occasionally causes mild pain

Good = a foot that occasionally limits activities of daily living or strenuous activities or is painful after strenuous activities.

Poor = a foot that limits daily activities or routine walking, or is painful in daily activities, walking, or at night

The outcome as defined earlier was not different between the control and Ponseti-treated patients with clubfoot. Dobbs and coworkers[43] administered these questions and compared them with quite different results (Box 36–1).

Several studies have used the Laaveg and Ponseti functional rating system for clubfoot as their only or

BOX 36–1					
	Excellent	**Good**	**Poor**	**Age (years)**	**% of Cohort Evaluated**
Control subjects	63%	22%	15%	21–50	—
Cooper/Dietz[17]	62%	16%	22%	34 average	36
Dobbs et al.[43]	4%	22%	73%	31 average	73

1 of several outcome measures. This rating scheme is not validated but combines reasonable elements of outcomes that are arbitrarily weighted and scored. Excellent was defined as 90 to 100 points, good as 80 to 89, fair as 70 to 79, and poor as less than 70. The rating scheme is presented in Table 36–3. Tables 36–4 and 36–5 summarize long-term follow-up articles.

What can be concluded from the available data? The single study using validated outcome measures and follow-up past skeletal maturity showed poor results for PMR. The single study using a control group of nonclubfoot subjects for comparison sho-wed equal quality of foot function between Ponseti method–treated patients and control subjects who were without congenital foot deformity. Comparison of these 2 studies, each with 30-year average follow-up, shows superior results for the Ponseti method over the PMR method that Dobbs described. The long-term Ponseti method studies are flawed by a relatively small percentage of eligible patients being evaluated.

Ippolito and researchers'[45] PMR cohort scored statistically significantly more poorly on the Laaveg and Ponseti scale than did their Ponseti with PR cohort. A detail that may be important is that Ippolito's PR was an ankle capsulotomy alone. Most of the other descriptions of PR that are reported here (Hutchins et al[38] and Haasbeek and Wright[46]) include a posterior subtalar joint and ligament release as well. The devil may be in the details—the more joints opened, the worse the results. In contrast, there was no significant difference between Haasbeek and Wright's PMR and PR group. Haasbeek and Wright's PMR group had significant numbers of skeletally immature subjects, as did Hutchins's group and Laaveg and Ponseti's group.

Summary

It is difficult to extrapolate firm conclusions from such a limited number of long-term follow-up studies. What available evidence suggests is that joint release surgery and Ponseti treatment give comparable results when evaluating patients whose average age is in the teenage years and the evaluation instrument is the Laaveg and Ponseti scale. The only 2 studies that compare patients who are all skeletally mature with average ages in the 30s strongly support the superiority of the Ponseti method over surgical release. Nonetheless, these are only 2 articles. The weight of evidence suggests that long-term results are better

TABLE 36-3. Functional Rating System for Club Foot[44]

CATEGORY	POINTS
Satisfaction (20 points)	
I am	
a. very satisfied with the end result	20
b. satisfied with the end result	16
c. neither satisfied nor unsatisfied with the end result	12
d. unsatisfied with the end result	8
e. very unsatisfied with the end result	4
Function (20 points)	
In my daily living, my clubfoot	
a. does not limit my activities	20
b. occasionally limits my strenuous activities	16
c. usually limits me in strenuous activities	12
d. limits me occasionally in routine activities	8
e. limits me in walking	4
Pain (30 points)	
My clubfoot	
a. is never painful	30
b. occasionally causes mild pain during strenuous activities	24
c. usually is painful after strenuous activities only	18
d. is occasionally painful during routine activities	12
e. is painful during walking	6
Position of heel when standing (10 points)	
Heel varus, 0 degrees or some heel valgus	10
Heel varus, 1–5 degrees	5
Heel varus, 6–10 degrees	3
Heel varus, greater than 10 degrees	0
Passive motion (10 points)	
Dorsiflexion	1 point per 5 degrees (up to 5 points)
Total varus-valgus motion of heel	1 point per 10 degrees (up to 3 points)
Total anterior inversion-eversion of foot	1 point per 25 degrees (up to 2 points)
Gait (10 points)	
Normal	6
Can toe-walk	2
Can heel-walk	2
Limp	−2
No heel-strike	−2
Abnormal toe-off	−2

TABLE 36–4. Characteristics of Long Term Follow-up Studies Using Laaveg-Ponseti Rating Scale

AUTHOR	TREATMENT	PATIENTS/FEET	FOLLOW-UP AVERAGE AND RANGE	% OF ELIGIBLE COHORT EVALUATED
Laaveg and Ponseti (1980)[44]	Ponseti method	70/104	18.5 (10–27)	56
Dobbs et al. (2006)[43]	PMR	45/73	30 (25–32)	73
Ippolito et al. (2003)[45]	PMR	32/47	25 (24–28)	78
Ippolito et al. (2003)[45]	Ponseti/PR	32/49	19 (17–22)	84
Hutchins et al. (1985)[38]	Early PR	170/252	16.4 (8–31)	70
Haasbeek and Wright (1997)[46]	PMR	29/44	16 (13–20)	85
Haasbeek and Wright (1997)[46]	PR	30/46	28 (25–30)	77

PMR, posteromedial release; PR, posterior release.

TABLE 36–5. Laaveg-Ponseti Rating Scale Outcomes for Long term Follow-up Studies

AUTHOR	TREATMENT	EXCELLENT (%)	GOOD (%)	FAIR (%)	POOR (%)	AVERAGE LAAVEG AND PONSETI SCORE
Laaveg and Ponseti (1980)[44]	Ponseti method	54	20	14	12	87.5
Dobbs et al. (2006)[43]	PMR	0	33	20	47	65
Ippolito et al. (2003)[45]	PMR	4	38	23	34	75
Ippolito et al. (2003)[45]	Ponseti with early PR	37	41	12	10	85
Hutchins et al. (1985)[38]	Early PR	17	39	24	19	
Haasbeek and Wright (1997)[46]	PMR					85
Haasbeek and Wright (1997)[46]	PR					81

PMR, posteromedial release; PR, posterior release.

TABLE 36–6. Summary of Recommendations

STATEMENT	LEVEL OF EVIDENCE/GRADE OF RECOMMENDATION	REFERENCES
1. The Ponseti method is the best currently described casting treatment for rapidly and safely obtaining correction of idiopathic clubfoot.	A	2
	B	3–5
	C	6–12
2. Relapse after Ponseti casting is associated with lack of compliance with bracing.	B	12, 39, 40
3. Relapse after complete subtalar release is less likely than after posteromedial release.	B	18–24
4. Ponseti-treated clubfeet have similar functional outcomes to normal feet at average of 34 years of follow-up.	B	17
5. Ponseti treated clubfeet have better long-term (30 years) functional outcomes that clubfeet treated by posteromedial release.	B	45
	C	43, 44

the fewer joints are surgically invaded, but the strength of the evidence is poor.

CONCLUSIONS

The Ponseti method is the best treatment for rapidly and safely obtaining correction of idiopathic clubfoot. Whether recurrence is more common with Ponseti method or various surgical methods is unclear from the literature. Treatment of recurrence by the Ponseti method is less invasive through either recasting or anterior tibial tendon transfer as compared with repeated joint releases, osteotomies, and arthrodeses.

The long-term evidence is extremely thin but supports Ponseti method over joint release surgery for the correction of clubfoot. Table 36–6 provides a summary of recommendations for the treatment of idiopathic clubfoot.

REFERENCES

1. Bensahel H, Csukonyi Z, Desgrippes Y, Chaumien JP: Surgery in residual clubfoot: One-stage medioposterior release "a la carte." J Pediatr Orthop 7:145–148, 1987.
2. Sud A, Tiwari A, Sharma D, Kapoor S: Ponseti's vs. Kite's Method in the Treatment of Clubfoot: A Prospective Randomized Study. International Orthopaedics (SICOT) 32:15–21, 2007.
3. Herzenberg JE, Radler C, Bor N: Ponseti versus traditional methods of casting for idiopathic clubfoot. J Pediatr Orthop 22:517–521, 2002.
4. Segev E, Keret D, Lokiec F, et al: Early experience with Ponseti method for the treatment of congenital idiopathic clubfoot. Israel Medical Assoc J 7:307–310, 2005.
5. Aurell Y, Andriesse H, Johansson A, Jonsson K: Ultrasound assessment of early clubfoot treatment: A comparison of the Ponseti method and a modified Copenhagen method. J Pediatr Orthop B 14:347–357, 2005.
6. Changulani M, Garg NK, Rajagopal Ts, et al: Treatment of idiopathic clubfoot using the Ponseti method. Initial experience. J Bone Joint Surg Br 88:1385–1387, 2006.
7. Colburn M, Williams M: Evaluation of the treatment of idiopathic clubfoot by using the Ponseti method. J Foot Ankle Surg 42:259–267, 2003.
8. Goksan SB, Bursali A, Bilgili F, et al: Ponseti technique for the correction of idiopathic clubfeet presenting up to 1 year of age. A preliminary study in children with untreated or complex deformities. Arch Orthop Trauma Surg 126:15–21, 2006.
9. Lehman WB, Mohaideen A, Madan S, et al: A method for the early evaluation of the Ponseti (Iowa) technique for the treatment of idiopathic clubfoot. J Pediatr Orthop B 12:133–140, 2003.
10. Tindall AJ, Steinlechner CWB, Lavy CBD, et al: Results of manipulation of idiopathic clubfoot deformity in Malawi by orthopaedic clinical officers using the Ponseti method: A realistic alternative for the developing world? J Pediatr Orthop 25:627–629, 2005.
11. Shack N, Eastwood DM: Early results of a physiotherapist-delivered Ponseti service for the management of idiopathic congenital talipes equinovarus foot deformity. J Bone Joint Surg Br 88:1085–1089, 2006.
12. Morcuende JA, Dolan LA, Dietz FR, Ponseti IV: Radical reduction in the rate of extensive corrective surgery for clubfoot using the Ponseti method. Pediatrics 113:376–380, 2004.
13. Van Campenhout A, Molenaers G, Moens P, Fabry G: Does functional treatment of idiopathic clubfoot reduce the indication for surgery? Call for a widely accepted rating system. J Pediatr Orthop B 10:315–318, 2001.
14. Richards BS, Johnston CE, Wilson H: Nonoperative clubfoot treatment using the French physical therapy method. J Pediatr Orthop 25:98–102, 2005.
15. Souchet P, Bensahel H, Themar-Noel C, et al: Functional treatment of clubfoot: A new series of 350 idiopathic clubfeet with long-term followup. J Pediatr Orthop B 13:189–196, 2004.

16. Stromqvist B, Johnsson R, Jonsson K, Sunden G: Early intensive treatment of clubfoot: 75 feet followed for 6-11 years. Acta Orthop Scand 63:183–188, 1992.

17. Cooper DM, Dietz FR: Treatment of idiopathic clubfoot: A thirty-year follow-up. J Bone Joint Surg Am 77:1477–1489, 1995.

18. Tschopp O, Rombouts JJ, Rossillon R: Comparison of posteromedial and subtalar release in surgical treatment of resistant clubfoot. Orthopedics 25:527–529, 2002.

19. Centel T, Bagatur AE, Out T, Aksu T: Comparison of the soft-tissue methods in idiopathic clubfoot. J Pediatr Orthop 20:648–651, 2000.

20. Nimityongskul P, Anderson LD, Herbert DE: Surgical treatment of clubfoot: A comparison of two techniques. Foot Ankle 13:116–124, 1992.

21. Pavlovcic V, Pecak F: Surgical treatment of clubfoot: The significance of talocalcaneonavicular malposition correction. J Pediatr Orthop B 8:1–4, 1999.

22. Wicart PR, Barthes X, Ghanem I, Seringe R: Clubfoot posteromedial release: Advantages of tibialis anterior tendon lengthening. J Pediatr Orthop 22:526–532, 2002.

23. Simons GW: Complete subtalar release in club feet: Part II—Comparison with less extensive procedures. J Bone Joint Surg Am 67:1056–1065, 1985.

24. Otremski I, Salama R, Khermosh O, Wientroub S: An analysis of the results of a modified one-stage posteromedial release (Turco Operation) for the treatment of clubfoot. J Pediatr Orthop 7:149–151, 1987.

24a. Thompson GH, Richardson AB, Westin WW: Surgical management of resistant congenital talipes equinovarus deformities. J Bone Joint Surg Am 64:652–665, 1982.

25. Turko VJ: Resistant congenital club foot—one stage posteromedial release with internal fixation. J Bone Joint Surg Am 61:805–813, 1979.

26. McKay DW: New concept of and approach to clubfoot treatment: Section III—evaluation and results. J Pediatr Orthop 3:141–148, 1983.

27. Moses W, Allen BL Jr, Pugh LI, Stasikelis PJ: Predictive value of intraoperative clubfoot radiographs on revision rates. J Pediatr Orthop 20:529–532, 2000.

28. Lau JHK, Meyer LC, Lau HC: Results of surgical treatment of talipes equinovarus congenital. Clin Orthop 248:219–226, 1989.

29. Levin MN, Kuo KN, Harris GF, Matesi DV: Posteromedial release for idiopathic talipes equinovarus. Clin Orthop 242:265–268, 1989.

30. Yngve DA, Gross RH, Sullivan JA: Clubfoot release without wide subtalar release. J Pediatr Orthop 20:473–476, 1990.

31. Blakeslee TJ, DeValentine SJ: Management of the resistant idiopathic clubfoot: The Kaiser experience from 1980-1990. J Foot Ankle Surg 34:167–176, 1995.

32. Esser RD: The medial sagittal approach in the treatment of the congenital clubfoot. Clin Orthop 302:156–163, 1994.

33. Dewaele J, Zachee B, De Vleeschauwer P, Fabry G: Treatment of the idiopathic clubfoot: Critical evaluation of different types of treatment programs. J Pediatr Orthop B 3:89–95, 1994.

34. Templeton PA, Flowers MJ, Latz KH, et al: Factors predicting the outcome of the primary clubfoot surgery. Can J Surg 49:123–127, 2006.

35. Uglow MG, Clarke NM: The functional outcome of staged surgery for the correction of talipes equinovarus. J Pediatr Orthop 20:517–523, 2000.

36. Singh BI, Vaishnavi AJ: Modified Turco procedure for treatment of idiopathic clubfoot. Clin Orthop 438:209–214, 2005.

37. Sobel E, Giorgini RJ, Michel R, Cohen SI: The natural history and longitudinal study of the surgically corrected clubfoot. J Foot Ankle Surg 39:305–320, 2000.

38. Hutchins PM, Foster BK, Paterson DC, Cole EA: Long-term results of early surgical release in club feet. J Bone Joint Surg Br 67:791–798, 1985.

39. Dobbs MB, Rudzki JR, Purcell DB, et al: Factors predictive of outcome after use of the Ponseti method for the treatment of idiopathic clubfeet. J Bone Joint Surg Am 86:22–27, 2004.

40. Haft GF, Walker CG, Crawford HA: Early clubfoot recurrence after use of the Ponseti method in a New Zealand population. J Bone Joint Surg Am 89:487–493, 2007.

41. Krauspe R, Vispo Seara JL, Lohr JF: Long-term results after surgery for congenital clubfoot. J Foot Ankle Surg 2:77–82, 1996.

42. Wynne-Davies R: Talipes Equinovarus—a review of eighty-four cases after completion of treatment. J Bone Joint Surg Br 46:464–476, 1964.

43. Dobbs MB, Nunley R, Schoenecker PL: Long-term follow-up of patients with clubfeet treated with extensive soft-tissue release. J Bone Joint Surg Am 88:986–996, 2006.

44. Laaveg SJ, Ponseti IV: Long-term results of treatment of congenital clubfoot. J Bone Joint Surg Am 62:23–30, 1980.

45. Ippolito E, Farsetti P, Caterini R, Tudisco C: Long-term comparative results in patients with congenital clubfoot treated with two different protocols. J Bone Joint Surg Am 85:1286–1294, 2003.

46. Haasbeek JF, Wright JG: A comparison of the long-term results of posterior and comprehensive release in the treatment of clubfoot. J Pediatr Orthop 17:29–35, 1997.

What Is the Optimal Treatment for Hip and Spine in Myelomeningocele?

LUCIANO DIAS, MD AND VINEETA T. SWAROOP, MD

SPINE

Should Children with Myelomeningocele and Scoliosis Undergo Spinal Surgery?

In children with myelomeningocele, scoliosis is a common and complicated problem. Most of the published literature on this topic addresses the technical correction of spinal deformities. Perhaps more important, however, are the functional consequences of such a serious surgery in this patient population.

Studies have clearly shown the ability to achieve significant reduction of the scoliotic curvature with surgical treatment in patients with myelomeningocele.[1–3] Progressive, untreated scoliosis often results in loss of truncal stability, which may endanger sitting balance. Thus, the main goals of surgical intervention should be prevention of progressive spinal deformity and improvement of sitting balance.[1,4]

It is important to note that a corresponding improvement in ambulation, motor skills, and activities of daily living (ADL) has not been demonstrated in the literature. In fact, studies evaluating ambulatory ability after spinal fusion have suggested ambulation may be more difficult after surgery.[1,2,4] Multiple studies have also shown no significant difference in the ability to perform ADL after surgical intervention.[1,2,4]

Evidence

One study by Schoenmakers and colleagues[1] assessed 10 children with myelomeningocele who underwent spinal surgery. They found that ambulation became more difficult for three of the four patients who had been able to ambulate before surgery. They also note no long-term effects on ability to perform ADL after surgery (Level IV).

Another study by Müller and coworkers[2] examined the influence of surgical treatment for scoliosis on both ambulation and motor skills. This study included 14 patients from different levels of dysraphism. They found that in the eight patients with preoperative hip flexion contractures, averaging 15.2 degrees, there was a significant increase after surgery to 38.4 degrees. No patients experienced improvement in hip flexion contracture after sur-

gery. In addition, seven patients lost the ability to ambulate with or without assistive devices after surgery. These authors did note three patients who gained better sitting balance. They also found no significant difference in the ability to manage ADL from before to after surgery. Of note, the authors found no significant difference in the postoperative changes with regard to motor skills, ambulation, and ADL between the different levels of dysraphism (Level IV).

A study by Mazur and researchers[4] examined the effect of spinal fusion on sitting balance and ambulatory ability in 49 patients. They grouped results according to whether patients underwent staged anterior and posterior fusion, posterior fusion alone, or anterior fusion alone. They found improved sitting balance in 70% of patients after anterior and posterior fusions, 67% after posterior only, and 28% after anterior only. The authors also report an adverse effect on ambulation in 67% of patients with combined fusions, 27% of posterior-only fusions, and 57% of anterior-only fusions. No patients in this study showed improvement in ambulatory status after surgery. The authors also note little change in ability to perform ADL after surgery (Level III).

In a study by Wai and investigators,[3] 80 children with myelomeningocele were assessed to determine the relation of spinal deformity to physical function and self-perception. They found no significant relation between spinal deformity and overall physical function or self-perception. The only aspect of spinal deformity that showed an effect on one aspect of physical function was coronal imbalance on sitting. The authors conclude that simple interventions such as chair modifications should be explored as a means to improve coronal balance and sitting function (Level IV).

It is important to keep in mind that the presence of infrapelvic pelvic obliquity can also contribute to the overall imbalance seen in patients with myelomeningocele with scoliosis. As an example, this could result from the combination of a unilateral hip adduction contracture with a contralateral hip abduction contracture. Patients should be assessed for infrapelvic obliquity, and if present, this should be addressed at the same time as correction of any spinal deformity.

TABLE 37–1. Grade of Recommendation for the Spine

GRADE	RECOMMENDATION
C	Children with myelomeningocele and scoliosis should have surgery if the aim is to improve sitting balance.
C	Children with myelomeningocele and scoliosis should not have surgery if the aim is to improve ambulatory ability.
C	Children with myelomeningocele and scoliosis should not have surgery if the aim is to improve motor skills.
C	Children with myelomeningocele and scoliosis should not have surgery if the aim is to improve ability to perform activities of daily living.

RECOMMENDATIONS

The current literature shows that surgical correction of scoliosis in the myelomeningocele population may be accompanied by impairment in functional status. It should be mentioned that the true underlying cause of loss of function has not been defined. Many patients with myelomeningocele who do not undergo spinal surgery also demonstrate a decrease in ambulatory ability over time.

It is imperative for surgeons to counsel patients and their families before surgery that although surgical treatment of scoliosis can reliably reduce spinal curvature, the functional consequences may be severe. The goals of surgery should be clearly understood by all parties. In patients who are functionally limited to sitting before surgery, surgery may actually improve sitting balance. But ambulating patients should understand that surgery may result in decreased ambulatory ability and motor skills and no change in ADL (See Table 37–1, Grade C).

In Children Who Undergo Surgery, Should Fusion Extend to the Sacrum?

In patients with spinal deformity and pelvic obliquity, the procedure of choice typically involves combined anterior and posterior surgery with fusion extending to the sacrum to achieve better curve correction and a lower pseudoarthrosis rate.[5] Indications for extension of fusion to the sacrum include progressive scoliosis with lumbar spine involvement, neuromuscular scoliosis, pelvic obliquity greater than 15 degrees, poor sitting balance, and posterior lumbar and sacral dysraphism.[6]

Including the sacrum in fusion results in better correction of pelvic obliquity and improves sitting balance. However, it is important to note that fusion of the spine to the pelvis creates a rigid trunk, mak-

ing walking more difficult.[4] This is especially true in patients with myelomeningocele accustomed to ambulating with a swinging gait. In addition, extension of fusion to the sacrum with the resulting loss of lumbosacral mobility can adversely affect ability to perform wheelchair transfer.[7] Another potential complication associated with fusion to the sacrum is the development of ischial pressure sores. Various studies have reported on this complication with a frequency varying from 3%[5] to 33%.[8]

Wild and coworkers[7] performed a prospective study on 11 patients with myelomeningocele who underwent two-stage anterior and posterior fusion without fixation to the sacrum to evaluate their functional outcome. With an average of 4 years 11 months of follow-up, they found that pelvic obliquity spontaneously corrected when scoliosis was adequately treated with instrumented fusion not including the sacrum. In their study, the achieved correction remained stable at follow-up. The authors believe that sparing the lumbosacral segment from primary fusion offered the patients better freedom of mobility. They also state that these patients were spared the risk for complications associated with lumbosacral fixation including hardware failure, loss of correction, pressure sores, high infection rate, and high pseudoarthrosis rate (Level IV).

Should the Technique Used for Fusion Involve Anterior Surgery Only, Posterior Surgery Only, or Combined Staged Procedures?

Multiple different surgical techniques have been used to treat children with myelomeningocele and spinal deformity who are deemed appropriate candidates for operative treatment. These techniques typically fall within three broad categories: single-stage anterior fusion, single-stage posterior fusion, and two-stage anterior and posterior fusion. Multiple studies exist with the goal of determining which of these techniques provides the best results whereas minimizing risk for complications.

In a classic study, Osebold and investigators[8] examined a group of 40 patients with myelomeningocele treated with either posterior fusion alone, anterior fusion alone, or combined anterior and posterior fusion. They found a high rate of pseudoarthrosis (46%) with posterior fusion alone and a loss of initial correction for an average final correction of scoliosis of only 12 degrees. In contrast, when anterior fusion with instrumentation was used in combination with instrumented posterior fusion, they report an average final correction of 45 degrees with a decrease in the pseudoarthrosis rate to 23% (Level III).

Banta[5] also reports on a series of 50 children treated with combined anterior and posterior fusion. He notes correction of scoliosis from an average of 73 degrees to average of 34 degrees, with a pseudoarthrosis rate of only 12%. He concludes that combining anterior fusion with posterior fusion leads to increased correction of both spinal deformity and pelvic obliquity whereas also contributing significant strength to the fusion mass (Level IV).

Ward and colleagues[9] performed a retrospective review of 38 patients with myelomeningocele who underwent surgical correction of scoliosis with at least 2 years of follow-up. Patients were treated with either one-stage anterior fusion, one-stage posterior fusion, or two-stage anterior and posterior fusion. The determination of success or failure was made on the basis of radiographic results only, assessing radiographic fusion, lack of curve progression, or both. The authors report a 50% failure rate with anterior or posterior fusion alone, compared with only an 8% failure rate with two-stage procedures (Level III).

Banit and coauthors[10] report on a series of 50 patients with myelomeningocele treated with posterior-only spinal fusion for scoliosis. The authors examined whether the use of modern segmental instrumentation systems could obviate the need for two-stage procedures. Using historical controls, they found an equivalent degree of correction of scoliosis, truncal decompensation, and pelvic obliquity in their study group. They also report a pseudoarthrosis incidence rate of 16% in their study group. The authors conclude that using segmental instrumentation decreases the pseudoarthrosis rate compared with that reported with nonsegmental instrumentation. However, regardless of the instrumentation used, they did not believe posterior-only techniques could match the fusion rates obtained with combined anterior and posterior surgery (Level IV).

In another study, Basobas and coworkers[11] assessed the results of selective anterior fusion with instrumentation for the treatment of neuromuscular scoliosis in 21 patients. The authors propose that certain carefully selected patients may benefit from preservation of motion segments whereas still achieving good curve correction. They report an average curve correction of 60.3 degrees with correction of pelvic obliquity from an average of 15.1 to 3.2 degrees. Of note, they also found no change in the ambulatory status of any patient. They had only one patient (4.7%) with pseudoarthrosis. The authors conclude that anterior fusion alone is a valuable alternative to posterior fusion alone or combined anterior and posterior techniques based on their demonstrated success with curve correction and low complication rate. However, they did not comment on selection criteria for patients to be treated appropriately with anterior fusion alone (Level IV).

In contrast, Sponseller and coauthors[12] report on a series of 14 patients treated with anterior fusion alone for myelomeningocele scoliosis to define appropriate selection criteria. They conclude that anterior-only fusion may offer significant advantages including less extensive surgery with lower infection rate than posterior fusion. However, they advocated this technique only in patients with thoracolumbar curves less than 75 degrees, compensatory curves less than 40 degrees, no increased kyphosis, and no syrinx (Level IV).

In summary, many authors have reported on the challenges, complications, and poor results associated with techniques of anterior fusion alone and posterior fusion alone.[8,9] The current literature widely supports the use of staged combined anterior and posterior fusion to adequately treat patients with myelomeningocele with scoliosis and achieve the highest rates of fusion (Grade C). Only in carefully selected patients should the option of anterior-only fusion be considered. However, in the appropriate population, anterior-only fusion can provide the advantage of preserving motion segments and maintaining the ability to perform ADL with a lower rate of infection.[11,12]

HIP

Does Hip Surgery in Patients with Myelomeningocele Provide Improved Functional Results?

Transfer of iliopsoas is a technique that has been used in patients with myelomeningocele to maintain reduction of paralytic hip dislocations. Numerous studies exist reporting on the results of iliopsoas tendon transfer; however, many of these studies classify success or failure on the basis of radiologic results only. Critical review of the literature is necessary to determine the functional implications of hip surgery in the myelomeningocele population. Concerns exist regarding whether stable hip reduction leads to restricted range of motion and pathologic fractures, which would compromise the functional result.[13]

Evidence

Sherk and Ames[13] reviewed a series of 36 patients with myelomeningocele with an average follow-up of 7 years who underwent iliopsoas transfers with open reduction and capsular plication for dislocated hips. They found that 47% maintained reduction of the hip, but 17.6% of those patients demonstrated loss of hip motion and difficulty with sitting. In all patients, the transferred muscle did not function as a strong abductor. In their series, 11% experienced a worsening of their neurologic deficit. They also report a high rate of pathologic fractures after surgery that they related to disuse osteoporosis. The authors conclude that other factors, such as level of spinal lesion, lower extremity alignment, and presence of scoliosis and pelvic obliquity, were more important in determining function rather than maintenance of hip reduction (Level IV).

In another study, Duffy and investigators[14] examined gait patterns in 28 children with myelomeningocele using three-dimensional gait analysis to determine whether ambulation was improved by tendon transfers. All of the patients who had undergone posterolateral iliopsoas tendon transfer had concentrically reduced hips at the time of the study. They found no significant difference in range of pelvic obliquity in those patients who had iliopsoas transfer as compared with those who had not. They also reported worse pelvic rotation and significantly worse range of hip abduction/adduction in those who had undergone psoas transfer. The authors conclude that gait was not improved by posterolateral iliopsoas transfer (Level III).

Feiwell and colleagues[15] reviewed a series of 76 patients with myelomeningocele to compare the functional results in those who had undergone surgical treatment to reduce the hip with those who had not had surgical treatment. They found that the presence of a concentric reduction did not lead to improved hip range of motion or ability to ambulate. They also did not find a decrease in need for bracing or decrease in pain with a stable reduction of the hip. Rather, the authors did report a high rate of complications in the surgically treated group including loss of motion (29%) and pathologic fractures (17%). They conclude that the most important factor in determining ability to walk is level of neural involvement and not the status of the hip (Level III).

In a retrospective, comparative review, Sherk and coworkers[16] compared 30 patients with no surgical treatment of hip dislocation with 11 patients who had surgical treatment. In agreement with the previously reported studies, they found the ability to walk was independent of hip reduction and instead depended on neurologic level. In the surgically treated group, four patients (36%) had worsened ambulatory capacity as a result of surgical complications. Of note, the authors report that patients in the group treated without surgery had no difficulty in sitting with either unilateral or bilateral dislocated hips (Level III).

Gabrieli and researchers[17] report on a series of 20 patients with low lumbar myelomeningocele who walked with crutches that underwent three-dimensional gait analysis to determine the influence of unilateral hip dislocation on gait. They report the walking speed of patients with dislocated hips was 60% of normal, a value that corresponds to the walking speed in low-lumbar patients without hip dislocation observed in previous studies from the same center. The authors also note that gait symmetry corresponded to either absence of hip contractures or bilateral symmetric contractures. They found no relation between gait symmetry and hip dislocation, and conclude that there is no indication for surgical relocation of the unilaterally unstable hip. Rather, they recommend correcting unilateral soft-tissue contractures to restore gait symmetry (Level IV).

RECOMMENDATIONS

In conclusion, the available literature supports level of neural deficit as the most important predictor of ambulatory ability Grade B (See Table 37–2).[13,15–18] Many authors agree that extensive surgery to reduce hip dislocations is not indicated in the myelomeningocele

population.[14,15] Treatment goals should include a level pelvis and free motion of the hips rather than radiographic reduction of the hip.[15] Especially in high dislocations and older children, the only recommended surgical treatment is contracture release.[15,17]

One important consideration that is not addressed in any existing studies is how to treat the rare patient with sacral level myelomeningocele and a dislocated hip who walks without support. These patients may demonstrate an increased lurch caused by the loss of a fulcrum as a result of the hip dislocation and consequently may benefit from surgical reduction. Further studies are necessary to examine this issue. Table 37–2 provides a summary of recommendations.

TABLE 37–2. Grade of Recommendation for the Hip

STATEMENT	LEVEL OF EVIDENCE/GRADE OF RECOMMENDATION
1. Children with myelomeningocele and bilateral hip dislocations should not have surgical reduction of the dislocated hips.	B
2. Children with myelomeningocele and unilateral hip dislocation should not have surgical reduction of the dislocated hip.	B
3. Children with myelomeningocele and hip contractures associated with a dislocation should have surgical treatment of the contractures only.	B
4. Children with sacral level myelomeningocele and a hip dislocation who walk without support may benefit from surgical reduction of the hip.	I

REFERENCES

1. Schoenmakers MAGC, Gulmans VAM, Gooskens RHJM, et al: Spinal fusion in children with spina bifida: Influence on ambulation level and functional abilities. Eur Spine J 14:415–422, 2005.
2. Müller EB, Nordwall A, von Wendt L: Influence of surgical treatment of scoliosis in children with spina bifida on ambulation and motoric skills. Acta Paediatr 81:173–176, 1992.
3. Wai EK, Young NL, Feldman BM, et al: The relationship between function, self-perception, and spinal deformity. J Pediatr Orthop 25:64–69, 2005.
4. Mazur J, Menelaus MB, Dickens DRV, et al: Efficacy of surgical management for scoliosis in myelomeningocele: Correction of deformity and alteration of functional status. J Pediatr Orthop 6:568–575, 1986.
5. Banta JV: Combined anterior and posterior fusion for spinal deformity in myelomeningocele. Spine 15:946–952, 1990.
6. Widmann RF, Hresko MT, Hall JE: Lumbosacral fusion in children and adolescents using the modified sacral bar technique. Clin Orthop 364:85–91, 1999.
7. Wild A, Haak H, Kumar M, et al: Is sacral instrumentation mandatory to address pelvic obliquity in neuromuscular thoracolumbar scoliosis due to myelomeningocele? Spine 26: E325–E329, 2001.

8. Osebold WR, Mayfield JK, Winter RB, et al: Surgical treatment of paralytic scoliosis associated with myelomeningocele. J Bone Joint Surg Am 64:841–856, 1982.
9. Ward WT, Wenger DR, Roach JW: Surgical correction of myelomeningocele scoliosis: A critical appraisal of various spinal instrumentation systems. J Pediatr Orthop 9:262–268, 1989.
10. Banit DM, Iwinski HJ, Talwalkar V, et al: Posterior spinal fusion in paralytic scoliosis and myelomeningocele. J Pediatr Orthop 21:117–125, 2001.
11. Basobas L, Mardjetko S, Hammerberg K, et al: Selective anterior fusion and instrumentation for the treatment of neuromuscular scoliosis. Spine 28:S245–S248, 2003.
12. Sponseller PD, Young AT, Sarwark JF, et al: Anterior only fusion for scoliosis in patients with myelomeningocele. Clin Orthop 364:117–124, 1999.
13. Sherk HH, Ames MD: Functional results of iliopsoas transfer in myelomeningocele hip dislocations. Clin Orthop 137:181–186, 1978.
14. Duffy CM, Hill AE, Cosgrove AP, et al: Three-dimensional gait analysis in spina bifida. J Pediatr Orthop 16:786–791, 1996.
15. Feiwell E, Sakai D, Blatt T: The effect of hip reduction on function in patients with myelomeningocele. J Bone Joint Surg Am 60:169–173, 1978.
16. Sherk HH, Uppal GS, Lane G, et al: Treatment versus nontreatment of hip dislocations in ambulatory patients with myelomeningocele. Dev Med Child Neur 33:491–494, 1991.
17. Gabrieli APT, Vankoski SJ, Dias LS, et al: Gait analysis in low lumbar myelomeningocele patients with unilateral hip dislocation or subluxation. J Pediatr Orthop 23:330–334, 2003.
18. Feiwell E: Surgery of the hip in myelomeningocele as related to adult goals. Clin Orthop 148:87–93, 1980.

Chapter 38

What Is the Best Treatment of Malignant Bone Tumors in Children?

ABHA GUPTA, MD, MSC, FRCPC AND SEVAN HOPYAN, MD, PhD, FRCSC

SYSTEMIC THERAPY

The two most common primary tumors of bone are osteosarcoma (OS) and Ewing's sarcoma (ES) with an incidence of 4.8 cases/million and 2.9 cases/million, respectively, in people younger than 20 years.[1] ES is part of a family of small, round, blue cell tumors whose exact cell of origin remains unknown. The mainstay of therapy includes multiagent cytotoxic chemotherapy and effective local control with surgery and/or radiation. The following section focuses on the medical therapy of localized OS. Improvement in the survival of patients with OS has been elusive since the therapeutic breakthroughs of the late 1970s to early 1980s, despite the efforts of large multinational cooperative groups.

CHEMOTHERAPY IN OSTEOSARCOMA

It is clear that with surgery alone, 80% of patients with malignant bone tumors will develop pulmonary metastases.[2] Therefore, the treatment of OS has evolved to include systemic chemotherapy in addition to surgical resection. OS is relatively resistant to radiotherapy, so this particular modality is not used with curative intent. With current chemotherapy regimens, event-free survival remains at approximately 70% at 5 years.

Multiple fundamental issues regarding the treatment of OS remain incompletely resolved:

1. Which drugs are most effective?
2. Should postsurgical chemotherapy be tailored to percentage necrosis at the time of resection?
3. What are the relative merits of intra-arterial versus intravenous chemotherapy?
4. Should patients be treated with chemotherapy before or after surgery?

Since the late 1980s, many centers have conducted trials to attempt to answer the above questions. However, many studies are uncontrolled case series that document the outcomes of a given treatment according to an institutional protocol.

Which Drugs Are Most Effective?

It is generally accepted that cisplatin, adriamycin, ifosfamide, and methotrexate are active against OS. Various combinations of chemotherapy have been tested in randomized, controlled trials, none of which has demonstrated robust superiority over another in improving survival. A recent large trial involving 677 patients demonstrated a 6-year event-free survival rate of 64% with the use of these agents; survival did not improve with the addition of ifosfamide.[3] Although it is widely used, the role of methotrexate in OS remains uncertain[4] and is currently under investigation[4a] (Table 38–1).

Does Tailoring Postsurgical Chemotherapy According to the Degree of Tumor Response Improve Survival?

One advantage to neoadjuvant (pre-operative) chemotherapy is the opportunity provided for assessment of the tumor's response to the drugs being administered. Histologic assessment of the tumor after resection is most commonly described as per the Huvos system. A major distinction is drawn between tumors in which there are fewer than 10% residual viable cells and those with more than 10%.[9] The degree of histologic response to chemotherapy is of prognostic relevance with "responders" (patients >90% necrosis) having significantly better outcome than "nonresponders" (patients <90% necrosis). It is less clear whether changing the therapeutic regimen in patients with poor response will improve survival. Unfortunately, all studies that have attempted to address this question have been single-arm case series. None of these studies demonstrated the ability to salvage patients who had a poor response by an alteration in postoperative therapy.[10–13] Currently, an international study is under way to address this question in a randomized fashion.[13a]

Is Intra-Arterial or Intravenous Chemotherapy Better?

Some investigators have advocated the use of intra-arterial cisplatin or adriamycin to increase the local response rate that was found to be predictive of survival. Although many centers have attempted intra-arterial chemotherapy in OS, only a few randomized studies exist. Histologic response at the time of surgery improved from 43%–46% good response to 64%–77% with intravenous cisplatin compared with intra-arterial administration, respectively.[14–16] However, there was no difference in survival.

TABLE 38–1. Randomized, Controlled Trials (Excluding Intra-arterial Chemotherapy)

REFERENCE	TRIAL NAME	N	ARM 1	ARM 2	EFS	P
Winkler et al., 1984[5]	COSS-80	158	M, A, P	M, A/BCD	2.5-year rate: 68%	NS
Krailo et al., 1987[6]*	CCG	166	M, A	LD M, A	4-year rate: 38%	NS
Bramwell et al., 1992[4]	EOI	198	A, P	M, A, P (8)	(1) 5-year rate: 57% (2) 5-year rate: 41%	0.02[†]
Souhami et al., 1997[7]	EOI	407	Preoperative A, P Postoperative A, P	M, A M, A, P	5-year rate: 44%	NS
Meyers et al., 1998[8]	T12	73	M, A, P/BCD	M, A, P	(1) 5-year rate: 78% (2) 5-year rate: 73%	NS
Meyers et al., 2008[3]		677	M, A, P	MAI-MAIP	(1) 6-year rate: 64% (2) 6-year rate: 58%	NS

A, adriamycin; BCD, bleomycin/cyclophosphamide/actinomycin-D; EFS, event-free survival; I, ifosfamide; LD, low dose; M, methotrexate; MAI, methotrexate /adriamycin/ifosfamide; MAIP, methotrexate/adriamycin/ifosfamide/cisplatinum; NS, not significant; P, cisplatin.
*Adjuvant chemotherapy only.
†No difference in overall survival.

Should Patients Be Treated with Chemotherapy before or after Surgery?

Neo-adjuvant chemotherapy, which is the current standard in the treatment of OS, initially evolved in order to allow time for the construction of endoprosthetic devices. The rationale for the administration of neo-adjuvant chemotherapy includes the early treatment of micrometastatic disease, optimization of the opportunity for limb salvage procedures, and the ability to gauge tumor response to therapy. The impact of timing of surgery was recently evaluated.[17] No difference was found in survival between patients randomized to immediate surgery or neoadjuvant chemotherapy.

LOCAL CONTROL

The current basic principles for the surgical management of malignant pediatric musculoskeletal tumors were developed approximately 25 to 30 years ago when limb salvage surgery became commonly feasible. The primary basis for these principles included case series, anecdotes, and expert opinion. These principles are not disputed in the main, so few comparative studies challenge them directly. Techniques developed in this manner include safe biopsy principles and the necessity for wide en bloc resection. Here, we consider only those issues relating to local control for which there is at least Level III evidence and where the study population at least substantially involves skeletally immature patients. Comparative studies in musculoskeletal tumor surgery are primarily focused on reconstruction of defects after en bloc resection.

General Issues

Biopsy. What constitutes a safe biopsy is taught by experts, and there is no prospective study to confirm the validity of expert opinion and anecdotal evidence in this regard. Nonetheless, a comparison of outcomes in patients who underwent appropriately or poorly performed biopsy as judged retrospectively by experts revealed the latter result in about a 10% incidence rate of otherwise unnecessary functional or anatomic loss.[18]

Limb Salvage Surgery. To investigate oncologic outcomes from the late 1970s through the 1980s when limb salvage surgery was supplanting amputation for local control of bone sarcoma, researchers performed retrospective comparative studies. Survival is equivalent between amputation and limb salvage cohorts of patients with OS.[19,20]

Surgical Margins. The incidence of local recurrence after limb salvage procedures of the distal femur is greater than that after above-knee amputation. Local recurrence is less likely with more proximal levels of amputation.[19,21,22] These findings imply that the magnitude of a negative surgical margin is related to the ability to obtain local control but cannot specify what constitutes an adequate margin. Contradictory findings regarding rates of local recurrence after limb salvage or amputation have also been published,[23] suggesting that surgical selection bias influences the outcome in these retrospective comparisons.

It takes great care to plan the distal resection margin of a malignant metaphyseal bone tumor in a skeletally immature individual. Preservation of the epiphysis, and therefore the native adjacent joint, would likely be a functionally optimal and durable option. However, it is often difficult to be certain of the distal extent of the tumor. It has been shown that the accuracy of magnetic resonance imaging (MRI) in detecting involvement of the epiphysis by tumor is 90.3% using histology of the same tumors as a reference. Importantly, there are no false-negative results by computed tomography or MRI.[24] The surgical margin is therefore likely to safely correlate with preoperative MRI findings.

Surgical Complications

Two comparative studies highlight the importance of primary wound healing in the setting of limb-sparing procedures. Risk factors for developing infection of an orthopedic implant were assessed in a retrospective comparative fashion.[25] The overall implant infection incidence rate was 21%, and multivariate analysis revealed that the only modifiable risk factor in those who experienced development of implant infections compared with those who did not was local wound infection. Those who experienced implant infection were more likely to undergo amputation and had poorer functional outcomes. A prospective comparison of patients who did and did not receive primary muscle flap coverage of a structural allograft reconstruction revealed that those in the former group were less likely to undergo reoperation for bone-related complications.[26]

Nonunion of a structural allograft that is used to reconstruct skeletal defects after resection of a sarcoma is another limb-threatening complication. In a retrospective comparison of a large number of patients, it was found that those who underwent chemotherapy were more likely to develop allograft nonunion than those who did not.[27] Of course, this risk factor is not readily modifiable, but it highlights the anticipated difficult course for limb salvage reconstructions. Other retrospective comparisons have shown that locking plates improve the union rate of host-allograft junctions compared with ordinary plates,[28] and that intramedullary cement can decrease the incidence of allograft fractures.[29] In a comparison of reconstructions that used allograft alone versus allograft-vascularized fibular composites, it was shown that complication rates were comparable.[30] The presence of a vascularized fibula, however, hastened the time to union.

Surgery versus Radiotherapy for Ewing's Sarcoma

Radiotherapy and surgery have been used individually or combined for the local control of ES. Multiple retrospective comparisons of these 2 modalities have been performed as part of large cooperative group studies. In these studies, the treating physicians chose the modality for local control. Most studies demonstrate superior local control after surgery alone or when surgery and radiation are combined compared with radiotherapy alone,[31] whereas others show equivalent results.[31,32] However, some of these findings may reflect bias in the selection of radiation for larger tumors. Intralesional debulking surgery combined with radiotherapy results in local recurrence rates similar to local treatment with radiotherapy alone.[31] The additional risks posed by the use of radiotherapy, such as development of a second malignant neoplasm,[33] need to be considered when making decisions to undertake local control. A comparison of large, prospective studies reveals that if radiotherapy is used, survival is better when it is administered earlier in the course of chemotherapy as opposed to later.[31]

SPECIFIC RECONSTRUCTIVE OPTIONS

Upper Extremity

Reconstructive options after extra-articular resection of the shoulder together with the abductor mechanism include suspension arthroplasty with a spacer (metal or bone graft) and allograft intercalary fusion of the remaining native scapula to the native distal humerus. In a retrospective comparison of patients who underwent one of these two types of reconstruction, it was shown that physician-administered functional outcome measures (Musculoskeletal Tumor Society) are superior in those with a fusion.[34] There are, of course, other factors to consider when choosing such a reconstruction, such as patient preference, the relative incidence of complications, and the planned strategy to manage anticipated limb-length discrepancy in young children.

Lower Extremity

When the articular surface of the distal femur or proximal tibia needs to be resected, the reconstructive options include replacement of the joint with a mega-endoprosthesis, an allograft-endoprosthetic composite, or an osteoarticular allograft; ablation of the joint by above-knee amputation or by rotationplasty; or arthrodesis of the joint. The use of an intercalary allograft to perform an arthrodesis of the knee as a limb-sparing reconstruction is associated with a greater rate of complications compared with allograft use in other settings.[27,35] Osteoarticular allografts were found to be less predictably successful than endoprostheses in a mixed-age population,[36] and allograft-endoprosthetic composites are less predictably successful than mega-endoprostheses in adults.[37]

Many pediatric cases are frequently amenable to what are likely the most reasonable two options: endoprosthetic replacement or rotationplasty. The decision to undertake one or the other is often individualized and is largely made by the patient and their family based on the anticipated relative functionality, appearance, durability, and risk for complications. Retrospective comparisons[38–40] have shown that the functional outcome and quality of life after rotationplasty is comparable with that of endoprosthetic reconstruction both with regard to physician-administered (Musculoskeletal Tumor Society) and patient-derived (Toronto Extremity Salvage Score, Short Form 36, European Organization for Research and Treatment of Cancer) scores. The outcome of both of these reconstructive options score modestly greater than that of above-knee amputation. In general, outcome scores are better with limb salvage compared with amputation, except when the amputation is below the knee.[41] Internal hemipelvectomy for pelvic tumors is also advantageous over hind-quarter amputation.[41] No reconstruction of the pelvis after resection is associated with lower complication rates and at least comparable function compared with reconstruction of pelvic defects in children.[42,43]

Expandable endoprostheses bear mention because of their increasing popularity. Multiple case series involving various generations of these implants seem to document a relatively high rate of complications such as implant fracture,[44] which are not common in adult series. No comparisons have been made yet to biological reconstruction or to reconstruction with a nonexpandable endoprosthesis combined with an alternative approach for the management of limb-length discrepancy from which to draw conclusions.

SUMMARY

- Poorly performed biopsy increases the incidence of unnecessary functional and anatomic loss (Level III).[18]

- Limb salvage surgery does not compromise survival compared with amputation (Level III).[19,20]
- Wide negative margins are required to avoid local recurrence (Level III).[19,21,22]
- Soft-tissue coverage is important to minimize complications (Level III).[25,26]
- Physician-assessed shoulder function is better with an arthrodesis compared with a suspension reconstruction (Level III).[34]
- Rotationplasty and endoprosthetic reconstruction are functionally favorable compared with above-knee amputation (Level III)[38–41]

Table 38–2 provides a summary of recommendations for treatment of malignant bone tumors in children.

TABLE 38–2. Summary of Recommendations

STATEMENT	LEVEL OF EVIDENCE/GRADE OF RECOMMENDATION	REFERENCES
1. Chemotherapy is essential to reduce development of metastatic disease in OS.	A	2
2. Cisplatin and adriamycin are essential drugs in OS.	A	3
3. Intra-arterial chemotherapy does not improve survival compared with intravenous chemotherapy.	B	14–16
4. Poorly performed biopsy increases the incidence of unnecessary functional and anatomic loss.	B	18
5. Limb salvage surgery does not compromise survival compared with amputation.	B	19,20
6. Wide negative margins are required to avoid local recurrence.	B	19,21,22
7. Soft-tissue coverage is important to minimize complications.	B	25,26
8. Physician-assessed should function is better with an arthrodesis compared with a suspension reconstruction.	B	34
9. Rotationplasty and endoprosthetic reconstruction are functionally favorable compared with above-kneed amputation.	B	38–41

REFERENCES

1. Gurney JG, Bulterys M: Malignant bone tumors. Cancer incidence and survival among children and adolescents: United States SEER Program 1975–1995. Ries LAG, Gurney JG (eds). Bethesda, MD, National Institutes of Health, 1999, pp 99–110.
2. Link MP, et al: The effect of adjuvant chemotherapy on relapse-free survival in patients with osteosarcoma of the extremity. N Engl J Med 314:1600–1606, 1986.
3. Meyers PA, Schwartz CL, Krailo MD, et al: Osteosarcoma: the addition of muramyl tripeptide to chemotherapy improves overall survival–a report from the Children's Oncology Group. J Clin Oncol 26(4):633-638, 2008.
4. Bramwell VH, et al: A comparison of two short intensive adjuvant chemotherapy regimens in operable osteosarcoma of limbs in children and young adults: The first study of the European Osteosarcoma Intergroup. J Clin Oncol 10:1579–1591, 1992.

4a. De Camargo B, Van den Berg H, Van Dalen EC: Methotrexate for high-grade osteosarcoma in children and young adults. Cochrane Database of Systematic Reviews 2, 2008. CD 006325
5. Winkler K, et al: Neoadjuvant chemotherapy for osteogenic sarcoma: Results of a Cooperative German/Austrian study. J Clin Oncol 2:617–624, 1984.
6. Krailo M, et al: A randomized study comparing high-dose methotrexate with moderate-dose methotrexate as components of adjuvant chemotherapy in childhood nonmetastatic osteosarcoma: A report from the Childrens Cancer Study Group. Med Pediatr Oncol 15:69–77, 1987.
7. Souhami RL, et al: Randomised trial of two regimens of chemotherapy in operable osteosarcoma: A study of the European Osteosarcoma Intergroup. Lancet 350:911–917, 1997.
8. Meyers PA, et al: Intensification of preoperative chemotherapy for osteogenic sarcoma: Results of the Memorial Sloan-Kettering (T12) protocol. J Clin Oncol 16:2452–2458, 1998.
9. Huvos AG, Rosen G, Marcove RC: Primary osteogenic sarcoma: Pathologic aspects in 20 patients after treatment

with chemotherapy en bloc resection, and prosthetic bone replacement. Arch Pathol Lab Med 101:14–18, 1977.

10. Rosen G, et al: Preoperative chemotherapy for osteogenic sarcoma: Selection of postoperative adjuvant chemotherapy based on the response of the primary tumor to preoperative chemotherapy. Cancer 49:1221–1230, 1982.

11. Winkler K, et al: Neoadjuvant chemotherapy of osteosarcoma: Results of a randomized cooperative trial (COSS-82) with salvage chemotherapy based on histological tumor response. J Clin Oncol 6:329–337, 1988.

12. Saeter G, et al: Treatment of osteosarcoma of the extremities with the T-10 protocol, with emphasis on the effects of preoperative chemotherapy with single-agent high-dose methotrexate: A Scandinavian Sarcoma Group study. J Clin Oncol 9:1766–1775, 1991.

13. Provisor AJ, et al: Treatment of nonmetastatic osteosarcoma of the extremity with preoperative and postoperative chemotherapy: A report from the Children's Cancer Group. J Clin Oncol 15:76–84, 1997.

13a. National Cancer Institute. Combination chemotherapy, PEG-interferon alfa-2b, and surgery in treating patients with osteosarcoma. http://www.cancer.gov/search/ViewClinicalTrials.aspx?cdrid=438714&version=patient&protocolsearchid=4812149. Accessed July 2008.

14. Bacci G, et al: Effect of intra-arterial versus intravenous cisplatin in addition to systemic adriamycin and high-dose methotrexate on histologic tumor response of osteosarcoma of the extremities. J Chemother 4:189–195, 1992.

15. Bacci G, et al: A comparison of methods of loco-regional chemotherapy combined with systemic chemotherapy as neo-adjuvant treatment of osteosarcoma of the extremity. Eur J Surg Oncol 27:98–104, 2001.

16. Ferrari S, et al: Nonmetastatic osteosarcoma of the extremity: Results of a neoadjuvant chemotherapy protocol (IOR/OS-3) with high-dose methotrexate, intraarterial or intravenous cisplatin, doxorubicin, and salvage chemotherapy based on histologic tumor response. Tumori 85:458–464, 1999.

17. Goorin AM, et al: Presurgical chemotherapy compared with immediate surgery and adjuvant chemotherapy for nonmetastatic osteosarcoma: Pediatric Oncology Group Study POG-8651. J Clin Oncol 21:1574–1580, 2003.

18. Mankin HJ, Mankin CJ, Simon MA: The hazards of the biopsy, revisited. Members of the Musculoskeletal Tumor Society. J Bone Joint Surg Am 78:656–663, 1996.

19. Rougraff BT, et al: Limb salvage compared with amputation for osteosarcoma of the distal end of the femur. A long-term oncological, functional, and quality-of-life study. J Bone Joint Surg Am 76:649–656, 1994.

20. Simon MA, et al: Limb-salvage treatment versus amputation for osteosarcoma of the distal end of the femur. J Bone Joint Surg Am 68:1331–1337, 1986.

21. Bacci G, et al: Predictive factors for local recurrence in osteosarcoma: 540 patients with extremity tumors followed for minimum 2.5 years after neoadjuvant chemotherapy. Acta Orthop Scand 69:230–236, 1998.

22. Picci P, et al: Relationship of chemotherapy-induced necrosis and surgical margins to local recurrence in osteosarcoma. J Clin Oncol 12:2699–2705, 1994.

23. Sluga M, et al: Local and systemic control after ablative and limb sparing surgery in patients with osteosarcoma. Clin Orthop Relat Res (358):120–127, 1999.

24. San-Julian M, et al: Indications for epiphyseal preservation in metaphyseal malignant bone tumors of children: Relationship between image methods and histological findings. J Pediatr Orthop 19:543–548, 1999.

25. Gaur AH, et al: Infections in children and young adults with bone malignancies undergoing limb-sparing surgery. Cancer 104:602–610, 2005.

26. Mastorakos DP, et al: Soft-tissue flap coverage maximizes limb salvage after allograft bone extremity reconstruction. Plast Reconstr Surg 109:1567–1573, 2002.

27. Hornicek FJ, et al: Factors affecting nonunion of the allograft-host junction. Clin Orthop Relat Res (382):87–98, 2001.

28. Buecker PJ, et al: Locking versus standard plates for allograft fixation after tumor resection in children and adolescents. J Pediatr Orthop 26:680–685, 2006.

29. Ozaki T, et al: Intramedullary, antibiotic-loaded cemented, massive allografts for skeletal reconstruction. 26 cases compared with 19 uncemented allografts. Acta Orthop Scand 68:387–391, 1997.

30. Belt PJ, Dickinson IC, Theile DR: Vascularised free fibular flap in bone resection and reconstruction. Br J Plast Surg 58:425–430, 2005.

31. Dunst J, Schuck A: Role of radiotherapy in Ewing tumors. Pediatr Blood Cancer 42:465–470, 2004.

32. Yock TI, et al: Local control in pelvic Ewing sarcoma: Analysis from INT-0091—a report from the Children's Oncology Group. J Clin Oncol 24:3838–3843, 2006.

33. Henderson TO, et al: Secondary sarcomas in childhood cancer survivors: A report from the Childhood Cancer Survivor Study. J Natl Cancer Inst 99:300–308, 2007.

34. O'Connor MI, Sim FH, Chao EY: Limb salvage for neoplasms of the shoulder girdle. Intermediate reconstructive and functional results. J Bone Joint Surg Am 78:1872–1888, 1996.

35. Donati D, et al: Allograft arthrodesis treatment of bone tumors: A two-center study. Clin Orthop Relat Res (400): 217–224, 2002.

36. Brien EW, et al: Allograft reconstruction after proximal tibial resection for bone tumors. An analysis of function and outcome comparing allograft and prosthetic reconstructions. Clin Orthop Relat Res (303):116–127, 1994.

37. Wunder JS, et al: Comparison of two methods of reconstruction for primary malignant tumors at the knee: A sequential cohort study. J Surg Oncol 77:89–100, 2001.

38. Cammisa FP Jr, et al: The Van Nes tibial rotationplasty. A functionally viable reconstructive procedure in children who have a tumor of the distal end of the femur. J Bone Joint Surg Am 72:1541–1547, 1990.

39. Hillmann A, et al: Malignant tumor of the distal part of the femur or the proximal part of the tibia: endoprosthetic replacement or rotationplasty. Functional outcome and quality-of-life measurements. J Bone Joint Surg Am 81:462–468, 1999.

40. Hopyan S, et al: Function and upright time following limb salvage, amputation, and rotationplasty for pediatric sarcoma of bone. J Pediatr Orthop 26:405–408, 2006.

41. Pardasaney PK, et al: Advantage of limb salvage over amputation for proximal lower extremity tumors. Clin Orthop Relat Res 444:201–208, 2006.

42. Hillmann A, et al: Tumors of the pelvis: complications after reconstruction. Arch Orthop Trauma Surg 123:340–344, 2003.

43. Schwameis E, et al: Reconstruction of the pelvis after tumor resection in children and adolescents. Clin Orthop Relat Res (402):220–235, 2002.

44. Gitelis S, et al: The use of a closed expandable prosthesis for pediatric sarcomas. Chir Organi Mov 88:327–333, 2003.

Chapter 39

What Is the Best Treatment for Simple Bone Cysts?

Suzanne Yandow, MD

Simple bone cysts (SBCs) are benign bone tumors with a thin, cystlike lining and a fluid-filled cavity.[1,2] They occur most commonly in the metaphyses of long bones in skeletally immature patients, although they have been reported in almost every bone of the skeleton.[3] The proximal humerus and femur are the most common locations, with 50% to 80% humeral and 20% to 30% femoral in several large studies.[4-6] Many cysts heal near skeletal maturity, thereby explaining the rarity in adults, but several large series have patients in their 40s and 50s.[4,7,8] Male-to-female ratios are varied, but two to three times greater in male than female individuals in most large series.[4-6,9] SBCs are one of the most common bone tumors in children, representing 3% of all bone lesion biopsies.[10-12] Many more lesions, however, have classic radiographic appearance and are never biopsied. The lesions, although characteristically metaphyseal and central, may rarely cross the physis.[13-16] Most SBCs are centrally located and thought to originate from or near a physis. Various theories of cyst origin include physeal aberrations, venous obstruction, and synovial entrapment, or "local disturbance of bone growth and development."[2,7,17-20] SBCs were also called *unicameral* or *solitary cysts.* Although normally solitary, multiple concomitant cysts have been reported.[21] Monolocular, or unicameral, is the common initial presentation, but fracture or treatment commonly results in septation and multiloculation. Rarely, SBC presents with more extensive ossification, confusing the diagnosis.[22,23] Extension into the diaphysis is commonly reported and may represent a large active lesion that extends from the physis to mid-diaphysis, or a small latent diaphyseal cyst that has grown away from the physis.[24,25] Cysts are radiolucent because of the fluid content, which is serous in nature but has some unique properties such as greater prostaglandin levels.[18,26-30] This fluid under pressure could cause the endosteal erosion and bone expansion that is characteristic of these lesions.[31] This expansion may also be due to bone weakness and the body's attempt to preserve strength by increasing bone diameter.[32,33] Cysts that occupy greater then 85% of the bone diameter are associated with increased risk for fracture.[34] This is supported by the fact that healing cysts tend to "tubulate", or narrow, and fragile cysts at risk for fracture are more expanded.[35] Fracture in this weakened bone is common and may produce the classic "fallen-fragment"

sign.[36-38] This small fleck of bone fractures and settles in the cystic content. Fracture initiates a healing response and may cause opacification and septation with the cyst.[39] Once the aggressive phase of fracture healing passes, however, the cyst, which appears to be healing, may again become more radiolucent and at risk for future fracture. Garceau and Gregory,[40] in 1954, reported 15% cyst healing after fracture, but the true natural history of cyst healing has not been reported because of frequent and varied interventions and treatments. Lesions are reported to recur up to 4 years after initial healing.[41] A natural history study was attempted by Neer and researchers[16] but abandoned because of frequent fractures. Fractures may result in limb shortening and angular deformity. Physeal involvement may also cause the limb length inequality and angular deformity. Perceived risk for fracture prevents many children from participation in physical activities until cyst resolution. This can be disruptive to childhood for extended periods and limit activities.[11,12]

Bone cysts were first recognized by Virchow in 1891 and delineated more clearly in a case series by Bloodgood in 1910.[42] Since these early times, numerous and various treatments have been proposed and combined. This chapter references more than 130 articles with greater than 20 treatment variations. The fact that so many variations and combinations of treatment for one bone lesion exists suggests the failure of any single current treatment for complete and permanent healing. Most articles are Level IV evidence and represent either single-center or multicenter case experiences with a single treatment. A few articles are comparison studies of two treatments and represent Level III evidence, but only one Level I evidence article is currently available. Another difficulty related to evaluation of cyst treatment is there is no universal system for defining a healed cyst. Neer proposed a classification that has been modified by many, but no study has outlined definitively what constitutes a healed cyst[5,8,11,43-49] (Table 39-1). Most practitioners agree that even if a small cyst is present, as long as it does not pose a significant fracture risk and is not increasing in size, then observation is reasonable.[4] Recent studies, however, have suggested that plain radiographs may be an inadequate measure of fracture risk and suggest computed tomographic (CT) scan as an alternative measure of fracture risk.[32] Magnetic resonance imaging (MRI) study is also promising for

TABLE 39–1. Summary of Criteria for Healing

Graham (1951)[43]	• Trabeculae traversing cyst cavity: "Obliteration of cyst" • Obliteration of cyst
Neer et al. (new) (1966)[4]	Proposed classification: • Excellent = complete obliteration • Residual defect = one or more static, cystlike residual with good bone strength suggested by the appearance of the roentgenogram • Reoperation = subsequent operation required by recurrence • True recurrence = cavity reappears, enlarges causing expansion and thinning of cortex Incomplete obliteration of the cyst after operation appears to be of little clinical significance, provided there is good bone strength
Spence et al. (new) (1969)[44]	• Healed = complete obliteration • Recurrence = any residual cystic defect
Baker (1970)[45]	• Healed: 2 categories • Incomplete healing: 3 categories • Recurrence
Capanna et al. (modification of Neer Criteria) (1982)[8]	• Healed: cyst completely filled with bone and cortical margins thickened • Healed with residual: cyst consolidated with bone and the cortical margins thickened, but still small residual areas of osteolysis within cyst • Recurrence: cyst initially consolidated; however, large areas of osteolysis and cortical thinning subsequently returned • No response: no evidence of response to treatments (3 and 4 are considered failures)
Chigara et al. (1983)[17]	• Good • Fair • Poor
Oppenheim and Galleno (1984)[11]	• Healed = complete obliteration or <1 cm radiolucent • Improved = 1–3-cm area of radiolucency, nonprogressive cortical thickening • Incomplete obliteration = nonprogressive radiolucent areas greater than 3 cm or thin cortical rim • Recurrence = reappearance of cystic area in prior obliterated/healed cyst, progressive cortical thinning
Lokiec et al. (1996)[114] Weintroub (1989)[104]	Features of healing: a. Consolidation b. Narrowing c. Decreased expansion d. Cortical thickening
Hashemi-Nejad and Cole (modification of Neer criteria; Reverse of Neer) (1997)[47]	• Grade 1: cyst clearly visible • Grade 2: cyst visible, but multilocular and opaque • Grade 3: sclerosis around or within a partially visible cyst • Grade 4: complete healing with obliteration of the cyst Grade 1–2 = unsatisfactory healing Grade 3–4 = satisfactory healing
Killian (modification of Neer criteria) (1998)[48]	• I: Complete = completely filled in with new bone, obliterating cyst • II: Incomplete = new bone, increased cortical width, small area of osteolysis 1–3 cm in diameter • III: Recurrence = cortical thinning or cyst >3 cm • IV: No response
Yandow et al. (1998)[49]	Substantial healing Partial healing Failure to respond • Enlargement • Expansion • Cortical thinning
Chang et al. (2002)[6]	Healed: cyst filled by formation of new bone with or without small static, radiolucent area(s) less than 1 cm in size Healing with defect: static, radiolucent area(s) less than 50% of the diameter of bone with enough cortical thickness to prevent fracture Persistent cyst: radiolucent areas greater than 50% of diameter of the bone and with a thin cortical rim; no increase in cyst size; continued restriction of activity or repeated treatment is required Recurrent cyst: cyst reappeared in a previously obliterated area or a residual radiolucent area has increased in size
Wright (modification of Neer and Cole criteria) (2008)[56]	Not healed: Grade 1: cyst clearly visible Grade 2: cyst visible, but multilocular and opaque Healed: Grade 3: sclerosis around or within a partially visible cyst Grade 4: complete healing with obliteration of cyst

Definition of healing: One of the single greatest difficulties in comparison of treatments and natural history is the definition of healing of simple bone cysts.

assessing the load-carrying capacity of bones with osteolytic lesions.[50] With poor outcome tools used for measurement of SBC healing, the comparison of treatment is arbitrary and difficult. Without having an accurate comparison of cysts before treatment, stratification for randomization is also arbitrary. Cysts are known to begin healing and then recur more than 2 to 4 years after healing.[41,51] This may represent reactivation of a smaller remaining cystic area or recurrence of a completely healed or resected cyst.[52] Capanna and coauthors[8] described 12 of 90 patients treated with steroid injection whose cysts recurred after initial consolidation. Most studies have less than 2-year minimum follow-up and, therefore, show early promise for cyst healing, but later extensive follow-up demonstrates recurrence or persistence, or both, of these lesions.[4,6,41] Few articles evaluate the angular deformity and limb-length inequality that results from cysts.[53–55] Some of this may be because of the presence of the cyst near the physis, and others may represent physeal damage secondary to treatment. Few studies evaluate whether patients have persistent pain or functional difficulties; however, one recent study does attempt to incorporate functional outcomes using the Activity Scale for Kids (ASK) and pain assessment using the OUCHER scale in a randomized prospective study of two treatments.[49,56]

FACTORS THAT AFFECT CYST HEALING

Many factors related to the location of the cyst and its host have been proposed to affect the rate of healing.[57,58] Most of the series that discuss cyst treatment qualify the results by separating these various factors, which are discussed later. This, however, does not separate the treatment groups before initiation of treatment and, therefore, does not provide equivalent groups for study purposes. More randomized prospective trials will be needed to clarify factors that may affect healing and then to compare head-to-head the various treatments.

Lesion Size

Cysts can vary from less than 1 cm^2 on two orthogonal views to large complex lesions extending from physis to mid-diaphysis, or more than 50% the length of the bone.[49] Cyst index based on size and geography of the lesion was described by Kaelin and McEwen[60] as a predictor for fracture risk, but a recent article suggests poor reliability for this technique as a predictor of fracture.[59] Others have demonstrated that larger cyst areas correlate with poorer healing.[8,56] Capanna and coauthors[8] defined small cysts as less than 24 cm^2. Spence and coworkers,[44] in 1969, in a large multicenter review, showed 80% healing of small lesions, 49% of medium lesions, and 53% of large cysts. This makes excellent sense because larger lesions theoretically have been present for a longer time and may be recalcitrant to the body's attempts at healing.

Patient Age and Sex

Cysts are uniformly reported in all series reviewed to occur more frequently in male than female individuals. The most common male-to-female ratio is 3:1.[9,44] The only exception is 1 smaller series by Dorman[121] in 2005 with a 1:1 ratio. The variation in number of male and female patients may affect the healing rates, as Spence suggested in his large multicenter series review of 177 cases. Cysts occur in all age groups. Originally, patients younger than 10 years were considered to have more active cysts.[31] Capanna and coauthors,[8] in 1982, found less recurrence of cysts after steroid treatment in patients 0 to 5 years of age and poorer healing in those older than 6. Spence and coworkers[5] confirm in his large review the adverse effect of younger age on healing. Spence and coworkers also report that female patients had healed cysts in 77% of cases, whereas only 48% of male patients had healed cysts in his review ($P < 0.001$).[44] Case series by Chigira[46], Garceau[40], Neer[4], and Capanna[8] include patients with cysts at older than 50 years. The overall lower frequency of this lesion in adulthood in many articles, however, helps us to understand that physeal closure and skeletal maturity does, in some unknown way, promote cyst healing.[61] This is important because many of the reviewed articles vary in average age from 6.9 to 17.3 years.[62,63] This variation of age may be the cause of variations in healing rates.

Proximity to Physis

Cysts were categorized as active and latent originally by Jaffe and Lichtenstein[7] in 1942, based on proximity to the physis. Lesions less than 1 cm from the physis are considered active. Variation of healing response of active verses latent cysts exists in numerous reported series since that time.[40,45,64] Neer, however, in a large series of 175 cases, found no difference in healing of active verses latent cysts.[4] Spence, in contrast, showed healing in 35% of active cysts and 67% of latent cysts.[5] The data are inconsistent regarding whether location of cyst affects healing. Many articles even fail to evaluate this before treatment.[65,66] No trials of similar treatment in randomized groups of active verses latent cysts have been reported to clearly compare location as a unique factor related to healing.

Cyst Fluid and Venous Outflow. An early study of cyst fluid was conducted by Cohen in 1960.[18] It was found to be either serous or bloody, but no correlation to healing was made. Needle perforation and measurement of manometric pressure was elucidated by Neer and coworkers[4] in 1966. Active cysts had pressures of 30 cm of H_2O and pulsated with Valsalva maneuver. Enneking,[31] using this technique, also performed cystograms with injections of radiopaque contrast material attempting to correlate active lesions with rapid outflow of contrast into the venous circulation, and puddling and slow outflow with latent cysts. These are Level IV, observational, and Level V expert opinion articles. Draining or venting the cystic cavity is described in various articles with K-wires, cannulated screws, and intramedullary rods, and these articles are reported and level of evidence reviewed in this summary separately.

Bone Location

SBCs are reported in almost every bone; however, jaw lesions have a different histologic appearance and may be a separate entity. For the purposes of this chapter, these are not included. Greater than 90% of cysts occur in long bones. The calcaneus represents an unusual location, and treatment series for this bone are reported separately in this chapter. The proximal humerus is the most common location. In 195 cases reviewed by Mirra,[10] 44% were proximal humerus, and the second most common condition was proximal femur with 26% of cases. Hands are a rare location for SBCs. Neer's series[4] showed the femur as the most common location for cyst in adulthood, but fractures of adult cyst were also rarer. Healing rates for treatment of femoral cysts may be higher because of the weight-bearing status of the bone initiating a healing response because of added load. This weight-bearing bone, however, makes this location more at risk for fracture. Angular deformities are reported in numerous studies and may lead to the benefit of intramedullary devices for load sharing or external support during healing.[65,67] Location also refers to the location of the cyst within the bone. Metaphysis is the most common initial presentation. Although called *simple cysts,* their geography and variability is extensive. Cross-sectional imaging (MRI and CT scan) is adding to a more detailed understanding of these lesions.[68,69]

Length of Follow-Up

Another of the significant difficulties in comparing healing rates of various treatments is the length of post-treatment follow-up. Follow-up varies from 6 months to 20 years in one series.[70] Enneking[31] states that fracture or intervention to the cyst initially stimulates an aggressive biologic fracture healing response. This promotes early bone formation and opacification of the cyst and "healing." Once this process becomes more quiescent, the tumor's biology may again become more active and cause "recurrence" or "visible reappearance" of the lesion.[71] Many series report recurrence more than 2 years after treatment in lesions that initially "healed."[5,72] Docquier and Delloye[73] had a recurrence at 89 months (7.4 years) after treatment. Therefore, uniform, longer length of follow-up may ruin early positive results. Lokiec and Wientroub[12] report 100% healing with bone marrow injection in his preliminary report, but follow-up in some patients was only 12 months. Neer's report carries such long-term value because of his insistence of a minimum 2-year follow-up period.

Capanna and coauthors describe an interesting phenomenon not studied by others since his articles in 1982.[8] Recurrences occurred at varying rates based on healing patterns:

1. If cyst consolidation was complete but further compartmentalization occurred with bony septae, 28.5% of cysts recurred.
2. If cyst consolidation was incomplete and areas of osteolysis persisted, the recurrence rate was 54%.
3. If cyst consolidation was complete but a rim of osteolysis persisted at the periphery, the recurrence rate was 100%.

Future randomized, prospective study must take the high risk for late recurrence into consideration. A minimum follow-up period of 2 years after final treatment of fracture is recommended. Longer follow-up time until complete skeletal maturity would add value to any cyst treatment or natural history study.

TRANSFORMATION OF SIMPLE BONE CYSTS

Six cases of malignant conversion of SBC to sarcoma have been reported, but 5 are unproved because of lack of biopsy confirmation of the SBC before transformation, and therefore a lesser level of certainty.[74] There is 1 report of malignant transformation to chondrosarcoma from a biopsy-proved SBC.[75] This biopsy confirmation of SBC, and later biopsy confirmation of sarcoma, is valuable for the understanding that malignant conversion is a true risk, but not for estimating its incidence, which must be low. SBC can transform into another benign lesion, aneurysmal bone cyst (ABC).[76,77] ABC may represent a spectrum of the same disease as SBC, as Neer and coauthors discussed in 1973.[78–81] Separation of the two may be difficult even with cross-sectional imaging. Biopsy may be indicated for definitive diagnosis.[13,82,83] Recognition of this possibility is important because ABC does not respond to many forms of treatment proposed for SBC.[84] Injections of steroids into ABC were tried by Scaglietti and investigators[85] and abandoned because of poor healing in the original series of patients in 1982.

HISTORICAL SUMMARY OF TREATMENT RECOMMENDATIONS AND LEVEL OF EVIDENCE COMPARISON

Although variation of characteristics of the SBC exists, variations of treatment recommended in the literature are also widely variable and difficult to compare.[86] There is only 1 Level I evidence article on the treatment of SBC; the remaining reports, no matter how large, are either case series Level IV or, at best, retrospective comparative Level III.[6,9,11,66] Lokiec's series[114] in 1996 is prospective but not comparative and may be considered Level II evidence regarding prognosis, but only Level IV evidence regarding selection of therapy because no comparison was made.

Early Case Series (Level IV)

The earliest articles were summaries of case descriptions by Bloodgood in 1910,[42] Phemister[20] and Gordon in 1926, James and colleagues[41] in 1942, Graham[43] in 1951, and Garceau and Gregory[40] in 1954. They focus on the pathology of the lesion, and Garceau states a 15% healing rate after fracture with observation alone. Blount[61] reports in *Fractures in Children* that most cysts heal during childhood. A natural history study following fracture of cysts was further attempted by Neer[4] in 1966 but abandoned during the study because of greater than 70% refracture in both humeral and femoral locations. Active verses latent cysts were compared with little variation of refracture rate. These case series are Level IV evidence, but they are important for historical significance.

Intralesional Curettage and Grafting (Level IV)

The largest group of articles in the literature on the treatment of SBC reports results for intralesional curettage and grafting. Graft materials were initially autograft, but subsequent series have recommended allograft and a host of other nonbiologic materials, which are discussed separately.[87,88] In early studies after curettage, the lining was removed; then the residual rim was treated with phenol or zinc chloride, followed by bone grafting. Curettage provided cyst lining to pathology, and detailed descriptions of findings by Geschickter and Copeland,[90] Jaffe,[89] and Jaffe and Lichtenstein[7] delineated the histologic findings of simple cysts. Some are cases series Level IV and others comparative and Level III. Neer and coworkers[4] showed no difference in those treated with or without adjuvant chemicals; therefore, this step was abandoned, but later series did advocate cryosurgery to ablate the lining.[91] Neer's series was the largest reported at that time and carefully outlined many variables contributing to treatment results including location, age, and proximity to the physis. He also proposed one of the first grading scales for cyst healing, which serves as the basis for most other authors. Variations of this are still used today, and a variation was utilized in the current randomized, prospective trial by Wright.[4,8,47,56] The problems with intralesional curettage and grafting are the need for a larger open procedure, the necessity of harvesting bone graft and its risk, the risk for physeal damage with curetting near the physis in active cysts, and universally, the reports of recurrence despite initial healing.[9,11,40,43,45,92–94] The complications of autograft harvesting and the shortage of bone available to fill the cyst led some authors to recommend allograft and bone substitutes. Peltier and Jones,[95] in 1978, reported a new technique of curettage followed by filling the lesion with sterile plaster of Paris(Ethicon). Ninety-two percent of these patients healed, but 8% recurred and 12% (3/26) either had post-operative drainage or infection. The technique did not spread widely into the literature. Spence and coworkers,[44] in 1969, reported a Level IV multicenter large series of 177 patients treated with freeze-dried allograft. Recurrence or failure of healing, however, was 45%, and this technique was not popularized, likely because of the high recurrence rate. Because of the recurrence seen with intralesional curettage and grafting with or without bone, radical or subtotal resection of the cysts were next historically recommended.

Radical or Subtotal Cyst Resection (Level IV)

Agerholm and Goodfellow[96] described the technique of subperiosteal diaphysectomy in 1965; the first 20 case series was published in 1973 by Fahey and O'Brien,[70] 12 cases by Gartland and Cole[62] in 1975, and another series of 21 patients was published by McKay and Nason[98] in 1977.[97] This technique was proposed because of the recurrence rate of 21% to 50% with intralesional curettage and grafting[70] (Table I summary from Fahey and O'Brien's[70] article). Despite this aggressive resection without grafting, McKay and Nason[98] had a 9% rate of recurrence. It would seem that aggressively removing the entire cyst subperiosteally could still result in later recurrences. It is important to understand that McKay's recurrences occurred greater than 1 year after initial treatment, and this aggressive surgery was also complicated by postoperative fractures and limb shortening.[98] These aggressive procedures, with their complications and recurrences, were the spawning ground of percutaneous injection techniques that would follow.

Percutaneous Injection with Steroid (Methylprednisolone Acetate)

A landmark article of innovative treatment appeared from Pisa, Italy, by Dr. Scaglietti and investigators[99] in 1979. It provided Level IV evidence of a new treatment utilizing percutaneous injection of methylprednisolone acetate (MPA) into 72 cysts. The initial article had up to six injections of MPA varying from 40 to 200 mg. Follow-up period was a minimum of 18 months; 60% of patients healed completely, and 36% healed "more or less complete," with only a 4% failure to heal rate. Campanacci and Capanna[9] from Rizzoli Institute in Bologna, Italy, reported results in 90 patients treated similarly and followed a minimum of 1 year (Level IV evidence) with 46 of 90 patients (51%) healed, 26 of 90 (29%) healed with small residual cysts, 12 of 90 (13%) with recurrence, and 6 of 90 (7%) had no response. They emphasize that smaller cyst size (<24 cm^2) and monoloculation positively affected the healing outcome ($P = 0.002$ and $P < 0.001$, respectively). Scaglietti and investigators reported final follow-up in 1982 and strongly cautioned that "patients must be observed until termination of their skeletal growth before evaluating the final results of the injection treatment. Otherwise, further extension of the cyst is possible."[85,100] Subsequent Level III articles comparing steroid with intralesional curettage and grafting showed only 74% healing with steroid and 54% healing with curettage and grafting.[11] Bovill et al,[86] also with Level III studies, compared steroid injection with open curettage and grafting, and found similar levels of efficacy for both treatments, but less complications in the injections group. Percutaneous injection offered the other advantage of a smaller intervention for residual or recurrent cysts, but the disadvantage of chemical injection near the physis and reports of local and systemic effects of the steroids and osseous necrosis of the femoral head after injection.[8,9,11,101–103]

Bone Marrow Aspiration and Percutaneous Injection. Bone marrow transplant for malignancy and bone-marrow aspiration and injection to promote fracture healing laid the groundwork for bone-marrow aspiration and percutaneous injection into SBCs to promote healing.[104–110] In 1985, Burwell[111] discussed the expanded understanding of the biology of bone marrow as an important osteoinductive factor in bone graft incorporation. Many subsequent articles furthered our understanding of the osteoinductive power of bone marrow.[106,109,112,113] The negative host effects of open bone graft harvesting added to the appeal of a less invasive technique of obtaining the osteogenic cells by aspiration.[92,94] A preliminary (Level of Evidence IV) prospective case series report by Lokiec and coworkers[114] of 10 patients with 100% healing of SBCs treated by bone marrow injection was published in 1996. This injection was combined with indirect venting of the cyst using a custom curved needle into the medullary canal.[114] A similar injection of bone marrow into cysts, but obtained by small 3-mL aliquot aspiration to potentiate osteoblast concentration and without venting into the medullary canal, showed similar positive results to Lokiec and Weintroub's initial reports, but 2 of 12 patients (17%) did not respond to marrow injection.[49,81,105] Because of these reports, marrow injection became a popular technique with minimal invasion to promote cyst healing.[115–117] Chang and coauthors,[6] in a Level III review of 79 patients treated with bone marrow (14 patients) verses steroid (65 patients) injection, showed no superiority of 1 technique over the other (*P* > 0.05). Docquier and Delloye[73,118] reported a Level IV series of 17 cases with 76% healing rate, 12% recurrence rate, and 12% failure of response rate. None of the bone marrow studies had uniform greater than 2-year follow-up until Wright's[56] study in 2007. Currently, this is the only Level I randomized, prospective, multicenter study that compares bone marrow with steroid injection. Seventy-seven of 90 patients completed 2-year follow-up. Radiologists, using Cole's modification of Neer's criteria for healing, demonstrated only 42% healing with steroids and 23% healing with bone marrow (*P* = 0.01). No cases were vented into the medullary canal before injection. The radiologists grading the healing were blind to treatment, and this is the first report of outside grading of the surgical outcome for cyst treatment. The great disparity to prior reports may be related to past evaluation bias, the longer length of follow-up in

this study, or the failure to vent cysts into the medullary canal in the recent study.

Mechanical Cyst Disruption with and without Fixation. Although the literature is full of exogenous materials that can promote cyst healing, many authors have outlined that simple mechanical disruption of the cyst can promote fracture-like biologic response and healing of cysts.[34,119,120] Chigira and colleagues,[17] in a 1983 Level IV study, utilized Kirschner-wire disruption of the cyst to decrease the pressure within the cyst, but their 1986 review reported recurrence if the K-wire was removed.[46] Komiya and coauthors'[27] 1991 Level IV study recommends "trepanation" of cysts percutaneously with a K-wire to promote healing. This article offers an evaluation of cyst fluid content and theory of its negative effect on bone formation. Although the first report of drainage of the cyst into the medullary canal was Ober's[122] in 1944, many subsequent articles offer drainage either intramedullary or cortically.[65,121,123] A Level III comparative study by Tsuchiya[66] in 2002 recommends continuous cyst decompression after curettage by either a cannulated screw or a hydroxyapatite cannulated pin, with 100% healing in the hydroxyapatite pin group. Follow-up, however, was 8 to 60 months in this group. Similar ideas of mechanical disruption with intramedullary rodding and the added advantage of fracture fixation and prophylaxis of possible future fracture were introduced by Catier and researchers[124] in 1981 and further by Santori and investigators[125] in 1988. These ideas were even further popularized by Roposch and colleagues[65] in 2000 and de Sanctis and Andreacchio[126] in 2006. Healing occurred in all 32 patients of this Level IV study, but 2 recurrences resulted from nail removal. Roposch and colleagues[65] emphasize in their review the tenacity and prevalence of cyst recurrence after treatment. Givon and coauthors,[127] in a technique article, utilizes a titanium elastic nail to indirectly open the cyst into the medullary canal but removes the nail and fills the defect with a bone substitute, Osteoset. Again, combinations of treatment obscure what actually is promoting cyst healing, and short follow-up negates the later recurrences seen throughout cyst treatment history.

Alternative Graft Materials for Treatment of Simple Bone Cysts. Gazdag and colleagues[88] wrote an excellent summary of alternatives to autogenous bone grafting. Many of the substitutes from hydroxyapatite cubes to demineralized bone matrix, Ethibloc and bioactive glass (Norion), have been utilized to encourage healing in bone cysts.[48,128–130] Demineralized bone matrix and bone marrow were combined with trephination in a percutaneous injection technique by Rougraff and Kling[87] reported in 2002. Twenty-three patients in this Level IV evidence study were observed for 30 to 81 months with 100% healing. In 2005, Kanellopoulos and coworkers[131] further amplified the technique with the addition of intramedullary perforation of the cyst and similar DBM and bone marrow injection. All patients healed, but 2 required repeat procedures to achieve this outcome. Follow-up period was 12 to 42 months, and Neer's criteria were used for healing. The historical return to calcium sulfate (Osteoset) but with a newer addition of venting into the medullary canal and indirect curettage, is reported in Dormans and researchers'[121] Level IV series. Twelve of 28 patients were managed for at least 24 months. Eleven of these achieved complete healing and 1 partial healing. In contrast with Peltier and Jones's[95] study in 1978 utilizing plaster of Paris, only 1 of Dormans's patients had a stitch abscess. A risk of alternative graft material is the possibility of rapid venous outflow from some active cysts.[31,132] Reports have demonstrated central Doppler flow disturbances from marrow and steroids injected into cyst with large venous outflow.[49,83,132] Smaller particulate materials used as graft substitutes could also exit these venous channels and pose a similar risk.

Calcaneal Bone Cysts

The calcaneus is the sixth most common location for SBCs, which are relatively rare. In large series reviewing SBCs, they represent a small percentage of overall cyst locations.[22] Behavior of calcaneal cysts related to fracture risk and treatment is somewhat unique. Pogoda and researchers[133] studied 50 cysts in 47 patients and found cysts reaching a critical size, defined as a 100% intracalcaneal cross section in the coronal plane and at least 30% in the sagittal plane, are at risk for fracture. Calcaneal cysts tend to occur in older patients and, because of the weight-bearing nature of the bone, when larger, cause pain with daily activities.[133] Radiologic assessment with plain films, CT scans, and/or MRI offer a characteristic pattern that aids with diagnosis. Radiographically, atypical cysts should undergo biopsy to prevent misdiagnosis and confusion with intraosseous lipomas, pseudocysts, or cysts secondary to other osseous or chondral lesions.[134] Intralesional curettage and bone grafting, either with allograft or autograft, has been the mainstay of treatment.[134-136] Curettage and grafting, in several studies, has shown superior healing to steroid injection.[137,138] Saraph's[117,134] articles include an excellent table providing a comprehensive overview of the literature to date with methods of treatment for calcaneus cysts. All of the articles are Level IV evidence and are retrospective summaries of techniques used with outcomes of healing reported. This summary Level IV evidence article outlines their excellent result with continuous decompression of the cyst using titanium cannulated screws and no curettage or grafting. Eight of nine healed completely with a minimum of 2-year follow-up. Patients healed with a residual cyst. This technique supports the theory that cyst fluid decompression facilitates and/or promotes healing in all cyst locations.

SUMMARY

Clearly, numerous treatments and combinations of treatment have been utilized for treatment of SBCs. The unique features of the host, such as age, sex, and activity, have been reported to affect healing. Tumor variables such as lesion size, proximity to the physis, and venous outflow are also reported to affect response to treatment and healing. Surgical treatment variables of curettage, septation disruption, medullary or cortical venting, and fixation have been shown to affect healing. Graft materials, both biologic and nonbiologic, osteoinductive and conductive, are important factors. A standardized scale for healing and clear risk for fracture must be determined. Length of follow-up, ideally to skeletal maturity, is important in outcome success. Unless these variables are controlled in a randomized, prospective study, the levels of evidence will remain as multiple case series and be difficult, if not impossible, to compare. Level IV evidence supports injection or venting techniques using a variety of specific procedures as outlined earlier. The only Level I evidence reports a greater healing rate with steroid injection than with bone marrow injection, but fewer than 50% of the cysts in either arm of the randomized trial healed. More randomized, prospective, multicenter studies are needed to guide treatment recommendations for patients and families. Table 39–2 provides a summary of recommendations for calcaneal SBC treatment.

TABLE 39-2. Summary of Recommendations for Calcaneal Simple Bone Cyst Treatment

STATEMENT	LEVEL OF EVIDENCE/GRADE OF RECOMMENDATION	REFERENCES
1. Calcaneal SBC reaching a "critical size" is at risk for fracture.	B	133
2. Intralesional curettage and bone grafting for treatment of calcaneal SBC is superior to observation.	B	136, 139, 140
	C	135, 141–145
3. Alternative products to bone graft can promote healing of calcaneal SBC.	C	146, 147
4. Intralesional curettage and bone grafting is superior to steroid injection for treatment of calcaneal SBC.	B	137, 138
	C	148
5. Multiple drilling and/or continuous decompression of calcaneal SBC results in healing.	C	134, 149

SBC, simple bone cyst.

REFERENCES

1. Campanacci M: Pseudotumors of bone. Bone and Soft Tissue Tumors. New York, Springer-Verlag Wien, 1990, pp 709–724.
2. Cohen J: Etiology of simple bone cyst. J Bone Joint Surg Am 52:1493–1497, 1970.
3. Johnson L, Kindred R: The anatomy of bone cysts. J Bone Joint Surg Am 40:1440, 1958.
4. Neer CN, Francis K, Marcove R: Treatment of unicameral bone cyst. A follow-up study of one hundred seventy-five cases. J Bone Joint Surg Am 48:731–745, 1966.
5. Spence KJ, Bright R, Fitzgerald S: Solitary unicameral bone cyst: Treatment with freeze-dried crushed cortical-bone allograft. A review of one hundred and forty-four cases. J Bone Joint Surg Am 58:636–641, 1976.
6. Chang C, Stanton R, Glutting J: Unicameral bone cysts treated by injection of bone marrow or methylprednisolone. J Bone Joint Surg Am 84:407–412, 2002.
7. Jaffe H, Lichtenstein L: Solitary unicameral bone cyst with emphasis on the roentgen picture, the pathologic appearance and the pathogenesis. Arch Surg 44:288–293, 1942.
8. Capanna R, Dal Monte A, Gitelis S: The natural history of unicameral bone cyst after steroid injection. Clin Orthop Relat Res 166:204–211, 1982.
9. Campanacci M, Capanna R, Picci P: Unicameral and aneurysmal bone cysts. Clin Orthop Relat Res (204)25–36, 1986.
10. Mirra J: Bone Tumors Diagnosis and Treatment. Philadelphia, J.B. Lippincott, 1980.
11. Oppenheim W, Galleno H: Operative treatment versus steroid injection in the management of unicameral bone cysts. J Pediatr Orthop 4:1–7, 1984.
12. Lokiec F, Wientroub S: Simple bone cyst: Etiology, classification, pathology and treatment modalities. J Pediatr Orthop B 7:262–273, 1998.
13. Malawer MM, Markle B: Unicameral bone cyst with epiphyseal involvement: Clinicoanatomic analysis. J Pediatr Orthop 2:71–79, 1982.
14. Ovadia D, Ezra E, Segev E: Epiphyseal involvement of simple bone cysts. J Pediatr Orthop 23:222–229, 2003.
15. Gupta A, Crawford A: Solitary bone cyst with epiphyseal involvement: Confirmation with magnetic resonance imaging. J Bone Joint Surg Am 78:911–915, 1996.
16. Nelson J, Foster R: Solitary bone cyst with epiphyseal involvement. Clin Orthop Relat Res 118:147–150, 1976.
17. Chigira M, Maehara S, Arita S: The aetiology and treatment of simple bone cysts. J Bone Joint Surg Am 65:633–637, 1983.
18. Cohen J: Simple bone cysts. Studies of cyst fluid in six cases with a theory of pathogenesis. Am J Orthop 42-A:609–616, 1960.
19. Allredge R: Localized fibrocystic disease of bone. Results of treatment in one hundred and fifty-two cases. J Bone Joint Surg Am 24:795–804, 1942.
20. Phemister: The etiology of solitary bone cyst. JAMA 87:1429–1433, 1926.
21. Abdel-Wanis ME, Tsuchiya H, Minato H, et al: Bilateral symmetrical cysts in the upper tibiae in a skeletally mature patient: Might they be simple bone cysts? J Orthop Sci 6:595–600, 2001.
22. Mirra J, Bernard G, Bullough P: Cementum-like bone production in solitary bone cysts (so-called "cementoma" of long bones). Report of three cases. Electron microscopic observations supporting a synovial origin to the simple bone cyst. Clin Orthop Relat Res (135):295–307, 1978.
23. Amling M, Werner M, Pösl M, et al: Calcifying solitary bone cyst: Morphological aspects and differential diagnosis of sclerotic bone tumours. Virchows Arch 426:235–242, 1995.
24. Cohen J: Unicameral bone cysts. A current synthesis of reported cases. Orthop Clin North Am 8:715–736, 1977.
25. Makley J, Joyce M: Unicameral bone cyst (simple bone cyst). Orthop Clin North Am 20:407–415, 1989.
26. Komiya S, Inoue A: Development of a solitary bone cyst: A report of a case suggesting its pathogenesis. Arch Orthop Trauma Surg 120:455–457, 2000.
27. Komiya S, Minamitani K, Sasaguri Y: Simple bone cyst. Treatment by trepanation and studies on bone resorptive factors in cyst fluid with a theory of its pathogenesis. Clin Orthop Relat Res 204–211, 1993.
28. Komiya S, Tsuzuki K, Mangham DC, et al: Oxygen scavengers in simple bone cysts. Clin Orthop Relat Res (308):199–206, 1994.
29. Gerasimov A, Toporova S, Furtseva L: The role of lysosomes in the pathogenesis of unicameral bone cysts. Clin Orthop Relat Res 266:53–63, 1991.
30. Shindell R, Connolly JF, Lippiello L: Prostaglandin levels in a unicameral bone cyst treated by corticosteroid injection. J Pediatr Orthop 7:210–212, 1987.
31. Enneking W: Lesions of Uncertain Origin Originating in Bone. Musculoskeletal Tumor Surgery, vol. 2. New York, Churchill Livingston, 1983.
32. Snyder BD, Hauser-Kara DA, Hipp JA, et al: Predicting fracture through benign skeletal lesions with quantitative computed tomography. J Bone Joint Surg Am 88:55–70, 2006.
33. Hong J, Cabe GD, Tedrow JR, et al: Failure of trabecular bone with simulated lytic defects can be predicted non-invasively by structural analysis. J Orthop Res 22:479–486, 2004.
34. Ahn JI, Park JS: Pathological fractures secondary to unicameral bone cysts. Int Orthop 18:20–22, 1994.
35. Hipp JA, Springfield DS, Hayes WC: Predicting pathologic fracture risk in the management of metastatic bone defects. Clin Orthop Relat Res (312):120–135, 1995.
36. McGlynn F, Mickelson M, El-Khoury G: The fallen fragment sign in unicameral bone cyst. Clin Orthop Relat Res 157–159, 1981.
37. Reynolds J: "The fallen fragment sign" in the diagnosis of unicameral bone cyst. J Radiol 92:949–953, 1969.
38. Struhl S, Edelson C, Pritzker H, et al: Solitary (unicameral) bone cyst. The fallen fragment sign revisited. Skeletal Radiol 18:261–265, 1989.
39. Suei Y, Tanimoto K, Wada T: Simple bone cyst. Evaluation of contents with conventional radiography and computed tomography. Oral Surg Oral Med Oral Pathol 77:296–301, 1994.
40. Garceau G, Gregory C: Solitary unicameral bone cyst. J Bone Joint Surg Am 36:267–280, 1954.
41. James A, Coley B, Higinbotham N: Solitary (unicameral) bone cyst. Arch Surg 57:137–147, 1942.
42. Bloodgood J: Benign bone cysts, ostitis fibrosa, giant-cell sarcoma and bone aneurism of the long pipe bones. Ann Surg 52:145–185, 1910.
43. Graham J: Solitary unicameral bone cyst. A follow-up study of thirty-one cases with proven pathological diagnosis. Bull Hosp Joint Dis 13(1):106–130, 1952.
44. Spence KJ, Sell K, Brown R: Solitary bone cyst: Treatment with freeze-dried cancellous bone allograft. J Bone Joint Surg Am 51:87–96, 1969.
45. Baker D: Benign unicameral bone cyst. A study of forty-five cases with long-term follow up. Clin Orthop Relat Res 71:140–151, 1970.
46. Chigira M, Shimizu T, Arita S, et al: Radiological evidence of healing of a simple bone cyst after hole drilling. Arch Orthop Trauma Surg 105:150–153, 1986.
47. Hashemi-Nejad A, Cole W: Incomplete healing of simple bone cysts after steroid injections. J Bone Joint Surg Br 79:727–730, 1997.
48. Killian J, Wilkinson L, White S: Treatment of unicameral bone cyst with demineralized bone matrix. J Pediatr Orthop 18:621–624, 1998.
49. Yandow SM, Lundeen GA, Scott SM, Coffin C: Autogenic bone marrow injections as a treatment for simple bone cyst. J Pediatr Orthop 18:616–620, 1998.
50. Hong J, et al: Magnetic resonance imaging measurements of bone density and cross-sectional geometry. Calcif Tissue Int 66:74–78, 2000.
51. Kleinberg S: The solitary bone cyst. A report of a case of twenty years' duration. J Bone Joint Surg Am 26:337–344, 1944.
52. Bowen RE, Morrissy RT: Recurrence of a unicameral bone cyst in the proximal part of the fibula after en bloc resection. A case report. J Bone Joint Surg Am 86:154–158, 2004.
53. Stanton R, Abdel-Motá al M: Growth arrest resulting from unicameral bone cyst. J Pediatr Orthop 18:198–201, 1998.
54. Violas P, Salmeron F, Chapuis M, et al: Simple bone cysts of the proximal humerus complicated with growth arrest. Acta Orthop Belg 70:166–170, 2004.

55. Norman-Taylor FH, Hashemi-Nejad A, Gillingham BL, et al: Risk of refracture through unicameral bone cysts of the proximal femur. J Pediatr Orthop 22:249–254, 2002.
56. Wright JG, Yandow S, Donaldson S, et al: A randomized trial comparing intralesional bone marrow and steroid injections for simple bone cysts. J Bone Joint Surg Am 90(4):722–730, 2008.
57. Wilkins RM: Unicameral bone cysts. J Am Acad Orthop Surg 8:217–224, 2000.
58. Biermann JS: Common benign lesions of bone in children and adolescents. J Pediatr Orthop 22:268–273, 2002.
59. Vasconcellos D, Yandow SM, Grace AM, et al: Cyst index: A nonpredictor of simple bone cyst fracture. J Pediatr Orthop 27:307–310, 2007.
60. Kaelin AJ, MacEwen GD: Unicameral bone cysts. Natural history and the risk of fracture. Int Orthop 13:275–282, 1989.
61. Blount W: Fractures in Children. Philadelphia, Lippincott Williams & Wilkins, 1955, pp 251–252.
62. Gartland J, Cole F: Modern concepts in the treatment of unicameral bone cysts of the proximal humerus. Orthop Clin North Am 6:487–498, 1975.
63. Inoue O, Ibaraki K, Shimabukuro H: Packing with high-porosity hydroxyapatite cubes alone for treatment of simple bone cyst. Clin Orthop Relat Res 287–292, 1993.
64. Farber J, Stanton R: Treatment options in unicameral bone cysts. Orthopedics 13:25–32, 1990.
65. Roposch A, Saraph V, Linhart W: Flexible intramedullary nailing for the treatment of unicameral bone cysts in long bones. J Bone Joint Surg Am 82:1447–1453, 2000.
66. Tsuchiya H, Abdel-Wanis M, Uehara K: Cannulation of simple bone cysts. J Bone Joint Surg Br 84:245–248, 2002.
67. Taroni A, Faccini R, Ventre T: Pathologic fracture on bone cyst of the femoral neck treated by external fixator. Chirurgia Degli Organi di Movimento 82:91–94, 1997.
68. Margau R, Babyn P, Cole W, et al: MR imaging of simple bone cysts in children: Not so simple. Pediatr Radiol 30:551–557, 2000.
69. Woertler K: Benign bone tumors and tumor-like lesions: Value of cross-sectional imaging. Eur Radiol 13:1820–1835, 2003.
70. Fahey J, O'Brien E: Subtotal resection and grafting in selected cases of solitary unicameral bone cyst. J Bone Joint Surg Am 55:59–68, 1973.
71. Enneking W, Yandow SM: (personal communication) Editor. 1990.
72. James A, Coley B, Higinbotham N: Solitary (unicameral) bone cyst. Arch Surg 137:144, 1948.
73. Docquier P, Delloye C: Treatment of simple bone cysts with aspiration and a single bone marrow injection. J Pediatr Orthop 23:766–773, 2003.
74. Johnson L, Vetter H, Pautschar WG: Sarcomas arising in bone cysts. Virchows Arch Path Anat 335:428–451, 1962.
75. Grabias S, Mankin H: Chondrosarcoma arising in histologically proved unicameral bone cyst. J Bone Joint Surg Am 56:1501–1509, 1974.
76. Vergel De Dios A, et al: Aneurysmal bone cyst: A clinicapathologic study of 238 cases. Cancer 69:2921–2931, 1992.
77. Dahlin D, Unni K: Bone Tumors: General Aspects and Data on 8,542 Cases. Springfield, IL, Charles C. Thomas, 1986.
78. Neer C, Francis K, Johnston A: Current concepts on the treatment of solitary unicameral bone cyst. Clin Orthop Relat Res 97:40–51, 1973.
79. Hillerup S, Hjorting-Hansen E: Aneurysmal bone cyst—simple bone cyst, two aspects of the same pathologic entity? Int J Oral Surg 7:16–22, 1978.
80. Abdel-Wanis M, Tsuchiya H: Simple bone cyst is not a single entity: Point of view based on a literature review. Med Hypotheses 58:87–91, 2002.
81. Yandow SM, Coffin C, Perkins S, et al: Aneurysmal (ABC) & Solitary (SBC) Bone Cyst. Separate Entities or a Pathologic Continuum? POSNA (Poster Presentation). Salt Lake City, UT, May 4, 2002.
82. Woertler K, Brinkschmidt C: Imaging features of subperiosteal aneurysmal bone cyst. Acta Radiol 43:336–339, 2002.
83. Yandow SM, Crim J, Donaldson S, et al: The Not So Simple Bone Cyst: Appearance on MRI. POSNA (Poster Presentation). Ottawa, Ontario, Canada, May 13–15, 2005.
84. Cole W: Treatment of aneurysmal bone cysts in childhood. J Pediatr Orthop 6:326–329, 1986.
85. Scaglietti O, Marchetti P, Bartolozzi P: Final results obtained in the treatment of bone cysts with methylprednisolone acetate (depo-medrol) and a discussion of results achieved in other bone lesions. Clin Orthop Relat Res (165):33–42, 1982.
86. Bovill DF, Skinner HB: Unicameral bone cysts. A comparison of treatment options. Orthop Rev 18:420–427, 1989.
87. Rougraff B, Kling T: Treatment of active unicameral bone cysts with percutaneous injection of demineralized bone matrix and autogenous bone marrow. J Bone Joint Surg Am 84:921–929, 2002.
88. Gazdag A, Lane J, Glaser D: Alternatives to autogenous bone graft: Efficacy and indications. J Am Acad Orthop Surg 3:1–8, 1995.
89. Jaffe H: Tumors and tumorous conditions of the bones and joints. Philadelphia, Lea & Febiger, 1958, 629.
90. Geschickter C, Copeland M: Tumors of Bone, 3rd ed. Philadelphia, JB Lippincott, 1949.
91. Schreuder HB, Conrad EU 3rd, Bruckner JD, et al: Treatment of simple bone cysts in children with curettage and cryosurgery. J Pediatr Orthop 17:814–820, 1997.
92. Goulet JA, Senunas LE, DeSilva GL, Greenfield ML: Autogenous iliac crest bone graft. Clin Orthop Relat Res 339:76–81, 1997.
93. Lane J, Sandhu H: Current approaches to experimental bone grafting. Orthop Clin North Am 18:213–225, 1987.
94. Younger E, Chapman M: Morbidity at bone graft donor sites. J Orthop Trauma 3:192–195, 1989.
95. Peltier L, Jones R: Treatment of unicameral bone cysts by curettage and packing with plaster-of-Paris pellets. J Bone Joint Surg Am 60:820–822, 1978.
96. Agerholm J, Goodfellow J: Simple cysts of the humerus treated by radical excision. J Bone Joint Surg Br 47:714–717, 1965.
97. MacKenzie D: Treatment of solitary bone cysts by diaphysectomy and bone grafting. S Afr Med J 58:154–158, 1980.
98. McKay D, Nason S: Treatment of unicameral bone cysts by subtotal resection without grafts. J Bone Joint Surg Am 59:515–518, 1977.
99. Scaglietti O, Marchetti P, Bartolozzi P: The effects of methylprednisolone acetate in the treatemtn of bone cysts. Results of three years follow-up. J Bone Joint Surg Br 61:200–204, 1979.
100. Yu C, D'Astous J, Finnegan M: Simple bone cysts. The effects of methylprednisolone on synovial cells in culture. Clin Orthop Relat Res 34–41, 1991.
101. Colville M, Aronson DD, Prcevski P, Crissman JD: The systemic and local effects of an intramedullary injection of methylprednisolone acetate in growing rabbits. J Pediatr Orthop 7:412–414, 1986.
102. Taneda H, Azuma H: Avascular necrosis of the femoral epiphysis complicating a minimally displaced fracture of solitary bone cyst of the neck of the femur in a child. Clin Orthop Relat Res 304:172–175, 1994.
103. Nakamura T, Takagi K, Kitagawa T, Harada M: Microdensity of solitary bone cyst after steroid injection. J Pediatr Orthop 8:566–568, 1988.
104. Weintroub S, Goodwin D, Khermosh O: The clinical use of autologous marrow to improve osteogenic potential of bone grafts in pediatric orthopedics. J Pediatr Orthop 9:186–190, 1989.
105. Batinić D, Marusić M, Pavletić Z, et al: Relationship between differing volumes of bone marrow aspirates and their cellular composition. Bone Marrow Transplant 6:103–107, 1990.
106. Majors A, Boehm C, Nitto H: Characterization of human bone marrow stromal cells with respect to osteoblastic differentiation. J Orthop Res 15:546–557, 1997.
107. Connolly J, Guse R, Lippiello L: Development of an osteogenic bone-marrow preparation. J Bone Joint Surg Am 71:684–691, 1989.
108. Connolly J, Guse R, Tiedeman J: Autologous marrow injection as a substitute for operative grafting of tibial nonunions. Clin Orthop Relat Res 266:259–270, 1991.
109. Beresford JN: Osteogenic stem cells and the stromal system of bone and marrow. Clin Orthop Relat Res 240:270–280, 1989.

110. Healey J, Zimmerman P, McDonnell J: Percutaneous bone marrow grafting of delayed union and nonunion in cancer patients. Clin Orthop Relat Res 256:280–285, 1990.

111. Burwell R: The function of bone marrow in the incorporation of a bone graft. Clin Orthop Relat Res 125–141, 1985.

112. Muschler G, Boehm C, Easley K: Aspiration to obtain osteoblast progenitor cells from human bone marrow: The influence of aspiration volume. J Bone Joint Surg Am 79:1699–1709, 1997.

113. Maniatopoulos C, Sodek J, Melcher A: Bone formation in vitro by stromal cells obtained from bone marrow of young adult rats. Cell Tissue Res 254:317–330, 1988.

114. Lokiec F, Ezra E, Khermosh O: Simple bone cysts treated by percutaneous autologous marrow grafting. A preliminary report. J Bone Joint Surg Br 78:934–937, 1996.

115. Arazi M, Senaran H, Memik R, Kapicioglu S: Minimally invasive treatment of simple bone cysts with percutaneous autogenous bone marrow injection. Orthopedics 28:108–112, 2005.

116. Köse N, Göktürk E, Turgut A, et al: Percutaneous autologous bone marrow grafting for simple bone cysts. Bull Hosp Jt Dis 58:105–110, 1999.

117. Saraph V: Treatment of simple bone cyst using bone marrow injection. J Pediatr Orthop 24:449, 2004.

118. Docquier P, Delloye C: Autologous bone marrow injection in the management of simple bone cysts in children. Acta Orthop Belg 70:204–213, 2004.

119. Badgley C: Unicameral cyst of the long bones. Treatment by crushing cystic walls and onlay grafts. In Proceedings of the AOA. J Bone Joint Surg Am 39:1429–1430, 1957.

120. Kuboyama K, et al: Therapy of solitary unicameral bone cyst with percutaneous trepanation. Rinsho Seikei Geka (Japanese) 16:288, 1981.

121. Dormans J, et al: Percutaneous intramedullary decompression, curettage, and grafting with medical-grade calcium sulfate pellets for unicameral bone cysts in children: A new minimally invasive technique. J Pediatr Orthop 25:804–811, 2005.

122. Ober FR: Discussion of the solitary bone cyst by Samuel Kleinberg. J Bone Joint Surg Am 26:343, 1944.

123. Linhart W, Roposch A, Reitinger T: Flexible but stable intramedullary nailing for unicameral bone cysts of the humerus in juveniles. Orthop Traumatol 10:60–69, 2002.

124. Catier P, Bracq H, Canciani JP, et al: The treatment of upper femoral unicameral bone cysts in children by Ender's nailing technique. Rev Chir Orthop Reparatrice Appar Mot 67:147–149, 1981.

125. Santori F, Ghera S, Castelli V: Treatment of solitary bone cysts with intramedullary nailing. Orthopedics 11:873–878, 1988.

126. de Sanctis N, Andreacchio A: Elastic stable intramedullary nailing is the best treatment of unicameral bone cysts of the long bones in children? Prospective long-term follow-up study. J Pediatr Orthop 26:520–525, 2006.

127. Givon U, Sher-Lurie N, Schindler A: Titanium elastic nail—A useful instrument for the treatment of simple bone cyst. J Pediatr Orthop 24:317–318, 2004.

128. Sponer P, Urban K: Treatment of juvenile bone cysts by curettage and filling of the cavity with BAS-0 bioactive glass-ceramic material. Acta Chir Orthop Traumatol Cech 71:214–219, 2004.

129. Adamsbaum C, Kalifa G, Seringe R, Dubousset J: Direct Ethibloc injection in benign bone cysts: Preliminary report on four patients. Skeletal Radiol 22:317–320, 1993.

130. Wilkins RM, Kelly CM, Giusti DE: Bio-assayed demineralized bone matrix and calcium sulfate: Use in bone-grafting procedures. Ann Chir Gynaecol 88:180–185, 1999.

131. Kanellopoulos A, Yiannakopoulos C, Soucacos P: Percutaneous reaming of simple bone cysts in children followed by injection of demineralized bone matrix and autologous bone marrow. J Pediatr Orthop 25:671–675, 2005.

132. Yandow SM, Galloway K, Fillman R, et al: Precordial Doppler evaluation of simple bone cyst injections. POSNA (Poster Presentation). St. Louis, MO, April 28-May 4, 2004. J Pediatr Orthop (accepted).

133. Pogoda P, Priemel M, Linhart W: Clinical relevance of calcaneal bone cysts: A study of 50 cysts in 47 patients. Clin Orthop Relat Res 202–210, 2004.

134. Saraph V, Zwick E, Maizen C: Treatment of unicameral calcaneal bone cysts in children: Review of literature and results using a cannulated screw for continuous decompression of the cyst. J Pediatr Orthop 24:568–573, 2004.

135. Moreau G, Letts M: Unicameral bone cyst of the calcaneus in children. J Pediatr Orthop 14:101–104, 1994.

136. Smith R, Smith C: Solitary unicameral bone cyst of the calcaneus. A review of twenty cases. J Bone Joint Surg Am 56:49–56, 1974.

137. Fantini A, Ruggieri P, Biagini R: Cisti ossee di calcagno (studio di 14 osservazioni). Chir Org Mov 70:315–320, 1985.

138. Glaser D, Dormans J, Stanton R: Surgical management of calcaneal unicameral bone cysts. Clin Orthop Relat Res 231–237, 1999.

Chapter 40

Legg–Calve–Perthes Disease: How Should It Be Treated?

John Anthony Herring, MD

The necessity for evidenced-based investigation is nowhere better illustrated than in the case of the treatment of Legg–Calve–Perthes disease. In the United States, as well as around the world, an amazing variety of treatment methods are used for this condition. These vary from long-term relief from weight bearing, to months and months of abduction cast treatment, to combined femoral and pelvic surgical procedures, to ignoring the disease altogether. Even more striking is the degree with which orthopedists defend their chosen method.

The literature reflects this unique situation. Most studies have no control subjects and numbers too small for statistical validity. Different methods are used to determine severity and outcome, and until recently, few were subjected to validation by interobserver trials. It is abundantly clear that, in this instance, Level I and II studies are needed. Although many believe that the pressure for evidence-based knowledge is an academic exercise, I fully disagree, for it is the confused parent seeking treatment for a child who will benefit from this discipline. Time and again, orthopedists must dispel absurd treatment measures that other physicians have presented to the parent as an absolute necessity.

This chapter first reviews the investigations that reach Levels I, II, and III. It then briefly covers the information from other recent studies that have useful retrospective information.

Some years ago, I critically reviewed the literature up to 1994.[1] Although much has been written since that date, some principles of importance came out of that review that apply specifically to Legg–Perthes disease.

1. It is well known that the severity of the disorder is closely related to the age at onset. A study that does not adequately control for age at onset cannot reach useful conclusions.
2. The severity of femoral head involvement has been shown to be an even more important variable in outcome within all age groups up to 10 years of age at onset. Classification of outcome and severity of disease must be standardized by interobserver trials based on clear definitions. The Catterall classification and the associated risk factors were widely used in earlier works, but interobserver studies failed to show agreement among observers, even when well-versed in the

details. The lateral pillar classification has had good interobserver reliability and has been shown to strongly correlate with outcome. The Stulberg classification of outcome has also been shown to have reliable reproducibility when detailed descriptors are used.

STUDIES THAT REACH LEVEL I OR II

In 1993, Fulford, Lunn, and Macnicol's[2] comparison of 2 groups of patients randomized by source of referral was published. The children treated at Royal Hospital for Sick Children were compared with those treated at the Princess Margaret Rose Orthopaedic hospital. The children at the first hospital were treated with an ischial-bearing patten-ended caliper. Those at the second hospital had a varus, derotational proximal femoral osteotomy. This study can be considered a controlled, prospective study. The authors identified no differences in outcome between the groups. Outcome in their study was found to correlate with femoral head shape at presentation and the age at onset. They note that of the heads with severe deformity at the initial arthrogram, only 4 of 25 hips improved to have a good result, and all were younger than 5 years at onset. Two of these patients were receiving brace therapy, and two had surgery. Compared with historical control subjects, the authors believe that both methods are effective. Because of the wide variation in reporting of historical control subjects, I do not believe that such comparisons are useful in this disorder.

Another difficulty is that the authors do not state what stage of disease was present when the patient first presented. Those who presented with severe head deformity must have been beyond the stage of increased density. Others presenting before head deformation had occurred may still go on to severe deformity, so this factor has questionable validity as a predictor.

Harrison and Bassett[3] performed a double-blind trial of pulsed electromagnetic field treatment in patients also being treated with a non–weight-bearing Birmingham orthosis. This study shows no discernible effect of the electromagnetic field treatment. The effectiveness of the orthosis was not elucidated by this study because the study did not include a control or comparative group.

Herring and colleagues[4] report on the results of a long-term, controlled study performed by the Legg Perthes Study Group. Thirty-nine pediatric orthopedists from North America and New Zealand agreed to a "best-effort" study in lieu of randomization. In this paradigm, each surgeon agreed to apply a single treatment method to each patient who met the study criteria. The presumption of this type of study is that so large a sample will likely override local selection factors and provide comparable treatment groups. The treatment groups were no treatment, range of motion treatment in which the patient did exercises once a day, Atlanta brace treatment, femoral varus osteotomy, and Salter innominate osteotomy. Within each treatment group, except the no treatment group, Petrie casts could be used up to two times to overcome hip stiffness.

Part one of the study provides detailed classifications that were tested in interobserver and intraobserver trials that showed good reliability[5]. The classifications evaluated were the lateral pillar classification in the early stages of disease and the Stulberg classification at skeletal maturity. The outcomes were analyzed relative to age at onset and severity of disease. Patients were managed to skeletal maturity and assessed independently by an observer not involved in patient treatment.

This study came to the following conclusions: First, the lateral pillar classification was the strongest predictor of outcome. Those in lateral pillar groups A and B were much more likely to have a favorable outcome than those in lateral pillar group C. Those classified as B/C border had an outcome intermediate between groups B and C. The second strongest factor in outcome was age at onset. Those whose age at onset was older than 8 years had a less favorable outcome than those 8 years and younger. An identical effect was found when the outcome of those with onset at skeletal age of 6 years and younger was compared with those with onset beyond skeletal age of 6. (The mean delay of skeletal age in the boys was 2 years.)

Treatment methods were also significantly related to outcome. In the entire cohort, the patients treated surgically had better outcome compared with the nonsurgical groups ($P = 0.02$). The improved outcome with surgery was found in the lateral pillar groups B and B/C border, whose age at onset was greater than 8.0 years. In lateral pillar group B hips with an age at onset of more than 8.0 years, 73% of the operated hips had a Stulberg I or II result compared with 44% of the nonoperated hips ($P = 0.02$). The group B hips with onset at 8.0 years or younger had a favorable outcome profile, and there was no advantage demonstrated for the surgical group. This is an important finding given that 63% of the hips in the study were classified as group B. The group C hips, the most severely involved, were not shown to benefit from surgical treatment overall or in either age group when compared with the nonsurgical groups. No difference in outcome was reported between the Salter and varus osteotomy groups. Neither were there any

differences among no treatment, range-of-motion treatment, and brace treatment.

The strength of this study lies in the prospective comparison among many surgeons in many centers. Longitudinal follow-up to maturity adds to the strength of the study, but the loss of follow-up of some patients before maturity weakens it. Exclusion forms were required for patients not enrolled to help reduce selection bias. A small number of hips (16) were excluded because of protocol violation. A total of 345 hips remained at final follow-up of 451 initially enrolled.

In conclusion, the evidence produced by this study supports a treatment concept based on age at onset and lateral pillar classification. Patients older than 8 years classified as lateral pillar B or B/C border are likely to benefit from femoral varus or Salter pelvic osteotomy compared with nonoperative treatment. Because lateral pillar classification is not evident for 6 to 9 months after onset, an osteotomy may be justified on presentation for those children older than 8 in the initial phase of disease. Those with lateral pillar C disease would not likely benefit, but these cases occur infrequently, representing only 13% of hips with onset after age 8 in this study.

One could also conclude from this study that none of the nonoperative methods was effective in altering outcome. A trend appeared that was not statistically significant for patients undergoing brace therapy to have more Stulberg I and II results in patients 8.0 years or younger compared with the nontreatment group. However, the small number of patients in the nontreatment group (19) limits the power of this study to answer this question. It is also difficult to assess any nonoperative treatment when there is no objective monitoring for compliance with the method, be it bracing or range-of-motion exercise protocol. Not only should a study assess hours of brace wear, but ideally, it should monitor position of the femoral head within the acetabulum throughout the treatment period. This study monitored femoral head position at initiation of treatment, but subsequent monitoring was incomplete.

STUDIES WITH LESSER LEVELS OF EVIDENCE

Varus Osteotomy or Salter Osteotomy

Aksoy and colleagues[6] retrospectively compared 23 patients receiving therapy with 26 hips not treated with braces or surgery. The patients' ages were similar. No difference in outcome was found between the 2 groups, suggesting that brace treatment did not alter outcome. In this series, the braced group had 30% lateral pillar C hips compared with 18% in the nonbraced group. The authors found that the lateral pillar classification was useful in predicting outcome. The small numbers of patients in this study did not allow the authors to consider age at onset in the analysis. These issues limit the strength of the conclusions.

Aksoy and colleagues[7] also evaluated the results of femoral varus osteotomy in 26 lateral pillar group C patients. Group C hips in patients older than 9 all had outcomes in Stulberg III, IV, and V categories. Six of 14 treated before age 9 had Stulberg II results. Their conclusion was that this surgery did not improve results for hips with lateral pillar group C involvement, especially if older than 9 when treated.

Friedlander and Weiner[8] reviewed 116 hips treated with varus osteotomy without a control group. They found that those patients with lateral pillar B involvement had Stulberg I and II results in 86% when they were younger than 9 years at onset. Those older than 9 years with lateral pillar class B had Stulberg I and II results in 67% of cases. The hips of patients older than 9 years with lateral pillar C involvement had Stulberg II results in only 30% of cases. These results mirror those of Herring and colleagues[4] but with better results for the group C hips in patients older than 9.

Grzegorzewski and colleagues[9] retrospectively compared hips among five treatment groups, which included traction with abduction, Petrie casting, abduction bracing, pelvic osteotomy, and femoral osteotomy. They found that lateral pillar C hips fared less well than the others. They found no difference in outcome related to the treatment groups. They conclude that containment treatment was effective by any of the methods studied. The lack of a control group renders that conclusion unwarranted.

Ishida and colleagues[10] reviewed results in 37 hips treated with Salter osteotomy without a control group. The younger patients fared better than the older patients. Those patients older than 7 years at onset had 3 Stulberg I or II, 10 Stulberg III, and 5 Stulberg IV results, but these were not stratified by lateral pillar classification.

Kim and coworkers[11] report on a large, multicenter study of patients in Japan. They compared 6 treatment methods and found no difference in outcome among the groups. The lateral pillar classification and age at onset were the most important predictors of outcome. The overall outcome was similar to other studies in the Western literature.

Studies of Augmented Acetabuloplasty

Domzalski and colleagues demonstrated the occurrence of acetabular growth stimulation after a modified shelf arthroplasty in a Level III study.[12] These hips were compared with hips treated with varus osteotomy. The authors hypothesize that the increase in acetabular depth will prevent hip subluxation and encourage acetabular growth. The stage of disease in which the operation was performed is not stated in the study. This study does not report or compare the Stulberg outcome between the 2 treatment groups. This omission leaves the clinical efficacy of this operation unproven.

Bursal and Erkula[13] reviewed 19 hips without a control group and showed that acetabulum–head index and center-edge angles were improved. This finding, which is a direct effect of acetabular augmentation, appears in all studies of this operation. The clinical effectiveness of this change has not been demonstrated.

Jacobs and colleagues[14] report on 43 hips treated with shelf acetabuloplasty. They show increased acetabular depth, but no comparative outcome data were presented.

Kuwajima and colleagues[15] compare the Salter procedure with and without acetabular augmentation. Acetabular depth was improved, but outcome was similar between the 2 groups.

Studies of Valgus Osteotomy for Late Cases with Hinge Abduction

Bankes and colleagues[16] found mixed results after valgus, extension osteotomy for hips with hinge abduction. Of 52 hips, 4 had total hip replacement and 1 had arthrodesis. Twelve had favorable remodeling. Younger hips, those in earlier stages of the disease, and those with open triradiate cartilages had better outcomes. No control data were presented.

Raney and colleagues[17] also studied hips treated with valgus osteotomy for hinge abduction and pain. Twenty-one of 31 hips had Iowa hip scores averaging 93 points, but 10 failed to return for follow-up. No comparative group was studied.

Yoo and colleagues[18] varied the extension and valgus of their osteotomy depending on the morphology of the involved hip. They report an improvement in the Iowa hip score from 66 before surgery to 92 after surgery. No control data were presented.

OTHER STUDIES

Fabry and colleagues[19] report 36 hips in patients younger than 5 years at onset. They found that one third of patients had a poor result, and that the lateral pillar classification was useful in predicting outcome. Treatment methods were not related to outcome.

Rowe and colleagues[20] studied the effect of cheilectomy in patients with Legg–Perthes disease over a 25-year follow-up. In this series, the extruded portion of the femoral head was excised in patients who had collapse of the femoral head and hinge abduction. Patients were between 9 and 11 years of age at onset. Early results showed improvement in range of motion and a decrease in symptoms. The 25-year follow-up showed 3 hips with poor results, 1 with fair results, and 1 with good outcome. All hips showed degenerative changes radiographically and patients were mildly symptomatic. This study is timely because femoral head reshaping procedures, usually done with surgical dislocation, are being done in a number of centers. The absence of a control group makes conclusions difficult. To the optimist, these hips responded better than they would have without treatment, whereas the

TABLE 40–1. Summary of Recommendations for the Treatment of Legg–Calve–Perthes Disease

STATEMENT	LEVEL OF EVIDENCE/GRADE OF RECOMMENDATION	REFERENCES
1. The lateral pillar classification (prognostic) and the Stulberg classification (outcome) have good interobserver reliability.	B	5
2. Radiographic outcome at maturity is better with younger age at presentation and worse with increasing radiographic extent of disease at presentation.	B B	2, 4 6, 7, 9, 10
3. Operation (Salter innominate or femoral varus osteotomy) improved radiographic outcome compared with nonoperative treatments in patients 8 years and older at presentation with lateral column B or B/C hips.	B	4
4. Valgus osteotomy improved Iowa hip scores in patients with hinge abduction.	C	15–17
5. Hinge distraction prevented femoral head collapse compared with historical control subjects.	B	20

pessimist concludes that they are still facing progressive degenerative arthropathy.

Maxwell and colleagues[21] studied arthrodiastasis of the hip and compared the treated hips with a historical control group. The distraction treatment was done in the early phase of disease, before any collapse, in boys older than 8 and girls older than 7 years. One of 15 treated hips showed collapse, whereas 9 of 30 control hips collapsed. Pretreatment classification for severity was not done, and final outcome data were not available. Other studies of distraction treatment have focused on hips that have already had collapse with or without hinge abduction. In these patients, the operation is considered as salvage for severe disease.

SUMMARY

Based on strong evidence, that being Level II studies, we can conclude that surgical treatment is best for patients with Legg–Perthes disease in certain specific instances. Patients with lateral pillar B and B/C border involvement whose onset is after their eighth birthday are likely to benefit from femoral varus osteotomy or Salter innominate osteotomy. The surgery is best performed early in the course of the disease, either in the initial stage or in the early portion of the fragmentation stage. Studies to date have not shown benefit of surgery for children younger than 8 at onset. The evidence is strong that without specific treatment, the lateral pillar B hips in the younger age group have a high likelihood of a favorable outcome; for example, in one study, results were 76% Stulberg I or II and only 3% Stulberg IV. This group represents about one third of a population of children with Legg–Perthes disease older than 6 years.

To perform surgery in the earliest stage of disease, surgeons may choose to perform these procedures before being able to classify the severity of involvement. If all children older than 8 were to be offered surgical treatment, the group A and C hips would not

likely benefit. These groups combined represent only 13% of hips presenting at age older than 8, and this approach may be justified.

Unfortunately, these studies have not shown benefit for lateral pillar C hips with either surgical procedure, or with any of the treatment methods studied. One Level III study suggests that early distraction with hinged external fixation may alter the likelihood of the hip being classified as a lateral pillar C. A clear need now exists for Level I and II studies evaluating this and other innovative treatment methods for this more severe form of the disease.

Studies with lesser levels of evidence have suggested benefit from acetabular augmentation surgery in early stages of disease. In later stages, benefit has been suggested for femoral valgus osteotomy and for joint distraction. Cheilectomy may provide short-term benefit, but long-term benefit is unproven. Table 40–1 provides a summary of recommendations.

REFERENCES

1. Herring JA: The treatment of Legg-Calve-Perthes disease. A critical review of the literature. J Bone Joint Surg Am 76:448–458, 1994.
2. Fulford GE, Lunn PG, Macnicol MF: A prospective study of nonoperative and operative management for Perthes' disease. J Pediatr Orthop 13:281–285, 1993.
3. Harrison MH, Bassett CA: The results of a double-blind trial of pulsed electromagnetic frequency in the treatment of Perthes' disease. J Pediatr Orthop 17:264–265, 1997.
4. Herring JA, Kim HT, Browne R: Legg-Calve-Perthes disease. Part II: Prospective multicenter study of the effect of treatment on outcome. In: J Bone Joint Surg Am 86-A:2121–2134, 2004.
5. Herring J, Kim H, Browne R: Legg–Calve–Perthes disease: Part 1. Classification of radiographs with use of the modified lateral pillar and stulbereg classification. J Bone Joint Surg Am 26:2103, 2004.
6. Aksoy MC, Caglar O, Yazici M, Alpaslan AM: Comparison between braced and non-braced Legg-Calve-Perthes-disease patients: A radiological outcome study. J Pediatr Orthop B 13:153–157, 2004.
7. Aksoy MC, Cankus MC, Alanay A, et al: Radiological outcome of proximal femoral varus osteotomy for the treatment of lateral pillar group-C Legg-Calvé-Perthes disease. J Pediatr Orthop B 14:88–91, 2005.

8. Friedlander JK, Weiner DS: Radiographic results of proximal femoral varus osteotomy in Legg-Calve-Perthes disease. J Pediatr Orthop 20:566–571, 2000.

9. Grzegorzewski A, Bowen J, Guille J, Glutting J: Treatment of the collapsed femoral head by containment in Legg-Calve-Perthes disease. J Pediatr Orthop 23:15–19, 2003.

10. Ishida A, Kuwajima SS, Laredo Filho J, Milani C: Salter innominate osteotomy in the treatment of severe Legg-Calve-Perthes disease: Clinical and radiographic results in 32 patients (37 hips) at skeletal maturity. J Pediatr Orthop 24:257–264, 2004.

11. Kim WC, Hiroshima K, Imaeda T: Multicenter study for Legg-Calve-Perthes disease in Japan. J Orthop Sci 11:333–341, 2006.

12. Domzalski ME, Glutting J, Bowen JR, Littleton AG: Lateral acetabular growth stimulation following a labral support procedure in Legg-Calve-Perthes disease. J Bone Joint Surg Am 88:1458–1466, 2006.

13. Bursal A, Erkula G: Lateral shelf acetabuloplasty in the treatment of Legg-Calvé-Perthes disease. J Pediatr Orthop B 13: 150–152, 2004.

14. Jacobs R, Moens P, Fabry G: Lateral shelf acetabuloplasty in the early stage of Legg-Calve-Perthes disease with special emphasis on the remaining growth of the acetabulum: A preliminary report. J Pediatr Orthop B 13:21–28, 2004.

15. Kuwajima SS, Crawford AH, Ishida A, et al: Comparison between Salter's innominate osteotomy and augmented acetabuloplasty in the treatment of patients with severe Legg-Calve-Perthes disease. Analysis of 90 hips with special reference to roentgenographic sphericity and coverage of the femoral head. J Pediatr Orthop B 11:15–28, 2002.

16. Bankes MJ, Catterall A, Hashemi-Nejad A: Valgus extension osteotomy for 'hinge abduction' in Perthes' disease. Results at maturity and factors influencing the radiological outcome. J Bone Joint Surg Br 82:548–554, 2000.

17. Raney EM, Grogan DP, Hurley ME, Ogden JA: The role of proximal femoral valgus osteotomy in Legg-Calve-Perthes disease. Orthopedics 25:513–517, 2002.

18. Yoo WJ, Choi IH, Chung CY, et al: Valgus femoral osteotomy for hinge abduction in Perthes' disease. Decision-making and outcomes. J Bone Joint Surg Br 86:726–730, 2004.

19. Fabry K, Fabry G, Moens P: Legg-Calve-Perthes disease in patients under 5 years of age does not always result in a good outcome. Personal experience and meta-analysis of the literature. J Pediatr Orthop B 12:222–227, 2003.

20 Rowe SM, Jung ST, Cheon SY, et al: Outcome of cheilectomy in Legg-Calve-Perthes disease: Minimum 25-year follow-up of five patients. J Pediatr Orthop 26:204–210, 2006.

21. Maxwell SL, Lappin KJ, Kealey WD, et al: Arthrodiastasis in Perthes' disease. Preliminary results. J Bone Joint Surg Br 86:244–250, 2004.

What Is the Best Treatment for Hip Displacement in Nonambulatory Patients with Cerebral Palsy?

Tim Theologis, MD, MSc, PhD, FRCS and Andrew Wainwright, BSc (Hons), MB, ChB, FRCS (Tr and Orth)

Hip displacement in cerebral palsy (CP) is a common problem, particularly in nonambulant patients.[1] Depending on age and severity of involvement, the incidence rate of hip displacement varies between 10% and 70%.[2] Lack of stimulation to the femoral head and acetabulum by weight bearing, muscle spasticity, and asymmetrical posture may explain the greater incidence of displacement in the nonambulant children. The displacement is gradual, and secondary changes occur on both sides of the joint. The femoral head becomes oval-shaped, whereas acetabular dysplasia develops gradually with the formation of a grove-shaped deformity proximally. The direction of the displacement is superoposterior in the majority of patients. Posterior acetabular defects are more often seen in patients who progress to subluxation, whereas global defects are more common in patients with fully dislocated hips.[3]

It has been recommended that the migration percentage should be used to quantify the severity of the displacement,[4] but the acetabular index has also been used.[5] However, problems with the reliability of both measurements have been reported.[1,6] Three-dimensional imaging, particularly as part of preoperative planning may be appropriate in investigating the direction of instability and acetabular deficiency.[3]

Indications for treatment of hip displacement in CP include pain during the displacement process and prevention of pain from secondary degenerative changes in chronic, established displacement. Correction of posture and improvement in the range of hip movement may facilitate better sitting, as well as easier care and hygiene. The indications for early screening and any preventative interventions are unclear. The role of soft-tissue surgery is also controversial. Finally, the choice of surgical procedure to treat displacement or to salvage the painful, chronically dislocated hip remains controversial. These issues of controversy are discussed in this chapter.

SCREENING FOR HIP DISPLACEMENT IN CEREBRAL PALSY

A retrospective review of the notes and radiographs of 462 patients with CP showed an overall dislocation rate of 10%. Measurement of the acetabular index by a method that allowed for rotation of the pelvis was the single-most important predictor of dislocation. A normal index at the age of 3 years would predict normal development of the hips, provided that clinical examination remained normal and no scoliosis developed[5] (Level of Evidence 2).

A similar finding was presented in a prospective, population-based study of hip displacement in CP.[4] Migration percentage was thought, however, to be the best guide to hip surveillance. The recommendation was that all children with bilateral CP should undergo a standardized position radiograph of their hips at the age of 30 months, to predict the risk for dislocation (Level of Evidence 2).

A population-based study in southern Sweden claimed that, with adequate screening and early intervention, the incidence of dislocation declined significantly, when compared with historical controls (Level IV evidence).[7] The screening was based on a register of children with CP and, therefore, relied on its efficacy.

Radiologic surveillance of children with hips at risk was recommended by a retrospective (Level III evidence) study, which demonstrated a high incidence of dislocation in Gross Motor Function Classification System (GMFCS) level IV and V patients.[1] Similarly, a greater risk for dislocation was identified in quadriplegic children who were not walking by the age of 5 years, when compared with diplegic patients.[8]

In conclusion, two of the studies[4,5] suggest that a radiograph of the hips should be taken around the age of 2 to 3 years to assess the risk for hip dislocation. The presence of an abnormal acetabular index of more than 30 degrees or an abnormal migration percentage of more than 15% would indicate a significant risk for dislocation. A normal radiograph at this age would be reassuring, provided no changes occur on clinical examination of the hips over time. There is consensus in these articles that nonambulant children (GMFCS levels IV and V) are at greater risk and should be screened thoroughly (grade C).

Natural History and Indications for Treatment

Hip displacement in CP is a slow process, which allows secondary structural changes in the femoral head and the acetabulum.[9] It has been suggested that these secondary changes occur early and, in some cases, before the evolution of hip instability.[10]

Pain, poor sitting balance, as well as prevention of windswept posture and the resulting pain have been suggested as indications for treatment of the displaced hip in CP.[11] Loss of mobility in ambulant children, as well as decubitus ulceration and secondary deformity of the spine in the nonambulant ones, have also been suggested as indications.[12] However, a comparison between quadriplegic children with scoliosis and hip displacement and children with the same diagnosis and spinal deformity but no hip displacement showed no effect of the hip displacement on the progression of the spinal curvature (Level III evidence). This was despite the greater incidence of pelvic obliquity in the group with hip displacement.[13]

Preventing dislocation, or reducing dislocated hips, requires that the treated hip represent an improvement on the natural history of the untreated hip. In 1990, Pritchett[14] reported a cross-sectional study of 100 mature patients with total body involvement CP. Fifty had had hip surgery, and 50 had had no treatment. No differences were found in the level or frequency of pain, the sitting ability, pelvic obliquity, scoliosis, or nursing care between the groups. Nursing care difficulties and the ability to sit did not depend on the status of the hip. The conclusion drawn was that the surgical treatment of already dislocated hips of patients with severe CP is not helpful (Level of Evidence III).

A similar cross-sectional study of 77 patients older than 21 years with total body involvement CP attempted to correlate the radiographic status of the hip (dislocated, subluxed, arthritic) with clinical symptoms of hip pain, seating difficulty, and contractures.[15] Clinical symptoms were obtained by caregiver interview and physical examination. Hip status was determined by radiographs with evaluators blinded to clinical status. The Ashworth scale of knee muscle spasticity was strongly correlated with hip pain, and with radiographic dislocation and osteoarthritis. The overall incidence rate of hip pain was low with only 18% definitely painful. The radiographic status of the hip (dislocated, subluxed, or osteoarthritic) was a poor predictor of which hips were painful. The authors conclude that surgical treatment of the hip be based on the presence of pain or contractures, and not on the radiographic status of the hip. This study can be considered Level II evidence regarding prognosis because it did not directly address the results of therapy.

PREVENTION OF HIP DISPLACEMENT AND THE ROLE OF SOFT-TISSUE SURGERY

It has been suggested that soft-tissue surgery around the hips can result in long-term radiographic stability in previously displaced hips.[16–19] Preventative surgery in a cohort of 22 children followed up prospectively for a minimum of 5 years showed that 39 hips remained enlocated, whereas 5 were subluxed. None of the hips that was radiographically normal before surgery deteriorated in the follow-up period[20] (Level of Evidence 4). The effectiveness of adductor tenotomy alone compared with more extensive releases and obturator neurectomy remains a controversial issue.[21,22] However, agreement exists that a preoperative migration percentage of less than 40% would predict successful outcome[22–24] (Level of Evidence 2). It has also been suggested that early surgery, before the age of 6 years, and postoperative bracing contribute to good results[24,25] (Level of Evidence 4). Finally, nonsurgical postural control has also been claimed to limit hip displacement.[26] These studies are limited by the small numbers of patients assessed, the lack of control subjects, and their retrospective design (Level IV evidence).

In a retrospective study of 65 children treated within a well-defined surgical protocol and followed up for a minimum of 8 years, it was found that prevention of dislocation was achieved in 67% of patients. Migration percentage at 1 year after surgery was a good predictor of outcome. Diplegic pattern and the ability to walk were also positive prognostic factors.[27] A similar study of 78 patients followed-up for a mean of 10 years showed a favorable outcome in two thirds of the patients. Preoperative migration percentage of less than 50% was associated with a good result.[28] However, a failure rate of 58% with continuing or recurrent subluxation was found in another retrospective study with 8 years of mean follow-up[29] (Level of Evidence 4).

Iliopsoas transfer has also been suggested for the treatment of hip instability. A study of 39 patients over a mean of 8 years demonstrated that 45 of the 47 displaced hips remained enlocated. However, sitting ability had deteriorated in 50% of the patients.[30] Disappointing results of the same operation have also been reported[31] (Level of Evidence 4).

In a population-based study from Sweden, it was shown that the introduction of preventative measures to treat spasticity or dystonia reduced the incidence of hip dislocation, compared with historical control subjects. Preventative measures included selective dorsal rhizotomy, continuous intrathecal Baclofen infusion, botulinum toxin injections, and nonsurgical treatment of contractures.[7,32] A prospective, open-label case series has also demonstrated that controlling spasticity with continuous intrathecal Baclofen infusion led to improvement or no deterioration of more than 90% of displaced hips within the first 12 months from implantation of the baclofen pump. The observed changes were not associated with age or severity of involvement[33] (Level of Evidence 4). A retrospective study of patients with spastic diplegia before and after selective dorsal rhizotomy showed that 93% of all hips were stable after surgery. However, the follow-up time was short, and no control subjects were used.[34]

An American Academy of Cerebral Palsy and Developmental Medicine evidence report concludes that the published evidence on the effects of adductor surgery in CP should be "regarded as preliminary at best."[35] The lack of long-term studies and comparison with control subjects was highlighted. The need to study the reliability and validity of the radiographic methods was also discussed (grade I).

The existing literature suggests that soft-tissue surgery may prevent hip displacement in young children with bilateral CP. Low preoperative migration index and young age may be associated with good results. Approximately two thirds of patients maintain hip stability at 8 to 10 years from surgery. The evidence supporting these interventions is generally of low quality (case series) and primarily reports radiographic rather than patient-related results. In light of the natural history studies showing that radiographic results are not predictive of either pain or function,[14,15] the clinician is left uncertain whether "preventive" treatment is warranted by the current information available.

BONE PROCEDURES FOR HIP DISPLACEMENT: CHOICE AND RESULTS

Surgical correction of hip displacement in CP may include a combination of femoral and/or pelvic procedures. The choice and combination of these procedures and the results to be expected are discussed in this chapter. Furthermore, whether to treat the contralateral hip is addressed.

Femoral varus/derotation osteotomy was shown to lead to improvement of hip displacement in 20 patients (20 hips) with CP followed up for a minimum of 7 years. However, some degree of subluxation persisted in 4 hips and 1 remained dislocated.[36] A retrospective study of 65 patients treated with 79 varus femoral osteotomies showed that 72% of those were still stable at 5.2 years of follow-up. Age at surgery and degree of preoperative displacement determined the postoperative results.[15] Another retrospective study of 99 patients (144 hips) showed good results in 43% of patients at 7.7 years of follow-up. Pain was still present in 8% of patients, and 8% of hips redislocated.[37] Prolonged rehabilitation should be expected after femoral osteotomy, and patients take a mean of 7 months to achieve preoperative functional level.[38]

A retrospective review of 42 patients (58 hips) treated with open reduction, femoral osteotomy, and a variety of acetabular osteotomies showed a redislocation rate of 11% at 5.9 years of follow-up when a Pemberton or Salter osteotomy was used. This compared favorably with patients treated with a Chiari osteotomy.[9] However, another study of 11 patients (12 hips) treated by femoral and Chiari osteotomies and soft-tissue releases, and followed up for 14.1 years showed significant improvement in radiographic parameters. Two hips showed early degenerative changes.[39] A further study of 44 patients (5 hips) treated by femoral varus rotational and Pemberton pelvic osteotomies showed redisplacement in 1 hip at 4 years of follow-up. All hips remained asymptomatic.[40] Another study using a similar surgical protocol showed improvement of the migration index at 10 years of follow-up.[41] A study of 21 patients (23 hips) treated with a variety of pelvic osteotomies showed that 4 hips had redisplaced at 6.1 years of follow-up.[42]

A combination of femoral osteotomy with a triple pelvic osteotomy to improve acetabular coverage has also been suggested. The results were evaluated in 11 ambulant patients with CP. All hips remained enlocated at follow-up, and the migration index improved significantly.[43] Satisfactory results were also reported after shelf acetabuloplasty. Twenty hips in 17 patients with CP were followed up for 41.5 months. Only 1 failure, requiring reoperation, was reported.[44]

Dega's transiliac osteotomy performed in isolation or combined with open reduction led to satisfactory early results in 25 patients (30 hips). However, at 12 years of follow-up, 7 hips had displaced. The authors conclude that the procedure should be performed in combination with varus shortening derotation femoral osteotomy.[45] Several modifications of the Dega procedure have been suggested in combination with femoral varus shortening derotation osteotomy to treat hip displacement in CP. The common principle of these procedures is based on leaving the medial cortex of the ilium intact and centering the osteotomy on the center of the triradiate cartilage. The claimed advantage of the procedure includes the reduction in volume of the acetabulum, the provision of posterolateral cover by articular cartilage, and the preservation of the medial wall of the ilium. Consistent satisfactory results in more than 90% of patients at 5 to 10 years of follow-up were reported in retrospective series that examined clinical and radiographic outcomes.[46–48]

Unilateral surgery to treat hip displacement in nonambulant patients with CP was shown to be associated with progressive deformity and displacement of the contralateral nonoperated hip.[49] A further study of 35 patients with CP treated for unilateral hip displacement and followed up for 4.2 years demonstrated dislocation in 10 contralateral hips and subluxation in a further 16 hips. The authors recommend bilateral surgery for the majority of patients.[15] Bilateral pelvic and femoral osteotomies were shown to carry similar risk for postoperative complications compared with unilateral pelvic and bilateral femoral operations. Postoperative anemia and respiratory problems were the most common early postoperative complications observed.[50]

Nonambulant patients with CP and particularly those with reflux, absent gag reflex, and respiratory problems are more at risk for perioperative complications, particularly respiratory problems, and risk for perioperative death. It has been suggested that 25% of patients with CP undergoing hip osteotomies suffer at least 1 complication.[51] Complications of bony hip reconstruction include heterotopic ossification (HO). In a study of 219 patients with CP who underwent a combination of femoral and pelvic osteotomies for hip displacement, HO was observed in 16%. However, only 2% were symptomatic. Spastic quadriplegia was highly associated with HO, compared with diplegia or hemiplegia.[52] Another study showed greater incidence rates of skin sores, instrumentation failure, reoperation, and infection in patients who were casted after surgery compared with those who were not.[53] Epiphyseal changes suggestive of osteonecrosis were reported in 10% of patients who underwent femoral osteotomy and 46% of those who underwent a combination of pelvic and femoral osteotomy. The clinical significance of those radiographic changes were unclear.[54]

The untreated established hip displacement in CP may progress to the development of secondary degenerative changes and pain. This may, in turn, result in further functional compromise and affect quality of life. However, severe and definite hip pain is a relatively rare outcome among adults with CP and correlates poorly with radiographic status of the hip.[15] Furthermore, cross-sectional studies find little difference in pain or quality of life among totally involved adults regardless of whether the hips have been treated with surgery.[14] Hip replacement surgery, excision/interposition arthroplasty with or without valgus femoral osteotomy, and hip arthrodesis have been suggested.[55–57] However, the existing reports in the literature include small numbers of patients, no control subjects, and limited follow-up. Therefore, it is not possible to draw any useful conclusions on the optimal management of these patients.

In conclusion, comparing Level IV studies suggests that combined femoral and pelvic osteotomies claim better results in the mid term compared with femoral osteotomy in isolation. Level IV evidence has been reported that hip stability and clinical improvement, including improved pain, hip mobility, and sitting balance, should be expected at 5 to 10 years of follow-up. The Dega osteotomy and its modifications address posterolateral instability and may carry advantages over conventional pelvic osteotomies performed for developmental hip displacement. Limited evidence exists that postoperative cast immobilization is associated with a greater risk for complications. In the majority of children, the contralateral hip should be treated if the goal is to prevent progressive deformity and displacement. This additional treatment was shown not to significantly increase perioperative risk compared with staged surgery. A high risk rate for complications, suggested at 25%, is expected from hip osteotomies in children with CP. Perioperative death, respiratory problems, anemia, infection, failure of fixation, skin sores, HO, osteonecrosis, and recurrence have been reported. Salvage surgery for the untreated arthritic hip displacement remains controversial.

Deciding on the best treatment for the dislocated or at-risk hip in severe CP is difficult given the current state of the literature. Most of the available material regarding treatment consists of uncontrolled case series, and radiographic outcomes predominate over

TABLE 41–1. Summary of Recommendations

STATEMENT	LEVEL OF EVIDENCE/GRADE OF RECOMMENDATION	REFERENCES
Surveillance		
Nonambulant children with CP should be screened for hip displacement with a pelvic radiograph at the age of approximately 3 years. A normal radiograph at this age would rule out hip pathology, provided no changes occur on clinical examination of the hips over time.	B	4
Natural History		
Hip displacement in CP is a slow process, which allows secondary changes to the femoral head and acetabulum to develop.	B	9, 11, 12
Hip dislocation does not increase the risk for progression of scoliosis.	B	13
Hip pain, seating function, and contractures are unrelated to the radiographic status of the hip (dislocated, subluxed, or osteoarthritic)	B	14, 15
Soft-Tissue Surgery		
Soft-tissue surgery prevents hip displacement at 8 to 10 years in approximately two thirds of young children with bilateral CP.	C	27
Low preoperative migration index and young age are associated with good results.	B	22–25
Bony Surgery		
Combined femoral and pelvic osteotomies lead to better results in the mid term, compared with femoral osteotomy or soft-tissue surgery in isolation.	C	9, 42–44
The Dega osteotomy and its modifications address posterolateral instability and carry advantages over conventional pelvic osteotomies performed for developmental hip displacement.	C	45–48
In the majority of children, the contralateral hip should be treated to prevent progressive deformity and displacement.	C	15
A high risk for complications is associated with this type of surgery.	C	50, 51

CP, cerebral palsy.

clinical ones. The only prognostic studies of high quality[14,15] suggest that, among adult patients, the radiographic status of the hip is a poor predictor of clinical outcome, the incidence of severe pain is low, and the clinical status of patients is no better among those with operated hips than those without. The complication rates are high in all the reported series. Some consensus exists in the Level IV literature regarding the particular techniques to soft-tissue releases (for prevention) and open reductions with femoral and pelvic osteotomies (for treatment). However, from the current literature, we cannot confidently conclude whether patients with severe CP should have hip operations. Table 41–1 provides a summary of recommendations.

REFERENCES

1. Morton RE, Scott B, McClelland V: Dislocation of the hips in children with bilateral spastic cerebral palsy, 1985-2000. Dev Med Child Neurol 48:555–558, 2006.
2. Murray AW, Robb JE: The hip in cerebral palsy. Curr Orthop 20:286–293, 2006.
3. Chung CY, Park MS, Choi IH, et al: Morphometric analysis of acetabular dysplasia in cerebral palsy. J Bone Joint Surg Br 88B:243–247, 2006.
4. Scrutton D, Baird G: Surveillance measures of the hips of children with bilateral cerebral palsy. Arch Dis Child 56: 381–384, 1997.
5. Cooke P, Cole W, Carey R: Dislocation of the hip in cerebral palsy. J Bone Joint Surg Br 71B:441–446, 1989.
6. Spencer JD, Sait MS: The 'true' acetabular index in children with cerebral palsy. Ann R Coll Surg Engl 86:371–374, 2004.
7. Hägglund G, Andersson S, Düppe H, et al: Prevention of severe contractures might replace multilevel surgery in cerebral palsy: Results of a population-based health care programme and new techniques to reduce spasticity. J Pediatr Orthop B 14:269–273, 2005.
8. Terjesen T: Development of the hip joints in unoperated children with cerebral palsy: 3a A radiographic study of 76 patients. Acta Orthop 77:125–131, 2006.
9. Brunner R, Baumann JU: Clinical benefit of reconstruction of dislocated or subluxated hip joints in patients with spastic cerebral palsy. J Pediatr Orthop 14:290–294, 1994.
10. Heinrich SD, MacEwen GD, Zembo MM: Hip dysplasia, subluxation, and dislocation in cerebral palsy: An arthrographic analysis. J Pediatr Orthop 11:488–493, 1991.
11. Bos CF, Rozing PM, Verbout AJ: Surgery for hip dislocation in cerebral palsy. Acta Orthop Scand 58:638–640, 1987.
12. Cigala F, Marmo C, Lotito FM, et al: Hip surgery in cerebropalsy. Chir Organi Mov 88:23–32, 2003.
13. Senaran H, Shah SA, Glutting JJ, et al: The associated effects of untreated unilateral hip dislocation in cerebral palsy scoliosis. J Pediatr Orthop 26:769–772, 2006.
14. Pritchett JW: Treated and untreated unstable hips in severe cerebral palsy. Dev Med Child Neurol 32:3–6, 1990.
15. Noonan KJ, Jones J, Pierson J, et al: Hip function in adults with severe cerebral palsy. J Bone Joint Surg Am 86-A: 2607–2613, 2004.
16. Bowen JR, MacEwen GD, Mathews PA: Treatment of extension contracture of the hip in cerebral palsy. Dev Med Child Neurol 23:23–29, 1981.
17. Schultz RS, Chamberlain SE, Stevens PM: Radiographic comparison of adductor procedures in cerebral palsied hips. J Pediatr Orthop 4:741–744, 1984.
18. Spruit M, Fabry G: Psoas and adductor release in children with cerebral palsy. Acta Orthop Belg 63:91–93, 1997.
19. Wheeler ME, Weinstein SL: Adductor tenotomyobturator neurectomy. J Pediatr Orthop 4:48–51, 1984.
20. Moreau M, Cook PC, Ashton B: Adductor and psoas release for subluxation of the hip in children with spastic cerebral palsy. J Pediatr Orthop 15:672–676, 1995.
21. Cobeljic G, Vukasinovic Z, Djoric I: Surgical prevention of paralytic dislocation of the hip in cerebral palsy. Int Orthop 18:313–316, 1994.
22. Cornell MS, Hatrick NC, Boyd R, et al: The hip in children with cerebral palsy. Predicting the outcome of soft tissue surgery. Clin Orthop 340:165–171, 1997.
23. Cottalorda J, Gautheron V, Metton G, et al: Predicting the outcome of adductor tenotomy. Int Orthop 22:374–379, 1998.
24. Onimus M, Allamel G, Manzone P, Laurain JM: Prevention of hip dislocation in cerebral palsy by early psoas and adductors tenotomies. J Pediatr Orthop 11:432–435, 1991.
25. Houkom JA, Roach JW, Wenger DR, et al: Treatment of acquired hip subluxation in cerebral palsy. J Pediatr Orthop 6:285–290, 1986.
26. Pountney T, Green EM: Hip dislocation in cerebral palsy. BMJ 332:772–775, 2006.
27. Presedo A, Oh CW, Dabney KW, Miller F: Soft-tissue releases to treat spastic hip subluxation in children with cerebral palsy. J Bone Joint Surg Am 87A:832–841, 2005.
28. Terjesen T, Lie GD, Hyldmo AA, Knaus A: Adductor tenotomy in spastic cerebral palsy. A long-term follow-up study of 78 patients. Acta Orthop 76:128–137, 2005.
29. Turker RJ, Lee R: Adductor tenotomies in children with quadriplegic cerebral palsy: Longer term follow-up. J Pediatr Orthop 20:370–374, 2000.
30. Erken EH, Bischof FM: Iliopsoas transfer in cerebral palsy: The long term outcome. J Pediatr Orthop 14:295–298, 1994.
31. Uematsu A, Bailey HL, Winter WG Jr, Brower TD: Results of posterior iliopsoas transfer for hip instability caused by cerebral palsy. Clin Orthop Relat Res (126):183–189, 1977.
32. Hägglund G, Andersson S, Düppe H, et al: Prevention of dislocation of the hip in children with cerebral palsy. The first ten years of a population-based prevention programme. J Bone Joint Surg Br 87:95–101, 2005.
33. Krach LE, Kriel RL, Gilmartin RC, et al: Hip status in cerebral palsy after one year of continuous intrathecal baclofen infusion. Pediatr Neurol 30:163–168, 2004.
34. Park TS: Selective dorsal rhizotomy: An excellent option for spastic cerebral palsy. Clin Neurosurg 47:422–439, 2000.
35. Stott NS: Effects of surgical adductor releases for hip subluxation in cerebral palsy: An AACPDM evidence report. Dev Med Child Neurol 46:628–645, 2004.
36. Hoffer MM, Stein GA, Koffman M, Prietto M: Femoral varus-derotation osteotomy in spastic cerebral palsy. J Bone Joint Surg Am 67:1229–1235, 1985.
37. Settecerri JJ, Karol LA: Effectiveness of femoral varus osteotomy in patients with cerebral palsy. J Pediatr Orthop 20: 776–780, 2000.
38. Stasikelis PJ, Davids JR, Johnson BH, Jacobs JM: Rehabilitation after femoral osteotomy in cerebral palsy. J Pediatr Orthop B 12:311–314, 2003.
39. Debnath UK, Guha AR, Karlakki S, et al: Combined femoral and Chiari osteotomies for reconstruction of the painful subluxation or dislocation of the hip in cerebral palsy: A long-term outcome study. J Bone Joint Surg Br 88B:1373–1378, 2006.
40. Gordon JE, Capelli AM, Strecker WB, et al: Pemberton pelvic osteotomy and varus rotational osteotomy in the treatment of acetabular dysplasia in patients who have static encephalopathy. J Bone Joint Surg 78:1863–1871, 1996.
41. Shea KG, Coleman SS, Carroll K, et al: Pemberton pericapsular osteotomy to treat a dysplastic hip in cerebral palsy. J Bone Joint Surg Am 79:1342–1351, 1997.
42. Pope DF, Bueff HU, De Luca A: Pelvic osteotomies for subluxation of the hip in cerebral palsy. J Pediatr Orthop 14: 724–730, 1994.
43. Jerosch J, Senst S, Hoffstetter I: Combined realignment procedure (femoral and acetabular) of the hip joint in ambulatory patients with cerebral palsy and secondary hip dislocation. Acta Orthop Belg 61:92–99, 1995.
44. Zuckerman JD, Staheli LT, McLaughlin JF: Acetabular augmentation for progressive hip subluxation in cerebral palsy. J Pediatr Orthop 4:436–442, 1984.

45. Jozwiak M, Marciniak W, Piontek T, Pietrzak S: Dega's transiliac osteotomy in the treatment of spastic hip subluxation and dislocation in cerebral palsy. J Pediatr Orthop B 9:257–264, 2000.
46. Roposch A, Wedge JH: A modified periacetabular osteotomy to treat spastic hip dysplasia. J Bone Joint Surg Br 90B (supp I):53–54, 2003.
47. Miller F, Girardi H, Lipton G, et al: Reconstruction of the spastic hip with peri-ilial pelvic and femoral osteotomy followed by immediate mobilization. J Pediatr Orthop 17:592–602, 1997.
48. Mubarak SJ, Valencia FG, Wenger DR: One stage correction of the spastic dislocated hip. J Bone Joint Surg Am 74A: 1347–1357, 1992.
49. Carr CR, Boyd BM: Correctional osteotomy for metatarsus primus varus and hallux valgus. J Bone Joint Surg Am 50: 1353–1367, 1968.
50. Inan M, Harma A, Ertem K, et al: Successful treatment of high congenital dislocated hips in older children by open reduction, pelvic and femoral osteotomy with external fixator stabilization (average 8.2 years of age). J Pediatr Orthop B 14:405–409, 2005.
51. Stasikelis PJ, Lee DD, Sullivan CM: Complications of osteotomies in severe cerebral palsy. J Pediatr Orthop 19:207–210, 1999.
52. Inan M, Chan G, Dabney K, Miller F: Heterotopic ossification following hip osteotomies in cerebral palsy: Incidence and risk factors. J Pediatr Orthop 26:551–556, 2006.
53. Lubicky JP, Bernotas S, Herman JE: Complications related to postoperative casting after surgical treatment of subluxed/dislocated hips in patients with cerebral palsy. Orthopedics 26:407–411, 2003.
54. Stasikelis PJ, Ridgeway SR, Pugh LI, Allen BL Jr: Epiphyseal changes after proximal femoral osteotomy. J Pediatr Orthop B 10:25–29, 2001.
55. Blake SM, Kitson J, Howell JR, et al: Constrained total hip arthroplasty in a paediatric patient with cerebral palsy and painful dislocation of the hip: A case report. J Bone Joint Surg Br 88B:655–657, 2006.
56. de Moraes Barros Fucs PM, Svartman C, de Assumpcao RM, Kertzman PF: Treatment of the painful chronically dislocated and subluxated hip in cerebral palsy with hip arthrodesis. J Pediatr Orthop 23:529–534, 2003.
57. McHale KA: Bilateral spontaneous arthrodesis of the hip after combined shelf acetabular augmentation and femoral varus osteotomies. J Pediatr Orthop 11:108–111, 1991.

Muscular Dystrophy: How Should It Be Treated?

SHAHRYAR NOORDIN, MBBS, FCPS

Improvements in healthcare have resulted in longevity for patients with muscular dystrophies. Until a cure is found, therapeutic and supportive care is essential in preventing complications and improving the affected child's quality of life (QOL). This chapter reviews the available evidence from a surgeon's perspective to guide in the management of this condition.

STEROID THERAPY

Currently, corticosteroids are the only class of drug that has been extensively studied in this condition. In 1989, a large, multicenter, randomized, placebo-controlled study in the United States showed an unequivocal improvement in muscle force with prednisone in patients with Duchenne muscular dystrophy (DMD), and that a low-dose (0.75 mg/kg) daily regimen was as effective as the standard 1.5 mg/kg.[1] The improvement in muscle force seemed to be fairly rapid, within a matter of weeks, and followed by a plateau. However, the substantial side effects, particularly weight gain, weighed heavily against the potential benefits, and the authors recommended further research regarding use of steroids as a long-term therapy for muscular dystrophy. After the initial trial, another randomized study examined the use of alternate dosing regimens, and duration of therapy was reported.[2] Although many studies provided Level III and IV evidence,[3-8] they showed that use of a relatively high dose of deflazacort resulted in long-term maintenance of pulmonary function, and the age at which boys became full-time wheelchair users increased by several years over boys who did not take deflazacort. Some debate remains as to the exact dosage regimen (daily vs. alternative schedules) of steroids to compare both efficacy and adverse effects.[9,10] Long-term steroid effects on quality and length of life are not yet known. Nevertheless, current Level III and IV evidence suggests that all boys with DMD should be given the opportunity to start these medications early in their disease course, well before they reach the stage of full-time wheelchair use.

NECK HYPEREXTENSION

Neck hyperextension with progressive increase of lordosis associated with a limitation in flexion of the cervical spine forces these patients to assume awkward compensatory postures to maintain balance and level vision, worsening their QOL significantly. Level IV evidence suggests posterior interspinous cervical fusion in seven patients led to a better sitting position, to easier nursing, and better cosmesis.[11] The mean angle between C2-C7 decreased from an average of 30 degrees before surgery to an average of 19 degrees at 1-year of follow-up. Clinically, these patients had more control over their head position after surgery.

SHOULDER

Orthopedic intervention for the shoulder is mainly confined to fascioscapulohumeral dystrophy. Surgical indications that have been described include inability to abduct or elevate arms and loss of power with inability to hold arm sustained in abduction and elevation. As the muscles stabilizing the scapula become involved, the scapula starts to wing, leading to issues with cosmesis and problems with garment wear particularly in female patients.[12] Surgery should be performed only if the deltoid strength is 4/5 or better. Furthermore, although improvement in appearance and diminution of pain and fatigue can be maintained over the long term, the gains in motion may be lost over time.

Scapulothoracic Fusion

Copeland and colleagues[12] reported Level IV evidence with average 16-year follow-up period (range, 14 months to 44 years) of scapulothoracic arthrodesis in patients aged 16 to 35 years. From the 13 initial patients (20 fusions), 10 patients (14 shoulders) were available for long-term follow-up. Complications included pleuritic pain (resolved spontaneously within 1 week), hemopneumothorax (requiring drainage), rib and scapula fractures, screw pullout, and painful nonunion requiring revision surgery. These patients had an average flexion of 123 degrees and an average abduction of 103 degrees. All patients eventually had improved function, activities of daily living, and cosmesis.

Diab and coauthors[13] report their Level IV evidence of 11 scapulothoracic arthrodesis in 8 patients with adolescent and infantile forms of fascioscapulohumeral muscular dystrophy. They fused the scapula to the thorax in 25 degrees of abduction using 16-gauge wires, a plate, or washers on the posteromedial scapular surface to prevent wire pullout and iliac crest autograft. In all cases, scapular winging and shoulder fatigue and pain initially were eliminated. Active abduction and forward flexion improved to an average of 145 and 144 degrees, respectively. At 6.3 years after surgery, seven shoulders retained motion, whereas four lost motion because of progressive weakness of deltoid with no evidence of failure of the arthrodesis. No short- or long-term respiratory compromise was reported.

Scapulopexy

Scapulopexy has been proposed as an alternative to theoretically avoid the problems of reduced respiratory function, and the shoulder can be mobilized almost immediately after surgery, reducing the risk for muscle atrophy and complications such as stress fractures and nonunion. Giannini and coworkers[14] have reported their case series (Level 4 evidence) with 9 patients (18 shoulders). The scapula was repositioned over the rib cage and fixed to the ribs with metal wires. Arm abduction increased from an average of 68 degrees before surgery to 96 degrees after surgery. Arm flexion increased from an average of 57 degrees before surgery to 116 degrees after surgery. The position of the scapula obtained at the time of surgery was maintained, and the patients had satisfactory cosmetic results at 9.9 years of follow-up. This technique does not require grafts and reduces postoperative complications such as pneumothorax or hemothorax.

SPINE

Steroid Treatment and the Development of Scoliosis

Alman and researchers[15] reported Level 2 evidence showing that steroid treatment slows the progression of scoliosis in male patients with DMD. This was a nonrandomized, comparative study with 7- to 10-year-old boys who were able to walk. Thirty patients were treated with deflazacort (treatment group), and 24 were not (control group). Patients were matched for age and pulmonary function at baseline, and were managed for at least 5 years. A curve of 20 degrees or greater developed during the follow-up period in 16 (67%) of the 24 patients in the control group, but in only 5 (17%) of the 30 patients in the treatment group. Fifteen of the 24 patients in the control group underwent spine surgery, at a mean age of 13 years, whereas only 5 of the 30 patients in the treatment group underwent spine surgery, at a mean age of 15 years. Kaplan–Meier analysis demonstrated a significant difference between the two groups with regard to development of scoliosis of 20 degrees or more ($P < 0.001$). Adverse effects with steroids included cataract (10 patients, none of which interfered with visual acuity or required surgical treatment), stress fractures (3 patients treated with immobilization and/or rest), and weight gain (patients in the treatment group weighed a mean of 3.7 kg more than did those in the control group). Because the families rather than the physician chose the treatment, there may be an inherent selection bias because it is possible that the families who saw more physical deterioration in their child decided against steroid treatment, resulting in the selection of a less severely affected treatment group. These patients were continued on steroid therapy even while the patients were using the wheelchair full time. The future of spines of these patients once skeletal maturity is reached is currently unclear and warrants further study.

Prediction of Spinal Deformity

Several studies have shown that scoliosis develops in almost all patients with DMD, with the exception of those who have a stable, hyperextended spine.[16–18] The progression of spinal deformity leads to a deterioration in pulmonary function in patients with DMD. Yamashita and colleagues[19] reported a case series (Level IV evidence) showing the correlation of age at and value of the plateau of vital capacity (VC) with the severity of progression of spine deformity. They show in a retrospective study of 36 patients that rapid and severe progression of spinal deformity could be expected in patients whose VC plateau was less than 1900 mL and in those in whom it occurred before age 14 years.

To further refine their criteria, Yamashita and colleagues[20] published their results on a cohort of 11 patients (Level IV) using multiple discriminant analysis on the basis of 4 predictors: (1) VC at age 10 years, (2) age at which ambulation ceased, (3) curve pattern of spinal scoliosis, and (4) Cobb angles at age 10 years. In these 11 patients, multiple discriminant analysis correctly predicted the severity of the clinical course of 91.7% of patients with DMD. VC at age 10 was found to be the strongest predictor among the variables. These patients could be identified earlier on as candidates for surgical intervention of spinal deformity.

Surgical Management

Spinal fusion surgery with instrumentation remains the mainstay of treatment for patients with DMD with scoliosis. Cheuk and investigators[21] reviewed the available evidence in the literature for spinal surgery in patients with DMD. They evaluated publications from 1861 to January 2006, and because there were no randomized or quasi-randomized clinical trials to evaluate the effectiveness of scoliosis surgery in patients with DMD, they were unable to make any evidence-based recommendation for clinical practice. They recommend that patients should be informed about the uncertainty of benefits and potential risks of surgery for scoliosis.

The potential advantages of spinal surgery described in the literature are to obtain and maintain sitting balance and correction of pelvic obliquity to preserve the ability of the patient to be mobile in a wheelchair for the remainder of his life. In addition, cosmetic improvement, no need for orthopedic braces, easier nursing care, and pain relief are other mentioned factors. Nevertheless, the effects of spinal surgery on respiratory function and life expectancy are still controversial. Velasco and coauthors[22] recommend posterior spinal fusion for scoliosis in nonambulatory patients with DMD earlier in the course of progression based on Level III evidence. They found that in 20 patients with a minimum of 2 pulmonary function tests (PFTs) before surgery and 2 after surgery, posterior spinal fusion for scoliosis in DMD slowed the rate of respiratory decline in percentage forced VC from 8% per year before surgery to 3.9% per year after surgery ($p < 0.0001$). In an expanded group of 56 patients with DMD with variable numbers of PFTs, the rate of decline also slowed after surgery from 4% per year to 1.75% per year as determined by within-subjects mixed-model regression analysis ($P < 0.0001$).

Quality of Life

Mercado and coworkers[23] report a systematic literature review pertaining to QOL in patients with neuromuscular scoliosis who underwent spinal fusion. The need to operate early in the course of the deformity frequently when curves are relatively mild, as well as the change in the course of the disease caused by steroids, makes measuring the impact of scoliosis surgery on QOL in patients with muscular dystrophy more complex. Based on self-report, the surgery may improve sitting ability, posture, simplify nursing care, and improve self-esteem. The effect on the respiratory and cardiac function is unknown.[24] The authors conclude that given the large emotional family investment in surgery, and the uncontrolled nature of the surgical series, the evidence in support of improving QOL of these patients is weak (grade C recommendation[25]).

Intraoperative Blood Loss

Intraoperative blood loss is high in patients with DMD who are undergoing posterior spinal fusion for scoliosis. Shapiro and coworkers[26] have reported their results of a cohort of 56 patients divided into 2 groups: 1 group received tranexamic acid (TXA) whereas the other did not (Level III evidence). The groups were comparable in relation to surgical technique, age at surgery, number of levels fused, preoperative deformity, and surgical time. Blood loss with TXA decreased by 42% compared with those not treated with TXA. Accounting for patient weight and estimated blood volume, mean percentage blood loss with and without TXA was 47% ± 28% versus 112% ± 67% ($P < 0.001$). This physiologic indicator shows that blood loss with TXA decreased by 58% compared with those patients not treated with TXA. TXA was also showed to significantly reduce intraoperative blood loss after accounting for surgical time. Intraoperative homologous blood replacement by whole blood and packed red blood cells and autologous cell saver replacement are also significantly reduced with TXA.

Distal Extent of Fusion

Most authors previously recommended fixation to the sacrum or pelvis for scoliosis in DMD to correct pelvic obliquity. However, this has been questioned because the curve size and pelvic obliquity are small in early cases, and pelvic fixation has a greater complication rate. Mubarak and colleagues[27] published Level III evidence comparing pelvic versus lumbar fixation for scoliosis in 22 wheelchair-mobilized patients with DMD. They found that in small curves with minimal preoperative pelvic obliquity (15 degrees or less), instrumentation and fusion to L5 was adequate at the time of a 34-month follow-up. However, in a later study, comparing pelvic and lumbar fixation in 48 cases of DMD, Alman and Kim[28] disagreed (Level III evidence). Using Luque instrumentation and following Mubarak and colleagues' criteria[27] (fixation to L5 when Cobb angle < 40 degrees and pelvic obliquity < 10 degrees), they found progression of pelvic obliquity in 32 of 38 cases in their lumbar fixation group (with 2 cases requiring revision), but no progression at all in 10 cases in the sacral fixation group. They recommend sacral fixation in general and especially when the apex of the curve is below L1. They recognized, however, that sublaminar wire instrumentation in the lumbar spine could be responsible for the failure in the lumbar fixation group, and suggested that the use of screws or hooks into the lumbar spine may avoid this problem.

Sengupta and coworkers[29] report on their cohort of 50 patients (Level III evidence) with DMD using newer constructs with lumbar pedicle screws. They divided their patients into two groups who were observed for a minimum of 3 years. The first group consisted of 31 patients with an average age of 14 years. This group underwent a spinal fusion that extended to the pelvis. The average preoperative Cobb angle was 48 degrees, and the average preoperative pelvic obliquity was 20 degrees. The second group consisted of 19 patients with an average age at surgery of 11.7 years. The patients in this group were treated with thoracic sublaminar wires and lumbar pedicle screws. The average preoperative Cobb angle was 19.8 degrees, and the average preoperative pelvic obliquity was 9 degrees. The authors document improved correction and maintenance of correction in the group that underwent fusion with pedicle screw fixation to L5. They acknowledge that the pre-operative deformity was greater in the patients who had fusion to the pelvis and conclude that lumbar pedicle screw fixation that stops short of the pelvis is adequate in patients who have minimal deformity and pelvic obliquity.

HIP AND KNEE FLEXION CONTRACTURES

Contractures and progressive weakness of the lower extremities render walking increasingly difficult for patients with DMD. Extensive rehabilitation and orthopedic measures, in addition to medical treatment, have been directed toward prolongation of the ability to walk. Manzur and coauthors[30] reported a randomized, controlled trial (Level II evidence) in 1992 to evaluate the role of early surgical treatment of contractures in 20 boys with DMD. Their entry criteria were designed to recruit a cohort of boys with a relatively uniform clinical severity, in the age range of 4 to 6 years. These boys were divided into two groups. The 10 boys in the surgical treatment group had the operation within 1 month of randomization by a single surgeon. Surgery was standardized and consisted of open release at the hip of sartorius, superficial head of rectus femoris and tensor fascia lata. A long incision was made along the lateral aspect of the thigh to expose the deep fascia, which was incised anterior to the lateral intermuscular septum, and a strip of fascia approximately 2 cm wide was removed. The tendo-Achilles (TA) was routinely lengthened percutaneously. Hamstring tendons were released percutaneously if there were knee flexion contractures. They were discharged 4 to 6 days after surgery, walking without any orthotic support. No passive stretching or physiotherapy was prescribed. The second control group continued with routine management including regular passive stretching of TA, iliotibial bands (ITBs), and hip flexors. The stretching was performed daily by parents after demonstration by the physiotherapist and was kept under surveillance at each follow-up attendance. Regression analysis showed no significant difference between the two groups in any of the parameters measured. No measurable difference was found between the surgical and control groups. Surgery was effective in reducing the TA contractures in all of the boys who underwent surgery. However, freedom from the need for regular passive stretching was short-lived, and 7 of the 10 boys had recurrence of the TA contractures within 1 to 2 years after surgery. Based on these results, the authors did not recommend surgery as standard treatment.

Bakker and de Groot[31] did a structured literature review on the effects of knee-ankle-foot orthosis (KAFO) for patients with DMD. They searched the literature from 1966 to 1997 based on their inclusion criteria. No RCT had been performed to determine the effectiveness of KAFO. Only four nonrandomized, controlled studies were described. They suggest the possibility of a publication bias (only best results published), patient selection bias (only motivated families), and the absence of blinding with measurement bias leading to a positive influence on the results. All reviewed studies described surgical Achilles tenotomy. The scientific strength of the studies reviewed was poor. Results showed that the KAFO can prolong assisted walking, but it is uncertain whether it can prolong functional walking. The boys that benefit most have a relatively low rate of deterioration, are capable of enduring an operation, and are well motivated.

FOOT AND ANKLE

Equinus and equinovarus deformity of the ankle are serious problems associated with DMD. Hyde and colleagues[32] reported Level II evidence, a randomized, prospective, multicenter trial, looking at passive stretching techniques with or without the use of below-knee night splints early in the course of the disease on the evolution of ankle equinus. Twenty-seven boys were evaluated and randomized using an incomplete block design using age and muscle strength as variables for stratification. The authors show that boys who wore night splints in addition to performing passive stretching of the TA benefited by an annual delay of 23% in the development of contractures compared with those who did not.

Main et al.[33] published Level III evidence regarding serial casting of ankles in DMD to reduce TA contractures and to allow fitting of KAFOs at the end of functional walking. TA range and age at loss of standing with KAFOs were prospectively assessed in 9 patients who underwent serial casting before rehabilitation into KAFOs and compared with a group of 20 patients with DMD who had TA (group II) or TA and ITB surgical resection (group III). Mean age at loss of functional ability to walk and rehabilitation with KAFOs was 10.3 years (8.7–11.7 years) in group I, 9.3 years (7.7–12 years) in group II, and 9.5 years (8.3–11.7 years) in group III. The authors conclude that although further studies will be required to evaluate the effect of all these variables in a larger prospective, randomized cohort, the results of this pilot study suggest that serial casting can be considered in patients with DMD with moderate TA contractures and in whom there is no significant ITB tightness. The results of this study have to be interpreted with caution because the number of patients is too small. Furthermore, this was not a prospective study, and the groups could not be randomized or matched for age at intervention, use of steroids, and other relevant factors that may have contributed to the duration of ambulation in KAFOs.

Scher and Mubarak[34] reported Level 3 evidence for the use of posterior tibial tendon transfer in patients with DMD with regard to foot deformity and ambulation. Fifty-seven patients were divided into three treatment groups. Group I contained patients who had surgery to maintain or resume ambulation. Group II included patients who had stopped walking and did not have the potential to resume ambulation or had no desire to do so. They had surgery to correct and maintain foot position. Group III (*n* = 25) patients did not have any surgery. All 32 patients in groups I and II had posterior tibial tendon transfer and Achilles tendon lengthening as part of the procedure. The mean age at cessation of ambulation for those who had surgery was 11.2 years versus 10.3 years for those who did not have surgery (*P* < 0.005). Thirty-four available patients (20 in groups I and II, and 10 in group III) were assessed for outcomes and foot position. Of the 24 patients who had lower extremity surgery, 23 (96%) were comfortable in any shoes or sneakers versus 6 (60%) in the group who did not have surgery. The authors indicate a positive role of foot surgery for these patients.

In contrast, Leitch and coworkers[35] presented their Level III evidence with 88 full-time wheelchair patients with DMD divided into 2 groups. The first group comprised 30 boys with DMD who had had foot surgery including an open or percutaneous TA lengthening or tenotomy, and 26 of the 30 patients in this group also had a tibialis posterior tendon transfer. The second group consisted of boys who did not have surgery. A self-report questionnaire was used to assess difficulty with shoe wear, foot pain, foot hypersensitivity, and cosmetic concerns with regard to the feet, and a foot examination was performed. No significant differences were found between patients who did and did not receive foot surgery with respect to shoe wear (*P* > 0.05), pain (*P* > 0.05), hypersensitivity (*P* > 0.05), or cosmesis (*P* > 0.05). Hindfoot motion was significantly better in patients who did not have surgery (*P* < 0.05). Equinus contractures were significantly worse in patients who did not have surgery (*P* < 0.05). The authors conclude that surgery changes the position of the feet. However, all patients, regardless of whether they had surgery, had minimal concerns about their feet cosmesis, minimal difficulty with shoe wear, and infrequent pain. They recommend that full-time wheelchair users with DMD do well with or without surgery. Therefore, given the greater risks for surgery in this population, foot surgery should be performed only in children with specific foot problems that surgery can definitely address. The main caveat was that the patients were not randomized, and preoperative data for all patients were not available. Therefore, it is possible that patients who had more severe pain, concerns about the appearance of their feet, or difficulty with shoe wear may have been more likely to receive surgery.

Based on the current level of evidence available, full-time wheelchair sitters can be advised that the frequency of poor outcome is low in patients who do not receive surgery and that surgery can change the shape of their feet, but the outcomes of treatment appear to be roughly similar with or without surgery. Table 42–1 summarizes the current available evidence for surgery in patients with DMD.

TABLE 42–1. Summary of Recommendations

STATEMENT	LEVEL OF EVIDENCE/GRADE OF RECOMMENDATION	REFERENCES
1. Steroid treatment results in better maintenance of muscle strength, improves pulmonary function, and delays boys becoming full-time wheelchair users.	B	1, 2
2. Steroid treatment delays the development of scoliosis and need for spinal surgery.	B	15
3. Surgical correction of scoliosis results in better sitting position, correction of pelvic obliquity, and easier nursing care with no long-term obvious benefits in terms of respiratory function, QOL, or life expectancy.	B	21–23
4. Early release of hip, knee, and ankle contractures have not shown to benefit by surgery in the long term.	B	30
5. Night splints in addition to passive stretching of TA are effective in controlling TA contractures.	B	32

QOL, quality of life; TA, tendo-Achilles.

REFERENCES

1. Mendell JR, Moxley RT, Griggs RC, et al: Randomized, double-blind six-month trial of prednisone in Duchenne's muscular dystrophy. N Engl J Med 320:1592–1597, 1989.
2. Beenakker EA, Fock JM, Van Tol MJ, et al: Intermittent prednisone therapy in Duchenne muscular dystrophy: A randomized controlled trial. Arch Neurol 62:128–132, 2005.
3. Alman BA: Duchenne muscular dystrophy and steroids: Pharmacologic treatment in the absence of effective gene therapy. J Pediatr Orthop 25:554–556, 2005.
4. Biggar WD, Gingras M, Fehlings DL, et al: Deflazacort treatment of Duchenne muscular dystrophy. J Pediatr 138:45–50, 2001.
5. Biggar WD, Harris VA, Eliasoph L, Alman B: Long-term benefits of deflazacort treatment for boys with Duchenne muscular dystrophy in their second decade. Neuromuscul Disord 16:249–255, 2006.
6. Biggar WD, Politano L, Harris VA, et al: Deflazacort in Duchenne muscular dystrophy: A comparison of two different protocols. Neuromuscul Disord 14(8-9):476–482, 2004.
7. Carter GT, McDonald CM: Preserving function in Duchenne dystrophy with long-term pulse prednisone therapy. Am J Phys Med Rehabil 79:455–458, 2000.
8. Fenichel GM, Florence JM, Pestronk A, et al: Long-term benefit from prednisone therapy in Duchenne muscular dystrophy. Neurology 41:1874–1877, 1991.
9. Bushby K, Muntoni F, Urtizberea A, et al: Report on the 124th ENMC International Workshop. Treatment of Duchenne

muscular dystrophy; defining the gold standards of management in the use of corticosteroids. 2-4 April 2004, Naarden, The Netherlands. Neuromuscul Disord 14(8-9):526–534, 2004.

10. Dubowitz V: Prednisone for Duchenne muscular dystrophy. Lancet Neurol 4:264, 2005.

11. Giannini S, Faldini C, Pagkrati S, et al: Surgical treatment of neck hyperextension in duchenne muscular dystrophy by posterior interspinous fusion. Spine 31:1805–1809, 2006.

12. Copeland SA, Levy O, Warner GC, Dodenhoff RM: The shoulder in patients with muscular dystrophy. Clin Orthop Relat Res (368):80–91, 1999.

13. Diab M, Darras BT, Shapiro F: Scapulothoracic fusion for facioscapulohumeral muscular dystrophy. J Bone Joint Surg Am 87:2267–2275, 2005.

14. Giannini S, Ceccarelli F, Faldini C, et al: Scapulopexy of winged scapula secondary to facioscapulohumeral muscular dystrophy. Clin Orthop Relat Res 449:288–294, 2006.

15. Alman BA, Raza SN, Biggar WD: Steroid treatment and the development of scoliosis in males with duchenne muscular dystrophy. J Bone Joint Surg Am 86-A:519–524, 2004.

16. Wilkins KE, Gibson DA: The patterns of spinal deformity in Duchenne muscular dystrophy. J Bone Joint Surg Am 58:24–32, 1976.

17. Smith AD, Koreska J, Moseley CF: Progression of scoliosis in Duchenne muscular dystrophy. J Bone Joint Surg Am 71:1066–1074, 1989.

18. Oda T, Shimizu N, Yonenobu K, et al: Longitudinal study of spinal deformity in Duchenne muscular dystrophy. J Pediatr Orthop 13:478–488, 1993.

19. Yamashita T, Kanaya K, Yokogushi K, et al: Correlation between progression of spinal deformity and pulmonary function in Duchenne muscular dystrophy. J Pediatr Orthop 21:113–116, 2001.

20. Yamashita T, Kanaya K, Kawaguchi S, et al: Prediction of progression of spinal deformity in Duchenne muscular dystrophy: A preliminary report. Spine 26:E223–E226, 2001.

21. Cheuk DK, Wong V, Wraige E, et al: Surgery for scoliosis in Duchenne muscular dystrophy. Cochrane Database Syst Rev (1):CD005375, 2007.

22. Velasco MV, Colin AA, Zurakowski D, et al: Posterior spinal fusion for scoliosis in Duchenne muscular dystrophy diminishes the rate of respiratory decline. Spine 32:459–465, 2007.

23. Mercado E, Alman B, Wright JG: Does spinal fusion influence quality of life in neuromuscular scoliosis? Spine 32(19 suppl):S120–S125, 2007.

24. Andersson GB, Bridwell KH, Danielsson A, et al: Evidence-based medicine summary statement. Spine 32(19 suppl):S64–S65, 2007.

25. Wright JG, Einhorn TA, Heckman JD: Grades of recommendation. J Bone Joint Surg Am 87:1909–1910, 2005.

26. Shapiro F, Zurakowski D, Sethna NF: Tranexamic acid diminishes intraoperative blood loss and transfusion in spinal fusions for duchenne muscular dystrophy scoliosis. Spine 32:2278–2283, 2007.

27. Mubarak SJ, Morin WD, Leach J: Spinal fusion in Duchenne muscular dystrophy—fixation and fusion to the sacropelvis? J Pediatr Orthop 13:752–757, 1993.

28. Alman BA, Kim HK: Pelvic obliquity after fusion of the spine in Duchenne muscular dystrophy. J Bone Joint Surg Br 81:821–824, 1999.

29. Sengupta DK, Mehdian SH, McConnell JR, et al: Pelvic or lumbar fixation for the surgical management of scoliosis in duchenne muscular dystrophy. Spine 27:2072–2079, 2002.

30. Manzur AY, Hyde SA, Rodillo E, et al: A randomized controlled trial of early surgery in Duchenne muscular dystrophy. Neuromuscul Disord 2(5-6):379–387, 1992.

31. Bakker JP, de Groot IJ, Beckerman H, et al: The effects of knee-ankle-foot orthoses in the treatment of Duchenne muscular dystrophy: Review of the literature. Clin Rehabil 14:343–359, 2000.

32. Hyde SA, Filytrup I, Glent S, et al: A randomized comparative study of two methods for controlling Tendo Achilles contracture in Duchenne muscular dystrophy. Neuromuscul Disord 10(4-5):257–263, 2000.

33. Main M, Mercuri E, Haliloglu G, Baker et al: Serial casting of the ankles in Duchenne muscular dystrophy: can it be an alternative to surgery? Neuromuscular Disord 17(33):227–230, 2007.

34. Scher DM, Mubarak SJ: Surgical prevention of foot deformity in patients with Duchenne muscular dystrophy. J Pediatr Orthop 22:384–391, 2002.

35. Leitch KK, Raza N, Biggar D, et al: Should foot surgery be performed for children with Duchenne muscular dystrophy? J Pediatr Orthop 25:95–97, 2005.

TRAUMA TOPICS

Chapter 43

What Is the Best Treatment for Open Fractures?

DONALD WEBER, MD, BSc, FRCSC

A fracture is considered open if the bone or the fracture hematoma communicates with the outside environment. These injuries often occur in conjunction with high-energy trauma. It is imperative not be distracted by the potentially gross injury and initiate an Advanced Trauma Life Support protocol. Stabilization of the patient can prevent secondary injury from hypoxia, hypothermia, and reduced tissue perfusion. The treatment of open fractures is a multifactorial and longitudinal endeavor. As with most orthopaedic algorithms the evidence for each step of treatment has a differing level of supporting literature. An exhaustive discussion of each anatomic location and grade of open fracture is neither practical nor supported in the literature. Most studies group all open fractures together or concentrate on tibia fractures when assessing different treatment protocols. Tibias are among the most common location of open fractures, as well as the ones plagued with the highest rates of infection and nonunion. With this in mind most of the treatment recommendations for the tibia can be considered as worst-case scenario for other fractures regardless of their location. Preservation of blood supply is of paramount importance in the treatment of any fracture. This is what allows fracture healing and prevents infection.

OPTIONS

After appropriate ATLS management of the patient, the basic principles of open fracture management include reduction of the fracture, application of a wound dressing and splinting of the involved extremity.

A careful neurological and vascular assessment should be completed and documented. A photograph of the open injury prior to dressing and splint application reduce repeated exposures of the open wound by multiple examiners leading to potential contamination, as a large number of infections are nosocomial.[1] Rapid transportation to the nearest trauma center may reduce the overall rate of long term complications, especially in grade III B open fractures requiring specialty care from orthopaedic and plastic surgeons.[2] Tetanus status must be established early in the course of treatment. Tetanus toxoid should be administered if the patient's immune status is uncertain or the last booster was more than 10 years previous. The administration of human tetanus immune globulin will depend on the patient's injury and immunization status.

Subsequent issues that must be considered include: timing of surgical intervention, the type and duration of antibiotic treatment, what type of irrigation fluid should be used during debridement, how the fracture should be stabilized, and when definitive soft tissue closure should be undertaken. Open fractures are associated with a high rate of nonunion and infection. Ancillary techniques such as bone grafting and various forms of bone stimulation have been tried to minimize the risk of nonunion. The purpose of this chapter is to review the evidence regarding these issues to help guide clinicians and to outline areas where further study is required.

EVIDENCE

Timing of Surgical Intervention

Open fractures have traditionally been considered orthopaedic emergencies, however, there is some evidence that operative treatment within six hours of injury versus treatment after six hours has no effect on ultimate infection rates.[11] Definitive guidelines are not yet established for all open fractures. It is known that the location and grade of injury has a significant bearing on complication rates.[12] As the severity of the fracture increases so does the infection rate. With the tibial location of the open fracture the complication rate is highest. Current evidence with regards to delayed initial treatment is Level II.

Quality radiographs are important to determine the extent of injury and to plan both the temporary and definitive fracture management.

Type and Duration of Antibiotic Administration

Prophylactic antibiotics play a key role in the prevention of one of the most dreaded complications of open fractures; that of infection.[3] It is well established that antibiotics reduce the risk of infection.[4]

Numerous studies have looked at antibiotic selection and duration. There is evidence that when infection does become established the organism is usually one that is resistant to the original antibiotic chosen.[1,5]

Protocols for antibiotic selection are based upon the grade of open fracture and the degree of contamination. Although the open fracture grading system has poor interobserver reliability it still provides guidelines for treatment.[6] There are numerous randomized control trials studying different antibiotic protocols and their conclusions are all very similar. The use of a broad spectrum antibiotic, such as cefazolin, or the use of clindamycin or cloxacillin has been proven to reduce infection rates in grade I and grade II open fractures up to seven fold.[7,8,9] In grade III fractures, additional coverage is needed for gram-negative organisms with an aminoglycocide or fluoroquinolone.[8] Gross contamination or "farm injuries" necessitate the addition of clostidial coverage and this usually means adding penicillin or metronidazole. Once daily high dose gentamicin (5-6 mg/kg) has been proven to be as effective as conventional divided dosing.[10] In severe open wounds the use of an antibiotic bead pouch has been shown to reduce infection rates.[20,21] Gentamicin beads are available commercially or tobramycin beads can be made by hand. Add 1.2 grams of powdered tobramycin to each package of cement. Round beads of 5 to fifteen millimeters are formed, strung on a wire, and placed in the open wound. The wound is sealed over with an adhesive, impermeable film such as Opsite or Ioban until the second debridement in 48 to 72 hours.

Irrigation Fluid during Debridement

Once the patient has been stabilized, the extremity reduced and splinted, and antibiotics and tetanus status addressed, definitive wound and possibly definitive fracture management should occur.

With the patient under anaesthetic the extremity is carefully exposed and a wound scrub is generally recommended to remove gross debris prior to preparation and draping of the fracture. Maintaining control of both sides of the fracture is imperative throughout the process. A tourniquet is applied but used only if absolutely necessary (level V). One of the most important steps in the optimization of outcomes is a meticulous layer-by-layer debridement of the open wound. An extensile exposure should be used taking care to minimize further soft tissue injury. Skin resection should be limited, knowing that questionable integument can be resected at the time of secondary debridement. Fat and fascia are generally expendable and poorly vascular. Muscle viability is evaluated along the lines of consistency, contractility, color, and capillary perfusion (4 C's). Bone ends are delivered into the wound and cleaned and all non-viable bone is resected. Retained devascularized bone in the wound, even as a structural

piece, can lead to a fifty percent increase in infection rates.[13] Fasciotomies may be required in open fractures.

Throughout and following the surgical debridement six to twelve litres of warm isotonic irrigation should be run through the wound. The use of detergents such as castile soap as well as antibiotic solutions such as bacitracin has been studied. One large Level I prospective study concluded that neither fluid affected fracture healing or infection rates but the antibiotic solution cases had an increased rate of wound healing problems.[14] Lavage fluid should be delivered by open gravity flow cystoscopy tubing or with low pressure pulsed lavage. High-pressure lavage has been shown to cause damage to bone.[15] There is at least one well-designed in-vitro study showing increased effectiveness of 1% liquid soap in removing adherent bacteria from bone and preservation of osteoblast activity when applied with low-pressure lavage.[16]

Fracture Stabilization

Stabilization of the fracture is the next step. Depending on the grade and location of the injury different treatment methods are recommended. In general, unless a wound is highly contaminated and/or in the tibia, definitive fixation can occur after the irrigation and debridement is completed with the fixation method of choice. The use of both reamed and unreamed nails (level 1) has been proven safe in all grades of open tibia fractures.[16,17,18] Although considered quite safe and probably preferable in the upper extremity, plate fixation is generally not recommended in open tibia fractures.[19] In some cases with extensive contamination and soft tissue injury an external fixator may be chosen for temporary or definitive stabilization.

Timing of Definitive Wound Closure

By convention most open wounds are dressed open or loosely closed with repeat debridements completed every 48 hours until the wound is clean. Antibiotics coverage should continue for 24 hours after definitive closure as greater than 24 hours imparts no greater protection from infection.[22]

A large prospective randomized study is currently underway to look at primary closure of open fracture wounds. It appears that simple, low energy grade one injuries in highly vascular areas may be safe to close primarily. At least one study has shown no difference in infection rates with wound closure at the initial debridement compared to delayed closure.[5] This does not however eliminate the risk of infection with common organisms or a clostridial infection.

In the case of soft tissue loss or high-energy gunshot wounds, early emergency treatment is extremely important. In order to optimize patient outcomes rapid re-establishment of blood supply and limb stabilization is mandatory. Vascular reconstruction needs to take place in less than six hours if there is any hope of limb salvage. In some cases this means rapid transportation of a patient to an appropriate trauma center. Immediate coverage with flaps has been used with success in some centers having microvascular surgeons available. Soft tissue coverage with local tissue, wound vacuums, grafts, or flaps should be completed within 7 to 10 days to significantly reduce overall infection rates.[23]

Additional Techniques to Promote Bone Healing

Reconstruction of bony defects can take place as a planned bone grafting at 6 weeks post injury or using a bone transport system such as an Ilizarov fixator early on. Bone grafting prior to six weeks can lead to resorption of the graft in the inflammatory wound bed or an increased infection rate.[24]

At least 1 large, prospective, multi-centered trial has been completed to study the use of bone morphogenic protein in open fractures. A collagen sponge was soaked with rhBMP-2 and placed in the open fracture at the time of definitive closure. The conclusion of this randomized trial was that the technique was safe and that both wound and fracture healing were accelerated.[25]

Another technology that has been tested in open fractures is the use of Ultrasound to stimulate bone healing. This is controversial as one study in closed fractures revealed no difference in healing rates in tibias.[26] A second study in open tibia fractures concluded accelerated fracture healing with the use of ultrasound.[27]

AREAS OF UNCERTAINTY

Although open fractures are relatively common there are still some gray areas in terms of definitive guidelines. Areas for further evaluation include timing of initial surgery, duration of antibiotics, type of irrigation fluid, and stimulants to bone healing such as ultrasound or bone morphogenic proteins.

AUTHORS RECOMMENDATIONS

Timing of Surgery

Open fractures in association with vascular injury require emergent management within 6 hours to repair the circulation, debride, and stabilize the fracture. For the more common Grade 1 and 2 open fractures there is level 2 evidence to support definitive surgical

treatment that begins more than 6 hours after the initial injury. This means that the extremity needs to be stabilized, antibiotic prophylaxis initiated, and tetanus status verified upon initial presentation. Surgical debridement should be completed at the first opportunity. Higher energy injuries should be taken to the operating room emergently to avoid secondary damage and to ascertain the true degree of soft tissue injury.

Type and Duration of Antibiotic Administration

Grade 1 and 2 fractures should be given a broad-spectrum antibiotic, such as cefazolin. An alternative is clindamycin, cloxacillin, or vancomyacin if allergies exist. In grade III fractures additional coverage is needed for gram-negative organisms with an aminoglycocide or fluoroquinolone.[8] Gross contamination or "farm injuries" necessitate the addition of clostidial coverage and this usually means adding penicillin or metronidazole we administer antibiotics until 24 hours after definitive wound closure.

Type of Irrigation Fluid

We irrigate with warmed normal saline but a detergent solution would also be acceptable and with further study may prove superior.

Fracture Stabilization

Once a wound has been debrided there are only 3 situations in which we would not proceed to immediate definitive fixation. If the patient is unstable, there was gross contamination and questionable tissue viability, or the fracture pattern is complex requiring prolonged surgery and a fresh surgical team. In these situations a temporary spanning fixator is ideal.

Timing of Closure

In general we feel that low energy injuries with no contamination or non-viable tissue in highly vascular areas such as the upper extremity can be safely closed at the first surgery. Anything beyond this requires further evaluation and would be treated with a second debridement and closure.

Ancillary techniques to obtain bone healing: Currently we do not employ any ancillary techniques such as ultrasound or bone-morphogenic proteins in the face of primary treatment of open fractures. On a rare occasion or with a particularly difficult case of nonunion we may add 1 of the ancillary techniques to a standard approach (Table 43–1).

TABLE 43–1. Summary of Recommendations

RECOMMENDATION	LEVEL OF EVIDENCE /GRADE OF RECOMMENDATION
1. Adults with Grade 1 and 2 open fractures should be given a broad-spectrum antibiotic, such as cefazolin. An alternative is clindamycin, cloxacillin, or vancomyacin if allergies exist. This should be started immediately upon presentation and continued for 24 hours after definitive wound closure.	Grade A
2. Adults with grade III fractures require additional coverage for gram-negative organisms with an aminoglycocide or fluoroquinolone. (8). Gross contamination or "farm injuries" necessitate the addition of clostidial coverage and this usually means adding penicillin or metronidazole.	Grade A
3. Open fractures should be taken to the operating room emergently within 6 hours. Differentiation of fracture grade and further study may allow for more refinement of this recommendation.	Grade B
4. There is level II evidence to support the use of warmed saline or detergent for irrigation of open fractures with volume being undefined but 3 to 6 litres being the minimum.	Grade B
5. Adults with open fractures that have been adequately debrided should undergo immediate fracture stabilization. Internal fixation is safe in all fracture types. The decision regarding the type of fracture stabilization should be dictated in part by patient status. If the patient is unstable or the soft tissue injury is not fully declared external fixation is more appropriate.	Grade B
6. Adults with grade I and II open fractures should have immediate wound closure following adequate debridement	Grade B
7. Wounds requiring flaps or grafts should be covered within 7 days.	
8. Adults with grade IIIA open fractures can safely be treated with immediate wound closure following adequate debridement.	Grade C
9. Immediate flap coverage for grade IIIB open fractures has been shown to be safe in some institutions.	Grade C
10. Bone grafting should be carried out after 6 weeks.	Grade C
11. Ultrasound may be beneficial to enhance early fracture healing.	
12. Bone-morphogenic proteins at the time of wound closure may be beneficial.	

REFERENCES

1. Carsenti-Etesse H, Doyon F, Desplaces N, et al: Epidemiology of bacterial infection during management of open leg fractures. Eur J Clin Microbiol Infect Dis 18:315–323, 1999.
2. Naique SB, Pearse M, Nanchahal J: Management of severe open tibial fractures. The need for combined orthopaedic and plastic surgical treatment in specialist centres. J Bone Joint Surg Br 88:351–357, 2006.
3. Braun R, Enzler MA, Rittmann WW: A double-blind clinical trial of prophylactic cloxacillin in open fractures. J Orthop Trauma 1:12–17, 1987.
4. Gosselin RA, Roberts I, Gillespie WJ: Antibiotics for preventing infection in open limb fractures. Cochrane Database Syst Rev (1):CD003764, 2004.
5. Benson DR, Riggins RS, Lawrence RM, et al: Treatment of open fractures: A prospective study. J Trauma 23:25–30, 1983.
6. Brumback RJ, Jones AL: Interobserver agreement in classification of open fractures of the tibia. J Bone Joint Surg Am 76:1162–1166, 1994.
7. Patzakis MJ, Bains RS, Lee J, et al: Prospective, randomized, double-blind study comparing single-agent antibiotic therapy, ciprofloxacin, to combination antibiotic therapy in open fracture wounds. J Orthop Trauma 14:529–533, 2000.
8. Vasenius J, Tulikoura I, Vainionpaa S, Rokkanen P: Clindamycin versus cloxacillin in the treatment of 240 open fractures. A randomized prospective study. Ann Chir Gynaecol 87:224–228, 1998.
9. Patzakis MJ, Harvey JP Jr, Ivler D: The role of antibiotics in the management of open fractures. J Bone Joint Surg Am 56:532–541, 1974.
10. Sorger JI, Kirk PG, Ruhnke CJ, et al: Once daily, high dose versus divided, low dose gentamicin for open fractures. Clin Orthop Relat Res 366:197–204, 1999.
11. Charalambous CP, Siddique I, Zenios M, et al: Early versus delayed surgical treatment of open tibial fractures: Effect on the rates of infection and need of secondary surgical procedures to promote bone union. J Injury 36:656–661, 2005.
12. Harley BJ, Beaupre LA, Jones CA: The effect of time to definitive treatment on the rate of non-union and infection in open fractures. J Orthop Trauma 16:484–490, 2002.
13. Edward CC, Simmons SC, Browner BD, et al: Severe open tibial fractures: Results treating 202 injuries with external fixation. Clin Orthop 230:98–115, 1988.
14. Anglen JO: Comparison of soap and antibiotic solutions for irrigation of lower-limb open fracture wounds. A prospective, randomized study. J Bone Joint Surg Am 87:1415–1422, 2005.

15. Bhandari M, Schemitsch EH, Adili A, et al: High and low pressure lavage of contaminated tibial fractures: An in vitro study of bacterial adherence and bone damage. J Orthop Trauma 13:526–533, 1999.
16. Bhandari M, Adili A, Schemitsch EH: The efficacy of low-pressure lavage with different irrigating solutions to remove adherent bacteria from bone. J Bone Joint Surg Am 83-A: 412–419, 2001.
17. Dervin GF: Skeletal fixation of grade IIIB tibial fractures. The potential of metaanalysis. J Clin Orthop Relat Res 332:10–15, 1996.
18. Keating JF, O'Brien PJ, Blachut PA, et al: Locking intramedullary nailing with and without reaming for open fractures of the tibial shaft. A prospective, randomized study. J Bone Joint Surg Am 79:334–341, 1997.
19. Tornetta P, Bergman M, Watnik N, et al: Treatment of grade-IIIb open tibial fractures. A prospective randomised comparison of external fixation and non-reamed locked nailing. J Bone Joint Surg Br 76:13–19, 1994.
20. Bach AW, Hansen ST Jr: Plates versus external fixation in severe open tibial shaft fractures. A randomized trial. Clin Orthop Relat Res 241:89–94, 1989.
21. Ostermann PA, Seligson D, Henry SL: Local antibiotic therapy for severe open fractures: A review of 1085 consecutive cases. J Bone Joint Surg Br 77:93–97, 1995.
22. Moehring HD, Gravel C, Chapman MW, Olson SA: Comparison of antibiotic beads and intravenous antibiotics in open fractures. Clin Orthop Relat Res 372:254–261, 2000.
23. Dellinger EP, Caplan ES, Weaver LD, et al: Duration of preventive antibiotic administration for open extremity fractures. Arch Surg 123:333–339, 1988.
24. Godina M: Early microsurgical reconstruction of complex trauma of the extremities. Plast Reconst Surg 78:285–292, 1986.
25. Johnson KD, Bone LB, Scheinberg R: Severe open tibial fractures: A study protocol. J Orthop Trauma 2:175–180, 1988.
26. Govender S, Csimma C, Genant HK, et al: Evaluation in Surgery for Tibial Trauma Study: Recombinant human bone morphogenetic protein-2 for treatment of open tibial fractures: A prospective, controlled, randomized study of four hundred and fifty patients. J Bone Joint Surg Am 84-A:2123–2134, 2002.
27. Emami A, Petren-Mallmin M, Larsson S: No effect of low-intensity ultrasound on healing time of intramedullary fixed tibial fractures. J Orthop Trauma 13:252–257, 1999.
28. Heckman JD, Ryaby JP, McCabe J, et al: Acceleration of tibial fracture-healing by non-invasive, low-intensity pulsed ultrasound. J Bone Joint Surg Am 76:26–34, 1994.

Mangled Extremity:
Are Scoring Systems Useful?

DAVID W. SANDERS, MD, MSc, FRCSc

The decision to proceed with amputation or salvage of a mangled extremity is one of the most challenging decisions in orthopedic trauma. Orthopedic trauma surgeons are highly skilled at exercising heroic attempts at limb salvage. However, unsuccessful attempts at salvage are extremely costly and carry with them high morbidity and prolonged rehabilitation. Amputation, on the other hand, is commonly feared by patients. In an attempt to aid in the decision-making process regarding the need for amputation or salvage, a number of predictive indices have been proposed. All of these indices attempt to identify limbs for which salvage or amputation would be preferred.

Advances in care of the traumatized patient including microvascular surgery, nerve reconstruction, tissue transfer, and fracture management continue to expand the orthopedic trauma surgeon's ability to preserve limbs. However, prolonged, costly, and morbid attempts at preservation may, indeed, be worse than the results of early amputation. As suggested by prominent experts in limb reconstruction,[1] this may leave the patient "demoralized, divorced and destitute."

Many considerations must be factored in when making the difficult decision regarding amputation versus limb salvage. These include vascular status, infection risk, tissue devitalization, fracture instability, social impact, physical healing potential, and probably psychological healing potential.[2]

Predictive indices have been created to assist with the decision-making process. These are predominately related to important physical findings that may be associated with the mangled extremity. In many instances, promising results of initial retrospective reports regarding the utility of individual scoring systems are not maintained under the objective scrutiny of higher levels of evidence. These scoring systems, as well as the evidence supporting and validating them, are considered in this chapter.

OPTIONS: SCORING SYSTEMS

Surgeons intuitively recognize that some limbs are frankly beyond salvage, whereas in other cases, a reasonable possibility of limb salvage and restoration of function exists. For centuries before the development of scoring systems, surgical indications for amputation were considered. Kirk,[3] in 1943, noted indications for amputation included any injury or disease rendering limb salvage incompatible with function. Absolute and relative indications for amputation after open tibial fractures with vascular injury were described by Lange and colleagues[4] in 1985. Absolute indications included anatomically complete disruption of the posterior tibial nerve and a crush injury with a warm ischemic time greater than 6 hours. Relative indications included serious associated polytrauma, severe ipsilateral foot trauma, and an anticipated protracted reconstructive course. The authors specify that their indications for primary amputation included either of the absolute indications or two to three relative indications. Although never validated, this type of classification scheme illustrates several crucial elements of decision making used by experienced surgeons.

Mangled Extremity Syndrome Index

In 1985, Gregory and coworkers'[5] severity grading system for multisystem extremity injury entitled "The Mangled Extremity Syndrome Index" (MESI) was published. This scale uses a point score system including the degree of injury severity score to reflect polytrauma, skin injury, nerve injury, vascular injury, bone injury, lag time to surgery and age in years, as well as preexisting disease and shock. In retrospective work, 100% of patients with an MESI of greater than 20 required amputation. However, the patient mix was heterogeneous. Concerns surrounding the MESI include the complexity and the subjectivity of the scoring system. In Roessler and coauthors' retrospective study[6] using this scoring system, the MESI predicted amputation incorrectly in five patients and incorrectly predicted salvage in four patients.

In a second study, Bonanni and colleagues[7] note that the sensitivity of the MESI to predict amputation was low at only 6%; specificity was 90%. Both Bonanni and colleagues[7] and Roessler and coauthors[6] note that many variables included as part of the MESI were unavailable at the time of the initial assessment of the patient, making it impossible to apply this scoring system accurately.

Predictive Salvage Index

The predictive salvage index (PSI) system was introduced by Howe and researchers.[8] Patients with combined orthopedic and vascular injuries were studied. Only patients with lower extremity injuries were included. The PSI system is a simplified variation of the MESI. Points are given for the level of arterial injury, the degree of bone injury, the degree of muscle injury, and the interval from injury to the operating room. An initial retrospective analysis of the PSI was performed in 21 patients. All patients who achieved salvage had a PSI < 8. In contrast, seven of nine patients who required amputation scored 8 or greater. Conclusions from this retrospective study suggest that the sensitivity of the PSI was 78% and specificity was 100%. Bonanni and colleagues[7] applied the PSI retrospectively to their data as well. They found that the PSI predicted amputation with a specificity of 70%, but sensitivity of only 33%. Roessler and coauthors[6] also found that the PSI predicted amputation for two patients who ultimately had their limb salvaged and predicted salvage for five patients who ultimately required amputation.

Mangled Extremity Severity Score

The mangled extremity severity score (MESS) may be the most commonly applied and heavily researched lower extremity scoring index. The MESS system[9] was introduced by Johansen and investigators[9] in 1990. Only five criteria are included in the MESS: skeletal and soft-tissue injury, limb ischemia, shock, and age. The initial MESS analysis was based on a retrospective review of 26 mangled lower extremities. It was subsequently validated in a prospective trial at a different trauma center involving 26 patients.[10] In both the original retrospective analysis and the prospective trial, a MESS score of less than 7 predicted salvage with 100% accuracy. Advantages of the MESS system include simplicity and a relatively more thorough validation compared with the PSI or MESI. However, it remains subjective and includes, in particular, consideration of contamination as a relevant issue surrounding the degree of energy.

MESS data retrospectively applied by Robertson[11] to 152 patients with open fractures that required vascular or soft-tissue reconstruction were also considered. All patients with a MESS score of 7 or more eventually underwent amputation. Forty-three patients whose limbs were ultimately salvaged had a score of less than 7. Sixty-five patients underwent delayed amputation. Of these, 16 had a MESS of greater than 7 at the time of initial amputation. Based on the results of this study, the authors conclude that the MESS system had 100% specificity but lacked sensitivity.

Bonanni and colleagues[7] applied the MESS system to their patients and found that the sensitivity of the scoring system to predict amputation was 22% and specificity was 53%. In contrast with the good specificity reported by Robertson[11] and Johansen and investigators,[9] Bonanni and colleagues[7] believe that the reduced complexity used in the MESS system reduces sensitivity.

McNamara and investigators[12] applied the MESS system to 33 patients, all of whom had severe open tibial fractures. The authors note a significant difference between the mean MESS of the amputation group compared with the salvage group. A score of greater than 7 accurately predicted amputation. The authors conclude that the MESS system was an objective and somewhat useful guide to assist in predicting the ultimate viability of the mangled lower extremity.

Slauterbeck and coauthors[13] have considered application of the MESS to the upper extremity. Forty-three patients with mangled upper extremities were considered. All nine patients with a MESS of greater than 7 underwent amputation. Thirty-four patients with a MESS of less than 7 underwent successful salvage. The authors advocate the use of the MESS as an aid to augment the surgeon's clinical experience.

Limb Salvage Index

Russell and colleagues proposed[14] the limb salvage index (LSI). These authors retrospectively reviewed 70 lower extremity injuries. The authors consider factors such as arterial injury, nature of arterial injury, nature of nerve injury, type of bone injury, type of skin injury, nature of the muscle injury, degree of deep vein injury, and warm ischemic time. Fifty-one patients with successful limb salvage had an LSI of less than 6, and 19 patients who underwent amputation had a LSI of greater than 6. Approximately 95% of amputated limbs included disruption of the sciatic, tibial, or perineal nerves.[14] Bonanni and colleagues[7] apply the LSI retrospectively and conclude that it had a sensitivity of 61% and a specificity of 43%. The authors believe that the degree of detail of the LSI required application to be done in the operating room, and that accurate scoring was difficult at the time of initial assessment.

Nerve Injury, Ischemia, Soft-Tissue Injury, Skeletal Injury, Shock, and Age of Patient Scoring System

The Nerve Injury, Ischemia, Soft-Tissue Injury, Skeletal Injury, Shock, and Age of Patient Score (NISSSA), a modification of the MESS score, was introduced by McNamara and investigators[12] and includes nerve injury, ischemia, soft-tissue injury and contamination, skeletal injury, blood pressure, and age. This system is a modification of the MESS system. The skeletal and soft-tissue components are separated, and nerve injury is added. The authors retrospectively compare the MESS score with the NISSSA system and note an improvement in sensitivity and specificity. Concerns about the NISSSA system relate to its additional complexity compared with the MESS system.

Current Evidence

The best current evidence related to the outcome of limb salvage or reconstruction is provided by the Lower Extremity Assessment Project (LEAP) study. LEAP considers civilian injuries in the U.S. population exposed to severe lower extremity trauma. The LEAP study is the largest study of its kind and includes patients managed up to 7 years. The LEAP study was designed to compare functional outcome in patients with limb-threatening injuries treated with either amputation or limb salvage. The authors in particular note no difference in functional outcome between patients who underwent limb salvage surgery or amputation, but note overall poor functional outcomes in both groups.[15–17]

The LEAP study provides grade 1 evidence and large patient numbers to use in comparing injury severity scores.[18] A total of 556 patients with high-energy injuries were prospectively evaluated. Sixty-three patients had immediate amputations and 86 had delayed amputations such that 407 patients were treated with definitive limb salvage. The authors considered five injury severity scoring systems: The MESS, the LSI, the PSI, the NISSSA Scale, and the Hanover Fracture Scale 97. In all of the patient subgroups, low scores successfully predicted a high potential for limb salvage. However, the converse was not true; a high score was unable to predict amputation. The results suggest that use of these scores alone, in the absence of clinical judgment, was insufficient. The authors conclude that lower extremity scores at or above the amputation threshold should be used with caution in determining the fate of a lower extremity with a high-energy injury.

The same group also considers whether an insensate foot is an indicator for amputation.[19] A subset of 55 patients from the larger LEAP group was found to have an insensate extremity at the time of presentation. Twenty-six were treated with amputation, and 29 with salvage. Overall, the patients treated with limb salvage who presented with an insensate extremity had no difference in functional outcomes at 12 or 24 months, compared with patients treated with limb salvage who had sensation in the sole of the foot. Furthermore, in the group of patients with a lack of sensation, no difference was found when comparing patients with limb salvage with those treated with amputation. The authors suggest that outcome in a patient with an insensate foot at the time of presentation could not be predicted accurately. Surprisingly, more than 50% of the patients who presented with an insensate foot who were treated with primary limb reconstruction ultimately regained sensation. As a result, the authors determined that initial plantar sensation was not prognostic of long-term plantar sensory status or functional outcome (Level I evidence).

A recent prospective study from Egypt assessed the results of arterial reconstruction on 62 patients.[20] Overall limb salvage rates were 93.5%. Salvage rates were high even in the presence of high MESS and MESI scores. Limbs with MESS scores greater than 7 and MESI scores greater 20 were salvaged in 91% of cases (Level 1 evidence). These results agree with those of the LEAP study; that is, salvage can often be achieved even in limbs with high mangled extremity scores.

The evidence comparing outcome after limb salvage or amputation suggests that, overall, the results of the two treatment strategies may be similar. In the end, outcomes are generally poor and comparable with serious chronic illness.[15–17,21] In a recent study by Dagum and coworkers,[21] 92% of patients preferred an attempt at salvage.

AREAS OF UNCERTAINTY

Scoring systems do, however, have significant intrinsic utility. They are a useful ancillary tool to clinical judgment and provide a valuable teaching tool in discussing the elements of the limb salvage decision-making process. Many tools have been developed, reflecting the complexity and individuality of this critical decision-making process. To date, the focus of all scoring tools has been physical findings predictive of limb salvage. This oversimplifies what is ultimately a complex decision, which must include personal, psychological, social, and institutional resources, as well as the critical physical elements that the creators of the scoring systems described have trained us to recognize. Two different individuals with the same injury may require different approaches depending on their personality, social support system, educational and vocational situation, among other factors. This area requires much more study so that the treatment matches a particular individual's needs rather than being dictated entirely by the injury characteristics.

RECOMMENDATIONS

In cases of limb-threatening trauma, the critical decision of salvage versus amputation is challenging to the surgeon and fraught with concern for the patient. Careful judgment, experience, and a consideration of patient and institutional resources are required. The exclusive use of mangled extremity scoring systems, in the absence of clinical judgment, is not supported by the literature.

Most of the best evidence comparing limb salvage with amputation is derived from the LEAP studies. From these studies, it is reasonable to make the following conclusions: (1) limb-threatening injuries severely impair functional outcome; (2) the outcome of amputation and limb salvage is generally equivalent between 1 and 5 years; (3) scoring systems are a useful ancillary tool but do not replace clinical judgment; and (4) lack of plantar sensation does not predict a poor outcome after salvage (Tables 44–1 and 44–2).

TABLE 44–1. Summary of Recommendations

RECOMMENDATION	LEVEL OF EVIDENCE/GRADE OF RECOMMENDATION
1. Adults with limb-threatening injuries can expect a severely impaired functional outcome regardless of whether limb salvage or amputation is undertaken.	B
2. In adults with limb-threatening injuries, lack of plantar sensation is NOT predictive of poor outcome after limb salvage.	A
3. In adults with limb-threatening injuries, scoring systems alone are insufficient to make a decision regarding limb salvage versus amputation.	B

TABLE 44–2. Mangled Extremity Scoring Systems

SCORING SYSTEM	CRITERIA	SCORES	SCORE PREDICTIVE OF AMPUTATION	EVIDENCE
MESI	ISS	1–3	>20	• 100% accuracy (Level IV; $n = 17$)[5]
	Skin injury	1–3		• Sensitivity 6%, specificity 90% (Level II; $n = 58$)[7]
	Nerve injury	1–3		
	Vascular injury	1–3		
	Bone injury	1–6		
	Age	0–3		
	Preexisting disease	1		
	Shock	2		
PSI	Arterial injury	1–3	8	• Sensitivity 78%, specificity 100% (Level IV; $n = 21$)[8]
	Bone injury	1–3		
	Muscle injury	1–3		• Sensitivity 33%, specificity 70% (Level II; $n = 58$)[7]
	Time from injury to surgery	0–4		
MESS	Injury (skeletal, soft tissue)	1–4	7	• Sensitivity/specificity 100% (Level IV; $n = 26$)[9]
	Ischemia	1–3		• Sensitivity/specificity 100% (Level II; $n = 26$)[10]
	Shock	0–2		
	Age	0–2		• Specificity 100% (Level IV; $n = 152$)[11]
				• Sensitivity 22%, specificity 53% (Level II; $n = 58$)[7]
				• Specificity 100% (Level IV; $n = 33$)[12]
LSI	Arterial injury	0–2	6	• Sensitivity/specificity 100% ($n = 70$; Level IV)[14]
	Nerve injury	0–2		
	Bone injury	0–2		• Sensitivity 61%, specificity 43% (Level II; $n = 58$)[7]
	Skin injury	0–1		
	Muscle injury	0–1		
	Deep vein injury	0–1		
	Warm ischemia time	0–4		
NISSSA	Nerve injury	0–3	7	
	Ischemia	0–3		
	Soft-tissue contamination	0–3		
	Skeletal injury	0–3		
	Shock	0–2		
	Age	0–2		

ISS, injury severity score; LSI, limb salvage index; MESI, mangled extremity syndrome index; MESS, mangled extremity severity score; NISSSA, Nerve Injury, Ischemia, Soft-Tissue Injury, Skeletal Injury, Shock, and Age of Patient Score; PSI, predictive salvage index.

REFERENCES

1. Hansen ST Jr: The type-IIIC tibial fracture: Salvage or amputation. J Bone Joint Surg Am 69:799–800, 1987.
2. Cole P: Case controversy open tibial fracture: Amputation versus limb salvage. J Orthop Trauma 21:67–69, 2007.
3. Kirk NT: Amputations. Clin Orthop 243:3–16, 1989.
4. Lange RH, Bach AW, Hansen ST Jr, et al: Open tibial fractures with associated vascular injuries: Prognosis for limb salvage. J Trauma 25:203–208, 1985.
5. Gregory RT, Gould RJ, Peclet M, et al: The mangled extremity syndrome (M.E.S.): A severity grading system for multisystem injury of the extremity. J Trauma 25:1147–1150, 1985.
6. Roessler MS, Wisner DH, Holcroft JW: The mangled extremity: When to amputate? Arch Surg 126:1243–1249, 1991.
7. Bonanni F, Rhodes M, Lucke JF: The futility of predictive scoring of mangled lower extremities. J Trauma 34:99–140, 1993.

8. Howe HR Jr, Poole GV Jr, Hansen ST Jr, et al: Salvage of lower extremities following combined orthopaedic and vascular trauma: A predictive salvage index. Am Surg 53:205–208, 1987.
9. Johansen K, Daines M, Howey T, et al: Objective criteria accurately predict amputation following lower extremity trauma. J Trauma 30:568–573, 1990.
10. Helfet DL, Howey T, Sanders R, et al: Limb salvage versus amputation: Preliminary results of the Mangled Extremity Severity Score. Clin Orthop 256:80–86, 1990.
11. Robertson, PA: Prediction of amputation after severe lower limb trauma. J Bone Joint Surg Br 73:816–818, 1991.
12. McNamara MG, Heckman JD, Corley FG: Severe open fractures of the lower extremity: A retrospective evaluation of the Mangled Extremity Severity Score (MESS). J Orthop Trauma 8:81–87, 1994.
13. Slauterbeck JR, Britton C, Moneim MS, et al: Mangled Extremity Severity Score: An accurate guide to treatment of the severely injured upper extremity. J Orthop Trauma 8:282–285, 1994.

14. Russell WL, Sailors DM, Whittle TB, et al: Limb salvage versus traumatic amputation: A decision based on a seven-part predictive index. Ann Surg 213:473–481, 1991.

15. Bosse MJ, MacKenzie EJ, Kellam J, et al: An analysis of outcomes of reconstruction or amputation of leg threatening injuries. N Engl J Med 347:1924–1931, 2002.

16. MacKenzie EJ, Bosse MJ, Castillo RC, et al: Functional outcomes following lower extremity amputation for trauma. J Bone Joint Surg Am 86:1636–1645, 2004.

17. MacKenzie EJ, Bosse MJ, Pollak AN, et al: Disability persists long-term following severe lower limb trauma: Results of a seven year follow-up. J Bone Joint Surg Am 87:1801–1809, 2005.

18. Bosse MJ, MacKenzie EJ, Kellam JF, et al: A prospective evaluation of the clinical utility of lower extremity injury severity scores. J Bone Joint Surg Am 83:3–14, 2001.

19. Bosse MJ, McCarthy ML, Jones AL, et al; Lower Extremity Assessment Project (LEAP) study group: The Insensate foot following severe lower extremity trauma: An indication for amputation? J Bone Joint Surg Am 87:2601–2608, 2005.

20. Elsharawy MA: Arterial reconstruction after mangled extremity: Injury severity scoring Systems are not predictive of limb salvage. Vascular 13:114–119, 2005.

21. Dagum AB, Best AK, Schemitsch EH, et al: Salvage after severe lower-extremity trauma: Are the outcomes worth the means? Plast Reconstr Surg 103:1212–1220, 1999.

Chapter 45

What Is the Appropriate Timing of Prophylactic Stabilization of Osseous Metastases?

David John Garth Stephen, MD, FRCS(C)

Metastatic bone disease continues to challenge even the most experienced orthopedic surgeon. The increased survival rate of patients with carcinoma has led to an increasing population of patients with osseous metastases. Bone is the third most common site of metastasis after lung and liver.[1] In up to 25% of patients, metastatic bone disease is the first presentation of carcinoma. Metastasis to bone is common, with 50% of newly diagnosed cancers eventually spreading to bone.[2] The most common primary tumors that metastasize to bone are prostate (36%), breast (32%), and lung (14%).[2] The most common sites for metastasis to bone are vertebrae, pelvis, ribs, femur, and skull. In as many as 10% of patients with metastases, the primary site is never found. Survival after diagnosis of bone metastasis is related to the primary bone tumor: breast, 34 months; prostate, 24 months; cervix, 18 months; colorectal, 13 months; lung, less than 12 months; and melanoma, 3 months.[2] A variation exists in survival related to types and grades of primary tumor.

Plain radiographs of the involved limb in at least two planes form the initial investigation. The metastatic lesion must destroy 30% to 50% of bone and reach a size of 1 cm to be seen on plain radiographs. The characteristic features seen include radiolucent (osteolytic) lesion, although the lesion can be osteoblastic, radiodense, or mixed; minimal periosteal reaction; epicenter in the intramedullary canal; and intracortical/juxtacortical locations are rare. A bone scan demonstrates metastatic lesions on average 3 months before plain radiographs, and it can detect a lesion as small as 2 mm. McNeil[3] reviewed 273 patients with known primaries and a positive bone scan. He found that 55% had actual metastases, whereas the other 45% had other reasons: trauma in 25%, infection in 10%, and miscellaneous in 10% of patients. Overall, the diagnosis of metastatic bone disease can be made in 66% of patients with a careful history and physical examination, chest radiograph, and computed tomography (CT) of the chest. An additional 13% can be diagnosed with a CT scan of the abdomen. A biopsy of the skeletal lesion adds a further 8% and allows confirmation in 28% of patients.

OPTIONS

The treatment of metastatic bone disease involves a multidisciplinary approach that includes orthopedic surgery, radiation oncologists, and medical oncologists. The indication for nonoperative management is controversial and is dependent on the extent and location of metastatic involvement, as well as patient factors. The goal is to identify those patients who are at high risk for progressing from an impending fracture to a pathologic fracture. The rationale for this approach relates to the improved results in those patients treated before fracture. The purpose of this chapter is to help guide clinicians regarding when to consider prophylactic fixation of a metastatic lesion in bone based on the best available evidence.

EVIDENCE

Ward and colleagues[4] compared the results of 97 impending fractures compared with 85 complete fractures. In the impending group, there was less blood loss (438 vs. 636 mL), shorter hospital stays (7 vs. 11 days), greater likelihood of discharge home as opposed to an extended care facility (79% vs. 56%), and a greater likelihood of resuming support-free ambulation (35% vs. 12%).[4]

It has been recommended that femoral metastases can be treated without surgery if they are small (<2.5 cm), less than 50% of the diameter of the cortex, and are in a low-risk location (i.e., not in the pertrochanteric region of the femur)[5,6] (Level V). Often, a CT scan of the affected area is valuable in determining the exact size and location of the lesion. These recommendations are controversial, serving only as guidelines, and treatment should be individualized.

Fidler[7] examined the concept of greater than 50% cortical diameter as a criterion for operative intervention (Level II). The fracture risk was low (2%) when the lesion size was less than 50% of the diameter. The fracture risk was high (80%) when the lesion was greater than 75% of the diameter. Finally, when the lesion was 50% to 75% of the diameter, there was a 61% incidence rate of fracture.

Beals and coauthors[8] reviewed 338 patients with 94 femoral metastases; 8 of 19 with a pathologic fracture had a lesion smaller than 2.5 cm on radiographs (Level II). This was a false-negative rate of 42% for the concept of 2.5 cm being a guideline.

Finally, Keene and coworkers[9] could not use the criteria to predict which pathologic fractures would occur in patients with metastatic breast carcinoma to the proximal femur (Level II). The ranges of sizes and percentages of the cortical involvement on plain radiographs were the same for patients with and without fractures.

Several biomechanical studies have been completed to resolve the issue of pathologic fracture risk. Sprujit and researchers[10] used finite element models from quantitative CT scans of cadaveric femora with lesions created in the subtrochanteric region. The model was able to successfully predict torsional failure in 82% of cases. Lee also developed a model using quantitative CT combined with engineering beam analysis to predict the load-carrying capacity of femurs with metastatic defects.[10a]

Roth and colleagues[11] used biomechanically based models to predict metastatic burst fracture risk. They examined 92 vertebrae with osteolytic spinal metastases. Specific burst fracture risk was calculated incorporating load-bearing capacity (tumor volume, trabecular bone density, disc quality, and pedicle involvement) and load-bearing requirement (pressure load, loading rate). The models were able to predict fracture in patients at high risk and predict stability in patients at low risk.

Tschirhart and investigators[12] were able to use parametric finite element modeling to determine the effects of vertebral level, geometry, and metastatic compromise to the cortical shell on the risk for burst fracture in the thoracic spine. Their findings demonstrate that upper thoracic vertebrae are at greater risk whereas kyphotic motion segments are at a lower risk for burst fracture. In addition, transcortical lesions are at up to 30% less likely to lead to burst fracture.

Mirels[13] has proposed a scoring system for diagnosing the risk for impending pathologic fracture. This system objectively analyzes and combines four radiographic and clinical risk factors (that score is 1–3 independently, then added) into a single score. The variables include location (upper, lower extremity, and pertrochanteric); nature of the lesion (blastic, mixed, osteolytic); size of the lesion (<1/3, 1/3 2/3, >2/3 of the diameter of the bone); and pain (mild, moderate, functional). Using the system in a retrospective review of 78 patients (Level II), Mirels[13] found that as the score increased to greater than 7, so did the risk for fracture. The actual occurrence of pathologic fracture was 5% with a score of 7 or less, 15% with a score of 8, and 33% with a score of 9 or greater. However, this means that two thirds of the patients will undergo stabilization that will not eventually sustain a pathologic fracture. Mirels[13] recommends that patients with scores of 8 or higher should be treated with prophylactic stabilization before irradiation.

Damron performed a critical evaluation of Mirels's[13] criteria for impending pathologic fractures, which involved 53 medical participants of varying degrees of specialty and experience[14] (Level II). The participants reviewed 12 actual clinical cases. The pooled odds ratio favored Mirels' criteria over clinical judgment regardless of experience level. Overall sensitivity was 91%, but the specificity was only 35%.

Van der Linden and coworkers,[15] using the randomized Dutch bone metastasis study, followed 102 patients to identify lesional risk factors for fracture who were undergoing irradiation of femoral metastases. The authors conclude that if the axial cortical involvement is greater than 30 mm, prophylactic surgery should be performed (Level I).

PREOPERATIVE EMBOLIZATION OF BONE METASTASES

Once the diagnosis of osseous metastasis is made, any suspicion of hypervascularity should be investigated and treated. Most commonly, the primary tumor renal cell carcinoma, but other primaries such as bronchogenic carcinoma can be associated with neovascularization. Preoperative embolization (POE), used 48 to 72 hours before peripheral or spinal surgery, is a method of reducing potential blood loss at the time of stabilization and can result in dramatic reduction of neovascularization[16] (Level IV).

Sun and Lang[17] found that blood loss was significantly less when POE resulted in obliteration of more than 70% of the tumor stain (blush on angiogram). Roscoe and researchers,[18] as well as Manke and coworkers,[19] found that POE was an effective way of significantly reducing blood loss before spinal stabilization for metastatic renal cell carcinoma[18] (Level IV).

VENTING BEFORE PROPHYLACTIC STABILIZATION OF FEMORAL METASTASES WITH AN INTRAMEDULLARY NAIL

Most of the research regarding techniques to reduce marrow embolization during femoral manipulation is based on total hip arthroplasty. Heinrich and coauthors,[20] in 26 patients undergoing total hip arthroplasty, used a 4.5-mm lateral cortical drill hole ("vent") distal to the tip of the prosthesis. A significant reduction in air and fat embolism, as well as no change in end-expiratory carbon dioxide, were observed in the vented group[20] (Level III). Martin and investigators[21] found that proximal and distal vents reduced intramedullary pressure by up to 90% in a cadaveric model. Roth and colleagues[11] used a cadaveric model to show a greater than 50% reduction in intramedullary pressure with distal venting in a cadaveric model with proximal metastatic defects. The creation of a distal vent before prophylactic stabilization for femoral metastases is a safe, easy method of reducing marrow embolization[22] (Table 45–1).

TABLE 45–1. Summary of Literature Regarding Prophylactic Stabilization

AUTHOR	LEVEL OF EVIDENCE	NO. OF PATIENTS/METHOD	OUTCOME	COMMENTS
Ward et al. (CORR, 1993)	II	97 impending fracture 85 complete fracture	Blood loss (438 vs. 636 mL) Shorter hospital stay (7 vs. 11 days) Discharge home (79% vs. 56%) Support-free ambulation (35% vs. 12%)	Improved outcome in impending cases after stabilization
Fidler et al. (Acta Orth Scand, 1983)	II	Examined the fracture risk according to the size of lesion as a percentage of the cortical diameter	Fracture risk: 2% if lesion <50% diameter 61% if lesion 50–75% 80% if lesion >75%	High risk for fracture if lesion greater than 50% of cortical diameter
Beals (Cancer, 1971)	II	94 femoral metastases: concept of lesion >2.5 cm being at high risk for fracture	8/19 pathologic fractures had lesions <2.5 cm (42% false-negative rate)	The concept of size of lesion (>2.5 cm) is not reliable in decision making for prophylactic stabilization
Keene (CORR, 1986)	II	Size and percentage of lesion as a risk for pathologic fracture	The size and percentage of lesions were similar in the fracture and nonfracture groups	Could not predict which lesions will cause fracture
Mirels (CORR, 1993)	II	Reviewed 78 patients to develop a scoring system based on 4 radiographic criteria (3 points for each category): location of lesion, nature of lesion, lesion size, and presence of pain	Risk for pathologic fracture was 5% with score ≤7, 15% with score of 8, and 33% with score ≥9	Patients with scores greater than 8 should undergo prophylactic stabilization before irradiation
Damron (CORR, 1993)	I	Evaluation of Mirels's criteria to predict pathologic fracture risk with 53 medical participants reviewing 12 cases	Mirels's criteria: sensitivity of 91% and specificity of 35%	The pooled odds ratio favored Mirels's criteria regardless of medical experience
Van der Linden (Radiotherapy and Oncology, 2003)	I	102 patients undergoing irradiation from a prospective database to evaluate lesional risk factors		If the axial cortical involvement is greater than 30 mm, prophylactic surgery should be performed
Sprujit (Acta, 2006)	N/A*	Biomechanic study using 11 matched pairs of cadaveric femora	Used finite element models from quantitative computed tomographic scans of cadaveric femora with lesions created in the subtrochanteric region	The model was able to successfully predict torsional failure in 82% of cases
Tschirat et al. (J Biomechanics, 2007)	N/A*	Parametric finite element modeling	Comparison of effects of cortical shell compromise by comparing scenarios ranging from transcortical to contained defects	Upper thoracic vertebrae are at greater risk, whereas transcortical lesions are up to 30% lower risk for burst fracture

*Biomechanic study.

AREAS OF UNCERTAINTY/CONTROVERSY

General guidelines are difficult in this patient population as a result of many variables including the primary tumor, the location and size of the metastatic lesion, the current medical status of the patient, and the life expectancy of the patient. Determination of the optimal surgical candidate and the method of stabilization remain controversial, especially in the setting of an impending pathologic fracture.[23]

A low threshold exists for operative intervention of impending pathologic fractures or lesions of the proximal femur. This is related to the high stresses to which the proximal femur is subjected and, therefore, the high risk for fracture.[24] The exact method of stabilization is controversial. Lesions or fractures of the femoral neck or head or intertrochanteric fractures are usually managed with hemiarthroplasty. If any pathologic involvement of the acetabulum occurs, then a total hip arthroplasty is indicated. Rarely, lesions in the pertrochanteric region can be stabilized with a hip screw and side-plate device augmented with polymethylmethacrylate (PMMA) cement.

No studies have compared the use of intramedullary nail to plate for stabilization. However, Yazawa and coworkers[25] report a 23% failure rate in cases treated with compression screw and plate[25] (Level IV). The potential complication of plate fixation is a stress riser at the end of the plate. For this reason, intramedullary nail fixation should be considered when possible to span the entire length of the femur. Most often a nail is utilized that allows screw fixation into the femoral head.[24]

RECOMMENDATIONS

When metastases involve the femoral diaphysis, lesions greater than 3 cm or more than 75% of the cortical diameter should undergo stabilization. Intramedullary stabilization is the optimal method. Distal femoral venting should be used in prophylactic intramedullary nailing. The proximal femur is subject to tremendous loads, both compressive and tensile, and for this reason, lesions are treated more aggressively with early stabilization independent of the size of the lesion.

Preoperative embolization should be undertaken 24 to 72 hours before stabilization of metastases associated with renal cell carcinoma or other hypervascular tumors to reduce the risk for blood loss. Table 45–2 provides a summary of recommendations.

TABLE 45–2. Summary of Recommendations

RECOMMENDATION	LEVEL OF EVIDENCE/ GRADE OF RECOMMENDATION
1 A patient with known or suspected renal cell metastases (or any other hypervascular tumor) to bone should have preoperative embolization to decrease blood loss 24 to 72 hours before surgery.	C
2. Patients with a cortical long-bone lesion that is greater than 3 cm or 50% of the cortical diameter, or involves the pertrochanteric region should have prophylactic stabilization.	B
3. During prophylactic stabilization, distal venting should be used to reduce fat and tumor embolization.	C

REFERENCES

1. Aaron AD: Treatment of metastatic adenocarcinoma of the pelvis and extremities. J Bone Joint Surg Am 79-A:917–932, 1997.
2. Campanacci M: Bone and soft tissue tumors. New York, Springer-Verlag, 1999.
3. McNeil BJ: Value of bone scanning in neoplastic disease. Semin Nucl Med 14:277–286, 1984.
4. Ward WG, Holsenbeck S, Dorey FJ, et al: Metastatic disease of the femur: Surgical treatment. Clin Orthop 415(suppl):230–244, 2003.
5. Harrington KD: New trends in the management of lower extremity metastases. Clin Orthop (169):53–61, 1982.
6. Harrington KD: Impending pathologic fractures from metastatic malignancy: Evaluation and management. Instr Course Lect 35:357–381, 1986.
7. Fidler M: Incidence of fracture through metastases in long bones. Acta Orthop Scand 52:623–627, 1981.
8. Beals RK, Lawton GD, Snell WE: Prophylactic internal fixation of the femur in metastatic breast cancer. Cancer 28:1350–1354, 1971.
9. Keene JS, Sellinger DS, McBeath AA, et al: Metastatic breast cancer in the femur. A search for the lesion at risk of fracture. Clin Orthop (203):282–288, 1986.
10. Spruijt S, van der Linden JC, Dijkstra PD, et al: Prediction of torsional failure in 22 cadaver femora with and without simulated subtrochanteric metastatic defects: A CT scan based finite element analysis. Acta Orthop 77:474–481, 2006.
10a. Lee T. Predicting failure load of the femur with simulated osteolytic defects using noninvasive imaging technique in a simplified load case. Ann Biomed Eng 35(4):642-650, 2007. Epub 2007 Feb 8.
11. Roth SE, Mousavi P, Finkelstein J, et al: Metastatic burst fracture risk prediction using biomechanically based equations. Clin Orthop (419):83–90, 2004.
12. Tschirhart CE, Finkelstein JA, Whyne CM: Biomechanics of vertebral, geometry, and transcortical tumours in the metastatic spine. J Biomech 40:46–54, 2007.
13. Mirels H: Metastatic disease in long bones: A proposed scoring system for diagnosing impending pathologic fractures. Clin Orthop 415(suppl):S4–S13, 2003.
14. Damron TA, Ward WG: Risk of pathologic fracture: Assessment. Clin Orthop 415S:S201–S207, 2003.
15. Van der Linden YM, Kroon HM, Dijkstra PD, et al: Simple radiographic parameter predicts fracturing in metastatic femoral bone lesions: Results from a randomized trial. Radiother Oncol 69:21–31, 2003.
16. Stephen DJG: Preoperative embolization of bone metastases. Tech Orthop 19:49–52, 2004.
17. Sun S, Lang EV: Bone metastases from renal cell carcinoma: Preoperative embolization. J Vasc Interv Radiol 9:263–269, 1998.
18. Roscoe MW, McBroom RJ, St. Louis, et al: Preoperative embolization in the treatment of osseous metastases from renal cell carcinoma. Clin Orthop 238:302–307, 1989.
19. Manke C, Bretschneifer T, Lenhart M, et al: Spinal metastases from renal cell carcinoma: Effect of preoperative particle embolization on intraoperative blood loss. AJNR Am J Neuroradiol 22:997–1003, 2001.
20. Heinrich H, Kremer P, Winter H, et al: Transesophageal 2-dimensional echocardiography in hip endoprostheses. Anaesthesist 34:118–123, 1985.
21. Martin R, Leighton RK, Petrie D, et al: Effect of proximal and distal venting during intramedullary nailing. Clin Orthop 332:80–89, 1996.
22. Stephen DJG: Venting the femoral canal. Tech Orthop 19:49–52, 2004.
23. Jacofsky DJ, Papagelopoulos PJ, Sim FH: Advances and challenges in the surgical treatment of metastatic bone disease. Clin Orthop 415(suppl):S14–S18, 2003.
24. Edwards SA, Pandit HG, Clarke HJ: The treatment of impending and existing pathological femoral fractures using the long gamma nail. Injury 32:229–306, 2001.
25. Yazawa Y, Frassica FJ, Chao EY, et al: Metastatic bone disease. A study of the surgical treatment of 166 pathologic humeral and femoral fractures. Clin Orthop Relat Res (251):213–219, 1990.
26. Jung ST, Ghert MA, Harrelson JM, et al: Treatment of osseous metastases in patients with renal cell carcinoma. Clin Orthop (409):223–231, 2003.
27. Roth SE, Rebello MM, Kreder HJ, et al: Pressurization of the metastatic femur during prophylactic intramedullary nail fixation. J Trauma 57:333–339, 2004.

Chapter 46

What Is the Role of Splinting for Comfort?

Hans J. Kreder, MD, MPH, FRCSC

External immobilization is used in three situations: the provisional (and sometimes the definitive) nonoperative treatment of unstable bone and soft-tissue injuries, the treatment of stable bone and soft-tissue injuries, and after surgical fracture or soft-tissue stabilization.

Unstable injuries involve bone or soft-tissue discontinuity to the extent that the pieces move independently with minimal force. Immobilizing unstable limb injuries is a basic principle of emergency fracture management designed to decrease pain and to minimize additional soft-tissue damage and hemorrhage. Provisional immobilization of unstable injuries may be followed by surgical intervention or definitive nonoperative treatment. External immobilization such as casting for the definitive treatment of unstable injuries usually requires that at least one adjacent joint near the injury is immobilized to prevent displacement during healing. When the decision is made to treat an unstable injury (e.g., a displaced tibia fracture) without surgery, the deleterious effects of joint immobilization,[1] such as muscle atrophy, weakness, and joint stiffness, are generally unavoidable. For unstable injuries, some form of immobilization is mandatory.

In the treatment of stable soft tissue or bone injuries such as sprains and undisplaced or impacted fractures, uncertainty exists regarding the role of rigid versus dynamic immobilization or, indeed, whether any immobilization is necessary and for how long immobilization should continue. The goal of treatment is to maximize patient function and to prevent a stable injury from becoming unstable because of reinjury or excessive loading. Thus, immobilization may be considered for comfort and for protection.

The goal of surgical fracture fixation is to provide absolute or relative stability that is biomechanically sufficient to allow the adjacent joints to be mobilized. However, many clinicians routinely immobilize a limb, including one or more joints, after surgery with the intention of minimizing pain and soft-tissue contractures caused by persistent painful joint positioning (e.g., ankle equinus), and promoting soft-tissue healing by preventing shear stress across the incision. Given the known deleterious effects of joint immobilization, especially when the articular surface is involved, the need for postoperative immobilization has been questioned. This debate is complicated by issues of weight bearing or not, the type of fixation that was used, and patient factors such as the ability to use crutches or to participate actively in range-of-motion exercises.

OPTIONS

The treatment of unstable fractures and soft-tissue injuries does involve provisional external immobilization or traction, which occasionally becomes the definitive treatment; however, the main point of debate for these injuries is operative versus nonoperative care because clearly some form of immobilization is required for controlling an unstable injury. This topic is addressed separately under the chapters relevant to a specific type of injury and is not considered further here.

When a bone or soft-tissue injury is stable, treatment options include either no immobilization or some form of static or dynamic immobilization. Does immobilization improve patient comfort and return to activities? Does immobilization reduce the risk for a stable injury becoming unstable? How long should a stable injury be immobilized? The same questions of patient comfort and return to function apply to the postoperative immobilization of joints adjacent to a surgically fixed bone or soft-tissue injury. Additional concerns include the following: Does immobilization prevent complications related to the incision such as wound dehiscence and infection? Is immobilization necessary to prevent deformity in some situations (e.g., ankle fractures with a concern of possible equinus deformity)?

The purpose of this chapter is to provide guidance to the clinician with respect to the immobilization of stable injuries and postoperative patients, and to highlight areas where further study would be helpful in strengthening the evidence base for treatment.

EVIDENCE

A number of randomized clinical trials of varying quality have been undertaken to address the issue of immobilization versus functional treatment for stable injuries and after open reduction and internal fixation of ankle fractures. Most of these studies have been summarized in meta-analyses (Table 46–1). Most studies have dealt with ankle injuries.[2–10] Few studies have addressed upper extremity injuries.[11–13]

TABLE 46–1. Summary of Evidence

REFERENCE	LEVEL OF EVIDENCE	TYPE OF STUDY	N	PATIENT POPULATION	INTERVENTIONS	OUTCOMES	RESULTS	COMMENTS
Beynnon et al. (2006)[2]	I	RCT funded by "aircast"	212	Acute ankle sprains (grades 1–3)	• Wrap • Stirrup brace • Wrap and brace • Cast	Return to normal walking and stair climbing	Grade 1: wrap plus stirrup better than either alone Grade 2: cast worst Grade 3: no difference	• 19% dropout rate • Treatment options varied by grade: Grade 1: wrap, stirrup, both together Grade 2: wrap + stirrup, cast Grade 3: stirrup, cast • Both studies from same center different patients
de Vries et al. (2006)[3]	II	Meta-analysis (2 RCTs)	70	Postoperative chronic ankle instability repair	• Early mobilization • Cast	Pain, function, return to work and sports, ROM	Early mobilization was better for return to work and sports	
Nash et al. (2004)[13]	II	Meta-analysis (49 RCTs)	NA	Stable fractures, soft-tissue injuries and postoperative patients (upper and lower extremities)	• Early mobilization • Cast	Function, pain, swelling, return to work and sport, complications, cost	Early mobilization better for all results when weight-bearing status same in both groups In one study, post ankle ORIF, WBAT in cast gave better 6-week ADL versus non–weight bearing with crutches[10]	• No difference in complications • No loss of reduction in stable fractures

Continued

TABLE 46–1. Summary of Evidence—cont'd

REFERENCE	LEVEL OF EVIDENCE	TYPE OF STUDY	N	PATIENT POPULATION	INTERVENTIONS	OUTCOMES	RESULTS	COMMENTS
Kerkhoffs et al. (2002)[6]	II	Meta-analysis (21 RCTs)	2184	Acute lateral ankle ligament rupture (N = 2184)	• Early mobilization • Cast	Return to work and sport, satisfaction, swelling and instability (stress films)	Early mobilization better for all outcomes	• Many low-quality studies among the 21 trials; when excluded, no difference noted across treatments
Kerkhoffs et al. (2002)[7]	I	Meta-analysis (9 RCTs)	892	Acute lateral ankle ligament rupture	• Taping • Elastic wrap • Semirigid support	Swelling, return to work and sport, function, complications	Semi-rigid support faster return to work and sport versus wrap or tape Lace-up support best at reducing swelling	• Taping: most complications (skin)
Egol et al. (2000)[5]	I	RCT	60	Postoperative ankle ORIF	• Functional brace • Cast	Ankle grading scale and SF-36	Function scores better at all times for functional brace but only significant at 6 weeks	• All non-weight bearing for 6–8 weeks • No complications in either group
Dogra and Rangan (1999)[4]	II	RCT	52	Postoperative ankle ORIF	• 2 weeks free + • 4 weeks cast • 6 weeks cast	3-month assessment only; pain, ROM, ankle score, gait assessment	2 weeks of immediate mobility improved gait assessment	• Both groups non-weight bearing for first 2 weeks

ADL, activities of daily living; ORIF, open reduction with internal fixation; RCT, randomized clinical trial; ROM, range of motion; SF-36, 36-Item Short Form Health Survey; WBAT, weight bearing as tolerated.

Ankle Sprain

Faster return to normal activities such as work and sport with functional mobilization versus rigid immobilization has been the most consistent finding across trials. An industry-sponsored randomized clinical trial[2] (Level I) graded the degree of ankle sprain and then randomized grade 1 sprains to an elastic wrap, an ankle stirrup brace, or a combination of both[2] (Fig. 46–1). Grade 2 sprains were randomized to the same groups as grade 1 sprains or a cast, and grade 3 sprains were allocated to either a stirrup brace or cast. For grade 1 sprains, the combination of an elastic wrap under an ankle stirrup resulted in a return to normal walking and stair climbing that was roughly twice as fast as either alone (4–6 vs. 10–12 weeks; $P < 0.01$). For grade 2 sprains, the combination of elastic wrap beneath an ankle stirrup brace was similar to a wrap alone or a brace alone, with these functional treatments all resulting in a significant decrease in the time to normal weight bearing and stair climbing versus cast immobilization (10–12 vs. 24–28 weeks; $P < 0.01$). There was no difference in return to these activities for grade 3 sprains treated with either stirrup bracing or cast immobilization (18–21 weeks for both groups with grade 3 sprains). When comparing the different types of functional treatments, Kerkhoff and colleagues[7] note that a semirigid brace led to faster return to work (4.2 days; 95% confidence interval [CI]: 2.4–6.1 days) and sport

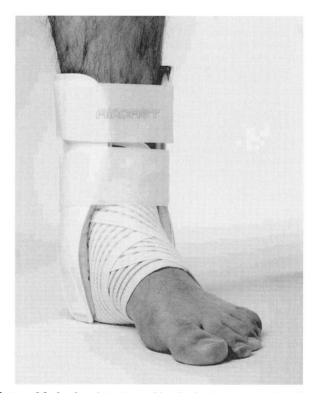

FIGURE 46–1. Combination of both elastic wrap and ankle stirrup brace. (From Beynnon BD, et al: A prospective, randomized clinical investigation of the treatment of first-time ankle sprains. Am J Sports Med 34:1401–1412, 2006, reprinted with permission of SAGE Publications.)

(relative risk [RR], 9.6; 95% CI, 6.3–12.9) than an elastic bandage alone. Lace-up ankle supports were best at decreasing swelling, with elastic bandages the worst for swelling (RR, 5.5; 95% CI, 1.7–17.8). Taping led to the most skin irritations.

Kerkhoff and colleagues' systematic review[6] (Level II) reports on early mobilization with "functional treatment" versus cast immobilization for ankle sprains. Functional treatment was defined as any treatment that did not rigidly immobilize the ankle joint, but that may involve elastic wraps, braces, or other support. All patients were allowed weight bearing as tolerated. A second review compared the various forms of functional treatment[7] (Level I). Return to work was faster (8.2 days; 95% CI, 6.3–10.2 days), as was return to sport (4.9 days; 95% CI, 1.5–8.3 days). Patients were also more likely to be satisfied with functional treatment (RR, 1.8; 95% CI, 1.1–3.1), and they suffered less swelling at 6 to 12 weeks of follow-up (RR, 1.7. 95% CI, 1.2–2.6). Instability on stress films was less likely at follow-up after functional treatment (RR, 2.6; 95% CI, 1.2–4.0). When only the highest quality studies were included, return to work remained significantly faster in functionally treated patients (12.9 days; 95% CI, 7.1–18.7 days).

Ankle Instability Surgery

de Vries and coauthors[3] summarize the results of two studies[6,7] that compared functional treatment versus immobilization after surgical repair for chronic ankle instability. Patients experienced faster return to work (1.8 days; 95% CI, 0.9–2.7 days) and earlier return to sport (3 days; 95% CI, 2–4 days) with functional treatment versus immobilization. Pain scores and Tegner function score favored functional treatment but did not reach significance.[3]

Ankle Fracture Fixation

The studies that address the issue of ankle fracture fixation are difficult to summarize.[4,5,10,13] Some immobilize both groups for varying periods, and some allow weight bearing in the casted group but not the functional treatment group, and still others exclude patients with osteoporosis and questionable fixation from randomization considering these patients ineligible for potential functional treatment. Is early functional treatment safe? None of the comparisons notes an increased rate of wound problems or loss of fixation, but the study issues noted earlier demand that this result be interpreted with caution. When similar weight-bearing protocols were used in the functional and the casted group after ankle fracture fixation, there is a consistent finding of faster return to work and to function with early mobilization[4,5,13] (Level II), with no difference in function noted across treatment groups by 3 months given the available sample sizes. Egol and researchers[5] note better vitality and general health scores (36-item short form [SF-36]) at 6 weeks with early functional treatment. These authors also note a significantly faster return to work in the functional group (53.8 vs. 106.5 days; $P = 0.007$).

Weight bearing after ankle fixation improved patient satisfaction and allowed faster return to activities of daily living[10,13] (Level II). Weight bearing was accompanied by cast immobilization. A 2-week period of non–weight bearing associated with range-of-motion exercises followed by 4 weeks of weight bearing in a cast gave similar results at 3 months as 6 weeks of continuous cast immobilization, except that the gait pattern was more symmetric in the early mobilization group.[4]

Other Injuries

Nash and coworkers[13] summarize the evidence from 49 randomized clinical trials regarding immobilization versus functional treatment for stable fractures or soft-tissue injuries and for postoperative treatment[14] (Level II). Early functional treatment was not associated with displacement of stable fractures and was not associated with increased wound problems. Patients generally preferred early mobilization and experienced earlier return to work and sport, decreased pain, swelling, and stiffness.[13,14]

AREAS OF UNCERTAINTY

Uncertainty exists because of lack of research involving many specific injuries, protocols that include varying periods of immobilization and varying rigidity of immobilization in both treatment arms, protocols that are confounded by weight-bearing status, and imprecise definitions of fracture stability or fixation quality.

Most studies have addressed injuries of the ankle joint and may not be generalizeable to other areas, especially the upper extremity, which is generally non–weight bearing. In many of the protocols discussed earlier, the so-called early functional treatment included a period of immobilization immediately after injury or surgery for up to 2 weeks, whereas some used a period of mobility followed by subsequent cast immobilization, potentially diluting the effects of early mobility. Studies were also confounded by weight bearing; usually restricting the "early function group" from weight bearing. This leads to confusing results regarding patient preferences, pain, and function, and it is difficult to know whether the outcome is due to early weight bearing versus early range of movement. The ability to weight bear seems to confer considerable functional benefits and is preferred by patients, but there has been insufficient evaluation of the safety and utility of early weight bearing without rigid immobilization.

Cast immobilization has been used to "protect" stable fractures from unexpected force such as a fall; however, there is little work to guide the clinician as to what the risk for displacement is without cast immobilization in specific injuries, how a stable fracture is defined, and what parameters render a nonoperative stable fracture or an injury treated with surgery vulnerable.

RECOMMENDATIONS

Patients generally benefit from being able to use their limbs after injury for weight bearing. Early mobility helps speed return to work and sports, and there appears to be little danger that "stable" injuries will become unstable if treated with mobilization and early function. Table 46–2 provides a summary of recommendations.

TABLE 46–2. Summary of Recommendations

RECOMMENDATION	LEVEL OF EVIDENCE/ GRADE OF RECOMMENDATION
1. Adult with lateral ankle ligament injury should be treated with WBAT in a semirigid brace in preference to a rigid cast and in preference to taping or an elastic wrap alone.	A
2. Adult with surgical repair for chronic lateral ankle instability should be treated with early mobilization.	B
3. Adults after ankle ORIF should be treated with support that allows early range of motion as opposed to a rigid cast.	B
4. Adults after ankle ORIF: There is insufficient evidence to recommend for or against immediate mobilization versus an initial period of a few days in a splint immediately after surgery.	I
5. Adults after ankle ORIF: There is insufficient evidence to recommend for or against immediate weight bearing after ankle ORIF (with or without immobilization).	I
6. Adults and children with stable fractures and soft-tissue injuries can be treated with early functional mobilization.	C

ORIF, open reduction with internal fixation; WBAT, weight bearing as tolerated.

REFERENCES

1. Pathare NC, et al: Deficit in human muscle strength with cast immobilization: Contribution of inorganic phosphate. Eur J Appl Physiol 98:71–78, 2006.
2. Beynnon BD, et al: A prospective, randomized clinical investigation of the treatment of first-time ankle sprains. Am J Sports Med 34:1401–1412, 2006.
3. de Vries JS, et al: Interventions for treating chronic ankle instability. Cochrane Database Syst Rev 4:CD004124, 2006.
4. Dogra AS, Rangan A: Early mobiliation versus immobiliation of surgically treated ankle fractures. Prospective randomised control trial. Injury 30:417–419, 1999.
5. Egol KA, Dolan R, Koval KJ: Functional outcome of surgery for fractures of the ankle. A prospective, randomised comparison of management in a cast or a functional brace. J Bone Joint Surg Br 82:246–249, 2000.

6. Kerkhoffs GM, et al: Immobiliation and functional treatment for acute lateral ankle ligament injuries in adults. Cochrane Database Syst Rev 3:CD003762, 2002.
7. Kerkhoffs GM, et al: Different functional treatment strategies for acute lateral ankle ligament injuries in adults. Cochrane Database Syst Rev 3:CD002938, 2002.
8. Margo K: The Air-Stirrup brace with elastic wrap improved function in first incident grade 1 or 2 lateral ankle ligament sprain. Evid Based Med 12:48, 2007.
9. Swiontkowski MF, et al: Interobserver variation in the AO/OTA fracture classification system for pilon fractures: Is there a problem? J Orthop Trauma 11:467–470, 1997.
10. van Laarhoven CJ, Meeuwis JD, van der Werken C: Postoperative treatment of internally fixed ankle fractures: A prospective randomised study. J Bone Joint Surg Br 78:395–399, 1996.
11. Plint AC, et al: A randomized, controlled trial of removable splinting versus casting for wrist buckle fractures in children. Pediatrics 117:691–697, 2006.
12. Handoll HH, Pearce PK: Interventions for isolated diaphyseal fractures of the ulna in adults. Cochrane Database Syst Rev 2: CD000523, 2004.
13. Nash CE, et al: Resting injured limbs delays recovery: A systematic review. J Fam Pract 53:706–712, 2004.
14. Kreder HJ: Commentary: Review; early mobilisation is better than cast immobilisation for injured limbs. Evid Based Med 10:118, 2000.

Does the Type of Hospital in Which a Patient Is Treated Affect Outcomes in Orthopaedic Patients?

Iris Weller, MSc, PhD

Although healthcare systems differ around the world, there is currently nearly universal political and financial pressure for change to create greater efficiencies in delivery while maintaining favorable patient outcomes. Hospitals are an important part of the healthcare system, and the services and quality of care in different types of hospitals are currently the subject of much debate.[1,2]

Hospitals can be broadly classified by their teaching status (teaching or nonteaching), funding status (for-profit or not for-profit), or ownership (public or private),[1,2] or in some jurisdictions, by their specialty services (orthopedic, cardiovascular, etc.).[3]

Evidence has been reported that the type of hospital in which a patient is treated can affect both his or her outcome and healthcare costs.[1,4] This is an important issue that could have a large impact on health policy decisions at the government and hospital levels. Unfortunately, a paucity of evidence exists in the literature in general and in the orthopedic literature in particular to inform this debate.

EVIDENCE

This chapter evaluates the evidence in the literature around four questions: (1) Are outcomes better in teaching hospitals versus nonteaching hospitals? (2) Is there a difference in outcomes between for-profit and not-for-profit hospitals? (3) Is there a difference in outcome between urban and rural hospitals? (4) How do we interpret the evidence for patients undergoing orthopedic procedures within the context of the first three questions?

Several issues must be considered to resolve these questions, with the major one being the considerable heterogeneity of studies with respect to diseases and procedures, risk adjustment, types of data, and settings.[2,5]

Studies report outcomes for patients with a variety of conditions; however, most studies are on cardiovascular disease, mainly congestive heart failure, acute myocardial infarction (AMI), or stroke.[3,4,6-9] Only five studies included patients undergoing orthopedic procedures, and these were in patients who had received surgery for total joint replacement[10] or hip fractures.[4,7,11,12] No studies of outcome in patients with fractures as a result of major trauma have been reported.

No randomized, controlled trials have been identified, and it is unlikely that this will happen in the future. All studies have been observational because this is the most feasible design to address these questions.[1] Although this level of evidence may be considered weak, a well-conducted observational study can contribute valuable information. Many studies are retrospective cohort studies, a relatively robust observational design, not as subject to bias as some other study designs, and these have an important part to play in medical research.[13] The main concern with cohort studies is residual confounding by unmeasured variables related to the patients and the outcome. This is problematic with the use of administrative data, because usually only demographic information and some measures of comorbidities are available for risk adjustment in the analyses.

Nearly all of the evidence available is based on either clinical chart reviews or administrative data.[2] Because administrative data are collected for billing, rather than research purposes, problems with coding are an issue.[14] These problems may differ among databases. Nevertheless, although those such as the Health Care Financing Administration data, which has been used in many U.S. studies,[7,10,15] and the Canadian Institutes of Health Information data, which has been used in many Canadian studies,[11,16,17] have been validated,[14,18] to some extent, this remains a problem inherent in all studies. The administrative data in the U.S. studies are mainly for Medicare patients,[4,10] and this could introduce some bias, if these patients are older and sicker than the average patient. This is less of a problem in countries with universal healthcare, such as Canada, where administrative databases contain information on all patients.

Another challenge in evaluating the evidence is that most of the studies that examine these issues have been done in the United States, where the hospital system is more complex, compared with Canada, for example. In the United States, all teaching hospitals are not-for-profit; however, nonteaching hospitals can be either for-profit or not-for-profit. Thus, the issue of whether teaching hospitals are different from nonteaching hospitals may be confounded by their funding status (for-profit or not for-profit). For example, some studies have compared not-for-profit teaching hospitals with not-for-profit nonteaching hospitals,[11] whereas others have compared not-for-profit teaching hospitals with for-profit nonteaching hospitals.[4] This could lead to inconsistent conclusions.

Two recent meta-analyses have attempted to resolve the questions of whether outcomes are better in teaching hospitals versus nonteaching hospitals[2] and whether mortality rates differ between private for-profit and private not-for-profit hospitals.[1]

The first analysis identified 132 eligible studies that included 93 on mortality and 61 on other outcomes.[2] Twenty-two of these assessed both. A wide range of patient groups were represented by these studies; most were patients with cardiovascular disease, and only two involved orthopedic patients. Most studies were done in U.S. hospitals. Ten studies were done in Canada, 9 in the United Kingdom, 4 in Norway, and 12 in other countries. Using all adjusted mortality data, the authors report a relative risk (RR) for teaching hospitals of 0.96 (95% confidence interval [CI], 0.93–1.00). Subgroup analyses involving data sources (clinical or administrative) and location of study (United States or other) yielded no important differences. The authors report some evidence that teaching hospitals performed better for certain diagnoses (breast cancer, cerebrovascular accidents, and mixed diagnoses). Because of the small numbers of studies, no information could be calculated for orthopedic procedures. This was an extensive and thorough meta-analysis that suggests that differences between teaching and nonteaching hospitals are minimal.

The second meta-analysis by Devereaux and colleagues[1] compares mortality rates between private for-profit and private not-for-profit hospitals. Fifteen studies were included in this analysis. In an attempt to remove hospital teaching status as a confounding influence, they included results from for-profit nonteaching and not-for-profit teaching hospitals when they were available. They also avoided adjusting for variables under the control of hospital administrators that could be influenced by a profit motive and affect mortality, such as nursing staffing levels. Three of the studies in their analysis included orthopedic patients (hip fractures, lower extremity fractures, hip replacement).[7,10,15] One of the three included all patients in the dataset but did not differentiate diagnoses in the analysis.[15] They reported a RR for for-profit hospitals of 1.020 (95% CI, 1.003–1.038). These results also suggest minimal differences between private for-profit and private not-for-profit hospitals.

The evidence for a difference between rural or urban hospitals is even more tenuous, because few studies are reported in the literature. Keeler and coauthors[7] reviewed the medical records of 14,008 patients aged 65 years or older in 297 hospitals in the United States and compared them with mortality data from an administrative database. Patients had either congestive heart failure, cerebrovascular disease, AMI, pneumonia, or hip fracture; however, subgroup analyses on each diagnosis were not reported. Their results, adjusted for comorbidities, showed that rural hospitals consistently provided below-average care, and patients treated there had a slightly increased chance of dying compared with the average for all hospitals. Patients treated in larger urban hospitals, including teaching hospitals, had a slightly smaller chance of dying.

Another study of patients with heart failure in Germany found that adherence to heart failure guidelines was less in rural hospitals; however, there was no significant difference in mortality after adjustment for age and sex.[3]

A Canadian study[11] found a trend to increased mortality at 3, 6, and 12 months after hip fracture surgery in rural hospitals compared with urban community hospitals; however, this did not reach statistical significance. This study is discussed in greater detail in the next section.

In contrast, Glenn and Jijon[19] found that risk-adjusted death rates for small hospitals with unspecialized services were similar between urban and rural areas,[19] leading the authors to conclude that small rural hospitals make appropriate decisions to transfer severely ill patients and provide quality care for retained patients.

Thus, the evidence examining urban/rural differences is so sparse that it is difficult to evaluate. It appears, however, that there is no strong suggestion that major differences in outcomes exist.

Some evidence does show that delay to surgery for fractures resulting from major trauma is related to a poorer outcome.[20–22] One study that took place in a rural trauma center found an incidence of delay to diagnosis of 3%, and that this was related to patient outcome. Whether this accounts for some of the differences observed between urban and rural institutions remains to be determined.

EVIDENCE IN ORTHOPEDIC PATIENTS

A consistent theme in this chapter is the lack of evidence in orthopedic patients. The studies that have been reported are summarized in Table 47–1. One did not specify hospital type.[12] Hip fractures were included in the sample of another study, but no subgroup analyses were presented.[7]

Yuan and coworkers[10] studied the association between hospital type and mortality and length of stay in 16.9 million Medicare beneficiaries in the United States. Hospitals were categorized as for-profit, not-for-profit, osteopathic, public, teaching not-for-profit, and teaching public. They report results, adjusted for comorbidities associated with mortality, for nonspecified lower extremity fractures and hip replacements separately. No differences among hospitals were found for lower extremity fractures; however, they report in the text that mortality rates for hip replacement were greater at teaching not-for-profit hospitals than at for-profit, not-for-profit, and public hospitals. Unfortunately, the graphs presented indicate the opposite; therefore, it is not possible to interpret their data.

TABLE 47–1. Effect of Hospital Type on Outcomes in Orthopedic Patients

STUDY	DESIGN	PATIENT GROUP	HOSPITAL COMPARISON	OUTCOME	RISK ADJUSTMENT	RESULTS
Keeler et al.,[7] United States	Retrospective Medical records HFCA data	HFx, CHF, MI, stroke, pneumonia	Teaching status Urban vs. rural Profit vs. non-profit	30-day mortality Quality of care	Comorbidities	Higher quality of care and decreased all-cause mortality in teaching and larger urban vs. rural No difference between for-profit and not-for-profit hospitals
Hannan et al.,[12] United States	Medical records, interviews (N = 571)	HFx	4 hospitals in NY—unspecified	Mortality need for assistive devices	Comorbidities	1 Hospital—↑ mortality OR, 1.95 (1.04–3.57) ↑ mortality or ↑ devices OR, 2.59 (1.55–3.34)
Weller et al.,[11] Canada	Cohort Administrative Ontario Health Insurance Plan Canadian Institute of Health Information Hospital Discharge Abstract data Registered Persons data (n = 57,315 patients)	HFx	Urban teaching, urban nonteaching, rural	Mortality Major complications	Charlson Comorbidy Index Age Sex	Lower HFx mortality, fewer complications in teaching vs. nonteaching hospitals Lower mortality in urban vs. rural hospitals
Taylor et al.,[4] United States	Administrative & Survey National Longterm Care Survey Medicare claims data (N = 2674 patients) (N = 1378 hospitals)	HFx, MI, stroke, CHF	Teaching status (major, minor, nonteaching) Financial status (profit/non-profit)	Mortality Cost	Comorbidities Age, sex SES	Major teaching lower all-cause and HFx mortality than for-profit hospitals
Hartz et al.,[15] United States	Retrospective Cohort Administrative HFCA data (N = 3100 hospitals)	All patients	Teaching status Financial status Public Private	All-cause mortality	Illness severity	Mortality higher in for-profit & public vs. private not-for-profit hospitals Mortality lower in private teaching vs. private nonteaching hospitals
Yuan et al.,[10] United States	Retrospective Cohort HFCA data (N = 16.9 million patients) (N = 5127 hospitals)	10 common surgical procedures included lower extremity fractures, hip replacement	Teaching status and financial structure Profit/non-profit	30-day mortality, 6-month mortality, LOS	Comorbidities	Major teaching not-for-profit had decreased mortality For each diagnosis increased LOS
Shortell et al.,[26] United States	MEDPAR (N = 214,839 patients)	16 procedures including THR, TKR	Profit/not-for-profit	Age, sex, LOS, comorbidities	No difference between profit/not-for-profit Market penetration by HMOs associated with increased mortality Five conditions associated with effects of certificate of need had greater mortality rates	

CHF, congestive heart failure; HCFA, Health Care Financing Administration; HFx, hip fractures; LOS, length of hospital stay; MEDPAR, Health Care Financing Administration's Medical Provider Analysis and Review; MI, myocardial infarction; SES, socioeconomic status; THR, total hip replacement; TKR, total knee replacement.

Two studies have examined mortality in hip fracture patients, one in the United States[4] and one in Canada.[11] Both studies use administrative data.

Taylor and investigators[4] used the National Long Term Care Survey, which was representative of Medicare beneficiaries in the United States 65 years or older, linked to Medicare claims data, to study the relation of hospital type to outcome in 3206 patients with hip fracture, stroke, coronary heart disease, or congestive heart failure. Hospitals were classified according to teaching status (major or minor) and ownership using the American Hospital Association's annual hospital survey. Comorbid conditions were assessed using the Hierarchical Coexisting Conditions DxCG model.[24]

In a survival analysis, which included controlling for comorbidities, the mortality rate was noted to be 25% lower for patients treated at a teaching hospital than those treated at for-profit institutions (hazard ratio, 0.75; 95% CI, 0.62–0.91; $P < 0.004$). Interestingly, this significant association appears to have been driven by the inclusion of patients with hip fracture.

The hazard ratio of mortality after hip fracture at major teaching hospitals was 0.54 (95% CI, 0.37–0.79). Moreover, a gradient of decreasing risk was noted through the categories of for-profit nonteaching hospitals, government, nonprofit, minor teaching and major teaching hospitals. The results for the cardiovascular disease diagnoses were much less striking (stroke: hazard ratio, 0.89; 95% CI, 0.64–1.24; $P = 0.49$; coronary heart disease: hazard ratio, 0.76; 95% CI, 0.55–1.07; $P = 0.11$; congestive heart failure: hazard ratio, 0.95; 95% CI, 0.64–1.41; $P = 0.81$) and were similar to results reported from the meta-analysis reported by Papanikolaou and colleagues.[2]

In a Canadian study by Weller and coworkers,[11] 57,315 patients with hip fracture aged 50 years or older were identified from the Canadian Institute for Health Information Discharge Abstracts Database. The modified Charlson–Deyo index, a well-validated scale that can be calculated from administrative data, was used to adjust for comorbidity.[25] Hospitals were classified as teaching or nonteaching. Nonteaching (community) hospitals were further classified as urban (located in communities with population > 10,000) or rural (located in communities with population ≤ 10,000). The cohort was linked to a registry containing information on all deaths in Ontario.

Results showed, after adjustment for delay to surgery, sex, age, and comorbidities in a logistic regression analysis, that teaching hospitals had lower mortality compared with urban community hospitals. The odds ratios (ORs) were as follows: in-hospital death, 0.89 (95% CI, 0.83–0.97); death within 3 months, 0.86 (95% CI, 0.81–0.91); death within 6 months, 0.86 (95% CI, 0.82–0.91), and at 1 year, 0.88 (95% CI, 0.83–0.92).

Teaching hospitals in the United States are not-for-profit institutions and were compared with private for-profit hospitals in the U.S. study, suggesting that a profit motive may explain the strong association observed in the patients with hip fracture. Nevertheless, a profit motive cannot explain the outcomes observed in the Canadian study because 95% of Canadian hospitals are private not-for-profit institutions.[1] The difference in the strength of the association observed in the U.S. data (OR, 0.54)[4] compared with the Canadian study (ORs ranging from 0.86–0.89) suggests that, although a profit motive may be the most important factor in explaining the increased mortality observed in for-profit hospitals, other hospital characteristics may also play a role in patients with hip fracture.

It is interesting that the results for breast cancer and cerebrovascular accident in the meta-analysis by Papanikolaou and colleagues[2] were similar in magnitude and significance to those observed for hip fracture (breast cancer: OR, 0.85; 95% CI, 0.78–0.93; cerebrovascular accident: OR, 0.96; 95% CI, 0.90–0.99), whereas those for heart disease outcomes other than stroke are similar to the overall ORs. Perhaps because the heart disease studies predominate, they are masking relations for other conditions.

UNCERTAINTIES

Although the evidence is not strong, there appears to a difference between teaching hospital status and outcome in orthopedic patients, especially for some diagnoses, including hip fracture. It is possible that this may be even stronger for fractures as the result of a major trauma because they need timely specialized care. Perhaps treatment guidelines for common conditions such as myocardial infarction or congestive heart failure have been more widely adopted across different settings, minimizing differences among institutions.

GUIDELINES

Insufficient evidence is available to inform health policy and system-wide decisions.

RECOMMENDATIONS

The decreased mortality rates after hip fracture surgery in teaching hospitals compared with community hospitals has important implications. An urgent need exists for research to understand which factors associated with hospital teaching status lead to differences in outcome after surgery in patients with hip fracture. Also, more good quality studies should be done on a variety of orthopedic conditions to establish the consistency of literature. It is of significant concern that no information has been reported on patients with major orthopedic trauma.

More advanced statistical methods such as hierarchical modeling may help clarify some of the questions around clustering of certain types of patients in particular hospitals and regions. The use of propensity scores would also help in the interpretation of the data. Table 47–2 provides a summary of recommendations.

TABLE 47–2. Summary of Recommendations

RECOMMENDATION	LEVEL OF EVIDENCE/GRADE OF RECOMMENDATION
1. Adults with fractures may have a lower mortality rate when treated in a teaching versus non-teaching hospital.	C
2. There is insufficient evidence to determine whether there is a difference in mortality between for profit and not for profit institutions.	I

REFERENCES

1. Devereaux PJ, Choi PTL, Lacchetti C, et al: A systematic review and meta-analysis of studies comparing mortality rates of private for-profit and private not-for-profit hospitals. Can Med Assoc J 166:1399–1406, 2002.
2. Papanikolaou PN, Christidi GD, Ioannidis JP: Patient outcomes with teaching versus nonteaching healthcare: A systematic review. PLoS Med 3:e341, 2006.
3. Taubert G, Bergmeier C, Andresen H, et al: Clinical profile and management of heart failure: Rural community hospital vs. metropolitan heart center. Eur J Heart Fail 3:611–617, 2001.
4. Taylor DH, Whellan DJ, Sloan FA: Effects of admission to a teaching hospital on the cost and quality of care for medicare beneficiaries. N Engl J Med 340:293–299, 1999.
5. Ayanian JZ, Weissman JS: Teaching hospitals and quality of care: A review of the literature. Milbank Q 80:569–593, v, 2002.
6. Allison JJ, Kiefe CI, Weissman NW, et al: Relationship of hospital teaching status with quality of care and mortality for Medicare patients with acute MI. JAMA 284:1256–1262, 2000.
7. Keeler EB, Rubenstein LV, Kahn KL, et al: Hospital characteristics and quality of care. JAMA 268:1709–1714, 1992.
8. Polanczyk CA, Lane A, Coburn M, et al: Hospital outcomes in major teaching, minor teaching, and nonteaching hospitals in New York State. Am J Med 112:255–261, 2002.
9. Rosenthal GE, Harper DL, Quinn LM, Cooper GS: Severity-adjusted mortality and length of stay in teaching and nonteaching hospitals. Results of a regional study. JAMA 278:485–490, 1997.
10. Yuan Z, Cooper GS, Einstadter D, et al: The association between hospital type and mortality and length of stay: A study of 16.9 million hospitalized Medicare beneficiaries. Med Care 38:231–245, 2000.
11. Weller I, Wai EK, Jaglal S, Kreder HJ: The effect of hospital type and surgical delay on mortality after surgery for hip fracture. J Bone Joint Surg Br 87:361–366, 2005.
12. Hannan EL, Magaziner J, Wang JJ, et al: Mortality and locomotion 6 months after hospitalization for hip fracture: Risk factors and risk-adjusted hospital outcomes. JAMA 285:2736–2742, 2001.
13. Doll R: Cohort studies: History of the method. II. Retrospective cohort studies. Soz Praventivmed 46:152–160, 2001.
14. Fisher ES, Whaley FS, Krushat WM, et al: The accuracy of Medicare's hospital claims data: Progress has been made, but problems remain. Am J Public Health 82:243–248, 1992.
15. Hartz AJ, Krakauer H, Kuhn EM, et al: Hospital characteristics and mortality rates. N Engl J Med 321:1720–1725, 1989.
16. Alter DA, Austin PC, Tu JV: Community factors, hospital characteristics and inter-regional outcome variations following acute myocardial infarction in Canada. Can J Cardiol 21:247–255, 2005.
17. Alter DA, Tu JV, Austin PC, Naylor CD: Waiting times, revascularization modality, and outcomes after acute myocardial infarction at hospitals with and without on-site revascularization facilities in Canada. J Am Coll Cardiol 42:410–419, 2003.
18. Hawker GA, Coyte PC, Wright JG, et al: Accuracy of administrative data for assessing outcomes after knee replacement surgery. J Clin Epidemiol 50:265–273, 1997.
19. Glenn LL, Jijon CR: Risk-adjusted in-hospital death rates for peer hospitals in rural and urban regions. J Rural Health 15:94–107, 1999.
20. Naique SB, Pearse M, Nanchahal J: Management of severe open tibial fractures: The need for combined orthopaedic and plastic surgical treatment in specialist centres. J Bone Joint Surg Br 88:351–357, 2006.
21. Solan MC, Molloy S, Packham I, et al: Pelvic and acetabular fractures in the United Kingdom: A continued public health emergency. Injury 35:16–22, 2004.
22. Bircher M, Giannoudis PV: Pelvic trauma management within the UK: A reflection of a failing trauma service. Injury 35:2–6, 2004.
23. Tepper J, Pollett W, Jin Y, et al: Utilization rates for surgical procedures in rural and urban Canada. Can J Rural Med 11:195–203, 2006.
24. Ellis RP, Pope GC, Iezzoni L, et al: Diagnosis-based risk adjustment for Medicare capitation payments. Health Care Financ Rev 17:101–128, 1996.
25. Deyo RA, Cherkin DC, Ciol MA: Adapting a clinical comorbidity index for use with ICD-9-CM administrative databases. J Clin Epidemiol 45:613–619, 1992.
26. Shortell SM, Hughes EFX: The effects of regulation, competition, and ownership on mortality rates among hospital inpatients. N Engl J Med 318:1100–1107, 1988.

How Does Surgeon and Hospital Volume Affect Patient Outcome after Traumatic Injury?

Hans J. Kreder, MD, MPH, FRCSC

For many orthopedic conditions, a clear association exists between patient outcome and the volume of similar cases treated by the hospital or surgeon providing care in Canada,[1-4] the United States,[5-12] and other countries.[13-15] After traumatic injury, patient factors such as age, comorbidity, and the severity of injury are by far the most important determinants of mortality, although provider volume and availability of appropriate resources and care protocols do have an important influence on survival. For survivors of multisystem injuries, functional outcome is in large part determined by the residual impact of musculoskeletal and neurologic injuries. The experience and expertise of the hospital and the surgical team managing such injuries may well have a profound impact on the risk for complications, the rate of return to maximal function, the cost of care, and the ultimate functional outcome achieved. Provider experience may affect not only the excellence of procedural execution, but may be a factor at all stages of management, including preoperative decision making, the availability of optimal implants, monitoring equipment and support staff, and the adherence to optimized postoperative management protocols. Few studies have attempted to delineate the underlying mechanisms that might be driving the volume–outcome relation.[2] Although the mechanism may be that high-volume providers have developed mature systems of care and expertise from exposure to a high volume of cases, there is also some evidence that vulnerable populations in the United States with elective conditions such as total knee replacement are preferentially selecting or being forced to select low-volume institutions.[16] A similar finding was noted for patients with hip fracture.[17]

OPTIONS

The demonstration of a systematic variation in patient outcome should be followed by strategies to eliminate suboptimal results, thereby minimizing outcome variation near the high end of the scale. Strategies to achieve this fall into three categories: (1) mandating minimum provider volumes; (2) regionalizing care to specialized centers; and (3) trying to understand the internal mechanisms involved and providing support, education, and best practice advice to those with inferior results (regardless of whether that given provider is low or high volume). The problem with simply mandating a minimum volume for a provider is that there is no scientific evidence to support the existence of a threshold volume below which outcomes are likely to suffer.[14,18] Furthermore, a given low-volume provider might have excellent results, and a specific high-volume provider could have a high complication rate. Alternative strategies may include monitoring provider outcomes and following up on significant variances (in a negative or positive direction) to learn from good results and to work to improve poor results. Regionalization for specific conditions to specialized high-volume "centers of excellence" has been proposed for a number of conditions including trauma[7] and total joint arthroplasty.[19] Regionalization allows for a critical mass of specialists with access to specialized equipment, care protocols, and a variety of medical and support staff available to support the care of resource-intensive, specific conditions; but for common conditions that require no specialized staff or equipment, the inconvenience and expense of patient travel needs to be considered. If a volume–outcome relation were demonstrated for a less resource-intensive injury, an alternative strategy to regionalization for such conditions might involve linking low- and high-volume providers together to share in preoperative surgical decision making, provide advice regarding the development of care protocols for perioperative care, and to monitor the execution of surgery itself.

The purpose of this chapter is to determine whether a volume–outcome relation exists for traumatic orthopedic conditions, with the aim of assisting clinicians and policy makers in developing strategies to improve patient outcomes, and helping researchers to strengthen the evidence base used to refine these strategies.

EVIDENCE

Specialized hospitals and surgeons have specific qualifications and interest in the subject of their subspecialty area. They also tend to be high-volume providers for the conditions of interest. Both specialized trauma providers and total joint arthroplasty centers have been studied.

Specialized Hospitals

In a Level I prospective cohort study, MacKenzie and colleagues[7] compared patient outcomes for those treated in specialized trauma hospitals versus nontrauma hospitals. The most severely injured complex patients (with one or more system Abbreviated Injury Scale scores of 5 or 6) were significantly more likely to survive when treated in specialized trauma centers (RR of hospital death, 0.70; 95% confidence interval [CI], 0.51–0.96). Young trauma victims younger than 55 years also had a lower in-hospital mortality rate when treated in specialized trauma centers (RR, 0.66; 95% CI, 0.48–0.89). For older patients, the mortality rate was driven largely by comorbidity and age with less noticeable influence on risk for death for specialized versus nonspecialized trauma center care. These findings are consistent with data from the United Kingdom. Freeman and coauthors[13] (Level II) note that the relation between volume and outcome for trauma centers in the United Kingdom was significant only for patients with complex multiple traumatic injuries; however, even the highest volume trauma hospital studied had volumes of only 96 patients per year, which is well below the volumes seen in many North American centers.[7,11,20]

Specialized centers for total joint surgery have also been evaluated. Cram and coauthors[19] (Level II) compared total joint replacement surgery in specialty and general hospitals using Medicare data from 1999 to 2003, which included 51,788 total hip and 99,765 total knee replacements. The profile of patients treated at specialized centers differed from that of general hospitals. Patients attending specialized centers tended to be from wealthier neighborhoods and had fewer comorbid conditions. After adjusting for patient comorbidity and hospital volume, the risk for adverse events was lower in specialty hospitals (odds ratio [OR], 0.64; 95% CI, 0.56–0.75) for primaries and much lower for more complex revision operations (OR, 0.49; 95% CI, 0.36–0.66).

Specialized Surgeons

Haut and coworkers[21] (Level II) compared the outcome for patients treated in the same center (Johns Hopkins) but by dedicated specialized trauma surgeons versus nonspecialist surgeons. The institutional protocols were the same regardless of which surgeon was on call. Despite this, the authors note a 50% increase in mortality rates for patients treated by nonspecialist surgeons in patients with severe injuries (Injury Severity Scale [ISS] > 15; OR of death, 1.45; 95% CI, 1.04–2.02) compared with specialized surgeons. Unexpected survivors were twice as common in the full-time trauma surgeon group (approximately 8 vs. 4 unexpected survivors per 1000 patients). Although surgeon factors certainly played a role in patient outcome, the largest driver of mortality was the severity of injury. Patients with an ISS greater than 15 were much less likely to survive regardless of surgeon specialization (OR, 36.8; 95% CI, 20.7–65.6). Severe head injury was the factor with the second greatest OR for risk for death (15.9; 95% CI, 10.1–25.2).

In summary, outcomes are better for patients with complex traumatic injuries and arthroplasty-related conditions when they are treated in specialized centers by specialized surgeons. This effect is reduced for less complex conditions.

Provider Volume and Outcome

Numerous studies have evaluated the relation between provider volume and outcome without necessarily evaluating the subspecialty qualifications of the providers in high- versus low-volume categories. Only the highest quality recent studies of interest are discussed here. Few studies have included specific traumatic conditions, although trauma care in general has been evaluated, and the bulk of evidence concerns arthroplasty outcomes.

Shah and researchers[8] (Level II) analyzed Nationwide Inpatient Sample (NIS) data for patients who underwent hemiarthroplasty for femoral neck fracture. Volume quartiles were generated from the data, which included 173,508 patients. For hospitals, the lowest quartile treated fewer than 20 patients compared with more than 61 for the highest quartile, and for surgeons, the lowest quartile treated fewer than 4 patients compared with more than 11 for the highest quartile. Low-volume hospitals had a greater rate of complications including pulmonary embolus, urinary tract infection, and pneumonia, and a greater rate of prolonged length of stay beyond 10 days (OR, 1.56; 95% CI, 1.46–1.66). Low-volume surgeons had a greater mortality rate (OR, 1.18; 95% CI, 1.03–1.34) and a greater chance of prolonged (>10 days) length of stay (OR, 1.37; 95% CI, 1.29–1.45).

Marcin and Romano[22] (Level II) were interested to know whether volume changes over time within an institution might affect outcome. They studied only patient mortality and readmission rates for patients treated at designated trauma centers (Levels I-III). The authors did not compare results by trauma level designation. In contrast with other trauma studies that could not identify a significant association between mortality and provider volume in elderly patients,[7] Marcin and Romano[22] note lower mortality rates for patients older than 64 years treated in high-volume centers (OR, 0.79; 95% CI, 0.71–0.87). They also note that for every 10 patients added to a particular institution's monthly caseload, the odds of readmission for elderly patients older than 64 years increased (OR, 1.11; 95% CI, 1.01–1.21). The authors suggest that perhaps systems became overloaded, resulting in greater readmissions. These findings are in contrast with work by Hamilton and coworkers[4] (Level II), who found that, for hip fractures, changing hospital volume over time had no effect on outcome. The authors suggest, therefore, that the observed volume–outcome relation between high- and low-volume institutions reflects differences in the quality of care between high- and low-volume hospitals, and not volume fluctuations per se.

The main outcomes reported for provider volume–outcome relations have included mortality and other complications, but there has been little information available regarding functional outcome. Katz and investigators[5] (Level I) recently note that patients undergoing total joint replacement surgery who were treated by low-volume surgeons in low-volume hospitals were twice as likely to have a poor functional outcome score at 2 years compared with patients of high-volume surgeons in high-volume hospitals (OR of poor function, 2.1; 95% CI, 1.1–4.2). To the best of our knowledge, there are no reported studies of volume and functional outcome for patients with traumatic injuries.

In summary, patients with multiple traumatic injuries, hip fractures treated by hemiarthroplasty, and patients undergoing total joint replacement have fewer complications, and in the case of total joint replacement surgery, experience better functional outcomes when treated by high-volume hospital and surgeon providers. Contradictory evidence has been presented regarding the effect of temporal changes within a given institution as it relates to patient outcome. A positive relation would suggest that volume per se drives the outcome, whereas the absence of a relation implies that volume is merely a surrogate for identifying the quality of care rendered by a particular provider, and that this quality is stable over time (i.e., independent of minor within-provider volume fluctuations).

AREAS OF UNCERTAINTY

Volume–outcome research has been criticized for incomplete consideration of confounding factors.[18] Patient profile differs between high- and low-volume providers, making it difficult to adjust completely for differences in patient characteristics.[16,17] This may account for the fact that fewer prospective studies were found to have a strong positive volume outcome relation compared with retrospective studies.[23] Nonetheless, a randomized clinical trial allocating patients to low- or high-volume providers is unlikely ever to be conducted, and high-quality recent cohort studies have used innovative techniques to adjust for differences in patient case-mix across high- and low-volume providers.[7,21]

The identification of a volume–outcome relation is interesting, but much work needs to be done if patients are to benefit from these findings. Little information is available regarding the reasons for the observed better outcomes in higher volume or specialized centers.[2] High-volume surgeons may be more enthusiastic about a procedure and have different indications[24,25]; however, there are no data available regarding how high- and low-volume providers make decisions regarding care, how the execution of surgery might differ, and how postoperative protocols might affect patient outcome. This information is necessary if we are to devise ways of using volume outcome information to improve care by educating low-volume providers.

Although it is tempting to try and improve outcomes by simply mandating minimum volumes for specific procedures, or by regionalizing care to high-volume centers of excellence, the fact remains that there is no science to guide the setting of specific volume targets. How many cases are required to overcome the "learning curve"? And how many cases need to be performed on an ongoing basis after this period? The literature is not conclusive in this regard, with many studies using completely different volume categories, and none to date having provided clear evidence that a specific threshold exists beyond which results improve or decline.

Clearly, much more work is needed to understand the mechanisms that underlie volume–outcome relations. Moreover, these mechanisms may differ for specific conditions, and work needs to be extended to include many other areas within orthopedics and traumatology (Table 48–1).

RECOMMENDATIONS

Table 48–2 provides a summary of recommendations.

TABLE 48–1. Summary of Evidence

REFERENCE	LEVEL OF EVIDENCE	TYPE OF STUDY	N	PATIENT POPULATION	HOSPITAL EFFECT	SURGEON EFFECT	COMMENTS
Chowdhury et al. (2007)[23]	II	Meta-analysis	9.9 million	All surgical procedures including trauma and orthopedics	Inconclusive*	Complications Mortality	*Hospital effect strong only in retrospective studies, not prospective. Surgeon volume and specialization are both important.
Shervin et al. (2007)[6]	II	Meta-analysis	NA	Arthroplasty, spine general orthopedics and hip fractures (only hip fractures discussed here)	Mortality Complications	Inconclusive	See reference for procedures other than hip fracture.
Clark et al. (2007)[26]	II	Population cohort (Medicare 1999)	95,867	Age ≥ 65 with severe trauma	No relation	Not studied	Mortality was the only outcome studied. Trauma vs. nontrauma hospital was not analyzed.
Mackenzie et al. (2006)[7]	I	Prospective cohort	18,198	Age 18–84 with 2 or more AIS ≥ 3	Mortality (lower in trauma vs. nontrauma)	Not studied	Only high-volume trauma and nontrauma centers included to allow case-mix adjustment. Only urban and suburban areas (rural excluded).
Marcin and Romano (2004)[22]	II	Population cohort (CA Discharge Data 1995–1999)	54,352	Age ≥ 16 with ISS ≥ 9	Mortality in age ≥ 65	Not studied	Only designated trauma centers (Levels I-III) included, but outcomes by level were not compared.
Shah et al. (2005)[8]	II	Population cohort (NIS 1988-2000)	173,508	Age ≥ 65 with hemiarthroplasty for femoral neck fracture	PE, UTI, pneumonia Prolonged LOS	Mortality Prolonged LOS	—

AIS, Abbreviated Injury Scale; ISS, Injury Severity Scale; LOS, length of stay; NIS Nationwide Inpatient Sample; PE, pulmonary embolism; UTI, urinary tract infection.

TABLE 48–2. Summary of Recommendations

RECOMMENDATION	LEVEL OF EVIDENCE /GRADE OF RECOMMENDATION	REFERENCES
1. Patients with complex trauma and with complex arthroplasty have better outcomes when treated by specialized surgeons in a specialized center.	B	7, 13, 18, 20
2. Conflicting evidence exists as to whether volume represents a surrogate marker for provider excellence or whether volume per se may affect outcome.	I	3, 4, 21
3. No scientific basis exists for recommending specific volume targets for orthopedic conditions at this time.	B	

REFERENCES

1. Kreder HJ, et al: Provider volume and other predictors of outcome after total knee arthroplasty: A population study in Ontario. Can J Surg 46:15–22, 2003.
2. Liberman M, et al: The association between trauma system and trauma center components and outcome in a mature regionalized trauma system. Surgery 137:647–658, 2005.
3. Hamilton BH, Ho V: Does practice make perfect? Examining the relationship between hospital surgical volume and outcomes for hip fracture patients in Quebec. Med Care 36:892–903, 1998.
4. Hamilton BH, Hamilton VH: Estimating surgical volume—outcome relationships applying survival models: Accounting for frailty and hospital fixed effects. Health Econ 6:383–395, 1997.
5. Katz JN, et al: Association of hospital and surgeon procedure volume with patient-centered outcomes of total knee replacement in a population-based cohort of patients age 65 years and older. Arthritis Rheum 56:568–574, 2007.
6. Shervin N, Rubash HE, Katz JN: Orthopaedic procedure volume and patient outcomes: A systematic literature review. Clin Orthop Relat Res 457:35–41, 2007.
7. Mackenzie EJ, et al: A national evaluation of the effect of trauma-center care on mortality. N Engl J Med 354:366–378, 2006.
8. Shah SN, Wainess RM, Karunakar MA: Hemiarthroplasty for femoral neck fracture in the elderly surgeon and hospital volume-related outcomes. J Arthroplasty 20:503–508, 2005.
9. Vitale MA, et al: The contribution of hospital volume, payer status, and other factors on the surgical outcomes of scoliosis patients: A review of 3,606 cases in the state of California. J Pediatr Orthop 25:393–399, 2005.
10. Katz JN, et al: Association between hospital and surgeon procedure volume and outcomes of total hip replacement in the United States medicare population. J Bone Joint Surg Am 83:1622–1629, 2001.
11. Nathens AB, et al: The effect of organized systems of trauma care on motor vehicle crash mortality. JAMA 283:1990–1994, 2000.
12. Kreder HJ, et al: Relationship between the volume of total hip replacements performed by providers and the rates of postoperative complications in the state of Washington. J Bone Joint Surg Am 79:485–494, 1997.
13. Freeman J, Nicholl J, Turner J: Does size matter? The relationship between volume and outcome in the care of major trauma. J Health Serv Res Policy 11:101–105, 2006.
14. Halm EA, Lee C, Chassin MR: Is volume related to outcome in health care? A systematic review and methodologic critique of the literature. Ann Intern Med 137:511–520, 2002.
15. Davoli M, et al: [Volume and health outcomes: An overview of systematic reviews]. Epidemiol Prev 29(suppl):3–63, 2005.
16. Losina E, et al: Neighborhoods matter: Use of hospitals with worse outcomes following total knee replacement by patients from vulnerable populations. Arch Intern Med 167:182–187, 2007.
17. Liu JH, et al: Disparities in the utilization of high-volume hospitals for complex surgery. JAMA 296:1973–1980, 2006.
18. Clark CR, Heckman JD: Volume versus outcomes in orthopaedic surgery: A proper perspective is paramount. J Bone Joint Surg Am 83:1619–1621, 2001.
19. Cram P, et al: A comparison of total hip and knee replacement in specialty and general hospitals. J Bone Joint Surg Am 89:1675–1684, 2007.
20. Nathens AB, et al: Relationship between trauma center volume and outcomes. JAMA 285:1164–1171, 2001.
21. Haut ER, et al: Injured patients have lower mortality when treated by "full-time" trauma surgeons vs. surgeons who cover trauma "part-time." J Trauma 61:272–278, 2006.
22. Marcin JP, Romano PS: Impact of between-hospital volume and within-hospital volume on mortality and readmission rates for trauma patients in California. Crit Care Med 32:1477–1483, 2004.
23. Chowdhury MM, Dagash H, Pierro A: A systematic review of the impact of volume of surgery and specialization on patient outcome. Br J Surg 94:145–161, 2007.
24. Dunn WR, et al: Variation in orthopaedic surgeons' perceptions about the indications for rotator cuff surgery. J Bone Joint Surg Am 87:1978–1984, 2005.
25. Marx RG, et al: Beliefs and attitudes of members of the American Academy of Orthopaedic Surgeons regarding the treatment of anterior cruciate ligament injury. Arthroscopy 19:762–770, 2003.
26. Clark DE, et al: Initial presentation of older injured patients to high-volume hospitals is not associated with lower 30-day mortality in Medicare data. Crit Care Med 35:1829–1836, 2007.

Are Bone Substitutes Useful in the Treatment and Prevention of Nonunions and in the Management of Subchondral Voids?

Ross K. Leighton, BSc, MD, FRCSC, FACS, Mohit Bhandari, MD, MSc, FRCSC, Thomas A. Russell, MD, and Kelly Trask, MSc

Bone substitutes can be considered in two circumstances: (1) as an agent for the prevention and treatment of nonunions, and (2) as a "void filler" to maintain joint or metaphyseal alignment, usually in a periarticular or intra-articular fracture.

The prevention and treatment of nonunions remains a conundrum in orthopedic surgery. Despite the best treatment protocols and attention to detail, nonunions still occur. The acute care of a fracture does not usually involve the use of bone graft or bone substitutes. However, the treatment of nonunions involves consideration of a bone substitute that induces (osteoinductive substance) or facilitates (osteoconductive substance) bone ingrowth, particularly if the nonunion is located in the diaphysis.

Periarticular fractures are common injuries that result from indirect coronal and/or direct axial compressive forces. The usual surgical guidelines for treating depressed articular fractures with joint instability include anatomic reduction, re-establishment of the long bone alignment, subchondral bone grafting to support the articular cartilage, and stable internal fixation.[1] In this situation, a substance that withstands compressive forces and provides structural support is of primary importance, with osteoinductive properties being secondary.

OPTIONS

Cancellous bone graft retrieved from an iliac crest donor site has been the traditional substance of choice used both to promote healing and to fill voids and provide structural support. This procedure involves making a separate incision over the crest to obtain the graft, which can cause morbidity such as pain, nerve injury, arterial injury, and infection.[2,3] Allograft bone can be used to avoid the morbidity associated with autograft harvesting; however, allograft bone acts mainly as an osteoconductive substance, and there is a risk for disease transmission. In recent years, new bone alternatives have become commercially available to act as "substitute" bone graft.

These consist of various forms of ceramics such as tricalcium phosphate and hydroxyapatite.[4–7]

Bone graft substitutes can be either osteoinductive (inducing existing cells to make new bone) or osteoconductive (acting as a scaffold along which existing cells can lay down new bone), or a combination of the two. They may have a consistency similar to cancellous bone or corticocancellous chips, or they may harden into a solid structural mass.

The purpose of this chapter is to provide evidence-based guidance to the reader regarding the use of bone substitutes for the prevention and treatment of nonunions and for the management of subchondral voids.

Evidence

Based on the method that Bajammal and colleagues[8] used for their recent meta-analysis, we primarily identified articles with the following features: (1) the target population was skeletally mature patients with a fracture of a bone of the appendicular skeleton; (2) the intervention was the use of calcium phosphate bone cement, calcium sulfate bone cement, or a recombinant human bone morphogenetic protein (rhBMP) compared with alternative or no treatment in the management of these fractures; (3) the outcome measure was either functional (pain or impairment) or radiographic (fracture healing or subsidence) outcome, or infection rate; and (4) the study was a published or unpublished randomized, controlled trial. We secondarily also included other less rigorous studies in this review because of the paucity of articles with Level I evidence.

Osteoconductive Bone Graft Substitutes

Allograft Bone. Allograft bone harvested from living or deceased donors as cancellous, or corticocancellous chips, has a wide application as an osteoconductive filler for metaphyseal defects typically at the proximal and distal end of the tibia (Table 49–1). McKee and coworkers[9] report on a case series of six humeral

TABLE 49–1. Characteristics of Studies Included in the Meta-analysis

FIRST AUTHOR (YEAR OF PUBLICATION)	NO. OF CENTERS, COUNTRY	NO. OF PATIENTS (INT, CONT)	FEMALES INT, CONT	MEAN AGE INT, CONT*	POPULATION	INTERVENTION Vs. CONTROL	MAJOR OUTCOME MEASURES	FUNDING
Chapman et al. (1997)[15]	18, USA	345† (176, 169)	N/R	37, 37	Multiple† types, 18–70 years	Collagraft vs. AIBG	Pain, ADL function; Fracture healing; Deformity	Industry
Kopylov et al. (1999)[47,48]	1, Sweden	40 (20, 20)	18, 18	69, 66	Distal radius, 50–80 years	CR, Norian and cast vs. CR and ExFix	Pain, ROM, grip strength; Radiographic parameters; RSA measurement	Industry and peer-reviewed
Sanchez-Sotelo et al. (2000)[20]	1, Spain	110 (55, 55)	48, 49	65, 67	Distal radius, 50–85 years	CR, Norian and cast vs. CR and cast	Pain, ROM, grip strength; Radiographic parameters; Malunion	No industry
Jeyam et al. (2002)[49]	1, UK	18 (9, 9)	9, 9	71, 74	Distal radius, >60 years	CR, BoneSource and cast vs. CR, K-wires and cast	ROM, grip strength; Radiographic parameters	Industry
Kopylov et al. (2002)[50]	1, Sweden	20 (9, 11)	9, 11	65, 67	Distal radius, 50–80 years	CR, Norian and cast vs. retain original cast (no reduction)	Pain, ROM, grip strength; Radiographic parameters	Industry and peer-reviewed
Cassidy et al. (2003)[16]	23, USA	323 (161,162)	129, 143	64, 64	Distal radius, ≥45 years	CR, Norian and (cast or ExFix) vs. CR and (cast or ExFix)	Pain, ROM, grip strength; Radiographic parameters; Loss of reduction, SF-36	Industry
Dickson et al. (2002)[18]	3, USA	40† (21, 19)	7, 6	45, 40	Multiple types,† 18–80 years	Both groups ± K-wires BoneSource vs. AIBG	Pain, regain of function; Fracture healing; Loss of reduction	N/R
Mattsson and Larsson (2003)[51]	1, Sweden	40 (20, 20)	18, 15	78, 78	Low-energy femoral neck	CR, 2 screws and Norian vs. CR and 2 screws	RSA measurement	Industry
Zimmermann et al. (2003)[17]	1, Austria	52 (26, 26)	26, 26	63, 57	Distal radius, menopausal women	CR, Norian, K-wires and cast vs. CR, K-wires and cast	ROM, grip strength; Radiographic parameters; Fracture healing, DASH	N/R
Mattsson and Larsson (2004)[52]	1, Sweden	26 (14, 12)	12, 10	84, 82	Unstable trochanteric†	DHS and Norian vs. DHS	RSA measurement	Industry
Russell et al. (2004)[14]	12, USA, Canada	119† (82, 38) 1 bilateral	Overall 46	43, 43	Tibial plateau,† 16–77 years	ORIF and α-BSM vs. ORIF and AIBG	ROM; Fracture healing; Loss of reduction	Industry
Larsson et al. (2004)[19‡]	1, Sweden	26§ (13, 13)	N/R	50, 52	Tibial plateau,† 18–60 years§	ORIF and Norian vs. ORIF and AIBG	Pain, weight bearing; RSA measurement; Lysholm knee score	Industry and peer-reviewed
Mattsson et al. (2005)[53]	3, Sweden	112 (55, 57)	44, 47	81, 82	Unstable trochanteric† Age > 65 years	DHS and Norian vs. DHS	Pain, ADL functions, muscle strength, SF-36, radiographic parameters	Industry and peer-reviewed
Mattsson et al. (2006)[54]	1, Sweden	118 (58, 60)	46, 49§	77, 77§	Displaced femoral neck, age > 60 years	CR, 2 screws and Norian vs. CR and 2 screws	Pain, ADL functions, muscle strength, radiographic parameters	Industry and peer-reviewed
Reed et al. (2005)[55]	1, Canada	48 fractures (21, 27)§	1, 1§	36, 37§	Displaced calcaneal fractures, age > 16 years	ORIF and α-BSM vs. ORIF	Radiographic parameters; SF-36, LEM score	N/R

*Mean age in years (rounded to integer).
†Fractures.
‡Unpublished.
§Author contact.

α-BSM, bioabsorbable calcium phosphate paste; ADL, activities of daily living; AIBG, autogenous iliac crest bone graft; CR, closed reduction; DASH, Disability of Arm Shoulder and Hand Questionnaire; DHS, dynamic hip screw; ExFix, external fixation; K-wires, Kirschner wires; no. of patients (int, cont), number of patients in the intervention group and control group; N/R, not reported; ORIF, open reduction and internal fixation; ROM, range of motion; RSA, radiostereometric analysis; SF-36, 36-Item Short Form Health Survey.
Data from Sohail S, Bajammal SS, Zlowodski M, Schmitz-Lelwicka AE, et al: The use of calcium phosphate bone cement in fracture treatment: A meta-analysis of randomized trials. J Bone Joint Surg Am 90:1186–1196, 2008.

nonunions treated with a combination of compression plate fixation and cortical onlay grafts. All six nonunions had united at a median of 3.4 months. Hornicek and coauthors[10] report a series of nine humeral nonunions treated in a similar fashion; union was achieved in all patients at an average of 2.9 months. Haddad and researchers[11] report on a retrospective case series of 40 patients using cortical onlay strut grafts together with well-fixed prosthetic femoral stems; 39 of the 40 patients united. Herrera and investigators[12] report on distal radial fractures treated with external fixation and internal fixation together with cancellous bone grafts and concluded that allograft was a useful adjunct for treatment of unstable distal radial fractures. An article that prospectively compared autologous graft versus allograft, delivered at the Orthopaedic Trauma Association (OTA) in 2005, demonstrated that allograft was not equal to autograft. However, autograft did have associated donor morbidity.[13] No Level I evidence supports corticocancellous allografts in reconstructive trauma surgery, but Level II and IV evidence does exist, as noted earlier.

Calcium Phosphate Synthetic Substitutes. The calcium phosphate synthetic substitutes have been investigated as devices by the FDA and by industry over the last 8 years. Initial studies were done with critical defects in rats, sheep, and dogs. Subsequent biomechanical studies suggested that bioabsorbable calcium phosphate paste (α-BSM) in tibias was stronger than cancellous bone graft used to repair periarticular fractures[14] (Fig. 49–1). Trenholm and coworkers[14] illustrate that the initial stiffness was

significantly better in the α-BSM group (calcium phosphate cement) as compared with autograft under a 1000-newton load. Russell and investigators[1] in a prospective, randomized, multicenter trial compared the treatment of subarticular bone defects in tibial plateau fractures with conventional autogenous iliac bone graft (AIBG) with α-BSM. One hundred nineteen acute closed tibial plateau fractures were prospectively enrolled, and randomization occurred at surgery with a 2:1 ration of the α-BSM to autogenous bone graft. Russell and investigators[1] found both a significant increase in graft-related adverse effects on the AIBG group, and a statistically significantly greater rate of articular subsidence in the 3- to 12-month period in the AIBG group (Fig. 49–2). Thus, Level I evidence supports the use of bioabsorbable calcium phosphate material, such as α-BSM, as the treatment of choice for subarticular defects in tibial plateau fractures.

Three of these six studies in the meta-analysis by Bajammal and colleagues[8] report significantly improved functional outcome scores with the use of calcium phosphate versus autograft, and in evaluating them separately, Chapman and researchers[15] found a difference in functional repair in favor of the calcium phosphate group. Cassidy and investigators[16] found significant greater scores representing better function in bodily pain, role physical, role emotional, social function, and mental health subdomains of the 36-Item Short Form Health Survey (SF-36). Zimmermann and colleagues[17] found significantly better DASH (disability of the arm, shoulder, and hand) scores in distal radius fractures for the calcium phosphate group. Six of the studies also reported loss-of-reduction outcome, and calcium phosphate significantly reduced the incidence of loss of fracture reduction compared with controls.[1,15,16,18–20] Thus, loss of fracture alignment was 48% less likely when calcium phosphate was used. For every 17 patients treated with calcium phosphate, one loss of fracture reduction could be prevented.[8]

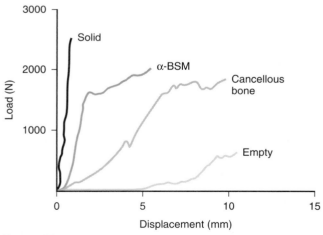

FIGURE 49–1. Higher compressive strength of calcium phosphate bone substitute in a biomechanical study of tibial plateau fractures. α-BSM, subchondral defect filled with calcium phosphate bone substitute; cancellous bone, subchondral defect filled with cancellous bone chips; empty, repair of fracture with no filling of subchondral defect; solid, no defect in tibial plateau. Adapted from Bajammal SS, Zlowodski M, Schmitz-Lelwicka AE, et al.: The use of calcium phosphate bone cement in fracture treatment: a meta-analysis of randomized trials. Hamilton, ON, McMaster University, 2007, unpublished.

Calcium Sulfate Synthetic Substitutes

Evidence for the use of calcium sulfate is extremely poor. In a study done by Petruskevicius and coworkers[21] looking at OsteoSet (Wright Medical Technology, Arlington, TN) on bone healing and tibial defect in humans, OsteoSet was compared with no bone graft in the substitution of anterior cruciate ligament repairs. Computed tomographic scans of the defect were taken on the first day after the operation, at 6 weeks, 3 months, and 6 months. No difference was found in the amount of bone in the defect in the OsteoSet and control groups, and indeed, in the control group (no bone graft or pellets), the bone volume increased from 6 weeks to 3 months. A study looking at the use of calcium sulfate in nonunions, presented at the OTA in 2004,

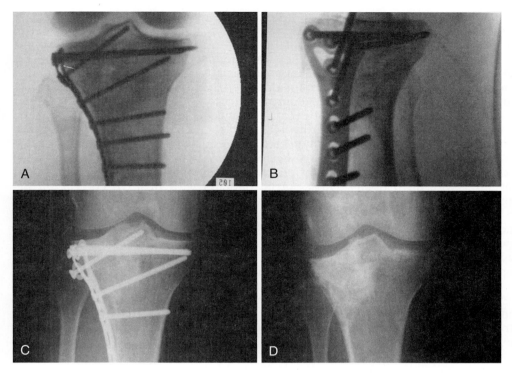

Figure 49–2. Late collapse of the tibial plateau after fracture fixation using autogenous iliac bone graft (AIBG) to support the articular surface. *A,* Initial fixation of the Schatzker II fracture. *B,* Three months after surgery. *C,* Twelve months after surgery. *D,* Eighteen months after surgery, articular surface has collapsed after hardware removal at 1 year.

demonstrated no improvement in bone healing, an increased infection rate, and increased wound drainage.[22] The authors' conclusion was to suggest calcium sulfate should not be used in the treatment of nonunions. Despite excellent efforts, there is no Level I or II evidence that the healing is enhanced, and indeed, healing may be worse in periarticular injuries or nonunions with the addition of calcium sulfate.

With the increasing popularity of calcium sulfate, there have been some cases of severe inflammatory response particularly in tumor cases. It has been hypothesized that the rapid absorption of the calcium sulfate pellets into a calcium-rich fluid stimulates inflammation.[23]

Demineralized Bone Matrix

No studies have been reported in which the investigators carefully evaluated the osteoconductive properties of allograft bone per se. Demineralized bone matrix (DBM) is produced by acid extraction of allograft that contains type I collagen, noncollagenous proteins, and osteoconductive growth factors. Tiedeman and coauthors[24] report on an uncontrolled case series of 48 patients in whom DBM had been used in conjunction with bone marrow for the treatment of skeletal injuries. Because there was no control group, the role of DBM in the 30 patients who had healing remains unknown. One prospective, controlled study showed equivalent rates of spinal fusion between sides in patients who had been treated with autograft on one side and a 2:1 ratio

composite of Grafton DBM gel and autograft on the other, suggesting the potential use of Grafton DBM as a bone graft extender in spine fusions.[25] Only anecdotal information is available regarding similar applications in diaphyseal and metaphyseal bone injuries.

Osteoinductive Bone Graft Substitutes

Human Bone Morphogenetic Protein. The two most widely studied osteoinductive bone substitutes are rhBMP-2 and rhBMP-7. The use of bone morphogenetic protein (BMP) to improve the healing of open tibial shaft fractures has been the focus of several prospective clinical studies. Swiontkowski and investigators[26] analyzed two prospective, clinical, randomized studies that recruited a total of 510 patients with open tibial fractures. They were randomized to receive the control treatment, intramedullary nail fixation, and routine soft-tissue management versus treatment with an absorbable collagen sponge impregnated with one of two concentrations of rhBMP-2. Fifty-nine trauma centers in 12 countries participated, and the patients were followed for 12 months after surgery. Two subgroups were analyzed: (1) 131 patients with Gustilo–Anderson type IIIA or IIIB open tibial fractures not treated with internal fixation, and (2) 113 patients treated with reamed intramedullary nailing. The first subgroup demonstrated significant improvements in the rhBMP-2 group with fewer bone grafting procedures and fewer patients requiring invasive secondary interventions. The subgroup analysis of fractures treated with reamed, intramedullary nailing demonstrated no significant difference between the control and the rhBMP-2 groups. Both groups illustrated a trend in reduction of the infection rate in those patients who received rhBMP-2. Therefore, the following conclusion can be reached: If intramedullary nailing is not utilized, the addition of rhBMP-2 to open tibial fractures can significantly reduce the frequency of bone grafting procedures and other secondary interventions. There seems to be no improvement in outcome when IM nailing is used.

Govender and coauthors[27] also presented evidence on a prospective, randomized, controlled, single-blind study with 450 patients presenting with open tibial fractures. They were randomized to receive either intramedullary nail fixation and routine soft-tissue management or the same care plus rhBMP-2. A trend suggested better healing and faster bone growth in the rhBMP-2 group that did not reach statistical significance, and the final nonunion rate was similar between the two groups.

McKee and coworkers[28] evaluated rhBMP-7 (also known as OP-1) by randomizing 122 patients with 124 open tibial shaft fractures. All patients received an initial débridement plus open reduction and internal fixation with a locked intramuscular nail within 48 hours of injury. At the time of secondary closure, the patients either received no additional treatment, except for wound closure, or wound closure with the addition of OP-1. They were followed up for 1 year. The results did not demonstrate any difference in union rate. The number of nonunions was not decreased with the addition of rhBMP-7. However, the amount of bone created was greater with the treatment group, and the time to healing was reduced, but the study was underpowered and did not reach statistical significance. In addition to the trend to improve bone healing, there was also a corresponding improvement in patient function, with 80% of the OP-1 group having no pain or mild pain with activity at 12 months after injury compared with 65% of the control group ($P = 0.04$).

Given the weaknesses of the studies noted earlier, there is still no Level I evidence that rhBMP in combination with the usual internal fixation will reduce the nonunion rate in these patients. The infection rate may be reduced in the patients treated with rhBMP. Further multicenter, randomized, prospective studies are indicated because at this time there is only Level II evidence that BMPs can be useful in areas other than spine fusion. It appears that when rigid internal fixation is not utilized at the initial onset of these terrible grade IIIA and IIIB injuries, that the use of a BMP could help reduce secondary procedures and seems to have a reduction in the infection rate in these huge soft-tissue injuries.

Clinical Application of Autologous Bone Marrow. Bone marrow aspirate has been utilized as another way of applying connective tissue progenitors intraoperatively to enhance bone growth and repair. Garg and coworkers[29] and Healey and researchers[30] were able to show low-level evidence of improvement with bone marrow aspirate. Goel and coauthors[31] report that they used bone marrow injections with the use of local anesthesia for patients who are on waiting lists for open repair of a nonunion. They used this procedure in an attempt to provide a low-cost alternative and claimed success in 15 of 20 patients. Hernigou and colleagues[32] report on 60 patients with noninfected nonunions who had undergone bone marrow aspiration of both iliac crests followed by injection at the nonunion site. Results showed union in 53 of 60 patients with positive correlation between the volume of mineralized callous at 4 months and the number and concentration of colony-forming units. This study provided the best evidence (Level III) for the use of autologous bone marrow. An article presented at the 2006 OTA annual meeting in Phoenix demonstrated no benefit of autologous bone marrow in a randomized, controlled study.[33] Currently, no level I or II evidence documents the effectiveness of bone marrow for the enhancement of bone healing.

Use of Platelet-Rich Plasma and Related Peripheral Blood Concentrations. Several strategies for platelet concentration delivery have been developed on the basis of the assumption that delivery of a concentrated amount of platelets would contribute to the early stages of bone repair, thus initiating a fracture healing cascade.[34,35] However, to date, indications are based only on longitudinal case series, multiple case reports, and abstracts documenting the effects of platelet gels and concentrates.[36] Therefore, at this time, the use of platelet-rich plasma and related peripheral blood concentrates seem to function best as a physiologic carrier for other graft materials.

AREAS OF UNCERTAINTY

If bone substitutes provide equivalent results to bone autograft, is the increased cost justified to avoid the morbidity associated with autogenous bone harvesting? Jones[56] presents data to suggest that in severe open tibia fractures the addition of BMP might be cost saving depending on the payor model; however, there are no prospective costing data available to address this issue.

Autogenous iliac graft procurement requires a second surgical procedure with loss of tissues from the body, the induction of pain at a previously uninjured site, and presents the possibility of iatrogenic infection.[37,38] Younger and Chapman[3] document the relative rates of major and minor complications after an autogenous bone graft harvest procedure. Goulet and coauthors[39] report the functional disturbances from the harvest of autogenous iliac bone. Autogenous graft is not a homogenous material; there are significant differences in the hosts, and this problem is exacerbated in osteoporotic donors. Thus, osteoporotic autograft is less useful; however, it is unknown whether bone substitutes are as effective in the setting of an elderly osteoporotic individual as they might be in a younger host with more active osteoprogenitor cells that can respond to the potential osteoinductive properties of a substitute, or that can populate the scaffold provided by an osteoconductive bone substitute.

Acknowledgments

We are grateful to Dr. Russell and his coauthors for proving the full unpublished manuscript of their meeting abstract, and Drs. Bhandari and Bajammal for providing the full unpublished manuscript for their meta-analysis.

RECOMMENDATIONS

Prevention of Nonunion in Fresh Fractures

No evidence supports the use of bone substitutes in addition to internal fixation as an agent or device to reduce the occurrence of nonunions. rhBMP may reduce the infection rate when used in fresh open tibia fractures. Level II evidence exists that if no internal fixation is utilized at initial treatment, then the addition of rhBMP-2 may reduce the need for subsequent surgical procedures.

Treatment of Established Nonunions

The treatment of nonunions is always difficult. Finkemeier and Chapman[46] in 2002 achieved a 97% union rate in diaphyseal nonunions by following the usual protocol, as noted earlier, without the use of rhBMPs. To date, the power in the studies performed has not been able to demonstrate a significant difference between the usual treatment (débridement, stabilization, and bone graft) and those treated in the usual way plus the addition of an rhBMP. The trend for improved healing in the rhBMP group has been documented, but the cause of nonunions remains multifactorial, and it remains a difficult group to obtain clean Level I evidence.

Management of a Subchondral Void

Calcium phosphate is significantly stronger in compression than in cancellous bone graft,[14] and it should be considered the treatment of choice for subchondral void management of tibial plateau fractures. Use in other areas requires additional study. Table 49–2 provides a summary of recommendations.

TABLE 49–2. Summary of Recommendations

RECOMMENDATION	LEVEL OF EVIDENCE /GRADE OF RECOMMENDATION
1. Adults with open tibia fractures do not require bone grafting or bone substitutes if nailing or internal fixation is used.	B
2. Adults with type III open tibia fractures where no internal fixation is used should be considered for treatment with human bone morphogenetic protein to minimize the risk of requiring secondary procedures.	B
3. Adults with established nonunions: The use of bone substitutes may be similar to autogenous bone graft but without the morbidity associated with autograft iliac crest harvesting but more evidence is needed before a clear recommendation can be made.	I
4. Adults with compressed articular surfaces and a contained subchondral void after reduction should be managed with a calcium phosphate bone substitute to minimize the risk for joint collapse.	A

REFERENCES

1. Russell TA, Leighton RK, Bucholz RW, et al: The gold standard in tibial plateau fractures? A prospective multicenter randomized study of AIBG vs. alpha-BSM. Presented at the Orthopaedic Trauma Association Annual Meeting; 2004 Oct 8–10; Hollywood, FL. J Bone Joint Surg 2008 (in press).
2. De Long WG Jr, Einhorn TA, Koval K, et al: Bone grafts and bone graft substitutes in orthopaedic trauma surgery. A critical analysis. J Bone Joint Surg Am 89:649–658, 2007.
3. Younger EM, Chapman MW: Morbidity at bone graft donor sites. J Orthop Trauma 3:192–195, 1989.
4. Ladd AL, Pliam NB: Use of bone-graft substitutes in distal radius fractures. J Am Acad Orthop Surg 7:279–290, 1999.
5. Larsson S, Bauer TW: Use of injectable calcium phosphate cement for fracture fixation: A review. Clin Orthop Relat Res 23–32, 2002.
6. Moore WR, Graves SE, Bain GI: Synthetic bone graft substitutes. ANZ J Surg 71:354–361, 2001.
7. Szpalski M, Gunzburg R: Applications of calcium phosphate-based cancellous bone void fillers in trauma surgery. Orthopedics 25:s601–s609, 2002.
8. Bajammal SS, Zlowodski M, Schmitz-Lelwicka AE, et al: The Use of Calcium Phosphate Bone Cement in Fracture Treatment: A Meta-analysis of Randomized Trials. Hamilton, Ontario, Canada, McMaster University, 2007.
9. McKee MD, Miranda MA, Riemer BL, et al: Management of humeral nonunion after the failure of locking intramedullary nails. J Orthop Trauma 10:492–499, 1996.
10. Hornicek FJ, Zych GA, Hutson JJ, et al: Salvage of humeral nonunions with onlay bone plate allograft augmentation. Clin Orthop Relat Res 203–209, 2001.
11. Haddad FS, Duncan CP, Berry DJ, et al: Periprosthetic femoral fractures around well-fixed implants: Use of cortical onlay allografts with or without a plate. J Bone Joint Surg Am 84-A:945–950, 2002.
12. Herrera M, Chapman CB, Roh M, et al: Treatment of unstable distal radius fractures with cancellous allograft and external fixation. J Hand Surg 24:1269–1278, 1999.
13. Volgas D, Emblom B, Stannard JP, et al: A randomized controlled prospective trial of autologous bone graft versus iliac crest bone graft for nonunions and delayed unions.

Presented at the Orthopaedic Trauma Association Annual Meeting; 2004 Oct 8–10; Hollywood, FL.

14. Trenholm A, Landry S, McLaughlin K, et al: Comparative fixation of tibial plateau fractures using a-BSM, a calcium phosphate cement, versus cancellous bone graft. J Orthop Trauma 19:698–702, 2005.

15. Chapman MW, Bucholz R, Cornell C: Treatment of acute fractures with a collagen-calcium phosphate graft material. A randomized clinical trial. J Bone Joint Surg Am 79:495–502, 1997.

16. Cassidy C, Jupiter JB, Cohen M, et al: Norian SRS cement compared with conventional fixation in distal radial fractures. A randomized study. J Bone Joint Surg Am 85-A:2127–2137, 2003.

17. Zimmermann R, Gabl M, Lutz M, et al: Injectable calcium phosphate bone cement Norian SRS for the treatment of intra-articular compression fractures of the distal radius in osteoporotic women. Arch Orthop Trauma Surg 123:22–27, 2003.

18. Dickson KF, Friedman J, Buchholz JG, et al: The use of BoneSource hydroxyapatite cement for traumatic metaphyseal bone void filling. J Trauma 53:1103–1108, 2002.

19. Larsson S, Berg P, Sagerfors M: Augmentation of tibial plateau fractures with calcium phosphate cement: A randomized study using radiostereometry. Presented at the Orthopaedic Trauma Association Annual Meeting; 2004 Oct 8–10; Hollywood, FL.

20. Sanchez-Sotelo J, Munuera L, Madero R: Treatment of fractures of the distal radius with a remodellable bone cement: A prospective, randomised study using Norian SRS. J Bone Joint Surg Br 82:856–863, 2000.

21. Petruskevicius J, Nielsen S, Kaalund S, et al: No effect of Osteoset, a bone graft substitute, on bone healing in humans: A prospective randomized double-blind study. Acta Orthop Scand 73:575–578, 2002.

22. Ziran BH, Smith WR, Lahti Z, et al: Use of calcium-based demineralized bone matrix (DBM) allograft product for nonunions and posttraumatic reconstruction of the appendicular skeleton: Preliminary results and complications. Presented at the Orthopaedic Trauma Association Annual Meeting; 2004 Oct 8–10; Hollywood, FL.

23. Robinson D, Alk D, Sandbank J, et al: Inflammatory reactions associated with a calcium sulfate bone substitute. Ann Transplant 4:91–97, 1999.

24. Tiedeman JJ, Garvin KL, Kile TA, et al: The role of a composite, demineralized bone matrix and bone marrow in the treatment of osseous defects. Orthopedics 18:1153–1158, 1995.

25. Cammisa FP Jr, Lowery G, Garfin SR, et al: Two-year fusion rate equivalency between Grafton DBM gel and autograft in posterolateral spine fusion: A prospective controlled trial employing a side-by-side comparison in the same patient. Spine 29:660–666, 2004.

26. Swiontkowski MF, Aro HT, Donell S, et al: Recombinant human bone morphogenetic protein-2 in open tibial fractures. A subgroup analysis of data combined from two prospective randomized studies. J Bone Joint Surg Am 88:1258–1265, 2006.

27. Govender S, Csimma C, Genant HK, et al: Recombinant human bone morphogenetic protein-2 for treatment of open tibial fractures: A prospective, controlled, randomized study of four hundred and fifty patients. J Bone Joint Surg Am 84-A:2123–2134, 2002.

28. McKee MD, Wild LM, Schemitsch EH, et al: The use of an antibiotic-impregnated, osteoconductive, bioabsorbable bone substitute in the treatment of infected long bone defects: Early results of a prospective trial. J Orthop Trauma 16:622–627, 2002.

29. Garg NK, Gaur S, Sharma S: Percutaneous autogenous bone marrow grafting in 20 cases of ununited fracture. Acta Orthop Scand 64:671–672, 1993.

30. Healey JH, Zimmerman PA, McDonnell JM, et al: Percutaneous bone marrow grafting of delayed union and nonunion in cancer patients. Clin Orthop Relat Res 280–285, 1990.

31. Goel A, Sangwan SS, Siwach RC, et al: Percutaneous bone marrow grafting for the treatment of tibial non-union. Injury 36:203–206, 2005.

32. Hernigou P, Poignard A, Beaujean F, et al: Percutaneous autologous bone-marrow grafting for nonunions. Influence of the number and concentration of progenitor cells. J Bone Joint Surg Am 87:1430–1437, 2005.

33. Watson JT, Quigley KJ, Mudd CD: Percutaneous injection of iliac crest aspirate for the treatment of long bone delayed union and nonunion. Phoenix, AZ, 2006.

34. Marx RE, Carlson ER, Eichstaedt RM, et al: Platelet-rich plasma: Growth factor enhancement for bone grafts. Oral Surg Oral Med Oral Pathol Oral Radiol Endod 85:638–646, 1998.

35. Slater M, Patava J, Kingham K, et al: Involvement of platelets in stimulating osteogenic activity. J Orthop Res 13:655–663, 1995.

36. Bibbo C, Bono CM, Lin SS: Union rates using autologous platelet concentrate alone and with bone graft in high-risk foot and ankle surgery patients. J Surg Orthop Adv 14:17–22, 2005.

37. Fowler BL, Dall BE, Rowe DE: Complications associated with harvesting autogenous iliac bone graft. Am J Orthop 24:895–903, 1995.

38. Seiler JG 3rd, Johnson J: Iliac crest autogenous bone grafting: Donor site complications. J South Orthop Assoc 9:91–97, 2000.

39. Goulet JA, Senunas LE, DeSilva GL, et al: Autogenous iliac crest bone graft. Complications and functional assessment. Clin Orthop Relat Res 76–81, 1997.

40. Cornell CN, Lane JM, Chapman M, et al: Multicenter trial of Collagraft as bone graft substitute. J Orthop Trauma 5:1–8, 1991.

41. Horstmann WG, Verheyen CC, Leemans R: An injectable calcium phosphate cement as a bone-graft substitute in the treatment of displaced lateral tibial plateau fractures. Injury 34:141–144, 2003.

42. Keating JF, Hajducka CL, Harper J: Minimal internal fixation and calcium-phosphate cement in the treatment of fractures of the tibial plateau. A pilot study. J Bone Joint Surg Br 85:68–73, 2003.

43. Yetkinler DN, McClellan RT, Reindel ES, et al: Biomechanical comparison of conventional open reduction and internal fixation versus calcium phosphate cement fixation of a central depressed tibial plateau fracture. J Orthop Trauma 15:197–206, 2001.

44. Knaack D, Goad ME, Aiolova M, et al: Resorbable calcium phosphate bone substitute. J Biomed Mater Res 43:399–409, 1998.

45. Welch RD, Zhang H, Bronson DG: Experimental tibial plateau fractures augmented with calcium phosphate cement or autologous bone graft. J Bone Joint Surg Am 85-A:222–231, 2003.

46. Finkemeier CG, Chapman MW: Treatment of femoral diaphyseal nonunions. Clin Orthop Relat Res 223–234, 2002.

47. Kopylov P, Aspenberg P, Yuan X, et al: Radiostereometric analysis of distal radial fracture displacement during treatment: A randomized study comparing Norian SRS and external fixation in 23 patients. Acta Orthop Scand 72:57–61, 2001.

48. Kopylov P, Runnqvist K, Jonsson K, et al: Norian SRS versus external fixation in redisplaced distal radial fractures. A randomized study in 40 patients. Acta Orthop Scand 70:1–5, 1999.

49. Jeyam M, Andrew JG, Muir LT, et al: Controlled trial of distal radial fractures treated with a resorbable bone mineral substitute. J Hand Surg 27:146–149, 2002.

50. Kopylov P, Adalberth K, Jonsson K, et al: Norian SRS versus functional treatment in redisplaced distal radial fractures: A randomized study in 20 patients. J Hand Surg 27:538–541, 2002.

51. Mattsson P, Larsson S: Stability of internally fixed femoral neck fractures augmented with resorbable cement. A prospective randomized study using radiostereometry. Scand J Surg 92:215–219, 2003.

52. Mattsson P, Larsson S: Unstable trochanteric fractures augmented with calcium phosphate cement. A prospective randomized study using radiostereometry to measure fracture stability. Scand J Surg 93:223–228, 2004.

53. Mattsson P, Alberts A, Dahlberg G, et al: Resorbable cement for the augmentation of internally-fixed unstable trochanteric fractures. A prospective, randomised multicentre study. J Bone Joint Surg Br 87:1203–1209, 2005.

54. Mattsson P, Larsson S: Calcium phosphate cement for augmentation did not improve results after internal fixation of displaced femoral neck fractures: A randomized study of 118 patients. Acta Orthop 77:251–256, 2006.

55. Reed J, Le ILD, Buckley RE, et al: A prospective randomized controlled trial of a bioresorbable calcium phosphate paste (a-BSM) in displaced intra-articular calcaneal fractures. Montreal, Quebec, Canada, 2005.

56. Jones AL: Recombinant human bone morphogenetic protein-2 in fracture care. J Orthop Trauma 19;S23–S25, 2005.

Fracture Healing: How Strong Is the Effect of Smoking on Bone Healing?

Michael D. McKee, MD, FRCS(C)

The negative sequelae of cigarette smoking on the musculoskeletal system and wound healing have become a popular topic of study.[1–4] A variety of specialties and institutions (especially those responsible for healthcare costs) have focused on smoking as a potentially remediable risk factor for negative outcome after a variety of medical interventions. For example, epidemiologic and experimental studies in the plastic surgery literature identify nicotine as a deleterious constituent of cigarette smoke, leading to increased rates of wound complications and pedicle flap necrosis secondary to vasoconstriction and microthrombus formation.[5–7]

For years, orthopedic experts have anecdotally described the negative impact of cigarette smoking on the musculoskeletal system. More recently, this effect has been the subject of a number of reports: cigarette smoking leads to an increased incidence of pseudarthrosis after spinal fusion,[8,9] increased time to union in tibial fractures[10–13] lower bone mineral density,[3] and poor outcome after treatment of chronic osteomyelitis.[11,14] In addition, clinical and experimental evidence suggests that cigarette smoking leads to decreased mineralization and mechanical strength of regenerate bone during tibial lengthening.[14–17]

The purpose of this chapter is to critically analyze the evidence available in the literature on the effect of smoking on fracture healing, outline areas of uncertainty, and provide some recommendations for future care. Because it is not a topic that lends itself well to randomization, or even prospective studies, most of the evidence available is contained in basic science studies and relatively low-quality Level III and IV retrospective clinical reviews.

EVIDENCE

Basic Science Research

Regenerate bone is vulnerable to the vasoconstrictive and hypoxic effects of cigarette smoke and nicotine.[14–17] In a model of tibial lengthening in rabbits, Ueng and colleagues[15] demonstrate decreased production, maturation, and torsional strength of regenerate bone formation in subjects exposed to cigarette smoke. The same group demonstrated improved mechanical strength of regenerate bone in animals treated with hyperbaric oxygen, suggesting

that local tissue oxygen tissue tension is of paramount importance.[16] El-zawawy and coworkers[17] show that the chondrogenic phase of tibial fracture healing in a mouse model was delayed by exposure to nicotine. Similarly, Skott and coauthors[18] studied the effect of tobacco extract on the healing of a closed femoral fracture model in the rat. They found that the rats given tobacco extract had a 20% to 26% decrease in the mechanical strength of the femur 21 days after fracture. In a rabbit model, Raikin and colleagues[19] conducted a study examining the effect of administration of nicotine on the mechanical strength of midshaft tibial osteotomies. They found a nearly identical 26% decrease in mechanical strength in the nicotine group with a corresponding decrease in callous size. In summary, abundant basic science evidence illustrates the negative effects of smoking in general and nicotine in particular on fracture healing (Table 50–1).

Clinical Research

Numerous clinical studies describe the effects of smoking on various aspects of fracture healing, regenerate bone formation, spinal fusion, arthrodeses, or osteotomy healing.[3,5,10–14,20,21] Because of the nature of the condition, it is not possible to randomize patients into smoking and nonsmoking groups; therefore, most reports are Level III retrospective reviews, although there are some studies with prospectively gathered information in a comparative study (Level II).[11,12,14] However, even though it is of relatively low quality, the clinical information that is available is overwhelming in its description of the negative effects of smoking on bone healing (Table 50–2).

In the upper extremity, Chen and colleagues[21] describe a 30% nonunion rate with a mean time to healing of 7.1 months in smokers versus a 0% nonunion rate and a mean healing time of 4.1 months in nonsmokers after ulnar shortening osteotomy. Similarly, in a series of 64 patients, Little and colleagues[22] found that smokers were 3.7 times more likely ($P = 0.005$) than nonsmokers to have failure of their scaphoid nonunion repair.

In the lower extremity, Hak and coauthors[23] found that all 8 smokers had a healed femoral nonunion after exchange reamed femoral nailing versus only

TABLE 50–1. Basic Science Studies on the Effect of Smoking on Bone Healing

AUTHOR (YEAR OF PUBLICATION)	STUDY TYPE	ANIMAL MODEL	OUTCOME
Daftari et al. (1994)[9]	Implanted cancellous bone cells	Rabbits	Exposure to nicotine delayed revascularization of implanted cancellous bone cells
Ueng et al. (1997)[15]	Tibial lengthening	Rabbits	Decreased mechanical strength ($P = 0.01$) in group exposed to smoke
El-zawawy et al. (2006)[17]	Surgical tibial fracture	Mouse	Chondrogenic phase of fracture healing delayed by exposure to smoke
Skott et al. (2006)[18]	Closed femoral fracture	Rat	20% decrease in torque strength in tobacco group at 3 weeks
Raikin et al. (1998)[19]	Midshaft tibial fracture	Rabbit	Nicotine-exposed tibia 26% weaker, as well as greater nonunion rate

TABLE 50–2. Clinical Studies on the Effect of Smoking on Bone Healing

AUTHOR (YEAR OF PUBLICATION)	STUDY TYPE	OUTCOME	LEVEL OF EVIDENCE
Chen et al. (2001)[21]	Retrospective comparative study	Patients who smoked took longer to heal ulnar osteotomy (4.1 vs. 7.1 weeks)	III
Harvey et al. (2002)[12]	Retrospective review of prospective data	Smoking increased time to union and complication rate in open tibial fractures	II-III
Castillo and the LEAP Study Group (2005)[11]	Prospective study	Smokers less likely to unite open tibia fractures ($P = 0.01$), much more likely (3.7 times) to experience development of osteomyelitis	II
Little et al. (2006)[22]	Retrospective cohort	Smokers 3.7 times ($P = 0.005$) more likely to have nonunion after scaphoid repair	III
McKee et al. (2003)[14]	Retrospective study of prospective data	Smokers risk for poor outcome is 38% compared with nonsmokers (10%) after Ilizarov reconstruction ($P = 0.003$)	III
Adams et al. (2001)[10]	Retrospective comparative study	Smoking increased time to union ($P < 0.05$), flap failure, and requirement for grafting (26% vs. 18%) compared with nonsmokers with open tibial shaft fractures	III
Cobb et al. (1994)[20]	Retrospective comparative study	Smokers had a 3.75 times greater rate of nonunion after ankle arthrodesis	III
Hak et al. (2000)[23]	Case series	8/8 nonsmokers healed after femoral exchange nailing versus 10/15 smokers	II
Schmitz et al. (1999)[13]	Retrospective comparative study	Patients with fractured tibia who smoke took 62% longer to achieve union compared with nonsmokers	III

10 of 15 smokers. Folk, Starr, and Early[5] found that smoking was a significant negative risk factor for wound complications in a series of 190 calcaneal fractures treated with surgery (relative risk, 1.2; $P = 0.03$). McKee and colleagues,[14] in a series of 84 adult patients treated with Ilizarov reconstruction, found that smokers had a 38% chance of a poor outcome versus 10% in nonsmokers ($P = 0.003$). Significantly, all five amputations in their series were in smokers.

Perhaps the most closely studied aspect of orthopedic trauma with respect to smoking is that of the fracture that continues to plague orthopedic surgeons with poor outcomes, nonunion, infection, and limb loss: the open tibia fracture. In retrospective reviews, Harvey and investigators,[12] Schmitz and researchers,[13] and Adams, Keating, and Court-Brown[10] all describe consistently longer times to union, greater complication rates, and greater rates of secondary intervention in smokers. In a prospective (Level II) report, the LEAP (Lower Extremity Assessment Project) Study group found that both current and former smokers had increased rates of nonunion (current smokers: 37%; $P = 0.01$; former smokers: 32%; $P = 0.04$) and osteomyelitis (current smokers: relative risk, 3.7; $P = 0.01$; former smokers: relative risk, 2.8; $P = 0.07$) compared with patients who had never smoked.[10–14]

AREAS OF UNCERTAINTY

Deleterious Physiologic Effects of Smoking as It Relates to Bone Healing

Basic science research shows that nicotine has a vasoconstrictive effect that inhibits tissue differentiation and the angiogenic response necessary in the early stages of fracture healing.[9] Chronically, this (reversible) effect can lead to accelerated atherosclerosis, arterial narrowing, platelet thrombi, and irreversible ischemic changes. At the cellular level, nicotine (among other components of cigarette smoke) is a toxin that also interferes with osteoblast function and alters skeletal metabolism.[17–19] Nicotine has also been shown to have an immunosuppressive effect, which may explain the greater rates of infection and delayed union described in some series.[4,11,14] Used even in isolation, orally or parenterally, it still demonstrates this effect.[18,19] What is unclear is the point at which reversible changes become irreversible, the effects of one type of tobacco product versus another, and why there appears to be considerable interpatient variability.

Definition of "Smoker"

The definition of "smoker" in the majority of available studies remains problematic.[1,2] Because most studies of this nature are retrospective, there is rarely an accurate history of the type of smoking material or the amount smoked. For most studies, a smoker is typically defined as a patient who was actively smoking cigarettes during the treatment period. Conversely, nonsmokers are defined as patients who were not actively smoking during the study period.[10–14] The deficiencies of such a definition are obvious: A person who smokes one or two cigarettes a day is not equivalent to one who smokes two or three packs a day, yet both are included as "smokers." Also, the inclusion of patients who use other tobacco products such as pipes, cigars, or chewing tobacco is not consistent: Because they are usually excluded from the "smoking" group, their inclusion as "nonsmokers" is problematic. As a result of poor quality retrospective data, no correlation can be established between quantity and duration of smoking and treatment outcomes; it may well be that such a relationship exists.

Smoking Cessation

Although there are some general data in the medical literature regarding when the medical risks associated with smoking return to a nonsmoking baseline level after cessation of smoking, there is little such information with regards to fracture healing.[11] Thus, the effect on bone healing in a heavy smoker who quits smoking 6 months before being included in a study is unknown. As stated, most reports include only patients actively smoking as "smokers," and this distinction may be artificial. Although active smoking is probably the least favorable environment, the chronic negative effects of long-standing smoking (i.e., vascular occlusion and ischemia) linger long past the point of smoking cessation. One prospective study divided patients with open tibial fractures into three groups: active smokers, former smokers, and nonsmokers. They found that former smokers had risks of delayed union and infection greater than nonsmokers but less than current smokers. This is the best evidence available that smoking cessation can decrease risk, although not to that of nonsmoking control subjects.[11]

A number of effective cessation programs are available including nicotine replacement therapy, psychotropic medications, education and motivational counseling, and skills training.[24,25] The reported smoking cessation rates after intervention vary from 20% to 60% at 1 year, with increased success rates in programs utilizing a focus on immediate complications. Moller and colleagues,[26] in a randomized clinical trial, described a prearthroplasty smoking cessation program and were able to get the majority of patients in the treatment group to stop or decrease their cigarette consumption. They also showed a significantly decreased postoperative complication rate compared with control subjects (18% vs. 52%; $P = 0.001$). Thus, the setting of an acute fracture may be an ideal opportunity for positive intervention in a patient's life with a greater long-term significance than simple fracture union. Ideally, in the elective setting (i.e., before osteotomy or arthrodesis), smoking should be considered a medical condition with a significant negative effect on outcome (not unlike diabetes) that can and should be "optimized" before surgery. It is rare for an orthopedic surgeon to have the time or skill for this intervention; it requires a multidisciplinary approach that typically involves the patient's primary care physician.

Confounding Variables

It can be stated with some certainty that smokers represent a unique group in society, in whom other confounding variables usually exist. For example,

---

RECOMMENDATIONS

Although the data available are of relatively low quality (Level III and IV studies), currently, cigarette smoking in a fracture or nonunion patient should be considered a potentially remediable risk factor for negative outcome (grade B evidence). Orthopedic patients should be questioned concerning smoking history and counseled regarding the potential effects on the orthopedic prognosis in an effort to decrease or cease their tobacco intake. Grade "A" evidence is available that smoking cessation programs using a variety of techniques can be routinely successful in ameliorating the effects of tobacco use.

In summary, grade B evidence exists that smoking has a consistent deleterious effect on bone healing (including fracture, osteotomy, and arthrodesis union rates and regenerate bone formation). Grade A evidence exists that smoking cessation programs have a success rate in the 50% range, and that success increases if there is a focus on an acute medical event (i.e., fracture or operation). Emerging prospective evidence reports that smoking cessation may lower complication rates after orthopedic procedures. Table 50–3 provides a summary of recommendations.

a prospective study at our institution found that 45% of patients admitted with an open tibial fracture were smokers, compared with 19% of the general Canadian population.[1] Similarly, a study on the effects of smoking on Ilizarov reconstruction revealed that alcoholism, drug addiction, and narcotic dependency were seen almost exclusively in the smoking group.[14] Therefore, even though a study may purport to compare "smokers" versus "nonsmokers," there are other variables (alcohol consumption, risk-taking behavior, drug dependency) that may be overrepresented in the "smoker" group that can confound results.

TABLE 50–3. Summary of Recommendations

RECOMMENDATIONS	LEVEL OF EVIDENCE/GRADE OF RECOMMENDATION
1. Adult smokers with an acute fracture and those requiring osteotomy or arthrodesis should be advised that they are twice as likely to acquire a bone infection and 1.6 times as likely to have a nonunion compared with a nonsmoker.	B
2. Adult smokers with an acute fracture and those requiring osteotomy or arthrodesis can successfully modify smoking behavior with appropriate expert multidisciplinary intervention.	A
3. Adult smokers with an acute fracture and those requiring osteotomy or arthrodesis should be advised to quit smoking to modify their risk for complications.	C

REFERENCES

1. Statistics Canada. Smoker's Report 1999. Government of Canada Publication. Ottawa, Canada.
2. Gilpin EA, Pierce JP, Cavin S, et al: Estimates of population smoking prevalence: Self vs proxy reports of smoking status. Am J Public Health 89:1576–1579, 1994.
3. Porter SE, Hanley EN Jr: The musculoskeletal effects of smoking. J Am Acad Orthop Surg 9:9–17, 2001.
4. Sopori M: Effects of cigarette smoke on the immune system. Nat Rev Immunol 2:372–377, 2002.
5. Folk JW, Starr AJ, Early JS: Early wound complications of operative treatment of calcaneal fractures: analysis of 190 fractures. J Orthop Trauma 13:369–374, 1999.
6. Kaufman T, Eichenlaub EH, Levin M, et al: Tobacco smoking: Impairment of experimental flap survival. Ann Plast Surg 13:468–472, 1984.
7. Nolan J, Jenkins RA, Schultz RC, et al: The acute effects of cigarette smoke exposure on experimental skin flaps. Plast Reconstr Surg 75:544–549, 1985.
8. Glassman SD, Anagnost SC, Parker A, et al: The effect of cigarette smoking and smoking cessation on spinal fusion. Spine 25:2608–2615, 2000.
9. Daftari TK, Whitesides TE, Hellen JG, et al: Nicotine on the revascularization of bone graft: An experimental study in rabbits. Spine 19:904–911, 1994.
10. Adams CI, Keating JF, Court-Brown CM: Cigarette smoking and open tibial fractures. Injury 32:61–65, 2001.
11. Castillo RC, Bosse MJ, MacKenzie Ej, Patterson BM; LEAP Study Group. Impact of smoking on fracture healing and risk of complications in limb-threatening open tibia fractures. J Orthop Trauma 19:151–157, 2005.
12. Harvey EJ, Agel J, Selznick HS, et al: Deleterious effect of smoking on healing of open tibia-shaft fractures. Am J Orthop 31:518–521, 2002.
13. Schmitz M, Finnegan M, Champine J: The effect of smoking on the clinical healing of tibial shaft fracture healing. Clin Orthop Relat Res 365:184–200, 1999.
14. McKee MD, Dipasquale D, Wild LM, et al: The effect of smoking on clinical outcome and complication rates following Ilizarov reconstruction. J Orthop Trauma 17:663–667, 2003.
15. Ueng SWN, Lee M, Li AFY, et al: Effect of intermittent cigarette smoke inhalation on tibial lengthening: Experimental study on rabbits. J Trauma Inj Infect Crit Care 42:231–238, 1997.
16. Ueng SWN, Lin SS, Wang CR, et al: Bone healing of tibial lengthening is delayed by cigarette smoking: Study of bone mineral density and torsional strength on rabbits. J Trauma 46:110–115, 1999.
17. El-zawawy HB, Gill CS, Wright RW, Sandell LJ: Smoking delays chondrogenesis in a mouse model of closed tibial fracture healing. J Orthop Res 249:2150–2158, 2006.
18. Skott M, Andreassen TT, Ulrich-Vinther M, et al: Tobacco extract but not nicotine impairs the mechanical strength of fracture healing in rats. J Orthop Trauma 24:1472–1479, 2006.
19. Raikin SM, Landsman JC, Alexander VA, et al: Effect of nicotine on the rate and strength of long bone fracture healing. Clin Orthop Relat Res (353):231–237, 1998.
20. Cobb TK, Gabrielsen TA, Campbell DC, et al: Cigarette smoking and nonunion after ankle arthrodesis. Foot Ankle 15:64–67, 1994.
21. Chen F, Osterman AL, Mahony K: Smoking and bony union after ulnar-shortening osteotomy. Am J Orthop 30:486–489, 2001.
22. Little CP, Burston BJ, Hopkinson-Woolley J, Burge P: Failure of surgery for scaphoid non-union is associated with smoking. J Hand Surg [B] 3193:252–255, 2006.
23. Hak DJ, Lee SS, Goulet JA: Success of exchange reamed intramedullary nailing for femoral shaft nonunion or delayed union. J Orthop Trauma 14:178–182, 2000.
24. Cinciripini PM, Lapitsky L, Seay S, et al: A placebo controlled evaluation of the effects of busipirone on smoking cessation. J Clin Psychopharmacol 15:182–191, 1995.
25. Fiore MC, Smith SS, Jorenby DE, et al: The effectiveness of the nicotine patch for smoking cessation. J Am Med Assoc 74:1347–1352, 1995.
26. Moller AM, Villebro N, Pedersen T, Tonnesen H: Effect of preoperative smoking intervention on postoperative complications: A randomized clinical trial. Lancet 359:114–117, 2002.

What Is the Best Way to Prevent Heterotopic Ossification after Acetabular Fracture Fixation?

Berton R. Moed, MD and Heidi Israel, PhD

Heterotopic ossification is common after acetabular fracture surgery. Occurring in only approximately 5% of conservatively treated patients,[1] it has been reported in as many as 90% of patients after fracture fixation, with severe involvement as high as 50% in some patient groups.[2-4] An association with poor results has been reported in many case series.[3,4] The specific cause of heterotopic ossification remains obscure, and numerous risk factors have been implicated. The most noted risk factor is stripping of the gluteal muscles from the external surface of the ilium.[2-7] Therefore, the use of an extended surgical approach (i.e., extended iliofemoral, triradiate, or modification thereof) in particular is thought to result in a high rate of heterotopic ossification.[2,3,5-7] The ilioinguinal approach has been associated with an extremely low rate of ectopic bone formation.[3,6]

The expressions "severe heterotopic ossification" and "significant heterotopic ossification" are commonly used to describe the amount of heterotopic ossification necessary to impair hip function. However, these terms have actually been defined in differing ways,[2,5,8] possibly causing confusion in the literature. Most reports have used the Brooker classification[9] (Table 51–1), which relies solely on the anteroposterior radiographic view of the hip, to grade the severity of heterotopic ossification and have defined Classes III and IV as severe.[2,5,7,8,10] Although this system is easy to use, its actual correlation to hip motion and function is questionable.[3,5,11,12] In fact, a study with Level II evidence has shown that the Brooker classification overestimates the functional importance of "severe heterotopic ossification."[11] Greater than 20% loss of total hip motion has been proposed as the deficit necessary to impair hip function (or the "gold standard") and heterotopic ossification causing this amount of loss has been defined as "significant."[5,6,13] In the clinical situation, however, there are many factors other than the presence of heterotopic ossification that can adversely affect hip motion. Therefore, a simple radiographic classification that accurately correlates the presence of heterotopic ossification with this amount of impaired hip motion (absent of any other motion-limiting factors) should be useful in evaluating the independent effect of heterotopic ossification on functional hip motion in patients after acetabular fracture fixation. Level II evidence research has shown that

using three radiographs to grade the severity of heterotopic ossification, with the addition of the two standard oblique (Judet) pelvic radiographs, rather than relying only on the anteroposterior view, accomplishes this goal.[11] Using this modified Brooker method would be helpful both for individual patient prognosis and general scientific study. Unfortunately, it is the standard Brooker technique that continues in general use. Therefore, the findings from any clinical research investigating heterotopic ossification after acetabular fracture fixation, no matter what its apparent "level of evidence" based on study design, may often be diminished by the limitations inherent in the Brooker diagnostic criteria.

NATURAL HISTORY

As noted earlier, a relation exists between the severity of heterotopic ossification and limitation of hip motion. In an analysis of any intervention to prevent heterotopic ossification, it is important to know the outcome expected without any prophylactic treatments. Substantial case series (Level IV evidence) data are available for both the standard Brooker radiographic outcome measure and the hip motion (more than 20% loss) diagnostic criterion.

In their series of 499 acetabulum fractures operated on without any prophylactic treatment and followed for at least 1 year, Letournel and Judet[3] found a 25% (123/499) overall prevalence of heterotopic ossification, using the standard Brooker classification. There were 4% (18/499) with Class I, 10% (50/499) with Class II, 8% (39/499) with Class III, and 3% (16/499) with Class IV ossification. Important distinctions were made among the different surgical approaches, which are thought to be related to differences in the relative extent of the stripping of the gluteal muscles from the external surface of the ilium: the more extensive the stripping, the greater the risk for heterotopic ossification. For the extended iliofemoral approach, there were 4% (1/26) with Class I, 23% (6/26) with Class II, 19% (5/26) with Class III, and 23% (6/26) with Class IV ossification. For the Kocher–Langenbeck approach, there were 4% (11/281) with Class I, 13% (37/281) with class II, 9% (25/281) with Class III, and 2% (6/281) with Class IV ossification. For the ilioinguinal approach,

TABLE 51–1. Radiographic Grading of Heterotopic Ossification

GRADE	DESCRIPTION
Class I	Islands of bone within the soft tissues about the hip
Class II	Bone spurs from the pelvis or proximal end of the femur, leaving at least 1 cm between opposing bone surfaces
Class III	Bone spurs from the pelvis or proximal end of the femur, leaving less than 1 cm between opposing bone surfaces
Class IV	Apparent bony ankylosis of the hip

From Brooker AF, Bowerman JW, Robinson RA, Riley LH Jr: Ectopic ossification following total hip replacement: Incidence and a method of classification. J Bone Joint Surg Am 55-A:1629–1632, 1973, by permission.

there were 1% (1/138) with Class I, 2% (3/138) with Class II, 1% (2/138) with Class III, and 1% (1/138) with Class IV ossification. Adding stripping of the gluteal muscles from the external surface of the ilium to the standard ilioinguinal approach drastically changed the outcome, resulting in 9% (1/11) with Class I, 9% (1/11) with Class II, 36% (4/11) with Class III, and 0% (0/11) with Class IV ossification. Therefore, the expectation is that without prophylaxis of any kind, "severe heterotopic ossification," defined as Class III or IV using the standard Brooker technique, will occur in 42% of patients treated through the extended iliofemoral approach, 11% of patients treated through the Kocher–Langenbeck approach, and 2% of patients treated through the ilioinguinal approach.

Matta[6] reported on his series of 259 patients with 262 acetabular fractures followed for at least 2 years and operated on without any prophylactic treatment. Moderate (standard Brooker Class II) or severe heterotopic ossification (standard Brooker Class III or IV) that was associated with greater than 20% loss of motion occurred in 9% (23/262) of fractures. This amount of heterotopic ossification was noted in 20% (12/59) of the extended iliofemoral approaches, 8% (9/112) of the Kocher–Langenbeck approaches, and 2% (2/87) of the ilioinguinal approaches.

PREVENTION OPTIONS

In a 1998 survey of 226 members of the Orthopaedic Trauma Association, Morgan and colleagues[14] report that prophylaxis for heterotopic ossification was used by 88.3% of the respondents. The stated rationale(s) for this preventative treatment included its effectiveness (39%), perception to be the standard of care (16%), and support in the literature (45%). More than one type of prophylaxis was used by 36.5% of the respondents. Indomethacin was used by 78.6%, low-dose irradiation by 46.5%, low-dose irradiation combined with nonsteroidal anti-inflammatory drugs (NSAIDs) by 15.1%, and NSAIDs other than indomethacin by 3.1%. Therefore, there are three basic preventative treatment options: NSAIDs, low-dose irradiation, and a combination of these two.

EVIDENCE

Indomethacin

The NSAID indomethacin has been shown to decrease the prevalence of heterotopic ossification in experimental animals[15–17] and in a number of Level III evidence clinical studies of patients with acetabular fracture.[7,8,10,18] Most of these clinical studies were retrospective in nature, having the attendant design limitations. More recently, there have been a number of clinical reports with Level I and II evidence, prospectively evaluating the efficacy of indomethacin prophylaxis as compared with a nontreatment control group.[19–21] Unfortunately, the data from these studies offer conflicting results. Therefore, critical review of these studies is required, taking into consideration the main important variable of the differing expected baseline prevalence of heterotopic ossification depending on surgical approach, as well as an analysis of the statistical method.

In a Level II study, Iotov[21] evaluated the results of prophylaxis with indomethacin in 52 patients operated for fractures of the acetabulum. Twenty-eight received indomethacin prophylaxis, consisting of 25 mg three times per day given orally or per rectum for 30 days after surgery, and 24 composed a control group. The grade of heterotopic ossification was assessed using the Brooker classification. The development of heterotopic ossification was analyzed depending on the type of surgical approach. The rate of severe ossification was 0% in the indomethacin-treated group and 21% in the control group ($P < 0.01$), mainly after extensile posterior and posterior approaches. One error in this study was including in the control group the one patient who could not tolerate indomethacin because of gastrointestinal symptoms. Ragnarsson and coworkers[22] in another level II study had similar findings in a group of 23 patients operated on through the triradiate surgical approach. Of the 14 patients receiving indomethacin prophylaxis (25 mg three times each day for 6 weeks), 10 had no heterotopic ossification, 2 had Brooker Class I, and 2 had Brooker Class II. In the control group, six had Brooker Class II, two had Brooker Class III, and one had Brooker Class IV ($P < 0.0001$). These Level II findings are consistent with those of the Level III studies.

In contradistinction, Matta and Siebenrock[19] report a Level I evidence, randomized, prospective trial indicating that indomethacin was not effective. However, this study was vastly underpowered to detect differences. This study included 107 consecutive patients. Patients with an even hospital number received 100 mg indomethacin by suppository at the end of the operation and then 25 mg by mouth or rectally three times a day for 6 weeks. Those with an odd hospital number received no prophylactic treatment. Patients with all three surgical approaches (extended iliofemoral, Kocher–Langenbeck, and ilioinguinal) were included. The ilioinguinal group (with an expected prevalence of only 2% for heterotopic ossification sufficient to cause impairment, whether by radiographs alone or in combination with measurement of joint motion) represented almost 50% (50/107) of the patients. Thirty-seven patients were in the Kocher–Langenbeck groups, and 20 were in the extended iliofemoral groups. The authors themselves did a power analysis and found low power in their numbers for the motion impairment criteria (24%), and discussed the large patient numbers they would have needed to find significant effects. A simple analysis will show the large sample sizes required in the design of a randomized, prospective study to provide the desired 80% power to minimize the risk for type II error at an alpha < 0.05. Assuming that the comparative change of clinical interest in this study would be a decrease from the expected 2% to 1% for the ilioinguinal approach, 8% to 3% for the Kocher–Langenbeck approach, and 20% to 10% for the extended iliofemoral approach, the sample sizes needed per group for the desired 80% power are approximately 2300, 325, and 200, respectively. The small clinical effect size (2%) and limited drug treatment benefit for the ilioinguinal approach indicates that there is limited value in proceeding with a prospective trial requiring such large patient numbers. In addition, although this was a Level I study, clearly there were not enough patients to answer the study question.

Karunakar and coauthors[20] completed a Level I evidence study designed to compare the effect of indomethacin with that of a placebo in reducing the incidence of heterotopic ossification in a prospective, randomized trial. A total of 121 patients with fractures of the acetabulum treated using a Kocher–Langenbeck approach were randomized to receive either indomethacin (once-a-day 75-mg sustained-release capsule) or a placebo once daily for 6 weeks. The extent of heterotopic ossification was evaluated on plain radiographs 3 months after operation using the standard Brooker classification. Fifty-nine patients were in the indomethacin group, and 62 were in the placebo group. Significant heterotopic ossification, defined as Brooker Class III to IV, occurred in 9 of 59 patients (15.2%) in the indomethacin group and 12 of 62 (19.4%) receiving the placebo (*P* = 0.722). On this basis, the authors recommend against the routine use of indomethacin for prophylaxis against heterotopic ossification after isolated fractures of the acetabulum treated using the Kocher–Langenbeck approach. Although this study appears to be well designed, it suffers from important deficiencies. Eighteen patients randomized to the indomethacin group did not complete their course of prophylactic therapy. These patients were maintained in the indomethacin treatment group for the statistical analysis, which on the surface seems a confounding variable. This approach is consistent with the "intent-to-treat" analysis design. However, what is also required, which was not provided by the authors, is a secondary analysis of these noncompliant patients. This secondary analysis is explanatory in nature, comparing compliant with noncompliant patients within the treatment group. This analysis is critical because it may change the overall findings by revealing a significant difference in compliant versus noncompliant patients. The sample size required to provide the desired 80% power to minimize the risk for type II error at an alpha < 0.05 is 80 per group for the Kocher–Langenbeck approach. This calculation assumes that 11% is the expected baseline prevalence with the Brooker classification and uses an 11% decrease to 0% (the maximum possible) to define the comparative change of clinical interest. With the standard drug study expectation of a 5% comparative change of clinical interest from 11% to 6%, 490 per group would be required. Ninety patients per group would be required to show a 10% treatment difference. The authors recognized the fact that their study was underpowered. However, they explained away the need to adequately power the study by stating that the clinical effect size is small. If that is truly the case, if the impairment from heterotopic ossification after acetabular fracture fixation through the Kocher–Langenbeck approach is minimal without any preventative treatment, then there was no point in doing this study based on the known natural history. In summary, the authors did not add the minimally required 20 to 30 patients per group or do the secondary analysis, and left the study question unanswered.

A consistent finding is that a certain number of patients will discontinue their prescribed course of indomethacin treatment.[20,21] Patients discontinue the drug either because of medication-related gastrointestinal symptoms or just failure to "follow the doctor's orders."

Therefore, based on the available evidence, it appears that indomethacin does effectively decrease the prevalence of heterotopic ossification in acetabular fracture patients as long as the patients actually take their medicine.

Other Nonsteroidal Anti-inflammatory Drugs

Experimental evidence exists to suggest that NSAIDs (including selective cyclooxygenase-2 inhibitors) other than indomethacin have effects similar to indomethacin in the prevention of heterotopic ossification.[23–25] However, there are limited clinical studies in patients with total joint arthroplasty[24,26,27] and essentially none for patients with acetabular fracture. Because all NSAIDs potentially have the same effects as indomethacin, uncontrolled use of NSAIDs other than indomethacin by study patients represents an important confounding variable investigators have not routinely addressed.

Low-Dose Irradiation

Some Level III evidence supports using low-dose irradiation to prevent heterotopic ossification after acetabular fracture fixation.[2,28,29] In a retrospective study of 37 patients treated with an extended or modified extended surgical approach, Bosse and colleagues[2] used prophylactic radiation, delivering 1000 cGy in 200-cGy increments, starting on the third postoperative day. They found a significant ($P < 0.01$) difference in severe (Brooker class III or IV) heterotopic ossification between the no-treatment control group and the irradiation group. In 1996, Anglen and Moore[28] showed similar findings in patients treated with 800 cGy as a single dose within 3 days of surgery. Childs and coworkers[29] found a 700-cGy single-dose regimen to be effective.

From our review of the English-language literature, no Level I or II evidence studies compare low-dose radiation therapy with a no-treatment control group for patients after acetabular fracture fixation. However, such evidence does exist comparing irradiation with indomethacin.[30,31] Moore, Goss, and Anglen[30] compared indomethacin (25 mg, given three times daily for 6 weeks) with irradiation with 800 cGy delivered within 3 days of operation.[30] Plain radiographs were evaluated using Brooker classification. The investigators found no difference between the two treatment methods. Once again, this study was grossly underpowered. The authors recognized this issue, stating that "for this approximate sample size and outcome effect, p = 0.05 with a power of 80% would require an outcome difference of 27% between the two groups."[30] In a follow-up to this study, Burd, Lowry, and Anglen[31] performed a comparable study in a larger group of patients with Level II evidence. Their findings were similar.[31] Although there are some issues with how the statistical data were presented, the methods appear adequate to support their findings of no difference between the indomethacin and irradiation treatment groups. These authors used the intent-to-treat method. Therefore, 16 patients who were randomized into either the indomethacin (8 patients) or irradiation (8 patients) treatment groups, but did not receive these treatments, were included. As has been discussed previously, these authors appropriately included a secondary analysis of the 16 patients who did not receive treatment. Interestingly, all 16 had heterotopic ossification, which was Class III or IV in 6 of them. In summary, based on the available evidence, it appears that low-dose irradiation does decrease the prevalence of heterotopic ossification in patients with acetabular fracture.

Combination Indomethacin and Low-Dose Irradiation

A theoretical basis exists for the use of combination therapy. Experimental evidence indicates that radiation therapy and indomethacin decrease heterotopic ossification by different pathways.[32] However, to the best of our knowledge, there is only Level IV evidence in support of using the combination of indomethacin and low-dose irradiation to prevent heterotopic ossification after acetabular fracture fixation.[33] In this series that Moed and Letournel reported,[33] the use of this regimen essentially eliminated postoperative heterotopic ossification and there was no progression, even

when early ossification was seen on preoperative radiographs. Childs and coworkers,[29] in an uncontrolled Level III portion of their study, were unable to show a significant difference between the 700-cGy single-dose regimen and the combination of indomethacin and low-dose irradiation.

AREAS OF UNCERTAINTY

Effectiveness of Preventative Therapies

From the studies available to us for review, as described earlier, it is clear that there is a scarcity of Level I and II evidence in support of treatments aimed toward the prevention of heterotopic ossification after acetabular fracture fixation. It is apparent that indomethacin does not completely eliminate heterotopic ossification. However, Level II and III studies indicate that its use does significantly decrease the occurrence of "clinically important" ossification. Unfortunately, these studies are limited by their use of the Brooker classification to define "clinically important." The Level I studies that conclude that indomethacin is not effective suffer from a multitude of design flaws. A Level I or II, randomized, prospective study in patients with acetabular fracture fixation comparing low-dose irradiation with 700 cGy delivered as a single dose within 3 days of surgery to a control no-treatment group is wanting. The Level III studies in support of low-dose irradiation have the limitations detailed earlier.

Timing and Dosing of Preventative Therapies

The standard prescription for indomethacin for acetabular fracture patients is 75 mg/day delivered either orally or per rectum as 25 mg in three divided doses (TID), instituted within 24 hours of surgery and continued for 6 weeks after surgery. In a Level II study, Iotov[21] used the medication for only 30 days with success. Evidence exists from other patient populations (notably, patients with total joint arthroplasty) that shorter treatment regimens can be used. However, no data support this decrease for patients with acetabular fracture. Karunakar and coauthors,[20] in their Level I study detailed earlier, used once-a-day 75-mg sustained-release capsules without success in preventing heterotopic ossification. Interestingly, this study was one of the few not to show a significant effect with indomethacin usage. Whether this dosing method affected the outcome is not known. The "effective preventative dose" of indomethacin is not known. Missing one or two of the three prescribed 25-mg doses in the TID regimen may not cause the loss of clinical effectiveness, as opposed to failing to take an entire day's medication by missing the single once-a-day 75-mg sustained-release capsule.

Currently, low-dose radiation therapy usually consists of 700 cGY delivered to the hip region as a single dose within 72 hours after surgery. Evidence in support of the various dosing regimens for patients with acetabular fracture is limited. Most of the reported Level I to III evidence studies in patients with acetabular fracture presented data based on using either 1000 cGy in increments over a number of days or 800 cGy as a single dose within 3 days of surgery. Childs and coworkers,[29] in a study with Level II evidence, evaluated the timing of postoperative irradiation using a 700-cGy single-dose regimen. They note no increase in heterotopic ossification with up to a 72-hour interval between surgery and radiation therapy.

Complications

Experimental animal studies have also shown that indomethacin will decrease the formation of new bone,[34,35] impair fracture healing,[36,37] and inhibit the remodeling of haversian bone.[38] In the rabbit, indomethacin decreased the torsional strength of healing bone.[39] In an in vitro study, NSAIDs have been shown to adversely affect human osteoblasts.[40] However, this effect on the osteoblasts is reversible after discontinuation of the drug.[40] Clinical correlation had been scarce,[34] and no problems with fracture healing had been noted in many reported Level III evidence series of patients with acetabular fracture.[7,8,10] However, a more recent Level II study in patients with acetabular fracture has shown that the use of indomethacin increases the risk for long-bone nonunion.[41] This potential complication is likely associated with all NSAID use.[40,42] As noted earlier, a certain number of patients will discontinue their prescribed course of indomethacin treatment either because of medication-related gastrointestinal symptoms or just failure to "follow the doctor's orders."[10,20,21,31] Several important risk factors predisposing patients to NSAID-induced gastrointestinal symptoms have been identified, including age, prednisone use, underlying severe illness, and a history of NSAID-induced gastrointestinal symptoms.[43] Length of therapy is also thought to be a factor with patients receiving short-term therapy (less than 1 month) at less risk.[44] Level I evidence suggests that the synthetic prostaglandin E_1 analog,

misoprostol, is preventative for NSAID-induced gastric and duodenal mucosal lesions and symptoms but does not interfere with the antirheumatic activity of the administered NSAID.[43,45] However, its use, or that of any other gastroduodenal mucosal protective agent, in patients with acetabular fracture receiving indomethacin for heterotopic ossification prophylaxis has not been studied.

The possibility of induced malignant disease is the main concern with low-dose radiation therapy, although genetic alterations in offspring may also be at issue. Radiation-induced malignancy is rare, and no case of malignancy caused by low-dose irradiation for heterotopic ossification prophylaxis has been reported.[46,47] However, pelvic low-dose irradiation with limited fields in the range of 260 to 530 cGy has been given for metropathia haemorrhagica.[48] Mortality was greater more than 30 years after radiotherapy than between 5 and 29 years after radiotherapy in this Level III epidemiologic study, suggesting that full risks for development of cancer may not be assessed for more than 30 years. Low-dose irradiation for heterotopic ossification prophylaxis has not been used that long, and unfortunately, study has shown that patients with acetabular fracture often fail to return for even short-term follow-up.[47] In one study of 25 patients with acetabular fracture fixation treated with low-dose irradiation for heterotopic ossification prophylaxis, not a single patient returned for follow-up beyond 5 years.[47]

Cost

A substantial cost difference exists between indomethacin and low-dose irradiation prophylaxis. Burd and colleagues,[31] in 2001, reported a radiation therapy cost of $2400 compared with $12 for a 6-week course of indomethacin at their institution. However, the costs will vary from institution to institution. In addition, costs for possible complication-related treatments have yet to be considered in the equation.

RECOMMENDATIONS

Given the baseline prevalence of heterotopic ossification after acetabular fracture fixation without the use of prophylactic treatment reported by Letournel and Judet[3] and Matta,[6] one may reasonably conclude that prophylaxis is not necessary for some patient groups. Patients treated using the ilioinguinal approach fit in this category. Patients treated using more extensive surgical approaches involving stripping of the gluteal muscles from the external surface of the ilium (i.e., extended iliofemoral, triradiate, or modification thereof) present the opposite end of the spectrum. Patients undergoing acetabular fracture fixation through the Kocher–Langenbeck approach

present an intermediate risk. In view of the levels of evidence gleaned from our review of the literature, patients with acetabular fracture treated using these approaches involving stripping of the gluteal muscles from the external surface of the ilium are candidates for preventative treatment (Table 51–2). The potential adverse effects of preventative treatments must be considered. Therefore, the question remains, which patients are at sufficient risk for acquiring an amount of heterotopic ossification necessary to impair hip function?

We recommend preventative treatment for heterotopic ossification after acetabular

Continued

RECOMMENDATIONS—CONT'D

fracture fixation using the extended iliofemoral surgical approach or similar extensive surgical approaches (see Table 51–2). However, care should be taken regarding patient selection and method of prophylaxis.

To minimize its side effects and maximize effective drug delivery, physicians should prescribe indomethacin as 25 mg TID taken for no more than 30 days. The elderly, infirm, those taking prednisone, and those with a history of NSAID-induced gastrointestinal symptoms should be excluded. Patients with an associated long-bone fracture should be recognized as at increased risk for impaired fracture healing. This factor should be considered in the decision-making process.

Low-dose irradiation with 700 cGy delivered as a single dose within 72 hours of surgery should be considered in patients who are not candidates for indomethacin use, patients who are believed to be unreliable regarding taking their medications, and patients with associated long-bone fractures. However, we believe that the unanswered long-term outcomes of low-dose irradiation should preclude routine prophylac-

tic irradiation in children, young adults, and women of childbearing age.

Preventative treatment for heterotopic ossification after acetabular fracture fixation using the ilioinguinal surgical approach or similar limited surgical approaches is not recommended.

We recommend preventative treatment with indomethacin for heterotopic ossification after acetabular fracture fixation through the Kocher–Langenbeck surgical approach or similar posterolateral surgical approaches. Despite the fact that there is conflicting evidence regarding this treatment (see Table 51–2), we believe that with careful patient selection, the potential benefit outweighs the overall risk. However, this is not the case for low-dose irradiation and we do not recommend its use.

In conclusion, routine prophylaxis against heterotopic ossification with indomethacin or low-dose irradiation appears be a useful adjuvant therapy for selected patients undergoing acetabular fracture fixation. However, the overall balance of risks and benefits continues to await assessment in a large-scale randomized trial.

TABLE 51–2. Summary of Recommendations

RECOMMENDATIONS	LEVEL OF EVIDENCE/GRADE OF RECIMMENDATION
1. HO prophylaxis should be used for acetabular fracture fixation in all patients.	I
2. HO prophylaxis should be used for patients operated on using the ilioinguinal approach.	I
3. HO prophylaxis should be used for patients operated using the Kocher–Langenbeck approach.	I
4. HO prophylaxis should be used for patients operated on using extended approaches.	B
5. Indomethacin is effective when given for at least 30 days after surgery in a 25-mg TID regimen.	B
6. Indomethacin is effective when given as a single daily 75-mg sustained-release dose or other regimens.	I
7. Indomethacin use is associated with impaired healing of long-bone fractures.	B
8. Other NSAIDs have similar HO prophylaxis effects as indomethacin in patients with acetabular fracture.	I
9. Low-dose irradiation is effective when given as a single 700-cGy dose within 3 days of surgery.	B
10. Indomethacin and low-dose irradiation are equally effective.	B
11. Adding indomethacin to low-dose irradiation improves the prophylactic effectiveness.	I

HO, heterotopic ossification; NSAID, nonsteroidal anti-inflammatory drug.

REFERENCES

1. Pennal GF, Davidson J, Garside H, et al: Results of treatment of acetabular fractures. Clin Orthop 151:115–123, 1980.
2. Bosse MJ, Reinert CM, Ellwanger F, et al: Heterotopic ossification as a complication of acetabular fractures: Prophylaxis with low-dose irradiation. J Bone Joint Surg Am 70-A:1231–1237, 1988.
3. Letournel E, Judet R: Fractures of the Acetabulum, 2nd ed. New York, Springer Verlag, 1993, pp. 541–563.
4. Mears DC, Rubash HE: Pelvic and Acetabular Fractures. Thorofare, NJ, Slack, 1986, pp. 411–414.
5. Ghalambor N, Matta J, Bernstein L: Heterotopic ossification following operative treatment of acetabular fracture: An analysis of risk factors. Clin Orthop 305:96–105, 1994.
6. Matta JM: Fractures of the acetabulum: Accuracy of reduction and clinical results in patients managed operatively within three weeks after injury. J Bone Joint Surg Am 78-A:1632–1645, 1996.
7. Moed BR, Maxey JW: The effect of indomethacin on heterotopic ossification following acetabular fracture surgery. J Orthop Trauma 7:33–38, 1993.
8. Moed BR, Karges DE: Prophylactic indomethacin for the prevention of heterotopic ossification after acetabular fracture surgery in high-risk patients. J Orthop Trauma 8:34–39, 1994.
9. Brooker AF, Bowerman JW, Robinson RA, Riley LH Jr: Ectopic ossification following total hip replacement: Incidence and a method of classification. J Bone Joint Surg Am 55-A:1629–1632, 1973.

10. McLaren AC: Prophylaxis with indomethacin for heterotopic bone after open reduction of fractures of the acetabulum. J Bone Joint Surg Am 72-A:245–247, 1990.
11. Moed BR, Smith ST: Three-view radiographic assessment of heterotopic ossification after acetabular fracture surgery: Correlation with hip motion in 100 cases. J Orthop Trauma 10:93–98, 1996.
12. Alonso J, Davila R, Bradley E: Extended iliofemoral versus triradiate approaches in management of associated acetabular fractures. Clin Orthop 305:81–87, 1994.
13. Matta JM, Mehne DK, Roffi R: Fractures of the acetabulum: Early results of a prospective study. Clin Orthop 205:241–250, 1986.
14. Morgan S J, Jeray KJ, Phieffer LS, et al: Attitudes of orthopaedic trauma surgeons regarding current controversies in the management of pelvic and acetabular fractures. J Orthop Trauma 15:526–532, 2001.
15. Moed BR, Resnick RB, Fakhouri AJ, et al: Effect of two nonsteroidal antiinflammatory drugs on heterotopic bone formation in a rabbit model. J Arthroplasty 9:81–87, 1994.
16. Nilsson OS, Bauer HCF, Brosjo O, Tomkvist H: Influence of indomethacin on induced heterotopic bone formation in rats: Importance of length of treatment and of age. Clin Orthop 207:239–245, 1986.
17. Tornkvist H, Bauer FCH, Nilsson OS: Influence of indomethacin on experimental bone metabolism in rats. Clin Orthop 193:264–270, 1985.
18. Johnson EE, Kay RM, Dorey FJ: Heterotopic ossification prophylaxis following operative treatment of acetabular fracture. Clin Orthop (305)88–95, 1994.
19. Matta JM, Siebenrock KA: Does indomethacin reduce heterotopic bone formation after operations for acetabular fractures? J Bone Joint Surg Br 79-B:959–963, 1997.
20. Karunakar MA, Sen A, Bosse MJ, et al: Indometacin as prophylaxis for heterotopic ossification after the operative treatment of fractures of the acetabulum. J Bone Joint Surg 88:1613–1617, 2006.
21. Iotov A: Heterotopic ossification in surgically treated patients with acetabular fractures and indomethacin prophylaxis for its prevention. Ortopediya i Travmatologiya 36:367–373, 2000.
22. Ragnarsson B, Danckwardt-Lilliestrom G, Mjoberg B: The triradiate incision for acetabular fractures: A prospective study of 23 cases. Acta Orthop Scand 63:515–519, 1992.
23. Tornkvist H, Nilsson OS, Bauer FCH, Lindholm TS: Experimentally induced heterotopic ossification in rats influenced by anti-inflammatory drugs. Scand J Rheumatol 12:177–180, 1983.
24. Elmstedt E, Lindholm TS, Nilsson OS, Tornkvist H: Effect of ibuprofen on heterotopic ossification after hip replacement. Acta Orthop Scand 56:25–27, 1985.
25. Banovac K, Williams JM, Patrick LD, Levi A: Prevention of heterotopic ossification after spinal cord injury with COX-2 selective inhibitor (rofecoxib). Spinal Cord 42:707–710, 2004.
26. Grohs JG, Schmidt M, Wanivenhaus A: Selective COX-2 inhibitor versus indomethacin for the prevention of heterotopic ossification after hip replacement: A double-blind randomized trial of 100 patients with 1-year follow-up. Acta Orthop 78:95–98, 2007.
27. Vielpeau C, Joubert JM, Hulet C: Naproxen in the prevention of heterotopic ossification after total hip replacement. Clin Orthop 279–288, 1999.
28. Anglen JO, Moore KD: Prevention of heterotopic bone formation after acetabular fracture fixation by single-dose radiation therapy: A preliminary report. J Orthop Trauma 10:258–263, 1996.
29. Childs HA 3rd, Cole T, Falkenberg E, et al: A prospective evaluation of the timing of postoperative radiotherapy for preventing heterotopic ossification following traumatic acetabular fractures. Int J Radiat Oncol Biol Phys 47:1347–1352, 2000.
30. Moore KD, Goss K, Anglen JO: Indomethacin versus radiation therapy for prophylaxis against heterotopic ossification in acetabular fractures: A randomised, prospective study. J Bone Joint Surg Br 80-B:259–263, 1998.
31. Burd TA, Lowry KJ, Anglen JO: Indomethacin compared with localized irradiation for the prevention of heterotopic ossification following surgical treatment of acetabular fractures. J Bone Joint Surg Am 83-A:1783–1788, 2001 [erratum appears in J Bone Joint Surg 84-A:100, 2002].
32. Ahrengart L, Lindgren U, Reinholt FP: Comparative study of the effects of radiation, indomethacin, prednisolone, and ethane-l-hydroxy-l,l-diphosphonate (EHDP) in the prevention of ectopic bone formation. Clin Orthop 229:265–273, 1988.
33. Moed BR, Letournel E: Low-dose irradiation and indomethacin prevent heterotopic ossification after acetabular fracture surgery. J Bone Joint Surg Br 76-B:895–900, 1994.
34. Sudmann E, Hagen T: Indomethacin-induced delayed fracture healing. Arch Orthop Unfalichir 85:151–154, 1976.
35. Tornkvist H, Bauer FCH, Nilsson OS: Influence of indomethacin on experimental bone metabolism in rats. Clin Orthop 193:264–270, 1985.
36. Allen HL, Wase A, Bear WT: Indomethacin and aspirin: Effect of nonsteroidal anti-inflammatory agents on the rate of fracture repair in the rat. Acta Orthop Scand 51:595–600, 1980.
37. Bo J, Sudmann E, Marton PF: Effect of indomethacin on fracture healing in rats. Acta Orthop Scand 47:588–599, 1976.
38. Sudmann E, Bang G: Indomethacin-induced inhibition of Haversian remodelling in rabbits. Acta Orthop Scand 50:621–627, 1979.
39. Tornkvist H, Lindholm TS, Netz P, et al: Effect of ibuprofen and indomethacin on bone metabolism reflected in bone strength. Clin Orthop 187:255–259, 1984.
40. Evans CE, Butcher C: The influence on human osteoblasts in vitro of non-steroidal anti-inflammatory drugs which act on different enzymes. J Bone Joint Surg Br 86-B:444–449, 2004.
41. Burd TA, Hughes MS, Anglen JO: Heterotopic ossification prophylaxis with indomethacin increases the risk of long-bone nonunion. J Bone Joint Surg Br 85-B:700–705, 2003.
42. Giannoudis PV, MacDonald DA, Matthews SJ, et al: Nonunion of the femoral diaphysis: The influence of reaming and Non-steroidal anti-inflammatory drugs. J Bone Joint Surg Br 82-B:655–658, 2000.
43. Graham DY, White RH, Moreland LW, et al: Duodenal and gastric ulcer prevention with misoprostol in arthritis patients taking NSAIDs. Misoprostol study group. Ann Intern Med 119:257–262, 1993.
44. Wilson DE, Galati JS: NSAID gastropathy: Prevention and treatment. J Musculoskel Med 8:55–70, 1991.
45. Saggioro A, Alvisi A, Blasi A, et al: Misoprostol prevents NSAID-induced gastroduodenal lesions in patients with osteoarthritis and rheumatoid arthritis. Ital J Gastroenterol 23:119–123, 1991.
46. Lo TCM: Radiation therapy for heterotopic ossification. Semin Radiat Oncol 9:163–170, 1999.
47. Cornes PGS, Shahidi M, Glees JP: Heterotopic bone formation: Irradiation of high risk patients. Br J Radiol 75:448–452, 2002.
48. Darby SC, Reeves G, Key T, et al: Mortality in a cohort of women given X-ray therapy for metropathia haemorrhagica. Int J Cancer 56:793–801, 1994.

When Is It Safe to Resect Heterotopic Ossification?

Terry S. Axelrod, MD, MSc, FRCS(C)

WHAT IS HETEROTOPIC OSSIFICATION AND WHAT CAUSES IT?

Heterotopic ossification (HO) is the development of bone in areas in which it is not normally found. This usually creates the most problems around joints, where the presence of the excess ossification can lead to blocks to motion, irritation of the soft tissues, and even bony ankylosis of the affected joints. Soft-tissue ossification in areas remote from joints will often be asymptomatic but can cause local muscle and fascial irritation, and with this, symptoms of pain and dysfunction.

The formation of HO is associated with many differing conditions. A direct cause-and-effect relation has not been established; however, the most common associations are with burns, spinal cord injury, and trauma. It is also a problem that can develop with elective joint replacement arthroplasty, specifically total hip and knee arthroplasty. Head injury in association with traumatic fractures or dislocations will significantly increase the chances of acquiring this problem. HO that develops in patients with head injuries usually affects only areas of musculoskeletal injury, although the trauma may be fairly minor. In burn victims and patients with spinal cord injury, HO may develop around joints that have not had any specific injury to them, often being quite extensive and frequently causing ankylosis by bridging across normal joints.

It is postulated that a circulatory factor, released from the brain, is the common factor in burn and trauma victims that leads to the growth of the HO. Much work is yet to be done to fully isolate this factor. The factors seem to be subtypes of bone morphogenetic protein (BMP), with BMP-1, -4, and -6 found in pathologic specimens.[1] A correlation exists between the severity of the head injury and the risk for development of ectopic bone. The occurrence of autonomic dysregulation may predict the chance of development of HO in patients with severe head injury.[2] The role of prostaglandin E_2 has recently been suggested as a mediator in the differentiation of the progenitor cells.[3]

CLINICAL PROBLEMS ASSOCIATED WITH HETEROTOPIC OSSIFICATION

The causative factor of pain associated with HO is unclear. Pain associated with neurologic or vascular entrapment, or functionally restricting joint stiffness

associated with HO, may be indications to consider HO resection.

As with many areas within orthopedic surgery, a full consideration of all of the clinical aspects of the problem is required before considering surgical intervention: Do the patient's symptoms fit with the radiographic findings? Is the HO in a location where it can be safely removed without undue risk for harm to the associated soft tissues, including critical neurologic and vascular structures? Is the bone sufficiently mature to allow resection and not simply immediately re-form after it is removed? These are but some of the questions that must be answered before embarking on this type of technically demanding surgery. The purpose of this chapter is to guide clinicians regarding the optimal timing of surgical resection based on the best available evidence.

OPTIONS

Preoperative radiographic assessment of the HO is critical in terms of the decision to operate and acts as a guide through the surgical session. The use of plain radiographs, oblique views, and tomograms are helpful, but a computed tomographic (CT) scan is important to fully assess the extent and pattern of the bone formation. A three-dimensional reconstruction is a major help to conceptualize the HO. On the CT scan, a halo of inflammatory tissue around the bone mass may indicate continued activity of bone formation. Magnetic resonance imaging scanning may play a role in defining the location of adjacent critical neurovascular structures adjacent to a mass of HO.

The timing of surgical HO resection is of critical importance. There is a balance to be found between the urge to intervene early, with the possibility that HO may simply re-form, versus delaying surgery, which prolongs the patient's symptoms of pain or joint stiffness, or both, with the associated functional impairments that this will cause. Moreover, waiting for a prolonged period can result in fixed contractures of the periarticular soft tissues, making restoration of movement after resection more difficult to achieve.

Classic teaching has been to wait until the HO tissue is mature, until there is no further evidence of bone formation before attempting to remove it, thus minimizing the risk for HO re-formation. This traditional approach is based on the following theoretical concept: If the bone has matured and is no longer in an active stage of formation, there will be less chance of it re-forming after the resection. Although reasonable in theory, no Level I or II studies have evaluated this concept. More recently, individual surgeons are moving to earlier resection to reduce the time of disability for the patient.[4]

The traditional methods for assessing the maturity of the HO are as follows:
1. Radiographic appearance
   a. Maturity of bone, trabecular patterns
   b. Lack of additional bone formation on serial radiographs
2. Blood tests
   a. A return of serum alkaline phosphatase (ALK) levels to normal
3. Nuclear medicine bone scans
   a. Progressively reduced new bone activity, falling to a "cold scan"

Classic orthopedic texts (Level V) recommend the following approach to HO resection: Wait at least 12 to 18 months after the HO has formed to guarantee that the tissue is mature and will not reoccur. Look at the quality of the bone on radiographs to look for the features of mature bone, density, trabecular patterns of bone, and cortical maturation. Always obtain a bone scan of the area. The bone scan must be cold—that is, showing no evidence of bone turnover or overt activity, thus assuring the surgeon that the tissue is mature and not likely to return once resected. In addition, the serum ALK should be followed until it normalizes before removing the bone.[5–7]

The reasons for these positions are largely anecdotal (Level V). No high level evidence exists to support any of the suggestions made in the classic literature. At best, the recommendations made are based on the clinical experience of senior authors and clinical experts in the field.

Currently, many authors believe that waiting until the radiographic appearance is reasonably mature and then proceeding with the resection is the best approach. They are hoping to reduce the morbidity of the prolonged delay to surgery and the problems of joint immobility that may not be correctable after resection. Tsionos, Leclercq, and Rochet,[8] from the Institut de la Main, Paris, France, advised early resection in burn patients at the elbow with a suggested reduction of the period of morbidity for the patients (Level IV). Their mean time between the burn and operation was 12 months, with the median being 9.5 months. This chapter analyzes the literature according to levels of evidence to attempt to answer the question posed: When is it safe to resect HO?

EVIDENCE

Radiographic Appearance of Maturity

The typical radiologic appearance of HO is circumferential ossification with a lucent center.[9] X-ray indicators of maturity—lesions with distinct margins and well-defined trabeculations—have not proved to be reliable predictors of nonrecurrence of HO after surgery[10] (Level III).

Really only one study has been widely quoted that looks at the level of bone maturity and attempts to correlate this to the risk for bone reformation after resection. In a small, retrospective review of 19 patients with spinal cord injuries, Garland and Orwin[10] found that 15 of 22 hips with a mature preoperative pattern of heterotopic bone had a recurrence after resection. No evidence was reported that a mature pattern of bone was less associated with a recurrence than one that was less mature. This is a Level III study.

As such, there is a lack of literature at an adequate level relating interpretation of the maturity of bone on x-ray film to reoccurrence after resection. It may be that areas of nonmature bone are obscured by overlying areas of mature bone. It may be that there is no direct correlation between maturity and recurrence after resection. Despite assumptions made in the past that to prevent recurrence, bone must be mature before resection, maturity and recurrence may be independent variables. No studies have been published on interobserver and intraobserver reliability in the assessment of bone maturity within HO. As such, we have no evidence to answer the question of what degree of bone maturity, as judged by radiographic appearance, is sufficient to allow safe resection with a low chance of reoccurrence.

Role of Alkaline Phosphatase in Assessing the Maturity of the Heterotopic Ossification

In situations in which there is the formation of large amounts of HO, ALK levels may become abnormal approximately 2 weeks after injury. In the typical case of HO, the ALK levels reached approximately 3.5 times the normal value 10 weeks after the inciting trauma, before returning to normal at approximately 18 weeks.[11] Although it may seem a logical conclusion that there is a direct correlation between the level of ALK and the activity of the HO, this is not always the case. The levels of ALK may be entirely normal with active HO.[10,11] Alternatively, the levels may remain increased for years after formation, yet the tissue appears completely mature on radiographs.[12]

The level of evidence is fair (Level II) for an association between increased ALK and the development of HO. In a prospective cohort analysis study by Tibone and coauthors,[12] in which the authors gathered data on a series of patients with spinal cord injuries with developing HO, a relation between increasing levels of ALK and the development of HO was established. This study did not look at surgical resection or recurrence of the lesions after resection. The authors also found persistently increased levels of ALK in several patients for years after the development of HO, indicating that, if the level of ALK was an important parameter for determining the maturity of the HO, it might be thought that the HO might take many years to mature. In some cases, it may never be mature.

Comparing the levels of ALK and the rates of recurrence, Garland and Orwin,[10] in their small retrospective series (Level III), found that serum ALK levels were normal in 9 of 13 hips that had a recurrence of bone formation after resection of the HO. Thus, little support exists for the routine use of serum ALK normalization as an indicator of the safety to proceed with resection of the HO.

BONE SCANS

Three-phase bone scans may be the most sensitive imaging modality for early detection of HO.[10,11,13–19] Specifically, flow studies and blood-pool images will detect the beginnings of HO approximately 2.5 weeks after injury, with findings on delayed scintigrams becoming positive approximately 1 week later. Activity on the delayed bone scans usually peaks a few months after injury, after which the intensity of activity on these scans progressively lessens, with a return toward normal at 6 to 12 months. The scans will usually return to normal within 12 months, hence the classic suggestions to wait the 1-year period before resecting the bone. Paradoxically, in some cases, activity on the scan remains slightly increased even though the underlying HO has become mature.[12]

Several authors report on the use of serial bone scans to successfully monitor the metabolic activity of HO and determine the appropriate time for surgical resection, if needed, and to predict postoperative recurrence.[14,15,20,21]

The studies evidence is summarized as follows:

- Although there appears to be value in serial bone scans to determine the level of maturity of the HO, there is no correlation between maturation on bone scan and nonrecurrence after resection.
- Tanaka and coworkers[21] recommend the following protocol if one uses serial bone scans to help decide the timing of heterotopic bone resection: The authors suggest obtaining a baseline quantitative bone scan as soon as possible after the onset of clinical symptoms of HO. This is done if the possibility of resecting the bone at some time in the future is being considered. Obtain serial scans at between 1- and 6-month intervals. More frequent serial scans improve the accuracy of the technique.
- Serial quantitative bone scans that show a sharply decreasing trend followed by a steady state over a 2- to 3-month period are the most reliable scintigraphic parameter for determining whether HO has reached maturity.
- This Level III evidence of maturity evidenced by decreasing bone scan activity does not indicate that it is safe to surgically remove the HO because recurrences occurred in the presence of a cold or a maturing bone scan[10,22] with substantial frequency.

Level of Neurologic Recovery

In a retrospective chart review of 25 adult patients with brain injury, Garland and coworkers[23] analyzed the extent of the brain injury and the degree of recovery of the involved limb after resection of the HO (Level III). The authors categorized the patients into Class I to V according to the cognitive and physical residua of the brain injury, with Class I being minimal disability in both areas. In addition, the authors looked at the bone scans, levels of ALK, radiographic evidence of bone maturity before surgery, and use of postoperative preventive measures such as diphosphonate.

The findings of this study were that the single best predictor of a good surgical result with the lowest recurrence rate was a rating of Class I or II in terms of neurologic recovery of the affected limb. In contrast, the Class V group with severe ongoing neurologic impairments had no improvement in function and had high recurrence rates. The authors found that normalized levels of ALK, mature radiographic appearance of the HO, or waiting more than 18 months after injury before surgery were not consistent in predicting a good functional outcome or a low recurrence rate. Bone scans were not routinely available, and as such, no conclusions could be drawn as to the predictive value of this test regarding recurrence of the HO.

Moreover, the study concludes that an increased level of ALK, evidence of immature bone on radiographs, and early surgery on Class V (poor neurologic recovery) patients were associated with high recurrence rates.

The authors postulate that the level of neurologic recovery may influence the success of surgery based on the ability of the patient to use the limb effectively after surgery and to participate in the rehabilitation process. In addition, recovery of the neurologic impairment would reduce the levels of circulatory central factors that would be active in causing a recurrence of the HO. This Level III study provides the strongest evidence available relating the level of neurologic recovery and the success of resection of HO.

Garland[13] has recommended different schedules for surgical intervention, depending on the cause of the condition underlying the HO: 6 months after direct traumatic musculoskeletal injury, 1 year after spinal cord injury, and 1.5 years after traumatic brain injury. This publication makes recommendations that the author describes as an estimate of timing without substantive evidence.

AREAS OF UNCERTAINTY

It is unclear whether what is required is a refinement of techniques to determine when the HO has matured, or whether there are other, more important factors that affect the likelihood of recurrence after surgical resection apart from the maturity of the bone mass. Little evidence is available to support the contention that radiographic assessment of HO maturity predicts the chance of reoccurrence after resection surgery[10] (Level III).

For several investigators,[14,20,21] serial preoperative bone scans that quantify the ratio of heterotopic to normal bone activity have successfully predicted postoperative nonrecurrence; a decreasing or stable scintigraphic activity ratio is considered the hallmark of mature HO. As HO becomes mature, there also is a significant decrease, often reaching a normal level, in both flow study and blood-pool activity. Other authors, again based on poor level evidence, have found that even in the presence of a quiescent bone scan, a postresection reoccurrence of HO can occur (Level III).[10,24]

Neurologic recovery of the affected limb seems to be an important factor in reducing the chance of recurrence after resection of the HO (Level III).[23] Although not specifically covered in this article, the use of appropriate postoperative measures to reduce the chances of recurrence, be this radiation treatment, use of anti-inflammatory drugs such as indomethacin or cyclo-oxygenase-2 inhibitors, or a combination of the two, may well be more important than the above preoperative indices in achieving a successful outcome from resection surgery.

Finally, atraumatic surgical technique should be important in reducing the amount of additional soft-tissue trauma to the local area, reducing the regional stimulus to bone reformation. This surgery is technically demanding and should be attempted only when the surgeon has excellent knowledge of the intricate local anatomy and can perform the surgery in an atraumatic fashion, respecting the soft tissues (Level V).

RECOMMENDATIONS

Based on a critical review of the available literature with an assessment of the quality of the studies, the assessment of when it is safe to resect HO remains difficult. Table 52–1 provides a summary of recommendations for the treatment of heterotopic ossification.

TABLE 52–1. Summary of Recommendations

RECOMMENDATION	LEVEL OF EVIDENCE/GRADE OF RECOMMENDATION
1. Adults awaiting surgical HO resection should delay surgery until plain radiographs and computed tomographic scan demonstrate a mature bone appearance to minimize recurrence rates.	C
2. Adults awaiting surgical HO resection may have lower recurrence rates if they wait until serial bone scans show that activity has reduced to a low level.	C
3. Adults awaiting surgical HO resection should achieve a high level of neurologic recovery of the affected limb before the procedure is undertaken.	C

HO, heterotopic ossification.

REFERENCES

1. Liu K, Tripp S, Layfield LJ: Heterotopic ossification: Review of histologic findings and tissue distribution in a 10-year experience. Pathol Res Pract 203:633–640, 2007.
2. Hendricks HT, Geurts AC, van Ginneken BC, et al: Brain injury severity and autonomic dysregulation accurately predict heterotopic ossification in patients with traumatic brain injury. Clin Rehabil 21:545–553, 2007.
3. Ho SSW, Stern PJ, Bruno LP, et al: Pharmacological inhibition of prostaglandin E-2 in bone and its effect on pathological new bone formation in a rat brain model. Trans Orthop Res Soc 13:536, 1988.
4. Freebourn TM, Barber DB, Able AC: The treatment of immature heterotopic ossification in spinal cord injury with combination surgery, radiation therapy and NSAID. Spinal Cord 37:50–53, 1999.
5. Canale ST: Campbell's Operative Orthopedics, 10th ed. St. Louis, Mosby, 2003.
6. Bucholz RW, Heckman JD: Rockwood and Green's Fractures in Adults, 6th ed. Philadelphia, Lippincott Williams & Wilkins, 2005.
7. Weinstein SL, Buckwalter JA: Turek's Orthopaedics: Principles and Their Application, 6th ed. Philadelphia, Lippincott William & Wilkins, 2005.
8. Tsionos I, Leclercq C, Rochet JM: Heterotopic ossification of the elbow in patients with burns: Results after early resection. J Bone Joint Surg Br 86-B:396–403, 2004.
9. Helms CA: "Skeletal don't touch" lesions. In Brant WE, Helms CA (eds): Fundamentals of Diagnostic Radiology. Baltimore, MD. Williams & Wilkins, 1994, pp 963–975.
10. Garland DE, Orwin JF: Resection of heterotopic ossification in patients with spinal cord injuries. Clin Orthop 242:169–176, 1989.
11. Orzel JA, Rudd TG: Heterotopic bone formation: Clinical, laboratory and imaging correlation. J Nucl Med 26:125–132, 1985.
12. Tibone J, Sakimura I, Nickel VL, Hsu JD: Heterotopic ossification around the hip in spinal cord-injured patients: A long-term follow-up study. J Bone Joint Surg Am 60:769–775, 1978.
13. Garland DE: A clinical perspective on common forms of acquired heterotopic ossification. Clin Orthop 263:13–29, 1991.
14. Rossier AB, Bussat P, Infante F, et al: Current facts on para-osteoarthropathy (POA). Paraplegia 11:36–78, 1973.
15. Freed JH, Hahn H, Menter R, Dillon T: The use of three-phase bone scan in the early diagnosis of heterotopic ossification (HO) and in the evaluation of Didronel therapy. Paraplegia 20:208–216, 1982.
16. Tyler JL, Derbekyan V, Lisbona R: Early diagnosis of myositis ossificans with Tc-99m diphosphonate imaging. Clin Nucl Med 9:256–258, 1984.
17. Drane WE: Myositis ossificans and the three phase bone scan. AJR Am J Roentgenol 142:179–180, 1984.
18. Szabo Z, Ritzl F, Chittima S, et al: Bone scintigraphy of myositis ossificans in apallic syndrome. Eur J Nucl Med 7:426–428, 1982.
19. Suzuki Y, Hisada K, Takeda M: Demonstration of myositis ossificans by 99mTc pyrophosphate bone scanning. Radiology 111:663–664, 1974.
20. Muheim G, Donath A, Rossier AB: Serial scintigrams in the course of ectopic bone formation in paraplegic patients. AJR Am J Roentgenol 118:865–869, 1973.
21. Tanaka T, Rossier AB, Hussey RW, et al: Quantitative assessment of para-osteo-arthropathy and its maturation on serial radionuclide bone images. Radiology 123:217–221, 1977.
22. Stover SL, Niemann KM, Tulloss JR: Experience with surgical resection of heterotopic bone in spinal cord injury patients. Clin Orthop 263:71–77, 1991.
23. Garland DE, Hanscom DA, Keenan MA, et al: Resection of heterotopic ossification in the adult with head trauma. J Bone Joint Surg Am 67:1261–1269, 1985.
24. Garland DE: Surgical approaches for resection of heterotopic ossification in traumatic brain-injured adults. Clin Orthop Relat Res (263):59–70, 1991.

Damage Control Trauma Care:
Does It Save Lives or Make No Difference?

RALF SCHOENIGER, MD AND PETER J. O'BRIEN, MD, FRCSC

Controversy still exists about the early definitive treatment of fractures in patients with multiple injuries. Several authors in the 1980s supported the benefit of early intramedullary nailing of femoral shaft fractures.[1–6] However, because of experimental and retrospective studies in the 1990s, concerns were raised about primary intramedullary nailing of the femur, sometimes referred to as early total care (ETC), especially in patients with associated chest and head injuries.[7–9] The concept of "damage control orthopedics" (DCO) was then developed in the large trauma centers. This technique involves primary external skeletal fixation of the femoral fracture followed in a few days by definitive intramedullary nailing when the patient's physiology has been completely corrected. Several authors have advocated delayed definitive treatment in the more recent literature.[10–13] Since the 1990s, there has been an ongoing debate about early versus delayed definitive fracture fixation in femoral shaft fractures in the setting of polytrauma and when treating femoral shaft fractures in patients with multiple injuries regarding whether the reamed or the unreamed technique should be used.

Since the late 1980s, the assessment and treatment of the patient with multiple injuries has markedly improved. The establishment of highly specialized trauma centers for early intervention of life-threatening injuries, such as intrathoracic, intraabdominal, and intracranial injuries, has led to greater survival rates in these patients.[14–17]

In light of ongoing controversy since the 1990s with regard to timing and type of definitive treatment of long bone fractures in patients with multiple injuries, the purpose of this review is to provide guidance to clinicians based on the best available evidence on this topic.

EVIDENCE

Timing of Fracture Care in Patients with Multiple Trauma Injuries

Initial Clinical and Basic Science Research. Several studies in the 1980s and 1990s found that early definitive care (less than 24 hours) leads to a decrease of morbidity and mortality.[1–4,18–21] Most of the studies claimed that prevention of adult respiratory distress syndrome (ARDS), reduction of inflammatory mediators, and lower fat embolism rate were associated with early intramedullary nailing. In contrast, Pape and colleagues,[7] in a retrospective review, found that although early intramedullary nailing of femoral shaft fractures in patients without chest injuries had a reduced risk for morbidity, the rates of ARDS and mortality were increased in patients with associated severe chest injuries treated with reamed intramedullary nailing within 24 hours of injury when compared with those who had delayed fracture fixation[7] (Level of Evidence 3). Their suggestion was to consider alternate forms of femur fracture fixation or delayed definitive fixation in patients with severe chest injuries (Abbreviated Injury Scale [AIS] > 2). This then led to the development of the DCO concept. Other centers have advocated delayed definitive treatment in the more recent literature.[10–13]

Experimental Animal Studies. Parallel to the clinical studies, several experimental animal studies investigated the effect of reamed or unreamed nailing of the femur and the tibia on the intramedullary pressure and the rate of fat embolization.[8,9,22–28] In addition, Duwelius and researchers[22] and Wolinsky and colleagues[28] examined the effect of intramedullary nailing on pulmonary function in normal and contused lungs.

Most of the studies showed that intramedullary nailing of the femur increases the intramedullary pressure.[8,9,22–24] No difference was found if a reamed or unreamed nailing procedure was used.[22,23] Opening of the canal with an awl leads to the highest intramedullary pressure in studies by Heim and investigators[24] and Duwelius and researchers.[22] Marrow element extravasation and fat emboli are clearly associated with reamed and unreamed nailing of the femur.[9,22–24,27,28]

Manning and coworkers[25] showed greater rates of fat release in intact femurs compared with fractured femurs and concluded that the fracture is responsible for the low incidence of pulmonary dysfunction in the clinical field. Duwelius and researchers[22] found minimal pulmonary dysfunction in normal and contused lung in their sheep model with reamed or unreamed nailing of the femur. However, the reamed technique had a greater rate of fat emboli in the histologic analysis. Wolinsky and his group[28] confirmed these results in 1998 in their sheep model with a reamed nailing procedure.

No evidence has been provided from this basic physiology research that reamed intramedullary nailing of the femur leads to greater pulmonary dysfunction than unreamed nailing. However, manipulation of the medullary canal does have a negative effect on pulmonary physiology.

Immunologic Response Studies. Another field of interest is the systemic inflammatory response syndrome (SIRS) score of patients with multiple injuries related to the time of treatment. Several studies since the early 1990s have shown that the inflammatory response correlates with the severity of the injury, patient outcome, and mortality.[29–36] However, only two studies have focused on the comparison of early versus delayed fixation.[32,35] Pape and colleagues[35] show in their prospective, randomized, multicenter study with 35 patients from 2003 that certain interleukin levels (IL-6 and IL-8) are significantly increased in the primary intramedullary fixation group. Both groups were similar regarding age, injury severity score (ISS), AIS, and Glasgow Coma Scale (GCS). However, no difference was found in the IL-1 level and in the incidence of ARDS, sepsis, and multiorgan failure (Level of Evidence 2).

The second study that is from the same group, reported by Harwood and colleagues[32] in 2005, looked retrospectively at 174 patients and found a greater SIRS score in the early fixation group despite having significantly lower ISSs, and fewer head and chest injuries. They also had longer intensive care unit (ICU) stays, higher ARDS rates, and more multiorgan failures. Although the authors' conclusion that DCO does not add additional detrimental inflammatory response to the patient seems clear, the study did not demonstrate that the greater SIRS score in the early definitive fixation group will lead to more complications (Level of Evidence III).

No clinical evidence exists from these results that high levels of interleukin or high SIRS scores lead to a significantly greater rate of complications when timing of the fracture care is within 24 hours.

Chest Injuries and Femur Fractures. The benefits of early definitive fracture fixation in patients with associated chest injuries have been demonstrated repeatedly.[1,4,18–21,37–43] In contrast, Pape and colleagues[7] were the first to demonstrate in their study from 1993 that early reamed intramedullary nailing in patients with severe chest injuries (AIS > 2) increased the risk for ARDS and death. In the same study, early fixation without chest injury was associated with decreased morbidity.

Comparison between studies is difficult. One main difficulty is the definition of the severity of chest trauma. In most studies, an AIS score of greater than 2 is considered to be a severe chest injury. In several studies, however, the AIS is either not mentioned or is indicated as 2 or lower.[1,19,38,44] Another difficulty is the great variety of the ISSs in the studies. Most studies use an ISS of greater than 18 as a criterion for inclusion.[1,3,7,20,37,40] However, often the ISS was significantly different across studies and across the two treatment groups.[39]

As mentioned previously and as shown in Table 53–1, most studies showed either no difference or better outcome in the early definitive fixation group.

Bone and coauthors[1] showed in their prospective, randomized clinical study from 1989 that the incidence of pulmonary complications such as ARDS, pneumonia, and fat embolism is greater when the fracture fixation is delayed (Level of Evidence 2). This study was a prospective, randomized, clinical trial, but there were some limitations regarding the definition of the severity of the chest injury. In a retrospective review, similar results were presented from this group[37] in 1995 with a chest AIS greater than 3 (Level of Evidence 3).

Interestingly, regarding Pape and colleagues'[7] study, Charash and colleagues[40] arrived at an opposite conclusion using the same study design in their study with 138 patients. A complication rate of 56% was observed in the patient group with delayed definitive fracture fixation, and associated severe chest injuries were compared with a rate of only 16% in the early fixation group (Level of Evidence 3).

In the more recent literature, Handolin and researchers[41] and Weninger and colleagues[43] compared

TABLE 53–1. Chest Injuries

STUDY	DESIGN	CASES (N)	RESULT	LEVEL OF EVIDENCE	GRADE OF RECOMMENDATION*
Bone et al.[1]	Prospective	178	ETC	II	B
Pape et al.[7]	Retrospective	106	DCO	III	C
Charash et al.[40]	Retrospective	138	ETC	III	C
Bone et al.[37]	Retrospective	97	ETC	III	C
Reynolds et al.[20]	Retrospective	105	No difference	IV	C
Boulanger et al.[19]	Retrospective	149	No difference	IV	C
Bosse et al.[18]	Retrospective	453	No difference	III	C
Carlson et al.[39]	Retrospective	593	No difference	IV	C
Brundage et al.[38]	Retrospective	1362	ETC	IV	C
Nau et al.[44]	Retrospective	148	ETC	IV	C
Handolin et al.[41]	Retrospective	61	ETC	III	C
Weninger et al.[43]	Retrospective	152	ETC	III	C
COTS	Prospective	109	Reamed	II	B

*A = good evidence (Level I studies with consistent finding) for or against recommending intervention; B = fair evidence (Level II or III studies with consistent findings) for or against recommending intervention; C = poor quality evidence (Level IV or V with consistent findings) for or against recommending intervention; I = there is insufficient or conflicting evidence not allowing a recommendation for or against intervention.
COTS, Canadian Orthopaedic Trauma Society. DCO, damage control orthopedics; ETC, early total care.

patients with severe chest injuries (AIS $\geq$ 3) and femoral fractures treated with early intramedullary nailing with a group with severe chest injury but without long bone fractures (Level of Evidence 3). Both studies found that intramedullary nailing of the femur did not add any additional risk for ARDS, multiorgan failure syndrome, and mortality. The strength of Weninger and colleagues'[43] study is the equal distribution in the ISS (39.5 vs. 38.3), the chest AIS (4.2 vs. 4.1), and the distribution of thoracic injuries.

The Canadian Orthopaedic Trauma Society[45] report on a prospective, randomized, clinical trial that compared the rates of ARDS in patients with multiple trauma injuries who had their femur fractures treated primarily with either a reamed or an unreamed nail. The society found that there was no significant difference in the rate of ARDS (reamed, 4.8%; unreamed, 4.3%) or mortality between the two groups. The number of subjects was small and the event rate was low, indicating that further study may be necessary (Level of Evidence 2).

In summary, the literature is inconclusive regarding the optimal timing and type of fixation for femoral shaft fractures in association with severe chest injuries. It would appear from the early retrospective studies and from the Bone and coauthors'[1] prospective randomized trial that early (within 24 hours) femur fracture fixation is advantageous in terms of morbidity and perhaps mortality. It is not clear whether the primary fixation should be external skeletal fixation (DCO) or definitive fixation (ETC). For patients treated with early definitive fixation, it would appear from the Canadian prospective randomized trial that there is no advantage to the unreamed technique over the reamed technique for pulmonary complication or mortality.

Timing of Fracture Care in Patients with Multiple Trauma Injuries: Head Injuries. Patients with multiple injuries with associated head trauma must be evaluated carefully regarding early fracture fixation. Early fracture fixation may expose the patient to additional hypotension, hypoxemia, increased intracranial pressure, and reduced intracranial perfusion, potentially exacerbating the existing brain injury. Furthermore, because it may be difficult to monitor these patients intraoperatively regarding fluid management, careful anesthesia management is mandatory to avoid potential detrimental neurologic effects of fracture surgery.

Both early and delayed femur fracture fixation in polytrauma victims with head injury has been supported (Table 53–2). Jaicks and investigators[46] and Townsend and coworkers[47] postulate that early fracture fixation exposed the patient to an unacceptable risk for secondary brain damage.

Jaicks and investigators[46] retrospectively reviewed 33 patients with significant closed head injuries who were treated either with early ($\leq$ 24 hours) or late fixation (>24 hours). He found that patients with early fixation received significantly more fluids in the first 48 hours, had a greater rate of intraoperative hypotension and hypoxia, and had an average discharge GCS that was lower compared with the delayed fixation group. In contrast, the neurologic complication rate, ICU stay, and hospital time was slightly higher in the delayed fixation group[46] (Level of Evidence 3).

Sixty-one patients with moderate-to-severe closed head injuries in the retrospective review from Townsend and coworkers[47] received intramedullary nailing of the femur in the first 2 hours, within 24 hours, or after 24 hours of admission to hospital. Compared with fracture fixation after 24 hours, the authors note an eight-fold increased risk for becoming hypotensive during fracture fixation when treated within the first 2 hours. The risk for hypotension was twice as high when fracture fixation occurred within 24 hours compared with treatment after 24 hours. The authors conclude that the risk for low intraoperative cerebral perfusion pressure remains important for at least 24 hours[47] (Level of Evidence 3).

In contrast with these studies, there are numerous studies that not only shown no risk for early fracture fixation,[38,48–54] but also show benefit in patients with ancillary chest trauma.[38,53] Hofman and Goris[48] found a better neurologic outcome based on the Glasgow Outcome Scale score and Brundage and colleagues[38] based on a greater GCS score in the early fixation

TABLE 53–2. Head Injuries

STUDY	DESIGN	CASES (N)	RESULT	LEVEL OF EVIDENCE	GRADE OF RECOMMENDATION
Kotwica et al.[49]	Retrospective	100	ETC	III	C
Hofman and Goris[48]	Retrospective	58	ETC	III	C
Poole et al.[52]	Retrospective	114	No difference	III	C
Jaicks et al.[46]	Retrospective	33	DCO	III	C
McKee et al.[50]	Retrospective	145	No difference	III	C
Starr et al.[53]	Retrospective	32	ETC	III	C
Velmahos et al.[54]	Retrospective	47	No difference	III	C
Townsend et al.[47]	Retrospective	61	DCO	III	C
Brundage et al.[38]	Retrospective	1362	ETC	III	C
Nau et al.[51]	Retrospective	175	ETC	III	C

DCO, damage control orthopedics; ETC, early total care.

group in their studies from 1991 and 2002, respectively. None of the reviewed studies showed poorer neurologic outcome in the early fixation group. Hofman and Goris[48] showed a three-fold greater mortality rate, and also Kotwica and colleagues[49] and Riemer and coauthors[55] demonstrate greater rates of mortality in the delayed fixation group. Several authors present no difference in the mortality rate.[38,50,51,54]

Velmahos and associates[54] in their study from 1998 showed in 47 patients no difference of intraoperative hypotension and hypoxia in the early fixation group and found a trend to longer hospital and ICU stays after delayed treatment (Level of Evidence III). Also, Brundage and colleagues[38] detected longer hospital stay and ICU length in the delayed fixation group, where McKee and coworkers[50] and Nau and colleagues[51] could not find a difference between the two groups.

Starr and colleagues[53] found that delayed fixation was a strong predictor of pulmonary complications in 32 patients with mild-to-severe head injuries. Pulmonary complications were 48 times more likely in the delayed treatment group compared with early fixation. For each point increment in the chest AIS and head/neck AIS, the risk for pulmonary complications increased by 300% and 500%, respectively. The authors report no difference in the incidence of central nervous system complications with early or delayed treatment (Level of Evidence 3). Poole and coauthors[52] state that the neurologic outcome is determined by the severity of the head injury, and that delayed fixation did not protect the injured brain.

All studies about fracture fixation in patients with head injury are retrospective and have only looked at timing of fracture fixation. None has examined specifically the type of fracture fixation. It is therefore not possible to derive a definitive conclusion regarding the timing and type of long bone fracture treatment in the context of severe head injury. It is more important in these patients to individualize clinical assessment and treatment to the patient's condition with careful attention to intraoperative monitoring and adequate resuscitation. Maintenance of cerebral perfusion pressure greater than 70 mm Hg is mandatory.

AREAS OF UNCERTAINTY

Tremendous work has been invested since the 1980s in the field of fracture care in patients with multiple injuries. Because of this research, treatment strategies for this delicate patient group were developed and have led to a large improvement in the clinical outcome of these patients. Many important questions remain unanswered.

Previous authors postulate that only a large, prospective, randomized trial could be helpful. The question arises if such a study is ethical and if it is possible to recruit patients with such severe injury for these trials.

Early definitive fracture fixation of long bone fracture is the common standard in most trauma centers. Chest injuries and head injuries are not contraindications for ETC. It is our duty to optimize the clinical assessment of these patients, and provide careful monitoring and appropriate resuscitation to reach the best possible outcome. DCO would appear to be a safe alternative. In many situations, it may be the best option for the patient. An obvious example is the uncommon instance when the patient cannot be adequately resuscitated; no one has ever recommended definitive fracture care in the setting of a patient who is hypotensive, acidotic, hypothermic, hypoxic, or coagulopathic. In that setting, initial emergent external skeletal fixation can be done quickly with minimal additional blood loss and still fulfill the need to provide early surgical stabilization of a femur fracture with limited additional stress to the patient. Another situation where DCO is practiced is in institutions that do not have the personnel, facilities, or experience to manage complex polytrauma victims and, therefore, DCO may provide some benefit if transfer to an appropriate institution may take more than a few hours.

RECOMMENDATIONS

From our perspective, treatment of femur fractures with early intramedullary nailing is a safe procedure in patients with multiple injuries with associated severe thoracic or head trauma, as long as these patients are adequately resuscitated. If hemodynamic stability and oxygenation with adequate monitoring can be achieved, we recommend early (<24 hours) definitive fracture care of long bone fracture with intramedullary nailing to simplify intensive care, reduce fracture pain, and provide early mobilization as soon as possible.

If hemodynamic stability cannot be reached within the first hours of admission, temporary external fixation should be considered. The possible restriction of organ function caused by any surgical intervention in the vulnerable phase of hypovolemia and shock should always be kept in mind. Patient populations, resuscitation protocols and teams, orthopedic expertise, anaesthesia capabilities, and ICU resources vary from institution to institution. All of these are important to consider when making the decision about whether a polytrauma patient should have his or her femur treated with primary intramedullary nailing or with the DCO protocol. It would appear from the literature that both techniques are acceptable if the patient has been adequately resuscitated. Table 53–3 provides a summary of recommendations.

TABLE 53–3. Summary of Recommendations

RECOMMENDATIONS	LEVEL OF EVIDENCE/GRADE OF RECOMMENDATION
1. Adult with multiple traumatic injuries should undergo femur fracture stabilization within 24 hours.	B
2. Femoral stabilization with a reamed nail is as safe as an unreamed nail in adult patients with multiple trauma injuries.	B
3. The evidence is insufficient to make a definitive recommendation regarding whether early femoral stabilization should follow the early total care (early nailing) or damage control orthopedics (early external fixation and delayed nailing) model. Currently, both appear to be safe, as long as the patient has been adequately resuscitated.	I (indeterminate)

REFERENCES

1. Bone LB, Johnson KD, Weigelt J, Scheinberg R: Early versus delayed stabilization of femoral fractures. A prospective randomized study. J Bone Joint Surg Am 71:336–340, 1989.
2. Goris RJ, Gimbrere JS, van Niekerk JL, et al: Early osteosynthesis and prophylactic mechanical ventilation in the multitrauma patient. J Trauma 22:895–903, 1982.
3. Johnson KD, Cadambi A, Seibert GB: Incidence of adult respiratory distress syndrome in patients with multiple musculoskeletal injuries: Effect of early operative stabilization of fractures. J Trauma 25:375–384, 1985.
4. Meek RN, Vivoda EE, Pirani S: Comparison of mortality of patients with multiple injuries according to type of fracture treatment—a retrospective age- and injury-matched series. Injury 17:2–4, 1986.
5. Riska EB, Myllynen P: Fat embolism in patients with multiple injuries. J Trauma 22:891–894, 1982.
6. Shapiro MB, Jenkins DH, Schwab CW, Rotondo MF: Damage control: Collective review. J Trauma 49:969–978, 2000.
7. Pape HC, Auf'm'Kolk M, Paffrath T, et al: Primary intramedullary femur fixation in multiple trauma patients with associated lung contusion—a cause of posttraumatic ARDS? J Trauma 34:540–548, 1993.
8. Sturmer KM, Schuchardt W: [New aspects of closed intramedullary nailing and marrow cavity reaming in animal experiments. II. Intramedullary pressure in marrow cavity reaming (author's transl)]. Unfallheilkunde 83:346–352, 1980.
9. Wozasek GE, Simon P, Redl H, Schlag G: Intramedullary pressure changes and fat intravasation during intramedullary nailing: An experimental study in sheep. J Trauma 36:202–207, 1994.
10. Nowotarski PJ, Turen CH, Brumback RJ, Scarboro JM: Conversion of external fixation to intramedullary nailing for fractures of the shaft of the femur in multiply injured patients. J Bone Joint Surg Am 82:781–788, 2000.
11. Roberts CS, Pape HC, Jones AL, et al: Damage control orthopaedics: Evolving concepts in the treatment of patients who have sustained orthopaedic trauma. Instr Course Lect 54:447–462, 2005.
12. Scalea TM, Boswell SA, Scott JD, et al: External fixation as a bridge to intramedullary nailing for patients with multiple injuries and with femur fractures: Damage control orthopedics. J Trauma 48:613–621, 2000.
13. Taeger G, Ruchholtz S, Waydhas C, et al: Damage control orthopedics in patients with multiple injuries is effective, time saving, and safe. J Trauma 59:409–417, 2005.
14. Feliciano DV, Mattox KL, Jordan GL Jr: Intra-abdominal packing for control of hepatic hemorrhage: A reappraisal. J Trauma 21:285–290, 1981.
15. Rotondo MF, Zonies DH: The damage control sequence and underlying logic. Surg Clin North Am Aug 77:761–777, 1997.
16. Schweiberer L, Dambe LT, Klapp F: [Multiple injuries: Severity and therapeutic measures]. Chirurg 49:608–614, 1978.
17. Trentz O, Oestern HJ, Hempelmann G, et al: [Criteria for the operability of patients with multiple injuries (author's transl)]. Unfallheilkunde 81:451–458, 1978.
18. Bosse MJ, MacKenzie EJ, Riemer BL, et al: Adult respiratory distress syndrome, pneumonia, and mortality following thoracic injury and a femoral fracture treated either with intramedullary nailing with reaming or with a plate. A comparative study. J Bone Joint Surg Am 79:799–809, 1997.
19. Boulanger BR, Stephen D, Brenneman FD: Thoracic trauma and early intramedullary nailing of femur fractures: Are we doing harm? J Trauma 43:24–28, 1997.
20. Reynolds MA, Richardson JD, Spain DA, et al: Is the timing of fracture fixation important for the patient with multiple trauma? Ann Surg 222:470–481, 1995.
21. Riska EB, von Bonsdorff H, Hakkinen S, et al: Prevention of fat embolism by early internal fixation of fractures in patients with multiple injuries. Injury 8:110–116, 1976.
22. Duwelius PJ, Huckfeldt R, Mullins RJ, et al: The effects of femoral intramedullary reaming on pulmonary function in a sheep lung model. J Bone Joint Surg Am 79:194–202, 1997.
23. Heim D, Regazzoni P, Tsakiris DA, et al: Intramedullary nailing and pulmonary embolism: Does unreamed nailing prevent embolization? An in vivo study in rabbits. J Trauma 38:899–906, 1995.
24. Heim D, Schlegel U, Perren SM: Intramedullary pressure in reamed and unreamed nailing of the femur and tibia—an in vitro study in intact, human bones. Injury 24(suppl 3):S56–S63, 1993.
25. Manning JB, Bach AW, Herman CM, Carrico CJ: Fat release after femur nailing in the dog. J Trauma 23:322–326, 1983.
26. Oztuna V, Ersoz G, Ayan I, et al: Early internal fracture fixation prevents bacterial translocation. Clin Orthop Relat Res 446:253–258, 2006.
27. Pape HC, Dwenger A, Regel G, et al: Pulmonary damage after intramedullary femoral nailing in traumatized sheep—is there an effect from different nailing methods? J Trauma 33:574–581, 1992.
28. Wolinsky PR, Banit D, Parker RE, et al: Reamed intramedullary femoral nailing after induction of an "ARDS-like" state in sheep: Effect on clinically applicable markers of pulmonary function. J Orthop Trauma 12:169–176, 1998.
29. Bochicchio GV, Napolitano LM, Joshi M, et al: Systemic inflammatory response syndrome score at admission independently predicts infection in blunt trauma patients. J Trauma 50:817–820, 2001.
30. Ertel W, Keel M, Bonaccio M, et al: Release of anti-inflammatory mediators after mechanical trauma correlates with severity of injury and clinical outcome. J Trauma 39:879–887, 1995.
31. Giannoudis PV, Abbott C, Stone M, et al: Fatal systemic inflammatory response syndrome following early bilateral femoral nailing. Intensive Care Med 24:641–642, 1998.
32. Harwood PJ, Giannoudis PV, van Griensven M, et al: Alterations in the systemic inflammatory response after early total care and damage control procedures for femoral shaft fracture in severely injured patients. J Trauma 58:446–454, 2005.
33. Malone DL, Kuhls D, Napolitano LM, et al: Back to basics: Validation of the admission systemic inflammatory response syndrome score in predicting outcome in trauma. J Trauma 51:458–463, 2001.
34. Napolitano LM, Ferrer T, McCarter RJ Jr, Scalea TM: Systemic inflammatory response syndrome score at admission independently predicts mortality and length of stay in trauma patients. J Trauma 49:647–653, 2000.

35. Pape HC, Grimme K, Van Griensven M, et al: Impact of intramedullary instrumentation versus damage control for femoral fractures on immunoinflammatory parameters: Prospective randomized analysis by the EPOFF Study Group. J Trauma 55:7–13, 2003.
36. Wanner GA, Keel M, Steckholzer U, et al: Relationship between procalcitonin plasma levels and severity of injury, sepsis, organ failure, and mortality in injured patients. Crit Care Med 28:950–957, 2000.
37. Bone LB, Babikian G, Stegemann PM: Femoral canal reaming in the polytrauma patient with chest injury. A clinical perspective. Clin Orthop Relat Res (318):91–94, 1995.
38. Brundage SI, McGhan R, Jurkovich GJ, et al: Timing of femur fracture fixation: Effect on outcome in patients with thoracic and head injuries. J Trauma 52:299–307, 2002.
39. Carlson DW, Rodman GH Jr, Kaehr D, et al: Femur fractures in chest-injured patients: Is reaming contraindicated? J Orthop Trauma 12:164–168, 1998.
40. Charash WE, Fabian TC, Croce MA: Delayed surgical fixation of femur fractures is a risk factor for pulmonary failure independent of thoracic trauma. J Trauma 37:667–672, 1994.
41. Handolin L, Pajarinen J, Lassus J, Tulikoura I: Early intramedullary nailing of lower extremity fracture and respiratory function in polytraumatized patients with a chest injury: A retrospective study of 61 patients. Acta Orthop Scand 75:477–480, 2004.
42. Riska EB, von Bonsdorff H, Hakkinen S, et al: Primary operative fixation of long bone fractures in patients with multiple injuries. J Trauma 17:111–121, 1977.
43. Weninger P, Figl M, Spitaler R, et al: Early unreamed intramedullary nailing of femoral fractures is safe in patients with severe thoracic trauma. J Trauma 62:692–696, 2007.
44. Nau T, Aldrian S, Koenig F, Vecsei V: Fixation of femoral fractures in multiple-injury patients with combined chest and head injuries. ANZ J Surg 73:1018–1021, 2003.
45. The Canadian Orthopaedic Trauma Society: Reamed versus unreamed intramedullary nailing of the femur: Comparison of the rate of ARDS in multiple injured patients. J Orthop Trauma 20:384–387, 2006.
46. Jaicks RR, Cohn SM, Moller BA: Early fracture fixation may be deleterious after head injury. J Trauma 42:1–6, 1997.
47. Townsend RN, Lheureau T, Protech J, et al: Timing fracture repair in patients with severe brain injury (Glasgow Coma Scale score <9). J Trauma 44:977–983, 1998.
48. Hofman PA, Goris RJ: Timing of osteosynthesis of major fractures in patients with severe brain injury. J Trauma 31:261–263, 1991.
49. Kotwica Z, Balcewicz L, Jagodzinski Z: Head injuries coexistent with pelvic or lower extremity fractures—early or delayed osteosynthesis. Acta Neurochir (Wien) 102(1-2):19–21, 1990.
50. McKee MD, Schemitsch EH, Vincent LO, et al: The effect of a femoral fracture on concomitant closed head injury in patients with multiple injuries. J Trauma 42:1041–1045, 1997.
51. Nau T, Kutscha-Lissberg F, Muellner T, et al: Effects of a femoral shaft fracture on multiply injured patients with a head injury. World J Surg 27:365–369, 2003.
52. Poole GV, Miller JD, Agnew SG, Griswold JA: Lower extremity fracture fixation in head-injured patients. J Trauma 32:654–659, 1992.
53. Starr AJ, Hunt JL, Chason DP, et al: Treatment of femur fracture with associated head injury. J Orthop Trauma 12:38–45, 1998.
54. Velmahos GC, Arroyo H, Ramicone E, et al: Timing of fracture fixation in blunt trauma patients with severe head injuries. Am J Surg 176:324–330, 1998.
55. Riemer BL, Butterfield SL, Diamond DL, et al: Acute mortality associated with injuries to the pelvic ring: The role of early patient mobilization and external fixation. J Trauma 35:671–677, 1993.

Chapter 54

Humeral Shaft Fractures: What Is the Best Treatment?

Gregory K. Berry, MD

Fractures of the humeral shaft represent approximately 5% of all fractures.[1] The majority of humeral shaft fractures are currently treated without surgery in North America and Europe, a fact reflected in the following quote: "Because closed methods of treatment for humeral shaft fractures have a high rate of success, open reduction is rarely indicated."[2] The indications for operative reduction and fixation of humeral diaphysis fractures, first defined by Bandi[3] in 1964 and now found in most articles and textbooks, include failed conservative management (unable to maintain adequate reduction), open fracture, bilateral humeral shaft fractures, fractures with vascular injury/compromise, polytrauma victim with humeral shaft fracture, pathologic fracture, ipsilateral humeral shaft and forearm fractures (floating elbow), and segmental fractures.[4] These recommendations are based on expert opinion rather than comparative outcome studies.

OPTIONS

Options for treatment of humeral diaphysis fractures include operative and nonoperative techniques. Nonoperative modalities include hanging cast, coaptation splint (also known as functional bracing), and plaster U splint ("sugar-tong splint"). No evidence exists to support one of these methods over the other. Once there is indication for operative intervention, the surgeon can choose between open reduction and internal fixation with plate and screws, intramedullary nailing (statically locked and nonlocked), and external fixation.

OPERATIVE VERSUS NONOPERATIVE MANAGEMENT

Currently, no prospective trials have compared the outcomes of operative and nonoperative treatment of these fractures. In one study, Ekholm and coauthors[5] report on a cohort of 78 patients evaluated retrospectively after conservative treatment of humeral shaft fractures with fracture brace treatment. The nonunion rate overall was 10% but increased to 20% for AO/OTA (Arbeitsgemeinschaft für Osteosynthesefragen/Orthopaedic Trauma Association) type A fractures of the midshaft and more proximal diaphysis. Outcome scores were worse for those who went on to nonunion and required open reduction and internal fixation. Even in those who healed successfully with

nonoperative care, only 50% reported full recovery. The authors conclude that plate fixation should be considered for some fracture subtypes (Level V).

Operative Management: Compression Plating versus Statically Locked Intramedullary Nail

Since the advent of intramedullary nails designed for humeral shaft fractures, controversy has existed regarding the superiority of compression plating versus statically locked nailing of these fractures.[6] Advantages of nailing include a remote entry point preserving the biological environment for fracture healing; intramedullary reaming and fixation, eliminating risk for injury to the radial nerve (as long as no nerve interposition occurs); load sharing by the device; and more rapid surgery with less blood loss and muscle damage. In contrast, the advantages of plate fixation include a direct approach to the fracture site with no violation of the proximal humerus and, more importantly, the rotator cuff; no risk of shoulder impingement from prominent subacromial hardware; direct visualization and protection of the radial nerve depending on fracture level and approach; the possibility of rigid compressive fixation; and the opportunity for bone grafting or radial nerve exploration, or both, if needed. Both options permit rapid mobilization of the shoulder and elbow.

A number of prospective, randomized studies have compared plating and nailing of humeral shaft fractures. Rodrigues-Merchan[7] compared open reduction and compression plating with closed reduction and intramedullary fixation with Hackethal nails in 40 patients who did not respond successfully to conservative treatment. Given the lack of interlocking, the nailing group required 6 months of postoperative bracing. All except one of the former group required reoperation for hardware removal. No nonunions occurred, and delayed union and functional results were identical in both groups. The author concludes that the treatments were equivalent in healing and functional outcome, but that the nailing group required systematic hardware removal and prolonged bracing.

Chiu and colleagues[8] randomized 91 patients to 3 groups: open reduction and plate fixation, with and without bone graft, and closed reduction and nailing with flexible Enders nails without interlocking. Surgical time, blood loss, and length of stay were lowest in the nailing group. Time to union was increased in the group undergoing plating without bone graft. Overall, complications were more likely to occur in the plating without bone graft and the nailing groups, including a statistically greater rate of nonunion when compared with plating with bone graft. Infection and iatrogenic nerve injury were similar in all three groups. All patients reported satisfactory results according to functional parameters set out by the authors. The authors conclude that, in cases where operative time was a consideration (e.g., patient with polytrauma injuries), Enders nailing appeared superior. Overall, union was best assured with plating plus bone graft.

In 2000, McCormack and coauthors[9] reported the first published prospective, randomized trial comparing plating with statically locked intramedullary nailing. A total of 44 patients were randomly assigned to plating or locked nailing. Initially, nailing was antegrade, but then it was switched to retrograde based on reports of shoulder complications with the former technique. No statistical difference was detected in terms of pain, shoulder function (using validated outcome measures), union, alignment, blood loss, and operative time. Complications were significantly more common in the nailing group, however (62% vs. 13% in the plating group), whereas secondary surgery was required in 33% of nailing patients compared with 4% of plating patients. Fewer complications occurred with retrograde nailing compared with antegrade nailing. Surprisingly, iatrogenic radial nerve injury occurred in 14% (3/21) of nailing patients, with none in the plating group. These findings led the authors to recommend plating as the standard for fixation of humeral shaft fractures, reserving nailing for specific situations such as pathologic and segmental fractures.

In a larger randomized study, Chapman and researchers[10] compared plating and antegrade locked intramedullary nailing in 84 patients. No difference in time to union and rate of nonunion was detected. Significantly more patients described shoulder pain and had decreased shoulder range of motion in the nailing group, whereas fixed flexion contracture of the elbow was more common in the plating group, especially in distal third fractures. The authors conclude that healing was comparable with the two techniques with more pain and stiffness in the shoulder secondary to nailing.

To improve the inferences from the small, prospective, randomized trials comparing plating and locked intramedullary nailing in humeral shaft fractures, Bhandari and investigators[11] undertook a systematic review and meta-analysis to assess their effects on rates of reoperation and other secondary outcomes. Three studies were pooled[9,10,12] after confirming overall study quality. The relative risk of reoperation with plating was determined to be 0.3 (95% confidence interval, 0.07–0.9; $P = 0.03$), translating into a relative risk reduction of 74% compared with nailing. The relative risk of shoulder impingement was also reduced with plating (0.1; 95% confidence interval, 0.03–0.4; $P = 0.002$), resulting in a relative risk reduction of 90%. Analysis of secondary outcomes such as nonunion, infection, and iatrogenic nerve injury revealed no increased risk with plating when compared

with nailing. The authors conclude that, given a total of only 155 randomized patients across 3 studies, these results need to be interpreted with care and called for a much larger definitive trial to determine the true treatment effects of intramedullary nails and compression plates in humeral shaft fractures.[11]

INTRAMEDULLARY NAILING: ANTEGRADE VERSUS RETROGRADE

The initial enthusiasm accompanying the advent of antegrade locked intramedullary nailing of humeral shaft fractures was dampened by reports of subsequent shoulder pain.[13,14] This was attributed to rotator cuff and/or humeral head injury during insertion, as well as potentially prominent hardware provoking subacromial impingement. A retrograde insertion technique was developed to avoid these complications.

In a nonrandomized, prospective cohort study, Blum and coauthors[15] compared the antegrade and retrograde insertion techniques using an identical implant. Eighty-four acute diaphyseal fractures underwent nailing, two thirds retrograde and one third antegrade, based on surgeon preference. Iatrogenic fracture at the insertion point was seen in 5% of retrograde patients, a well-recognized complication of this technique. Nonunion occurred in 9% (5/57) of the retrograde group, with none in the antegrade group. Of these, the majority (4/5) was "hypotrophic" in nature, and all resolved with secondary surgery. The second primary outcome evaluated was pain and function. Overall, 6% (5/84) of patients reported significant shoulder pain. Interestingly, two of these five patients had undergone retrograde nailing. One case of elbow pain occurred in each of the groups. In terms of shoulder function, 3.7% of antegrade patients described poor function compared with 1.8% of the retrograde group. However, this advantage was lost when the 1.8% rate of poor elbow function seen in the retrograde group was added. Overall, intraoperative complications and nonunion results were greater in the retrograde group, with overall rates of pain and poor function similar in both cohorts.

EXTERNAL FIXATION OF HUMERAL SHAFT FRACTURES

No comparative studies exist to clarify the role of external in the fixation of humeral shaft fractures. This technique is currently reserved for specific clinical situations.[16] These include temporary stabilization in the polytrauma patient while awaiting improved physiologic parameters for more definitive fixation. Contaminated open fractures can be stabilized with external fixation until soft-tissue decontamination is completed by serial debridements. Fractures involving nerve or arterial injury requiring reconstruction can also benefit from external fixation for stabilization. In the nonacute setting, nonunion (whether sterile or infected) can be successfully treated with this type of fixation.[17]

RECOMMENDATIONS

Currently, the preferred treatment for isolated humeral shaft fractures continues to be nonoperative given the lack of strong evidence supporting operative care (Level V). However, outcome studies suggest that union rates and particularly patient function are not as good as historically assumed. No recommendations can be made about which type of nonoperative treatment is best in the absence of good quality comparative studies.

When indications exist for operative care of a humeral shaft fracture, open reduction and compression plating appears to be superior to intramedullary fixation with regards to rate of reoperation and shoulder impingement, but not for nonunion, infection, and iatrogenic nerve injury. As Bhandari and investigators[11] point out, these recommendations are based on a low number of patients, and larger prospective trials are necessary to draw more certain conclusions.[11]

Intramedullary nailing does appear to retain a role in segmental and pathologic fractures. In these cases, antegrade nailing is associated with fewer intraoperative complications and greater union rates than retrograde nailing.

External fixation has a definite but limited role to play in humeral shaft fracture fixation. Currently, this technique is limited to provisional fixation in open fractures and patients with multiple trauma injuries, as well as in the treatment of nonunions. Table 54–1 provides a summary of recommendations for the treatment of humeral shaft fractures.

TABLE 54–1. Summary of Recommendations for the Treatment of Humeral Shaft Fractures

ISSUE	RECOMMENDATIONS	GRADE OF RECOMMENDATION	LEVEL OF EVIDENCE	REFERENCES
1. Operative vs. nonoperative treatment	Operative care limited to indications cited in text	C	V	3, 4
2. Intramedullary nail vs. plate fixation	Plate fixation to reduce rate of reoperation and shoulder impingement	A, B	I, II	7–11
3. Antegrade vs. retrograde nailing	Antegrade to reduce rate of nonunion and intraoperative complications	C		15
4. External fixation	Indications as cited in the text	C	V	4, 16, 17

REFERENCES

1. Crolla RM, de Vries LS, Clevers GJ: Locked intramedullary nailing of humeral fractures. Injury 24:403–406, 1993.
2. Rockwood CA, Green DP, Bucholz RW (eds): Rockwood and Green's Fractures in Adults, 3rd ed. Philadelphia, JB Lippincott, 1991, p 853.
3. Bandi W: Indikation und Technik der Osteosynthese am Humerus. Helv Chir Acta 31:89–100, 1964.
4. Sarmiento A, Waddell JP, Latta LL: Diaphyseal humeral fractures: Treatment options. Instr Course Lect 51:257–269, 2002.
5. Ekholm R, Tidermark J, Tornkvist H, et al: Outcome after closed functional treatment of humeral shaft fractures. J Orthop Trauma 20:591–596, 2006.
6. Haberneck H, Orthner E: A locking nail for fractures of the humerus. J Bone Joint Surg Br 73-B:651–653, 1991.
7. Rodrigues-Merchan EC: Compression plating versus hackethal nailing in closed humeral shaft fractures failing nonoperative reduction. J Orthop Trauma 9:194–197, 1995.
8. Chiu FY, Chen CM, Lin CF, et al: Closed humeral shaft fractures: A prospective evaluation of surgical treatment. J Trauma 43:947–951, 1997.
9. McCormack RG, Brien D, Buckley RE, et al: Fixation of fractures of the shaft of the humerus by dynamic compression plate or intramedullary nail. A prospective, randomised trial. J Bone Joint Surg Br 82B:336–339, 2000.
10. Chapman JR, Henley MB, Agel J, Benca PJ: Randomized prospective study of humeral shaft fracture fixation: Intramedullary nails versus plates. J Orthop Trauma 14:162–166, 2000.
11. Bhandari M, Devereaux PJ, McKee MD, Schemitsch EH: Compression plating versus intramedullary nailing of humeral shaft fractures—a meta-analysis. Acta Orthop 77:279–284, 2006.
12. Bolano LE, Iaquinto JA, Vasicek V: Operative treatment of humerus shaft fractures: A prospective randomized study comparing intramedullary nailing with dynamic compression plating. Presented at the Annual Meeting of the American Academy of Orthopaedic Surgeons, Orlando, Florida, Feb 15–19, 1995.
13. Chapman J, Weber TG, Henley MB, Benca PJ: Randomized prospective study of humerus fixation: nails versus plates. Proceedings of the Annual Meeting of the Orthopaedic Trauma Association, Tampa Bay, Florida, Sept 29–Oct 1, 1995, pp 104–105.
14. Wagner MS, Patterson BM, Wilber JH, Sontich JK: Comparison of outcomes for humeral diaphysis fractures treated with either closed intramedullary nailing or open reduction internal fixation using a dynamic compression plate in the multiple trauma patient. Proceedings of the Annual Meeting of the Orthopaedic Trauma Association, Tampa Bay, Florida, Sept 29–Oct 1, 1995, pp 102–103.
15. Blum J, Janzing H, Gahr R, et al: Clinical performance of a new medullary humeral nail: Antegrade versus retrograde insertion. J Orthop Trauma 15:342–349, 2001.
16. Ruland WO: Is there a place for external fixation in humeral shaft fractures? Injury 31(suppl):27–34, 2000.
17. Lammens J, Bauduin G, Driesen R, et al: Treatment of nonunion of the humerus using the Ilizarov external fixator. Clin Orthop Relat Res 353:223–230, 1998.

Supracondylar Humeral Fractures:
Is Open Reduction and Internal Fixation or Primary Total Elbow Arthroplasty Better in Poor Quality Bone?

MICHAEL D. MCKEE, MD, FRCS(C)

In young patients, open reduction and internal fixation (ORIF) with double-plate fixation is the gold standard for displaced intra-articular fractures of the distal humerus, regardless of comminution.[1] This procedure, however, can be technically challenging even when excellent bone quality is present, and elbow stiffness, malunion, nonunion, failure of fixation, and ulnar neuropathy are common sequelae.[1] In elderly patients, the complication rate is increased because of osteoporotic bone, metaphyseal comminution, poor soft-tissue quality, and limited tolerance for joint immobilization; this is important because although distal humeral fractures represent only a small proportion of adult upper extremity fractures, the incidence of osteoporotic fractures of the distal humerus is increasing.[1,2] According to the Finnish National Hospital Discharge Register, the current trend in the number and incidence of osteoporotic fractures of the distal humerus in Finnish women aged 60 or older is increasing rapidly.[3] The annual incidence of these types of fractures has escalated from 11 per 100,000 in 1970 to 30 per 100,000 in 1995 and 2000; the increase is greatest in the oldest age group (women > 80 years) where the age-specific incidence rates showed a nine-fold increase (8 in 1970 vs. 75 in 2000). These results (which reflect trends seen in Europe and North America) reinforce the need to identify the optimal type of treatment for comminuted distal humeral fractures in the elderly to reduce the risk for reoperation and maximize functional outcome and independence. It should also be pointed out that, in most studies on this topic, women predominate in a 5:1 or 6:1 ratio.

OPTIONS

The three main options available for dealing with displaced intra-articular fractures of the distal humerus are as follows: (1) conventional ORIF; (2) total elbow arthroplasty (TEA); and (3) nonoperative care, or the "bag of bones" technique. This chapter concentrates on the first two options. The third is considered of historical interest only and is reserved for undisplaced fractures or injuries in patients with dementia or those incapable of receiving an anesthetic.

When discussing results, it is important to recognize the distinction between different types of supracondylar humeral fracture: AO type "A," an extra-articular or transcondylar fracture; AO type "B," or partial articular fracture affecting one column only; and AO type "C," or complete articular fracture with an intrinsically poor prognosis.

Although semiconstrained TEA has been recognized as a standard treatment for the complications or failure of primary ORIF of intra-articular distal humeral fractures,[4,5] the role of primary TEA in the setting of acute supracondylar humeral fracture is more controversial. Although the advantages are obvious, including immediate stability and enhanced rehabilitation, no requirement for bone grafting or concern for delayed or nonunion, and possibly shorter operative times, the longevity of the prosthesis in the increasingly active elderly population remains a concern. In a landmark study, Cobb and Morrey[6] report a series of 21 elderly patients (mean age, 72 years) who had primary TEA for comminuted fractures of the distal humerus and described a 95% good or excellent result rate at a mean follow-up of 3.3 years with a reoperation rate of 5% (one elbow).[6] Several other similar single-institution reviews have described remarkably similar results in smaller series.[7–11] More recently, Frankle and colleagues[12] performed a retrospective comparison of ORIF with TEA, and the Canadian Orthopaedic Trauma Society (COTS)[13] conducted a randomized clinical trial comparing these two treatment methods in older individuals. Although there is now an increasing amount of data to guide the clinician in decision making for elderly patients with intrinsically poor bone quality who sustain an intra-articular fracture of the distal humerus, it must be emphasized that this is a technique restricted to older patients and is contraindicated for patients younger than 65 years unless there are special circumstances (i.e., preexisting elbow arthritis).

EVIDENCE

Outcome after Open Reduction and Internal Fixation

Although there is substantial evidence for the benefits of ORIF in younger patients with fractures of the distal humerus,[1,2] the evidence is less clear in older patients because only retrospective studies with small numbers have been reported (Table 55–1).[14–19] Several of these studies have suggested that the majority of elderly patients achieve good or excellent functional results with ORIF; however, critical analysis of these results indicates a large variability in outcome and less predictable results than optimal.

Huang and coauthors[14] report on 19 patients with a mean age of 72 years who required ORIF for AO type "C" distal humeral fractures. They describe good results with no hardware failures, a mean range of flexion-extension from 17 to 128 degrees, with 15 excellent and 4 good results (according to the Mayo elbow score). Imatani and coworkers[15] describe a technique in the Japanese population of using a small AO "T" plate for fixation of transcondylar fractures with good or excellent results in 14 of 17 patients older than 70 years. However, these "A"-type extra-articular fractures were not the more severe intra-articular injuries typically seen; results are usually worse in the "C"-type injuries. Srinivasan and researchers[16] report their results of treatment with ORIF for "C"-type fractures in 21 patients with a mean age of 85 years (range, 75–100 years) and found 43% fair or poor outcomes. Korner and investigators[17] report on the outcome of 45 patients with a median age of 73 years (range, 61–92 years) and a minimum follow-up of 2 years. Overall, 19 patients (42%) had a fair or poor outcome according to the Mayo elbow score. Fourteen of these patients (74%) had an AO/OTA type C fracture. In the subset of 29 patients with AO/OTA type C fractures, only 45% had an excellent or good outcome.[17] Postoperative complications were recorded in 13 patients (29%), and revision surgery was required in 7 patients. Pereles and colleagues[18] report more favorable results in 14 patients with a mean age of 71 years (mean Mayo elbow score, 89 points). John and coauthors[19] reviewed the results of 49 patients with an average age of 80 years (range, 75–93 years) treated with ORIF of the distal humerus after a mean of 18 months.[5] Twenty-eight fractures (57%) were classified as AO/OTA type C. Fair and poor functional results were observed

in 26% of patients with an overall complication rate of 18%.[19] Clearly, the results of ORIF for this type of fracture in the elderly do not match those seen for younger patients, especially for the more severe C-type fractures, and there is significant room for improvement.

Outcome after Total Elbow Arthroplasty

Several studies suggest that semiconstrained TEA may have a role to play in the primary treatment of severe intra-articular distal humeral fractures (Table 55–2). Cobb and Morrey[6] reported in 1997 their initial experience of primary TEA in 20 patients (21 elbows) with a mean age of 72 years (range, 48–92 years) and a mean follow-up of 3.3 years. A follow-up report on 43 patients was published in 2004 that revealed similar results. The mean flexion-extension arc was 24 to 131 degrees, and the mean Mayo elbow score was 93 points. Mean follow-up had increased to 7 years, although 9 elbows had required a total of 10 additional procedures, ranging from simple hematoma evacuation to revision arthroplasty for infection.[20] Gambirasio and coworkers[9] report the functional outcome at a minimum of 1 year for 10 women (mean age, 85 years) treated with primary TEA for a comminuted, intra-articular distal humeral fracture. Eight patients had an excellent outcome and two had a good outcome based on the Mayo elbow score.[9] Garcia and colleagues[10] evaluated 16 patients with a mean age of 73 years (range, 61–95 years) treated by primary TEA using the Coonrad–Morrey prosthesis at a mean follow-up period of 3 years (range, 1.5–5 years). No patients had inflammatory or degenerative arthritis of the elbow. OTA type C3 fractures were present in 11 patients. The mean DASH (a patient-based disability score) was 23 (range, 1–63), and the mean Mayo elbow score was 93 (range, 80–100).

Ray and colleagues[7] describe good results in seven elderly (mean age, 82 years) women treated with semiconstrained arthroplasty for intra-articular dis-

TABLE 55–1. Results of Open Reduction and Internal Fixation for Distal Humeral Fractures in Elderly Patients

AUTHOR (YEAR OF PUBLICATION)	PATIENTS (N)/MEAN AGE	MEAN ROM (DEGREES, FLEXION/EXTENSION)	MEAN MAYO ELBOW SCORE	COMMENTS
Huang et al. (2005)[14]	19/72 yr	111	15 E, 4 G	No nonunions
Imatani et al. (2005)[15]	17/all 70+ yr	Unknown	3 E, 11 G, 3 F	Transcondylar fractures
Srinivasan et al. (2005)[16]	28/85 yr	76	3 E, 9 G, 7 F, 2 P	43% "C"-type fair or poor
Pereles et al. (1997)[18]	14/71 yr	112	89 mean	2 patients lost fixation
John et al. (1993)[19]	49/80 yr	Unknown	89 mean	34% still had pain
Korner et al. (2005)[17]	45/73 yr	Unknown	Most good/excellent	55% "C"-type fair or poor
Frankle et al. (2003)[12]	12/74 yr	100	81 mean (excludes 3 failures)	3 required conversion to TEA
COTS and McKee (2007)[13]	15/77 yr	95	73	RCT: 5 patients converted intraoperatively to TEA from ORIF

COTS, Canadian Orthopaedic Trauma Society; E, excellent; F, fair; G, good; ORIF, open reduction and internal fixation; P, poor; RCT, randomized, controlled trial; ROM, range of motion; TEA, total elbow arthroplasty.

tal humeral fractures.[7] The mean range of motion was 20 to 130 degrees, and there were five excellent and one good results according to the Mayo elbow score. Lee and researchers[11] report nearly identical results in seven elderly Asian women (mean age, 73 years).[11]

Comparative Studies

In one of the few comparative studies, Frankle and colleagues[12] compared primary TEA versus ORIF for the treatment of distal humeral fractures in women older than 65 years (all comminuted type C fractures) (Table 55–3). They found that in the 12 patients in the TEA group, 11 had excellent results and 1 had good results; no fair and no poor results were reported.[12] Notably, eight patients (67%) had associated rheumatoid arthritis. Three patients (25%) required subsequent operations, one to reconnect an uncoupled prosthesis, one to drain a postoperative hematoma, and one to débride a su-

perficial infection. All of these complications resolved without subsequent sequelae, and no patient required revision implant surgery. The ORIF group had four excellent, four good, one fair and three poor results. The poor results were all salvaged by conversion to TEA (a difficult procedure with a high complication rate). The authors recommend primary TEA as a viable alternative in type C fractures of the distal humerus in elderly patients, especially in the setting of associated comorbidity such as rheumatoid arthritis, osteoporosis, and systemic steroid use.

In a study that has been presented at the 2007 Annual American Academy of Orthopedic Surgeons (AAOS) Meeting (*J Shoulder Elbow Surg*, accepted) the COTS randomized 42 elderly patients (mean age, 78 years) with comminuted intra-articular distal humeral fractures to either semiconstrained TEA (Coonrad–Morrey prosthesis) or conventional ORIF (two small fragment plates).[13] Twenty-one patients were randomized to each group: one patient in each group died, and five patients randomized to ORIF had to be

TABLE 55–2. Results of Total Elbow Arthroplasty for Distal Humeral Fractures in Elderly Patients

AUTHOR (YEAR OF PUBLICATION)	PATIENTS *(N)*/MEAN AGE	MEAN ROM (DEGREES, FLEXION/EXTENSION)	MEAN MAYO ELBOW SCORE	COMMENTS
Ray et al. (2000)[7]	7/82 yr	110	5 E, 2 G	No reoperations
Adolfsson and Hammer (2006)[8]	4/80 yr	Unknown	3 E, 1 G	Hemiarthroplasty
Lee et al. (2006)[11]	7/73 yr	89	94	Asian population
Garcia et al. (2002)[10]	19/73 yr	101	93	No reoperations, no loosening
Gambirasio et al. (2001)[9]	10/85 yr	102	94	No reoperations or loosening
Frankle et al. (2003)[12]	12/72 yr	110	95	TEA had shorter operative time, hospital stay
Kamineni and Morrey (2004)[20]	43/69 yr	107	93	5 revision TEA required at mean follow-up of 7 years
COTS and McKee (2007)[13]	25/78 yr	107	86	RCT with 5 intraoperative crossovers from ORIF to TEA

COTS, Canadian Orthopaedic Trauma Society; E, excellent; G, good; ORIF, open reduction and internal fixation; RCT, randomized, controlled trial; ROM, range of motion; TEA, total elbow arthroplasty.

TABLE 55–3. Comparative Studies

AUTHOR (YEAR OF PUBLICATION)	PATIENTS *(N)*	MEAN DURATION OF FOLLOW-UP	FUNCTIONAL OUTCOME	COMMENTS
Frankle et al. (2003)[12]	12 ORIF (mean age, 74), 12 TEA (mean age, 72)	ORIF: 57 mo TEA: 45 mo	Mean Mayo elbow score: ORIF 81, TEA 95 (NS)	ORIF: 3 late conversions to TEA TEA: 8 had RA, 3 reoperations (infection, hematoma, uncoupled prosthesis)
COTS and McKee (2007)[13]	21 in each group (mean age, 78)	24 mo	DASH at 6 months: ORIF 77, TEA 43 ($P = 0.02$), 1 yr NS* Mean Mayo elbow score at 6, 12, and 24 months: ORIF 73, TEA 86 ($P = 0.02$)*	5 immediate failures of ORIF; 4 additional reoperations; TEA 3 reoperations

*Crossovers not analyzed by intention to treat.
COTS, Canadian Orthopaedic Trauma Society; DASH, disability of the arm, shoulder, and hand; NS, not significant; ORIF, open reduction and internal fixation; RA, rheumatoid arthritis; TEA, total elbow arthroplasty.

converted to TEA during surgery because of the inability to stably fix the fracture. This was anticipated and allowed as part of the study protocol. This left 25 patients in the TEA group and 15 patients in the ORIF group for evaluation. Despite the fact that the TEA group theoretically had worse injuries (by inclusion of the five most severe cases from the ORIF group), they had superior outcome, especially early. At 6 months, the mean DASH score in the TEA group was 43 versus 77 in the ORIF group ($P = 0.02$), although this difference was not statistically significant at 1 year (TEA vs. ORIF: 32 vs. 47; $P = 0.10$). The Mayo elbow scores were better in the TEA group at 6, 12, and 24 months (TEA vs. ORIF: 86 vs. 73, $P = 0.015$). The reoperation rate was not statistically different (TEA vs. ORIF: 3/25 [12%] vs. 4/15 [27%]; $P = 0.20$), although it must be remembered the TEA group included five patients who did not respond successfully to operative fixation. The authors' conclusion was that TEA improved functional outcome compared with ORIF for these difficult fractures, and this was the treatment of choice, especially when comminuted, osteoporotic bone made fixation technically difficult. However, to date, only short-term results (2 years) are available, and these patients will require longer follow-up before establishing the ultimate superiority of replacement arthroplasty in this population.

AREAS OF CONTROVERSEY

Length of Follow-up

Prosthetic longevity is a significant concern whenever arthroplasty is used as a treatment for fracture. The mean life expectancy for a healthy North American woman aged 70 years is 15 more years. This is an important fact to remember, especially when one considers the increasingly active lifestyles (golf, tennis, etc.) of the modern retired population, and the increased demands that the prosthesis may experience. The majority of reports describing TEA for severe distal humeral fracture have follow-up that at best can be described as short term (2–5 years). The longest follow-up period in the literature is from Kamineni and Morrey's[20] 2004 article, averaging 7 years.[20] They describe five patients who required a revision arthroplasty; only one patient required revision in their original 1997 report that had a mean follow-up period of just more than 3 years. It is reasonable to assume that with longer follow-up more TEA patients will require revision. This emphasizes the fact that this procedure should be restricted to older (≥70 years) patients, and that a more sedentary lifestyle or at least some physical restrictions on elbow use is preferred.

Effect of Condylar Resection

The use of semiconstrained TEA for comminuted fractures of the distal humerus typically requires resection of the fracture fragments, which include the humeral condyles. Because the condyles serve as origin for the collateral ligaments, the common extensor origin and flexor-pronator mass, their resection could have a detrimental effect on a number of functions, including elbow stability and forearm and hand strength. McKee and coworkers'[21] study examined the effect of condylar resection by comparing 16 total elbow arthroplasties with intact condyles versus 16 with resected or absent condyles.[21] Comparing strength to the opposite normal arm in each patient, the authors found no difference in objectively measured hand, forearm, or elbow strength. Mayo elbow scores were also similar between the two groups (intact: 79; resected: 77), suggesting that practically, condylar resection did not have a clinically relevant effect on strength. It is important to note, however, that this study did not address the question of stability and longevity of the prosthesis after condylar resection.

Hemiarthroplasty versus Total Elbow Arthroplasty

Conventional wisdom dictates that the treatment of a severe distal humeral fracture by arthroplasty requires a semiconstrained total joint prosthesis to provide immediate stability and allow early motion. However, this mandates resection of a (usually normal) ulnar articulation, which may not be necessary. Some have advocated replacement of the fractured distal humerus alone with a hemiarthroplasty, in conjunction with a ligament repair or reconstruction. Adolfsson and Hammer[8] provide a preliminary report on four elderly (mean age, 80 years) female patients with an unreconstructable distal humeral fracture treated with distal humeral hemiarthroplasty. The described excellent results in three and a good result in one. Although this technique has promise and does make some sense on a theoretical level (only replacing what is broken, potentially better longevity of the prosthesis), it should be considered experimental at the present time until further data are available.

Open Fractures of the Distal Humerus

Infection is a devastating complication for patients with an implanted elbow arthroplasty, and it should be avoided at all costs. For this reason, the presence of an open wound has been considered a relative, if not absolute, contraindication to TEA after supracondylar humeral fracture. However, although there is no specific article on this topic, some information is available that suggests it may be reasonable to perform primary TEA in the presence of an open wound. It is a question of some relevance because the fractures with an open wound tend to be of the more severe variety that makes ORIF difficult or impossible. Kamineni and Morrey[20] describe two patients with grade I open wounds treated with immediate debridement and arthroplasty, and neither became infected; the COTS study had three similar cases treated in the same fashion, and none suffered any infectious complications.[13]

Although it appears that primary TEA in the presence of a grade I wound may be safe, it is important to emphasize proper technique. First, all the above cases were treated within 12 hours of injury: It may be prudent to temporize with patients presenting late for treatment. Second, the open wound tends to be posterior and is made as the condyles break away as the elbow hits the ground and the distal humeral shaft drives through the soft tissue and skin to impact the ground. Thus, although a thorough debridement and copious irrigation of the entire wound tract is mandatory, careful attention must be given to debriding and cleaning the distal humeral shaft and associated intramedullary canal, and antibiotics should be added to the cement.

RECOMMENDATIONS

Displaced intra-articular fractures of the distal humerus in elderly patients with osteoporosis are best treated surgically: Nonoperative treatment is reserved for those too demented to comply with a rehabilitation program or benefit from the functional improvement surgery provides, or those too medically unwell to receive an anaesthetic. Unfortunately, there is a paucity of high-quality (Level I or II) studies to use to decide whether ORIF or TEA is superior for those who do qualify for surgical intervention. However, relying on what studies are available, some general guidelines are applicable:

Grade C: TEA is reserved for those patients 65 years or older. Given the average longevity of the prosthesis in most retrospective series, and the loosening rate in comparative studies, this should be considered an absolute minimum age for considering TEA. All younger patients should have ORIF unless there are extenuating circumstances such as preexisting arthritic change or diminished life expectancy.

Grade C: TEA should be reserved for complex, multifragmentary, intra-articular fractures (types C2 and C3). Generally favorable results are reported for ORIF of the more simple fracture patterns, and all comparative studies exclude simple (A, B, simple C) fracture types. Given the techniques and implants currently available[22] (anatomic, precontoured plates, locking plates, etc.), ORIF should be feasible for most extra-articular (type A), partial articular (type B), and simple (C1) fractures.

Grade C: Some evidence exists that primary TEA is an option for fractures associated with grade I open wounds, if certain conditions are met. These include a grade I or II open wound without extensive contamination, operative intervention within 12 hours of injury, and extensive irrigation and debridement with proper technique (see earlier).

Grade B: Good quality evidence has been reported from one randomized multicenter trial (COTS study) and one comparative study (Frankle and colleagues[12]) that TEA is superior, at least in the short to mid term, to ORIF in the treatment of complex, multifragmentary, intra-articular fractures of the distal humerus (C, C3 types), especially when the surgeon is unable to restore articular congruity or obtain stable fixation such that early motion is feasible.[12,20] TEA in this setting provides shorter rehabilitation and improved function, and decreases the need for revision to secondary TEA. Both prospective studies and retrospective reviews from multiple centers describe consistently good results with this technique (see Table 55–2) including a Mayo elbow score between 90 and 95 points, a flexion/extension arc of 100 to 110 degrees, and a reoperation rate of 5% to 10%.

SUMMARY

Most of the literature on this topic consists of case series and retrospective reviews that describe the experience of single centers. Although there are some recent prospective and comparative studies, more high-quality studies are required before definitive statements can be made regarding ideal treatment methods. It must be remembered that with the techniques and implants currently available, ORIF remains the treatment of choice for the majority of these fractures including anyone younger than 65 to 70 years, extra-articular or partial-articular fractures, and simple-pattern complete articular fractures. In the setting of a complex, intra-articular fracture not amenable to stable fixation in an elderly (≥70 years) patient with osteoporosis, TEA has been shown to have significant advantages in terms of quicker rehabilitation, improved function, and a lower catastrophic failure rate compared with ORIF. Table 55–4 provides a summary of recommendations.

TABLE 55–4. Summary of Recommendations

RECOMMENDATION	LEVEL OF EVIDENCE/ GRADE OF RECOMMENDATION
1. ORIF is preferred for young healthy patients with good bone quality.	C
2. ORIF is preferred for all simple fracture patterns (AO types A and B).	C
3. TEA is preferred in older patients with osteoporotic bone and type C fractures.	B
4. TEA is safe in the presence of a type I or II open fracture.	C

ORIF, open reduction and internal fixation; TEA, total elbow arthroplasty.

REFERENCES

1. McKee MD, Jupiter JB: Fractures of the distal humerus. Browner B, Jupiter J, Levine A, Trafton P (eds): Skeletal Trauma, 3rd ed. Philadelphia, Lippincott, 2002, pp 765–782.
2. Sodergard J, Sandelin J, Bostman O: Postoperative complications of distal humeral fractures. 27/96 adults followed up for 6 (2-10) years. Acta Orthop Scand 63:85–89, 1992.
3. Palvanen M, Kannus P, Niemi S, Parkkari J: Secular trends in the osteoporotic fractures of the distal humerus in elderly women. Eur J Epidemiol 14:159–164, 1998.
4. Morrey BF, Adams RA: Semiconstrained elbow replacement for distal humeral nonunion. J Bone Joint Surg Br 77:67–72, 1995.
5. Morrey BF, Adams RA, Bryan RS: Total replacement for post-traumatic arthritis of the elbow. J Bone Joint Surg Br 73:607–612, 1991.
6. Cobb TK, Morrey BF: Total elbow arthroplasty as primary treatment for distal humeral fractures in elderly patients. J Bone Joint Surg Am 79:826–832, 1997.
7. Ray PS, Kakarlapudi K, Rajsejhar C, Bhamra MS: Total elbow arthroplasty as primary treatment for distal humeral fractures in elderly patients. Injury 31:687–692, 2000.
8. Adolfsson L, Hammer R: Elbow hemiarthroplasty for acute reconstruction of intra-articular distal humerus fractures. Acta Orthop 77:785–787, 2006.
9. Gambirasio R, Riand N, Stern R, Hoffmeyer P: Total elbow replacement for complex fractures of the distal humerus. An option for the elderly patient. J Bone Joint Surg Br 83:974–978, 2001.
10. Garcia JA, Mykula R, Stanley D: Complex fractures of the distal humerus in the elderly. The role of total elbow replacement as primary treatment. J Bone Joint Surg Br 84:812–816, 2002.
11. Lee KT, Lai CH, Singh S: Results of total elbow arthroplasty in the treatment of distal humeral fractures in elderly Asian patients. J Trauma 61:889–892, 2006.
12. Frankle MA, Herscovici D Jr, DiPasquale TG, et al: A comparison of open reduction and internal fixation and primary total elbow arthroplasty in the treatment of intraarticular distal humerus fractures in women older than age 65. J Orthop Trauma 17:473–480, 2003.
13. Canadian Orthopaedic Trauma Society, McKee MD: A multi-center prospective randomized controlled trial of ORIF versus TEA for displaced intra-articular distal humeral fractures in elderly patients. Proceedings of the 2007 AAOS.
14. Huang TL, Chiu FY, Chuang TY, Chen TH: The results of open reduction and internal fixation in elderly patients with severe fractures of the distal humerus: A critical analysis of the results. J Trauma 58:62–69, 2005.
15. Imatani J, Ogura T, Morito Y, et al: Custom AO small T plate for transcondylar fractures of the distal humerus in the elderly. J Shoulder Elbow Surg 14:611–615, 2005.
16. Srinivasan K, Agarwal M, Matthews SJ, Giannoudis PV: Fractures of the distal humerus in the elderly: Is internal fixation the treatment of choice? Clin Orthop Relat Res (434):222–230, 2005.
17. Korner J, Lill H, Muller LP, et al: Distal humerus fractures in elderly patients: Results after open reduction and internal fixation. Osteoporos Int 16(suppl 2):S73–S79, 2005.
18. Pereles TR, Koval KJ, Gallagher M, Rosen H: Open reduction and internal fixation of the distal humerus: Functional outcome in the elderly. J Trauma 43:578–584, 1997.
19. John H, Rosso R, Neff U, et al: Distal humerus fractures in patients over 75 years of age. Long-term results of osteosynthesis. Helv Chir Acta 60(1-2):219–224, 1993.
20. Kamineni S, Morrey BF: Distal humeral fractures treated with noncustom total elbow replacement. J Bone Joint Surg Am 86A:940–947, 2004.
21. McKee MD, Pugh DM, Richards RR, et al: Effect of humeral condylar resection on strength and functional outcome after semiconstrained total elbow arthroplasty. J Bone Joint Surg Am 85-A(5):802–807, 2003.
22. Korner J, Diederichs G, Arzdorf M, et al: A biomechanical evaluation of methods of distal humerus fracture fixation using locking compression plates versus conventional reconstruction plates. J Orthop Trauma 18:286–293, 2004.

Chapter 56

Acetabular Fractures:
Does Delay to Surgery Influence Outcome?

RICHARD J. JENKINSON, MD, FRCSC, MARCELLA MAATHUIS, HANS J. KREDER, MD, MPH, FRCSC, AND DAVID J. G. STEPHEN, MD, FRCS(C)

Fractures of the acetabulum can be devastating injuries often associated with high-energy trauma. Patient outcome is adversely affected by many factors, some of which cannot be influenced by the treating surgeon. These include age, osteoporosis, obesity, and associated injuries. The fracture pattern and severity, as well as specific prognostic features such as marginal impaction and femoral head damage are also outside of the surgeon's control. However, the surgeon is able to influence factors such as the timing of surgery, choice of approach, accuracy of reduction, and the maintenance of that reduction.[1,2]

Historically, acetabular fractures were treated with traction and other nonoperative techniques. However, modern treatment now involves operative reduction and fixation of the acetabulum in most cases.[3] Acetabular fractures are classified as either elementary fractures involving one fracture line or associated fractures involving multiple fracture elements.[4,5] Anatomic reduction has been consistently identified as an important prognostic indicator of a good clinical outcome in acetabular fractures.[5–11]

Acetabular fracture surgery is demanding and requires a specialized surgeon and team (Level V). Surgical treatment strategies often involve partial fracture exposure and reduction via indirect means because of anatomic constraints of the pelvis. These indirect reduction strategies rely on mobility between the fracture fragments especially when treating associated fracture types. As the fracture begins to heal, organized hematoma and callus can interfere with fracture mobility. This decreased mobility makes anatomic reduction difficult, allowing imperfect reductions to become more prevalent.[9,10,12] A strategy to deal with decreased fracture mobility involves the use of more direct fracture reduction techniques; however, this often requires multiple or extensile exposures with their associated morbidity.[13–15]

The reasons for delay to treatment can vary from patient to patient. In some cases, the patient's traumatic or medical comorbidities may necessitate a delay until the patient is suitable for prolonged surgery. Availability of specialized surgeons and surgical resources can also be a cause for delay. In some medical systems, shortage of hospital bed resources can significantly delay transfer to specialized centers.[16] Few surgeons will argue that treatment of these injuries should be excessively delayed. The purpose of this chapter is to guide clinicians using the best available evidence as to the optimal timing for surgery and to evaluate the evidence regarding a potential threshold beyond which further delay to surgery adversely affects outcome.

EVIDENCE

Delay to surgery is mentioned as a contributing factor influencing outcome in several studies summarized in Table 56–1.[9,10,12,13,17–20] These studies are retrospective in design and usually originate from a single center. Most of these studies are small and do not achieve statistical significance.[9,13,17–20] However, they consistently note a trend of delay to surgery being associated with less favorable radiographic or functional outcome.

A retrospective review from Mears and researchers[10] catalogues their experience treating 411 patients with acetabular fractures (Level III). This study used Harris hip scores for functional outcomes and radiographs to measure postsurgical reduction. The authors identified several factors associated with poor outcome including articular impaction/abrasion, concomitant femoral neck fracture, elderly age, obesity, osteoporosis, and extensile exposure. The most important variable they identified was the quality of reduction. Time to surgery was categorized by the authors as before 3 days, 3 to 10 days, and 11 or more days. They found the rate of anatomic reduction to be decreased from 70% in those operated on within 10 days to 54% in the group receiving surgery after a delay of 11 days or more ($P = 0.002$). Matta,[9] using similar methods, retrospectively reported his experience with 259 patients with acetabular fracture (Level III). Results were similar, identifying quality of reduction as a major indicator of outcome. In Matta's[9] study, delay to surgery was associated with a trend to poorer reduction after a delay of greater than 14 days ($P = 0.06$). Time categories in both studies are arbitrary. Neither study specifically examined the effect of delay on clinical outcome, and instead used rate of anatomic reduction as a proxy indicator.

TABLE 56–1. Summary of Literature Examining Delay to Fixation of Acetabular Fractures

REFERENCE (YEAR OF PUBLICATION)	NO. OF PATIENTS	RADIOGRAPHIC OUTCOME	CLINICAL OUTCOME	COMMENTS
Brueton et al. (1993)[17]	40 patients	Not reported	Good results: average delay of 11 days; poor results: average delay of 17 days	Low numbers, not statistically significant
Johnson et al. (1994)[13]	207 patients all with delay greater than 21 days	Lower rate of anatomic reductions than authors' other studies	Lower rate of good/excellent results and greater complication rate than authors' previous studies	Heterogeneous group including malunions; historic controls only
Matta (1996)[9]	259 patients	Greater rates of anatomic reduction if surgery before 14 days ($P = 0.06$)	Effect of delay not reported	Not statistically significant
Plasier et al. (2000)[19]	59 patients	Not reported	Early acetabular surgery associated with decreased hospital stay, increased rate of discharge to home, and lower rate of multiorgan dysfunction syndrome	Low numbers, no long-term follow-up, no functional outcome, associations with tenuous causal link
Deo et al. (2001)[18]	74 patients	Not reported	Of patients with good/excellent outcome: 91% had surgery within 14 days; of patients with fair/poor outcome, only 78% had surgery within 14 days	No P value reported
Mears et al. (2003)[10]	411 patients	Rate of anatomic reductions lower (70% vs. 54%) after delay of 11 days ($P = 0.002$)	Effect of delay not reported	Arbitrary time categories, no functional outcomes
Kumar et al. (2005)[20]	73 patients	Not reported	Higher Harris hip scores in group treated before 14 days	Not statistically significant
Madhu et al. (2006)[12]	237 patients	Odds of anatomic reduction declines by 18% per day. For elementary fractures: anatomic reduction less likely after 15 days. For associated fractures: anatomic reduction less likely after 5 days	Good/excellent results 15–19% less likely per day of delay. For elementary fractures: good/excellent result less likely after 15 days. For associated fractures: good/excellent results less likely after 10 days	

Johnson and coworkers[13] conducted a multicenter review of acetabular fractures treated between 21 and 120 days after injury. These represented extreme delays, with many fractures actually being intra-articular malunions. This article compared their results with historic controls only (Level IV). Their reported rate of 57% anatomic reductions and 65% good and excellent clinical results is lower than reported in other studies but impressive considering the nature of these injuries. This article, however, also notes a need for extensile exposures in 33.2% of the patients and significantly greater complication rates including infection (4%), heterotopic ossification (11%), sciatic nerve palsy (10.6%), osteonecrosis (13.8%), and osteoarthritis (24%).

An article from Madhu and coauthors[12] specifically analyzed the effect of delay on outcomes of acetabular fractures (Level IV). This is a retrospective study of 254 patients from a teaching center in the United Kingdom. The authors analyzed the effect of delay to surgery on radiologic and clinical outcomes in elementary and associated fracture types. Radiologic outcomes were based on radiographs, with an anatomic reduction defined as no articular step and a gap of 2 mm or less. Functional results were compiled based on Merle d'Aubigne and Postel's[21] system. Rates of anatomic reductions and good/excellent functional outcomes decreased significantly with increased surgical delay. When analyzed as a continuous variable, the odds of obtaining an anatomic reduction or a good/excellent functional outcome declined by between 15% and 19% per day of delay ($P < 0.01$). As a categoric variable, the authors demonstrate a significant decrease in both functional and radiographic results for elementary fractures after 15 days of delay. For associated fractures, radiologic results declined after 5 days, whereas functional results decreased after 10 days. Complication rates showed a trend to increase with surgical delay, but this did not reach statistical significance in this study.

AREAS OF CONTROVERSY AND UNCERTAINTY

The literature involving acetabular fractures generally consists of retrospective reviews of variable size usually from single institutions. Mears and researchers'[9]

and Matta's[10] large reviews support accuracy of reduction as an important predictor of outcome. They suggest delay to surgery decreases anatomic reduction rates; however, they do not associate delay directly with functional outcome. Madhu and coauthors'[12] review specifically analyzes delay to surgery and has several strengths including large numbers, high rates of follow-up, and convincing statistics. However, each of these studies suffers from similar limitations of retrospective design with a lack of blind assessment of radiographs and functional outcomes. The functional outcome measures used by each study include Harris hip scores and Merle d'Aubigne–Postel scores. These are older, nonvalidated scoring systems.

Many trauma systems suffer from scarcity of surgical and other patient care resources. This is identified by some authors as a source of delay.[16] It would be helpful for resource management and triage to identify a threshold where delay begins to threaten chances of obtaining good clinical results. This threshold cannot definitively be stated based on the current literature. However, Madhu and coauthors'[12] study shows a decrease of between 15% and 19% in the odds of a good radiographic or clinical result for every day of delay. For elementary fractures, clinical scores significantly decreased after 15 days, whereas associated types decreased after 10 days.

Ideally, these questions could be answered by randomized, controlled trials. Unfortunately, patients cannot ethically be randomized to unnecessary delay. As a result, future studies examining delay to surgery should include prospective studies with modern observational design using validated outcome measurement tools.

RECOMMENDATIONS

Table 56–2 provides a summary of recommendations for the treatment of acetabular fractures.

TABLE 56–2. Summary of Recommendationos

RECOMMENDATIONS	LEVEL OF EVIDENCE/GRADE OF RECOMMENDATION
1. Acetabular fractures requiring open reduction and internal fixation should be treated as soon possible after the patient is stabilized for surgery.	C
2. Results of open reduction and internal fixation of acetabular fractures deteriorate with increasing delay to surgery. Clinically significant changes may occur after 15 days for elementary fractures and 10 days for associated fractures.	C
3. Extreme delay past 21 days decreases functional and radiographic results, increases need for extensile exposures, and increases complication rates.	C

REFERENCES

1. Letournel E, Judet R: Fractures of the Acetabulum, 2nd ed. New York, Springer Verlag, 1993.
2. Tile M, Helfet DL, Kellam JF: Fractures of the Pelvis and Acetabulum, 3rd ed. Philadelphia, Lippincott Williams & Wilkins, 2003.
3. Giannoudis PV, Grotz MR, Papakostidis C, Dinopoulos H: Operative treatment of fractures of the acetabulum: A meta-analysis. J Bone Joint Surg Br 87-B:2–9, 2005.
4. Judet R, Judet J, Letournel E: Fractures of the acetabulum: Classification and surgical approaches for open reduction-a preliminary report. J Bone Joint Surg Am 46A:1615–1646, 1964.
5. Letournel E: Acetabulum fractures: Classification and management. Clin Orthop 151:81–106, 1980.
6. Chiu FY, Chen CM, Lo WH: Surgical treatment of displaced acetabular fractures. 72 cases followed for 10(6-14) years. Injury 31:181–185, 2000.
7. Cole JD, Bolhoffner BR: Acetabular fracture fixation via a modified Stoppa limited intra-pelvic approach: Description of operative technique and preliminary treatment results. Clin Orthop 305:112–123, 1994.
8. Moed BR, Wilson Carr SE, Watson JT: Results of treatment of posterior wall fractures of the acetabulum. J Bone Joint Surg Am 84-A:752–758, 2002.
9. Matta JM: Fractures of the acetabulum: Accuracy of reduction and clinical results in patients managed within 3 weeks after the injury. J Bone Joint Surg Am 78:1632–1645, 1996.
10. Mears DC, Velyvis JH, Chang CP: Displaced acetabular fractures managed operatively: Indicators of outcome. Clin Orthop 407:173–186, 2003.
11. Kreder HJ, Rozen N, Borkhoff CM, et al: Determinants of functional outcome after simple and complex acetabular fractures involving the posterior wall. J Bone Joint Surg Br 88:776–782, 2006.
12. Madhu R, Kotnis R, Al-Mousawi A, et al: Outcome of surgery for reconstruction of the acetabulum: The time dependant effect of delay. J Bone Joint Surg Br 88:1197–1203, 2006.
13. Johnson EE, Matta JM, Mast JW, Letournel E: Delayed reconstruction of acetabular fractures 21-120 days following injury. Clin Orthop 305:20–33, 2004.
14. Routt ML Jr, Swiontkowski MF: Operative treatment of complex acetabular: Combined anterior and posterior exposures during the same procedure. J Bone Joint Surg Am 72-A:897–904, 1990.
15. Griffin DB, Beaule PE, Matta JM: Safety and efficacy of the extended iliofemoral approach in the treatment of complex fractures of the acetabulum. J Bone Joint Surg Br 87: 1391–1396, 2005.
16. Bircher M, Giannoudis PV: Pelvic trauma management within the UK: Reflection on a failing trauma service. Injury 35:2–6, 2004.
17. Brueton RN: A review of 40 acetabular fractures: The importance of early surgery. Injury 24:171–174, 1993.
18. Deo SD, Tavares SP, Pandey RK, et al: Operative management of acetabular fractures in Oxford. Injury 32:581–586, 2001.
19. Plasier BR, Meldon SW, Super DM, Malangoni MA: Improved outcome after early fixation of acetabular fractures. Injury 31:81–84, 2000.
20. Kumar A, Shah NA, Kershaw SA, Clayson AD: Operative management of acetabular fractures: A review of 73 fractures. Injury 36:605–612, 2005.
21. Merle d'Aubigne R, Postel M: Functional results of hip arthroplasty with acrylic prosthesis. J Bone Joint Surg Am 36-A:451–475, 1954.

Chapter 57

Hip Dislocation:
How Does Delay to Reduction Affect Avascular Necrosis Rate?

Paul R. T. Kuzyk, BSc, MASc, MD, FRCS(C) and Emil H. Schemitsch, MD, FRCS(C)

A dislocated hip represents a true orthopaedic emergency and requires immediate attention. Reduction of any dislocated joint helps to reduce pain, improves circulation within the surrounding soft tissues, removes pressure on the chondral surfaces, and allows for better radiographic imaging. In the case of the hip joint, an associated risk for avascular necrosis of the femoral head is present. Time to reduction of the dislocated hip has been implicated as a factor in the development of avascular necrosis.

OPTIONS

Avascular necrosis is a devastating complication that results in death of the osteocytes in the femoral head, subsequent chondral collapse, and secondary degenerative osteoarthritis of the hip joint. Death of these osteocytes is thought to occur because of ischemia from damage to the blood supply to the femoral head.[1] Blood is supplied to the femoral head through both extraosseous and intraosseous vessels. Extraosseous vessels include the medial femoral circumflex, the ligamentum teres, and the retinacular vessels.[2,3] Several basic science studies have shown that traumatic dislocation of the hip places tension on the medial femoral circumflex artery and more proximally at the junction of the common femoral artery with the external iliac artery.[4-6] This leads to disruption of both the intraosseous and extraosseous vasculature. Does this disruption improve with early reduction of the hip?

Reduction of a dislocated hip is often delayed for several reasons. Significant trauma is required to produce a hip dislocation; thus, patients with a dislocated hip tend to have multiple severe injuries. Head or abdominal injuries may require treatment before the dislocated hip. In the setting of the patient with multiple injuries, the hip dislocation may be missed. The patient may be transferred a significant distance from a referring hospital. What is the prognosis for the patient with a hip dislocation whose reduction has been delayed?

A subset of hip dislocations (3–13% in the literature) are irreducible closed and require open reduction.[7-11] These irreducible hip dislocations are frequently associated with fracture of the femoral head or acetabulum with incarceration of a bony fragment in the hip joint. Alternatively, the head may have "buttonholed" through the hip capsule, the piriformis muscle may block relocation of the head, or the labrum may have torn and flipped into the joint.[12] Given this scenario, when should surgical relocation of the hip be preformed? Most general orthopedic surgeons can perform an open reduction of a hip dislocation; however, those associated with femoral head or acetabular fracture often necessitate referral to a trauma specialist for definitive fixation. Should the referring surgeon perform an open reduction and relocate the hip before transferring to the specialist for a second procedure to fix the fracture? Should relocation of the hip be deferred and managed definitively by the trauma specialist?

EVIDENCE

Animal studies suggest that the disruption of the vascular supply to the femoral head may improve with reduction within 12 hours. Duncan and Shim[4] found that early reduction of the dislocated hip improved early and complete recovery of blood supply to the femoral head in a rabbit model. Reduction of the dislocated hip delayed beyond 12 hours did not benefit the rate and extent of the circulatory recovery of the femoral head. Histologic avascular necrosis was observed in hips reduced early and late; however, it was less frequently observed and less severe in those reduced early. In a subsequent study using rabbits and canines, Shim[5] found that vascular damage was largely due to compression, traction, and spasm of the extraosseous vessels (only a minority of these was ruptured). This is reinforced by a human cadaveric study demonstrating that dislocation caused compression of the medial femoral circumflex and common femoral vessels.[6] These basic science studies suggest that the vascular disruption is reversible with reduction of the hip. Furthermore, early reduction may reverse ischemic changes that occur in the femoral head at a cellular level.

Clinical studies that explore the effect of timing of hip reduction on the rates of avascular necrosis are largely retrospective cohort studies. No study was identified that focused solely on the rate of avascular necrosis as a function of time to reduction. Rather, these studies explored several different outcome measures (e.g., avascular necrosis, patient satisfaction, degenerative osteoarthritis) and several different variables (e.g., type of dislocation, time to weight bearing). We have identified six Level II and three Level IV studies with regard to effect of reduction on rate of avascular necrosis (Table 57–1).

Brav[8] reviewed traumatic hip dislocations that presented to U.S. Army hospitals during a 12-year period from 1947 to 1958.[8] He found that the rate of avascular necrosis was 17.6% when reduction occurred before 12 hours and 56.9% when reduction was delayed over 12 hours. Although no statistical analysis was done to prove significance (no P value was reported), there is a definite trend to reduced avascular necrosis in the group treated early.

Subsequent Level II studies have presented similar results with respect to timing of reduction and rates of avascular necrosis. Şahin and colleagues[13] examined 62 cases of traumatic hip dislocation (5 anterior and 57 posterior with associated acetabular fracture) and found a trend for decreased avascular necrosis when the hip was reduced within 12 hours (2.9%) as compared with after 12 hours (14.8%). In addition, they found that there was no significant difference between hips reduced less than 6 hours and those reduced between 6 to 12 hours after injury. Moed and coworkers[14] also note a significant reduction in rates of avascular necrosis in hips reduced within 12 hours ($P < 0.001$) but did not comment on the absolute rates. Yang and coauthors[15] present a retrospective cohort of 96 hip dislocations that included both anterior and posterior dislocations with and without acetabular fractures. They found no avascular necrosis in dislocations reduced within 24 hours and a rate of 42.2% in those reduced after 24 hours. Hougaard and Thomsen[16] presented 100 posterior hip dislocations with and without associated fracture of the acetabulum. They found a decrease in avascular necrosis when the hip was reduced within 6 hours (4.8% at <6 hours, and 58.8% at ≥6 hours). They had insufficient data to comment on a difference between reduction less than 6 hours and reduction between 6 and 12 hours. This study also found an increase in avascular necrosis with severity of injury (5% with minor acetabular fracture and 52.6% with severe acetabular fracture and/or femoral head or neck fracture).

Dreinhöfer and investigators'[17] study was the only Level II study that suggested there was no difference in avascular necrosis with delayed reduction.[17] However, all 35 hip dislocations (anterior and posterior dislocations without associated fracture) in their series were reduced within 6 hours of injury. They focused on a difference in avascular necrosis in a group treated within 1 hour (8.3%) versus a group treated in 1 to 6 hours (13%) and found no significant difference.

In all the Level II studies identified, selection bias occurred in the delayed reduction group. This group includes the more severe dislocations that require open reduction or transfer to a specialist. This group includes those dislocations with more severe trauma (acetabular fracture and/or femoral head or neck fracture) and those that will ultimately receive surgery (i.e., hips that are irreducible closed). Both surgery and the extensive trauma to the hip negatively affect vascularity.

Three Level IV evidence articles were identified. These articles are case series because they present rates of avascular necrosis for dislocations reduced at a specific time. Two of these articles, by Jaskulka and colleagues[18] and McKee and coworkers,[11] conclude that there was an increase in avascular necrosis with time to reduction.[11,18] Jaskulka and colleagues[18] report a rate of 1.8% (i.e., 1 case) in their series of 47 posterior fracture dislocations and attributed this low rate to the fact that all hips were reduced within 6 hours.[18] McKee and coworkers[11] presented a series of 25 central and posterior dislocations with associated severe acetabular and femoral neck fractures. They attribute their high avascular necrosis rate (26%), in part, to the relatively long time to reduction (mean, 15.3 hours). However, patients in this series all sustained severe trauma, and this may be a more significant factor in the high rate of avascular necrosis. Bhandari and coauthors[19] report on 109 posterior hip dislocations with associated acetabular fracture and conclude that time to reduction was not a prognostic factor. Their reported rate of avascular necrosis was 3%, and their average time from injury to reduction was 18 hours. They did not use avascular necrosis as an outcome but rather used radiologic grade, clinical grade, or the development of arthritis as outcomes. Their multivariate analysis suggests that the quality of fracture reduction has the greatest impact on these outcomes, and that time to reduction has less of an impact. However, these outcome measures do not specifically address development of avascular necrosis and likely are better indicators of the development of secondary osteoarthritis in the hip.

AREAS OF UNCERTAINTY

Position of Hip Dislocation

Anterior dislocations of the hip are rare and account for 6.3% to 13% of reported hip dislocations.[13,15,18] These injuries are typically grouped together with posterior dislocations in studies. However, of the two studies that analyzed anterior dislocations as a separate group, no avascular necrosis was reported in one study, and a rate of 4.8% was reported in the other study.[8,17] This lower rate of avascular necrosis may be because of the position of the dislocated proximal femur and the resulting trauma to its vasculature.

Yue and researchers[6] showed in their cadaveric study that a posteriorly dislocated hip with the leg in external rotation (i.e., the hip was first posteriorly dislocated and then the leg was forced into external

TABLE 57–1. Studies That Examine Correlation of Time to Reduction with Rate of Avascular Necrosis

STUDY	LEVEL OF EVIDENCE	DESIGN	RATE OF FOLLOW-UP	DURATION OF FOLLOW-UP (RANGE), YR	MEAN AGE (RANGE), YR	TYPE OF DISLOCATION	ASSOCIATED HIP INJURY	TYPE OF REDUCTION	TIME TO REDUCTION	RATE OF AVASCULAR NECROSIS	CORRELATION
Brav[8]	II	Retrospective cohort	262/523 (50%)	6.7 (2–14)	27 (3–75)	228 Posterior 34 Anterior	91 Simple acetabular fracture 27 Complex fracture		204 < 12 hr 58 > 12 hr	17.6% < 12 hr 6.9% > 12 hr	Yes
Şahin et al.[13]	II	Retrospective cohort	62/107 (57.9%)	9.6 (3.6–18.4)	34.5 (14–72)	57 Posterior 5 Anterior	57 Acetabular fracture	50 Closed (80.6%)	35 < 12 hr 27 >12 hr	2.9% < 12 hr 14.8% > 12 hr	Yes
Dreinhöfer et al.[17]	II	Retrospective cohort	42/421 (10%)	4.5 (2.5–9)	29 (5–62)	38 Posterior 12 Anterior	No fracture	48 Closed (96%)	12 < 1 hr 23 in 1–6 hr	8.3% < 1 hr 13% in 1–6 hr	No
Yang et al.[15]	II	Retrospective cohort	96/125 (76.8%)	7.5 (1.25–18)	33.5 (7–81)	90 Posterior 6 Anterior	90 Acetabular fracture		69 < 12 hr 8 in 12–24 hr 19 > 24 hr	0 < 24 hr 42.1% > 24 hr	Yes
Moed et al.[14]	II	Retrospective cohort	100/108 (92.6%)	5 (2–14)	38 (16–74)		All had acetabular fracture	83 Closed (96.5%)	71 < 12 hr 8 in 12–24 hr 7 > 24 hr		Yes
Hougaard and Thomsen[16]	II	Retrospective cohort	100/137 (73.0%)	14 (5–26)	39 (16–89)	All posterior	All had acetabular fracture		83 < 6 hr 17 > 6 hr	4.8% < 6 hr 58.8% > 6 hr	Yes
Bhandari et al.[19]	IV	Case series	109/163 (66.9%)	5.9 (2–19)	42 (15–79)	All posterior	9 Femoral neck fracture 11 Acetabular fracture		18 hr (mean)	3%	No
McKee et al.[11]	IV	Case series	25		41.8 (17–81)	19 Posterior 6 Central	All had acetabular fracture	All open	15.3 hr (mean)	26%	Yes
Jaskulka et al.[18]	IV	Case series	47/54 (87%)	6.7 (2–11)	29.7 (17–56)	All posterior		All closed	All < 6 hr	1.8%	Yes

rotation) created filling defects in both the common femoral and medial femoral circumflex arteries. The filling defects in the common femoral artery were reversed when the leg was rotated internally (the hip remained posteriorly dislocated); however, the filling defects in the medial femoral circumflex arteries remained. Presumably, the filling defects in the medial femoral circumflex arteries are due to pressure exerted on the posterior hip capsule and overlying vasculature because of the posteriorly displaced head of the femur. Defects in the common femoral artery result from twisting of the artery because of the position of the leg (i.e., worse when the leg is externally rotated). Although not specifically tested, one may assume that an anteriorly dislocated hip would result in a reversible defect in the common femoral artery (because the leg is externally rotated) and no defect in the femoral circumflex arteries (because the femoral head is displaced anteriorly and the posterior hip capsule is not under tension).

Associated Acetabular and Proximal Femur Fractures

Brav[8] reports lower rates of avascular necrosis in anterior and posterior dislocation groups without associated acetabular fracture (13.9% < 12 hours and 47.8% > 12 hours), and quite high rates of avascular necrosis in those with severe associated acetabular and femoral head fractures (62.5% < 12 hours and 81.8% > 12 hours). Greater rates of avascular necrosis were observed in series that included acetabular and femoral head/neck fractures as compared with those that did not (see Table 57–1). This may be explained by the more significant trauma to the soft tissue and vasculature that is sustained with these injuries. These injuries also often require surgical management, and this may further damage the vasculature.

Letournel and Judet[20] suggest that time to reduction had little prognostic value. Their series of acetabular fracture dislocations demonstrates low rates of avascular necrosis despite a long interval of time between injury and reduction (5% < 6 hours, 8% between 6 and 24 hours, and 4% > 24 hours). Bhandari and coauthors'[19] results agree with this as they have reported a low rate of avascular necrosis (3%) with posterior dislocation and associated acetabular fracture. Their explanation is that the posterior acetabular fracture allows the femoral head to sit in a position that places less tension on the medial femoral circumflex and retinacular vessels than if the acetabulum was intact. If this is correct, the greater rates of avascular necrosis observed in other series (see Table 57–1) may be caused by associated surgical trauma or inclusion of femoral head/neck fractures in these series. However, we cannot discount the Level II studies that suggest greater rates of avascular necrosis in patients with associated acetabular fracture that experience delay in reduction beyond 12 hours.

TABLE 57–2. Grades of Recommendations for the Treatment of Hip Dislocation

RECOMMENDATIONS	LEVEL OF EVIDENCE/GRADE OF RECOMMENATION
1. Adult with dislocation of the hip joint should be reduced no later than 12 hours.	B
2. Adult with dislocation of the hip joint may benefit from reduction within 6 hours.	I
3. Reduction may be delayed beyond 12 hours when acetabular fracture is present.	I
4. Adult with anterior hip dislocation can expect a better outcome than posterior dislocation.	B

REFERENCES

1. Rodriguez-Merchan EC: Osteonecrosis of the femoral head after traumatic hip dislocation in the adult. Clin Orthop 377:68–77, 2000.
2. Sevitt S, Thompson RG: The distribution and anastomoses of arteries supplying the head and neck of the femur. J Bone Joint Surg Br 47-B:560–573, 1965.
3. Gautier E, Ganz K, Krügel N, et al: Anatomy of the medial femoral circumflex artery and its surgical implications. J Bone Joint Surg Br 82-B:679–683, 2000.
4. Duncan C, Shim S: Blood supply of the head of the femur in traumatic hip dislocation. Surg Gynecol Obstet 144:185–191, 1977.
5. Shim SS: Circulatory and vascular changes in the hip following traumatic hip dislocation. Clin Orthop 140:255–261, 1979.

6. Yue JJ, Wilber JH, Lipuma JP, et al: Posterior hip dislocations. A cadaveric angiographic study. J Orthop Trauma 10:447–454, 1996.
7. Thompson VP, Epstein HC: Traumatic dislocations of the hip. A survey of two hundred and four cases covering a period of twenty-one years. J Bone Joint Surg Am 33-A:746–778, 1951.
8. Brav EA: Traumatic dislocations of the hip. Army experience and results over a twelve-year period. J Bone Joint Surg Am 44-A:1115–1134, 1962.
9. Hunter GA: Posterior dislocation and fracture-dislocation of the hip. A review of fifty-seven patients. J Bone Joint Surg Br 51-B:38–44, 1969.
10. Proctor H: Dislocations of the hip joint (excluding "central" dislocations) and their complications. Injury 5:1–12, 1973.
11. McKee MD, Garay ME, Schemitsch EH, et al: Irreducible fracture-dislocation of the hip: A severe injury with a poor prognosis. J Orthop Trauma 12:223–229, 1998.
12. Canale ST, Manugian AH: Irreducible traumatic dislocations of the hip. J Bone Joint Surg Am 61-A:7–14, 1979.
13. Şahin V, Karakas ES, Aku S, et al: Traumatic dislocation and fracture-dislocation of the hip: A long-term follow-up study. J Trauma 54:520–529, 2003.
14. Moed BR, Willson Carr SE, Watson JT: Results of operative treatment of fractures of the posterior wall of the acetabulum. J Bone Joint Surg Am 84-A:752–758, 2002.
15. Yang RS, Tsuang YH, Hang YS, et al: Traumatic dislocation of the hip. Clin Orthop 265:218–227, 1991.
16. Hougaard K, Thomsen PB: Coxarthrosis following traumatic posterior dislocation of the hip. J Bone Joint Surg Am 69-A:679–683, 1987.
17. Dreinhöfer KE, Schwarzkopf SR, Haas NP, et al: Isolated traumatic dislocation of the hip: Long-term results in 50 patients. J Bone Joint Surg Br 76-B:6–12, 1994.
18. Jaskulka RA, Fischer G, Fenzl G: Dislocation and fracture-dislocation of the hip. J Bone Joint Surg Br 73-B:465–469, 1991.
19. Bhandari M, Matta J, Ferguson T, et al: Predictors of clinical and radiological outcome in patients with fractures of the acetabulum and concomitant posterior dislocation of the hip. J Bone Joint Surg Br 88-B:1618–1624, 2006.
20. Letournel E, Judet R: Fractures of the Acetabulum. Elson RA (ed). New York, Springer-Verlag, 1993.

Combined Fractures of the Hip and Femoral Shaft:
What Is the Best Treatment Method?

Paul R. T. Kuzyk, BSc, MASc, MD, FRSC(C) and Emil H. Schemitsch, MD, FRCS(C)

Ipsilateral fractures of the hip and femur are rare injuries that result from high-energy trauma. This injury pattern is most commonly seen in motor vehicle accidents.[1,2] The mechanism of injury is an axial force applied along the femur as the occupant's knee strikes the dashboard. If the hip is adducted when this force is applied, the resulting injury to the hip is usually a dislocation or acetabular fracture, or both. If the hip is in abduction, this will produce a femoral neck and shaft fracture.[3] Given the rarity of this injury (i.e., occurring in less than 9% of all femoral shaft fractures), no large series are reported in the literature.[1,2,4] Nearly 60 different implant combinations have been described for this fracture pattern.[5,6]

OPTIONS

The main complications associated with isolated femoral neck fractures are high rates of nonunion and avascular necrosis of the femoral head. Complications associated with isolated femoral shaft fractures include malunion (i.e., >2 cm shortening, >10-degree varus or valgus alignment, and >20 degrees malrotation) and nonunion. Many authors contend that the complications of the femoral neck trump those of the femoral shaft. They suggest that avascular necrosis is the most significant complication and, therefore, the femoral neck fracture should be treated first.[4,7,8] Others suggest that the femur should be treated initially to allow for ease of closed reduction of the femoral neck fracture.[3,5,9] What are the most common complications of this injury pattern? In what order should fixation of the fractures proceed?

A large number of the femoral neck fractures associated with shaft fractures are missed (approximately 30%).[1] Many of the femoral neck fractures are nondisplaced at the time of presentation (25–60%).[1] (This may occur because some of the energy that would normally result in a displaced femoral neck fracture is dissipated by the shaft fracture.) In addition, many of these patients have multiple injuries with numerous "distracting" injuries. What is the best method of imaging the hip to avoid missing a fracture?

A spectrum of different hip fractures has been reported with this injury pattern. Hip fractures vary from intertrochanteric fractures to different types of intracapsular neck fractures. The position of the hip (degree of abduction) at the time of injury has been suggested as the determinant of the pattern of hip fracture produced.[10] What is the most common type of hip fracture encountered with this injury? What is the most common type of femoral shaft fracture?

Many different implants and implant combinations have been used to treat this combination of fractures. Implant designs have changed over the time periods of many of the retrospective case series reported in the literature (Table 58–1). For example, the antegrade femoral intramedullary nail has evolved from the unlocked (Küntscher) nail, to the first-generation locked nail, to the second-generation cephalomedullary (or reconstruction) locked nail, and finally to the intramedullary hip screw device. Retrograde femoral nailing has also become increasingly popular since the late 1990s. However, the literature consists of small case series that involve a mixture of different implants from different periods. What are the optimal implants for this fracture pattern?

EVIDENCE

Alho[1] conducted a meta-analysis on 65 studies published between 1970 and 1996 that incorporated 722 cases of ipsilateral hip and shaft fractures. This represents the largest summary of case series reported in the literature. He identified 10 studies (240 fractures) that included useful demographic data. This injury typically occurs in young individuals (mean age, 33 years) and results from a high-energy mechanism (85% motor vehicle accidents). Only 1% of cases occurred in elderly individuals. Approximately 18% of the femoral shaft fractures were reported as open, with a large number of comminuted fractures (i.e., 42% were Winquist type III or IV).[11] The majority of shaft fractures occurred in the middle third of the femur (72%). For hip fractures, Alho[1] reports that the majority of cases were femoral neck fractures (61%), with the rest being trochanteric fractures. Shuler and colleagues[10] report on 52 cases of hip fracture with femoral shaft fracture and found 90% to be femoral neck fractures. They found that these hip fractures all tended to

TABLE 58–1. Studies That Examine Implants Used for Femoral Shaft Fixation in Ipsilateral Hip and Femoral Shaft Fractures

STUDY (YEAR OF PUBLICATION)	LEVEL OF EVIDENCE	DESIGN	AVERAGE DURATION OF FOLLOW-UP (YR)	N	SEX	AVERAGE AGE (YR)	TYPE OF IMPLANT (n)	RATE OF AVASCULAR NECROSIS	RATE OF NONUNION (HIP)	RATE OF NONUNION (SHAFT)	RATE OF MALUNION (HIP)	RATE OF MALUNION (SHAFT)	CLINICAL OUTCOME (%FAIR/POOR)
Alho et al. (1997)[1]	III	Meta-analysis of 20 studies	N/A	219	78% M	33 (3–76)	A: Plate and screws (82) B: Unlocked nails (73) C: Locked nail (28) D: Cephalomedullary nail (36)	A: 2.4% B: 2.7% C: 3.6% D: 0%	0%	A: 9.7% B: 2.7% C: 0% D: 0%	A: 1.2% B: 1.4% C: 3.6% D: 2.8%	A: 3.7% B: 8.2% C: 0% D: 0%	A: 20.7% B: 15.1% C: 3.6% D: 2.8%
Oh et al. (2006)[18]	IV	Case series	N/A	17	87.5% M	44 (25–77)	Unreamed retrograde intramedullary nail; dynamic hip screws or screws for hip	5.9%	5.9%	29.4%	5.9%	5.9%	5.9%
Jain et al. (2004)[6]	IV	Case series	2.6 (1–4.6)	23	95.7% M	34.5 (21–56)	Reamed cephalomedullary nail; screws for hip	4.3%	4.3%	17.4%	4.3%	17.4%	13.0%
Hossam et al. (2001)[19]	IV	Case series	2.1 (1–3)	9	100% M	28.5 (18–36)	Reamed cephalomedullary nail; screws for hip	0%	0%	11.1%	11.1%	0%	22.2%
Swiontkowski et al. (1984)[4]	IV	Case series	2.9 (1–8)	7	85.7% M	29.1 (22–43)	Retrograde unlocked nail; screws for hip	0%	0%	0%	0%	0%	N/A

extend into the inferomedial neck regardless of the fracture type (i.e., midcervical, basocervical, or pertrochanteric). The extension of the fracture into the inferomedial neck (i.e., femoral calcar) makes it prone to displacement with weight bearing.

Complication rates for femoral neck fractures with an associated femoral shaft fracture tend to be less than with this injury in isolation. Alho[1] quotes an avascular necrosis rate of 5% and no nonunions of 254 fractures (this includes displaced and nondisplaced fractures). For isolated displaced femoral neck fractures, the incidence rate of avascular necrosis is 22.5% and of nonunion is 6%.[12] The reduced rate of avascular necrosis and nonunion seen with the combined injury may result from a greater rate of nondisplaced fractures (up to 60% for the combined injury),[1] perhaps because much of the energy is dissipated through the femoral shaft fracture. Thus, the hip fracture tends to be less comminuted with less injury to the vasculature (i.e., posterior retinacular vessels).

An important consequence of the high rate of nondisplaced femoral neck fractures is that they tend to be missed on initial presentation. Alho[1] states that the diagnosis of the hip fracture was delayed (from 1 day to several months) in 30% of cases. Tornetta and investigators[13] conducted a Level II study on the effectiveness of a radiographic protocol to detect nondisplaced hip fractures in patients with femoral shaft fractures.[13] A standard protocol of computed tomographic (CT) scan, dedicated internal rotation hip radiographs, and lateral intraoperative fluoroscopic hip images for all femoral shaft fractures was instituted, and the rate of missed hip fractures was recorded. This was compared with rates before institution of this protocol (i.e., when imaging was left to the discretion of the treating surgical team). They found that this protocol significantly decreased the rates of missed hip fractures (57% before vs. 6.3% after institution of the protocol). Of these imaging modalities, the authors found the CT scan to be the most useful (a poor-quality CT scan resulted in the only fracture that was missed on CT and subsequently diagnosed on an internal rotation hip radiograph). Thus, all femoral shaft fractures resulting from a high-energy mechanism (especially motor vehicle accidents) should undergo a CT scan of the ipsilateral hip before definitive fixation.

No comparative studies exist in the literature with regard to method of fixation for combined femoral neck and shaft fractures. Alho's[1] meta-analysis took 219 individual cases from 20 studies and segregated them into 4 groups based on fixation of the femoral shaft fracture: (1) plate and screws, (2) unlocked intramedullary nail, (3) first-generation locked intramedullary nail, and (4) cephalomedullary nail. This is Level III evidence given that it is a meta-analysis consisting of small, retrospective, comparative studies and case series. Methods of hip fixation varied among the groups, making the results for complications of the hip fracture unreliable. Alho[1] concludes that the locked nailing treatment groups (i.e., first-generation and cephalomedullary nails) had significantly better overall clinical outcomes ($P < 0.001$) than the plate or unlocked nailing groups. Locked nails also had lower rates of femoral shaft nonunion and malunion (see Table 58–1) than either plating or unlocked nailing. No significant difference was found in rates of complications or clinical outcome noted between first-generation locked and cephalomedullary nails. Alho[1] concluded that the femoral shaft fracture was the "key component" to this injury because this fracture exhibited greater complication rates than the hip fracture. In a review of complications associated with ipsilateral hip and femur fractures (level IV evidence), Watson and Moed[9] found that 76% of identified complications were nonunion of the femoral shaft fracture. Among these cases of femoral shaft nonunion, they found that 86% were open fractures, 80% were treated with an unreamed nail, 100% had prolonged non–weight bearing, and 30% were treated with a cephalomedullary nail. They conclude that a reamed, second-generation, locked intramedullary nail was the optimal implant for treatment of the femoral shaft fracture in this combined injury.

AREAS OF UNCERTAINTY

Should a Displaced Femoral Neck Fracture Be Fixed before Fixation of the Femoral Shaft?

Numerous authors have advocated that the hip fracture be fixed before the femoral shaft fracture. The most common argument for this approach is that rates of avascular necrosis of the femoral head increase with time to reduction and fixation for displaced femoral neck fractures.[4,7,8] However, no clinical evidence suggests this is, indeed, the case (see Chapter 54). Level II clinical evidence suggests that the outcome of a displaced femoral neck fracture is dependent on anatomic reduction (i.e., no varus) and rigid fixation.[14–16] Manipulation of the hip fracture (either through an open or closed approach) is simplified by fixation of the femoral shaft. Thus, we recommend fixation of the femoral shaft before fixation of the displaced femoral neck fracture (Level V evidence). No clinical studies in the literature compare these two approaches.

What Type of Implant Should Be Used for the Femoral Shaft Fracture?

Swiontkowski and colleagues[4] advocate fixation of this injury with an unlocked retrograde nail. Treatment of femoral shaft fractures with locked retrograde nails has increased in popularity in recent years. Ricci and coworkers[17] conducted a retrospective comparative trial (Level II evidence) for locked antegrade and retrograde nailing of isolated femoral shaft fractures. They found that rates of nonunion and malunion were not significantly different between the two methods of treatment. The incidence of knee pain was significantly greater for the retrograde nail, whereas the incidence of hip pain was significantly greater for the antegrade nail. The authors conclude that these two implants provide similar clinical results for femoral shaft fractures.

The retrograde femoral nail offers theoretical advantages to the antegrade femoral nail for the treatment of ipsilateral hip and femoral shaft fractures. Use of a retrograde nail allows the surgeon to use either a sliding hip screw or cannulated screws to fix the hip fracture, whereas with the use of an antegrade nail, the surgeon is obligated to use screws. With a nondisplaced femoral neck fracture, there is the risk for displacing the fracture when the antegrade nail is introduced. When a retrograde nail is used, the nondisplaced femoral neck fracture can be fixed before nailing the femur. No clinical studies compare these two methods of treatment for this injury. Only case series that show good results for retrograde nailing have been reported (Level IV evidence).[4,18] It is our opinion that a retrograde nail should be used to fix the femoral shaft fracture with this injury. We believe that cannulated screws should be used for the femoral neck fracture in patients with adequate bone stock, and a sliding hip screw for patients with osteopenic bone or a combined intertrochanteric fracture (Level V evidence). For nondisplaced femoral neck fractures, the hip should be fixed before retrograde nailing the femur (Level V evidence). For displaced femoral neck fractures, the femur should be fixed before reducing and fixing the hip fracture (Level V evidence).

Do Cephalomedullary Nails Provide Improved Fixation?

Cephalomedullary nails have been advocated by some authors because they provide added fixation of the hip fracture.[6] However, recent case series suggest that the clinical results of this type of fixation are inferior to those provided by a retrograde nail for ipsilateral hip and femoral shaft fractures (see Table 58–1).[6,19] These case series have small sample sizes, and no trials directly compare these two types of implants for this injury pattern. Watson and Moed[9] found a high rate of complications with the use of cephalomedullary nails, and therefore conclude that this implant should not be used with this fracture pattern (Level IV evidence).

RECOMMENDATIONS

No large comparative studies have been conducted to critically examine the implants used to treat this injury pattern. Based on limited case series and expert opinion, we make the following recommendations (Table 55A–2):

- When there is a displaced femoral neck fracture, the femoral shaft should be treated first. When the femoral neck fracture is nondisplaced, this fracture should be treated first. Grade C evidence supports these statements.

- Retrograde femoral nailing should be used over antegrade nailing for this injury pattern. These two treatments provide equivalent results for treatment of the femoral shaft fracture. However, retrograde nailing of the femur allows either a sliding hip screw or cannulated screws to be used for the hip fracture. Grade C evidence supports this statement.
- All femoral shaft fractures resulting from high-energy trauma (especially motor vehicle accidents) should receive a high-quality CT scan of the hip. Grade B evidence supports this statement.
- Cephalomedullary implants in isolation should not be used to treat this injury pattern. Grade C evidence supports this statement.

TABLE 58–2. Summary of Recommendations for the Treatment of Ipsilateral Hip and Femoral Shaft Fractures

RECOMMENDATIONS	LEVEL OF EVIDENCE/GRADE OF RECOMMENDATION
1. Fixation of the femoral shaft fracture should precede fixation of the hip fracture for displaced femoral neck fractures.	C
2. Fixation of the hip fracture should precede fixation of the femoral shaft fracture for nondisplaced femoral neck fractures.	C
3. Retrograde femoral nailing is preferred to antegrade femoral nailing.	C
4. High-quality computed tomographic scan of the ipsilateral hip should be performed for all femoral shaft fractures resulting from high-energy trauma.	B
5. Cephalomedullary implants should not be used in isolation to treat this injury pattern.	C

REFERENCES

1. Alho A: Concurrent ipsilateral fractures of the hip and shaft of the femur. A systematic review of 722 cases. Ann Chir Gynaecol 86:326–336, 1997.
2. Alho A: Concurrent ipsilateral fractures of the hip and femoral shaft: A meta-analysis of 659 cases. Acta Orthop Scand 67:19–28, 1996.
3. Schatzker J, Barrington TW: Fractures of the femoral neck associated with fractures of the same femoral shaft. Can J Surg 11:297–305, 1968.
4. Swiontkowski MF, Hansen ST, Kellam J: Ipsilateral fractures of the femoral neck and shaft. A treatment protocol. J Bone Joint Surg Am 66-A:260–268, 1984.
5. Wolinsky PR, Johnson KD: Ipsilateral femoral neck and shaft fractures. Clin Orthop Relat Res (318):81–90, 1995.
6. Jain P, Maini L, Mishra P, et al: Cephalomedullary interlocked nail for ipsilateral hip and femoral shaft fractures. Injury 35:1031–1038, 2004.
7. Swiontkowski MF: Ipsilateral femoral shaft and hip fractures. Orthop Clin North Am 18:73–84, 1987.
8. Peljovich AE, Patterson BM: Ipsilateral femoral neck and shaft fractures. J Am Acad Orthop Surg 6:106–113, 1998.

9. Watson JT, Moed BR: Ipsilateral femoral neck and shaft fractures: Complications and their treatment. Clin Orthop Relat Res (399):78–86, 2002.
10. Shuler TE, Gruen GS, DiTano O, Riemer BL: Ipsilateral proximal and shaft femoral fractures: Spectrum of injury involving the femoral neck. Injury 28:293–297, 1997.
11. Winquist RA, Hansen ST: Comminuted fractures of the femoral shaft treated by intramedullary nailing. Orthop Clin North Am 11:633–648, 1980.
12. Damany DS, Parker MJ, Chojnowski A: Complications after intracapsular hip fractures in young adults. A meta-analysis of 18 published studies involving 564 fractures. Injury 36:131–141, 2005.
13. Tornetta P 3rd, Kain MS, Creevy WR: Diagnosis of femoral neck fractures in patients with a femoral shaft fracture. Improvement with a standard protocol. J Bone Joint Surg Am 89-A:39–43, 2007.
14. Upadhyay A, Jain P, Mishra P, et al: Delayed internal fixation of fractures of the neck of the femur in young adults. A prospective, randomised study comparing closed and open reduction. J Bone Joint Surg Br 86-B:1035–1040, 2004.
15. Asnis SE, Wanek-Sgaglione L: Intracapsular fractures of the femoral neck: Results of cannulated screw fixation. J Bone Joint Surg Am 76-A:1793–1803, 1994.
16. Chua D, Jaglal SB, Schatzker J: Predictors of early failure of fixation in the treatment of displaced subcapital hip fractures. J Orthop Trauma 12:230–234, 1998.
17. Ricci WM, Bellabarba C, Evanoff B, et al: Retrograde versus antegrade nailing of femoral shaft fractures. J Orthop Trauma 15:161–169, 2001.
18. Oh CW, Oh JK, Park BC, et al: Retrograde nailing with subsequent screw fixation for ipsilateral femoral shaft and neck fractures. Arch Orthop Trauma Surg 126:448–453, 2006.
19. Hossam ElShafie M, Adel Morsey H, Emad Eid Y: Ipsilateral fracture of the femoral neck and shaft, treatment by reconstruction interlocking nail. Arch Orthop Trauma Surg 121:71–74, 2001.

Femoral Neck Fractures:
When Should a Displaced Subcapital Fracture Be Replaced versus Fixed?

Mohit Bhandari, MD, MSc, FRCSC

WHAT IS THE GLOBAL BURDEN OF HIP FRACTURES?

Hip fractures occur in 280,000 Americans (>5000 per week) and 36,000 (>690 per week) Canadians annually. By the year 2040, the number of people aged 65 or older will increase from 34.8 million to 77.2 million. Demographic projections by Statistics Canada indicate that, by the year 2041, 1 in 4 Canadians will be older than 65 years. The number of hip fractures is likely to exceed 500,000 annually in the United States and 88,000 in Canada over the next 40 years.[1-3] By the year 2040, the estimated annual healthcare costs will reach $9.8 billion in the United States and $650 million in Canada.[4]

Hip fractures are associated with a 30% mortality rate at 1 year and profound temporary, and sometimes permanent, impairment of independence and quality of life. Furthermore, approximately 30% of surgically treated hip fractures require revision surgery.[5] These revisions are associated with a large burden of morbidity and mortality. The disability adjusted life-years lost as a result of hip fractures ranks in the top 10 of all causes of disability globally.

WHAT ARE CURRENT MANAGEMENT OPTIONS?

Although there is general consensus regarding the operative management of nondisplaced fractures of the femoral neck,[5] the optimal choice for the stabilization of displaced femoral neck fractures remains controversial.[5] Operative approaches for displaced femoral neck fractures include prosthetic replacement (arthroplasty) or internal fixation. Approaches to arthroplasty include unipolar hemiarthroplasty, bipolar hemiarthroplasty, and total hip arthroplasty. Options for internal fixation include multiple screws, a compression screw and side plate, or an intramedullary hip screw device.

WHAT IS THE CURRENT OPINION?

Surveys of surgeon opinions in Denmark, Canada, and the United Kingdom[6,7] have been limited by lack of generalizability to other countries and a failure to elicit surgeons' views of the impact of alternative management strategies on patient-important out-

comes. As a result of the limitations of prior surveys, knowledge of the opinions of surgeons managing hip fractures remains limited. Knowing the extent of variability in opinions and practice can identify factors that influence surgeons' preferences for a particular treatment, serve to educate the orthopedic community on issues regarding the treatment of hip fractures, and assist in the planning of future clinical trials addressing issues that remain unresolved among orthopedic traumatologists.

We conducted an international survey of practicing orthopedic surgeons with an interest in fracture care to clarify current opinion in the treatment of displaced femoral neck fractures.[5] Of 442 surgeons who received the questionnaire, 298 (68%) responded. The typical respondent was a North American resident older than 40 years and in academic practice who supervised residents, had fellowship training in trauma, worked in a low-volume center (<100 hip fractures per year), and treated an equal proportion of displaced and undisplaced femoral neck fractures. Most surgeons believed that internal fixation was the procedure of choice in younger patients (< 60 years) across displaced fracture types (Garden types III-IV). Among those patients older than 80 years with Garden type III and IV fractures, almost all surgeons preferred arthroplasty (94% and 96%, respectively). Respondents varied widely in their preferences for patients aged 60 to 80 years with displaced fractures (Garden III/IV) or active patients with Garden III fractures. Many surgeons believed there was no difference between arthroplasty and internal fixation when considering mortality (45%), infection rates (30%), and quality of life (37%).

The purpose of this chapter is to guide clinicians regarding the treatment of displaced femoral neck fractures in patients older than 65 years by evaluating the evidence comparing internal fixation versus arthroplasty on major outcomes (mortality, revision surgery).

WHAT IS THE EVIDENCE?

In the hierarchy of evidence for questions about a "therapy" (in this case, a surgical intervention), a meta-analysis of randomized, controlled trials is the standard when no single large definitive trial exists. Our search identified 4 meta-analyses and 58 randomized trials that provide information on surgical treatments for femoral neck fractures. Three meta-analyses directly address the question of internal fixation versus arthroplasty in patients with displaced femoral neck fractures.[8-10] Their results are consistent. Here, we present the current results of the single meta-analysis of randomized trials.[8]

Mortality

Nine trials (N = 1162 patients) provided postoperative mortality data at 4 months or less. The results of the pooled statistical analyses are listed in Table 59–1. Arthroplasty showed a trend toward increased mortality when compared with internal fixation (relative risk [RR], 1.27; 95% confidence interval [CI], 0.84–1.92; P = 0.25; homogeneity P = 0.45). Twelve trials (N = 1767 patients) provided 1-year mortality data. At 1 year, arthroplasty did not increase the risk for mortality when compared with internal fixation, with wide variability between studies (RR, 1.04; 95% CI, 0.84–1.29; P = 0.68; homogeneity P = 0.03) (Fig. 59–1).

Revision Surgery

All 14 studies (N = 1901) provided information on revision surgery (see Table 59–1). Arthroplasty substantially reduced the risk for revision, and the results were consistent from study to study (RR, 0.23; 95% CI, 0.13–0.42; P = 0.0003; homogeneity P < 0.01). Thus, arthroplasty reduced the RR of revision surgery by 77% when compared with internal fixation. The risk difference of 18% translated into a number needed to treat (NNT) of 5.6, which meant that for every 6 patients treated with arthroplasty, 1 revision surgery could be avoided.

Pain, Function, and Infection Rates. Information on secondary outcomes was available in 6 studies for pain relief and 12 studies for function. Six studies (N = 1153 pa-tients) reported on pain relief and 12 on function (N = 1179 patients). Pain relief and function were similar in patients treated with arthroplasty or internal fixation (RR of no/little pain, 1.12; 95% CI, 0.88–1.35; good function, 0.99; 95% CI, 0.90–1.10). Arthroplasty significantly increased the risk for infection (12 studies, N = 1822) compared with internal fixation (RR, 1.81; 95% CI, 1.16–2.85; P = 0.009; homogeneity P = 0.16). The risk difference between the two treatments was 3.4%. This meant that for every 29 patients treated with internal fixation, 1 infection could be prevented (NNT = 1/0.034 = 29.4).

Blood Loss and Surgical Time. Four studies (N = 343 patients) reported on estimated blood loss, and 5 (N = 447 patients) on surgical time. Patients who underwent arthroplasty experienced greater blood loss than those who were treated with internal fixation (weighted mean difference, 176.4 mL; 95% CI, 132.4–220.4; P < 0.05) . Similarly, surgical time in the patients treated with arthroplasty was greater than the patients treated with internal fixation (weighted mean difference, 29.0 minutes; 95% CI, 23.2–34.8; P < 0.05).

UNCERTAINTY AND FUTURE RESEARCH

What Is the Optimal Choice of Internal Fixation (Multiple Screws or Sliding Hip Screws) for Fixation of Hip Fractures?

Parker and colleagues'[11] meta-analysis evaluated 28 trials (N = 5547 patients) and reported no advantage of any internal fixation technique over any other. The trials were small (sample size range, 33–410) and methodologically limited.

What Is the Optimal Choice of Arthroplasty (Total Hip Arthroplasty or Hemiarthroplasty) for Treatment of Hip Fractures?

Current best estimates of treatment effect suggest that total hip arthroplasty reduces hip pain (RR reduction, 24%; 95% CI, 2–41%) and may reduce func-

TABLE 59–1. Mortality and Revision Surgery

| | | EVENTS | | | | |
	N	A	IF	RR*	95% CI	P
Mortality (<4 months)						
All arthroplasty vs. IF	1162	55/615	34/547	1.27	0.84–1.92	0.25
Mortality (at 1 year)						
All arthroplasty vs. IF	1767	226/984	160/783	1.04	0.84–1.29	0.68
Mortality (>1 year)						
All arthroplasty vs. IF	1596	412/895	251/701	1.12	0.90–1.43	0.30
Revision surgery						
All arthroplasty vs. IF	1901	111/1051	299/850	0.23	0.13–0.42	0.0003

*The relative risk (RR) of outcome (i.e., mortality or revision surgery) with arthroplasty compared with internal fixation (>1.0 favors internal fixation; <1.0 favors arthroplasty).
A, all arthroplasty; CI, confidence interval; IF, internal fixation.

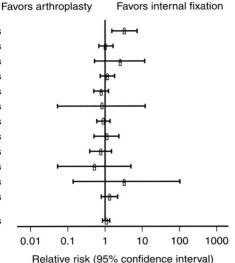

Favors arthroplasty   Favors internal fixation

Davison (2001) n = 280 patients
Ravikumar (2000) n = 271 patients
Van Vugt (1993) n = 43 patients
Parker (2000) n = 208 patients
Van Dortmont (2000) n = 60 patients
Tidermark (1999) n = 39 patients
Sikorski (1981) n = 218 patients
Soreide (1979) n = 104 patients
Johansson (2000) n = 100 patients
Neander (1997) n = 20 patients
Jonsson (1996) n = 47 patients
Rogmark (2002) n = 409 patients

Pooled estimate n = 1799 patients

0.01   0.1   1   10   100   1000

Relative risk (95% confidence interval)

FIGURE 59–1. A forrest plot depicting the treatment effect across multiple randomized trials comparing internal fixation and arthroplasty in patients with femoral neck fractures.

tional limitations (RR reduction, 10%; 95% CI, 24% to −6%) when compared with hemiarthroplasty. The reduction in pain and improvement in function may come at the cost of an increased risk for hip dislocation (RR, 2.95; 95% CI, 0.40–21.74). Despite the trend toward an increase in hip dislocation, the data (point estimate) shows a trend toward a decreased reoperation rate with hemiarthroplasty, though the sparse data are associated with wide CIs (RR reduction, 14%; 95% CI, 53% to −59%).[12,13]

Table 59–2 provides a summary of recommendations for the treatment of femoral neck fractures.

TABLE 59–2. Summary of Recommendations

RECOMMENDATIONS	LEVEL OF EVIDENCE/GRADE OF RECOMMENDATION
1. For patients 65 years or older with displaced femoral neck fractures, arthroplasty will reduce the need for revision surgery.	A
2. For patients 65 years or older with displaced femoral neck fractures, arthroplasty will increase operating time, blood loss, and the risk for infection.	A
3. For patients 65 years or older with displaced femoral neck fractures, arthroplasty and internal fixation have similar mortality rates.	B

RECOMMENDATIONS

In patients older than 65 years with displaced femoral neck fractures, evidence suggests:
- Arthroplasty significantly reduces the risk for revision surgery at 1 year compared with internal fixation (grade A recommendation: good evidence [Level I studies with consistent findings]).
- Arthroplasty does not increase the risk for mortality at 1 year compared with internal fixation (grade B recommendation: fair evidence [Level I studies with inconsistent findings and methodologic limitations]).
- Arthroplasty significantly increases the risk for infection, blood loss, and operating time at 1 year compared with internal fixation (grade A recommendation: good evidence [Level I studies with consistent findings).

REFERENCES

1. Cooper C, Campion G, Melton LJ: Hip fractures in the elderly: A world-wide projection. Osteoporos Int 2:285–289, 1992.
2. Cummings SR, Rubin SM, Black D: The future of hip fractures in the United States. Numbers, costs, and potential effects of postmenopausal estrogen. Clin Orthop Relat Res 252:163–166, 1990.
3. Johnell O, Kanis JA: An estimate of the worldwide prevalence, mortality and disability associated with hip fracture. Osteoporos Int 15:897–902, 2004.
4. Emmanuel A, Papadimitropoulos BSP, Coyte PC, et al: Current and projected rates of hip fracture in Canada. CMAJ 157:1357–1363, 1997.
5. Bhandari M, Devereaux PJ, Tornetta P 3rd, et al: Operative management of displaced femoral neck fractures in elderly patients. An international survey. J Bone Joint Surg Am 87:2122–2130, 2005.
6. Laursen JO: Treatment of intracapsular fractures of the femoral neck in Denmark: Trends over the past decade. Acta Orthop Belg 65:478–484, 1999.
7. Chua D, Jaglal SB, Schatzker J: An orthopedic surgeon survey on the treatment of displaced femoral neck fracture: Opposing views. Can J Surg 40:271–277, 1997.

8. Bhandari M, Devereaux PJ, Swiontkowski M, et al: Internal fixation compared with arthroplasty for displaced fractures of the femoral neck. J Bone Joint Surg Am 85A:1673–1681, 2003.

9. Lu-Yao GL, Keller RB, Littenberg B, Wennberg JE: Outcomes after displaced fractures of the femoral neck: A meta analysis of 106 published reports. J Bone Joint Surg Am 76A:15–25, 1994.

10. Masson M, Parker MJ, Fleischer S: Internal fixation versus arthroplasty for intracapsular proximal femoral fractures in adults. Cochrane Database Syst Rev (2):CD001708, 2003.

11. Parker MJ, Blundell C: Choice of implants for internal fixation of femoral neck fractures: Meta analysis of 25 randomized trials including 4,925 patients. Acta Orthop Scand 69:138–143, 1998.

12. Ravikumar KJ, Marsh G: Internal fixation versus hemiarthroplasty versus total hip arthroplasty for displaced subcapital fractures of femur—13 year results of a prospective randomised study. Injury 31:793–797, 2000.

13. Keating JF, Grant A, Masson M, et al: Displaced intracapsular hip fractures in fit, older people: A randomized comparison of reduction and fixation, bipolar hemiarthroplasty and total hip arthroplasty. Health Technol Assess 9:iii-iv, ix-x, 1–65, 2005.

Chapter 60

Intracapsular Femoral Neck Fracture: How Does Delay in Surgery Affect Complication Rate?

PAUL R. T. KUZYK, BSC, MASC, MD, FRCS(C) AND EMIL H. SCHEMITSCH, MD, FRCS(C)

Speed[1] termed the displaced intracapsular femoral neck fracture *the unsolved fracture* because of its high rate of complications and controversies in management at the time. Many years later, this fracture continues to challenge the treating orthopedic surgeon. Much of the difficulty lies in the precarious blood supply to the femoral neck and head. This leads to the two most common and devastating orthopedic complications: nonunion and avascular necrosis of the femoral head. These fractures have long been believed to represent an orthopedic emergency, requiring immediate intervention to prevent these complications. Displaced femoral neck fractures occur infrequently (only 3% of all hip fractures) in the young adult (i.e., younger than 60 years); therefore, it is difficult to obtain adequate power to conduct a study to determine whether timing of intervention actually impacts the rate of complications.[2,3] This fracture occurs much more frequently in the elderly population; however, epidemiology, mechanism of injury, rates of complications, and treatment options are different for this age group. This chapter examines the effect of time to surgery on complication rates for displaced femoral neck fractures in these two age groups.

OPTIONS

Displaced femoral neck fractures in the young adult patient tend to result from high-energy trauma. Typically, this produces a highly unstable vertical shear fracture and is often associated with other injuries (e.g., ipsilateral femoral shaft fracture).[3–5] This high-energy mechanism may also result in significant injury to the soft tissues surrounding the hip joint. Cadaveric injection studies and radioisotope scans of the femoral head show that there are both intraosseous and extraosseous vessels supplying the femoral head and neck.[6,7] The major extraosseous blood supply to the femoral head comes from the medial femoral circumflex artery and its retinacular branches (inferior, posterior, and superior). The artery of the ligamentum teres supplies a negligible volume of the femoral head in most of the population. In displaced femoral neck fractures, blood supply to the femoral head and neck is mainly dependant on the extraosseous retinacular branches of the medial femoral cir-

cumflex. Several questions become apparent: Does nonunion and avascular necrosis depend on the extent of damage to these vessels at the time of injury and not the time from injury to operative fixation in high-energy injuries? Do high-energy injuries have greater rates of nonunion and avascular necrosis than low-energy injuries?

Several authors have discussed the possibility that avascular necrosis of the femoral head is related to increased intracapsular pressure.[8,9] Increased intracapsular pressure may result in occlusion of the retinacular vessels. This has often been the argument for early surgical intervention or aspiration to "decompress" the hip capsule. Are rates of avascular necrosis affected by hip capsule decompression?

Low-energy injuries may occur in the young adult. Robinson and colleagues[3] and Swiontkowski and coauthors[4] comment on a subgroup of patients from this population who have longstanding medical problems and sustain this fracture from a simple fall. They found that these patients tended to have an increased prevalence of alcoholism, arthritis, cardiorespiratory problems, neuromuscular disorders, and epilepsy. Is this subgroup of patients best grouped with elderly patients because their fractures likely occur secondary to osteoporosis and result from low-energy trauma?

Displaced femoral neck fractures in the elderly have been examined mainly from the standpoint of treatment. A lack of agreement remains among surgeons regarding optimal treatment (internal fixation vs. arthroplasty) for those fractures in the young elderly group (i.e., 60–80 years of age).[10] Internal fixation of the fracture in this age group has several advantages compared with arthroplasty: shorter operative time, decreased blood loss, and reduced perioperative mortality.[11] Many of these patients have significant comorbidities and require medical management before surgery. Does time from injury to surgery affect the rates of nonunion and avascular necrosis in elderly patients with displaced femoral neck fractures?

EVIDENCE

Damany and coauthors[2] reported a meta-analysis on intracapsular femoral neck fractures in the young adult (15–50 years of age). This is Level II evidence because they incorporated the results of 18 retrospective cohort studies (547 fractures) published between 1976 and 2003. They found that displaced femoral neck fractures occurred more frequently than nondisplaced fractures (79.9% vs. 25.6%) in this age group. The overall rate of avascular necrosis for the displaced fractures was 22.5%, and the rate of nonunion was 6.0%. They identified 7 studies (170 fractures) that gave data regarding timing of surgery and development of complications. From their analysis of these data, they found no significant difference in the rate of avascular necrosis for fractures reduced within 12 hours of injury (13.6%) as compared with those reduced after 12 hours (15%) of injury. Similarly, there was no difference in nonunion rates between the 2 groups (11.8% before 12 hours and 5.0% after 12 hours). This study represents the best evidence on timing of surgery and complications for displaced femoral neck fractures (Table 60–1).

Upadhyay and investigators'[12] Level II study found no evidence of decreased complication rates with early intervention among 92 young adults with displaced femoral neck fractures. Rates of avascular necrosis were 14% in the group treated within 48 hours of injury and 19% in the group treated over 48 hours after injury. The nonunion rate was 18% in the early treatment group and 16.7% in the delayed group. Haidukewych and colleagues'[13] Level IV study also found no association between operative delay and complication rates.

Several Level II studies included in the meta-analysis by Damany and coauthors[2] conclude that the time interval between injury and surgery does affect complication rates. Swiontkowski and coauthors[4] conclude that their good results (no nonunions and 20% rate of avascular necrosis) were due to early intervention. However, their sample size was small (21 patients) and included 4 nondisplaced fractures and only 1 displaced fracture treated over 12 hours after injury. Jain and colleagues[14] found a significantly greater rate of avascular necrosis in patients treated 12 hours after injury (none in those treated before 12 hours and 26% after 12 hours). This study also had a small sample size (38 patients), 9 patients in the study had nondisplaced fractures, and only 7 patients in the early treatment group were followed for more than 2 years radiographically. Radiographic follow-up of more than 2 years is often suggested because approximately 20% of avascular necrosis cases present more than 2 years after injury.[7]

Two case series from the developing world give rates of avascular necrosis for neglected displaced femoral neck fractures in the young adult. Huang[15] found a rate of avascular necrosis of 25% for patients with displaced fractures seen for nonunion from 3 months to 2 years after injury. Roshan and Ram[16] treated 32 patients treated at 12 to 30 weeks after injury and recorded no cases of avascular necrosis after at least 2 years of follow-up. Both these studies conclude that avascular necrosis was not related to timing of surgery, given that the results were equal to or better than fractures fixed on an urgent basis.

Studies have examined the vascularity of femoral heads retrieved from patients undergoing arthroplasty within 2 weeks after sustaining a displaced femoral neck fracture. Calandruccio and Anderson[7] report that 22% of femoral heads were vascular, 47% were partially avascular, and 32% were avascular. Similarly, Catto[17] found that 17% of femoral heads were vascular, 50% were partially avascular, and 33% were avascular. These studies suggest that at the time of fracture, the majority of femoral heads (i.e., 79–83%) are at least partially avascular. Because reported rates of avascular necrosis are less than 30% (even with delayed fixation), there are two possible scenarios: (1) the femoral head undergoes revascularization with time, or (2) some patients have asymptomatic avascular necrosis without segmental collapse of the head. Calandruccio and Anderson[7] suggest that the latter was true, and that the fate of the femoral head was determined at the time of injury. We agree with this statement and believe that the vascularity of the femoral head is largely dependent on the degree of the initial injury.

AREAS OF UNCERTAINTY

Should the Intracapsular Hematoma Be Decompressed?

In young patients with displaced femoral neck fractures, time from injury to treatment does not appear to have a significant effect on avascular necrosis rates. This suggests that the fate of the femoral head is determined at the time of injury. Furthermore, decompression of the capsule (either through open reduction or aspiration) has not been shown clinically to affect development of avascular necrosis. Maruenda and coauthors'[18] Level I study showed no relation between intracapsular pressure (pressure above diastolic pressure) and development of avascular necrosis or reduction in blood supply to the femoral head (measured by the scintigraphy ratio). This study also included nondisplaced fractures and found no difference in intracapsular pressures between nondisplaced and displaced fractures with the leg in a resting position.

Upadhyay and investigators[12] also found no significant difference in rates of avascular necrosis and nonunion for displaced fractures treated with closed reduction and pinning compared with those treated with open reduction, capsulotomy, and pinning. This study found that quality of reduction, quality of fixation, and posterior comminution all influenced the rates of this complication. Posterior comminution has been cited by several as a poor prognostic indicator.[19–21] Posterior comminution may indicate significant damage to the posterior retinacular vessels (main blood supply to the femoral head) or may influence the ability to obtain a good quality reduction. Poor reduction, especially varus angulation, has also been cited by several authors as a factor for failure of fixation and development of nonunion.[12,20–22] Chua and coworkers[22] conducted a retrospective cohort study

TABLE 60–1. Studies That Examine Correlation of Complication Rates with Time from Injury to Surgery for Young Adults

STUDY	LEVEL OF EVIDENCE	DESIGN	RATE OF FOLLOW-UP	AVERAGE DURATION OF FOLLOW-UP (RANGE)	N	SEX	AVERAGE AGE (RANGE)	TIME TO OPERATION	RATE OF AVN	RATE OF NONUNION	CORRELATION WITH TIME TO SURGERY
Damany et al. (2005)[2]	II	Meta-analysis of 7 studies			170		16–50 yr	110 < 12 hr 60 > 12 hr	13.6% < 12 hr 25.0% > 12 hr	11.8% < 12 hr 5% > 12 hr	No
Upadhyay et al. (2004)[12]	II	Retrospective cohort	90.2%		92	82.6% M	37.72 (15–50)	50 < 48 hr 42 > 48 hr	14% < 48 hr 19% > 48 hr	18% < 48 hr 16.7% > 48 hr	No
Huang (1986)[15]	IV	Case series	100%	>2 yr	16	75% M	27.9 (16–43)	3–24 mo	25%	100%	No for AVN
Roshan and Ram (2006)[16]	IV	Case series	90.6%	6.1 (2–12) yr	32	78.1% M	33 (18–50)	12–30 wk	0	100%	No for AVN
Haidukewych et al. (2004)[13]	IV	Case series		6.6 yr (3 mo to 24 yr)	73	72.6% M	36 (15–50)	53 < 24 hr 20 > 24 hr	24.5% < 24 hr 20 > 24 hr	7% < 24 hr 10% > 24 hr	No

AVN, avascular necrosis.

TABLE 60–2. Studies That Examine the Rates of Complications in the Elderly Population

STUDY	LEVEL OF EVIDENCE	DESIGN	AVERAGE DURATION OF FOLLOW-UP (YR)	N	SEX	AVERAGE AGE (YR)	TIME TO OPERATION	RATE OF AVASCULAR NECROSIS	RATE OF NONUNION	CORRELATION WITH TIME TO SURGERY
Gerber et al. (1993)[26]	II	Retrospective cohort	>1	44	23.7% M	>60		4.5%	4.5%	No
Barnes et al. (1976)[23]	II	Prospective cohort	>3	848	15% M		148 < 24 hr 700 > 24 hr		27.7% < 24 hr 33.0% > 24 hr	No
Toh et al. (2004)[24]	II	Retrospective cohort		91	29% M		1.24–4.41 days	11%	13%	No
Bhandari et al. (2003)[11]	V	Meta-analysis of 14 studies		1933				9.7% (5–18%)	18.5% (5–28%)	Not discussed
Lu-Yao et al. (1994)[25]	V	Meta-analysis of 5 studies	>2	503		78–81		16%	33%	Not discussed

on 108 elderly patients with femoral neck fractures and found that difficulty in obtaining a reduction was associated with a significantly greater rate of failure of fixation (4.3 times).[22] If the reduction was difficult to obtain and the hip was fixed in varus, then the fixation was 13.6 times more likely not to be successful.

RECOMMENDATIONS

Displaced femoral neck fractures occur infrequently in the young adult population, and this has made clinical study of this fracture challenging. Studies in the literature have small sample sizes, require many years to obtain appropriate sample numbers, combine results from multiple surgeons and hospitals, and incorporate different methods of fixation. This makes interpretation of results difficult. Based on the results from Damany and coauthors'[2] meta-analysis (avascular necrosis rate of 13.6% and nonunion rate of 11.8% for fractures fixed within 12 hours), we calculated the sample size required to detect a difference in these complication rates between equal groups of fractures fixed within 12 hours and more than 12 hours after injury. Assuming a relative risk ratio of 2 (rate of complications is twice as frequent in the group of fractures fixed after 12 hours), these calculations suggest that at least 270 patients would be required to determine a significant difference ($\alpha = 0.05$; $\beta = 0.8$). (The actual relative risk ratio is likely less than 2, indicating that an even larger sample size is required.) No retrospective case-controlled studies in the literature have this sample size.

Studies on displaced femoral neck fractures in the elderly population have similar difficulties (Table 60–2). Although this fracture is much more common in this age group, many surgeons elect to replace the femoral head rather than attempt to save it. This also leads to relatively small sample sizes. As a result, we have had to rely on meta-analyses to extract data from the literature. Based on our review of the literature, we have made the following recommendations (Table 60–3):

- No good evidence has been reported that early intervention reduces complication rates for displaced femoral neck fractures. Best evidence actually suggests no difference in complication rates between fractures fixed before and after 12 hours after injury (grade C evidence). Overall rates of complication for this injury in the young adult are 22.5% for avascular necrosis and 6% for nonunion (grade B evidence).[2] No decrease in complication rates with decompression of the intracapsular hematoma occurs (grade B evidence).
- Poor reduction (i.e., coxa vara), difficulty in obtaining reduction, and posterior fracture comminution are correlated with greater rates of complication (grade B evidence).
- Despite a low-energy mechanism of injury, elderly patients have a greater incidence of nonunion (13–33%) after fixation of these fractures than young adults (grade B evidence).[11,23–25] This is likely because of poor fixation and difficulty obtaining reduction in osteopenic bone. Rates of avascular necrosis (10–16%) are similar to those seen in young adults (grade B evidence).[11,23–25] A decrease in time for fracture fixation in the elderly has not been shown to decrease rates of nonunion or avascular necrosis (grade B evidence).

TABLE 60–3. Grades of Evidence for Displaced Intracapsular Femoral Neck Fractures

RECOMMENDATIONS	LEVEL OF EVIDENCE/ GRADE OF RECOMMENDATION
1. Early intervention reduces rates of avascular necrosis, nonunion, or both.	I
2. No difference in complication rates between fractures fixed before and after 12 hours after injury.	C
3. Complication rates for this injury in the young adult are 22.5% for avascular necrosis and 6% for nonunion.	B
4. No role for decompression of intracapsular hematoma.	B
5. Complication rates increase with poor reduction, difficulty obtaining reduction, and degree of posterior comminution.	B
6. A decrease in time for fracture fixation in elderly patients has not been shown to decrease rates of nonunion or avascular necrosis.	B

REFERENCES

1. Speed K: The unsolved fracture. Surg Gynecol Obstet 60:341, 1935.
2. Damany DS, Parker MJ, Chojnowski A: Complications after intracapsular hip fractures in young adults. A meta-analysis of 18 published studies involving 564 fractures. Injury 36:131–141, 2005.
3. Robinson CM, Court-Brown CM, McQueen MM, et al: Hip fractures in adults younger than 50 years of age: Epidemiology and results. Clin Orthop 312:238–246, 1995.
4. Swiontkowski MF, Winquist RA, Hansen SH: Fractures of the femoral neck in patients between the ages of twelve and forty-nine years. J Bone Joint Surg Am 66-A:837–846, 1984.
5. Swiontkowski MF, Hansen ST, Kellam J: Ipsilateral fracture of the femoral neck and shaft. A treatment protocol. J Bone Joint Surg Am 66-A:260–268, 1984.
6. Sevitt S, Thompson RG: The distribution and anastomoses of arteries supplying the head and neck of the femur. J Bone Joint Surg Br 47-B:560–573, 1965.
7. Calandruccio RA, Anderson WE: Post-fracture avascular necrosis of the femoral head: Correlation of experimental and clinical studies. Clin Orthop 152:49–84, 1980.

8. Soto-Hall R, Johnson LH, Johnson R: Alterations in the intra-articular pressures in transcervical fractures of the hip. J Bone Joint Surg Am 46-A:662, 1963.

9. Bonnaire F, Schaefer DJ, Kuner EH: Hemarthrosis and hip joint pressure in femoral neck fractures. Clin Orthop 353:148–155, 1998.

10. Bhandari M, Devereaux PJ, Tornetta P, et al: Operative management of displaced femoral neck fractures in elderly patients. An international survey. J Bone Joint Surg Am 87-A:2122–2130, 2005.

11. Bhandari M, Devereaux PJ, Swiontkowski MF, et al: Internal fixation compared with arthroplasty for displaced fractures of the femoral neck. A meta-analysis. J Bone Joint Surg Am 85-A:1673–1681, 2003.

12. Upadhyay A, Jain P, Mishra P, et al: Delayed internal fixation of fractures of the neck of the femur in young adults. A prospective, randomised study comparing closed and open reduction. J Bone Joint Surg Br 86-B:1035–1040, 2004.

13. Haidukewych GJ, Rothwell WS, Jacofsky DJ, et al: Operative treatment of femoral neck fractures in patients between the ages of fifteen and fifty years. J Bone Joint Surg Am 86-A:1711–1716, 2004.

14. Jain R, Koo M, Kreder HJ, et al: Comparison of early and delayed fixation of subcapital fractures in patients sixty years of age or less. J Bone Joint Surg Am 84-A:1605–1612, 2002.

15. Huang CH: Treatment of neglected femoral neck fractures in young adults. Clin Orthop Relat Res 206:117–126, 1986.

16. Roshan A, Ram S: Early return to function in young adults with neglected femoral neck fractures. Clin Orthop Relat Res 447:152–157, 2006.

17. Catto M: A histological study of avascular necrosis of the femoral head after transcervical fracture. J Bone Joint Surg Br 47-B:749, 1965.

18. Maruenda JI, Barrios C, Gomar-Sancho F: Intracapsular hip pressure after femoral neck fracture. Clin Orthop Relat Res 340:172–180, 1997.

19. Scheck M: Intracapsular fractures of the femoral neck: Comminution of the posterior neck cortex as a case of unstable fixation. J Bone Joint Surg Am 41-A:1187–1200, 1959.

20. Asnis SE, Wanek-Sgaglione L: Intracapsular fractures of the femoral neck: Results of cannulated screw fixation. J Bone Joint Surg Am 76-A:1793–1803, 1994.

21. Bray TJ: Femoral neck fracture fixation. Clin Orthop Relat Res (339):20–31, 1997.

22. Chua D, Jaglal SB, Schatzker J: Predictors of early failure of fixation in the treatment of displaced subcapital hip fractures. J Orthop Trauma 12:230–234, 1998.

23. Barnes R, Brown JT, Garden RS, Nicoll EA: Subcapital fractures of the femur. A prospective review. J Bone Joint Surg 58-B:2–24, 1976.

24. Toh EM, Sahni V, Acharya A, et al.: Management of intracapsular femoral neck fractures in the elderly; is it time to rethink our strategy? Injury 35:125–129, 2004.

25. Lu-Yao GL, Keller RB, Littenberg B, et al.: Outcomes after displaced fractures of the femoral neck. A meta-analysis of one hundred and six published reports. J Bone Joint Surg 76-A:15–25, 1994.

26. Gerber C, Strehle J, Ganz R: The treatment of fractures of the femoral neck. Clin Orthop Relat Res 292:77–86, 1993.

Subtrochanteric Femoral Fractures:
Is a Nail or Plate Better?

Allan S. L. Liew, MD, FRCSC

Subtrochanteric fractures remain a problematic fracture for treatment because of the local biomechanics, deforming forces of the attached musculature, and fracture configuration. The combination of high-stress concentration in an area of dense, cortical, hypovascular bone results in a propensity for nonunion. The soft-tissue stripping from the fracture can be further exacerbated with surgical dissection, resulting in a greater risk for delayed union and nonunion.

The deforming forces of the muscular attachments on the fragments combined with the effect of weight bearing result in the typical deformity of varus, apex anterior angulation, shortening, and external rotation of the proximal fragment. When inadequately corrected, a significant malreduction can increase the stress on the implant, leading to further deformity and implant failure. If the implant selected has poor fixation, or if weight-bearing limits are not adhered to, delayed displacement, malunion, or nonunion are the usual results.

Several classification systems are currently in use, including the Russell–Taylor classification,[1] the Seinsheimer classification,[2] and the AO/OTA classification. Each has its own method of stratification and nomenclature; however, they have not been shown to be useful in predicting treatment and outcome.[3,4]

The treatment principles are similar to other nonarticular long bone fractures of the lower extremity. These include preoperative optimization, including smoking cessation, preoperative planning, surgical positioning, operative reduction and fixation emphasizing soft-tissue preservation, and postoperative rehabilitation protocols.

OPTIONS

The question of whether subtrochanteric femur fractures are best treated with an intramedullary nail device or an extramedullary plate device has been long debated and studied.[5,6] Devices currently in use include cephalomedullary nails, with either a piriformis or trochanteric start, and fixed-angle plating implants including blade plates, sliding hip screws, and locking plates. The purpose of this review is to guide surgeons in selecting the appropriate implant for this potentially troublesome fracture based on the best available evidence.

EVIDENCE

No Level I studies were available comparing treatment options for subtrochanteric fractures. The available Level II studies focused on pertrochanteric fractures, but few stratified for a subtrochanteric fracture group and even fewer specifically analyzed data for this fracture. Most of the studies were underpowered to show significant differences. Both biomechanical and clinical studies are available. However, extrapolating biomechanical results to the clinical situation must be done with caution because the most stable implant in the laboratory may not necessarily be optimal in a biological sense.

The available Level III and IV case series describing the treatment results with individual implants noted impressive success rates up to 100% and complication rates as low as 0%.[7-11] Although these studies may give some indication as to the success and pitfalls of various implants, they provide little help in guiding treatment considerations of one implant versus another.

Specific patient or fracture characteristics may limit the treatment options available. In patients with previous surgery or hardware distally in the femur, such as a total knee prosthesis,[12] with previous deformity, or in pediatric fractures with open proximal growth plates, a fixed-angle plate device may be preferred. In patients with a significant lateral soft-tissue injury, or with extensive comminution or a segmental injury extending down the femoral shaft, a cephalomedullary nail is less traumatic to the soft-tissue envelope. In the case of a pathologic fracture, a cephalomedullary nail treats the fracture and provides prophylactic support or fixation for distal lesions.[13] It would be difficult to produce randomized trials for each potential scenario comparing treatment strategy, and the level of evidence in this regard is therefore limited to Level V (expert opinion).

Biomechanics

The ideal fracture fixation device would be able to withstand the physiologic loads of postoperative rehabilitation. Typically, to stand in single-leg stance would axially load the femur with 750 N; however, walking or other activities of daily living would generate three to seven times that load.

Tencer and colleagues[14] compared seven devices in a cadaveric subtrochanteric fracture model tested in axial loading and found that the plate devices (compression hip screw and AO angled blade plate) failed between 1100 and 1500 N compared with a locked nail at 3000 N.

In a cadaveric study by Haynes and coworkers,[15] the short Gamma nail (GN) was tested against the dynamic hip screw (DHS) in an osteotomized proximal femur simulating a subtrochanteric fracture with intertrochanteric extension. The authors found that in the harder bone model, the GN had a failure load of 5761 N versus the DHS with a failure load of 4660 N in axial loading. In the soft bone model, the failure loads were 5725 N for the GN and 3225 N for the DHS. The modes of failure were fractures of the femoral shaft around the distal locking screws for the GN, and lateral plate and screw pullout with the DHS.

It can be concluded from these and other similar studies that intramedullary devices are able to withstand greater axial loads than plate devices in unstable subtrochanteric fractures with medial comminution. The effect of nonaxial muscular forces on the fragments and construct stiffness may be a factor in the development of a delayed union or nonunion; however, the differences between implants in this regard have not been adequately reported in the literature.

Clinical Trials

Few studies include the comparison of an intramedullary device versus a plate device for subtrochanteric fractures in a randomized controlled trial. Ekstrom and coworkers[16] conducted a pertrochanteric fracture fixation trial on 203 patients that included analysis of the subtrochanteric fracture data, 18 treated with the proximal femoral nail (PFN), and 13 treated with the Medoff sliding plate (MSP) (Level III). They found significant advantages in operating room time, blood loss, and earlier ability to walk 15 m at 6 weeks for those treated with the PFN. The MSP held the advantage for shorter fluoroscopy time. They also studied other functional parameters including intraoperative complications, walking ability at 4 and 12 months, hospital stay, transfusions, infection, and mortality, and they found no significant differences.

Goldhagen and colleagues[17] randomized 75 patients with pertrochanteric fractures to compare the GN and the compression hip screw (CHS), which included analysis of 12 subtrochanteric fractures. The GN was used in seven patients, and the CHS was used in five. The authors found a trend for shorter operative time with the GN (82 vs. 99 minutes); however, they were unable to show statistical significance. Other outcomes studied including fluoroscopy time, blood loss, transfusions, length of hospital stay, functional outcomes, and mortality showed no difference (Level II).

In another study by Miedel and coauthors,[18] 217 patients with pertrochanteric fractures were randomized to treatment with the standard Gamma nail (SGN) or a

MSP. Their analysis included stratification of some of the subtrochanteric fracture data: 16 patients treated with the SGN, and 12 treated with the MSP. They report a greater postoperative fixation complication rate with the MSP with loss of reduction in two patients. In their pooled data analysis of all the fractures, they report better operative reduction, less blood loss, and lower mortality for those treated with the SGN. Other outcomes examined including intraoperative fractures, operative time, transfusions, infections, length of hospital stay, and functional outcomes showed no significant differences.

Parker and Handoll[19] report in the Cochrane review on cephalomedullary versus extramedullary implants for the treatment of extra-articular pertrochanteric fractures that there were better intraoperative results and less fracture fixation complications in the subtrochanteric subgroup treated with a cephalomedullary device (Level I).

Of the available randomized trials that pooled subtrochanteric and intertrochanteric data, most of the outcomes studied showed no difference, except for a significant incidence of femoral shaft fracture with the use of a short intramedullary device, and a subsequent greater reoperation rate[20,21] (Level II).

RECOMMENDATIONS

Nails

The complication of femoral shaft fracture with short intramedullary devices has prompted further implant design and study. Kraemer and coworkers[22] used a cadaveric model to compare the Russell–Taylor reconstruction nail, the short intramedullary hip screw (IMHS), and the long IMHS in an unstable subtrochanteric fracture. In axial loading, the reconstruction nail and short IMHS were stiffer than the long IMHS in nondestructive cyclic loading. The reconstruction nail had the highest ultimate load to failure compared with either IMHS nails and failed by femoral head screw cutout, whereas the short IMHS failed by femoral shaft fracture.

In a cadaveric study by Wheeler and colleagues,[23] unstable subtrochanteric fractures were simulated and fixed with three different cephalomedullary nails, the Richards Russell–Taylor reconstruction nail, the Synthes spiral blade nail, and the Zimmer ZMS nail. The Richards and Zimmer constructs were significantly stiffer and had a higher failure load than the Synthes construct in axial loading. The Richards constructs typically failed by fracture of the distal femur at the interlocking screw holes. The Zimmer constructs failed by bending of the proximal end of the nail. The Synthes constructs failed by bending of the spiral blade and fracture of the femoral neck.

Starr and coauthors[24] report on a series of pertrochanteric fractures treated with a piriformis start or trochanteric start cephalomedullary nail. They found no difference in intraoperative or postoperative parameters studied (Level I). Thus, if a nail is to be used, a long cephalomedullary nail with either a piriformis or trochanteric start and appropriate proximal and distal locking should be selected.

Plates

There remains a wide variety of plates used for subtrochanteric fractures, including blade plates, 95- and 135-degree sliding hip screw constructs, biaxial sliding constructs, and locking plates. Many of these implants have not been tested in a comparative study either biomechanically or in a randomized clinical trial.

Tencer and colleagues[14] report a study of seven types of fixation in a stable and unstable subtrochanteric fracture model. In the stable fracture model, the 150-degree hip screw and 95-degree blade plate demonstrated similar stiffness in torsion, which was significantly greater than the intramedullary implants tested (none in current use). In axial loading, both plate systems were as rigid as the nails. In the unstable fracture model, both plate systems remained stiffer than the nails in rotation, but resistance to axial loading was poor.

In a clinical trial, Madsen and researchers[21] report on randomized pertrochanteric fractures that the DHS with trochanteric side plate (TSP) had less postoperative redisplacement and lag screw cutout compared with the CHS. They also report a longer hospital stay with the DHS with TSP compared with the CHS (Level I). Another study by Lunsjo and coworkers[25] reports that the MSP had less fixation failure than the DHS, dynamic condylar screw, and DHS with TSP (Level I).

With the advent of new plate designs, as well as improvements in indirect reduction and biologic plating techniques, it remains unclear which plate construct is best suited for subtrochanteric fractures, although a fixed angle device with adequate proximal fixation is recommended.

Nails versus Plates

With the change in practice to using long intramedullary devices, femoral shaft fracture complications are rare; however, the apparent shorter operating room time reported with short intramedullary nails compared with plates[16,17] may no longer be significant because of the extra time required to lock long nails distally. The disadvantage of greater intraoperative blood loss with plating is not seen clinically after surgery with the same transfusion rates as nailing.[16,18]

A potential advantage of earlier return to function in unstable fractures with intramedullary nailing exists, as supported by increased resistance to axial loading seen in biomechanical studies (14, 15) and clinically by Ekstrom and coworkers,[16] who reported better ability to walk 15 m at 6 weeks after surgery in those treated with an intramedullary nail. This difference is no longer seen at 4 and 12 months (Level III). This factor may be particularly important in patients who are unable to comply with postoperative weight-bearing restrictions.

Varus malreduction and inaccurate screw placement in the femoral head have been correlated with an increased risk for failure and further deformity.[16] Given the lack of clear evidence of the superiority of one implant over another, it is likely more important that the surgeon chooses the implant with which they are most facile, and able to get the most accurate reduction and appropriate implant position, whereas maximally preserving the local biology and soft-tissue envelope.

With the new armamentarium of current implants and soft-tissue–preserving techniques, further study is needed to determine what differences exist between nails and plates, and in which fracture types they are best applied. Table 61–1 provides a summary of recommendations.

TABLE 61–1. Summary of Recommendations

RECOMMENDATION	LEVEL OF EVIDENCE/GRADE OF RECOMMEDATION
1. Adults with subtrochanteric femur fractures can be treated with either a long intramedullary cephalomedullary device or a fixed-angle device.	B
2. A short intramedullary device should NOT be used for these fractures.	C

REFERENCES

1. Russell TA, Taylor JC: Subtrochanteric fractures of the femur. In Browner BD, Jupiter JB, Levine AM, Trafton PG (eds): Skeletal Trauma, 2nd ed. Philadelphia, WB Saunders, 1992, pp 1832–1878.
2. Seinsheimer F: Subtrochanteric fractures of the femur. J Bone Joint Surg Am 60:300–306, 1978.
3. Blundell CM, Parker MJ, Pryor GA, et al: Assessment of the AO classification of intracapsular fractures of the proximal femur. J Bone Joint Surg Br 80:679–683, 1998.
4. Parker MJ, Dutta BK, Sivaji C, Pryor GA: Subtrochanteric fractures of the femur. Injury 28:91–95, 1997.
5. Fielding JW: Subtrochanteric fractures. Clin Orthop Relat Res (92):86–99, 1973.
6. Thomas WG, Villar RN: Subtrochanteric fractures: Zickel nail or nail-plate? J Bone Joint Surg Br 68:255–259, 1986.
7. Alho A, Ekeland A, Stromsoe K: Subtrochanteric femoral fractures treated with locked intramedullary nails. Experience from 31 cases. Acta Orthop Scand 62:573–576, 1991.

8. Barquet A, Francescoli L, Rienzi D, Lopez L: Intertrochanteric-subtrochanteric fractures: Treatment with the long Gamma nail. J Orthop Trauma 14:324–328, 2000.

9. Bedi A, Toan Le T: Subtrochanteric femur fractures. Orthop Clin North Am 35:473–483, 2004.

10. Celebi L, Can M, Muratli HH, et al: Indirect reduction and biological internal fixation of comminuted subtrochanteric fractures of the femur. Injury 37:740–750, 2006.

11. Pai CH: Dynamic condylar screw for subtrochanteric femur fractures with greater trochanteric extension. J Orthop Trauma 10:317–322, 1996.

12. Althausen PL, Lee MA, Finkemeier CG, et al: Operative stabilization of supracondylar femur fractures above total knee arthroplasty: A comparison of four treatment methods. J Arthroplasty 18:834–839, 2003.

13. Weikert DR, Schwartz HS: Intramedullary nailing for impending pathological subtrochanteric fractures. J Bone Joint Surg Br 73:668–670, 1991.

14. Tencer AF, Johnson KD, Johnston DW, Gill K: A biomechanical comparison of various methods of stabilization of subtrochanteric fractures of the femur. J Orthop Res 2:297–305, 1984.

15. Haynes RC, Poll RG, Miles AW, Weston RB: An experimental study of the failure modes of the Gamma Locking Nail and AO Dynamic Hip Screw under static loading: A cadaveric study. Med Eng Phys 19:446–453, 1997.

16. Ekstrom W, Karlsson-Thur C, Larsson S, et al: Functional outcome in treatment of unstable trochanteric and subtrochanteric fractures with the proximal femoral nail and the Medoff sliding plate. J Orthop Trauma 21:18–25, 2007.

17. Goldhagen PR, O'Connor DR, Schwarze D, Schwartz E: A prospective comparative study of the compression hip screw and the gamma nail. J Orthop Trauma 8:367–372, 1994.

18. Miedel R, Ponzer S, Tornkvist H, et al: The standard Gamma nail or the Medoff sliding plate for unstable trochanteric and subtrochanteric fractures. A randomised, controlled trial. J Bone Joint Surg Br 87:68–75, 2005.

19. Parker MJ, Handoll HHG: Gamma and other cephalocondylic intramedullary nails versus extramedullary implants for extracapsular hip fractures. Cochrane Database Syst Rev CD000093, 2004.

20. Aune AK, Ekeland A, Odegaard B, et al: Gamma nail vs compression screw for trochanteric femoral fractures. 15 reoperations in a prospective, randomized study of 378 patients. Acta Orthop Scand 65:127–130, 1994.

21. Madsen JE, Naess L, Aune AK, et al: Dynamic hip screw with trochanteric stabilizing plate in the treatment of unstable proximal femoral fractures: A comparative study with the Gamma nail and compression hip screw. J Orthop Trauma 12:241–248, 1998.

22. Kraemer WJ, Hearn TC, Powell JN, Mahomed N: Fixation of segmental subtrochanteric fractures: A biomechanical study. Clin Orthop Relat Res 71–79, 1996.

23. Wheeler DL, Croy TJ, Woll TS, et al: Comparison of reconstruction nails for high subtrochanteric femur fracture fixation. Clin Orthop Relat Res 231–239, 1997.

24. Starr AJ, Hay MT, Reinert CM, et al: Cephalomedullary nails in the treatment of high-energy proximal femur fractures in young patients: A prospective, randomized comparison of trochanteric versus piriformis fossa entry portal. J Orthop Trauma 20:240–246, 2006.

25. Lunsjo K, Ceder L, Tidermark J, et al: Extramedullary fixation of 107 subtrochanteric fractures: A randomized multicenter trial of the Medoff sliding plate versus 3 other screw-plate systems. Acta Orthop Scand 70:459–466, 1999.

Femoral Shaft Fractures:
What Is the Best Treatment?

Rudolf W. Poolman, MD, PhD and Mohit Bhandari, MD, Msc, FRCSC

Intramedullary nailing remains the treatment of choice for femoral shaft fractures. However, some situations may direct surgeons to different treatment options. To guide the reader in making choices between these treatment options, we use the Evidence Cycle. This cycle systematically approaches clinical problems using evidence-based medicine.[1-4] The Evidence Cycle can be conceptualized to consist of five A's: assess, ask, acquire, appraise, and apply.

This chapter focuses on adult patients with traumatic femoral shaft fractures. The population of interest is skeletally mature patients with femoral shaft fractures.

Several treatment options can be considered in treatment of patients with femoral shaft fractures. Nonoperative treatment needs to be mentioned for its historical importance; however when operative management became available, this treatment modality was soon abandoned because of its high risk for complications. Traditionally, operative treatment consisted of open reduction and internal plate fixation. Intramedullary nails subsequently gained popularity and are the current standard of care in patients with shaft fractures, although recent minimally invasive plating techniques have revived femoral plating as an option in some circumstances. The purpose of this chapter is to assist the reader in making choices regarding the various treatment options for femoral shaft fractures in skeletally mature adults.

OPTIONS

Our review focuses on the following treatment options: plating or nailing. Specific technical issues that relate to intramedullary nails include the evidence surrounding fracture-table versus freehand reduction techniques, slotted versus solid intramedullary nailing, antegrade versus retrograde intramedullary nailing, trochanteric versus piriformis entry point, reamed versus undreamed nailing, and lastly, static versus dynamic locking of intramedullary nails. Timing of surgery is discussed in Chapter 50.

Our outcomes of interest are nonunion, malunion, including malrotation, and other adverse events. Each clinical question is addressed using a structured PICO (Patients, Intervention, Comparison, and Outcome) format.[3,5]

EVIDENCE

Plating or Intramedullary Nailing

Particularly in the patient with multiple injuries, plating was thought to have advantages in preventing brain damage in the patient with head injury.[6] Thus, our first question using the PICO format is: In patients with head injury and femoral shaft fracture (P), will plating (I) or intramedullary nailing (C) result in better neurologic outcome (O)? Bhandari and coworkers[6] evaluated this question in an observational study. The authors identified 21 patients with severe head injuries treated with a reamed femoral nail for a femoral fracture and 29 comparable patients treated by means of a femoral plate. In their series, severity of the head injury was the strongest predictor for outcome. Nailing was considered a safe procedure that did not worsen outcome, although the authors conclude that a large, sufficiently powered, randomized, controlled trial (RCT) is needed to definitively resolve this controversy[6] (grade C).

Bosse and coworkers'[7] retrospective study compares data from a trauma center using reamed nailing (I) for acute stabilization of femoral fractures with data from another North American center using plating (C). The rate of adult respiratory distress syndrome (O) in the patients who had a femoral fracture without a thoracic injury did not vary considerably according to whether the fracture had been nailed (118 patients) or plated (114 patients). Equally, the occurrence of adult respiratory distress syndrome, pneumonia, pulmonary embolism, failure of multiple organs, or mortality for the patients who had a femoral fracture and thoracic injury was comparable regardless of whether reamed nailing (117 patients) or plating (104 patients) had been used. The authors conclude that the use of intramedullary reamed nailing for acute fixation of fractures of the femur in patients with multiple injuries who have a thoracic injury without major comorbidity did not seem to increase the likelihood of development of adult respiratory distress syndrome, pulmonary embolism, failure of multiple organs, pneumonia, or mortality[7] (grade C).

Fracture-Table versus Freehand Reduction

After choosing intramedullary nailing as the treatment option for femoral shaft fractures, surgeons have different fracture reduction techniques in their toolbox. Stephen and coworkers[8] compared *fracture-table (I)* with *manual traction (C)* in femoral intramedullary nailing in a well-designed, sufficiently powered RCT.[8] The primary outcome was number of patients with 10 degrees or more malrotation. Also, the authors scored severity of rotational malalignment. Operative procedure time was a secondary outcome. Internal malrotation was exceedingly more frequent when the fracture table had been used: 12 (29%) of the 43 femora were internally rotated by more than 10 degrees compared with 3 (7%) of the 45 reduced with manual traction ($P = 0.007$). Total procedure time, from the beginning of the patient positioning to the finishing point of the skin closure, was reduced from a mean of 139 minutes (range, 100–212 minutes) when the fracture table was used to a mean of 119 minutes (range, 65–180 minutes) when manual traction was used ($P = 0.033$). No significant difference was found between the two treatment groups with regard to the number of assistants per case (mean, 2; range, 0–3), fluoroscopy time, other adverse events including femoral leg length discrepancy, or functional condition of the patient at 1-year follow-up[8] (grade A).

Slotted versus Solid Intramedullary Nail

After the fracture is manually well reduced and rotationally aligned options for nailing include using either a slotted or a solid nail. One European and one North American study evaluated this issue.[9,10] Alho and coauthors[10] randomized 22 nonslotted Gross–Kempf nails and 24 slotted AO/ASIF universal femoral nails. Although the nonslotted nails showed higher stiffness than the slotted nails, insertion resulted in splintering of the distal fragment, one resulting in a change of the implant to a condylar plate. Other complications were not implant related. No nonunions were observed in either group.

Cameron and coworkers[9] randomized patients with femoral shaft fractures into three groups: 32 were treated with a nonslotted Grosse–Kempf nail, 29 with a Russell–Taylor nail (nonslotted), and 27 with a Synthes nail (slotted). The operation took less time in the Grosse–Kempf nail group. Three proximal fractures could not be locked with the Synthes nail. At follow-up examination, the authors did not find important difference in pain, limp, range of motion, or time to union. On the other hand, the investigators removed fewer Synthes nails to resolve patient reports of pain. Three delayed unions were due to fracture distraction and were not implant related. The authors conclude that all three nails are suitable for the treatment of almost all femoral shaft fractures (grade I).

Antegrade versus Retrograde Nailing

Two studies compared antegrade versus retrograde reamed intramedullary nailing in RCTs with methodologic shortcomings. Tornetta and Tiburzi[11] used hospital chart numbers for patient allocation and randomized 38 fractures in the antegrade group and 31 in the retrograde group. A rotational deformity of greater than 10 degrees was seen on computed tomographic rotation studies in 3 of 18 (17%) of the antegrade and in 5 of 15 (33%) of retrograde nailings performed in cases with unstable patterns. Shortening occurred in five unstable fractures in the retrograde group, but in none of such injuries in the antegrade group. In these five patients, shortening averaged 12 mm (5–30 mm). Return to the operating room for acute lengthening and relocking was necessary for a patient with 3 cm of shortening. At union, four patients with retrograde nailing and five with antegrade nailing reported pain in the knee.

Ostrum and coworkers[12] compared 44 fractures (7 bilateral) treated with a retrograde nail and 46 (1 bilateral) with an antegrade nail. Discussing fracture results and not patients complicates making inferences when patients with bilateral fractures are compared with patients with single-site fractures.[5,13] Knee pain was equal in both groups (4 patients in the antegrade group; 5 patients in the retrograde group), but hip and thigh pain was in the majority in the antegrade-treated group (10 patients in the antegrade group; 2 patients in the retrograde group; $P = 0.0108$). Finally, three retrospective case series described this issue.[14–17]

Table 62–1 provides detailed information on the available data. Despite the potential for complications, most concerns have been unrealized in recent comparisons between antegrade and retrograde intramedullary nails in patients with femoral shaft fractures (see Table 62–1). In brief, retrograde nails achieve equal union rates and function at the expense of an increased need for nail dynamization. Shortening occurs at a greater rate with retrograde nail insertion but is seldom clinically significant (<1.5 cm). Thigh and hip pain, a common occurrence in antegrade nails, is significantly reduced with retrograde nail insertion. In conclusion, surgeons with experience in retrograde nailing techniques can achieve outcomes similar to those of antegrade nailing techniques. Retrograde nailing may be particularly useful in patients with multiple ipsilateral injuries and in obese patients. Based on our review, both antegrade and retrograde procedures can have acceptable results (grade B).

Trochanteric versus Piriformis Entry Point

Based on a prospective cohort study comparing 38 patients in the trochanteric starting point group with 53 in the piriformis fossa entry point, Ricci and coworkers[18] found reduced fluoroscopy time using a

TABLE 62–1. Antegrade versus Retrograde Nails

STUDY	YEAR	SAMPLE SIZE (N)	DESIGN	LOE	NONUNION (A/R)	ADDITIONAL OR NEEDED (A/R)	MALROTATION (A/R)	SHORTENING (A/R)	KNEE PAIN (A/R)	KNEEROM (A/R)	FUNCTION (A/R)
Tornetta and Tiburzi[11]*	2004	118	RCT	I	2%/3%	8%/16%	NS	1%/7%[†]	NS	NS	NS
Holmenschlager et al.[15]	2002	62	PCS	IV	—/2%	—	—/0%	—/2%	—	81%/ normal	—
Ricci et al.[17]	2001	283	RCS	III	6%/6%	—	NS	—	9%/36%[‡]	—	—
Ostrum et al.[12]	2000	100	RCT	I	0%/2%[§]	5%/17%	—	—	NS[¶]	NS/ normal	—
Ostrum et al.[16]	1998	57	PCS	IV	—/5%	—/12% dynamized	—	—	0%	—	—

*Updated series presented at 2004 Orthopaedic Trauma Association, October 2004.
[†]No patient had shortening >1.5 cm.
[‡]Hip pain more common in antegrade nailing (10% vs. 4%).
[§]Nail to canal diameter difference was a predictor of nonunion.
[¶]Thigh pain more common in antegrade nails.
A, antegrade group; LOE, level of evidence; NS, not significant; PCS, prospective case series; R, retrograde group; RCS, retrospective cohort study; RCT, randomized, controlled trial; ROM, range of motion.

trochanteric starting point and similar overall outcome (grade C).

Reamed versus Unreamed Nailing

The controversy surrounding reamed versus unreamed nailing is evaluated in several RCTs. Bhandari and coworkers[19] performed a systematic review published in 2000 comparing reamed versus unreamed nailing of lower extremity long bone fractures. Since this publication, new RCTs and a new systematic review have become available.[20]

Key outcomes of interest in these studies are delayed or nonunion and post-traumatic acute respiratory distress syndrome (ARDS). Pooling the data of four currently published studies showed a relative risk of 0.29 (95% confidence interval [CI], 0.14–0.57) for delayed or nonunion favoring reamed nails (Fig. 62–1).[21–24] Translated into number needed to treat (NNT) equals 7 (95% CI, 5–12); that is, with every 7 patients treated with a reamed nail, 1 delayed or nonunion result will be prevented.

The relative risk for ARDS in patients treated with a reamed nail was 1.91 (95% CI, 0.74–4.93) (Fig. 62–2).[21,24,25] The CIs crossing 1 indicate a nonsignificant result.

Data on reported adverse events as a composite end point showed a widespread range from patient-unimportant outcomes (e.g., a broken drill bit) to patient-important outcomes (such as pudendal nerve palsy), making pooling of these data futile as a single composite outcome measure.

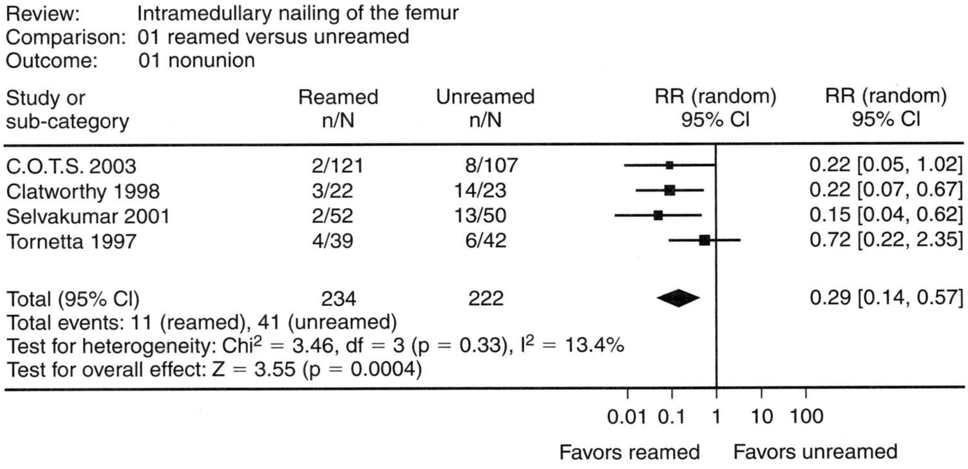

```
Review:        Intramedullary nailing of the femur
Comparison:  01 reamed versus unreamed
Outcome:      01 nonunion

Study or           Reamed   Unreamed     RR (random)       RR (random)
sub-category        n/N        n/N       95% CI            95% CI

C.O.T.S. 2003      2/121      8/107                         0.22 [0.05, 1.02]
Clatworthy 1998    3/22       14/23                         0.22 [0.07, 0.67]
Selvakumar 2001    2/52       13/50                         0.15 [0.04, 0.62]
Tornetta 1997      4/39        6/42                         0.72 [0.22, 2.35]

Total (95% CI)      234         222                         0.29 [0.14, 0.57]
Total events: 11 (reamed), 41 (unreamed)
Test for heterogeneity: Chi² = 3.46, df = 3 (p = 0.33), I² = 13.4%
Test for overall effect: Z = 3.55 (p = 0.0004)

              0.01  0.1   1   10  100
           Favors reamed   Favors unreamed
```

Figure 62–1. Pooled results reamed versus unreamed nailing in preventing nonunion.21–24 CI, confidence interval; RR, relative risk. Data from Canadian Orthopaedic Trauma Society: Nonunion following intramedullary nailing of the femur with and without reaming. Results of a multicenter randomized clinical trial. J Bone Joint Surg Am 85-A:2093-2096, 2003; Clatworthy MG, Clark DI, Gray DH, and Hardy AE: Reamed versus unreamed femoral nails. A randomised, prospective trial. [see comment]. J Bone Joint Surg Br 80:485-489, 1998; Selvakumar K, Saw KY, and Fathima M: Comparison study between reamed and unreamed nailing of closed femoral fractures. Med J Malaysia 56 Suppl D:24-28, 2001; and Tornetta P, III and Tiburzi D: Reamed versus nonreamed anterograde femoral nailing. J Orthop Trauma 14:15-19, 2000.

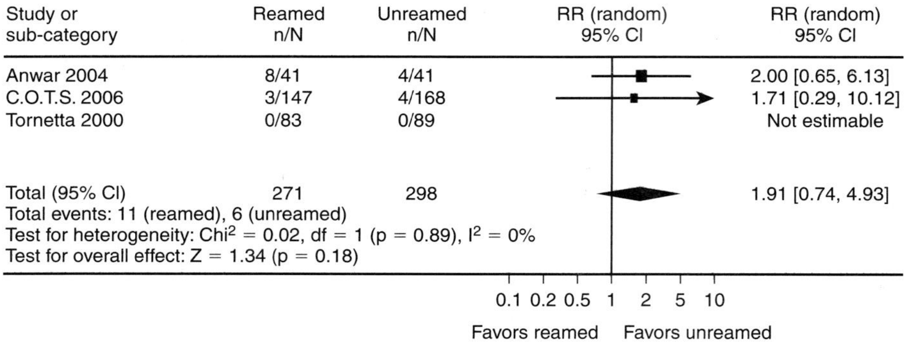

Figure 62–2. Pooled results reamed versus undreamed femoral nailing in preventing acute respiratory distress syndrome (ARDS).[24,25,29] CI, confidence interval; RR, relative risk. Data from Anwar IA, Battistella FD, Neiman R, Olson SA, Chapman MW, and Moehring HD: Femur fractures and lung complications: a prospective randomized study of reaming. Clin Orthop 71-76, 2004; and Canadian Orthopaedic Trauma Society: Nonunion following intramedullary nailing of the femur with and without reaming. Results of a multicenter randomized clinical trial. J Bone Joint Surg Am 85-A: 2093-2096, 2003.

Femoral shaft fractures can be treated safely using reamed intramedullary nails preventing delayed or nonunions without strong evidence for increasing risk for ARDS (grade B).

Static or Dynamic Locking

After the nail is inserted, static or dynamic locking of the nail is possible. One small RCT with methodologic shortcomings did not show a difference in union rates between static and dynamic locking; however, the authors did observe a trend to earlier union in the dynamically locked group.[26] Of the 26 femoral fractures in the dynamized group, union occurred between 13 and 28 weeks (average, 19.2 weeks) in 25 of 26 patients. Union rate was 96.2% in the dynamized group. Of the 24 patients with femoral fractures in the static group, union was achieved in 23 between 16 and 30 weeks (average, 23.45 weeks); union rate was 95.8%.

Conflicting information comes from a larger observational study comparing data from two Italian hospitals.[27] Time to union was significantly shorter in the 104 patients treated in the static group (103 days) compared with the 75 patients treated in the dynamized group (126 days)[27] (grade I conflicting data). Biomechanical data suggest that immediate weight bearing as tolerated is safe after static locking, even in comminuted fractures.[28] Dynamic locking of comminuted shaft fractures should be avoided because it would preclude immediate weight bearing without incurring shortening of the fracture.

AREAS OF UNCERTAINTY

Cost

In our literature search, we could not identify studies evaluating cost associated with treatment options for femoral shaft fractures. To our knowledge, economic analyses currently are lacking.

Patients with Multiple Injuries

Currently limited data are available to make inferences on the optimal treatment strategy for the patient with multiple injuries with a femoral shaft fracture.

RECOMMENDATIONS

Based on our review, our recommendations are as follows:

- In adult patients with femoral shaft fractures, a reamed nail is the implant of choice (grade B), reducing nonunion frequency, with insufficient data supporting theoretical adverse events such as increasing ARDS or worsening brain injury.
- Fracture reduction and nail insertion is ideally achieved on a radiolucent table using a free-hand technique, resulting in shorter operative time and reducing the likelihood of malrotation (grade A).
- Nails can be inserted either in an antegrade direction, at the cost of hip adverse events, or retrograde, increasing knee adverse events (grade B).
- Using a nail designed for a trochanteric starting point may reduce fluoroscopy time (grade C).

Table 62–2 provides a summary of recommendations for the treatment of femoral shaft fractures.

TABLE 62–2. Summary of Recommendations

RECOMMENDATIONS	LEVEL OF EVIDENCE/GRADE OF RECOMMENDATION
1. Adults with femoral shaft fractures should be treated with a reamed nail.	B
2. Femoral fracture reduction on a radiolucent table using manual traction is preferred.	A
3. Either antegrade or retrograde femoral nail insertion is acceptable.	B
4. A nail designed for a trochanteric starting point may reduce fluoroscopy time.	C

Conflicting Data

Based on published reports, we found conflicting data on slotted versus solid nails and static or dynamic locking.

REFERENCES

1. Guyatt GH, Rennie D, The Evidence-Based Medicine Working Group: Users' Guides to the Medical Literature, A Manual for Evidence-Based Clinical Practice. Chicago, AMA Press, 2002.
2. Hayward R: Centre for Health Evidence on line. Available at: http://www.cche.net/
3. Richardson WS, Wilson MC, Nishikawa J, Hayward RS: The well-built clinical question: A key to evidence-based decisions. ACP J Club 123:A12–A13, 1995.
4. Sackett DL, Straus SE, Richardson WS, et al: Evidence-Based Medicine. Edinburgh: Churchill Livingstone, 2000.
5. Poolman RW, Kerkhoffs GM, Struijs PA, et al: Don't be misled by the orthopedic literature: Tips for critical appraisal. Acta Orthop 78:162–171, 2007.
6. Bhandari M, Guyatt GH, Khera V, et al: Operative management of lower extremity fractures in patients with head injuries. Clin Orthop 187–198, 2003.
7. Bosse MJ, MacKenzie EJ, Riemer BL, et al: Adult respiratory distress syndrome, pneumonia, and mortality following thoracic injury and a femoral fracture treated either with intramedullary nailing with reaming or with a plate. A comparative study. J Bone Joint Surg Am 79:799–809, 1997.
8. Stephen DJG, Kreder HJ, Schemitsch EH, et al: Femoral intramedullary nailing: Comparison of fracture-table and manual traction: A prospective, randomized study. J Bone Joint Surg Am 84:1514–1521, 2002.
9. Cameron CD, Meek RN, Blachut PA, et al: Intramedullary nailing of the femoral shaft: A prospective, randomized study. J Orthop Trauma 6:448–451, 1992.
10. Alho A, Moen O, Husby T, et al: Slotted versus non-slotted locked intramedullary nailing for femoral shaft fractures. Arch Orthop Trauma Surg 111:91–95, 1992.
11. Tornetta P III, Tiburzi D: Antegrade or retrograde reamed femoral nailing. A prospective, randomised trial. J Bone Joint Surg Br 82:652–654, 2000.
12. Ostrum RF, Agarwal A, Lakatos R, Poka A: Prospective comparison of retrograde and antegrade femoral intramedullary nailing. J Orthop Trauma 14:496–501, 2000.
13. Bryant D, Havey TC, Roberts R, Guyatt G: How many patients? How many limbs? Analysis of patients or limbs in the orthopaedic literature: A systematic review. J Bone Joint Surg Am 88:41–45, 2006.
14. Blum J, Janzing H, Gahr R, et al: Clinical performance of a new medullary humeral nail: Antegrade versus retrograde insertion. J Orthop Trauma 15:342–349, 2001.
15. Holmenschlager F, Piatek S, Halm JP, Winckler S: [Retrograde intramedullary nailing of femoral shaft fractures. A prospective study]. Unfallchirurg 105:1100–1108, 2002.
16. Ostrum RF, DiCicco J, Lakatos R, Poka A: Retrograde intramedullary nailing of femoral diaphyseal fractures. J Orthop Trauma 12:464–468, 1998.
17. Ricci WM, Bellabarba C, Evanoff B, et al: Retrograde versus antegrade nailing of femoral shaft fractures. J Orthop Trauma 15:161–169, 2001.
18. Ricci WM, Schwappach J, Tucker M, et al: Trochanteric versus piriformis entry portal for the treatment of femoral shaft fractures. J Orthop Trauma 20:663–667, 2006.
19. Bhandari M, Guyatt GH, Tong D, et al: Reamed versus nonreamed intramedullary nailing of lower extremity long bone fractures: A systematic overview and meta-analysis. J Orthop Trauma 14:2–9, 2000.
20. Forster MC, Aster AS, Ahmed S: Reaming during anterograde femoral nailing: Is it worth it? Injury 36:445–449, 2005.
21. Canadian Orthopaedic Trauma: Nonunion following intramedullary nailing of the femur with and without reaming. Results of a multicenter randomized clinical trial. J Bone Joint Surg Am 85-A:2093–2096, 2003.
22. Clatworthy MG, Clark DI, Gray DH, Hardy AE: Reamed versus unreamed femoral nails. A randomised, prospective trial. J Bone Joint Surg Br 80:485–489, 1998.
23. Selvakumar K, Saw KY, Fathima M: Comparison study between reamed and unreamed nailing of closed femoral fractures. Med J Malaysia 56(suppl D):24–28, 2001.
24. Tornetta P III, Tiburzi D: Reamed versus nonreamed anterograde femoral nailing. J Orthop Trauma 14:15–19, 2000.
25. Anwar IA, Battistella FD, Neiman R, et al: Femur fractures and lung complications: A prospective randomized study of reaming. Clin Orthop 422:71–76, 2004.
26. Basumallick MN, Bandopadhyay A: Effect of dynamization in open interlocking nailing of femoral fractures. A prospective randomized comparative study of 50 cases with a 2-year follow-up. Acta Orthop Belg 68:42–48, 2002.
27. Tigani D, Fravisini M, Stagni C, et al: Interlocking nail for femoral shaft fractures: Is dynamization always necessary? Int Orthop 29:101–104, 2005.
28. Brumbach, et al: Immediate weight-bearing after treatment of a comminuted fracture of the femoral shaft with a statically locked intramedullary nail. J Bone Joint Surg Am 81:1538–1544, 1999.
29. Canadian Orthopaedic Trauma Society: Reamed versus unreamed intramedullary nailing of the femur: Comparison of the rate of ARDS in multiple injured patients. J Orthop Trauma 20(6):384–387, 2006.

Supracondylar Femoral Fractures:
Is a Locking Plate or a Nail Better?

Ross K. Leighton, BSc, MD, FRCSC, FACS and Kelly Trask, MSc

Supracondylar fractures of the femur have been a controversial topic over the years. As the literature indicates, the first attempt at minimally invasive surgery in this area was the intramedullary (IM) nail, first done antegrade, then later, more successfully, in a retrograde fashion.[1] Although the union rate seemed improved with the IM nail, the number of malunions appeared to increase as the fracture type became more complex. Eventually, the technique for a minimally invasive dynamic condylar screw (DCS)[2] and the advent of the locked plate with its minimally invasive tools and technique opened the door for biomechanical and prospective clinical studies to evaluate whether the increased cost of the new locked plate was associated with improved outcome.[3–7]

OPTIONS

Treatment options for fractures of the supracondylar femur in adults include nonoperative treatment and operative treatment. Nonoperative treatment is mainly of historical interest but may still have a role in special circumstances such as nonambulatory patients or those unable to undergo an anesthetic. This chapter focuses on operative treatment alternatives.

Operative management requires anatomic reduction of the articular surface, which is generally achieved with an open reduction and lag screw fixation. Arthroscopically or fluoroscopically assisted percutaneous reduction and fixation may be considered for simple fracture patterns but has not been studied systematically. Attaching the articular surface to the diaphysis can be achieved using IM nailing or plating with fixed-angle plates or regular plates and screws. Plates can be applied using an open technique or using minimally invasive techniques.

EVIDENCE

We identified primary articles with the following features: (1) the target population was skeletally mature patients with a fracture of the femur in the supracondylar region; (2) the intervention was the use of a fixed-angle plate (DCS, blade plate, or locked plate) or an IM nail in the management of these fractures; (3) the outcome measure was ei-

ther functional (pain or impairment) or radiographic (fracture healing or subsidence) outcome, or infection rate; and (4) the study was primarily based on published or unpublished randomized, controlled trials. However, because of the paucity of this data set, secondary articles were also reviewed.

Are Plates Better Than Nails in Supracondylar Fractures of the Femur?

Christodoulou and colleagues[11] examined the fixation methods of supracondylar fractures before the introduction of the locked plate. The objective of the study was to present the results of surgical management of supracondylar fractures of the femur (types A and C according to the Association for Osteosynthesis/Association for Research and Education Foundation [AO/ASIF] classification) in elderly patients with the use of two different methods of fixation: the mini open DCS fixation and the closed retrograde intramedullary nailing (RIN). Eighty patients with supracondylar fractures of the femur were treated from January 1994 to June 2000, and 72 of them followed up completely. The authors conclude that although the two methods appear to have the same percentage of excellent results and same time to bony union, RIN is preferable to DCS in terms of less blood loss and shorter operating time (Fig. 63–1).

Hartin and coauthors[12] studied the blade plate and the IM nail used in the treatment of supracondylar femoral fractures. The condylar blade plate relies on the principles of open reduction, absolute stability, and interfragmentary compression to achieve union. The technique of retrograde nailing uses indirect reduction of the metaphyseal fracture component, offering relative stability and a less invasive approach. Twenty-two patients with 23 supracondylar femur fractures were recruited from two regional trauma centers over a 26-month period and randomized to receive either a retrograde IM nail fixation (12 fractures) or a fixed-angle blade plate fixation (11 fractures). Both distal femoral nailing and blade plating gave good outcomes. There was a trend for patients undergoing retrograde nailing to report more pain and to require revision surgery for removal of implants.

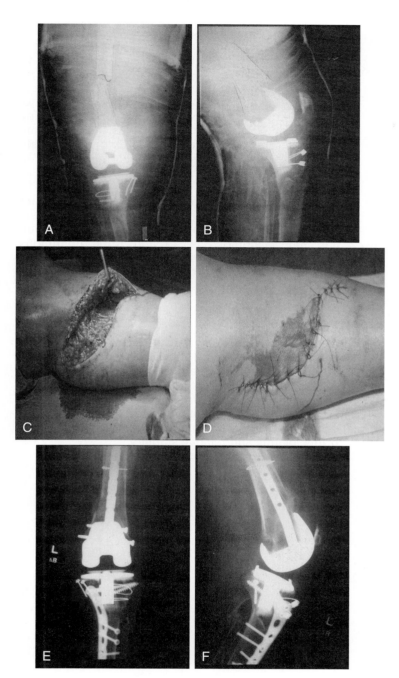

FIGURE 63–1. A retrograde intramedullary nail utilized to stabilize a compound periprosthetic supracondylar fracture of the femur with associated tibial fracture. *A–B,* Initial radiographs. *C–D,* Compound tibial wound. *E–F,* Postoperative radiographs.

Biomechanical Data on Nails versus Plates

Koval and investigators[5] performed a biomechanical cadaver study to compare the stability of three standard distal femoral fixation techniques. After initial mechanical characterization of intact femurs, a distal femoral osteotomy was created, reduced, and stabilized under compression using random assignment to one of three methods of fixation: (1) 6-hole 95-degree supracondylar plate; (2) retrograde inserted, statically locked, supracondylar IM nail; and (3) antegrade inserted, statically locked Russell–Taylor nail.

The 95-degree plate and Russell–Taylor nail had statistically significant greater loads to failure than the supracondylar IM nail. These results supported the use of a 95-degree plate when maximum rigidity of fixation or maximum compression is desired.

Koval and investigators[4] report on the biomechanical properties of the locked plate compared with the standard condylar buttress plate. The locked buttress plate provided significantly greater fixation stability than the standard plate both before and after cycling in axial loading. The locked buttress plate also proved significantly more stable in axial loading than the blade plate both before and

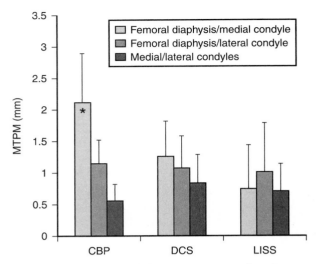

FIGURE 63–2. Permanent deformation reported as the mean maximum total point motion (MTPM) of each fracture segment pairing after cyclic loading. CBP, condylar buttress plate; DCS, dynamic condylar screw; LISS, less invasive stabilization system. *$P < 0.05$.

after cycling. The authors conclude that a condylar buttress plate with locked screws improves fixation stability.

Duffy and colleagues[13] also studied the biomechanical characteristics of the DCS, standard condylar buttress plate, and the limited invasive stabilization system (LISS). Both of these studies indicate the locked plate (LISS) was indeed stronger than the other two standard devices. Duffy and colleagues'[13] study used radiostereometric analysis to measure micromotion between bone segments. Permanent deformation was measured after cyclic axial loading, and elastic deformation was measured during a static load. The LISS plate proved to be more flexible and allowed some motion, which may explain the clinical impression of more exuberant callous formation at the fracture site (Figs. 63–2 and 63–3).

Prospective cohort studies suggest that the biomechanical properties of the locked plate seem to hold up clinically, although there are as yet no published prospective RCTs to compare implants. Fankhauser and coworkers[3] used the LISS to treat 30 distal femoral fractures in 29 patients. They found the LISS to be a safe and effective treatment. Schutz and researchers[6] managed 112 patients with 116 distal femoral fractures in a prospective multi-center study. All fractures were treated with the LISS plate. The study had a 93% follow-up rate with the follow-up period ranging from 7 to 33 months. The study showed that with a sound knowledge of the operative technique and careful preoperative planning, the LISS represents an excellent, safe procedure for the treatment of almost all distal femoral fracture types including periprosthetic fractures of the distal femur, generally without the need for primary cancellous bone grafting. Locked plates have

also demonstrated good results in the treatment of difficult fractures such as AO33 types A and C in patients with multiple trauma injuries with soft-tissue damage[7] (Fig. 63–4) and periprosthetic supracondylar femur fractures.[14]

Ly and coworkers[15] presented data at the Orthopaedic Trauma Association (OTA) general meeting indicating that, in a review of their last 124 supracondylar fractures treated in a standard nonlocked fashion, 20 were complicated by nonunion and required further surgical intervention to achieve union.

Large and colleagues[16] also presented at the OTA meeting a study of lateral locked plating versus other operative techniques. The locked plate group had six malunions (24%) and no nonunions. The other group had nine malunions (47%) and three nonunions (16%). Both approached clinical significance but remain underpowered to date.

AREAS OF CONTROVERSY

Although several of the implants have been compared biomechanically, clinical RCTs are needed to compare the functional outcome and complications associated with each treatment option. A biomechanically rigid system is required if a fracture is to be treated with absolute stability, but it may not be advantageous clinically in a multifragmentary fracture treated with bridge plating and relative stability.

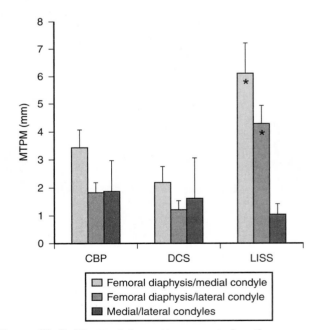

FIGURE 63–3. Elastic deformation reported as the mean maximum total point motion (MTPM) of each fracture segment pairing under static loading. CBP, condylar buttress plate; DCS, dynamic condylar screw; LISS, less invasive stabilization system. *$P < 0.05$.

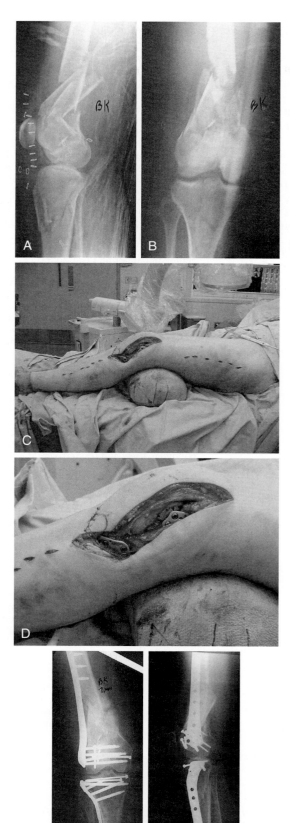

FIGURE 63–4. Locked plates inserted via a limited invasive approach are utilized to rigidly fix an associated supracondylar femoral fracture and a tibial fracture (floating knee) in a 32-year-old pregnant woman after a motor vehicle crash. *A–B,* Preoperative radiographs. *C–D,* Limited invasive approach. *E–F,* Seven months after surgery.

RECOMMENDATIONS

A fixed-angle device applied with the use of minimal soft-tissue stripping and indirect reduction techniques appears to lead to the best union rates. Subsequent movement of the fracture appears to be reduced with the use of a locked plate, particularly if the medial condyle is involved.

IM nails, usually retrograde, are utilized in supracondylar fractures where the fracture is extra-articular or an undisplaced intra-articular fracture is present. Given this fracture type, if a locked nail allows for axial and varus-valgus stability, the outcomes are satisfactory. If the fracture type is periarticular (within 5 cm of the joint), a fixed-angle device placed via a limited invasive approach appears to be the preferred method. This appears to reduce the risk for a malunion. If the fracture includes only one condyle or is axially stable, a standard plate without locking screws performs as well as or better than other implants tested. If the fracture involves both condyles or is axially unstable, a locked plate appears to provide the best fixation in both biomechanical and in clinical studies. Table 63–1 provides a summary of recommendations for the treatment of supracondylar femoral fractures.

TABLE 63–1. Summary of Recommendations for the Treatment of Supracondylar Femoral Fractures

RECOMMENDATIONS	LEVEL OF EVIDENCE/GRADE OF RECOMMENDATION
1. Adult with axially unstable supracondylar femur fracture within 5 cm of the joint should be treated with a lateral fixed angle device.	B
2. Adult with a unicondylar or an axially stable supracondylar femur fracture should be treated with compression screws and regular buttress/compression plating.	B
3. Adult with axially unstable supracondylar femur fracture more than 5 cm from the joint may be treated preferentially with a lateral fixed-angle device, but a retrograde statically locked femoral nail is also acceptable.	C

REFERENCES

1. Ostrum RF, Agarwal A, Lakatos R, et al: Prospective comparison of retrograde and antegrade femoral intramedullary nailing. J Orthop Trauma 14:496–501, 2000.
2. Krettek C, Schandelmaier P, Miclau T, et al: Minimally invasive percutaneous plate osteosynthesis (MIPPO) using the DCS in proximal and distal femoral fractures. Injury 28(suppl 1):A20–A30, 1997.
3. Fankhauser F, Gruber G, Schippinger G, et al: Minimal-invasive treatment of distal femoral fractures with the LISS (Less Invasive Stabilization System): A prospective study of 30 fractures with a follow up of 20 months. Acta Orthop Scand 75:56–60, 2004.
4. Koval KJ, Hoehl JJ, Kummer FJ, et al: Distal femoral fixation: A biomechanical comparison of the standard condylar buttress plate, a locked buttress plate, and the 95-degree blade plate. J Orthop Trauma 11:521–524, 1997.
5. Koval KJ, Kummer FJ, Bharam S, et al: Distal femoral fixation: A laboratory comparison of the 95 degrees plate, antegrade and retrograde inserted reamed intramedullary nails. J Orthop Trauma 10:378–382, 1996.
6. Schutz M, Muller M, Krettek C, et al: Minimally invasive fracture stabilization of distal femoral fractures with the LISS: A prospective multicenter study. Results of a clinical study with special emphasis on difficult cases. Injury 32(suppl 3): SC48–SC54, 2001.
7. Schutz M, Muller M, Regazzoni P, et al: Use of the less invasive stabilization system (LISS) in patients with distal femoral (AO33) fractures: A prospective multicenter study. Arch Orthop Trauma Surg 125:102–108, 2005.
8. Anwar IA, Battistella FD, Neiman R, et al: Femur fractures and lung complications: A prospective randomized study of reaming. Clin Orthop Relat Res 71–76, 2004.
9. Pape H-C, Grimme K, Van Griensven M, et al: Impact of intramedullary instrumentation versus damage control for femoral fractures on immunoinflammatory parameters: Prospective randomized analysis by the EPOFF Study Group. J Trauma 55:7–13, 2003.
10. Tornetta P 3rd, Tiburzi D: Antegrade or retrograde reamed femoral nailing. A prospective, randomised trial. J Bone Joint Surg Br 82:652–654, 2000.
11. Christodoulou A, Terzidis I, Ploumis A, et al: Supracondylar femoral fractures in elderly patients treated with the dynamic condylar screw and the retrograde intramedullary nail: A comparative study of the two methods. Arch Orthop Trauma Surg 125:73–79, 2005.
12. Hartin NL, Harris I, Hazratwala K: Retrograde nailing versus fixed-angle blade plating for supracondylar femoral fractures: A randomized controlled trial. ANZ J Surg 76:290–294, 2006.
13. Duffy P, Trask K, Hennigar A, et al: Assessment of fragment micromotion in distal femur fracture fixation with RSA. Clin Orthop Relat Res 448:105–113, 2006.
14. Ricci WM, Loftus T, Cox C, et al: Locked plates combined with minimally invasive insertion technique for the treatment of periprosthetic supracondylar femur fractures above a total knee arthroplasty. J Orthop Trauma 20:190–196, 2006.
15. Ly TV, Bong MR, Hamid N, et al: Results of operative intervention of supracondylar femur fractures. Available at: http://www.hwbf.org/ota/am/ota06/otapo/OTP06020.htm. Accessed May 2008.
16. Large TM, Norton J, Bosse MJ, et al: Locked plating of supracondylar periprosthetic femur fractures. Available at: http://www.hwbf.org/ota/am/ota06/otapa/OTA060212.htm. Accessed.
17. Canadian Orthopaedic Trauma Society: Nonunion following intramedullary nailing of the femur with and without reaming. Results of a multicenter randomized clinical trial. J Bone Joint Surg Am 85-A:2093–2096, 2003.

What Is the Relation Between Malunion and Function for Lower Extremity Tibial Diaphyseal Fractures?

BRAD A. PETRISOR, MSc, MD, FRCSC

Tibial diaphyseal fractures are one of the most common fractures of the long bones.[1] Controversy remains, however, over the best way to manage these fractures, with authors arguing not only over operative techniques but also between surgical and nonsurgical management. With any treatment, however, one thing is agreed on, there is an inherent risk for healing with some degree of residual malalignment. Indeed, in a recent systematic review of the treatment of distal-third tibial shaft fractures, for example, incidence rates of malunion (as defined by the authors of the included studies) ranged from 13.1% to 16.2% depending on treatment choice.[2]

Two major issues should be considered when discussing malunion. The first is what actually constitutes a malunion; that is, what are the limits of an acceptable reduction? Second, will a malunion result in any long-term adverse sequelae to the patient? If the malunion does not cause adverse sequelae, then does it actually matter? To make the argument completely circular, is it actually a malunion, radiographic issues aside? Surgeons' definition of angular malunion has been shown to range from less than 5 to 20 degrees, and a majority of surgeons defined significant shortening as greater than 15 mm.[3] However, some would argue that asymptomatic angulation be considered an anatomic deviation rather than malunion per se.[4]

This chapter discusses the literature that specifically focuses on the issue of how "malunion" of the tibial diaphysis potentially affects long-term function of the patient.

EVIDENCE

Prognostic studies address the possible outcomes of a disease or condition. In the hierarchy of evidence, a Level I prognostic study would be a prospective cohort with a ≥80% follow-up rate. One can understand it would be unethical (and difficult to obtain consent) to randomize patients into a malunion group.

For a number of reasons, reports are conflicting regarding the effect of malunion on the long-term functional outcome after tibial shaft fractures. These include a general lack of consensus as to what constitutes a malunion, retrospective reporting with incomplete follow-up and varying times of follow-up (from 10–40 years), a lack of standardized technique to radiographically measure malunion, and the use of multiple and varied functional outcome measures between studies (some that are nonstandardized and nonvalidated) (Table 64–1).

Before assessing whether malunion of the tibial shaft affects long-term functional outcome, it is important to understand the long-term outcome in those with a tibial shaft fracture in general. Greenwood and colleagues[5] retrospectively reviewed 398 patients with tibial shaft fractures (it was not stated how the fractures were all treated just that "most were treated with cast therapy") and compared these with a cohort of 1573 age- and sex-matched control subjects.[5] Outcome measures were subjective reporting of knee pain, ability to walk 100 yards, bend, kneel, and stoop, and a general practitioner's diagnosis of osteoarthritis. The 36-Item Short Form Health Survey (SF-36) outcome instrument was also used. Greenwood and colleagues[5] found that patients with a tibial shaft fracture had more knee pain (odds ratio, 1.23; 95% confidence interval [CI], 1.00–1.51) and an increase in having a diagnosis of osteoarthritis (odds ratio, 1.46; 95% CI, 1.08–1.97). They also found a statistically significant incidence of a decreased ability of the patients with fractures to climb stairs, bend, kneel, or stoop. Interestingly, even though the odds ratios themselves suggested a slightly increased risk for knee pain or diagnosis of osteoarthritis, the confidence intervals either include 1 or come close to 1, suggesting that these results are trends as opposed to true statistical differences. However, because the same trend was seen throughout all domains of the outcome measures, it may be that the study was underpowered and these trends are accurate estimates of the truth.

TABLE 64–1. Characteristics of Included Studies

STUDY (YEAR OF PUBLICATION)	DESIGN	N	TREATMENT	MEAN TIME FROM FRACTURE	MALUNION DEFINITION	OUTCOME MEASURES	OUTCOME
Obremskey and Medina (2004)[6]	Retrospective cohort	Group 1: 39 Group 2: 18	Group 1: IM nail by community surgeon Group 2: IM nail by orthopedic trauma surgeon	<2 yr	>5-degree angulation, >10-mm shortening, >10-degree rotation	**MODEMS lower limb module subsections:** Physical function, Physical limitations, Bodily pain	No difference between those with or without malunion in physical function ($P = 0.24$) or physical limitations ($P = 0.43$). Worse score for bodily pain in malunion group ($P = 0.42$)
Boucher et al. (2002)	Retrospective case series	13	IM nail	5.46 yr	≥10-degree rotation ≥5 degrees varus/valgus ≥10 degrees pro/recurvatum	**Functional Outcome:** WOMAC, LEFS **Physical Assessment:** ASLEF	**WOMAC:** No correlation with alignment in any plane and functional outcome. **LEFS:** No correlation with malunion in any plane and subject's response. **ASLEF:** No correlation between malunion in any plane and subject's response
Milner et al. (2002)[14]	Retrospective case series	164	Closed (cast)	36 yr	Lower-limb alignment: >6.25 degrees varus >4.75 degrees valgus ≥5 degrees angulation ≥10-mm shortening	**Functional Outcome:** WOMAC questionnaire Radiographic arthritis knee and ankle Clinical arthritis (pain with range of motion and joint stiffness)	No univariate associations between malunion and development of arthritis or functional scores. Some minor associations found within subgroup analysis
Kyro (1997)[17]	Retrospective case series	17	Intramedullary nail	N/A	>5-degree angulation >10-mm shortening No malrotation	**Subjective Functional Measures:** swelling, loss of knee extension, inability to squat, etc. **Subjective Complaints:** pain in knee, pain in leg, pain in ankle, etc.	Malunion group had 2-fold increase in subjective functional complaints. Malunion group had a 1.5-fold increase in subjective complaints. Worse outcomes in those with angulation >10 degrees and shortening >15 mm
Greenwood et al. (1997)[5]	Retrospective case–control	398 tibial shaft fractures	Majority closed (cast)	35 yr	N/A	Knee pain Self-reported diagnosis of knee OA Ability to climb stairs, walk 100 yards, bend, kneel, or stoop GP diagnosis of knee OA, SF-36	Patients with fractures are more likely to have knee pain (OR, 1.23; 95% CI, 1.00–1.51), Patients with fractures are more likely to report being given diagnosis of OA by GP (OR, 1.46; 95% CI, 1.08–1.97) Patients with fractures have lower SF-36 scores, less ability to climb stairs, walk 100 yards, bend, kneel, and stoop

Study	Design	Patients	Fracture type	Follow-up	Malalignment groups	Outcome measures	Results
van der Schoot et al. (1996)[15]	Retrospective case series	88 tibial fractures	Closed	15 yr	Three groups: 0–4 degrees, 5–10 degrees, and >10 degrees	Radiographic arthritis knee/ankle (author-derived rating scale)	Angular deformity of 5 degrees or more resulted in a greater proportion of ankle or knee arthritis compared with an angular deformity <5 degrees (58% vs. 31%; P = 0.02)
Puno et al. (1991)[16]	Retrospective case series	28 tibia fractures	24 closed (cast) 4 external fixation	8.2 yr	Author-derived joint malalignment Ankle mean: 1.3 degrees Knee mean: 6.6 degrees	Combined functional and radiographic score: author-derived for knee and ankle	Increased ankle malalignment correlated with poorer ankle score: no correlation seen with knee malalignment and knee score
Netz et al. (1991)[13]	Retrospective case series	25 tibia fractures	Closed (cast brace)	7 yr 8 mo	6 groups: <5 degrees varus 5–10 degrees varus >10 degrees varus <10 degrees other angulation 10–20 degrees other angulation >20 degrees other angulation	Patients' subjective complaints Clinical assessment Radiographic assessment Muscle force analysis	No association between residual angular deformity or shortening with outcomes
Merchant and Dietz (1989)[10]	Retrospective case series	37 tibia fractures	Closed (cast)	29 yr	3 groups: <5 degrees angulation (any plane) 5–10 degrees angulation >10 degrees angulation	**Knee/Ankle arthrosis:** author-developed rating scale **Functional: Knee**—Iowa knee evaluation **Ankle**—author-modified Iowa knee evaluation	No difference in outcome scores between any of the groups (both clinical and radiographic)
Kristensen et al. (1989)[8]	Retrospective case series	17 tibia fractures	Closed (cast)	28 yr	>10 degrees angular deformity	**Ankle arthrosis:** Magnusson's criteria **Functional measure:** Cedell criteria	**Arthritis:** 17 no ankle arthrosis (Magnusson's criteria) **Functional:** 15 asymptomatic 2 moderate symptoms (Cedell criteria)
Kettelkamp et al. (1988)[9]	Retrospective case series	14 patients 15 limbs (12 femora, 4 tibia)	Closed (cast)	31.7 yr	7–15 degrees tibial angular deformity in any plane	Radiographic signs of knee arthritis Biomechanical modelling of forces through knee	Increased forces through the medial or lateral tibial plateau correlated with a varus or valgus deformity at the knee

ASLEF, Assessment System of Lower Extremity Function; CI, confidence interval; IM, intramedullary; LEFS, Lower Extremity Functional Scale; MODEMS, Musculoskeletal Outcomes Data Evaluation and Management Scale; OR, odds ratio; SF-36, 36-Item Short Form Health Survey; WOMAC, Western Ontario and McMaster Osteoarthritis Index.

Malunion Does Not Affect Long-Term Functional Outcome

One retrospective cohort study was identified that attempted to correlate malunion with functional outcome[6] (Level of Evidence II, retrospective cohort). In this study, two different groups of surgeons (community surgeons and orthopedic trauma surgeons) each treated a cohort of patients with an intramedullary nail. Between the groups it was demonstrated that the community surgeon group had a greater malunion rate.[6] Using the Musculoskeletal Outcomes Data Evaluation and Management Scale (MODEMS) lower functional extremity score, they found no significant functional differences between those with a malunion as compared with those without within the subset scales of physical function and physical limitations. However, within the bodily function subscale, they found a slightly statistically significantly worse outcome in the malunion group ($P = 0.042$). This should be interpreted with caution, however, because multiple subgroup analysis may potentially result in spuriously positive findings.[7] Also, this study was primarily addressing the issue of whether orthopedic trauma surgeons had less malunions and was underpowered to detect a difference comparing those with a malunion and those without.

Smaller observational case series are available that suggest that the long-term effect of malunion of tibial shaft fractures does not affect functional outcome.[8-10] Merchant and Dietz[10] reviewed 37 tibial fractures with a mean follow-up period of 29 years[10] (Level of Evidence IV, retrospective case series). They assessed both clinical and radiographic outcome of both the knee and ankle. With the outcome scores used (Iowa knee evaluation and the Iowa knee evaluation modified by the authors for the ankle), 78% of the ankles and 92% of the knees of the study group were rated as good or excellent. With the radiographic outcome used (author derived from a synthesis of previously published scores), 76% of the ankles and 92% of the knees in the study group had a good or excellent result. When subgroup analysis was done, they found no statistically significant difference in function between those whose tibial angulation in any plane was less than 5 degrees compared with those whose angulation was 5 to 10 degrees or more than 10 degrees. Given their numbers, however, these statistical comparisons may be underpowered, potentially resulting in a beta or type II statistical error.

Kristensen and coworkers[8] examined 17 patients with a tibial angular deformity of more than 10 degrees a minimum of 20 years after their injury.[8] Using clinical outcome criteria according to Cedell[11] and radiographic criteria according to Magnusson,[12] they found no evidence of knee or ankle arthritis in their study population.[8] Netz and coauthors[13] reviewed their series of tibial fractures treated with cast application and found no correlation of patients' subjective complaints, clinical examination, or muscle force analysis with angular deformity or leg-length discrepancy.[13]

More recently, Milner and investigators[14] evaluated 167 subjects after an average follow-up period of 36 years from the initial injury. They used a validated functional outcome score (the Western Ontario and McMaster Osteoarthritis Index [WOMAC]) to assess knee function and an author-derived clinical and radiographic arthritis score. They found no significant association between the development of knee or ankle arthritis and tibial malalignment. There was, however, a trend for those limbs in varus malalignment to have more frequent evidence of medial compartment knee arthritis and for those limbs in either varus or valgus malalignment to be associated with subtalar stiffness.[14]

Malunion Does Affect Long-Term Functional Outcome

Observational case series have been identified that suggest that tibial malalignment does, in fact, correlate with the extent of knee or ankle arthritis and, therefore, the functional outcome of the patient. van der Schoot and coauthors[15] suggest that malaligned fractures show more degenerative changes with a correlation between symptoms in the knee and radiographic arthritis.[15] This correlation, however, did not hold for ankle symptoms and radiographic ankle arthritis. Puno and researchers[16] assessed 28 tibial fractures correlating joint malalignment and clinical outcome. They found that greater ankle malalignment correlated with poorer clinical results. However, this correlation did not hold for malalignment about the knee. Similar results have been associated with malunions after an intramedullary nail. Kyro[17] evaluated a group of 17 patients and found that those with a malunion had an increased number of subjective functional findings (such as swelling of the lower limb, loss of knee, ankle, or subtalar motion, or squatting difficulties) and subjective complaints (pain in the knee, leg, ankle or foot, swelling, and problems with walking, running, squatting or working).

ARE THE RESULTS OF THESE STUDIES VALID?

All studies are retrospective in nature, and the majority is case series reviews. This allows for the potential introduction of bias at a number of levels including a selection bias, recall bias, and measurement bias, among others. Indeed, it has been shown that observational studies can both overestimate and underestimate treatment effects.[18] Between the studies, the lack of standardized and fully validated outcome measures limits the inferences that can be made. Most of the studies had a small sample size, and thus could have been underpowered to detect differences between groups (type II error). As well, some of the studies performed a number of subgroup analyses with small numbers of patients that may lead to spuriously positive findings of statistical significance suggesting that these positive results should be interpreted with caution.[7]

TABLE 64–2. Level of Evidence and Overall Grade of Recommendation

STUDY	NEGATIVE CORRELATION BETWEEN MALALIGNMENT AND FUNCTIONAL OUTCOME?	LEVEL OF EVIDENCE (PROGNOSIS)	OVERALL GRADE OF RECOMMENDATION
Obremsky and Medina (2004)[6]	No (one minor subgroup with a negative correlation was identified)	II	I = Insufficient evidence and conflicting results of prognostic outcome of malunion in tibial shaft fractures
Boucher et al. (2002)[19]	No	IV	
Milner et al. (2002)[14]	No (one minor subgroup with a negative correlation was identified)	IV	
Greenwood et al. (1997)[5]	Yes	III	
Kyro (1997)[17]	Yes	IV	
van der Schoot et al. (1996)[15]	Yes	IV	
Puno et al. (1991)[16]	Yes	IV	
Netz et al. (1991)[13]	No	IV	
Merchant and Dietz (1989)[10]	No	IV	
Kristensen et al. (1989)[8]	No	IV	
Kettelkamp et al. (1988)[9]	No	IV	

EVIDENCE-BASED BOTTOM LINE

Based on the current available evidence, the following has been reported (Table 64–2):

1. No Level I (prospective cohort with ≥80% follow-up rate) data are available that address the long-term functional outcomes of tibial fracture malunion.
2. A number of retrospective observational studies with conflicting results have been identified, which limits the inferences that can be made regarding the long-term effects of malunion on functional outcome.
3. Prospective trials that focus specifically on the issue of malunion and functional outcome with well-validated functional outcome measures, validated measurement techniques, and long-term (>80%) follow-up will be necessary to accurately address this issue.

REFERENCES

1. Court-Brown C, McQueen MM, Tornetta P III: Tibia and fibula diaphyseal fractures. In Tornetta P III, Einhorn T (eds): Trauma. Philadelphia, Lippincott Williams & Wilkins, 2006, pp 339–353.
2. Zelle BA, Bhandari M, Espiritu M, et al: Treatment of distal tibia fractures without articular involvement: A systematic review of 1125 fractures. J Orthop Trauma 20:76–79, 2006.
3. Bhandari M, Guyatt GH, Swiontkowski MF, et al: A lack of consensus in the assessment of fracture healing among orthopaedic surgeons. J Orthop Trauma 16:562–566, 2002.
4. Sarmiento A: On the behavior of closed tibial fractures: Clinical/radiological correlations. J Orthop Trauma 14:199–205, 2000.
5. Greenwood DC, Muir KR, Doherty M, et al: Conservatively managed tibial shaft fractures in Nottingham, UK: Are pain, osteoarthritis, and disability long-term complications? J Epidemiol Community Health 51:701–704, 1997.
6. Obremskey WT, Medina M: Comparison of intramedullary nailing of distal third tibial shaft fractures: Before and after traumatologists. Orthopedics 27:1180–1184, 2004.
7. Bhandari M, Devereaux PJ, Li P, et al: Misuse of baseline comparison tests and subgroup analyses in surgical trials. Clin Orthop Relat Res 447:247–251, 2006.
8. Kristensen KD, Kiaer T, Blicher J: No arthrosis of the ankle 20 years after malaligned tibial-shaft fracture. Acta Orthop Scand 60:208–209, 1989.
9. Kettelkamp DB, Hillberry BM, Murrish DE, Heck DA: Degenerative arthritis of the knee secondary to fracture malunion. Clin Orthop Relat Res 234:159–169, 1988.
10. Merchant TC, Dietz FR: Long-term follow-up after fractures of the tibial and fibular shafts. J Bone Joint Surg Am 71:599–606, 1989.
11. Cedell CA: Supination-outward rotation injuries of the ankle. A clinical and roentgenological study with special reference to the operative treatment. Acta Orthop Scand (suppl 110):3+, 1967.
12. Magnusson R: On the late results in non-operated cases of malleolar fractures. clinical-roentgenological-statistical study: fractures by external rotation. Acta Chirugica Scandinavica 1:1-36;=1944.
13. Netz P, Olsson E, Ringertz H, Stark A: Functional restitution after lower leg fractures. A long-term follow-up. Arch Orthop Trauma Surg 110:238–241, 1991.
14. Milner SA, Davis TRC, Muir KR, et al: Long-term outcome after tibial shaft fracture: Is malunion important? J Bone Joint Surg Am 84-A:971–980, 2002.
15. van der Schoot DK, Den Outer AJ, Bode PJ, et al: Degenerative changes at the knee and ankle related to malunion of tibial fractures. 15-year follow-up of 88 patients. J Bone Joint Surg Br 78:722–725, 1996.
16. Puno RM, Vaughan JJ, Stetten ML, Johnson JR: Long-term effects of tibial angular malunion on the knee and ankle joints. J Orthop Trauma 5:247–254, 1991.
17. Kyro A: Malunion after intramedullary nailing of tibial shaft fractures. Ann Chir Gynaecol 86:56–64, 1997.
18. Bhandari M, Tornetta P III, Ellis T, et al: Hierarchy of evidence: Differences in results between non-randomized studies and randomized trials in patients with femoral neck fractures. Arch Orthop Trauma Surg 124:10–16, 2004.
19. Boucher M, Leone J, Pierrynowski M, Three-dimensional assessment of tibial malunion after intramedullary nailing: a preliminary study. J Orthop Trauma 16(7):473-483, 2002.

Chapter 65

Tibial Diaphyseal Fractures: What Is the Best Treatment?

NÄDER HELMY, MD AND PIOTR A. BLACHUT, MD, FRCSC

The management of tibia fractures has evolved over time from nonoperative treatment to operative treatment. Despite their common occurrence, the evidence base to direct the care of tibial shaft fractures is relatively poor. Moreover, there is little evidence to support the commonly recommended parameters of acceptable fracture alignment (less than 5–7 degrees of varus/valgus, less than 10 degrees of flexion/extension, less than 1.5 cm of shortening, and less than 15 degrees of rotational deformity). The characteristics of fractures amenable to nonsurgical management, stable fractures, are not well evidence based. It is generally accepted that nonpathologic, isolated, low-energy fractures, with little displacement, no significant soft-tissue injury, and having an associated fibular fracture can be treated without surgery. For the surgical management of tibial shaft fractures, a variety of implants is available, including external fixators, plates, and intramedullary (IM) nails.

This chapter summarizes the evidence to help guide the treatment of closed and open tibial shaft fractures, although details regarding open fracture management in general is presented elsewhere.

OPERATIVE VERSUS NONOPERATIVE TREATMENT OF DISPLACED TIBIA SHAFT FRACTURES

Minimally displaced, stable tibia shaft fractures are commonly treated without surgery with satisfactory results. Controversies, however, exist in the management of displaced tibial shaft fractures. Six studies have compared nonoperative treatment modalities with surgery for displaced closed tibia fractures.[1–7]

NONOPERATIVE TREATMENT VERSUS OPEN REDUCTION AND FIXATION WITH PLATES AND SCREWS

In a prospective randomized clinical trial by Abdel-Salam and colleagues,[1] 45 patients with closed tibial shaft fractures were treated with a long-leg plaster cast and compared with 45 patients managed with open reduction and internal fixation (ORIF).[1] Healing time and return to usual activity was significantly shorter in the ORIF group. The complication rate of secondary intervention for bone grafting or deep infection was lower in the ORIF cohort.

In a similar study by van der Linden and Larsson,[7] 100 patients were randomly assigned to ORIF with plates or closed treatment. Hospital stay seemed to be longer in the group treated by ORIF, and the complication rate was slightly greater. In accordance with Abdel-Salam and colleagues' study,[1] the healing time was significantly shorter in the ORIF group, and malalignment occurred more frequently in the nonoperative group.

A meta-analysis that included these studies reached the conclusion that the quality of the literature was poor. The risk for superficial infection was greater after ORIF versus cast treatment (odds ratio, 0.2; 95% confidence interval [CI], 0.08–0.50); however, there was no difference in the deep infection rate. Fractures treated with ORIF were more likely to be healed by 20 weeks than those treated in a cast (odds ratio, 0.02; 95% CI, 0.06–0.68).[8]

NONOPERATIVE TREATMENT VERSUS INTRAMEDULLARY NAIL

Hooper and coworkers'[4] prospective, randomized study of 62 patients with unstable tibial shaft fractures found that IM nailing reduced time to fracture union by 2 weeks ($P < 0.05$) compared with long leg casting. IM nailing was also associated with significantly less time off work (13.5 vs. 23 weeks; $P < 0.01$) and less time in the hospital (8.1 vs. 11.7 days; $P < 0.01$). Compared with IM nailing, more patients with cast treatment had angular deformity and shortening. One third of casted patients healed with more than 10 degrees of angular deformity, and two thirds with shortening of more than 1 cm. No significant differences were observed in regard to range of motion of the ankle or knee joints. Secondary interventions were necessary in five patients of the nonoperative group compared with only one patient in the ORIF group.

Toivanen and coauthors[6] note no delayed union in 33 patients treated with IM nailing compared with 8 of 54 patients treated with cast, representing a delayed union rate of 14.8% ($P < 0.05$). They did note anterior knee pain in 79% of patients treated with an IM nail compared with only 2% in the casted group ($P < 0.001$). Mean healing time, hospitalization time, and sick leave duration were significantly longer in the group treated with casting. A significant bias in this study was that patients initially treated without surgery who had a loss of reduction and needed revision surgery were excluded, so that the results in terms of final alignment were not statistically different between the groups. In a prospective, randomized trial, Karladani and researchers[5] studied 53 patients, with 27 being treated with IM nails and 26 receiving nonoperative care. The nonoperative group was divided into additional cohorts of 12 and 14 patients because some fractures were not considered stable enough to be treated in cast alone and underwent cerclage wire or screw fixation in addition to casting. In the analysis of the final outcome parameters such as quality of life, weight-bearing time, and union rate, these two groups were analyzed together and compared with the IM nail group. IM nailing resulted in a 6 weeks faster time to union (95% CI, 2.5–12 weeks), and a faster time to full weight bearing by 8 weeks (95% CI, 5–17 weeks). IM nailing was associated with a lower risk for delayed union (odds ratio, 0.36; 95% CI, 0.17–0.78) but an increased risk for anterior knee pain (12/27 vs. 0/26 patients). At 3 months after injury, patients who underwent IM nailing had significantly better mobility, social function, work function, and sexual function as measured on the Nottingham Health Profile ($P < 0.05$).

The current best evidence suggests that operative treatment is superior to nonoperative treatment with respect to healing time, alignment, nonunion rate, and working capacities in displaced tibia shaft fractures. Incidence rates of anterior knee pain and complications such as infection or secondary procedures for removal of the orthopedic implants are greater in patients treated with surgery (grade B).

OPERATIVE TREATMENT OF CLOSED TIBIA FRACTURES

Plate versus Intramedullary Nail

A prospective, randomized trial with a total of 64 patients was conducted by Im and Tae[9] to compare IM nailing to plate fixation of distal tibia fractures. Thirty-four patients were treated with an IM nail, and 30 patients underwent open reduction and plate fixation with a follow-up period of 2 years. In the group treated with IM nails, the average angulation was greater (2.8 vs. 0.9 degree; $P = 0.01$). Locked IM nails seem to be advantageous in regard to the length of operation, restoration of motion, and reduced soft-tissue complications, whereas open reduction and fixation with plate and screws can restore alignment better than IM nails.

A systematic review of the prospective literature by Coles and Gross[10] reports more superficial infection with plating (9% vs. <3% with reamed vs. unreamed nailing) but lower rates of malunion (0% vs. 3.2% with reamed and 11.8% with unreamed nailing). No evidence that assesses the utility of minimally invasive plating techniques in comparison with other treatment approaches is currently available.

Intramedullary Nail versus External Fixator

A total of 78 patients with 79 fractures was entered into Braten and coworkers'[11] study (41 external fixators, 38 IM nails). Time to radiographic union and full weight bearing did not differ significantly, but unprotected weight bearing was achieved earlier in the IM group (12 vs. 20 weeks; $P < 0.001$). Reoperation for secondary displacement was more frequent in the external fixator group. No differences were observed in the final alignment or in the amount of shortening. IM nailing was commonly associated with anterior knee pain.

Intramedullary Nail versus Ender Nail

In a study by Chiu and colleagues[12] that compares Ender nails with locked IM nails, IM nails were found to be superior for the treatment of comminuted, unstable tibial shaft fractures.

Reamed versus Unreamed Intramedullary Nails

Four Level II studies could be identified in which unreamed nailing was compared with reamed nailing.[13–16] Reamed nailing was consistently found to be superior compared with unreamed nailing. The incidence of delayed and nonunion, as well as malunion, was lower, secondary interventions were less frequent, and the overall healing time was shorter in the group treated with reamed IM nails. Implant failure was found to be more frequent with unreamed nailing, whereas no difference in infection rate was encountered.

The evidence suggests that the reamed locked IM nailing is the best operative treatment for unstable closed tibia shaft fractures. Standard plating may be advantageous in situations where achieving satisfactory alignment is expected to be problematic, but it is associated with increased risks for soft-tissue complications (grade B). The role of percutaneous, minimally invasive plating is yet to be determined.

OPEN FRACTURES

Early versus Late Treatment

Soft-tissue management is paramount to the successful management of all open fractures, particularly open tibial shaft fractures. Skeletal stabilization aids in the soft-tissue management, as well as being vital to the ultimate functional outcome.

Three retrospective cohort studies could be identified to determine the efficiency of early surgical treatment versus delayed treatment in open tibia fractures.[17–19] The final outcome measures included infection, secondary procedures, nonunion, and delayed union. Early surgery was defined as surgery less than 6 hours after the injury, whereas delayed surgery was defined as greater than 6 hours. In both groups, antibiotics were administered. No differences in the overall rate of infection, secondary procedures, nonunion, delayed union, or complications could be determined. Although the present consensus remains that open tibial shaft fractures be treated on an emergent basis (Level V), if unavoidable, delayed management does not seem to jeopardize the final outcome.

Plate Fixation versus External Fixator

In Bach and coauthors' study,[20] published in 1989, a total of 59 patients were randomized to undergo plate fixation or external fixation for grade 2 and 3 open fractures.[20] Their study showed a statistically significant greater rate of deep infections in the group treated with ORIF. Time to union and malalignment was not significantly different in both groups. Additional lag screws were used in 12 of 26 patients with external fixation for better alignment. This procedure did not seem to have any adverse effects in regard to the healing time or secondary procedures. This is in contrast with Krettek and colleagues'[21] study in which they recommend that additional lag screws not be used in open tibia fractures treated by external fixators because they seem to interfere with bone healing.

Locked Intramedullary Nail versus External Fixator

In the evolution of the treatment of open tibial fractures, a strategy of sequential locked IM nailing after external fixation was developed. Antich-Adrover and investigators[22] evaluated this strategy in a prospective, randomized study of 39 patients. Sequentially treated patients healed faster, with better alignment, and had a more predictable and rapid return to full function than patients treated with external fixation followed by casting.

In a prospective, randomized study of grade II, IIIA, and IIIB open fractures, Henley and coworkers[23] suggest that unreamed interlocked IM nailing was more efficacious than half-pin external fixation. IM nailing was associated with significantly better final alignment and significantly less operative interventions. Healing complications and infections were more associated with the severity of the soft-tissue injury than the method of skeletal stabilization.

Two Level III trials with a total of 65 patients and 1 Level III study with 41 patients evaluated unreamed nailing and external fixation in higher grade IIIB fractures.[24–26] Patients who underwent nailing were easier to manage, required less secondary procedures, and had more predictable anatomic outcomes, without having greater infection risks.

Reamed versus Unreamed Locked Intramedullary Nailing

Reaming has been the source of much debate in the management of tibial shaft fractures. An extensive body of basic science literature exists regarding this topic. Hupel and coauthors[27] conclude that "limited canal reaming before insertion of an intramedullary nail may result in the least damaging combination of insults to the cortical circulation."

Two trials, with a pooled 132 patients, have evaluated reamed versus unreamed nails in open tibial shaft fractures in a prospective, randomized fashion.[15,28] The outcomes in terms of nonunion or infection were not influenced by reaming. There was, however, a statistically greater rate of implant failure associated with the use of an unreamed nail.

Current best evidence would suggest that, in addition to aggressive soft-tissue management, open tibia fractures should be stabilized by locked IM nailing. Reamed and unreamed nails appear to have similar results, except for a greater rate of screw failure with the use of the unreamed device (grade B).

TECHNICAL CONSIDERATIONS

Having come to the conclusion that the majority of unstable tibial shaft fractures should be treated with locked IM nailing, some technical considerations are warranted. No good evidence has been reported to provide guidance as to the optimal timing for the intervention. However, the longer a fracture is left in a shortened, displaced position, the more difficult it becomes to regain anatomic length.

Fracture Table

Although early in the history of tibial nailing the use of a fracture table was usual, there has been a gradual move away from this. A prospective, randomized study[29] demonstrated that "free-draped" nailing was equally effective as using a fracture table and required less operative time. It also facilitated concomitant injury management. Although fluoroscopy time was no different, it may be that the surgeon exposure, not measured, was higher because of the requirement of being closer to the field in the free-draped technique. It should be pointed out that free-draped nailing generally requires an assistant, whereas fracture table nailing can usually be done without one. An external fixation device can be used as a temporary intraoperative reduction aid during nailing without a fracture table, but it has not been evaluated objectively.

Tourniquet

A generally held belief is that a tourniquet should not be used while reaming because it is theoretically postulated that the circulatory system acts as a radiator, dissipating the heat generated and preventing heat necrosis of the diaphysis, a devastating complication of reamed nailing. A prospective, randomized study by Giannoudis and coworkers[30] does not substantiate this concern. There was a slightly, but not statistically significant, higher temperature with the use of a tourniquet, but aggressive reaming was not carried out. The authors did, however, find that diaphyseal temperatures increased most with the larger reamers (11 and 12 mm) and in small medullary canals. Blood loss with IM reaming is usually small, so unless there are particular concerns, a tourniquet is not usually needed.

Approach and Starting Point

A move has been made to a less invasive, percutaneous technique of nail insertion, although no evidence demonstrates a benefit. The starting point for the insertion of a tibial IM nail has been the source of much discussion and debate. The two principle issues at play are the incidence of anterior knee pain and effects of start point on fracture alignment. Toivanen and coauthors[31] could demonstrate no difference in the incidence of late anterior knee pain or functional impairment with the use of a paratendinous versus a transtendinous approach. These findings are consistent with a body of evidence of lower quality.

The nailing of proximal-third tibial fractures has been associated with a significant incidence of malunion, valgus, and procurvatum. This has been related to the anatomy of the proximal tibia and to nailing with the knee in flexion. The oblique anteromedial face of the proximal tibia will direct a nail started medially and anteriorly in a posterolateral direction. Once centered in the canal of the distal segment, this will result in a valgus, procurvatum deformity. This malalignment can largely be avoided by a lateral and more posterior starting point. Indeed, the safe starting point has been delineated by McConnell and researchers[32] as being just medial to the lateral tibial spine, at the anterior edge of the articular surface of the tibial plateau.

Other strategies can be used to manage the tendency toward malalignment in difficult cases. This includes nailing in extension,[33] the use of "poller" blocking screws,[34] temporary limited plating, or entirely avoiding nailing and using definitive plating techniques.[35] Nailing in extension overcomes the tendency to flex the fracture, produce procurvatum, with nailing with the knee maximally bent. Blocking screws are screws (can also be pins) placed percutaneously across the tibia to narrow the medullary canal, thus directing the nail into proper alignment. These are effective only in the metaphyseal portion of the tibia where the nail is not constrained by the medullary canal. They are also unable to compensate for an entirely wrong starting point. Unicortical plating through a limited approach, preserving bone vascularity, can aid by maintaining fracture alignment while nailing and locking is undertaken. The plate can be left definitively or can be removed once locking has been accomplished. Leaving the plate is technically against basic principles because nails

generally provide relative stability, whereas these plates confer absolute stability. Surgeons with limited experience with nailing of proximal-third fractures may well consider using definitive plating techniques rather than nailing. No good evidence base exists for the selection of approaches to the management of proximal-third tibial fractures.

Locking

It is generally recommended that all tibial nails be locked proximally and distally. With stable transverse fracture patterns, the screws at one end can be placed in a dynamic mode, if the nail design allows, because one requires only rotational control and not axial control. In fractures in the midthird, one screw at each end of the nail is sufficient to control bony alignment. As the fracture approaches the metaphyseal area, because of the limited cortical bony contact, more than one locking screw in the short segment affords better angular stability. Kneifel and Buckley[36] prospectively evaluated the use of one versus two distal locking screws in diaphyseal tibial fractures treated with undreamed nails and showed a significantly greater screw failure rate with the use of only one screw. Heavier patients and longer locking screws (larger medullary canals) correlated with increased screw failure. This, however, had no impact on fracture union.

Although free-hand distal targeting is most commonly used for distal locking, two prospective, randomized studies compared the use of alternative devices. Gugala and coworkers[37] demonstrated no significant difference in operating time with the use of a distally based distal targeting device and no statistical difference in total fluoroscopy time. They did show a statistically shorter distal-locking fluoroscopy time with the distal device. Krettek and colleagues[38] showed a statistically shorter operative time and fluoroscopy time with their radiation-independent distal aiming device.

Fibular Plating

Some debate regards the merits of stabilization of an associated fibular fracture in distal-third tibial fractures. Clearly, if the fibular fracture represents an associated ankle fracture, the principles appropriate to ankle fractures should be applied. A retrospective, Level III study by Egol and coauthors[39] suggests a significantly lower rate of loss of alignment in nailed distal-third tibial shaft fractures when ORIF of the fibula was also undertaken.

Postoperative Management

In the postoperative management of nailed tibial fractures, there is little evidence base to direct care. The use of splints, the role of physiotherapy, and the time to weight bearing have not been evaluated. Although there is some support for the use of deep vein thrombosis prophylaxis in tibial fractures treated in cast, no evidence is available to direct prophylaxis in cases with surgical stabilization.

After fracture healing, implant removal is elective and usually indicated by significant symptoms. The routine removal of implants has no evidence base. If elected, the recommendations regarding the time to implant removal vary, but again are not evidence based.

Bone Healing Adjuncts

Smoking and the use of nonsteroidal anti-inflammatory drugs have been associated with an increased incidence of delayed and nonunion. It seems reasonable to counsel patient regarding these substances.

Several modalities have been investigated in an effort to accelerate bone healing. Studies conflict regarding the use of electrical stimulation in the management of tibial shaft fractures. Clinical studies all relate to the management of tibial delayed and nonunions, so there is no basis for its use in routine fracture care.

Low-intensity, pulsed ultrasound has been shown to be effective in accelerating tibial shaft fractures treated without surgery in well-constructed studies[40,41]; however, they found no effect in the use of this modality in tibial fractures treated by IM nailing in a prospective, randomized, double-blinded, placebo-controlled study of 32 patients. Interferential current treatment to reduce tibial shaft fracture healing time has also proved to be ineffective.[42]

RECOMMENDATIONS

Recommendations regarding the management of tibial shaft fractures are largely based on small Level II studies. Larger, higher-quality multicenter studies are required to consolidate these recommendations.

Current best evidence would suggest that locked IM nailing is the treatment of choice for most unstable tibial shaft fractures, with reaming being advantageous particularly in closed fractures. Special care needs to be devoted to proximal and distal fractures to avoid malalignment.

Anterior knee pain remains an issue with IM nailing. Rigorous evaluation of newer percutaneous plating techniques is required to determine its role in tibial shaft fracture management. Table 65–1 provides a summary of recommendations.

TABLE 65–1. Summary of Recommendations

RECOMMENDATIONS	LEVEL OF EVIDENCE/GRADE OF RECOMMENDATION
1. Adult with a closed unstable tibial shaft fracture should be treated with reamed, statically locked intramedullary nailing.	B
2. Adult with an open (all types) tibia fracture should be treated with statically locked intramedullary nailing after appropriate soft-tissue management.	B
3. Free-hand nailing shortens operative time.	B
4. Open fractures should be treated urgently.	C

REFERENCES

1. Abdel-Salam A, Eyres KS, Cleary J: Internal fixation of closed tibial fractures for the management of sports injuries. Br J Sports Med 25:213–217, 1991.
2. Ali SA, Mehboob G: Comparative study 'pin and plaster' and 'AO monoplane external fixator' in treatment of gustilo type I and II open fracture of tibia. J Coll Physicians Surg Pak 12:741–742, 2002.
3. Curtis JF, Killian JT, Alonso JE: Improved treatment of femoral shaft fractures in children utilizing the pontoon spica cast: A long-term follow-up. J Pediatr Orthop 15:36–40, 1995.
4. Hooper GJ, Keddell RG, Penny ID: Conservative management or closed nailing for tibial shaft fractures. A randomised prospective trial. J Bone Joint Surg Br 73:83–85, 1991.
5. Karladani AH, Granhed H, Edshage B, et al: Displaced tibial shaft fractures: A prospective randomized study of closed intramedullary nailing versus cast treatment in 53 patients. Acta Orthop Scand 71:160–167, 2000.
6. Toivanen JAK, Honkonen SE, Koivisto AM, Jarvinen MJ: Treatment of low-energy tibial shaft fractures: Plaster cast compared with intramedullary nailing. Int Orthop 25:110–113, 2001.
7. van der Linden W, Larsson K: Plate fixation versus conservative treatment of tibial shaft fractures. A randomized trial. J Bone Joint Surg Am 61(6A):873–878, 1979.
8. Littenberg B, Weinstein LP, McCarren M, et al: Closed fractures of the tibial shaft. A meta-analysis of three methods of treatment. J Bone Joint Surg Am 80:174–183, 1998.
9. Im G-I, Tae S-K: Distal metaphyseal fractures of tibia: A prospective randomized trial of closed reduction and intramedullary nail versus open reduction and plate and screws fixation. J Trauma 59:1219–1223, 2005.
10. Coles CP, Gross M: Closed tibial shaft fractures: Management and treatment complications. A review of the prospective literature. Can J Surg 43:256–262, 2000.
11. Braten M, Helland P, Grontvedt T, et al: External fixation versus locked intramedullary nailing in tibial shaft fractures: A prospective, randomised study of 78 patients. Arch Orthop Trauma Surg 125:21–26, 2005.
12. Chiu FY, Lo WH, Chen CM, et al: Treatment of unstable tibial fractures with interlocking nail versus ender nail: A prospective evaluation. Zhonghua Yi Xue Za Zhi (Taipei) 57:124–133, 1996.
13. Blachut PA, O'Brien PJ, Meek RN, Broekhuyse HM: Interlocking intramedullary nailing with and without reaming for the treatment of closed fractures of the tibial shaft. A prospective, randomized study. J Bone Joint Surg Am 79:640–646, 1997.
14. Court-Brown CM, Will E, Christie J, McQueen MM: Reamed or unreamed nailing for closed tibial fractures. A prospective

study in Tscherne C1 fractures. J Bone Joint Surg Br 78:580–583, 1996.

15. Finkemeier CG, Schmidt AH, Kyle RF, et al: A prospective, randomized study of intramedullary nails inserted with and without reaming for the treatment of open and closed fractures of the tibial shaft. J Orthop Trauma 14:187–193, 2000.

16. Larsen LB, Madsen JE, Hoiness PR, Ovre S: Should insertion of intramedullary nails for tibial fractures be with or without reaming? A prospective, randomized study with 3.8 years' follow-up. J Orthop Trauma 18:144–149, 2004.

17. Ashford RU, Mehta JA, Cripps R: Delayed presentation is no barrier to satisfactory outcome in the management of open tibial fractures. Injury 35:411–416, 2004.

18. Charalambous CP, Siddique I, Zenios M, et al: Early versus delayed surgical treatment of open tibial fractures: Effect on the rates of infection and need of secondary surgical procedures to promote bone union. Injury 36:656–661, 2005.

19. Khatod M, Botte MJ, Hoyt DB, et al: Outcomes in open tibia fractures: Relationship between delay in treatment and infection. J Trauma 55:949–954, 2003.

20. Bach AW, Hansen ST Jr: Plates versus external fixation in severe open tibial shaft fractures. A randomized trial. Clin Orthop Relat Res (241):89–94, 1989.

21. Krettek C, Haas N, Tscherne H: The role of supplemental lag-screw fixation for open fractures of the tibial shaft treated with external fixation. J Bone Joint Surg Am 73:893–897, 1991.

22. Antich-Adrover P, Marti-Garin D, Murias-Alvarez J, Puente-Alonso C: External fixation and secondary intramedullary nailing of open tibial fractures. A randomised, prospective trial. J Bone Joint Surg Br 79:433–437, 1997.

23. Henley MB, Chapman JR, Agel J, et al: Treatment of type II, IIIA, and IIIB open fractures of the tibial shaft: A prospective comparison of unreamed interlocking intramedullary nails and half-pin external fixators. J Orthop Trauma 12:1–7, 1998.

24. Schandelmaier P, Krettek C, Rudolf J, et al: Superior results of tibial rodding versus external fixation in grade 3B fractures. Clin Orthop Relat Res (342):164–172, 1997.

25. Tornetta P 3rd, Bergman M, Watnik N, et al: Treatment of grade-IIIb open tibial fractures. A prospective randomised comparison of external fixation and non-reamed locked nailing. J Bone Joint Surg Br 76:13–19, 1994.

26. Tu YK, Lin CH, Su JI, et al: Unreamed interlocking nail versus external fixator for open type III tibia fractures. J Trauma 39:361–367, 1995.

27. Hupel TM, Weinberg JA, Aksenov SA, Schemitsch EH: Effect of unreamed, limited reamed, and standard reamed intramedullary nailing on cortical bone porosity and new bone formation. J Orthop Trauma 15:18–27, 2001.

28. Keating JF, O'Brien PJ, Blachut PA, et al: Locking intramedullary nailing with and without reaming for open fractures of the tibial shaft. A prospective, randomized study. J Bone Joint Surg Am 79:334–341, 1997.

29. McKee MD, Schemitsch EH, Waddell JP, Yoo D: A prospective, randomized clinical trial comparing tibial nailing using fracture table traction versus manual traction. J Orthop Trauma 13:463–469, 1999.

30. Giannoudis PV, Snowden S, Matthews SJ, et al: Friction burns within the tibia during reaming. J Bone Joint Surg Br 84:492–496, 2002.

31. Toivanen JAK, Vaisto O, Kannus P, et al: Anterior knee pain after intramedullary nailing of fractures of the tibial shaft. A prospective, randomized study comparing two different nail-insertion techniques. J Bone Joint Surg Am 84-A:580–585, 2002.

32. McConnell T, Tornetta P 3rd, Tilzey J, Casey D: Tibial portal placement: The radiographic correlate of the anatomic safe zone. J Orthop Trauma 15:207–209, 2001.

33. Tornetta P 3rd, Collins E: Semiextended position of intramedullary nailing of the proximal tibia. Clin Orthop Relat Res (328):185–189, 1996.

34. Krettek C, Miclau T, Schandelmaier P, et al: The mechanical effect of blocking screws ("Poller screws") in stabilizing tibia fractures with short proximal or distal fragments after insertion of small-diameter intramedullary nails. J Orthop Trauma 13:550–553, 1999.

35. Matthews DE, McGuire R, Freeland AE: Anterior unicortical buttress plating in conjunction with an unreamed interlocking intramedullary nail for treatment of very proximal tibial diaphyseal fractures. Orthopedics 20:647–648, 1997.

36. Kneifel T, Buckley R: A comparison of one versus two distal locking screws in tibial fractures treated with unreamed tibial nails: A prospective randomized clinical trial. Injury 27:271–273, 1996.

37. Gugala Z, Nana A, Lindsey RW: Tibial intramedullary nail distal interlocking screw placement: Comparison of the free-hand versus distally-based targeting device techniques. Injury 32(suppl 4):SD-21–SD-25, 2001.

38. Krettek C, Konemann B, Farouk O, et al: Experimental study of distal interlocking of a solid tibial nail: Radiation-independent distal aiming device (DAD) versus freehand technique (FHT). J Orthop Trauma 12:373–378, 1998.

39. Egol KA, Weisz R, Hiebert R, et al: Does fibular plating improve alignment after intramedullary nailing of distal metaphyseal tibia fractures? J Orthop Trauma 20:94–103, 2006.

40. Emami A, Petren-Mallmin M, Larsson S: No effect of low-intensity ultrasound on healing time of intramedullary fixed tibial fractures. J Orthop Trauma 13:252–257, 1999.

41. Heckman JD, Ryaby JP, McCabe J, et al: Acceleration of tibial fracture-healing by non-invasive, low-intensity pulsed ultrasound. J Bone Joint Surg Am 76:26–34, 1994.

42. Fourie JA, Bowerbank P: Stimulation of bone healing in new fractures of the tibial shaft using interferential currents. Physiother Res Int 2:255–268, 1997.

Chapter 66

What Is the Best Treatment for Pilon Fractures?

Paul Vincent Fearon, BSc (Hons), MB, Bch, BAO, FRCS (Tr & Orth), MD and Peter J. O'Brien, MD, FRCSC

Intra-articular fractures of the distal tibia vary in regards to the amount of articular and metaphyseal damage. Pilon fractures are difficult injuries to manage and can be associated with high rates of complications, chronic pain, and disability. The underlying mechanism of injury and general physiology of the patient dictates the severity of the bony injury and, more importantly, the soft-tissue involvement. High-energy pilon fractures are the most challenging to manage.

IMAGING AND ANATOMY

After appropriate radiographs, computed tomography (CT) is important in operative planning (Table 66–1). Tornetta and Gorup[1] have shown that their operative plan was altered in 64% of patients, with additional information about fracture pattern gained in 82%, underlining the importance of appropriate imaging. Understanding the anatomy of the fracture should allow the development of appropriate steps in fracture fragment approach and reduction, improving surgical technique and ultimately outcome.

Recent work from Bristol[2] documents 126 pilon fractures, and defines 6 distinct fracture fragments (anterior, posterior, medial, anterolateral, posterolateral, and die-punch) and 2 fracture families (sagittal and coronal). Within each fracture group there was progression from a simple to a more complex type with increasing transfer of energy. Interestingly, a pilon fracture with an intact distal fibula was eight times more likely to have a functional disruption of the tibiofibular joint (separated lateral tibial fragments), and if not recognized, resulted in continued instability and its associated complications. The reproducibility of this fracture description was found by Topliss and colleagues[2] to be superior to the AO and Ruedi and Allgower's[3] classification concerning interobserver and intraobserver agreement. The authors conclude that the sagittal family fractures occur after high energy, with varus angulation in younger patients, whereas the coronal fractures occur with valgus angulation in older patients after less severe trauma. This work has implications for surgical approach, reduction of fracture fragments, and choice of implant.

TREATMENT OPTIONS

Pilon fractures, although not common, do cause considerable debate and controversy as to what surgical methods should be used and the timing of surgery in relation to soft-tissue status. The treating surgeon is faced with two competing priorities. The first priority is to achieve an anatomic reduction of the fracture with fixation sufficiently secure to allow early movement, and the second is to minimize iatrogenic disruption of the vulnerable soft-tissue envelope.

It has generally been accepted that for displaced pilon fractures, surgical management with reduction and fixation is appropriate as long as there is no contraindication to surgical intervention for the individual patient (Level IV).

The surgical strategies can be divided into three broad subsets:
1. Immediate open reduction and internal fixation (ORIF)
2. Primary closed reduction and external skeletal fixation (ExFix) with delayed ORIF—the staged protocol (Level IV)
3. Definitive ExFix with or without limited internal fixation

The optimal management of these difficult injuries remains controversial. The staged protocol has shown acceptable results and has gained a substantial level of support. Indeed, we are aware that the faculties at some recent international conferences and instructional courses have suggested that it is the only acceptable treatment option.

EVIDENCE

Several studies have been published that aim to compare the differing treatment modalities for pilon fractures, but all have their limitations when conclusions are drawn from limited sample size and variable patient conditions (Table 66–2).

Blauth and colleagues[4] retrospectively studied 51 patients. They had 3 treatment groups: primary ORIF (15 patients all with closed injuries), definitive ExFix with or without limited internal fixation (28 patients), and temporary ExFix with or without limited internal fixation followed by delayed minimally invasive medial plating (8 patients). The incidence of wound

TABLE 66–1. Imaging and Anatomy

STUDY	DESIGN	EVIDENCE	CASES *(N)*	RADIOGRAPHS ONLY	ENHANCED INFORMATION
Tornetta and Gorup[1]	Prospective	I	22	15 Ruedi II 7 Ruedi III	11 type II 11 type III increased fragments: 12 patients Impaction: 6 patients Increased comminution: 11 patients Additional information gained in 82% of patients
Topliss et al.[2]	Prospective	II	126	33 Ruedi I 38 Ruedi II 47 Ruedi III	6 distinct fracture fragments 2 fracture families Implications for surgical planning

TABLE 66–2. Evidence

STUDY	EVIDENCE	DESIGN	NO. OF FRACTURES	FRACTURE TYPES	TREATMENTS (NUMBER)	RESULTS
Blauth et al.[4]	III	Retrospective review	51	3 B2 1 B3 2 C1 26 C2 19 C3	ORIF (15) ExFix/limited ORIF (28) ExFix converted to ORIF (8)	Better ankle ROM in two-stage group
Pugh et al.[5]	III	Retrospective review	60	10 A 3 B1 4 B2 2 B3 8 C1 9 C2 24 C3	ORIF (24) Spanning ExFix (21) Nonspanning ExFix (15)	Malunions more common in fixator groups
Wyrsch et al.[6]	III	Prospective surgeon randomized	39	8 type I 14 type II 17 type III	ORIF (19) ExFix/limited ORIF (20)	Fewer soft-tissue complications with fixator group
Sirkin et al.[7]	IV	Retrospective	56	4 C1 10 C2 42 C3	Staged ORIF after ExFix	Effective in both open and closed injuries; reduced need for soft-tissue procedures
Patterson and Cole[8]	IV	Retrospective	22	23 C3	Staged ORIF after ExFix	Advantage of limited soft-tissue complications
Koulouvaris et al.[9]	III	Retrospective	55	19 B 36 C	Spanning ExFix (20) Nonspanning ExFix (22) Two-stage ORIF (13)	Delayed union and reduced activities more common with ExFix
Harris et al.[10]	III	Retrospective	79	11 B 68 C	Staged ORIF (63) Limited IF and ExFix (16)	ORIF fewer complications and less post-traumatic OA

ExFix, external skeletal fixation; IF, internal fixation; OA, osteoarthritis; ORIF, open reduction and internal fixation; ROM, range of motion.

infections did not differ significantly among the three groups. The range of ankle movement was greater in the two-stage treated group compared with the others. These patients also had less pain, more frequently continued working in their previous profession, and had fewer limitations in their leisure activities. On the basis of these findings, the authors recommend a two-stage procedure. However, the sample size is small in this retrospective review, and the groups are not well matched; therefore, definitive conclusions cannot be made.

Similar work by Pugh and coauthors[5] retrospectively assessed 60 pilon fractures. Again, there were 3 broad groups: 24 patients treated with ORIF, 21 patients treated with an ankle-spanning half-pin ExFix, and 15 patients with a single-ring hybrid ExFix. The severity of injuries was similar in all groups. No significant difference was reported in complications between groups, but a greater number of malunions occurred in fractures treated with ExFix compared with ORIF ($P = 0.03$). These findings were uninfluenced by whether the fracture was open or closed, was bone grafted, or had an associated fibula fracture stabilized. The authors conclude that external fixation had a lower risk for deep infection but a greater risk for malunion than did ORIF. No randomization, long-term follow-up, or functional outcome was performed in these patients.

A surgeon randomized, prospective study[6] evaluated 39 patients. Nineteen patients underwent ORIF of both tibia and fibula, and 20 patients had ExFix with or without limited internal fixation. The authors aimed to compare the rates of complications, the radiologic results, and the functional results between the two groups. In the ORIF group, there were 28 additional operations in 7 patients with 15 major complications compared with 5 additional operations in 4 patients with 4 major complications in the ExFix group. They found that nonvalidated clinical score (pain and range of motion) did not correlate well with type of fracture, and there was also no significant difference between treatment groups. The conclusion was that ExFix is a satisfactory method of treatment associated with fewer complications than ORIF. However, of note is the timing of surgery in the ORIF group, and this point should be highlighted. Operating in the presence of severe intradermal edema or fracture blisters can further compromise damaged soft tissues. On average, patients were operated on days 3 to 5, when soft-tissue swelling was well established. Therefore, it may well not be technique related but timing dependent.

This point has been examined by work from Sirkin and colleagues.[7] They retrospectively analyzed 56 pilon fractures (34 closed and 22 open fractures) from a single institution. All patients underwent immediate ORIF of the fibula and closed reduction with spanning ExFix for the distal tibia. Formal ORIF of the tibia was performed when soft-tissue swelling had subsided, on average, 14 days after injury. By following a staged protocol, they demonstrated that ORIF could be performed semielectively with a low risk for wound problem in both open and closed injuries. However, no functional outcome scoring of results with this effective soft-tissue–preserving procedure exists.

Similar retrospective work from Florida (Patterson and Cole[8]) examined 22 C3 distal tibia fractures treated with a comparable staged protocol. Anatomic reduction was possible in 73% of patients who underwent surgery, on average, 24 days after injury. Approximately 90% of patients had good/fair results on subjective and objective evaluation. The authors recognized difficulties with operating on 3-week-old fractures and the extended dissection needed.

Koulouvaris and coworkers[9] retrospectively compared ExFix with staged ORIF. The study population included 36 AO type C and 19 AO type B tibial plafond fractures. Of these fractures, 24 were open and 31 closed. Three surgical protocols were used. In 20 patients, group A, a half-pin ExFix with ankle spanning was used for fixation. In 22 patients, group B, a nonspanning ring hybrid ExFix was used. In 13 patients, group C, a two-staged ORIF was performed. Group A had union in 6.9 months, group B in 5.6 months, and group C in 5.1 months ($P = 0.009$). Six (group A), two (group B), and one (group C) patient had limitation of ankle motion ($P = 0.47$). One patient from group C acquired an infection, and the plate was removed. Four (group A), one (group B), and one (group C) pa-

tients have experienced development of post-traumatic arthritis (defined as loss of joint space and pain) ($P = 0.25$). Seven patients from group A have reduced their activities ($P = 0.004$). In this long-term follow-up study, the two-staged internal fixation and the hybrid fixation with small arthrotomy were equally efficacious in achieving bone union. Patients in external fixation with the ankle spanning had a significantly greater rate of delayed union. Also, more patients in this group had to reduce their activities.

Similar work from Cleveland (Harris and researchers[10]) retrospectively reviewed 79 pilon fractures. Patients were treated with ORIF (63 patients) or limited open articular reduction and wire-ring ExFix (16 patients). Tibial ORIF was performed at an average of 7.6 days after injury. Approximately 86% of patients with ORIF treatment underwent staged surgery, whereby initial surgery consisted of fibular fixation and temporary ankle-spanning ExFix or splinting. The patients treated definitively with ExFix had more complications ($P = 0.007$) and post-traumatic arthritis ($P = 0.01$) when compared with ORIF. However, this may be because of selection bias because more open injuries and more severely comminuted fractures were managed definitively with external fixation than with ORIF.

From the literature, the overall average rate of deep infection is approximately 5% after surgical management of pilon fractures regardless of the technique used. Definitive ORIF done at 2 to 5 days after injury would appear to be associated with more wound complications than delayed ORIF or definitive ExFix. Deep infection occurs more frequently in open fractures than it does in closed fractures. The risk for malunion and delayed union are more common in patients treated definitively with external fixation.

A number of other factors have been shown to be associated with risk for complications. Several authors have emphasized the importance of the level of experience of the surgeon and the quality of the reduction. Anatomic reduction of the articular segment and anatomic realignment of the nonarticular segment should intuitively be associated with a lower risk for malunion and post-traumatic osteoarthritis.

Although the optimal management of pilon fractures requires anatomic reduction and restoration of the alignment of the distal tibial articular surface, success or failure is often related more closely to the management of the vulnerable soft-tissue envelope around the fracture and the avoidance of wound complications. The natural history of the soft tissues overlying the distal tibia and ankle is that they are subject to swelling and blistering in the first few hours to days after injury, before gradually recovering some elasticity over a period of around 10 to 14 days. It is recognized that there is an early period after injury where the skin is pliant and is able to withstand open fracture surgery. However, this period is poorly quantified: Published graphs and guidelines continue to be based on anecdotal experience, and there remains considerable disagreement as to whether a "safe period" exists. Then there is a subsequent period of localized edema where the soft tissues are widely considered to be under too great a degree of tension, with compromised tissue perfusion, to allow predictable and safe wound closure and healing. Historically, the enthusiasm for open surgical treatment that followed Ruedi and Allgower's[3] seminal article in 1969 was tempered by subsequent reports of disconcerting rates of wound slough, infection, and osteomyelitis in other centers. Currently, a widespread preference exists for staged treatment whereby after temporary external fixation, definitive surgery is delayed until the end of the period of swelling. Several authorities and standard texts[6] advise against surgery in the "early" period.

Many studies outline the ability to treat pilon fractures with varying external skeletal fixation strategies with or without limited internal fixation. Comparative evidence, however, is lacking.

FUNCTIONAL OUTCOME RESULTS

The immediate management of pilon fractures is not the only area of concern for the patient. The long-term function and outcome after such injuries needs to be evaluated to give advice and counseling to patients (Table 66–3).

Although there is good documentation of the complications associated with pilon fractures, functional outcome studies using well-validated assessment tools are scarce in the literature. Ruedi and Allgower's[3] pivotal work with impressive outcomes has not been universally repeated in the current literature.

Pollak and colleagues[11] have shown that midterm outcome results after pilon fractures are not good. Their Level II evidence, retrospective, observational study of 103 patients, with a mean duration of follow-up of 3.2 years, showed of those used at time of injury, only 57% returned to work. Approximately one third of patients reported notable difficulty with ankle stiffness (35%), swelling (29%), or pain (33%). Thirteen percent reported that they usually used a walking aid. This was reflected in the Sickness Impact Profile ambulation scores, whereby up to 50% of patients were unable to ascend and descend stairs reciprocally or run on the spot for 30 seconds.

Patients treated with ExFix with or without limited internal fixation reported and demonstrated significantly poorer results for three of the five primary outcomes—walking ability, range-of-motion impairment, and pain—than did patients treated with ORIF. In addition to providing evidence about functional outcome, this study also provides strong support for the superiority of ORIF over ankle-spanning ExFix techniques.

More long-term studies related to fracture pattern of pilon fractures, which underwent ORIF, highlight the fact that post-traumatic arthritis is a progressive disease. Chen and coworkers[12] studied 128 patients with a mean follow-up period of 10 years (range, 6–15 years). All fractures were treated by ORIF; however, Ruedi and Allgower type II and III injuries underwent delayed surgery after 1 to 2 weeks of traction. At 2 years, the post-traumatic osteoarthritis rate was 5.1%, 9.7%, and 29.6% in types I, II, and III, respectively. There was progression of post-traumatic arthritis only in types II and III to 22.6% and 55.6%, respectively, at final follow-up (mean, 10 years). The average duration between initial injury and the development of severe arthritis was 6.7 years. Functional outcome was worse in patients with high-energy injuries. This study has important implications with regard to resources planning of subsequent patient follow-up, counseling, and possible salvage procedures.

Area of Uncertainty: Timing, Surgical Approach, and Plate Design

The techniques used in the treatment of pilon fractures often depend on the surgeon's preference and the associated soft-tissue trauma. When faced with a complex pilon fracture and considerable tissue trauma, the most widely accepted treatment option is to apply a spanning external fixator (with or without limited internal of the joint surface) and wait until the swelling abates before proceeding to definitive ORIF. However, intra-articular reduction in the presence of early callus and soft tissues with reduced elasticity further compromise an already challenging operation. Therefore, do we compromise articular

TABLE 66–3. Outcomes

STUDY	EVIDENCE	DESIGN	CASES (N)	OUTCOME MEASURES	MEAN FOLLOW-UP (RANGE)	FINDINGS
Chen et al.[2]	II	Retrospective	128	Adequacy of reduction, clinical rating of Teeny and Wiss[13]	10 yr (6–15 yr)	Average time to post-traumatic OA: 6.7 yr; post-traumatic OA progressive disease and requires long-term follow-up
Pollak et al.[6]	II	Retrospective observational	103	SF-36, Sickness Impact Profile, ROM impairment, pain on VAS, stair climbing	3.2 yr (2–5 yr)	Midterm pilon results not good; only 57% returned to work; poorer results with ExFix

ExFix, external skeletal fixation; ORIF, open reduction and internal fixation; ROM, range of motion; SF-36, 36-Item Short Form Health Survey; VAS, visual analogue pain scale.

reduction for soft-tissue preservation? And does this have a bearing on functional outcome? Insufficient evidence has been presented to make a recommendation about the timing of definitive ORIF, but most current studies advise delay until soft-tissue swelling subsides (7–14 days) by using the staged protocol.

It is generally agreed that surgical approaches used for ORIF should be designed to preserve the blood supply to bone to allow for rapid fracture healing. Elevation of large soft-tissue flaps is also thought to be associated with a risk for wound breakdown and subsequent infection. Minimally invasive surgical approaches with submuscular or subcutaneous plate placement and percutaneous screw placement have become popular. Ancillary equipment including radiolucent tables, image intensifiers, and distractors for reduction and temporary fixation are necessary for these techniques. No published evidence has documented the superiority of these techniques for pilon fractures.

New implants for ORIF have been utilized recently including low-profile plates and screws and locking plate designs. Despite theoretical advantages, no published evidence exists that precontoured low-profile plates or locking plate systems are associated with fewer complications or better outcomes than traditional implants for the treatment of tibial pilon fractures.

Guidelines

No guidelines have been published about the assessment of treatment of tibial pilon fractures.

RECOMMENDATIONS

Tibial pilon fractures frequently occur as a result of a high-energy mechanism of injury and can be associated with significant soft-tissue injury and a complex fracture pattern. Early surgical complications will occur if the patient is not carefully assessed and treated with appropriate surgical strategies. In general, the articular segment requires anatomic reduction and absolutely stable fixation, whereas the nonarticular segment requires anatomic realignment of the limb and adequate stabilization. The surgeon must consider the soft-tissue envelope and treat it carefully to allow fracture healing and to minimize the risk for infection. A variety of surgical techniques has been used to manage these complex injuries. The literature around this topic does not provide strong evidence about management.

We recommend that the patient be thoroughly assessed with clinical and radiographic evaluation including CT. The soft tissues are best assessed with clinical examination, whereas the bony injury requires plane radiographs and CT. The CT information is generally better obtained after fracture reduction.

Definitive management with ORIF is preferred to either spanning or nonspanning external fixation. Malunion and poorer functional outcome appear to be the main drawback to ExFix (Level IV).

Timing of surgical intervention is somewhat controversial. Low-energy injuries with little soft-tissue damage likely can be managed with early (within 24 hours) definitive ORIF as long as it is done by an experienced orthopedic trauma surgeon and a well-prepared team. If there is a question about the soft-tissue envelope, most surgeons advocate a staged procedure with ORIF of the fibula, limited ORIF of the articular surface, and external skeletal fixation of the tibia as the initial procedure. Definitive ORIF of the tibia is delayed until the soft-tissue swelling has subsided (7–14 days). No prospective comparative study of early versus delayed ORIF for tibial pilon fractures has been published.

Surgical approaches should be selected that will allow adequate exposure for fracture reduction whereas minimizing further injury to the soft tissue. Indirect reduction and minimally invasive fixation techniques are frequently used (Level V).

Precontoured, low-profile plates seem to be advantageous because of the soft-tissue envelope around the distal tibia. Locking plate technology is usually not necessary as long as both the tibia and the fibula are fixed (Level V).

In conclusion, the best treatment for tibial pilon fractures is anatomic reduction and stable fixation, whereas respecting the biology of the soft-tissue envelope and allowing early functional rehabilitation. Unfortunately, the literature does not contain good evidence-based studies to support overall superiority of one treatment method. Controversy will continue to exist about the optimum timing and surgical techniques, but the staged protocol for delayed ORIF has the most widespread support at this time. Table 66–4 provides a summary of recommendations for the management of tibial pilon fractures.

TABLE 66–4. Recommendations for the Management of Tibial Pilon Fractures

RECOMMENDATIONS	LEVEL OF EVIDENCE/ GRADE OF RECOMMENDATION
1. Preoperative computed tomographic scanning is an important aspect of patient assessment.	B
2. Patients should be advised that poor functional outcome may occur and is more common in high-energy injuries.	B
3. Displaced tibial pilon fractures should receive definitive surgical management with open reduction and internal fixation.	C
4. Timing: tibial pilon fractures require a staged protocol with delayed definitive fixation if open reduction and internal fixation is to be utilized.	I

REFERENCES

1. Tornetta P 3rd, Gorup J: Axial computed tomography of pilon fractures. Clin Orthop Relat Res (323):273–276, 1996.
2. Topliss CJ, Jackson M, Atkins RM: Anatomy of pilon fractures of the distal tibia. J Bone Joint Surg Br 87:692–697, 2005.
3. Ruedi TP, Allgower M: The operative treatment of intra-articular fractures of the lower end of the tibia. Clin Orthop Relat Res (138):105–110, 1979.
4. Blauth M, Bastian L, Krettek C, et al: Surgical options for the treatment of severe tibial pilon fractures: a study of three techniques. J Orthop Trauma 15:153–160, 2001.
5. Pugh KJ, Wolinsky PR, McAndrew MP, Johnson KD: Tibial pilon fractures: A comparison of treatment methods. J Trauma 47:937–941, 1999.
6. Wyrsch B, McFerran MA, McAndrew M, et al: Operative treatment of fractures of the tibial plafond. A randomized, prospective study. J Bone Joint Surg Am 78:1646–1657, 1996.
7. Sirkin M, Sanders R, DiPasquale T, Herscovici D Jr: A staged protocol for soft tissue management in the treatment of complex pilon fractures. J Orthop Trauma 18(8 suppl): S32–S28, 2004.
8. Patterson MJ, Cole JD: Two-staged delayed open reduction and internal fixation of severe pilon fractures. J Orthop Trauma, 13(2): 85–91, 1999.
9. Koulouvaris P, Stafylas K, Mitsionis G, et al: Long-term results of various therapy concepts in severe pilon fractures. Arch Orthop Trauma Surg, 2007. (Epub ahead of print)
10. Harris AM, Patterson BM, Sontich JK, Vallier HA: Results and outcomes after operative treatment of high-energy tibial plafond fractures. Foot Ankle Int 27:256–265, 2006.
11. Pollak AN, McCarthy ML, Bess RS, et al: Outcomes after treatment of high-energy tibial plafond fractures. J Bone Joint Surg Am, 85-A(10):1893–1900, 2003.
12. Chen SH, Wu PH, Lee YS: Long-term results of pilon fractures. Arch Orthop Trauma Surg 127:55–60, 2007.
13. Teeny SM, Wiss DA: Open reduction and internal fixation of tibial plafond fractures. Variables contributing to poor results and complications. Clin Orthop Relat Res (292):108–117, 1993.

FOOT AND ANKLE TOPICS

Chapter 67

What Is the Best Treatment for Plantar Fasciitis?

NELSON FONG SOOHOO, MD AND CALEB BEHREND, MD

Plantar fasciitis is a painful heel syndrome of unclear cause. Chronic or acute injury to the origin of the plantar fascia at the medial tubercle of the calcaneus is thought to produce a cycle of microtrauma and degenerative changes. Plantar fasciitis affects both active and sedentary adults with studies reporting that up to 10% of runners and a similar proportion of the general population are affected.[1-4] A significant occurrence also is reported in military personnel and professional athletes.[5,6] Increased body mass index, extended time standing, and limited ankle dorsiflexion are risk factors predisposing to plantar fasciitis.[7] The high prevalence, substantial pain, and decreased tolerance for activity result in large numbers of patients seeking treatment. The cumulative number of office visits in the United States is estimated to be nearly 1 million visits each year.[1]

TREATMENT

Plantar fasciitis tends to improve in most cases regardless of the treatment selected.[8-11] As a result, conservative management is effective for nearly 90% of patients.[12,13] The conservative treatments used in management of plantar fasciitis vary widely and are dependent on physician specialty.[1] Common treatments include nonsteroidal anti-inflammatory drugs (NSAIDs), stretching, insoles, taping, physical therapy, and night splints. If these simple and noninvasive modalities prove ineffective, additional treatment options include iontophoresis, injections, extracorporeal shock wave therapy (ESWT), and surgical treatment. This chapter reviews the various treatment methods for plantar fasciitis, and the effectiveness and safety of these treatments as supported by the best available evidence.

Stretching

Stretching protocols for the treatment of plantar fasciitis include stretching the Achilles tendon with or without stretching of the plantar fascia. Limited evidence is available from controlled trials to establish the effectiveness of stretching.[14] Prospective studies comparing a plantar fascia–specific stretching protocol before the first morning steps and Achilles tendon stretching for treating chronic plantar fasciitis

found a greater improvement in pain symptoms with the plantar fascia–specific stretching after 8 weeks (Level of Evidence II).[15] Long-term follow-up at 2 years was incomplete but suggested no difference between Achilles tendon stretching and the plantar fascia–specific groups, although both groups showed improvement (Level of Evidence III).[16]

Taping

Taping techniques are intended to alter the position and alignment of the calcaneus, and to support the longitudinal arch. The effectiveness of calcaneal taping was compared with stretching, no treatment, and sham taping in one small study. Taping produced greater improvement in reported pain on a visual analog scale (VAS) than sham taping, controls with no treatment, or stretching (Level II).[14] A larger study with 92 participants that examined taping with ultrasound compared with sham ultrasound reported a small improvement with taping in first step pain, one of four measured parameters (Level I).[17] Sensitivity or allergy to tape may cause skin irritation.[18]

Nonsteroidal Anti-inflammatory Drugs

NSAIDs are used extensively in the management of acute and chronic musculoskeletal pain. The mechanisms for the anti-inflammatory and analgesic effects of these drugs are well documented in an extensive body of basic science and clinical research. Despite this, limited evidence exists to support the efficacy of NSAIDs in shortening the course or decreasing the symptoms of plantar fasciitis. One small trial found a nonstatistically significant decrease in pain and disability with NSAID treatment of plantar fasciitis (Level II).[19] Other studies have quantified NSAID use as a measure of improvement with other therapies.[20] The use of NSAIDs is associated with known adverse effects, which have been reported extensively in the medical literature.

Orthoses

The use of orthoses is intended to change loading characteristics of the plantar aponeurosis. Studies using cadaveric limbs suggest that support of the medial longitudinal arch can decrease strain of the plantar aponeurosis.[21] Several randomized, controlled trials have examined the use of insoles in management of plantar fasciitis. A recent study comparing custom insoles, sham insoles, and prefabricated insoles found minor improvement in symptoms 3 months after treatment with prefabricated or custom insoles compared with sham (Level I).[22] Prefabricated insoles have been found to be as effective as custom insoles at a reduced total cost.[22–24] Insoles may be equally effective and offer improved patient compliance compared with night splints.[24,25] A randomized, placebo-controlled, double-blind study conducted with 101 patients compared magnetic insoles with sham magnetic insoles and found no statistically significant improvement in pain symptoms after 8 weeks of treatment (Level II).[26]

Night Splints

Tension night splints stretch the plantar fascia over several hours while the patient sleeps by maintaining a constant ankle dorsiflexion. A trial comparing night splints with conservative treatment with conservative treatment alone found no significant difference in symptoms (Level I).[27] Roos and coworkers[28] compared insoles with night splints and found no significant difference in pain reduction and improved compliance with insoles (Level II).[28] Three studies reported that patients find night splint treatment uncomfortable and difficult to maintain, resulting in decreased compliance.[24,28,29] A systematic review found that the evidence for the effectiveness of night splints is inconclusive (Level II).[3]

Casting

Limited evidence has been reported for the effectiveness of casting in treatment of plantar fasciitis. One case series of 32 patients reported improvement in pain symptoms after 6 months after treatment with casting (Level IV).[30] A fiberglass walking cast was used in the study.

Iontophoresis

Iontophoresis uses an electrical potential generated by bipolar electrodes to transfer charged ions and ionizable materials including some medications through the skin to provide anti-inflammatory or analgesic treatment.[31] Conflicting results have been published for the effectiveness of dexamethasone iontophoresis. In a double-blind study with 39 subjects comparing iontophoresis using dexamethasone with a placebo, significant improvement on the Maryland foot score was reported at the end of the 2-week treatment period (3.80; 95% confidence interval [CI], 0.76–6.84) but not after 1 month (0.30; 95% CI, −2.16 to 6.76) (Level I).[31] A second randomized, controlled trial with 31 subjects compared iontophoresis with taping and 0.4% dexamethasone, 5% acetic acid, or 0.9% NaCl placebo. The graphical data presented in the study indicate no statistically significant improvement with dexamethasone treatment in six measured outcomes at 4 weeks and less relief of pain symptoms compared with the control group at 2 weeks of treatment. In the group treated with acetic acid, there was a significant improvement in morning stiffness at 4 weeks with no reported statistically significant difference in three measures of pain at 4 weeks and no significant improvement compared with placebo in all six parameters at 2 weeks (Level I).[18]

Steroid Injection

Previously published reviews have found limited evidence to support the use of steroid injections in the treatment of plantar fasciitis.[3,8] Steroid injection with and without nerve block was compared with placebo in a double-blind, randomized, control trial with 91 participants (Level I).[32] The study found a statistically significant benefit at 1 month with steroid injection but not at 3 and 6 months. In addition, it was reported that tibial nerve block was not effective at relieving pain associated with steroid injection. A prospective study with 132 patients comparing steroid injection with ESWT or placebo found a statistically significant improvement in pain symptoms for the group receiving steroid injection over ESWT or placebo (Level II).[33] The participants in this study reported VAS pain scores that were significantly lower than for the control and ESWT groups at 3 and 12 months. Potential adverse side effects of steroid injection include fat pad atrophy and plantar fascia rupture.

Botulinum Toxin Type A Injection

Botulinum toxin is used in the treatment of a variety of pain syndromes, and its use in treatment of plantar fasciitis has been reported. A single randomized, placebo-controlled, double-blind study conducted with 27 patients and 43 treated feet found statistically significant improvement in pain symptoms 3 and 8 weeks after treatment (Level I).[34] Additional studies of the use of botulinum toxin in the treatment of plantar fasciitis are necessary to further define safety and efficacy.

Extracorporeal Shock Wave Therapy

ESWT utilizes application of mechanical waves similar to those used in lithotripsy but of lower energy density, usually less then 0.36 mJ/mm^2 per pulse. Therapy consists of 500 to 6000 pulses delivered at 2 to 4 Hz to treat plantar foot pain. The mechanism by which ESWT provides benefit is investigational. Current theories include stimulation of healing after increased release of growth factors and neovascularization in the environment of local tissue injury[35,36] or alteration in the chemical function of small axons producing analgesic effects.[37,38] The possibility of a noninvasive treatment for chronic plantar fasciitis has generated significant interest, and several studies investigating the effectiveness of this technique have been published. Many of these trials are not of sufficient quality to provide a reliable assessment of the effectiveness of ESWT.[3,8,39,40] The studies investigating ESWT have been in many cases sponsored by the equipment manufacturers, and the randomized control trials have produced conflicting results. Good quality, randomized, placebo-controlled, double-blind clinical trials have found no significant benefit to ESWT,[41–43] whereas other randomized, controlled trials[44–47] have found ESWT to be beneficial. The reasons for the discrepancy in reported results are unclear. A lack of uniformity of therapy exists from study to study, with differing methods for assessment of therapy, and in some studies, significant problems with study design have been reported.[3,40] Differences also exist in the definition of the terms *high energy* and *low energy,* as well as in the amount of energy used in various studies. No controlled trials adequately define and identify indications for high- or low-energy protocols for ESWT. In addition, differences in criteria for patient inclusion in the studies make it difficult to compare the trials directly. Table 67–1 summarizes double-blind, randomized studies comparing ESWT with placebo. The reported adverse reactions, including skin redness, bruising, pain, numbness, tingling, and local swelling,[42,44,46] likely do not pose serious health risks. However, clear evidence supporting the use of ESWT treatment in the treatment of plantar fasciitis has not been reported.

Surgery

No randomized, controlled trials compare patients undergoing surgical treatments with a control population. Surgical treatment is considered for the approximately 10% of patients who do not respond to conservative treatment. Surgical treatment options include percutaneous plantar fasciotomy, endoscopic plantar fasciotomy, or open fasciotomy.[48,49] Cryosurgery is another proposed treatment that was reported in one case series to result in improvement of symptoms.[50] Complications of surgical treatments include forefoot stress fracture, calcaneal fracture, medial or lateral column pain, nerve injury, infection, and instability.[51,52] For surgical treatments, published case series report that between 75% and 95% of patients responded with improvement in measured symptoms after surgical treatment, with up to 27% having residual pain symptoms and 20% reporting activity restriction.[8,49,53–56] Increasing body mass index is a risk factor for poorer response to surgical treatment.[57] A study comparing plantar fascia release of 25%, 50%, or 66% of the insertion by open or endoscopic procedures reports that increasing lateral column pain symptoms occurred with increased percentage of plantar fascia release.[51] Limited evidence is available to suggest

TABLE 67–1. Summary of Randomized, Controlled Trials of Extracorporeal Shock Wave Therapy Intervention

STUDY (YEAR OF PUBLICATION)	PATIENTS (N)	SYMPTOM DURATION	PULSES	FREQUENCY	ENERGY, mJ/mm²	TOTAL, mJ/mm²	RESULT	COMMENTS AND DISCLOSURES
Buchbinder (2004)[11]	166	>6 wks	>2000	<4 Hz	0.02–0.33	1406 × 3	No benefit	Manufacturer-supported study Variable treatment dose
Haake et al. (2003)[42]	272	>6 mo	4000		0.08	320 × 3	No benefit	Government-supported study
Ogden et al. (2001)[44]	260	>6 mo	100 1400	2 Hz	0.12–0.22 0.22	>308 × 1	Effective	Manufacturer-supported study Intention-to-treat analysis not used Unclear randomization procedure Results in the original disclosed to FDA where not significant
Rompe et al. (2003)[45]	45	>12 mo	2100	4 Hz	0.16	336 × 3	Effective	Population: running athletes
Speed et al. (2003)[43]	88	>3 mo	1500		0.12	180 × 3	No benefit	Study supported by charity
Theodore et al. (2004)[47]	150	>6 mo	3800		0.36	1300 ×1	Effective	Manufacturer-supported study
Kudo (2006)[66]	114	>6 mo	3800		0.36	1300 × 1	Some benefit	Manufacturer-supported study; one parameter was statistically significant
Malay et al. (2006)[46]	172	>6 mo	3800	2.5 Hz			Effective	Manufacturer-supported study

when surgical treatment should be recommended or to guide the choice of surgical treatment.

Open Fasciotomy. Medial fasciotomy can be performed with local or general anesthesia. The plantar fascia is approached through an incision beginning medially and extending to the plantar aspect of the foot to allow exposure and release of the deep and superficial fascia of the abductor hallucis brevis muscle. Further dissection is used to identify and transect the medial aspect of the central plantar fascial band.[58] For patients with neurologic symptoms resulting from suspected compression of the first branch of the lateral plantar nerve, which innervates the abductor digiti quinti (Baxter's nerve), fasciotomy is accompanied by decompression of the nerve through release of the deep fascia of the abductor hallucis.[59] Other authors advocate proximal release of the tarsal tunnel when neurologic symptoms suggest that refractory heel pain is associated with both plantar fasciitis and tarsal tunnel syndrome.[60] No controlled trials adequately compare isolated plantar fasciotomy with techniques that incorporate release of Baxter's nerve or the tarsal tunnel. The open technique also allows for the removal of a prominent plantar heel spur when present. No controlled trials have determined whether removal of a spur improves outcomes when compared with soft-tissue release only.

Endoscopic Fasciotomy. Endoscopic fasciotomy may be conducted with regional nerve blocks for anesthesia. One or two ports have been used with ideal port placement being 1 to 2 mm distal to the medial calcaneal tubercle at the level of the inferior aspect of the plantar fascia. After careful cannula placement, the plantar fascia is identified and the medial third is released with a hook knife. Patients can be fully weight bearing after the procedure with moderate activity. Prospective studies of endoscopic release of the plantar fascia have reported relief of symptoms in up to 97% of treated patients (Level II).[61] Other studies have reported shortened recovery time compared with open procedures (Level IV).[62] No large-scale trials have directly compared outcomes in patients undergoing open as opposed to endoscopic treatment for plantar fasciitis.

Other Treatments

The application of topical wheat-grass cream has been proposed in treatment of plantar fasciitis. A randomized, placebo-controlled double-blind study conducted with 80 patients found no statistically significant improvement resulting from treatment at 6 and 12 weeks. Primary outcome measures were a VAS for first-step pain in the morning and the Foot Health Status Questionnaire.[63] No further studies on this treatment have been reported.

Irradiation of skin or soft tissue with low-power lasers has been proposed as an agent for pain management in plantar fasciitis.[64] A single randomized, placebo-controlled, double-blind study conducted with 32 patients found no statistically significant improvement in 6 measured parameters during a series of treatments or 1 month after therapy. Adverse reactions were minimal (Level I).[65]

RECOMMENDATIONS

Limited evidence supports the recommendation of any one therapy in the treatment of plantar fasciitis.[40] As a result, the use of less costly and less invasive treatment modalities such as stretching, taping, NSAIDs, orthoses, and night splints remain first-line therapies for plantar fasciitis. The failure of these conservative modalities may lead to the need for more costly or invasive treatments including casting, iontophoresis, injection, ESWT, or open or endoscopic plantar fasciotomy.

Studies for several of these treatments have produced conflicting results. Recommendations with grade of evidence for specific treatments and references are summarized in Table 67–2. Problems with study design have been recognized for several published trials and include description of randomization procedures, concealment of allocation, use of intention-to-treat analysis, absent or ineffective blinding, and duplicate publication of previously published results.[2,3]

Plantar fasciitis tends to improve spontaneously, and in most of the comparative studies of treatment for plantar fasciitis, it was found that both the treatment groups and the control groups improved with time.[3,8,11] Conservative treatment is effective for nearly 90% of patients.[12,13] No evidence supports the use of rest and ice, and limited evidence supports NSAID use in the treatment of plantar fasciitis. These treatments are effective general measures used in conservative management of many musculoskeletal complaints and may be considered for adjunctive therapy for treatment of plantar fasciitis in absence of contraindications. Prefabricated insoles, plantar fascia–specific stretching, and taping techniques should be considered as part of conservative treatment for short-term improvement in symptoms, but evidence for their efficacy is also limited.

The optimal period of conservative treatment before considering more invasive treatments has not been determined. Most studies examined the effectiveness of conservative treatments at 3 months, 6 months, or 1 year. When symptoms persist despite conservative treatment, steroid injections may be considered for short-term relief of symptoms but are associated with plantar fascia rupture and fat pad atrophy. Botulinum toxin injection and acetic acid iontophoresis may be considered, but the effectiveness of each is supported by only a single, small randomized trial. Casting and cryosurgery are additional proposed therapies, but evidence is lacking to establish effectiveness of these treatments. Available evidence does not provide convincing support for the effectiveness of night splints, steroid iontophoresis, ESWT, magnetic insoles, laser therapy, or topical application of wheat grass. Patient who do not respond to nonoperative management may consider surgical treatment with endoscopic or open release of 50% or less of the plantar fascia. Reported complications of surgery include persistent pain, fracture, nerve injury, infection, and instability. No randomized controlled trials compare surgical treatment with a control population, but there have been several reports of series of patients achieving satisfactory results with either open or endoscopic plantar fasciotomy.

TABLE 67–2. Summary of Recommendations

RECOMMENDATIONS	LEVEL OF EVIDENCE/GRADE OF RECOMMENDATION	REFERENCES
1. Plantar fascia stretching exercises should be used for conservative management of plantar fasciitis.	B	14, 15
2. Taping techniques improve pain symptoms and should be considered for conservative management of plantar fasciitis.	B	14, 17
3. Nonsteroidal anti-inflammatory medications may shorten the course or decrease the symptoms of plantar fasciitis.	I	19
4. Prefabricated insoles are as effective as custom-made insoles and may decrease costs.	B	22–24
5. Prefabricated insoles are as effective as night splints and may improve patient compliance.	B	14, 28
6. Night splints have not been shown to be effective.	I	24, 29, 65
7. Magnetic insoles are not effective.	I	26
8. Casting may be considered for symptoms not responding to other treatment modalities.	I	30
9. Iontophoresis has not been shown to be effective.	I	18, 31
10. Steroid injections may shorten the course but have not been shown to change long-term outcomes for plantar fasciitis.	B	32, 33
11. Botulinum toxin A injection may improve symptoms, but limited data are available.	I	34
12. Topical wheat-grass treatment is not effective.	I	63
13. Laser treatment is not effective.	I	64
14. Extracorporeal shock wave therapy has shown conflicting results, and its effectiveness has not been definitively shown.	I	41–46
15. Open or endoscopic fasciotomy may be indicated for patients who do not respond to conservative management.	C	49, 51, 53–57

REFERENCES

1. Riddle DL, Schappert SM: Volume of ambulatory care visits and patterns of care for patients diagnosed with plantar fasciitis: A national study of medical doctors. Foot Ankle Int 25:303–310, 2004.
2. Atkins D, Crawford F, Edwards J, et al: A systematic review of treatments for the painful heel. Rheumatology 38:968–973, 1999.
3. Crawford F, Atkins D, Edward J: Interventions for treating plantar heel pain (Cochrane Review). In Cochrane Library, Issue 3. Oxford, Update Software, 2000.
4. DeMaio M, Paine R, Mangine RE, et al: Plantar fasciitis. Orthopedics 16:1153–1163, 1993.
5. Moseley JB Jr, Chimenti BT: Foot and ankle injuries in the professional athlete. The Foot and Ankle in Sport. St. Louis, Mosby, 1995, pp 321–328.
6. Sadat-Ali M: Plantar fasciitis/calcaneal spur among security forces personnel. Mil Med 163:56–57, 1998.
7. Riddle DL, Pulisic M, Pidcoe P, et al: Risk factors for plantar fasciitis: A matched case control study. J Bone Joint Surg Am 85-A:872–887, 2003.
8. Cole C, Seto C, Gazewood J: Plantar fasciitis: Evidence-based review of diagnosis and therapy. Am Fam Physician 72:2237–2242, 2005.
9. Berkowitz JF, Kier R, Rudicel S: Plantar fasciitis: MR imaging. Radiology 179:665–667, 1991.
10. Kane D, Greaney T, Shanahan M, et al: The role of ultrasonography in the diagnosis and management of idiopathic plantar fasciitis. Rheumatology (Oxford) 40:1002–1008, 2001.
11. Buchbinder R: Clinical practice. Plantar fasciitis. N Engl J Med 350:2159–2166, 2004.
12. Gill L, Kiebzak G: Outcome of non-surgical treatment for plantar fasciitis. Foot Ankle 18:821–822, 1997.
13. Wolgin M, Cook C, Graham C, Mauldin D: Conservative treatment of plantar heel pain: Long term follow-up. Foot Ankle Int 15:97–102, 1994.
14. Hyland MR, Webber-Gaffney A, Cohen L, et al: Randomized controlled trial of calcaneal taping, sham taping, and plantar fascia stretching for the short-term management of plantar heel pain. J Orthop Sports Phys Ther 36:364–371, 2006.
15. DiGiovanni BF, Nawoczenski DA, Lintal ME, et al: Tissue-specific plantar fascia-stretching exercise enhances outcomes in patients with chronic heel pain. A prospective, randomized study. J Bone Joint Surg Am 85-A:1270–1277, 2003.
16. Digiovanni BF, Nawoczenski DA, Malay DP, et al: Plantar fascia-specific stretching exercise improves outcomes in patients with chronic plantar fasciitis. A prospective clinical trial with two-year follow-up. J Bone Joint Surg Am 88:1775–1781, 2006.
17. Radford JA, Landorf KB, Buchbinder R, et al: Effectiveness of low-Dye taping for the short-term treatment of plantar heel pain: A randomised trial. BMC Musculoskelet Disord 7:64, 2006.
18. Osborne HR, Allison GT: Treatment of plantar fasciitis by LowDye taping and iontophoresis: Short term results of a double blinded, randomised, placebo controlled clinical trial of dexamethasone and acetic acid. Br J Sports Med 40:545–549, 2006.
19. Donley BG, Moore T, Sferra J, et al: The efficacy of oral non-steroidal anti-inflammatory medication (NSAID) in the

treatment of plantar fasciitis: A randomized, prospective, placebo-controlled study. Foot Ankle Int 28:20–23, 2007.

20. Turlik MA, Donatelli TJ, Veremis MG: A comparison of shoe inserts in relieving mechanical heel pain. Foot 9:84–87, 1999.

21. Kogler GF, Solomonidis SE, Paul JP: Biomechanics of longitudinal arch support mechanisms in foot orthoses and their effect on plantar aponeurosis strain. Clin Biomech (Bristol, Avon) 11:243–252, 1996.

22. Landorf KB, Keenan A-M, Herbert RD: Effectiveness of foot orthoses to treat plantar fasciitis: A randomized trial. Arch Intern Med 166:1305–1310, 2006.

23. Pfeffer G, Bacchetti P, Deland J, et al: Comparison of custom and prefabricated orthoses in the initial treatment of proximal plantar fasciitis. Foot Ankle Int 20:214–221, 1999.

24. Martin JE, Hosch JC, Goforth WP, et al: Mechanical treatment of plantar fasciitis. A prospective study. J Am Podiatr Med Assoc 91:55–62, 2001.

25. Roos E, Engstrom M, Soderberg B: Foot orthoses for the treatment of plantar fasciitis. Foot Ankle Int 27:606–611, 2006.

26. Winemiller MH, Billow RG, Laskowski ER, et al: Effect of magnetic vs sham-magnetic insoles on plantar heel pain: A randomized controlled trial [erratum appears in JAMA. 2004 Jan 7;291(1):46]. JAMA 290:1474–1478, 2003.

27. Probe RA, Baca M, Adams R, et al: Night splint treatment for plantar fasciitis. A prospective randomized study. Clin Orthop Relat Res 190–195, 1999.

28. Roos E, Engstrom M, Soderberg B: Foot orthoses for the treatment of plantar fasciitis. Foot Ankle Int 27:606–611, 2006.

29. Powell M, Post WR, Keener J, et al: Effective treatment of chronic plantar fasciitis with dorsiflexion night splints: A crossover prospective randomized outcome study. Foot Ankle Int 19:10–18, 1998.

30. Tisdel CL, Harper MC: Chronic plantar heel pain: Treatment with a short leg walking cast. Foot Ankle Int 17:41–42, 1996.

31. Gudeman SD, Eisele SA, Heidt RS Jr, et al: Treatment of plantar fasciitis by iontophoresis of 0.4% dexamethasone. A randomized, double-blind, placebo-controlled study. Am J Sports Med 25:312–316, 1997.

32. Crawford F, Atkins D, Young P, et al: Steroid injection for heel pain: Evidence of short-term effectiveness. A randomized controlled trial. Rheumatology 38:974–977, 1999.

33. Porter MD, Shadbolt B: Intralesional corticosteroid injection versus extracorporeal shock wave therapy for plantar fasciopathy. Clin J Sport Med 15:119–124, 2005.

34. Babcock MS, Foster L, Pasquina P, et al: Treatment of pain attributed to plantar fasciitis with botulinum toxin A: A short-term, randomized, placebo-controlled, double-blind study. Am J Phys Med Rehabil 84:649–654, 2005.

35. Perez M, Weiner R, Gilley JC: Extracorporeal shockwave therapy for plantar fasciitis. Clin Podiatr Med Surg 20:323–334, 2003.

36. Haake M, Wessel C, Wilke A: [Effects of extracorporeal shockwaves (ESW) on human bone marrow cell cultures]. Biomed Tech (Berl) 44:278–282, 1999.

37. Plaisier PW, van der Hul RL, Terpstra OT, et al: Current role of extracorporeal shockwave therapy in surgery. Br J Surg 81:174–181, 1994.

38. Wilner JM, Strash WW: Extracorporeal shockwave therapy for plantar fasciitis and other musculoskeletal conditions utilizing the Ossatron—an update. Clin Podiatr Med Surg 21:441–447, 2004.

39. Trebinjac S, Muji-Skiki E, Ninkovi M, et al: Extracorporeal shock wave therapy in orthopaedic diseases. Bosn J Basic Med Sci 5:27–32, 200.

40. Thomson CE, Crawford F, Murray GD: The effectiveness of extra corporeal shock wave therapy for plantar heel pain: A systematic review and meta-analysis. BMC Musculoskelet Disord 6:19, 2005.

41. Buchbinder R, Ptasznik R, Gordon J, et al: Ultrasound-guided extracorporeal shock wave therapy for plantar fasciitis: A randomized controlled trial. JAMA 288:1364–1372, 2002.

42. Haake M, Buch M, Schoellner C, et al: Extracorporeal shock wave therapy for plantar fasciitis: Randomised controlled multicentre trial. BMJ 327:75, 2003.

43. Speed CA, Nichols D, Wies J, et al: Extracorporeal shock wave therapy for plantar fasciitis. A double blind randomised controlled trial. J Orthop Res 21:937–940, 2003.

44. Ogden JA, Alvarez R, Levitt R, et al: Shock wave therapy for chronic proximal plantar fasciitis. Clin Orthop Relat Res 47–59, 2001.

45. Rompe JD, Decking J, Schoellner C, et al: Shock wave application for chronic plantar fasciitis in running athletes. A prospective, randomized, placebo-controlled trial. Am J Sports Med 31:268–275, 2003.

46. Malay DS, Pressman MM, Assili A, et al: Extracorporeal shockwave therapy versus placebo for the treatment of chronic proximal plantar fasciitis: Results of a randomized, placebo-controlled, double-blinded, multicenter intervention trial. J Foot Ankle Surg 45:196–210, 2006.

47. Theodore GH, Buch M, Amendola A, et al: Extracorporeal shock wave therapy for the treatment of plantar fasciitis. Foot Ankle Int 25:290–297, 2004.

48. Schepsis AA, Leach RE, Gorzyca J: Plantar fasciitis. Etiology, treatment, surgical results, and review of the literature. Clin Orthop 266:185–196, 1991.

49. Davies MS, Weiss GA, Saxby TS: Plantar fasciitis: How successful is surgical intervention? Foot Ankle Int 20:803–807, 1999.

50. Allen BH, Fallat LM, Schwartz SM: Cryosurgery: An innovative technique for the treatment of plantar fasciitis. J Foot Ankle Surg 46:75–79, 2007.

51. Brugh AM, Fallat LM, Savoy-Moore RT: Lateral column symptomatology following plantar fascial release: A prospective study. J Foot Ankle Surg 41:365–371, 2002.

52. Woelffer KE, Figura MA, Sandberg NS, et al: Five-year follow-up results of instep plantar fasciotomy for chronic heel pain. J Foot Ankle Surg 39:218–223, 2000.

53. Brown JN, Roberts S, Taylor M, et al: Plantar fascia release through a transverse plantar incision. Foot Ankle Int 20:364–367, 1999.

54. Boyle RA, Slater GL: Endoscopic plantar fascia release: A case series. Foot Ankle Int 24:176–179, 2003.

55. Fishco WD, Goecker RM, Schwartz RI: The instep plantar fasciotomy for chronic plantar fasciitis. A retrospective review. J Am Podiatr Med Assoc 90:66–69, 2000.

56. Vohra PK, Giorgini RJ, Sobel E, et al: Long-term follow-up of heel spur surgery. A 10-year retrospective study. J Am Podiatr Med Assoc 89:81–88, 1999.

57. Saxena A: Uniportal endoscopic plantar fasciotomy: A prospective study on athletic patients. Foot Ankle Int 25:882–889, 2004.

58. Fishco WD, Goecker RM, Schwartz RI: The instep plantar fasciotomy for chronic plantar fasciitis. A retrospective review. J Am Podiatric Med Assoc 90:66–69, 1998.

59. Baxter DE, Pfeffer GB: Treatment of chronic heel pain by the surgical release of the first branch o the lateral plantar nerve. Clin Orthop 279:229–236, 1992.

60. Labib SA, Gould JS, Rodriguez-del-Rio FA, Lyman S: Heel pain triad (HPT): The combination of plantar fasciitis, posterior tibial tendon dysfunction and tarsal tunnel syndrome. Foot Ankle Int 23:212–220, 2002.

61. Barrett SL, Day SV, Pignetti TT, et al: Endoscopic planter fasciotomy: A multi-surgeon prospective analysis of 652 cases. J Foot Ankle Surg 34:400–407, 1995.

62. Tomczak RL, Haverstock BD: A retrospective comparison of endoscopic plantar fasciotomy to open plantar fasciotomy with heel spur resection for chronic plantar fasciitis/heel spur surgery. J Foot Surg 34:305–311, 1995.

63. Young MA, Cook JL, Webster KE: The effect of topical wheatgrass cream on chronic plantar fasciitis: A randomized, double-blind, placebo-controlled trial. Complement Ther Med 14:3–9, 2006.

64. Basford JR, Malanga GA, Krause DA, et al: A randomized controlled evaluation of low-intensity laser therapy: Plantar fasciitis. Arch Phys Med Rehabil 79:249–254, 1998.

65. Batt ME, Tanji JL, Skattum N: Plantar fasciitis: A prospective randomized clinical trial of the tension night splint. Clin J Sport Med 6:158–162, 1996.

66. Kudo P, Dainty K, Clarfield M, et al.: Randomized, placebo-controlled, double-blind clinical trial evaluating the treatment of plantar fasciitis with an extracoporeal shockwave therapy (ESWT) device: a North American confirmatory study. J Orthop Res 24(2):115–123, 2006.

Chapter 68

What Is the Best Treatment for Posterior Tibial Tendonitis?

Praveen Yalamanchili, MD, Stephen Pinney, MD, FRCSC, and Sheldon S. Lin, MD

Posterior tibial tendonitis, also known as posterior tibial tendon dysfunction (PTTD), is a well-recognized clinical entity that encompasses a spectrum of disease ranging from inflammation to frank insufficiency and rupture of the tendon. Dysfunction of the posterior tibial tendon (PTT) has been found to be the leading cause of a flatfoot deformity[1] and can cause significant impairment of the affected extremity.[2] The diagnosis of PTT dysfunction is often delayed or missed. Increased awareness and knowledge of the presentation of this disease entity can help improve rates of diagnosis. The treatment of PTTD is an evolving area with several potential treatment options. Although both surgical and nonsurgical options have been investigated, controversy still exists regarding the ideal treatment for PTTD. This chapter aims to simplify some of the debate surrounding this topic.

STAGING

PTT dysfunction is classically divided into three clinical stages corresponding to the progression of the disease and used to guide treatment.[3,4] This classification system was modified to include a fourth stage by Myerson.[5] Stage I is characterized by mild swelling and medial ankle pain but no deformity when compared with the unaffected side. The patient retains the ability to single-leg heel rise. Stage II is characterized by progressive flattening of the arch, with a flexible valgus heel deformity. In this stage, the patient is unable to perform single-leg heel rise or invert against resistance. Stage III includes the signs of stage II, but the hindfoot deformity is fixed in valgus with forefoot abduction. Degenerative changes of the midfoot and subtalar joint are also present on radiographs. Stage IV is characterized by valgus tilt of the talus in the ankle mortise leading to lateral tibiotalar degeneration.

STAGE I

Nonoperative Therapy

Nonoperative therapy (Table 68–1) is an appropriate initial intervention in almost all cases of PTTD. The goals of treatment are pain relief and the return of PTT function when possible. In a flexible deformity, the aim is to control the progressive valgus deformity of the

hindfoot. In a rigid deformity, the goal is to support the position of the foot in situ with a brace that accommodates the bony deformities. In addition, symptomatic relief can be addressed with the use of nonsteroidal anti-inflammatory drugs, activity modification, and encouraging weight loss.

Few studies exist on the nonoperative treatment of PTT dysfunction, but it is believed that a well-fitted, custom-molded orthosis can be effective at relieving symptoms, and can delay and sometimes prevent surgical intervention[6] (Level of Evidence V). Chao and colleagues[7] performed a study of 49 patients with the diagnosis of PTTD treated with either a molded ankle-foot orthosis (AFO) or University of California Biomechanics Laboratory (UCBL) brace with medial posting (Level IV). Nonobese patients with flexible deformities and less than 10-degree residual forefoot varus with the heel in a neutral position received the UCBL brace. The remaining patients received the molded AFO. In total, 40 feet were treated with a molded AFO, and 13 were treated with a UCBL brace. Patients were divided into three groups based on a functional scoring system, and 67% of patients were found to have excellent to good results. Unfortunately, this study cannot be used to make a comparison between different disease stages because of the nonuniformity of treatment.

Augustin and coworkers[6] studied the nonoperative treatment of various stages of PTTD with an Arizona AFO brace, a custom-molded leather and polypropylene orthosis (Level IV). Twenty-one patients with PTTD were evaluated just before brace use and after a minimum of 3 months of use using questionnaires and clinical examination. American Orthopaedic Foot and Ankle Society (AOFAS) Hindfoot Scores, Foot Function Index scores, and 36-Item Short Form Health Survey (SF-36) scores all increased significantly except for the change in health perception area of the SF-36. Six of six patients with stage I PTTD showed improvement attributable to the brace. The authors suggest that the Arizona AFO brace is effective at relieving symptoms and either obviating or delaying any surgical intervention, especially in earlier stages. Further studies are needed to determine whether an orthosis can prevent disease progression together with providing symptomatic relief.

Alvarez and coauthors[8] studied the treatment of stage I and II PTTD in 47 patients with a nonoperative management protocol consisting of physical therapy,

TABLE 68–1. Nonoperative Treatment Levels of Evidence

AUTHOR	LEVEL OF EVIDENCE	TREATMENT	OUTCOME
Chao et al.[7]	IV	UCBL	33 of 49 (67%) of patients were found to have excellent to good results; 4 patients required surgery
Augustin et al.[6]	IV	Arizona AFO	18 of 20 (90%) patients demonstrated a statistically significant improvement of symptoms; 1 patient required surgery
Alvarez et al.[8]	IV	Physical therapy, Home exercise program, orthosis	39 of 47 (83%) patients had successful subjective and functional outcomes; 42 (89%) patients were satisfied; 5 patients required surgery

AFO, ankle-foot orthosis; UCBL, University of California Biomechanics Laboratory.

an aggressive home exercise program, and an orthosis (Level IV). Over a 4-month period, 39 (83%) patients had successful subjective and functional outcomes, and 42 (89%) patients were satisfied, with 5 (11%) patients requiring surgery.

Operative Treatment

A variety of surgical options exists for patients who do not respond to a trial of conservative treatment. The principal of operative treatment is to perform the least invasive procedure that will decrease pain and improve function.[9] For stage I PTTD exploration and debridement of the PTT and soft tissue is often a recommended option. (Table 68–2). All tenosynovial tissue should be excised, with debridement of degenerated tendon areas and repair of any tears. Crates and Richardson[10] report on a series of seven patients with stage I PTT dysfunction who were treated with debridement after failure of conservative treatment (Level IV). Six of the seven patients were pain free at 11-month follow-up examination. In Teasdall and Johnson's study,[11] 14 of 19 patients had complete relief of pain after a synovectomy and debridement for stage I PTTD (Level IV). Sixteen patients had a return of function of the PTT as evidenced by the ability to perform a single-limb heel-rise test. Significant pathology within the substance of the tendon may require aggressive resection followed by flexor digitorum

longus (FDL) transfer and Achilles lengthening to augment the PTT.

STAGE II

Nonoperative Treatment

Initially, stage II PTTD is treated similarly to stage I, but there are a few studies for nonoperative treatment of more advanced PTTD. Because the foot is flexible, corrective orthoses are utilized to prevent or correct deformity and control pain.[12] Alvarez and coauthors[8] showed improvement in functional and subjective outcomes in patients with stage II PTTD with physical therapy, an aggressive home exercise program, and an orthosis (Level IV). If corrective orthoses are unable to correct the deformity, a medial posted UCBL device, as suggested by Chao and colleagues,[7] may be used. Augustin and coworkers[6] showed that all 12 patients using an Arizona brace showed pain relief referable to the brace and improvement in multiple clinical measurement instruments. If the deformity is severe, an AFO may be needed.[7] As in stage I, stage II is given a 3- to 6-month trial before advocating surgical intervention.

Operative Treatment

A variety of options exists for the operative treatment of stage II PTT dysfunction. An FDL transfer is an accepted option,[13] but isolated FDL transfer has failed to demonstrate long-term durability despite short-term success.[14] A bony procedure will oftentimes be necessary to supplement the FDL transfer to improve its longevity. Bony procedures can be divided by position and include medial osteotomy, lateral column lengthening, or a combined procedure.

Medial Osteotomy with Flexor Digitorum Longus Transfer

A medial calcaneal slide osteotomy and FDL tendon transfer is one surgical option that has been shown to provide acceptable results for stage II disease (Table 68–3).[15] Myerson and researchers[16] performed a radiographic analysis of 18 patients 12 to 26 months after such a procedure (Level IV). They found improved radiographic values of the talar-first metatarsal angle and the distance from the medial cuneiform to the floor, concluding that the procedure may offset the weakness of isolated FDL transfer. Myerson and researchers[16] also found high patient satisfaction and functional improvement in 32 patients treated with this procedure for stage II disease at a mean of 20 months after surgery (Level IV).[5] Guyton and coworkers[17] performed a review of 26 patients who underwent the procedure at a mean of 32 months follow-up (Level IV). All patients except three were able to perform a single-leg toe raise, which none could perform before surgery. Pain relief was rated as excellent by 75% of patients. Patients felt a prolonged period of steady

TABLE 68–2. Debridement Levels of Evidence

AUTHOR	LEVEL OF EVIDENCE	TREATMENT	OUTCOME
Crates and Richardson[10]	IV	Debridement	6 of 7 patients with type I pain free at 11 months
Teasdall and Johnson[11]	IV	Debridement	14 of 19 patients with type I had complete relief of pain

TABLE 68–3. Medial Osteotomy

AUTHOR	LEVEL OF EVIDENCE	TREATMENT	OUTCOME
Myerson et al.[16]	IV	Medial calcaneal slide osteotomy with FDL tendon transfer	Patients showed improvement in multiple radiographic values after surgery
Myerson and Corrigan[5]	IV	Medial calcaneal slide osteotomy with FDL tendon transfer	30 of 32 (94%) of patients were satisfied with the outcome of surgery, had improved function, and exhibited radiographic correction of the foot deformity
Guyton et al.[17]	IV	Medial displacement calcaneal osteotomy with FDL tendon transfer	23 of 26 (88%) patients could perform single-leg toe raise at follow-up and felt function was markedly improved; 75% of patients reported excellent pain relief
Rosenfeld et al.[18]	II	Medial displacement calcaneal osteotomy with FDL tendon transfer either retaining or excising the PTT	No difference in clinical outcome based on excision or retention of PTT
Sammarco and Hockenbury[20]	IV	Medial displacement calcaneal osteotomy with FHL tendon transfer	No statistically significant improvement of the medial longitudinal arch but high patient satisfaction rate

FDL, flexor digitorum longus; FHL, flexor hallucal longus; PTT, posterior tibial tendon.

improvement in symptoms and function over time. Radiographic improvement in the alignment of the foot was noted but did not correlate to self-reported improvement in appearance. These early clinical studies suggest that FDL transfer and medial displacement calcaneal osteotomy provide good functional outcome and symptomatic relief.

The decision to remove or retain the PTT when performing a FDL tendon transfer and medial displacement calcaneal osteotomy has been examined. Rosenfeld and investigators[18] performed a prospective study randomizing 12 patients into 2 groups depending on excision or retention of the PTT, and assessed muscle volume and AOFAS scores at 1-year follow-up (Level II). Though the intact tendon group lost posterior tibial muscle volume, all of the posterior tibial muscles in the excised tendon group were replaced by fatty infiltration. The FDL muscle hypertrophied to a greater extent in the excised tendon group, but there was no difference in AOFAS scores between the two groups after surgery. The authors conclude that the FDL undergoes greater hypertrophy and the posterior tibia undergoes fatty infiltration with excision of the PTT, but this does not affect clinical outcome.

Medial Osteotomy with Flexor Hallucal Longus Transfer

Commonly, the FDL tendon has been used in tendon transfer for PTT dysfunction, but this choice has been questioned. The FDL is only 28% of the relative strength of PTT and only 69% of the strength of the antagonistic peroneal brevis (PB). The flexor hallucis longus (FHL) has 50% of the relative strength of the PTT and exceeds the strength of the PB.[19] Sammarco and Hockenbury[20] hypothesize that using a stronger muscle would lead to a greater arch correction (Level IV). They retrospectively analyzed a series of 19 patients undergoing an FHL tendon transfer and medial calcaneal osteotomy for stage 2 PTTD. The clinical outcomes using this technique were comparable with those observed in a series of FDL tendon transfer and calcaneal osteotomy, and no improvement was shown in radiographic appearance of the medial longitudinal arch. Despite the new interest in FHL transfer procedures, short-term results have failed to reveal superiority of the FHL to FDL transfer with calcaneal osteotomy. In addition, the FHL tendon requires a more complicated dissection, which places the neurovascular bundle under greater risk.

Lateral Osteotomy

Another option for stage II dysfunction is lateral column lengthening in conjunction with a tendon transfer (Table 68–4). The lengthening can be performed using an osteotomy of the neck of the calcaneus and interposing bone graft or through the calcaneocuboid (CC) joint itself. A version of the procedure by Evans recommends the osteotomy be done 1.5 cm proximal to the CC joint. Sangeorzan and researchers[21] studied the effect of Evans-type calcaneal lengthening on relations among the hindfoot, midfoot, and forefoot in seven patients who underwent the procedure for symptomatic pes planus (Level IV). The authors note an improvement in the flatfoot deformity. Kitaoka and investigators[22] performed a study using a dynamic flatfoot deformity model of nine fresh-frozen foot specimens to investigate their mechanical behavior after CC distraction arthrodesis. Three-dimensional tarsal bone positions were determined using a magnetic tracking system. Arch alignment in simulated toe-off phase of gait was found to be improved significantly but was not reduced anatomically.

No consensus has been reached on the ideal method of lateral column lengthening. Thomas and colleagues[23] analyzed 27 feet treated with lateral column lengthening for painful pes planus at 1-year follow-up examination (Level III). Ten feet underwent Evans-type open-wedge osteotomy with tricortical iliac crest graft, and 17 feet underwent CC distraction arthrodesis. Both groups underwent debridement of PTT with FDL transfer. Radiographic results documented marked improvement in all parameters, with no statistically significant difference between the two groups. Postoperative AOFAS rating score also did not show a statistically significant difference. Twenty of 25 patients in both groups were satisfied, and 96% stated they would have the same surgery again. Of note was a high rate of complications for both groups, specifically the rate of nonunion or delayed union in the CC distraction arthrodesis group. The authors conclude that both procedures offered marked improvement in radiographic parameters and AOFAS score, but both were also associated with a high rate of complications.

Particular concern regarding arthritis of the CC joint with Evans-type procedure has led several authors to recommended abandoning the procedure. The literature, however, is conflicting. A cadaver study demonstrated increased CC joint pressures after an Evans osteotomy with wedge graft.[24] In a study from 1983, Phillips and coauthors[25] report degenerative changes in CC joint in 6 of the 23 feet (Level IV). A more recent study by Hintermann and coworkers[26] reviewed 19 patients who underwent lateral column lengthening by calcaneal osteotomy in conjunction with medial soft-tissue procedures (Level IV). At an average follow-up of 23 months, 2 patients had radiographic signs of CC degeneration, and all 19 patients had satisfactory restoration of the medial arch height. One patient required arthrodesis of the CC joint after 5 months because of painful degenerative joint disease. In addition, Momberger and coworkers[27] examined the change in pressure across the CC joint after an Evans-type calcaneal osteotomy using a cadaveric adult flatfoot model. Joint pressures were compared among the normal foot, the created flatfoot, and the corrected flatfoot. Peak pressure across the joint increased significantly from the normal to the created flatfoot but did not change significantly from the flatfoot to the corrected flatfoot model. In some cases, the peak pressure in the flatfoot decreased with correction. These findings led the authors to conclude

TABLE 68–4. Lateral Osteotomy

AUTHOR	LEVEL OF EVIDENCE	TREATMENT	OUTCOME
Sangeorzan et al.[21]	IV	Evans-type calcaneal lengthening	Improvement in flatfoot deformity measured using weight-bearing radiographs
Thomas et al.[23]	III	FDL tendon transfer, PTT debridement with either Evans-type calcaneal lengthening or CC distraction arthrodesis	Improvement in radiographic parameters in both groups; no statistically significant difference in AOFAS score between groups; 20 of 25 (80%) total patients were satisfied; high rates of complications in both groups
Phillips et al.[25]	IV	Evans-type calcaneal lengthening	6 of 23 (26%) patients had degenerative changes at CC joint at long-term follow-up, with the remainder having good or good results
Hintermann et al.[26]	IV	Evans-type calcaneal lengthening and medial soft-tissue procedures	19 of 19 (100%) of patients had satisfactory restoration of their medial longitudinal arch, reduction of abduction in the forefoot, and restored height in the arch; one patient had to undergo arthrodesis of the calcaneocuboid joint after 5 months because of painful degenerative joint disease

AOFAS, American Orthopaedic Foot and Ankle Society; CC, calcaneocuboid; FDL, flexor digitorum longus; PTT, posterior tibial tendon.

TABLE 68–5. Combined Medial and Lateral Osteotomies

AUTHOR	LEVEL OF EVIDENCE	TREATMENT	OUTCOME
Pomeroy and Manoli[28]	IV	FDL tendon transfer, lateral column lengthening, medial displacement calcaneal osteotomy and heel-cord lengthening	Improved AOFAS score; statistically significant correction of the pes planovalgus deformity on radiographic measurements
Moseir-LaClair et al.[29]	IV	FDL tendon transfer, lateral column lengthening, medial displacement calcaneal osteotomy, and heel-cord lengthening	Improvement in radiographic parameters and AOFAS score

AOFAS, American Orthopaedic Foot and Ankle Society; FDL, flexor digitorum longus.

that the Evans-type osteotomy does not increase pressure across the CC joint. The literature provides an inconclusive picture of the superior method and precludes abandonment of the Evans-type osteotomy.

Combined Medial and Lateral Osteotomies

A technique of combining medial displacement calcaneal osteotomy, lateral column lengthening, FDL transfer, and heel cord lengthening has gained interest (Table 68–5). Pomeroy and Manoli[28] performed this procedure in 20 cases of stage II PTT dysfunction, and analyzed the patients radiographically and with the AOFAS scale at an average follow-up of 17.5 months (Level IV). The average foot rating improved from 51.4 to 82.8, and radiographic measurements demonstrated statistically significant correction of the pes planovalgus deformity. Moseir-LaClair and researchers[29] analyzed the effect of a similar procedure in 26 patients with 28 stage II feet at a mean follow-up of 5 years (Level IV). The AOFAS score was high after surgery, and there was radiographic improvement of the deformity. Four patients (14%) demonstrated signs of CC arthrosis, but the authors contend that half of these patients had preexisting CC joint arthritis. The authors of both studies suggest that the double osteotomy technique provides symptomatic relief and acceptable correction of pes planovalgus deformity associated with stage 2 PTTD.

Subtalar Fusion

Another proposed operative procedure for stage II PTTD consists of subtalar fusion in conjunction with soft-tissue rebalancing (Table 68–6). Johnson and investigators[30] performed a retrospective review of 17 feet with stage II PTT dysfunction treated with subtalar arthrodesis combined with spring ligament repair/reefing and FDL transfer at an average follow-up period of 27 months (Level IV). All patients had successful subtalar joint fusion with an average time to radiographic union of 10.1 weeks. Standing radiographic analysis demon-

strated an improvement in the anteroposterior talo-first metatarsal angle, the talonavicular coverage angle, and the medial cuneiform distance to the floor. These early results suggest that FDL transfer with medial soft-tissue reconstruction and subtalar fusion have comparable results with other extra-articular sparing procedures. The authors suggest that this procedure can be an effective and reliable alternative procedure in the treatment of stage II PTT dysfunction.

STAGES III AND IV

Nonoperative Treatment

In stage III and IV, the foot is rigid, and the goal is to provide support, reduce pain, and prevent further progression. Augustin and coworkers[6] showed that three of five patients with stage III PTTD had relief of symptoms referable to the use of an Arizona brace. The foot may be braced in situ with a custom-molded orthosis. Although a solid AFO may sometimes prove useful, often an articulated device is better tolerated. In stage IV disease, a solid device is usually required because orthoses usually provide little control of the deformity.[31] With the use of braces, particular care must be taken to avoid skin ulceration, which can be caused by the rigidity of the deformity. Although various conservative modalities have been described, advanced PTTD is difficult to manage without surgery.[31]

TABLE 68–6. Subtalar Arthrodesis Levels of Evidence

AUTHOR	LEVEL OF EVIDENCE	TREATMENT	OUTCOME
Johnson et al.[30]	IV	Subtalar arthrodesis combined with spring ligament repair/ reefing and flexor digitorum longus transfer to the navicular	17 of 17 (100%) feet had successful fusion; overall improvement in radiographic parameters and questionnaire scores

Operative Treatment

The standard treatment for stage III PTTD remains arthrodesis, although there is debate over the extent of fusion (Table 68–7). Traditionally, the gold standard for treatment of stage III PTTD has been triple arthrodesis[32,33] (Level V). Multiple studies have shown satisfactory results with this procedure, although there is the long-term risk for adjacent ankle arthritis.[34,35] Fortin and Walling[36] studied 32 patients who underwent triple arthrodesis for advanced PTTD and found that Foot and Ankle Society Hindfoot scores improved an average of 36 points with high patient satisfaction (Level IV). Jarde and colleagues[35] performed a retrospective review of 20 cases of flatfoot deformity secondary to PTTD and found good to excellent results in 70%, although follow-up radiographs showed progression of osteoarthritis (Level IV). The fusion technique should be meticulous and preceded with an anatomic reduction because an in situ fusion carries the risk for future arthrosis at the adjacent joints.[14] Isolated subtalar fusion has been suggested as an alternative in selected groups, but data are limited and it requires further study.[37]

Stage IV dysfunction is a rare anatomic condition with no specific gold standard. Described treatment modalities include tibiotalocalcaneal arthrodesis or pan-talar fusion, although few reports with these techniques in patients with PTTD have been published.[31,38] Experience with these procedures in other patient populations, such as arthritic or post-traumatic conditions, has shown that they are viable salvage procedures when there is disease involving both the subtalar and tibiotalar compartments.[39,40]

TABLE 68–7. Triple Arthrodesis Level of Evidence

AUTHOR	LEVEL OF EVIDENCE	TREATMENT	OUTCOME
Fortin and Walling[36]	IV	Triple arthrodesis	32 feet underwent triple arthrodesis for advanced PTTD and were evaluated at an average of 4.3 years; postoperative AOFAS scores improved an average of 36 points
Jarde et al.[35]	IV	Triple arthrodesis	70% of 20 cases of valgus flatfoot deformity secondary to PTTD treated with triple arthrodesis reported good to excellent results

AOFAS, American Orthopaedic Foot and Ankle Society; PTTD, posterior tibial tendon dysfunction.

SUMMARY

The PTT is a vital component of the lower extremity, and its dysfunction can lead to significant deformity and pain. PTT dysfunction is a clinical diagnosis in which the physical examination can help differentiate the disease into its various stages, depending on the presence and flexibility of deformity. Nearly all cases initially can be managed without surgery, but progression of disease or continuing pain will many times necessitate a surgical intervention. A variety of surgical procedures exists for the treatment of PTT dysfunction, and often there is no definitive standard of treatment. Both the conservative and surgical options are evolving areas with ample opportunity for future research. (Table 68–8).

TABLE 68–8. Summary of Recommendations

RECOMMENDATIONS	STAGE	LEVEL OF EVIDENCE/GRADE OF RECOMMENDATION
Activity modification, anti-inflammatories, immobilization alone	I	C
Orthosis		C
Surgical exploration with soft tissue debridement		C
AFO/UCBL	II	C
Medial osteotomy with FDL/FHL transfer		C
Lateral lengthening with FDL transfer		C
Combined procedures		C
Subtalar arthrodesis with soft-tissue procedures		C
Custom-molded orthosis	III	C
Triple arthrodesis		C
Custom-molded orthosis	IV	I
Tibiocalcaneal arthrodesis		C

AFO, ankle-foot orthosis; FDL, flexor digitorum longus; FHL, flexor hallucal longus; UCBL, University of California Biomechanics Laboratory.

REFERENCES

1. Geideman WM, Johnson JE: Posterior tibial tendon dysfunction. J Orthop Sports Phys Ther 30:68–77, 2000.
2. Mann RA: Acquired flatfoot in adults. Clin Orthop Relat Res (181):46–51, 1983.
3. Johnson KA, Strom DE: Tibialis posterior tendon dysfunction. Clin Orthop Relat Res (239):196–206, 1989.
4. Beals TC, Pomeroy GC, Manoli A 2nd: Posterior tendon insufficiency: Diagnosis and treatment. J Am Acad Orthop Surg 7:112–118, 1999.
5. Myerson MS, Corrigan J: Treatment of posterior tibial tendon dysfunction with flexor digitorum longus tendon transfer and calcaneal osteotomy. Orthopedics 19:383–388, 1996.
6. Augustin JF, et al: Nonoperative treatment of adult acquired flat foot with the Arizona brace. Foot Ankle Clin 8:491–502, 2003.
7. Chao W, et al: Nonoperative management of posterior tibial tendon dysfunction. Foot Ankle Int 17:736–741, 1996.
8. Alvarez RG, et al: Stage I and II posterior tibial tendon dysfunction treated by a structured nonoperative management

protocol: an orthosis and exercise program. Foot Ankle Int 27:2–8, 2006.

9. Myerson MS: Adult acquired flatfoot deformity: Treatment of dysfunction of the posterior tibial tendon. Instr Course Lect 46:393–405, 1997.

10. Crates JM, Richardson EG: Treatment of stage I posterior tibial tendon dysfunction with medial soft tissue procedures. Clin Orthop Relat Res (365):46–49, 1999.

11. Teasdall RD, Johnson KA: Surgical treatment of stage I posterior tibial tendon dysfunction. Foot Ankle Int 15:646–648, 1994.

12. Wapner KL, Chao W: Nonoperative treatment of posterior tibial tendon dysfunction. Clin Orthop Relat Res (365):39–45, 1999.

13. Funk DA, Cass JR, Johnson KA: Acquired adult flat foot secondary to posterior tibial-tendon pathology. J Bone Joint Surg Am 68:95–102, 1986.

14. Early J: Issues relating to failure in the treatment of posterior tibial tendon dysfunction. Foot Ankle Clin 8:637–645, 2003.

15. Hockenbury RT, Sammarco GJ: Medial sliding calcaneal osteotomy with flexor hallucis longus transfer for the treatment of posterior tibial tendon insufficiency. Foot Ankle Clin 6:569–581, 2001.

16. Myerson MS, et al: Tendon transfer combined with calcaneal osteotomy for treatment of posterior tibial tendon insufficiency: A radiological investigation. Foot Ankle Int 16:712–718, 1995.

17. Guyton GP, et al: Flexor digitorum longus transfer and medial displacement calcaneal osteotomy for posterior tibial tendon dysfunction: A middle-term clinical follow-up. Foot Ankle Int 22:627–632, 2001.

18. Rosenfeld PF, Dick J, Saxby TS: The response of the flexor digitorum longus and posterior tibial muscles to tendon transfer and calcaneal osteotomy for stage II posterior tibial tendon dysfunction. Foot Ankle Int 26:671–674, 2005.

19. Silver RL, de la Garza J, Rang M: The myth of muscle balance. A study of relative strengths and excursions of normal muscles about the foot and ankle. J Bone Joint Surg Br 67:432–437, 1985.

20. Sammarco GJ, Hockenbury RT: Treatment of stage II posterior tibial tendon dysfunction with flexor hallucis longus transfer and medial displacement calcaneal osteotomy. Foot Ankle Int 22:305–312, 2001.

21. Sangeorzan BJ, Mosca V, Hansen ST Jr: Effect of calcaneal lengthening on relationships among the hindfoot, midfoot, and forefoot. Foot Ankle 14:136–141, 1993.

22. Kitaoka HB, et al: Calcaneocuboid distraction arthrodesis for posterior tibial tendon dysfunction and flatfoot: A cadaveric study. Clin Orthop Relat Res (381):241–247, 2000.

23. Thomas RL, et al: Preliminary results comparing two methods of lateral column lengthening. Foot Ankle Int 22:107–119, 2001.

24. Cooper PS, Nowak MD, Shaer J: Calcaneocuboid joint pressures with lateral column lengthening (Evans) procedure. Foot Ankle Int 18:199–205, 1997.

25. Phillips GE: A review of elongation of os calcis for flat feet. J Bone Joint Surg Br 65:15–18, 1983.

26. Hintermann B, Valderrabano V, Kundert HP: Lengthening of the lateral column and reconstruction of the medial soft tissue for treatment of acquired flatfoot deformity associated with insufficiency of the posterior tibial tendon. Foot Ankle Int 20:622–629, 1999.

27. Momberger N, et al: Calcaneocuboid joint pressure after lateral column lengthening in a cadaveric planovalgus deformity model. Foot Ankle Int 21:730–735, 2000.

28. Pomeroy GC, Manoli A 2nd: A new operative approach for flatfoot secondary to posterior tibial tendon insufficiency: a preliminary report. Foot Ankle Int 18:206–212, 1997.

29. Moseir-LaClair S, Pomeroy G, Manoli A 2nd: Intermediate follow-up on the double osteotomy and tendon transfer procedure for stage II posterior tibial tendon insufficiency. Foot Ankle Int 22:283–291, 2001.

30. Johnson JE, et al: Subtalar arthrodesis with flexor digitorum longus transfer and spring ligament repair for treatment of posterior tibial tendon insufficiency. Foot Ankle Int 21:722–729, 2000.

31. Bohay DR, Anderson JG: Stage IV posterior tibial tendon insufficiency: The tilted ankle. Foot Ankle Clin 8:619–636, 2003.

32. Kelly IP, Easley ME: Treatment of stage 3 adult acquired flatfoot. Foot Ankle Clin 6:153–166, 2001.

33. Maskill MP, et al: Triple arthrodesis for the adult-acquired flatfoot deformity. Clin Podiatr Med Surg 24:765–778, 2007.

34. Graves SC, Mann RA, Graves KO: Triple arthrodesis in older adults. Results after long-term follow-up. J Bone Joint Surg Am 75:355–362, 1993.

35. Jarde O, et al: [Triple arthrodesis in the management of acquired flatfoot deformity in the adult secondary to posterior tibial tendon dysfunction. A retrospective study of 20 cases]. Acta Orthop Belg 68:56–62, 2002.

36. Fortin PT, Walling AK: Triple arthrodesis. Clin Orthop Relat Res (365):91–99, 1999.

37. Laughlin TJ, Payette CR: Triple arthrodesis and subtalar joint arthrodesis. For the treatment of end-stage posterior tibial tendon dysfunction. Clin Podiatr Med Surg 16:527–555, 1999.

38. Kelly IP, Nunley JA: Treatment of stage 4 adult acquired flatfoot. Foot Ankle Clin 6:167–178, 2001.

39. Chou LB, et al: Tibiotalocalcaneal arthrodesis. Foot Ankle Int 21:804–808, 2000.

40. Papa JA, Myerson MS: Pantalar and tibiotalocalcaneal arthrodesis for post-traumatic osteoarthrosis of the ankle and hindfoot. J Bone Joint Surg Am 74:1042–1049, 1992.

What Is the Best Treatment for Achilles Tendon Rupture?

Mark Glazebrook, MSc, PhD, MD, FRCS(C)

Achilles tendon ruptures (Fig. 69–1) are a catastrophic event that occurs when forces that are placed on the Achilles tendon exceed its tensile limits (approximately strain >8%).[1] This event is likely a result of a preexisting Achilles tendon disease[2-4] if the forces are relatively low. The histopathology of the diseased human Achilles tendon has been previously described on the basis of biopsies from the Achilles tendons of patients with subcutaneous rupture[3,5-9] and chronic, localized Achilles tendon symptoms.[6,10,11] These studies suggest that a common pathologic process may predispose individuals to rupture.[3,6]

The most common patient profile for human Achilles tendon rupture would be that of a man in his third or fourth decade of life who plays sports occasionally. Men-to-women rupture ratios have been reported from 2:1 to 12:1.[2,4,12] The mean age has been estimated between the 30s and 40s,[13] with the left Achilles rupture more common than the right probably reflecting right-side dominance with left leg pushing off.[14] Leppilahti and colleagues[13] report on an increasing incidence of rupture in 1994 in Oulu, Finland, to be 18 per 100,000, whereas Suchak and coworkers[15] report the incidence to be between 5.5 and 9.9 ruptures per 100,000 in North America. Subjects have been participating in sports during rupture at rates from 44.4% to 83%,[16,17] with 52.3% of ruptures playing badminton. The site of rupture has been reported to occur in the myotendinous junction in 12.1%, the insertion in 4.6%, and 3.5 cm proximal to the insertion in 83% of patients.[4]

The intention of this chapter is to provide the best evidence available for the treatment of Achilles tendon ruptures. It is divided into four sections including operative versus nonoperative treatment, percutaneous versus open operative treatment, and postoperative functional rehabilitation. Final treatment recommendations are based on the literature presented combined with clinical experience of overall patient care needs.

TREATMENT

Level I and II evidence evaluating operative and nonoperative treatment of Achilles tendon rupture are based on healthy patients. The surgical approaches of open repair and percutaneous repair are consistent. However, the specific surgical technique for open and percutaneous repairs may vary by suture technique and suture material. The variation in suture technique and material is not believed to be clinically significant because the strength of the repair is equivalent.

Operative versus Nonoperative Treatment

In an attempt to gather the best evidence available to guide treatment recommendations for Achilles tendon rupture, a literature search was performed using the search terms "Achilles," "tendon," "rupture," "treatment," "operative," and "nonoperative." Literature was then screened for Level I and II evidence comparing operative and nonoperative treatments of Achilles tendon ruptures. The search was narrowed to six studies (Table 69–1).

Three of the studies meet the criteria for Level 1 original evidence articles including randomized, control trials (RCT) by Cetti and investigators,[16] Moller and researchers,[21] and Nistor.[22] Cetti and investigators[16] randomized 111 healthy subjects, of which 90% were reported to regularly participate in sports, to operative repair ($n = 56$) or nonoperative treatment ($n = 55$) of their ruptured Achilles tendons. This study cites a rerupture rate of 5.4% and 14.5% for operative and nonoperative cohorts, respectively. The deep infection rate was 3.6% and 0% in favor of the nonoperative cohort. Furthermore, many complications rates were cited to be lower in the nonoperative group, as was the return to sport rate.

In the second Level I study, Moller and researchers[21] cite similar results with a rupture rate of 1.7% versus 20.8% in the operative and nonoperative cohorts, respectfully. This study also cites decreased complications with a slower return to work time in the patients treated without surgery. The patients in both cohorts had similar demographic characteristics and were healthy, reporting a high level (70–80%) of regular participation in sports.

In the third Level I original evidence article, Nistor[22] randomized 115 patients of similar health demographic characteristics to operative repair or nonoperative treatment of their ruptured Achilles tendon. Results reported included a 3% rerupture rate for both operative and nonoperative treatments, whereas the infection rate was 4.4% and 0% favoring nonoperative treatment. The minor complication rate was much greater (68.8% vs. 0%) in the nonoperative group.

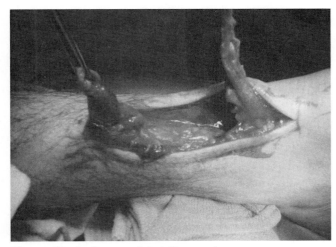

Figure 69–1. Ruptured Achilles tendon.

The final three studies reviewed included Level I meta-analysis studies by Bhandari and colleagues[23] and Khan and coauthors,[24] and a Level II quantitative review of the literature by Wong and coauthors.[25] The most recent study by Khan combined the results of four studies,[16,21,22,26] which included 356 patients. The cumulative rerupture rate was greater (12.6% vs. 4.6%) in the nonoperative group, but the infection (4.0% vs. 0%) and minor complication rates (33.5% vs. 2.7%) were lower.

In Bhandari and colleagues'[23] Level I meta-analysis study, six original articles were identified to meet all eligibility criteria.[16,21,22,27–29] The cumulative rerupture rate was greater in the nonoperative group (13% vs. 3.1%; $n = 448$; $P = 0.005$), but the infection rate was lower (0% vs. 4.7%; $n = 421$; $P = 0.03$). No difference was cited in the return to function and the spontaneous complaints cumulative data.

Finally, Wong and coauthors'[25] quantitative review of the literature pooled data gathered from 125 articles including 5370 patients. This study identifies no difference in the rerupture rate between operative and nonoperative cohorts (1.4% vs. 1.5%) but does cite an increased wound complication rate in the operative cohort (14.6% vs. 0.5 %).

Percutaneous versus Open Operative Repair

A literature search was performed using the search terms "Achilles," "tendon," "rupture," "treatment," and "operative," "open," "percutaneous," and "surgery." Literature was then screened for Level I and II evidence comparing percutaneous and open operative treatments of Achilles tendon ruptures; three studies were found[30–32] (see Table 69–1).

The best article currently available is a Level I RCT with a patient population of 66 (33 patients in each of the open and percutaneous cohorts) by Lim and coauthors.[32] Patients in these cohorts were described as more sedentary (30% regular participation in sports) with no information on health status. Results cited a lower rerupture rate in patients treated with percutaneous repair versus open repair (6% vs. 2%); however, the differences in these results were not statistically significant. However, a statistically significant increase in the infection rate for patients treated with open repair (21% vs. 0%) was reported. Sural nerve complications, adhesions, and perceived functional outcomes were greater in the percutaneous repair, although again they were not statistically significant.

The second Level I study by Goren and researchers[31] was an RCT comparing isokinetic strength and range of motion after percutaneous ($n = 10$) and open ($n = 10$) surgical repair of a ruptured Achilles tendon. The study cites no difference in health status of the two cohorts. Results indicate that isokinetic strength and range of motion were equal in the two cohorts; however, there was an increased incidence of Sural nerve injury (40% vs. 0%) in the percutaneous-treated cohort.

Cretnik and colleagues'[30] Level II, prospective, nonrandomized study compares 237 patients with an Achilles tendon rupture treated with open ($n = 105$) versus percutaneous ($n = 132$) surgical repair. The results revealed slight increases in rerupture (3.7% vs. 2.8 %) and sural nerve injury (4.5% vs. 2.8%) rates in the percutaneous cohorts, but these differences were not statistically significant. However, fewer major (4.5% vs. 12.4%) and total complications (9.7% vs. 21%) were reported in the percutaneous cohort. Functional assessment using Foot and Ankle society score and the Holtz score demonstrated no differences between the two cohorts.

TABLE 69–1. Summary of the Evidence Available That Should be Considered When Choosing Treatment Options for a Ruptured Achilles Tendon

PRINCIPAL AUTHOR	YEAR PUBLISHED	LEVEL OF EVIDENCE	STUDY TYPE
Operative versus Nonoperative Treatment			
Cetti[16]	1993	I	RCT original article
Moller[21]	2001	I	RCT original article
Bhandari[23]	2002	I	Meta-analysis
Khan[24]	2005	I	Meta-analysis
Nistor[22]	1981	I	RCT original article
Wong[25]	2002	II	Quantitative review
Percutaneous versus Open Operative Repair			
Lim[32]	2001	I	RCT original article
Goren[31]	2005	I	RCT original article
Cretnik[30]	2000	II	Prospective nonrandomized
Postoperative Rehabilitation			
Saleh[41]	1992	I	RCT original article
Cetti[33]	1994	I	RCT original article
Mortensen[38]	1999	I	RCT original article
Kerkhoffs[36]	2002	I	RCT original article
Kauranen[35]	2002	I	RCT original article
Petersen[39]	2002	I	RCT original article
Maffulli[37]	2003	I	RCT original article
Costa[34]	2003	I	RCT original article
Suchak[40]	2006	I	Meta-analysis

RCT, randomized, controlled trial.

Postoperative Rehabilitation

A literature search was undertaken to compare postoperative rehabilitation methods for treatment outcomes of patients with cast immobilization versus "functional rehabilitation" using the search terms "Achilles," "tendon," "rupture," "treatment," "operative," "cast," "immobilization," "rehabilitation," "functional," and "postoperative." Literature was then screened for Level I and II evidence, identifying nine articles[33-40] (see Table 69–1). Eight Level 1 original articles were RCTs, which were all in favor of early functional rehabilitation when compared with more traditional means of cast immobilization. The ninth article was a Level I meta-analysis pooling the results of six of the above articles.

Cetti and colleagues'[33] article was the first Level I article to compare the outcomes of patients using a mobile cast ($n = 30$) versus a rigid below-knee cast ($n = 30$). No significant difference in rerupture and infection rates was found in the two cohorts, but the mobile cast cohort was reported to have fewer minor complications, improved functional outcome, less elongation of the tendon, and was more likely to return to work.

Saleh and investigators[41] report results from a Level I study of functional rehabilitation with a full weight-bearing brace that holds the foot in 15 degrees of plantar flexion. The authors report a more rapid return of ankle dorsiflexion and return to normal activities.

Mortensen and researchers'[38] Level I study randomized 71 patients with an acute Achilles rupture to either cast immobilization for 8 weeks or early restricted motion of the ankle in a below-the-knee brace for 6 weeks. They also found that the increased motion cohort had improved functional outcome with respect to range of motion and a quicker return to sports or work.

Kerkhoffs and coworkers'[36] Level I study randomized a total of 39 consecutive patients with complete ruptures of the Achilles tendon to a walking cast or a wrap and showed that the wrap cohort allowed a significantly shorter hospital stay, as well as return to preinjury sports level compared with treatment with a walking cast. No increased risk of rerupture or wound healing problems were reported.

Costa and colleagues'[34] Level I study randomized 28 patients to either immediate loading in an orthosis or traditional serial plaster casting and showed improved clinical functional outcomes in the immediate loading group.

Kangas and coauthors'[42] level I study randomized 50 patients treated surgically for an acute Achilles tendon rupture to receive either early movement or immobilization. The calf muscle strength results were somewhat better in the early motion group, whereas other outcome results obtained in the two cohorts were similar.

Finally, Maffulli and coworkers'[37] Level I study showed that patients who were randomized to an early weight-bearing protocol had shortened the time of recovery without increased complications.

In contrast with the studies detailed earlier, Kauranen and researchers'[35] and Petersen and investigators'[39] Level I study showed no improvement in outcome for patients treated with and with an active brace and CAM walker versus a plaster cast after surgical repair of acute Achilles tendon ruptures.

A Level I meta-analysis by Suchak and colleagues[40] included six prospective RCTs[33,34,37,38,42,43] that were pooled to include 315 patients treated with surgical repair and postoperative immobilization ($n = 156$) or early functional rehabilitation ($n = 159$). The pooled results showed no difference in the rerupture rate in the immobilized and functional rehabilitation cohorts (3.8% vs. 2.5%, respectively) and no difference in the infection rates (3.8% vs. 3.1%, respectively). However, the functional rehabilitation cohort had improved subjective responses (88% vs. 62%) and less complications (e.g., scar adhesions and transient sural nerve deficits) (5.8% vs. 13.5%). The authors conclude that early functional rehabilitation for postoperative care of Achilles tendon ruptures treated with surgery improves patient satisfaction with reduced minor and major complications.

RECOMMENDATIONS

With respect to the choice of operative versus nonoperative care, one must consider patient factors that are detrimental to healing, infection, and a patient's ability to undergo surgery. If patients have such factors, then the recommended treatment should be nonoperative care based on increased complication rates such as infection and wound healing (Levels of Evidence I and II, grade A recommendation), which are summarized earlier. If patients are free of such factors, then faster return to normal activities and less chance of rerupture is likely with operative care (Levels of Evidence I and II, grade A recommendation).

With respect to a recommendation on the type of surgical repair (open vs. percutaneous), one must consider patient factors that are detrimental to healing or infection. Thus, with patient factors that are absent for healing or infection concerns, one should choose open operative repair to avoid excessive risk to the sural nerve (Levels of Evidence I and II, grade A recommendation). If patient factors that affect healing or infection rates adversely are present, one may recommend percutaneous over open surgical repair to avoid wound healing and infectious complications (Levels of Evidence I and II, grade A recommendation). However, to make recommendations on operative percutaneous repair of a ruptured Achilles versus nonoperative care, then direct Level I or II studies comparing the two would be necessary.

Finally, it is strongly recommended with support from the existing literature (Levels of

Evidence I and II, grade A recommendation) that that early functional rehabilitation for postoperative care of Achilles tendon ruptures treated with surgery improves patient function and satisfaction, and in some cases, reduces minor and major complications. Table 69–2 provides a summary of recommendations for the treatment of Achilles tendon rupture.

TABLE 69–2. Summary of Recommendations

STATEMENT	LEVEL OF EVIDENCE/ GRADE OF RECOMMENDATION	REFERENCES
1. Patients free of factors that are detrimental to healing, infection, and ability to undergo surgery then operative treatment will provide faster return to normal activities and less chance of re-rupture.	Level I & II Grade A	16,21,22,23, 24,25
2. Patients with factors that are detrimental to healing and infection should have percutaneous over open surgical repair to avoid wound healing and infectious complications.	Level I & II Grade A	30,31,32
3. Early functional rehabilitation is recommended for postoperative care of all patients treated with surgery.	Level I & II Grade A	33, 34,35,36, 37,38,39, 40,41

REFERENCES

1. Kastelic J, Baer E: Deformation in tendon collagen. Symp Soc Exp Biol 34:397–435, 1980.
2. Puddu G, Ippolito E, Postacchini F: A classification of Achilles tendon disease. Am J Sports Med 4:145–150, 1976.
3. Kannus P, Jozsa LG: Histopathological changes preceding spontaneous rupture of a tendon. A controlled study of 891 patients. J Bone Joint Surg Am 73:1507–1525, 1991.
4. Jozsa LG, Kannus P: Tendon pathology: Injuries, diseases and other disorders. Jozsa LG and Kannus P, eds. Human Tendons: Anatomy, Physiology, and Pathology. Champaign, IL, Human Kinetics, pp.161-254, 1997.
5. Arner O, Lindholm A, Orell SR: Histologic changes in subcutaneous rupture of the Achilles tendon; a study of 74 cases. Acta Chir Scand 116:484–490, 1959.
6. Jozsa L, Balint BJ, Reffy A, Demel Z: Fine structural alterations of collagen fibers in degenerative tendinopathy. Arch Orthop Trauma Surg 103:47–51, 1984.
7. Jozsa L, Reffy A, Balint JB: Polarization and electron microscopic studies on the collagen of intact and ruptured human tendons. Acta Histochem 74-2:209–215, 1984.
8. Maffulli N, Barrass V, Ewen SW: Light microscopic histology of Achilles tendon ruptures. A comparison with unruptured tendons. Am J Sports Med 28:857–863, 2000.
9. Cetti R, Junge J, Vyberg M: Spontaneous rupture of the Achilles tendon is preceded by widespread and bilateral tendon damage and ipsilateral inflammation: A clinical and histopathologic study of 60 patients. Acta Orthop Scand 74:78–84, 2003.
10. Astrom M, Rausing A: Chronic Achilles tendinopathy. A survey of surgical and histopathologic findings. Clin Orthop 316:151–164, 1995.
11. Movin T, Gad A, Reinholt FP, Rolf C: Tendon pathology in long-standing achillodynia. Biopsy findings in 40 patients. Acta Orthop Scand 68:170–175, 1997.
12. Carden DG, Noble J, Chalmers J, et al: Rupture of the calcaneal tendon. The early and late management. J Bone Joint Surg Br 69:416–420, 1987.
13. Leppilahti J, Puranen J, Orava S: Incidence of Achilles tendon rupture. Acta Orthop Scand 67:277–279, 1996.
14. Stein SR, Luekens CA Jr: Closed treatment of Achilles tendon ruptures. Orthop Clin North Am 7:241–246, 1976.
15. Suchak AA, Bostick G, Reid D, et al: The incidence of Achilles tendon ruptures in Edmonton, Canada. Foot Ankle Int 26:932–936, 2005.
16. Cetti R, Christensen SE, Ejsted R, et al: Operative versus nonoperative treatment of Achilles tendon rupture. A prospective randomized study and review of the literature. Am J Sports Med 21:791–799, 1993.
17. Postacchini F, Puddu G: Subcutaneous rupture of the Achilles tendon. Int Surg 61:14–18, 1976.
18. Deleted in proof.
19. Deleted in proof.
20. Deleted in proof.
21. Moller M, Movin T, Granhed H, et al: Acute rupture of tendon Achillis. A prospective randomised study of comparison between surgical and non-surgical treatment. J Bone Joint Surg Br 83:843–848, 2001.
22. Nistor L: Surgical and non-surgical treatment of Achilles tendon rupture. A prospective randomized study. J Bone Joint Surg Am 63:394–399, 1981.
23. Bhandari M, Guyatt GH, Siddiqui F, et al: Treatment of acute Achilles tendon ruptures: A systematic overview and meta-analysis. Clin Orthop Relat Res (400):190–200, 2002.
24. Khan RJ, Fick D, Keogh A, et al: Treatment of acute achilles tendon ruptures. A meta-analysis of randomized, controlled trials. J Bone Joint Surg Am 87:2202–2210, 2005.
25. Wong J, Barrass V, Maffulli N: Quantitative review of operative and nonoperative management of Achilles tendon ruptures. Am J Sports Med 30:565–575, 2002.
26. Schroeder D, Lehmann M, Steinbreuch K: Treatment of acute Achilles tendon ruptures: Open versus percutaneous repair vs. conservative treatment. A prospective randomized study. Orthopedic Transcripts 21:1228, 1997.
27. Coombs R: Prospective trial of conservative and surgical treatment of Achilles tendon rupture. J Bone Joint Surg Br 63B:288, 1981.
28. Majewski M, Rickert M, Steinbruck K: [Achilles tendon rupture. A prospective study assessing various treatment possibilities]. Orthopade 29:670–676, 2000.
29. Thermann H, Zwipp H, Tscherne H: [Functional treatment concept of acute rupture of the Achilles tendon. 2 years results of a prospective randomized study]. Unfallchirurg 98:21–32, 1995.
30. Cretnik A, Zlajpah L, Smrkolj V, Kosanovic M: The strength of percutaneous methods of repair of the Achilles tendon: A biomechanical study. Med Sci Sports Exerc 32:16–20, 2000.
31. Goren D, Ayalon M, Nyska M: Isokinetic strength and endurance after percutaneous and open surgical repair of Achilles tendon ruptures. Foot Ankle Int 26:286–290, 2005.
32. Lim J, Dalal R, Waseem M: Percutaneous vs. open repair of the ruptured Achilles tendon—a prospective randomized controlled study. Foot Ankle Int 22:559–568, 2001.
33. Cetti R, Henriksen LO, Jacobsen KS: A new treatment of ruptured Achilles tendons. A prospective randomized study. Clin Orthop Relat Res (308):155–165, 1994.

34. Costa ML, Shepstone L, Darrah C, et al: Immediate full-weight-bearing mobilisation for repaired Achilles tendon ruptures: A pilot study. Injury 34:874–876, 2003.

35. Kauranen K, Kangas J, Leppilahti J: Recovering motor performance of the foot after Achilles rupture repair: A randomized clinical study about early functional treatment vs. early immobilization of Achilles tendon in tension. Foot Ankle Int 23:600–605, 2002.

36. Kerkhoffs GM, Struijs PA, Raaymakers EL, Marti RK: Functional treatment after surgical repair of acute Achilles tendon rupture: Wrap vs walking cast. Arch Orthop Trauma Surg 122:102–105, 2002.

37. Maffulli N, Tallon C, Wong J, et al: Early weightbearing and ankle mobilization after open repair of acute midsubstance tears of the achilles tendon. Am J Sports Med 31:692–700, 2003.

38. Mortensen HM, Skov O, Jensen PE: Early motion of the ankle after operative treatment of a rupture of the Achilles tendon. A prospective, randomized clinical and radiographic study. J Bone Joint Surg Am 81:983–990, 1999.

39. Petersen OF, Nielsen MB, Jensen KH, Solgaard S: [Randomized comparison of CAM walker and light-weight plaster cast in the treatment of first-time Achilles tendon rupture]. Ugeskr Laeger 164:3852–3855, 2002.

40. Suchak AA, Spooner C, Reid DC, Jomha NM: Postoperative rehabilitation protocols for Achilles tendon ruptures: A meta-analysis. Clin Orthop Relat Res (445):216–221, 2006.

41. Saleh M, Marshall P, Senior R, et al: The Shefield splint for controlled early mobilization after rupture of the calcaneal tendon. A prospective randomised comparison with plaster treatment. J Bone Joint Surg Br 74-B:206–209, 1992.

42. Kangas J, Pajala A, Siira P, et al: Early functional treatment versus early immobilization in tension of the musculotendinous unit after Achilles rupture repair: A prospective, randomized, clinical study. J Trauma 54:1171–1181, 2003.

43. Maffulli N, Tallon C, Wong J, et al: No adverse effect of early weight bearing following open repair of acute tears of the Achilles tendon. J Sports Med Phys Fitness 43:367–379, 2003.

Chapter 70

What Is the Best Treatment for End-Stage Ankle Arthritis?

Tim R. Daniels, MD, FRCSC and Mohamed Maged Mokhimer, FRCS, Tr&Orth, MCh

Hip and knee arthroplasties are two of the most successful operations in the past century. For management of end-stage ankle arthritis, however, arthrodesis continues to be the mainstay of an orthopedic practice. This is in part due to the early catastrophic failures of the "first-generation" ankle arthroplasties and the high patient satisfaction after an ankle arthrodesis. Despite the initial failures of ankle arthroplasties, several individuals remained committed to the possibilities of replacing the ankle joint, and their persistence has resulted in the introduction of "second- and third-generation" ankle implants.[1,2] Preliminary clinical results are promising, again giving rise to total ankle arthroplasty as an option for managing end-stage arthritis. These developments have prompted the current debate at many national and international meetings regarding the role of ankle arthroplasty in the management of end-stage ankle arthritis. This chapter briefly reviews the evidence that exists in the literature for all treatment options available for the operative management of end-stage ankle arthritis; however, the primary focus is to assess the level of evidence regarding ankle fusion versus arthroplasty and to provide the reader with treatment guidelines for their patients.

OVERVIEW

An extensive literature search was performed in preparation for this chapter. The majority of the articles assessing operative management of patients with end-stage ankle arthritis are of poor scientific quality. Most of the studies provide Level III and IV evidence. Only a handful of Level I and II studies exist, many of which assess the outcomes of total ankle arthroplasty or compare different methods by which to obtain an ankle fusion. Also, no comparative studies exist for ankle fusion versus ankle arthroplasty.

The two latest techniques described for surgical management of end-stage ankle arthritis are ankle joint distraction and fresh total ankle allografts. The literature published on these new techniques includes Level IV evidence only. Consequently, best treatment recommendations of end-stage ankle arthritis are based on expert opinion and conclusions drawn from comparing the outcomes of different studies.

ANKLE ARTHRODESIS

Ankle arthrodesis for end-stage arthritis was first described by Albert in 1879,[3] and for almost 100 years, this was the only option offered to patients with severe ankle pathology. Little information has been published on the topic. Since the 1960s, numerous studies have looked at various aspects of ankle arthrodesis: techniques of fusion, fusion rates, open versus arthroscopic fusion, position of fusion, patient satisfaction, functional outcomes, gait analysis, long-term results with focus on the health of the ipsilateral hindfoot joints, and more recently, comparison with normal control populations. These studies are largely based on Level III and IV evidence.

With regard to technique of arthrodesis, the classic Level IV retrospective study authored by J. Charnley[4] and published in 1951 was the first to demonstrate that compression across a fusion site optimizes bone healing. Charnley[4] describe compression with external fixation, and this technique was used for more than two decades. During the late 1970s and 1980s, the use of internal fixation increased in frequency. In 1991, Moeckel and colleagues,[5] in a Level III study, compared external fixation with internal fixation and demonstrated an increased incidence of nonunion, delayed union, and infection in the external fixation group. More recently, circular external fixators with fine wires under tension are being used with increased frequency. The proponents of this technique suggest that the advantages are earlier weight bearing, ability to correct deformities during the postoperative follow-up phase, respect for soft tissues, more stable fixation, and fewer problems with prominent internal fixation.[6,7] Opponents argue that the procedure is more complex, more expensive, and more labor intensive, with increased complications such as pin-tract infections. To date, no comparative or cost analysis studies have been published. Level III studies have suggested that external fixation is advantageous in the presence of infection, bone loss, talar avascular necrosis, or severe deformity[6–8]; however, no comparative studies have been performed.

Studies comparing screw versus plate fixation have found an improved rate of union with screws.[9–14] Screw fixation can be obtained with less soft-tissue stripping. This, combined with better compression at the fusion site, may account for the difference. Holt and coauthors[10] describe a technique using three screws for fixation whereas preserving the medial and lateral malleoli. A fibular osteotomy is performed and, after denuding the cartilage, it is secured to the tibia and talus with compression screws. A second screw is placed from the medial malleolus into the talus, and then a third screw, the so-called home-run screw, is inserted from the posterior malleolus into the neck of the talus. This screw is of primary importance because it stabilizes plantarflexion and dorsiflexion forces (Fig. 70–1). Laboratory studies have shown that two crossed screws create a more rigid construct than two parallel screws.[15] Cadaveric studies have shown that the use of three screws has the advantage of increased compression and better resistance to torque.[16] These variations aside,[9–11,13,14,16] most surgeons would agree that a minimum of two screws is necessary for adequate stability. Stability can be improved further by adding a fibular strut graft[17]; the use of a T-plate has been shown on cadavers to provide the stiffest construct when compared with other types of fixation, but it requires more soft-tissue dissection.[18,19]

Arthroscopic ankle arthrodesis was introduced in 1983 by Schneider and popularized by others.[20,21] Since then, numerous articles have been published with the primary focus on surgical technique, time to fusion, duration of admission to hospital, and fusion rates.[20–34] Proponents of arthroscopic ankle arthrodesis advocate shorter operating room time, equivalent fusion rates to open methods, shorter hospital stay, and decreased wound healing problems. Again, these observations are based on Level III and IV evidence. Only two comparative studies,[22,34] both of which are retrospective (Level III), offer only marginal support for the aforementioned advantages of arthroscopic ankle arthrodesis. All agree that the procedure requires familiarity with arthroscopic skills for small joints and is indicated only in patients with minimal deformity at the ankle joint level.

Optimal position of ankle fusion has been studied closely in several Level III retrospective comparative clinical series.[35–38] These studies have demonstrated that patients fused in greater than 10 degrees of equinus have a vaulting gait, increased knee extension and recurvatum, laxity of the medial collateral ligament of the knee, and slower walking speeds. These abnormalities were not observed in patients whose ankles were fused in a neutral position.[36–38] It was also observed that when the hindfoot was in varus, patients reported increased pain and callus formation along the lateral border of the foot.[36] Current recommendations are to position the hindfoot in neutral dorsiflexion, slight valgus, external rotation equal to the opposite side, and position the talus directly under or slightly posterior to the midline of the tibia.

Overall patient satisfaction after ankle arthrodesis was good. A number of articles published between

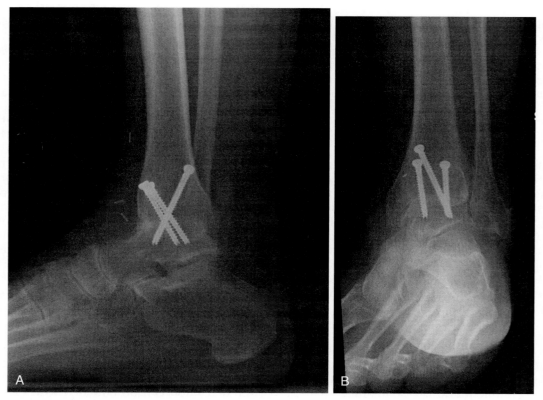

FIGURE 70–1. Recommended position of fusion is neutral dorsiflexion in the lateral plane and neutral alignment of the ankle in the coronal plane, slight valgus of the calcaneus. Equinus and varus positioning should be avoided.

1960 and 2006 demonstrated a high satisfaction rate, good relief of pain, and improved function. Most of these articles were retrospective case series studies with no control group. One Level III intermediate follow-up study compared outcomes of ankle arthrodesis with a normal control population, and it demonstrated that there were substantial differences between the two groups with regard to physical function and pain[39]; however, many of the patients treated with arthrodesis remained satisfied with their results.

Several Level III long-term studies demonstrated a high incidence of ipsilateral hindfoot arthritis after ankle arthrodesis, particularly of the subtalar joint (Fig. 70–2).[35,40–45] Two articles with more than a 20-year follow-up period demonstrated that more than 60% of the patients continue to be satisfied with their results despite the high prevalence of ipsilateral hindfoot arthritis.[40,46] Only two studies have assessed the preoperative radiographs to determine the presence of preexisting ipsilateral hindfoot arthritis.[46,47] Sheridan and coworkers[46] demonstrated the presence of preexisting subtalar arthritis in 77.5% of patients with end-stage ankle arthritis and suggested that ankle arthrodesis does not necessarily lead to progressive ipsilateral hindfoot arthritis because it is often present before surgery. Daniels and researchers[47] identified progression of subtalar arthritis in 4 of 26 (15%) patients in an intermediate follow-up study and progression of calcaneocuboid arthritis from stage 2 to 5 in one patient. Trauma has been identified as the most common causative factor of ankle arthritis.[48] What is not known is whether the preexisting ipsilateral hindfoot arthritis is the result of the stiffness of the arthritic ankle or is caused by the original trauma, or a combination of both. Regardless of the causative factor, it can be concluded that long-term patients with ankle arthritis or ankle arthrodesis, or both, have a high incidence of ipsilateral hindfoot arthritis with the subtalar joint most commonly affected. Level III evidence exists that the presence of ipsilateral hindfoot arthritis does compromise the functional outcome of the patient after ankle arthrodesis.[45,49] None of the long-term studies demonstrated an increased incidence of knee or metatarsophalangeal arthritis on either the ipsilateral or contralateral extremities.[40,46]

Articles that have assessed the effects of an ankle arthrodesis on gait have indicated that the abnormal kinetics and kinematics are most evident through the hindfoot, midfoot, and forefoot, with lesser effects on the knee, hip, and pelvis.[35–38,47,50,51] All the studies cited earlier are retrospective reviews and considered Level III evidence. Although some variability exists in the results of gait analysis, patients with hindfoot fusions generally have the following gait characteristics: shortened stride length, decreased cadence, slower walking speeds, earlier heel raise during stance phase, increased anterior tilt of the tibia during midstance, increased forefoot plantar pressures with the forefoot ground reactive forces (GRF) shifted posterior during terminal stance, increased hip flexion, earlier knee extension during stance, diminished hindfoot motion, and increased midfoot motion. Studies that have assessed the effects of footwear on gait have indicated that the gait pattern further normalizes with footwear, particularly if there is a slight elevation in the heel and a forefoot rocker[36–38]; however, what continues to persist are early heel rise, posterior shift of the GRFs, and early extension of the knee.[50] Beyaert and colleagues[50] have suggested that the early heel rise and increased anterior tibial tilt during midstance increases the shear forces to the midtarsal joints and is a possible reason for the increased incidence of ipsilateral hindfoot arthritis after ankle arthrodesis. Weiss and coworkers,[52] in a prospective, Level II, comparative study, assessed the effects of ankle/hindfoot arthrodesis on the function of the knee and hip. This study was not isolated to arthrodesis of the ankle alone, but it is the only prospective gait study that focused on the kinetic and kinematic outcomes of the ipsilateral hip and knee joints. It demonstrated that the overlying leg joints experience an improvement in joint motion, muscle-generated joint moments, and work during walking after arthrodesis.

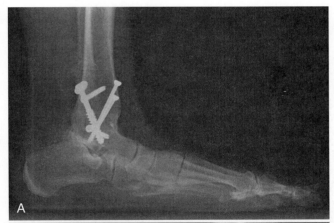
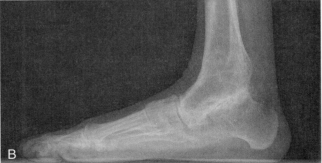

FIGURE 70–2. (*A*) Lateral radiograph of a patient that had an ankle fusion six years ago presenting with a one year history of increasing lateral hindfoot pain. Note the end-stage arthritis of the posterior facet of the subtalar joint. (*B*) Lateral radiograph of a patient that had undergone an ankle fusion 60 years ago. The talonavicular and the calcaneocuboid joints were fused 30 years ago due to the development of arthritis. Patient currently presents with painful subtalar and navicular-cuneiform arthritis.

ANKLE ARTHROPLASTY

Though the role of ankle arthroplasty remains controversial, interest in the procedure as a viable alternative to arthrodesis has increased substantially in the last decade because of the accumulative effect of several factors: (1) the development of foot and ankle surgery as a subspecialty, (2) improved ankle implants, and (3) the success of arthroplasties in other joints such as the hip, knee, shoulder, and elbow.

As is evident from the previous discussion, ankle arthrodesis is considered by many experts to provide a good functional outcome for their patients. However, the long-term consequences of ankle fusion consist of subtalar arthritis, which produces poor functional outcomes because of the stiff and painful subtalar joint complex. A pantalar fusion to address painful hindfoot arthritis below an ankle fusion produces significant functional limitations.[54,55]

It is beyond the scope of this article to assess in detail the types of ankle implants utilized today. In brief, there are fixed bearing (two-component) and mobile bearing (three-component) designs. The two-component designs have the polyethylene that locks into the tibial component, whereas three-component designs have a polyethylene that articulates with the tibial and talar component allowing for motion at both surfaces (Fig. 70–3).

There has been a gradual trend toward a three-component, mobile-bearing implant that requires minimal bone resection.[56–58] The disadvantages of the two-component design are that more bone resection is required and there is less room for error in positioning of the components.[59,60] However, no studies

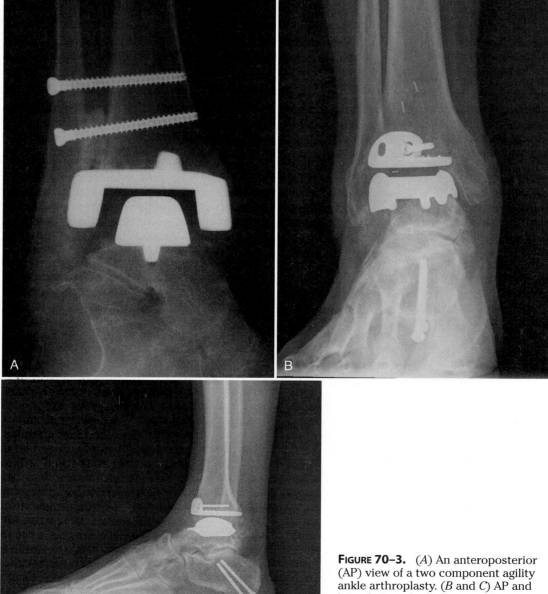

FIGURE 70–3. (*A*) An anteroposterior (AP) view of a two component agility ankle arthroplasty. (*B* and *C*) AP and lateral view of a 3-component Hintegra total ankle arthroplasty.

have compared the outcomes of three-component and two-component designs.

The evidence in assessing outcomes for ankle joint arthroplasty is actually superior to that of ankle arthrodesis because ankle arthroplasty studies are more recent. An increased number of prospective studies with validated outcomes and gait analysis are available. However, there are still no comparative prospective studies, long-term outcome studies, and randomized trials comparing ankle arthroplasty with fusion or different types of ankle arthroplasty. Furthermore, sufficient data are not available to compare differences between two- and three-component ankle replacements. Thus, the clinical results of meta-analysis are based on combining the results of two- and three-component designs.

Current clinical outcome studies of the newer ankle arthroplasties have determined the following: patients have a substantial relief of pain, improvement in their function and gait, and the implant 5- to 10-year survival rates are acceptable but not equivalent to knee or hip arthroplasty.[1,2,56,61–84] The most current and comprehensive review is a Level III meta-analysis of 10 total ankle arthroplasty articles published between 1998 and 2005 that meet a strict inclusion criteria.[85] The 5- and 10-year implant survival rates after total ankle arthroplasty were 78% (95% confidence interval, 69.0–87.6%) and 77% (95% confidence interval, 63.3–90.8%), respectively.

A revision during the follow-up period was required in 7% (95% confidence interval, 3.5–10.9%) of the patients who had undergone a total ankle arthroplasty. The most common reason for revision was loosening, subsidence, or both (28%). Five percent (95% confidence interval, 2.0–7.8%) of the total ankle arthroplasties were converted to arthrodeses, with the main reason for conversion being loosening, subsidence, or both (50% of all conversions). Below-the-knee amputation was performed in 1% of the patients treated with total ankle arthroplasty. When compared with 39 comparable ankle arthrodesis articles published between 1990 and 1997, nonunion was observed in 10% (95% confidence interval, 7.4–12.1%) of the patients treated with ankle arthrodesis. Nine percent (95% confidence interval, 5.5–11.6%) of the arthrodesis group underwent revision, primarily because of nonunion (the indication for 65% of all revisions of arthrodeses). Five percent of the patients treated with ankle arthrodesis underwent a below-the-knee amputation.

To date, all of the ankle arthroplasty articles assess the short- and mid-term results. The longest follow up is on the two-component Agility design by Knecht and colleagues[75] with an average follow-up period of 9 years. Long-term follow-up of the first-generation total ankle arthroplasties showed extremely poor results and prompted a period when ankle joint arthroplasties were rarely performed.[86–92] It is not known yet whether a similar fate awaits the second- and third-generation ankle joint arthroplasties.

Several Level IV retrospective articles have been published on the feasibility of salvaging a failed total ankle arthroplasty with arthrodesis,[93–96] all of which

have demonstrated an increased complication rate such as nonunion and infection with a prolonged recovery. This further emphasizes the cautious approach that should be taken when considering a young patient for ankle arthroplasty.

If ankle arthroplasty is to truly offer the patient an advantage over an ankle arthrodesis, it would have to allow for enough motion to normalize gait. Several studies have assessed the gait of patients who have undergone total ankle arthroplasty with the more recent two- and three-component designs.[64,67,83,97] Two of these studies provide Level II evidence[83,97] and two provide Level III evidence[64,67] that gait after this surgery is improved and approaches more normal kinetic and kinematic parameters. There is improved dorsiflexion of the ankle during the stance phase, improved muscle function, and increased cadence and stride length. GRF at midstance are improved, but patients continue to demonstrate decreased vertical peak pressures during the terminal stance phase.[67] The improved dorsiflexion during the stance phase may help decrease the abnormal shear forces to the subtalar joint complex, thereby decreasing the incidence of progressive ipsilateral hindfoot arthritis. A Level III meta-analysis by Soohoo and coworkers[98] assessed reoperation rates after ankle arthrodesis versus arthroplasty and demonstrated a decreased incidence of patients requiring subtalar fusion after ankle arthroplasty.

It is important to note that none of the gait parameters was completely normalized, and comparative studies to ankle arthrodesis do not exist. Valderrabano and researchers'[83] Level II study assessing muscle function and rehabilitation before and after ankle arthroplasty determined that total ankle arthroplasty improved muscle function (torque, electromyographic intensity). However, after 1 year, patients did not reach the level of the contralateral healthy leg and the electromyographic frequency remained unchanged.

Fresh Ankle Osteochondral Allografts

The outcomes of fresh ankle osteochondral allografts for end-stage ankle arthritis have been reported in a retrospective Level IV review by Brage and investigators,[99,100] where 11 patients were managed for an average of 33 months, and a successful outcome was identified in 6 of the 11 patients. The author concludes that this procedure is indicated in young patients with end-stage ankle arthritis as an alternative to ankle joint arthroplasty. To date, this procedure is highly experimental and should be restricted to a tertiary care practice with a close and continuous follow-up.

Ankle Joint Distraction

Articular distraction of the ankle joint with an external fixation device[101–106] has been advocated for patients with severe end-stage arthritis who are candidates for arthrodesis. The procedure involves application of a ringed external fixator to the distal tibial and foot after open or arthroscopic debridement. The joint is distracted a total of 5 mm, at 1-mm increments per day. Weight bearing is allowed, and hinges are applied to the fixator at 6 to 12 weeks to allow ankle flexion and extension. The fixator is removed at an average of 15 weeks after application. Marijnissen and coworkers[105] report on 46 patients with an average follow-up of 2.8 ± 0.3 years: 13 patients withdrew from the study and underwent an arthrodesis. The remaining patients reported a significant reduction in pain ($P < 0.0001$), and improvement in function ($P < 0.0001$) and clinical condition ($P < 0.0001$). The ankle range of motion improved, but not significantly. Radiographically, the joint space increased by 17% at the 1-year and 27% at the 3-year follow-up examination ($P < 0.05$). The functional and clinical outcome scores were significantly better at the 3-year follow-up examination ($P < 0.05$), suggesting that the clinical picture improved with time. A more recent Level IV long-term retrospective clinical series of 25 patients with more than 7 years of follow-up determined a 73% success rate.[106]

Acevedo and Myerson[107] report on a group of nine patients who underwent debridement and acute distraction (average, 5.8 mm; range, 4.5–8 mm). The fixator was removed at an average of 11 weeks. Only three patients reported functional improvement at the 1-year follow-up mark, and three underwent arthrodesis of the ankle at an average of 12 months after the distraction procedure. Although this treatment holds promise, data supporting a successful outcome are limited to Level III retrospective reviews published by a single group of physicians.

SUMMARY

Current literature highlights a paucity of comparative, prospective, and long-term studies for the various surgical options available to patients with end-stage ankle arthritis. Currently, the most common procedures performed are ankle arthrodesis and arthroplasty. Though the option of ankle arthroplasty is relatively new, no comparative studies are available to help the treating surgeons determine which procedure to choose and what advice to give their patients.

Problems with assessing outcomes of arthroplasty are that outcomes of greater than 5 years are required and some questions can be answered only with 15- to 20-year outcomes. By the time these results are published, the technology has changed substantially, making the outcomes obsolete.

RECOMMENDATIONS

After thorough review of the literature, the only expert advice we can offer is that the short-term outcomes of ankle fusion and arthroplasty are equivalent. Does the motion allowed for by an ankle arthroplasty offer sufficient benefits to the patient to make the risks for a difficult revision worthwhile? Does it decrease the incidence of symptomatic ipsilateral hindfoot arthritis? Does the improved gait over arthrodesis offer any long-term benefits to the patient? None of these questions can be answered by the current literature. Table 70–1 provides a summary of recommendations for the treatment of end-stage ankle arthritis.

TABLE 70–1. Summary of Recommendations

STATEMENT	LEVEL OF EVIDENCE/GRADE OF RECOMMENDATION	REFERENCES
1. Position of fusion – neutral dorsiflexion, slight valgus and 15° external rotation	B	6, 16, 17, 15,19
2. Less complications with internal fixation and compression compared to standard external fixation methods	B	23
3. High incidence of ipsilateral hindfoot arthritis in long-term reviews of patients that have undergone an ankle fusion	B, C	5, 12
4. Patient satisfaction, pain relief and improved function satisfactory following ankle fusion for end-stage ankle arthritis	B, C	4, 5, 6, 12, 13, 29, 35, 38, 58,
5. Outcomes and union rates of open vs. arthroscopic ankle fusions comparable	B	40, 52
6. Gait characteristics following ankle fusion are: shortened stride length, decreased cadence, slower walking speeds, earlier heel raise during stance phase, increased anterior tilt of the tibia during mid-stance, increased forefoot plantar pressures with the forefoot Ground Reactive Forces (GRF) shifted posterior during terminal stance, increased hip flexion, earlier knee extension during stance, diminished hindfoot motion and increased midfoot motion	B	6, 13, 16-20
7. Five-year and ten-year implant survival rates following total ankle arthroplasty were 78% and 77%, respectively	B	85
8. Average non-union rate following ankle fusion is 10%	B	85
9. Incidence of below knee amputation following failed ankle replacement is 1% compared to 5% following failed ankle fusion	B	85
10. Gait following total ankle replacement is improved and approaches more normal kinetic and kinematic parameters	B	64, 67, 83, 97
11. Short-term outcomes of ankle fusion and arthroplasty are equivalent	C	Current article

REFERENCES

1. Pyevich MT, Saltzman CL, Callaghan JJ, Alvine FG: Total ankle arthroplasty: A unique design. Two to twelve-year follow-up. J Bone Joint Surg Am 80:1410–1420, 1998.
2. Kofoed H, Lundberg-Jensen A: Ankle arthroplasty in patients younger and older than 50 years: A prospective series with long-term follow-up. Foot Ankle Int 20:501–506, 1999.
3. Albert E: Zur resektion des kniegelenkes. Wien Med Press 20:705–708, 1879.
4. Charnley J: Compression arthrodesis of the ankle and shoulder. J Bone Joint Surg 33-B:180–191, 1951.
5. Moeckel B, Patterson BM, Inglis AE, Sculco TP: Ankle arthrodesis. A comparison of internal and external fixation. Clin Orthop 268:78–83, 1991.
6. Eylon S, Porat S, Bor N, Leibner ED: Outcome of Ilizarov ankle arthrodesis. Foot Ankle Int 288:73–79, 2007.
7. Salem K, Kinzl L, Schmelz A: Ankle arthrodesis using Ilizarov ring fixators: A review of 22 cases. Foot Ankle Int 27:764–770, 2006.
8. Eralp L, Kocaoglu M, Yusof NM, Bulbul M: Distal tibial reconstruction with use of a circular external fixator and an intramedullary nail. The combined technique. J Bone Joint Surg Am 89:2218–2224, 2007.
9. Chen Y-J, Huang TJ, Shih HN, Hsu KY, Hsu RW: Ankle arthrodesis with cross-screw fixation. Acta Orthop Scand 67:473–478, 1996.
10. Holt E, Hansen ST, Mayo KA, Sangeorzan BJ: Ankle arthrodesis using internal screw fixation. Clin Orthop 268:56–64, 1991.
11. Mann RA, Rongstad KM: Arthrodesis of the ankle: A critical analysis. Foot Ankle Int 19:3–9, 1998.
12. Maurer R, Cimino WR, Cox CV, Satow GK: Transarticular cross-screw fixation: A technique of ankle arthrodesis. Clin Orthop 268:56–64, 1991.
13. Sward L, Hughes JS, Howell CJ, Colton CL: Posterior internal compression arthrodesis of the ankle. J Bone Joint Surg Br 74:752–756, 1992.
14. Morgan C, Henke JA, Bailey RW, Kaufer H: Long-term results of tibiotalar arthrodesis. J Bone Joint Surg Am 67-A:546–549, 1985.
15. Friedman RL, Glisson RR, Nunley JA 2nd: A biomechanical comparative analysis of two techniques for tibiotalar arthrodesis. Foot Ankle Int 15:301–305, 1994.
16. Ogilvie-Harris DJ, Fitsialos D, Hedman TP: Arthrodesis of the ankle. A comparison of two versus three screw fixation in a crossed configuration. Clin Orthop (304):195–199, 1994.
17. Thordarson DB, Markolf KL, Cracchiolo A 3rd: Arthrodesis of the ankle with cancellous-bone screws and fibular strut graft. Biomechanical analysis. J Bone Joint Surg Am 72:1359–1363, 1990.
18. Dohm MP, Benjamin JB, Harrison J, Szivek JA: A biomechanical evaluation of three forms of internal fixation used in ankle arthrodesis. Foot Ankle Int 15:297–300, 1994.
19. Scranton PE Jr, Fu FH, Brown TD: Ankle arthrodesis: A comparative clinical and biomechanical evaluation. Clin Orthop (151):234–243, 1980.
20. Ferkel R, Hewitt M: Long-term results of arthroscopic ankle arthrodesis. Foot Ankle Int 26:275–280, 2005.
21. Collman D, Kaas M, Schuberth J: Arthroscopic ankle arthrodesis: Factors influencing union in 39 consecutive patients. Foot Ankle Int 27:1079–1085, 2006.
22. Myerson M, Quill G: Ankle arthrodesis. A comparison of an arthroscopic and an open method of treatment. Clin Orthop Relat Res (268):84–95, 1991.
23. Corso S, Zimmer T: Technique and clinical evaluation of arthroscopic ankle arthrodesis. Arthroscopy 11:585–590, 1995.
24. Gougoulias N, Agathangelidis F, Parsons S: Arthroscopic ankle arthrodesis. Foot Ankle Int 28:695–706, 2007.
25. Glick JM, Morgan CD, Myerson MS, Sampson TG, Mann JA: Ankle arthrodesis using an arthroscopic method: Long-term follow-up of 34 cases. Arthroscopy 12:428–434, 1996.
26. Kats J, van Kampen A, de Waal-Malefijt M: Improvement in technique for arthroscopic ankle fusion: Results in 15 patients. Knee Surg Sports Traumatol Arthrosc 11:46–49, 2003.
27. Dent C, Patil M, Fairclough J: Arthroscopic ankle arthrodesis. J Bone Joint Surg Br 75:830–832, 1993.
28. Rippstein P, Kumar B, Muller M: Ankle arthrodesis using the arthroscopic technique. Oper Orthop Traumatol 17(4-5):442–456, 2005.
29. Turan I, Wredmark T, Fellander-Tsai L: Arthroscopic ankle arthrodesis in rheumatoid arthritis. Clin Orthop Relat Res (320):110–114, 1995.
30. Wasserman L, Saltzman C, Amendola A: Minimally invasive ankle reconstruction: Current scope and indications. Orthop Clin North Am 35:247–253, 2004.
31. Winson I, Robinson D, Allen P: Arthroscopic ankle arthrodesis. J Bone Joint Surg Br 87:343–347, 2005.
32. Zvijac J, Lemak L, Schurhoff MR, Hechtman KS, Uribe JW: Analysis of arthroscopically assisted ankle arthrodesis. Arthroscopy 18:70–75, 2002.
33. Cameron S, Ullrich P: Arthroscopic arthrodesis of the ankle joint. Arthroscopy 16:21–26, 2000.
34. O'Brien TS, Hart TS, Shereff MJ, Stone J, Johnson J: Open versus arthroscopic ankle arthrodesis: A comparative study. Foot Ankle Int 20:368–374, 1999.
35. Mazur J, Schwartz E, Simon S: Ankle arthrodesis. Long-term follow-up with gait analysis. J Bone Joint Surg 61:964–975, 1979.
36. Buck P, Morrey B, Chao E: The optimum position of arthrodesis of the ankle. A gait study of the knee and ankle. J Bone Joint Surg Am 69:1052–1062, 1987.
37. King HA, Watkins TB Jr, Samuelson KM: Analysis of foot position in ankle arthrodesis and its influence on gait. Foot Ankle 1:44–49, 1980.
38. Hefti FL, Baumann JU, Morscher EW: Ankle joint fusion—determination of optimal position by gait analysis. Arch Orthop Trauma Surg 96:187–195, 1980.
39. Thomas R, Daniels T, Parker K: Gait analysis and functional outcomes following ankle arthrodesis for isolated ankle arthritis. J Bone Joint Surg Am 88:526–535, 2006.
40. Coester L, Saltzman CL, Leupold J, Pontarelli W: Long-term results following ankle arthrodesis for post-traumatic arthritis. J Bone Joint Surg Am 83-A:219–228, 2001.
41. Lynch A, Bourne R, Rorabeck C: The long-term results of ankle arthrodesis. J Bone Joint Surg Am 70:113–116, 1988.
42. Morrey B, Wiedman G: Complications and long-term results of ankle arthrodesis following trauma. J Bone Joint Surg Am 62-A(5):777–784, 1980.
43. Ahlberg A, Henricson A: Late results of ankle fusion. Acta Orthop Scand 52:103–105, 1981.
44. Boobbyer G: The long-term results of ankle arthrodesis. Acta Orthop Scand 52:107–110, 1981.
45. Fuchs S, Sandmann C, Skwara A, Chylarecki C: Quality of life 20 years after arthrodesis of the ankle. A study of adjacent joints. J Bone Joint Surg Br 85:994–998, 2003.
46. Sheridan BD, Robinson DE, Hubble MJ, Winson IG: Ankle arthrodesis and its relationship to ipsilateral arthritis of the hind- and mid-foot. J Bone Joint Surg Br 88:206–207, 2006.
47. Daniels TR, Thomas RH, Parker K: Gait Analysis and Functional Outcomes of Isolated Ankle Arthrodesis. Presented at International Federation of Foot and Ankle Societies Triennial Scientific Meeting. San Francisco, CA, 2002.
48. Saltzman CL, Salamon ML, Blanchard GM, Huff T, Hayes A, Buckwalter JA, Amendola A: Epidemiology of ankle arthritis: Report of a consecutive series of 639 patients from a tertiary orthopaedic center. Iowa Orthop J 25:44–46, 2005.
49. Buchner M, Sabo D: Ankle fusion attributable to posttraumatic arthrosis: A long-term followup of 48 patients. Clin Orthop Relat Res 406:155–164, 2003.
50. Beyaert C, Sirveaux F, Paysant J, Molé D, André JM: The effect of tibio-talar arthrodesis on foot kinematics and ground reaction force progression during walking. Gait Posture 20:84–91, 2004.
51. Wu WL, Su FC, Cheng YM, Huang PJ, Chou YL, Chou CK: Gait analysis after ankle arthrodesis. Gait Posture 11:54–61, 2000.
52. Weiss R, Broström E, Stark A, Wick MC, Wretenberg P: Ankle/hindfoot arthrodesis in rheumatoid arthritis improves kinematics and kinetics of the knee and hip: A prospective gait analysis study. Rheumatology (Oxford) 46:1024–1028, 2007.

53. Deleted in proof.
54. Acosta R, Ushiba J, Cracchiolo A 3rd: The results of a primary and staged pantalar arthrodesis and tibiotalocalcaneal arthrodesis in adult patients. Foot Ankle Int 21:182–194, 2000.
55. Papa J, Myerson M: Pantalar and tibiotalocalcaneal arthrodesis for post-traumatic osteoarthritis of the ankle and hindfoot. J Bone Joint Surg 74:1042–1049, 1992.
56. Alvine FG: Total ankle arthroplasty. In Myerson MS (eds): Foot and Ankle Disorders, Vol. 2. Philadelphia, WB Saunders Company, 2000, p 1087.
57. Saltzman C, McIff TE, Buckwalter JA, Brown TD: Total ankle replacement revisited. J Orthop Sports Phys Ther 30:56–67, 2000.
58. Thomas RH, Daniels TR: Ankle arthritis. J Bone Joint Surg Am 85-A:923–936, 2003.
59. Saltzman C, Tochigi Y, Rudert MJ, McIff TE, Brown TD: The effect of agility ankle prosthesis misalignment on the peri-ankle ligaments. Clin Orthop Relat Res 424:137–142, 2004.
60. Tochigi Y, Rudert MJ, Brown TD, McIff TE, Saltzman CL: The effect of accuracy of implantation on range of movement of the Scandinavian total ankle replacement. J Bone Joint Surg Br 87:736–740, 2005.
61. Bonnin M, Judet T, Colombier JA, Buscayret F, Graveleau N, Piriou P: Midterm results of the Salto Total Ankle Prosthesis. Clin Orthop Relat Res 424:6–18, 2004.
62. Buechel FF, Pappas MJ: Survivorship and clinical evaluation of cementless, meniscal-bearing total ankle replacements. Semin Arthroplasty 3:43–50, 1992.
63. Buechel FF, Pappas MJ, Iorio LJ: New Jersey low contact stress total ankle replacement: Biomechanical rationale and review of 23 cementless cases. Foot Ankle 8:279–290, 1988.
64. Conti S, Lalonde K, Martin R: Kinematic analysis of the agility total ankle during gait. Foot Ankle Int 27:980–984, 2006.
65. Conti SF: Gait before and after total ankle arthroplasty with a comparison to arthrodesis. Presented at International Federation of Foot and Ankle Societies Triennial Scientific Meeting. San Francisco, CA, IFFAS, 2002.
66. Doets H, Brand R, Nelissen R: Total ankle arthroplasty in inflammatory joint disease with use of two mobile-bearing designs. J Bone Joint Surg Am 88:1272–1284, 2006.
67. Doets H, van Middelkoop M, Houdijk H, Nelissen RG, Veeger HE: Gait analysis after successful mobile bearing total ankle replacement. Foot Ankle Int 28:313–322, 2007.
68. Haskell A, Mann R: Ankle arthroplasty with preoperative coronal plane deformity: Short-term results. Clin Orthop Relat Res 424:98–103, 2004.
69. Hintermann B, Valderrabano V: Total ankle replacement. Foot Ankle Clin 8:375–405, 2003.
70. Hintermann, B, Valderrabano V, Dereymaeker G, Dick W: The HINTEGRA ankle: Rationale and short-term results of 122 consecutive ankles. Clin Orthop Relat Res (424):57–68, 2004.
71. Hintermann B, Valderrabano V, Knupp M, Horisberger M: The HINTEGRA ankle: short- and mid-term results. Orthopade 35:533–545, 2006.
72. Hurowitz E, Gould JS, Fleisig GS, Fowler R: Outcome analysis of agility total ankle replacement with prior adjunctive procedures: Two to six year followup. Foot Ankle Int 28:308–312, 2007.
73. Jensen NC, Kroner K: Total ankle joint replacement: A clinical follow up. Orthopedics 15:236–239, 1992.
74. Kirkup J: Richard Smith ankle arthroplasty. J R Soc Med 78:301–304, 1985.
75. Knecht SI, Estin M, Callaghan JJ, Zimmerman MB, Alliman KJ, et al: The agility total ankle arthroplasty. Seven to sixteen-year follow-up. J Bone Joint Surg Am 86-A:1161–1171, 2004.
76. Kofoed H: Ankle arthroplasty: Indications, alignment, stability and gain in mobility. In Kofoed H (ed): Current Status of Ankle Arthroplasty. Heidelberg, Springer, 1998, p 20.
77. Kofoed H, Sorensen TS: Ankle arthroplasty for rheumatoid arthritis and osteoarthritis: Prospective long-term study of cemented replacements. J Bone Joint Surg Br 80:328–332, 1998.
78. Kopp F, Patel MM, Deland JT, O'Malley MJ: Total ankle arthroplasty with the Agility prosthesis: Clinical and radiographic evaluation. Foot Ankle Int 27:97–103, 2006.
79. San Giovanni T, Keblish DJ, Thomas WH, Wilson MG: Eight-year results of a minimally constrained total ankle arthroplasty. Foot Ankle Int 27:418–426, 2006.
80. Su EP, Kahn B, Figgie MP: Total ankle replacement in patients with rheumatoid arthritis. Clin Orthop Relat Res (424):32–38, 2004.
81. Takakura Y, Tanaka Y, Kumai T, Sugimoto K, Ohgushi H: Ankle arthroplasty using three generations of metal and ceramic prostheses. Clin Orthop Relat Res (424):130–136, 2004.
82. Tanaka Y, Takakura Y: The TNK ankle: Short- and mid-term results. Orthopade 35:546–551, 2006.
83. Valderrabano V, Nigg BM, von Tscharner V, Frank CB, Hintermann B: Total ankle replacement in ankle osteoarthritis: An analysis of muscle rehabilitation. Foot Ankle Int 28:281–291, 2007.
84. Wood PL, Deakin S: Total ankle replacement. The results in 200 ankles. J Bone Joint Surg Br 85:334–341, 2003.
85. Haddad S, Coetzee JC, Estok R, Fahrbach K, Banel D, Nalysnyk L: Intermediate and long-term outcomes of total ankle arthroplasty and ankle arthrodesis. A systematic review of the literature. J Bone Joint Surg Am 89:1899–1905, 2007.
86. Bolton-Maggs BG, Sudlow RA, Freeman MA: Total ankle arthroplasty. A long-term review of the London Hospital experience. J Bone Joint Surg Br 67:785–790, 1985.
87. Kitaoka HB, Patzer GL, Ilstrup DM, Wallrichs SL: Survivorship analysis of the Mayo total ankle arthroplasty. J Bone Joint Surg Am 76:974–979, 1994.
88. McGuire MR, Kyle RF, Gustilo RB, Premer RF: Comparative analysis of ankle arthroplasty versus ankle arthrodesis. Clin Orthop Relat Res (226):174–181, 1988.
89. Newton SE 3rd: Total ankle arthroplasty. Clinical study of fifty cases. J Bone Joint Surg Am 64:104–111, 1982.
90. Stauffer RN: Salvage of painful total ankle arthroplasty. Clin Orthop Relat Res (170):184–188, 1982.
91. Stauffer RN, Segal NM: Total ankle arthroplasty: Four years' experience. Clin Orthop Relat Res (160):217–221, 1981.
92. Wynn AH, Wilde AH: Long-term follow-up of the Conaxial (Beck-Steffee) total ankle arthroplasty. Foot Ankle 13:303–306, 1992.
93. Groth HE, Fitch HF: Salvage procedures for complications of total ankle arthroplasty. Clin Orthop Relat Res (224):244–250, 1987.
94. Hopgood P, Kumar R, Wood P: Ankle arthrodesis for failed total ankle replacement. J Bone Joint Surg Br 88:1032–1038, 2006.
95. Kitaoka HB, Romness DW: Arthrodesis for failed ankle arthroplasty. J Arthroplasty 7:277–284, 1992.
96. Kotnis R, Pasapula C, Anwar F, Cooke PH, Sharp RJ.: The management of failed ankle replacement. J Bone Joint Surg Br 88:1039–1047, 2006.
97. Dyrby C, Chou LB, Andriacchi TP, Mann RA: Functional evaluation of the scandinavian total ankle replacement. Foot Ankle Int 25:377–381, 2004.
98. Soohoo N, Zingmond D, Ko C: Comparison of reoperation rates following ankle arthrodesis and total ankle arthroplasty. J Bone Joint Surg Am 89:2143–2149, 2007.
99. Kim C, Jamali A, Tontz W Jr, Convery FR, Brage ME, Bugbee W: Treatment of post-traumatic ankle arthrosis with bipolar tibiotalar osteochondral shell allografts. Foot Ankle Int 23:1091–1102, 2002.
100. Meehan R, McFarlin S, Bugbee W, Brage M: Fresh ankle osteochondral allograft transplantation for tibiotalar joint arthritis. Foot Ankle Int 26:793–802, 2005.
101. Van Valburg AA, van Roermund PM, Marijnissen AC, van Melkebeek J, Lammens J, et al: Joint distraction in treatment of osteoarthritis: A two-year follow-up of the ankle. Osteoarthritis Cartilage 7:474–479, 1999.
102. van Valburg AA, van Roermund PM, Marijnissen AC, Wenting MJ, Verbout AJ, Lafeber FP, Bijlsma JW: Joint distraction in treatment of osteoarthritis (II): Effects on cartilage in a canine model. Osteoarthritis Cartilage 8:1–8, 2000.
103. van Valburg AA, van Roermund PM, Lammens J, van Melkebeek J, Verbout AJ, et al: Can Ilizarov joint distraction delay the need for an arthrodesis of the ankle? A preliminary report. J Bone Joint Surg Br 77:720–725, 1995.

104. van Roermund PM, Lafeber FP: Joint distraction as treatment for ankle osteoarthritis. Instr Course Lect 48:249–254, 1999.

105. Marijnissen AC, van Roermund PM, van Melkebeek J, Schenk W, Verbout AJ, et al: Clinical benefit of joint distraction in the treatment of severe osteoarthritis of the ankle: Proof of concept in an open prospective study and in a randomized controlled study. Arthritis Rheum 46:2893–2902, 2002.

106. Ploegmakers J, van Roermund PM, van Melkebeek J, Lammens J, Bijlsma JW, et al: Prolonged clinical benefit from joint distraction in the treatment of ankle osteoarthritis. Osteoarthritis Cartilage 13:582–588, 2005.

107. Acevedo JI, Myerson M: Reconstructive alternatives for ankle arthritis. Foot Ankle Clin 4:409–430, 1999.

What Is the Best Treatment for Ankle Osteochondral Lesions?

Victor Valderrabano, MD, PhD and André Leumann, MD

Osteochondral lesions (OCLs) are focal articular injuries of the subchondral bone and the cartilage with a multifaceted cause (trauma, ligament instability, ischemic necrosis, malalignment, endocrine diseases, and others). The knee and the ankle joint are the most commonly involved joints for OCLs in the lower extremity. In the ankle joint, OCLs are mostly seen in the talus, at the posteromedial and anterolateral talar dome, closely related to the top of the curvature. Talus OCLs most often affect sports active young individuals and becomes symptomatic through persistent pain, joint swelling, and sometimes blocking of the joint. OCLs are known to have a significant impact on patients' quality of life and sports activity, or even their sports careers. In recent years, diagnosis of OCL increased substantially with the widespread use of modern diagnostic tools, such as computed tomography (CT), arthrocomputer tomography, magnetic resonance imaging (MRI), single-photon emission computed tomography (SPECT)-CT, and other tools. With improved diagnostics, treatment options also changed. Currently, ankle arthroscopy allows beside direct diagnostic visualization and palpable assessment, as well as simultaneous minimally invasive osteochondral treatment (debridement, drilling, microfracturing, and others). Based on the severity and location of the disease, open surgery and extensive techniques might be applied (mosaicplasty, autologous chondrocytes implantation, and others). Despite the large number of publications (Level II-IV evidence), to date, no strong evidences and guidelines are available in the literature. The orthopedic surgeon has to choose the treatment of choice based on different variables, such as age, size, location of the OCLs, and other factors.

DEFINITION, STAGING, CLINICS

OCLs are articular injuries of the subchondral bone and the overlaying cartilage. Because of the still unclear natural history of OCLs, several terms can be found for this entity to date in the literature, for example, osteochondritis dissecans, osteochondral fracture, flake fracture, and others. Because currently there is no proof for an underlying inflammation, the traditional term osteochondritis dissecans introduced by König[1] in 1888 should be abandoned. Furthermore, the term transchondral/osteochondral/flake fracture may be meaningful only in traumatic cases. To include all these causes and others, for example, idiopathic osteonecrosis, the term osteochondral lesions (OCLs) provides the most cautious terminology.

The traditional staging system for OCLs of the talus is the Berndt and Harty[2] classification based on radiographic findings. This classification consists of the following stages of an osteochondral talus fragment: stage I, small compression area; stage II, incomplete avulsion of a fragment; stage III, complete avulsion without displacement; and stage IV, avulsed fragment displaced within the joint. The Berndt and Harty classification has the advantage of being popular, but it does not accurately reflect the integrity of the articular cartilage. The Ferkel and Sgaglione[3] classification is a CT-based classification describing fragmentation, osteonecrosis, and cyst formations (stage I-IV). Anderson and colleagues[4] described an MRI-based classification including the bone marrow edema. Last, a commonly used arthroscopic classification is the OCL classification of the International Cartilage Repair Society.[5]

Epidemiologically, the ankle registers 4% of all the human osteochondral defects.[6] The cause of OCLs of the talus has multiple facets. However, it can be subdivided into a traumatic and nontraumatic cause. Trauma plays the most important role in the pathomechanism of talus OCLs. Overall, more than 80% of the talus OCLs are of traumatic origin.[7,8] In such traumatic cases, the acute OCLs are frequently located on the lateral dome of the talus (anterolateral) (Table 71–1). Hereby, the most common reasons are a severe inversion ankle sprain, chronic ankle instability (CAI; causing in 5–9% of the cases a lateral talar OCL),[9,10] or a fracture mechanism. However, medial lesions are more common than lateral OCLs. In these cases, the most affected area is the posteromedial talar dome (see Table 71–1). On the basis of repetitive microtraumas, avascular necrosis, genetics, endocrinic reasons, or systemic reasons, the nontraumatic causative agent with osteonecrosis represents to date still an unclear pathomechanism of chronic OCLs (longer than 2 months). Here, one should be alert on not missing a radiologically correlating hindfoot malalignment (hindfoot varus or valgus) that could explain the overload on the painful OCL joint region. In many cases, a causative agent cannot be traced and remains "idiopathic."

TABLE 71–1. Characteristics of Lateral and Medial Osteochondral Lesions of the Talus

CHARACTERISTICS	LATERAL TALUS OCL	MEDIAL TALUS OCL	REFERENCES
Traumatic causative factor	100%	64%	Canale and Kelly[66]
	98%	70%	Flick and Gould[16]
Location	43% lateral anterolateral	57% medial posteromedial	Berndt and Harty[2] Canale and Belding[18]
Depth	Deep	Shallow	Schachter et al.[13]
Shape	Wafer shaped	Egg shaped	Schachter et al.[13]
Displacement	Usually nondisplaced	Usually displaced	Schachter et al.[13]

OCL, osteochondral lesions.

An untreated OCL represents a local osteoarthritis model because of the altered joint biomechanics. Hereby, a traumatic osteochondral defect (flake fracture) or pathologic chronic shear forces (CAI[11]) cause damage of the superficial layer of the cartilage, and with time deep cracks and degeneration of the cartilage. Subsequently, joint fluid pumps into the subchondral bone and creates painful cysts and large-area cartilage lifting. At the end, OCL fragments can break off and dislocate all over the joint.

Patients with OCLs of the talus typically report chronic ankle pain, joint stiffness, ankle swelling, snapping, giving way, and weakness. The patients, usually of young age (mean age in a meta-analysis on 734 patients, 26.9 years),[12] are substantially limited in their daily life, in their sports activities, and have a reduced sports level. Many of them lose their sports career or even jobs by disability.

Clinical examination should document patient history and include physical examination. Patients may report ankle sprain or CAI. Other predisposing factors may be a periarticular fracture or severe ankle trauma. Patient history should further include systemic risk factors, as causative factors of avascular necrosis, systemic diseases, and others. Clinically, OCL ankle joints show, in almost all cases, a swelling and effusion. Tenderness may be triggered on the affected ankle side (lateral, medial) or periarticular. Regarding the ligament instability, one may find pathologic signs for lateral ankle instability (anterior drawer test, inversion tilt test), medial ankle instability (eversion tilt test), or a combination of both (rotational ankle instability). Furthermore, hindfoot malalignment (hindfoot varus or valgus) and foot deformity (pes planovalgus, cavovarus, etc.) should be checked.

The diagnostics of OCLs of the talus include first conventional weight-bearing radiographs of the ankle joint, anteroposteriorly and laterally. Radiographs provide information on the OCL location and stage only if the x-rays hit the OCL perpendicular, that is, if the OCL lies on the highest point of the talar dome. Radiographs further provide information on possible osseous predisposition for CAI, which represents a possible causative factor of OCL in the ankle joint.

With CT, the stages described by Berndt and Harty can be better defined, OCL cysts and fragments better visualized, and the integrity of the subchondral bone better analyzed. The CT scan is therefore a valuable diagnostic for preoperative planning. MRI provides complementary information, for example, the status of the OCL overlaying cartilage, information on bony edema, and the situation of the ligaments. Scintigraphy showed to be useful in evaluating OCLs when radiographs appear to be normal.[4,13] Addressing the lack of anatomic accuracy of the classic scintigraphy, a new diagnostic tool for OCLs emerged: the SPECT-CT. The SPECT-CT combines data of the scintigraphy and CT scan and fuses it to one picture: SPECT providing the activity and metabolic rate of the OCL surrounding bone, and the CT the precise anatomic localization (Fig. 71–1). Lastly, diagnostic ankle arthroscopy remains a reliable diagnostic tool, allowing direct and dynamic examination of the talus OCLs and the ankle-stabilizing ligaments.[14]

TREATMENT OPTIONS

The conservative treatment of OCLs of the talus is limited for stages I and II only. Success rates for nonoperative treatment with sports restriction and nonsteroidal anti-inflammatory drug or cast immobilization differ from 0% to 100% (review article[12]). A meta-analysis on 201 patients proved a 45% success rate of conservative treatment for stages I and II, as well as medial stage III talus OCLs.[15] Whereas acute lesions seem to do worse (0% success rates in acute transchondral fractures[16]), chronic lesions show different success rates between 41% (cast immobilization[12]) and 59% for restriction of activities, but free range of motion.[17,18] Young patients seem to do better with conservative treatment than aged patients. Bruns and Rosenbach[19] showed 85% excellent and good results in patients 16 years and younger in comparison with 65% in adults, with 8% failure in each group only (Level IV evidence).[19] These results are also confirmed by Higuera and coworkers (Level IV).[20] In long-term, persistent, radiologic irregularities were found in 38% (Level IV).[21] Shearer and coworkers[22] managed even high-grade cystic lesions nonsurgically (Level IV).[22] However, after 38 months of follow-up, 18% of patients had to be transferred to ankle arthrodesis.

In most of the conservatively treated OCL cases, the pain remains untreated and the disease advances to further stages. Berndt and Harty[2] reported in 1959

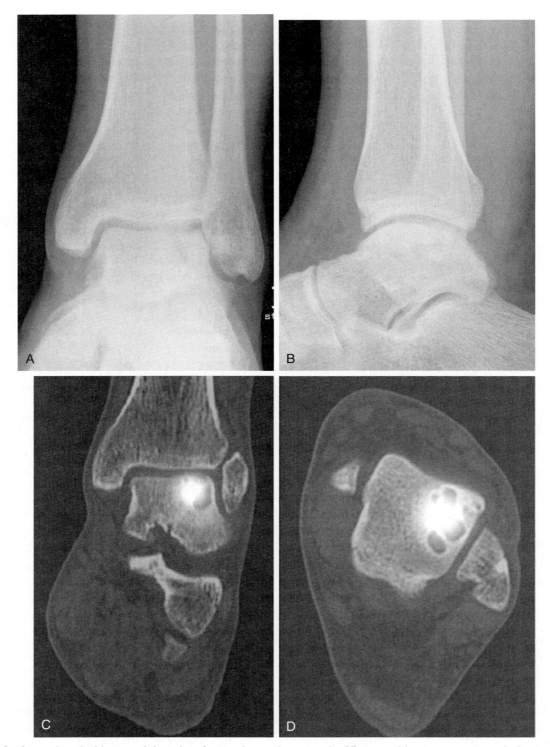

FIGURE 71–1. Osteochondral lesion of the talus. Series shows the case of a 25-years-old man, a sports and physically active patient, with chronic ankle pain, a lateral talus osteochondral lesion (OCL), and chronic ankle instability. Radiographs *(A, B)* showed a suspicious area on the lateral talar dome. Further diagnostic was performed using the single-photon emission computed tomography-computed tomography (SPECT-CT; combination of scintigraphy and CT) *(C–E).*

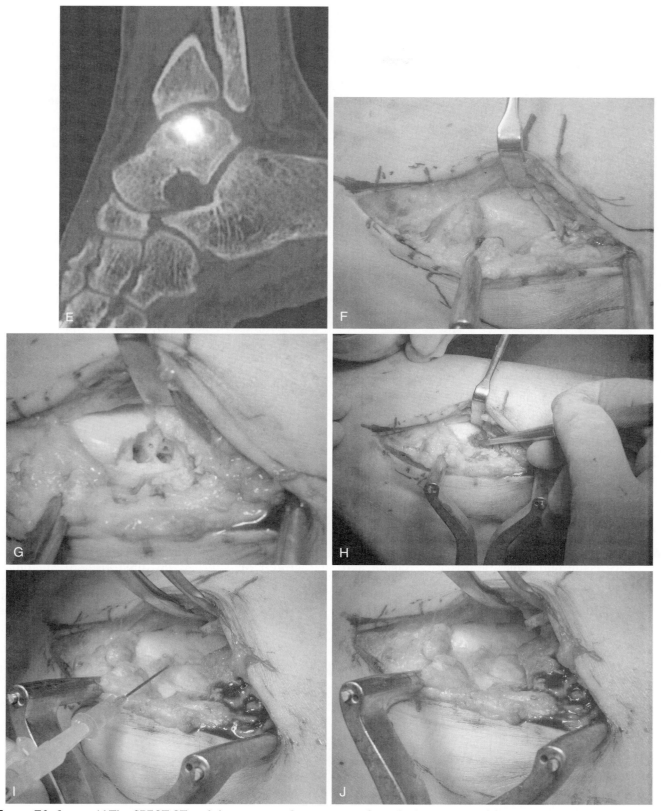

Figure 71–1. *cont'd* The SPECT-CT and diagnostic arthroscopy confirmed a lateral talus OCL stage III-IV with cystic lesions *(C–F). (C–F,* if in color, the SPECT-CT would have a red spot over the OCL) Therapy consisted of debridement, microfracturing *(G),* autologous bone transplantation *(H),* and treatment by "autologous matrix-induced chondrogenesis" (AMIC; bilayer collagen membrane; Geistlich Pharma AG, Wolhusen, Switzerland) *(I, J).* Further surgical treatment included the elimination of the OCL risk factor, chronic ankle instability, by lateral and medial ligament repair. About 6 months after osteochondral reconstruction, the patient is pain free, has an excellent function, and is back to daily life (job, sports).

that nonoperatively treated patients obtained poor results, and that good results were registered in 84% of the cases after surgical treatment (Level IV). Surgical treatment of OCLs traditionally includes excision of loose bodies, debridement of the area, and drilling or microfracturing. This surgery may be performed open or arthroscopically. The arthrotomy may sometimes require a medial or lateral malleolar osteotomy, grooving of the anteromedial distal tibia, or an osteotomy of the anterolateral tibia to reach the involved OCL talus region. As an alternative or as an addition to the open technique, ankle arthroscopy allows, beside a good diagnostic visualization of the OCLs, a minimal invasive therapy avoiding the high morbidity of an extensive arthrotomy or malleolar osteotomy. The treatment of OCLs of the talus includes a primary (as fixation of a flake fracture in traumatic cases) or a secondary repair (surgical treatment of chronic OCLs). The different options for secondary repairs depend on whether the OCL is predominantly a problem of the chondral layer, the osseous part, or a combination of both, on the age of the patient and the size of the OCL (Tables 71–2 and 71–3).

Primary Fixation of Acute Osteochondral Lesions

In case of an osteochondral fracture of the talus, the fragment can be fixed by low-profile screws, bioabsorbable materials, or other methods, for example, cortical bone peg fixation (89% success rate)[23] or fibrin fixation (75% success rate).[24] With this therapy, about 73% of the patients reach a satisfactory result[12,23] (all evidence Level IV).

Debridement, Abrasion

With the debridement, the surgeon removes the necrotic tissue and loose bodies by excision and curettage. Excision and curettage (76% overall success rate) in combination show better results than excision alone (38% overall success rate).[12] With

the simultaneous lavage, catabolic enzymes and inflammation mediators are also removed. This surgical option is adequate only for small OCL and gives only good results on a short-term basis. Hereby, arthroscopic results seem to be slightly better in comparison with open procedures[12,25,26] (all Level IV evidence). Surprisingly, the only Level of Evidence II study on OCL treatment, reported by Gobbi and coauthors,[27] describes arthroscopic excision and shaving to show no significant difference to microfracture and osteochondral autograft transfer system (OATS) in 33 patients after 12 and 24 months.

Retrograde Drilling

Retrograde drilling is reserved for stage I and II of the talus OCLs. Hereby, the sclerotic subchondral bone of the OCL cysts are minimally invasive opened up and filled with autologous spongiotic bone (as, for example, from the iliac crest) or osteoinductive and osteoconductive materials. This technique allows an ingrowing of marrow cells and blood vessels to build a healthy, stable subchondral bone and overlying fibrocartilaginous tissue. Retrograde drilling showed an 81% success rate by drilling through the sinus tarsi (Level IV).[28]

Kono and researchers[29] showed that in Pritsch O or I classified OCL (grade O: cartilage layer intact; grade I: cartilage soft, but stable in place), retrograde drilling reaches significantly better results than transmalleolar (anterograde) drilling (Level III).

Microfracturing

With microfracturing, the sclerotic subchondral bone is removed and the OCL area is multiply microfractured or alternatively microdrilled. Steadman and colleagues[30] first described the technique of microfracturing. Through the created bony holes, bone-marrow stem cells are expected to nest on the

---

TABLE 71–2. Treatment Options for Osteochondral Lesions of the Talus with Tissue Repair Potential (Cartilage and Bone)

TECHNIQUE	CARTILAGE	BONE	PUBLICATION OF HIGHEST LEVEL OF EVIDENCE
Fragment refixation	++	++	Kumai et al.[23] (Level IV)
Debridement/curettage	+	+	Gobbi et al.[27] (Level II)
Microfracturing	+	+	Gobbi et al.[27] (Level II)
Drilling	+	++	Draper and Fallat[42] (Level III)
			Kono et al.[29] (Level III)
Osteochondral autologous transplantation system (OATS)/mosaicplasty	++	++	Gobbi et al.[27] (Level II)
			Draper and Fallat[42] (Level III)
Autologous chondrocyte implantation (ACI)	++	−	Whittaker et al.[58] (Level IV)
Matrix-associated autologous chondrocyte Implantation (MACI)	++	−	—
			Bartlett et al.[67] (Level II)
Autologous matrix-induced chondrocytogenesis (AMIC)	++	−	—
			Bartlett et al.[68] (Level IV)
Autologous cancellous bone grafting	−	++	Kolker et al.[64] (Level IV)
Retrograde drilling	−	++	Kono et al.[29] (Level III)

TABLE 71–3. Surgical Principles of Osteochondral Lesions of the Talus

	TECHNIQUE	REFERENCES
OCL Stage		
Berndt and Harty stages I and II	Retrograde drilling Microfracturing Chondral reconstruction (ACI, MACI, AMIC)	Kono et al.[29] Gobbi et al.[27] Whittaker et al.[58]

Berndt and Harty stages III and IV	OATS/Mosaicplasty
	Chondral and osseous reconstruction (ACI, MACI,
	   or AMIC with or without microfracturing or
	   bone grafting)
		Kreuz et al.[51]
		Gobbi et al.[27]
		Kolker et al.[64]
		Whittaker et al.[58]

OCL Size		
<1.5 cm^2	Retrograde drilling Microfracturing Debridement	Taranow et al.[28] Becher and Thermann[35] Robinson et al.[63]

>1.5 cm^2	OATS/Mosaicplasty
	Chondral and osseous reconstruction (ACI, MACI,
	   or AMIC with or without microfracturing or
	   bone grafting)
		Scranton et al.[43]
		Kolker et al.[64]
		Whittaker et al.[58]

Patient Age		
≤50 years	Chondral reconstruction (ACI, MACI, AMIC)	Koulalis et al.[59]
>50 years	Retrograde drilling Microfracturing TAR, ankle arthrodesis	Kumai et al.[37] Becher and Thermann[35]

ACI, autologous chondrocyte implantation; AMIC, autologous membrane-induced chondrogenesis; MACI, matrix-membrane autologous chondrocyte implantation; OATS, osteochondral autograft transfer system; OCL, osteochondral lesions; TAR, total ankle replacement.

fibrin clot in the OCL defect and develop into chondroblasts, chondrocytes, and fibroblast, which produce a nonhyaline fibrocartilaginous matrix. However, fibrocartilage is known to have a pathologic viscoelastic property.[31] One limitation of microfracturing is the use only for cartilage defect smaller than 1.5 cm^2 and with a maximal depth of 7 mm (see Table 71–3).[32]

Currently, microfracturing of the talus has demonstrated good or excellent results,[6,33] with success rates of 77% to 96%[34,35] (all Level IV evidence). Saxena and Eakin[34] showed a significant shorter recovery time for microfracture in comparison with autogenous bone grafting (Level IV). Becher and Thermann[35] showed that after microfracturing in follow-up arthroscopies, the cartilage cannot be distinguished from the surrounding cartilage (Level IV).

Anterograde drilling, arthroscopically, percutaneous, or transmalleolar performed, shows in combination with excision and curettage better results than excision and curettage alone[7,16,36–40] (all Level IV), with success rates in a meta-analysis of 76% and 87%, respectively.[12] Angermann and Jensen[25] found in a follow-up of 9 to 15 years that only 1 of 18 patients had new signs of osteoarthritis (Level IV).

Osteochondral Autograft Transfer System

The OATS or mosaicplasty technique is based on harvesting full-thickness osteochondral grafts from a donor site such as the lateral supracondylar or the intercondylar notch area of the femur. This technique is indicated for grades III and IV of substantially large OCL defects of the talus. The reported results are believed to be good to excellent (Level IV).[41] However, the donor-site morbidity of knee-to-talus mosaicplasty is not negligible, and the cartilage properties of knee and talus are known to not biomechanically and biochemically match together.[6] Furthermore, with OATS, the precise restoration of the curvature and congruency of the talus is technically demanding. Gobbi and coauthors[27] (Level II) and Draper and Fallat[42] (Level III) showed that OATS and microfracturing/drilling show no significant differences in follow-up. Success rates of 89 to 100% are published (all Level IV).[43–50] Kreuz and investigators[51] showed that OATS offers a successful opportunity in OCL revisions (Level IV). Only recently were concerns about donor-site morbidity reported.[52]

Osteochondral Allograft Transplantation

The transplantation of an osteochondral allograft is indicated for large OCLs of the talus. In a long-term prospective study, Gross and colleagues[53] confirmed the value of fresh osteochondral allografts to reconstruct articular defects of joints in young active patients (knee joint study; Level II; success rate of 85% for femur and 80% for tibial plateau). Unlike for the knee, few reports are available for osteochondral allograft talus reconstruction in the literature (all evidence Level IV).[54–56] Gross and colleagues[54] report a 66% survivorship rate of talus osteochondral allografts after 11 years (Level IV).

TABLE 71–4. Original Peer-Reviewed Articles in the Area of Osteochondral Lesions of the Talus

FIRST AUTHOR (YEAR OF PUBLICATION)	CASES (N)	TYPE OF OSTEOCHONDRAL DEFECT	INTERVENTION	MEAN FOLLOW-UP TIME (MO)	METHODS OF FOLLOW-UP	RESULTS GOOD AND EXCELLENT (%)	FAILURES (%)	CONCLUSION	STUDY TYPE	LEVEL OF EVIDENCE
Gobbi et al. (2006)[27]	33	Ferkel 2b, 3, 4	Chondroplasty vs. microfracture vs. OATS	53	MRI	NK	12	No significant differences after 12 and 24 months Persistent edema and chondral lesion in the MRI	Randomized controlled trial	2 (no blinded groups, only blinded radiologic analysis)
Kono et al. (2006)[29]	30	Modified Pritsch grade 0 and I	TMD (19) vs. RD (11)	12	Rearthroscopy	TMD 0, RD 27.2	TMD 42.1, RD 0	RD significantly better	Case-control study	3
Draper and Fallat (2000)[42]	31	Mixed	BG (14) vs. CD (17)	71.5	Clinical examination radiographs	BG 6.9 vs. CD 4.5 points	NK	BG significantly better	Case-control study	3
Alexander and Lichtman (1980)[62]	49	NK	DC	18–216	Clinical examination	44	2	Improvements after surgery for 18 months, stable long-term results	Case series	4
Kelberine and Frank (1999)[36]	48	Acute osteochondral fractures vs. chronic osteochondral defects	Removal, curettage, transchondral drilling, loose body fixation	60	X-ray	Acute: 91, chronic: 67	NK	Significantly better results for acute lesions; incomplete bony healing; mixture of interventions	Case series	4
Kumai et al. (1999)[37]	18	Intact cartilage layer	Arthroscopic transmalleolar drilling	55 (24–114)	X-ray	72	0	Age dependence of results	Case series	4
Taranow et al. (1999)[28]	16	NK	Retrograde drilling	24	MRI	NK	NK	Significantly improved results	Case series	4
Hangody et al. (2001)[46]	36	ICRS grade III and IV	Mosaicplasty (OATS) from the knee	24–84	X-ray, histology	94	0	No long-term donor-site morbidity	Case series	4
Al-Shaikh et al. (2002)[50]	19	NK	OATS from the knee	16	X-ray	89	0	2 with mild knee pain, good graft ingrowth in all cases	Case series	4
Kumai et al. (2002)[23]	27	Unstable fragment	Cortical bone peg fixation	84	X-ray	89	0	Radiologic improvement in 89%	Case series	4
Shearer et al. (2002)[22]	34	Cystic modified Berndt and Harty type V lesions	Nonsurgical management	38	X-ray	54	18	6 converted to surgery; stable lesion, mild signs of OA, no correlation of x-ray, clinical outcome and joint degeneration, clinically 54% improved significantly	Case series	4

Study	Classification	No.	Treatment	Follow-up (mo)	Assessment	%	No.	Results	Study design	Level
Lee et al. (2003)[45]	Berndt and Harty types III-IV	18	Mosaicplasty (OATS) from the knee	36	Rearthroscopy	100	0	Good results in rearthroscopy	Case series	4
Robinson et al. (2003)[63]	Anderson I-IV	65	Arthroscopic excision and curettage or drilling	42	X-ray	52	22	Curettage is better than drilling; medial cystic lesions with poor outcome	Case series	4
Kolker et al. (2004)[64]	Berndt and Harty types III-IV	13	Autologous bone grafting	51.9	X-ray, CT scan	46	46	31% converted to ankle arthrodesis	Case series	4
Baltzer and Arnold (2005)[49]	Berndt and Harty types III-IV and focal osteoarthritis	43	OATS from the knee	0-54	MRI, rearthroscopy	95	5	Good integration of the grafts	Prospective case series	4
Becher and Thermann (2005)[35]	Osteochondral defects vs. local osteoarthritis	30	Microfracture	24	MRI	83	0	Cartilage repair in MRI, no limitation to age	Case series	4
Whittaker et al. (2005)[58]	1.95 m²	10	Autologous chondrocyte implantation	23	Rearthroscopy	90	10	Filled defects, biopsies showing fibrocartilage with some hyaline-like cartilage	Case series	4
Baums et al. (2006)[48]	NK	12	OATS	63	MRI		8	Full return to sports achieved	Case series	4
Han et al. (2006)[65]	Osteochondral defects with vs. without subchondral cysts	38	Microfracture and or abrasion (arthroscopic)	24-36	X-ray	77	5	No significant differences, small cysts without influence on outcome	Case series	4
Kreuz et al. (2006)[51]	Berndt and Harty types III and IV after primary treatment	35	Mosaicplasty (OATS) from the talus	48.9	MRI	91	0	Recommended option for revisions	Case series	4
Scranton et al. (2006)[43]	Cystic modified Berndt and Harty type V lesions	50	OATS from the knee	36	Clinical examination	90	7	No morbidity for medial malleolar osteotomy, 1 with donor-site morbidity for 3 months	Case series	4
Reddy et al. (2007)[52]	NK Revisions after primary treatment	15	Mosaicplasty (OATS) from the knee	47	Clinical examination	47	13	Donor-site morbidity: poor outcome in 27%	Case series	4
Saxena and Eakin (2007)[34]	Hepple II-V	46	Microfracturing (Hepple II-IV) and autogenous bone grafting (Hepple V)	24-96	Clinical examination	96	0	ABG needs more time for return to activity than MF	Prospective case series	4

ABG, autologous bone grafting; BG, bone grafting; CD, curettage and drilling; CT, computed tomography; ICRS, International Cartilage Repair Society; MF, microfracture; MRI, magnetic resonance imaging; NK, not known; OA, osteoarthritis; OATS, osteochondral autologous transplantation system; RD, retrograde drilling; TMD, transmalleolar drilling.

Autologous Chondrocyte Implantation

The principle of autologous chondrocyte implantation (ACI) is based on harvesting of autologous chondrocytes (knee, talus, detached OCL fragment), culturing of the cells in vitro for 2 to 5 weeks, and finally reimplantation of the proliferated cells. This technique was first described in knee OCLs[57] and also is currently used in talus OCLs successfully.[32] Whittaker and coworkers[58] report 90% good and excellent results and in rearthroscopies lesions completely disappeared (Level IV). Koulalis and coauthors[59] even report success in 100% of cases (Level IV). The ACI can be implanted under a periosteal flap (ACI), in a matrix-membrane, or under a collagen membrane cover. These chondrocyte transplantation techniques are indicated in large defects of OCL stages III and IV with cystic formations or failed previous surgery (after debridement, drilling, etc.). The defect should be greater than 1.5 cm^2, and the age of the patients is limited to younger than 55 years.[6,60] Kissing talus-tibia lesions and osteoarthritis are contraindications for ACI. In cases of larger bone defects, ACI can be used together with debridement and bone grafting. In cases of hindfoot malalignment and CAI, additional surgeries (osteotomies, ligament repair, etc.) should be added at the time of ACI surgery for restoration of normal ankle biomechanics. The first mid-term results of ACI are promising (Level IV).[32] ACI techniques, however, produce hyaline-like cartilage only. Furthermore, the duration of recovery and the treatment costs are substantially longer and greater compared with other methods.

A new method for autologous chondrocyte regeneration is the so-called autologous membrane-induced chondrogenesis (AMIC; see Table 71–2; see Fig. 71–1). The AMIC technique is a one-stage procedure consisting of debridement, microfracturing, or drilling (without or with bone transplantation), and coverage of the treated area by a bilayer collagen membrane that is fixed to the site by fibrin glue (see Fig. 71–1).

SUMMARY

In summary, based on the diagnostic tools (x-ray, CT, MRI, scintigraphy, SPECT-CT, arthroscopy) specifically used in the different publications, currently, several classifications are available for talus OCLs. Because OCLs of the talus have multiple causative factors and still an unclear pathomechanism and natural history, no classification so far has managed to provide satisfactory evidence for a proper therapeutic principle and outcome prediction. Despite the large number of publications, the evidence for treatment of OCL of the talus is still poor. To our knowledge, no publication to date shows Level I evidence for specific treatments. Only few publications show Level II and III evidence (Table 71–4) with small cohorts and, therefore, low

scientific power. The majority of the articles published on talus OCL state Level IV evidence (see Table 71–4). Accurate description of the causative factor, size, location of OCL lesions, and exact treatment and after-treatment are not provided in the majority of the studies. The indications for nonoperative and operative treatment of OCL of the talus are still quite controversial. Only a few treatment tendencies do crystallize out. A few variables, such as stage, size, location, tissue involved (cartilage/bone), and chronicity of the OCL lesion, as well as the age of the patient, are decisive for the treatment of choice and best outcome (see Tables 71–2 and 71–3). Most of the authors and reports recommend as a first attempt nonoperative treatment with non–weight bearing or immobilization, or both; this provides good results in patients especially of young age and those with stage I and II talus OCLs. In case of lack of pain relief after 1 year of conservative treatment or in cases with stage III and IV talus, OCL surgical treatment is indicated. Hereby a few rules can be followed based on a few variables: involved tissue (cartilage, bone; see Table 71–2), as well as OCL stage, OCL size, and patient age (see Table 71–3).

GUIDELINES

Currently, few review articles provide the best guidelines for treatment of OCL of the talus.[12,13,15,61] Guidelines and algorithms are also presented yearly in symposia and instructional courses of several societies, such as American Foot and Ankle Society, American Academy of Orthopaedic Surgeons, ICRS, and others. The current valid guidelines are summarized in this chapter.

RECOMMENDATIONS

Based on the actual evidence of the literature and our own clinical experience, we recommend following the therapeutic principles described in this chapter, specifically in Tables 71–2 and 71–3. In general, early grades of OCL (stage I or II) may be treated by conservative treatment first; more severe grades of OCL (stage III or IV) or failures of conservatively managed stage I or II OCL need a surgical approach. Because the half-life of the published talus OCL articles is short, and new publications and treatment modifications emerge almost monthly, we recommend acquiring continuing education through high evidence level articles, systematic reviews, meta-analyses, and specific high-quality symposia and courses. Table 71–5 provides a summary of recommendations.

TABLE 71–5. Summary of Recommendations

STATEMENT	LEVEL OF EVIDENCE/GRADE OF RECOMMENDATION	REFERENCE
1. Conservative treatment of OCLs of the talus are restricted to stage I and II.	C	17, 18, 22, 30
2. No significant difference in outcome was found between excision and debridment, microfracturing and OATS.	B	27
3. Fragment refixation for acute transchondral fractures is recommended.	C	23
4. Therapies that address the cartilage in first line: ACI, MACI, AMIC, microfracturing, OATS.	B, C	27, 33, 58, 67, 68
5. Therapies that address the osseous level in first line: OATS, autologous bone grafting, retrograde drilling.	B	27, 29, 33, 42

REFERENCES

1. König F: On the presence of loose bodies in joints. Deutsche Zeitschrift für Chirurgie 27:90–109, 1888.
2. Berndt AL, Harty M: Transchondral fractures (osteochondritis dissecans) of the talus. J Bone Joint Surg Am 41-A:988–1020, 1959.
3. Ferkel RD, Sgaglione NA, DelPizzo W: Arthroscopic treatment of osteochondral lesions of the talus: Long-term results. Orthop Trans 14:172–173, 1990.
4. Anderson IF, Crichton KJ, Grattan-Smith T, et al: Osteochondral fractures of the dome of the talus. J Bone Joint Surg Am 71:1143–1152, 1989.
5. Mainil-Varlet P, Aigner T, Brittberg M, et al: Histological assessment of cartilage repair: A report by the Histology Endpoint Committee of the International Cartilage Repair Society (ICRS). J Bone Joint Surg Am 85-A(suppl 2):45–57, 2003.
6. Zengerink M, Szerb I, Hangody L, et al: Current concepts: Treatment of osteochondral ankle defects. Foot Ankle Clin 11:331–359, vi, 2006.
7. Pritsch M, Horoshovski H, Farine I: Arthroscopic treatment of osteochondral lesions of the talus. J Bone Joint Surg Am 68:862–865, 1986.
8. Chin TW, Mitra AK, Lim GH, et al: Arthroscopic treatment of osteochondral lesion of the talus. Ann Acad Med Singapore 25:236–240, 1996.
9. Bosien WR, Staples OS, Russell SW: Residual disability following acute ankle sprains. J Bone Joint Surg Am 37-A:1237–1243, 1955.
10. Lippert MJ, Hawe W, Bernett P: [Surgical therapy of fibular capsule-ligament rupture]. Sportverletz Sportschaden 3:6–13, 1989.
11. Schimmer RC, Dick W, Hintermann B: The role of ankle arthroscopy in the treatment strategies of osteochondritis dissecans lesions of the talus. Foot Ankle Int 22:895–900, 2001.
12. Verhagen RA, Struijs PA, Bossuyt PM, van Dijk CN: Systematic review of treatment strategies for osteochondral defects of the talar dome. Foot Ankle Clin 8:233–242, 2003.
13. Schachter AK, Chen AL, Reddy PD, Tejwani NC: Osteochondral lesions of the talus. J Am Acad Orthop Surg 13:152–158, 2005.
14. Hintermann B, Boss A, Schafer D: Arthroscopic findings in patients with chronic ankle instability. Am J Sports Med 30:402–409, 2002.
15. Tol JL, Struijs PA, Bossuyt PM, et al: Treatment strategies in osteochondral defects of the talar dome: A systematic review. Foot Ankle Int 21:119–126, 2000.
16. Flick AB, Gould N: Osteochondritis dissecans of the talus (transchondral fractures of the talus): Review of the literature and new surgical approach for medial dome lesions. Foot Ankle 5:165–185, 1985.
17. Huylebroek JF, Martens M, Simon JP: Transchondral talar dome fracture. Arch Orthop Trauma Surg 104:238–241, 1985.
18. Canale ST, Belding RH: Osteochondral lesions of the talus. J Bone Joint Surg Am 62:97–102, 1980.
19. Bruns J, Rosenbach B: Osteochondrosis dissecans of the talus. Comparison of results of surgical treatment in adolescents and adults. Arch Orthop Trauma Surg 112:23–27, 1992.
20. Higuera J, Laguna R, Peral M, et al: Osteochondritis dissecans of the talus during childhood and adolescence. J Pediatr Orthop 18:328–332, 1998.
21. Wester JU, Jensen IE, Rasmussen F, et al: Osteochondral lesions of the talar dome in children. A 24 (7-36) year follow-up of 13 cases. Acta Orthop Scand 65:110–112, 1994.
22. Shearer C, Loomer R, Clement D: Nonoperatively managed stage 5 osteochondral talar lesions. Foot Ankle Int 23:651–654, 2002.
23. Kumai T, Takakura Y, Kitada C, et al: Fixation of osteochondral lesions of the talus using cortical bone pegs. J Bone Joint Surg Br 84:369–374, 2002.
24. Angermann P, Riegels-Nielsen P: Fibrin fixation of osteochondral talar fracture. Acta Orthop Scand 61:551–553, 1990.
25. Angermann P, Jensen P: Osteochondritis dissecans of the talus: Long-term results of surgical treatment. Foot Ankle 10:161–163, 1989.
26. Ogilvie-Harris DJ, Sarrosa EA: Arthroscopic treatment after previous failed open surgery for osteochondritis dissecans of the talus. Arthroscopy 15:809–812, 1999.
27. Gobbi A, Francisco RA, Lubowitz JH, et al: Osteochondral lesions of the talus: Randomized controlled trial comparing chondroplasty, microfracture, and osteochondral autograft transplantation. Arthroscopy 22:1085–1092, 2006.
28. Taranow WS, Bisignani GA, Towers JD, Conti SF: Retrograde drilling of osteochondral lesions of the medial talar dome. Foot Ankle Int 20:474–480, 1999.
29. Kono M, Takao M, Naito K, et al: Retrograde drilling for osteochondral lesions of the talar dome. Am J Sports Med 34:1450–1456, 2006.
30. Steadman JR, Rodkey WG, Rodrigo JJ: Microfracture: Surgical technique and rehabilitation to treat chondral defects. Clin Orthop Relat Res (391 suppl):S362–S369, 2001.
31. Peterson L, Brittberg M, Kiviranta I, et al: Autologous chondrocyte transplantation. Biomechanics and long-term durability. Am J Sports Med 30:2–12, 2002.
32. Giannini S, Vannini F: Operative treatment of osteochondral lesions of the talar dome: Current concepts review. Foot Ankle Int 25:168–175, 2004.
33. Thermann H, Becher C: [Microfracture technique for treatment of osteochondral and degenerative chondral lesions of the talus. 2-year results of a prospective study]. Unfallchirurg 107:27–32, 2004.
34. Saxena A, Eakin C: Articular talar injuries in athletes: Results of microfracture and autogenous bone graft. Am J Sports Med 35:1680–1687, 2007.
35. Becher C, Thermann H: Results of microfracture in the treatment of articular cartilage defects of the talus. Foot Ankle Int 26:583–589, 2005.
36. Kelberine F, Frank A: Arthroscopic treatment of osteochondral lesions of the talar dome: A retrospective study of 48 cases. Arthroscopy 15:77–84, 1999.
37. Kumai T, Takakura Y, Higashiyama I, Tamai S: Arthroscopic drilling for the treatment of osteochondral lesions of the talus. J Bone Joint Surg Am 81:1229–1235, 1999.
38. Lahm A, Erggelet C, Steinwachs M, Reichelt A: Arthroscopic management of osteochondral lesions of the talus: Results of drilling and usefulness of magnetic resonance imaging before and after treatment. Arthroscopy 16:299–304, 2000.

39. Loomer R, Fisher C, Lloyd-Smith R, et al: Osteochondral lesions of the talus. Am J Sports Med 21:13–19, 1993.

40. Schuman L, Struijs PA, van Dijk CN: Arthroscopic treatment for osteochondral defects of the talus. Results at follow-up at 2 to 11 years. J Bone Joint Surg Br 84:364–368, 2002.

41. Hangody L, Kish G, Karpati Z, et al: Treatment of osteochondritis dissecans of the talus: Use of the mosaicplasty technique—a preliminary report. Foot Ankle Int 18:628–634, 1997.

42. Draper SD, Fallat LM: Autogenous bone grafting for the treatment of talar dome lesions. J Foot Ankle Surg 39:15–23, 2000.

43. Scranton PE Jr, Frey CC, Feder KS: Outcome of osteochondral autograft transplantation for type-V cystic osteochondral lesions of the talus. J Bone Joint Surg Br 88:614–619, 2006.

44. Sammarco GJ, Makwana NK: Treatment of talar osteochondral lesions using local osteochondral graft. Foot Ankle Int 23:693–698, 2002.

45. Lee CH, Chao KH, Huang GS, Wu SS: Osteochondral autografts for osteochondritis dissecans of the talus. Foot Ankle Int 24:815–822, 2003.

46. Hangody L, Kish G, Modis L, et al: Mosaicplasty for the treatment of osteochondritis dissecans of the talus: Two to seven year results in 36 patients. Foot Ankle Int 22:552–558, 2001.

47. Gautier E, Kolker D, Jakob RP: Treatment of cartilage defects of the talus by autologous osteochondral grafts. J Bone Joint Surg Br 84:237–244, 2002.

48. Baums MH, Heidrich G, Schultz W, et al: Autologous chondrocyte transplantation for treating cartilage defects of the talus. J Bone Joint Surg Am 88:303–308, 2006.

49. Baltzer AW, Arnold JP: Bone-cartilage transplantation from the ipsilateral knee for chondral lesions of the talus. Arthroscopy 21:159–166, 2005.

50. Al-Shaikh RA, Chou LB, Mann JA, et al: Autologous osteochondral grafting for talar cartilage defects. Foot Ankle Int 23:381–389, 2002.

51. Kreuz PC, Steinwachs M, Erggelet C, et al: Mosaicplasty with autogenous talar autograft for osteochondral lesions of the talus after failed primary arthroscopic management: A prospective study with a 4-year follow-up. Am J Sports Med 34:55–63, 2006.

52. Reddy S, Pedowitz DI, Parekh SG, et al: The morbidity associated with osteochondral harvest from asymptomatic knees for the treatment of osteochondral lesions of the talus. Am J Sports Med 35:80–85, 2007.

53. Gross AE, Shasha N, Aubin P: Long-term followup of the use of fresh osteochondral allografts for posttraumatic knee defects. Clin Orthop Relat Res (435):79–87, 2005.

54. Gross AE, Agnidis Z, Hutchison CR: Osteochondral defects of the talus treated with fresh osteochondral allograft transplantation. Foot Ankle Int 22:385–391, 2001.

55. Kim CW, Jamali A, Tontz W Jr, et al: Treatment of post-traumatic ankle arthrosis with bipolar tibiotalar osteochondral shell allografts. Foot Ankle Int 23:1091–1102, 2002.

56. Rodriguez EG, Hall JP, Smith RL, et al: Treatment of osteochondral lesions of the talus with cryopreserved talar allograft and ankle distraction with external fixation. Surg Technol Int 15:282–288, 2006.

57. Brittberg M, Lindahl A, Nilsson A, et al: Treatment of deep cartilage defects in the knee with autologous chondrocyte transplantation. N Engl J Med 331:889–895, 1994.

58. Whittaker JP, Smith G, Makwana N, et al: Early results of autologous chondrocyte implantation in the talus. J Bone Joint Surg Br 87:179–183, 2005.

59. Koulalis D, Schultz W, Heyden M: Autologous chondrocyte transplantation for osteochondritis dissecans of the talus. Clin Orthop Relat Res (395):186–192, 2002.

60. Martin JA, Buckwalter JA: Aging, articular cartilage chondrocyte senescence and osteoarthritis. Biogerontology 3:257–264, 2002.

61. Giannini S, Buda R, Faldini C, et al: Surgical treatment of osteochondral lesions of the talus in young active patients. J Bone Joint Surg Am 87(suppl 2):28–41, 2005.

62. Alexander AH, Lichtman DM: Surgical treatment of transchondral talar-dome fractures (osteochondritis dissecans). Long-term follow-up. J Bone Joint Surg Am 62:646–652, 1980.

63. Robinson DE, Winson IG, Harries WJ, Kelly AJ: Arthroscopic treatment of osteochondral lesions of the talus. J Bone Joint Surg Br 85:989–993, 2003.

64. Kolker D, Murray M, Wilson M: Osteochondral defects of the talus treated with autologous bone grafting. J Bone Joint Surg Br 86:521–526, 2004.

65. Han SH, Lee JW, Lee DY, Kang ES: Radiographic changes and clinical results of osteochondral defects of the talus with and without subchondral cysts. Foot Ankle Int 27:1109–1114, 2006.

66. Canale ST, Kelly FB Jr: Fractures of the neck of the talus. Long-term evaluation of seventy-one cases. J Bone Joint Surg Am 60:143–156, 1978.

67. Bartlett W, Skinner JA, Gooding CR, et al: Autologous chondrocyte implantation versus Matrix-induced autologous chondrocyte implantation for osteochondral defects of the knee: A prospective, randomized study. J Bone Joint Surg Br 87:640–645, 2005.

68. Bartlett W, Gooding CR, Carrington RW, et al: Autologous chondrocyte implantation at the knee using a bilayer collagen membrane with bone graft. A preliminary report. J Bone Joint Surg Br 87:330–332, 2005.

Chapter 72

What Is the Best Treatment for End-Stage Hallux Rigidus?

Johnny Tak-Choy Lau, MD, MSc, FRCSC

Hallux rigidus is the commonest form of osteoarthritis in the foot with an incidence of 1 in 40 adults older than 50 years, and it is the second commonest complaint of the great toe behind hallux valgus.[1–3]

Patients generally report pain and stiffness over the first metatarsophalangeal (MTP) joint. The pain is aggravated with walking, particularly during terminal heel rise in the gait cycle. They also describe a dorsal prominence over the joint that may cause mechanical symptoms from pressure against the top of the shoe. During clinical examination, a dorsal exostosis is generally present, and the overlying skin can be erythematous and tender secondary to local irritation. Physical examination reveals a restricted range of motion of the first MTP, particularly in dorsiflexion.

Radiographic evaluation reveals findings consistent with osteoarthritis, which includes joint space narrowing, osteophyte formation (particularly dorsally), subchondral cysts, and sclerosis. Hattrup and Johnson[4] developed a radiographic classification of hallux rigidus, which was divided into three grades. In grade I, mild-to-moderate osteophytes are present; however, there is preservation of the joint space. In grade II, there is moderate osteophyte formation with narrowing of the joint space and subchondral sclerosis. Grade III is characterized by marked osteophyte formation, loss of the joint space, and subchondral cysts may be present.

Initial treatment should constitute nonsurgical management that attempts to reduce the inflammation and restrict the painful movement through the first MTP joint. Nonsteroidal anti-inflammatory drugs can help to improve the synovitis of the joint and alleviate other inflammatory processes. Cautious use of intraarticular corticosteroid injections can also be considered. Shoe modifications such as a high toe box help reduce mechanical pressure over the dorsal prominence, whereas a rocker bottom sole or an extended rigid shank will reduce the painful dorsiflexion. Similar principles are applied utilizing a rigid insole or orthotic with a toe extension covering the first ray. Activity modification can also be recommended to the patient to minimize high-impact loading of the foot (e.g., running). However, once these measures have failed to provide any significant relief of symptoms, operative intervention should be offered.

SURGICAL TREATMENT

Noncomparative Studies (Case Series; Level IV)

Cheilectomy. A cheilectomy entails excision of the dorsal osteophyte together with a portion of the dorsal degenerative articular surface. It is recommended to remove up to a third of the articular surface with the goal to obtain a minimum of 70 degrees of dorsiflexion. Usually included with the procedure is the resection of any dorsal osteophytes off the proximal phalanx, debridement of the joint, loose body removal, and synovectomy.[5,6]

Cheilectomy has been shown to have good results in early stages of hallux rigidus.[4,7] Some authors have reported good clinical results for cheilectomy irrespective of radiographic grade.[4–6] No study exists that isolates the subset of patients with advanced hallux rigidus. The largest published series is reported by Coughlin and Shurnas[7] where 93 feet of all stages of hallux rigidus underwent a cheilectomy and were reviewed retrospectively, with an average follow-up period of 9.6 years. Of the nine feet that had end-stage radiographic changes, five did not respond to treatment and underwent arthrodesis at a mean of 6.9 years after cheilectomy.[7] Easley and coworkers[8] conducted a retrospective review of 68 feet of all stages treated with cheilectomy at an average follow-up period of 5 years. A 90% satisfaction rate was achieved in the entire group. Of the nine feet that remained symptomatic; eight of those had end-stage grade 3 changes. It was noted that all nine demonstrated pain at the midrange of the motion arc, which would be suggestive of more global and advanced degenerative changes in the hallux MTP joint. The authors conclude that this was a negative prognosticator after cheilectomy.[8] Based on these two Level IV studies, a cheilectomy cannot be recommended for treatment of end-stage hallux rigidus (grade C level of recommendation).

Keller Resection Arthroplasty. In 1904, Keller described a procedure that involved excision of a portion of the proximal phalanx of the hallux for the treatment of hallux valgus and associated osteoarthritis of the first MTP joint. Although this procedure decompresses the joint, excessive resection can lead to instability secondary to loss of both bone and soft-tissue restraints. Shortening of the great toe occurs, and the plantar aponeurosis is disrupted, which

473

impairs the windlass mechanism contributing to the decreased stability of the medial column. Commonly described complications include transfer metatarsalgia, weak push off, and a cock-up deformity of the toe, which has led many investigators to recommend this procedure for low-demand and older patients.[9,10]

When reviewing the results of the Keller arthroplasty, variable outcomes are found with few being prospective or comparative trials. No studies review the subset of younger or higher demand patients. In addition, many studies also include hallux valgus deformities and lack any uniformity on grading or outcome measures, particularly older studies. Love and coworkers[10] performed a prospective trial studying 75 feet in patients with hallux valgus and hallux rigidus. Inclusion criteria included age older than 50 years, symptomatic osteoarthritis of the first MTP joint, and relatively low demand as defined by occupation and lifestyle. No differentiation was reported in radiographic grade of the osteoarthritis present in the first MTP joint. Mean follow-up period was 31 months. The authors report that joint pain was alleviated in 40 of 44 patients with an overall satisfaction rate of 77%. No increased incidence of postoperative metatarsal callosities occurred. However, they report a cock-up deformity after surgery in 28 feet compared with 8 before surgery, as well as a slight decrease in first MTP joint motion after surgery.[10]

Biologic Interpositional Arthroplasty. Biologic interpositional arthroplasties have been described for treatment of severe hallux rigidus. The technique involves performing both a cheilectomy and proximal phalanx excision with insertion of a biologic interpositional spacer. Different donor tissues have been used that include the extensor hallucis brevis (EHB), gracilis, and plantaris tendons. The goal of this procedure is to maintain motion through the joint, and with requirement of less bone resection, stability of the joint is improved, thereby avoiding some of the complications related to a traditional Keller arthroplasty.

Hamilton and colleagues[12] performed a retrospective review on 30 patients with advanced hallux rigidus who were treated with an EHB tendon and capsular interpositional arthroplasty collected over 10 years. However, the follow-up time is unknown. Subjectively, 93.3% of patients reported that they would undergo the same procedure. The American Orthopaedic Foot and Ankle Society (AOFAS) pain scores improved from 23.2 points before surgery to 37.4 points after surgery, and the average dorsiflexion improved from 10 to 50 degrees. No patients described weakness in push off or lateral metatarsalgia, and no calluses were found underneath the metatarsal heads.[12] Kennedy and coworkers[13] retrospectively reviewed 18 patients (21 feet) over a mean follow-up period of 38 months who underwent capsular interpositional arthroplasty utilizing the EHB tendon. Eighteen of 21 feet were grade 3 radiographically, whereas the remainder were grade 2. All 18 patients had pain relief, whereas 17 reported they would have the same procedure repeated. The mean postoperative increase in dorsiflexion was 37

degrees. One patient reported transfer metatarsalgia. The authors[13] conclude that interpositional arthroplasty was indicated for treatment of advanced hallux rigidus, and the technique as described by Hamilton and colleagues[12] had reproducible outcomes. However, Lau and Daniels[1] used a similar technique and retrospectively reviewed a series of 11 patients with a mean follow-up period of 2 years. Ten of 11 patients were grade III radiographically, whereas the other patient was grade II. Patient satisfaction was 72.7%. However, weakness of the great toe was reported in 72.7% of patients, whereas 27.3% reported lateral metatarsalgia. The investigators conclude that interpositional arthroplasty should be considered a salvage procedure with less reliable results.[1]

Barca[14] reports on the use of the plantaris tendon as the biologic spacer that was combined with a 20- to 30-degree dorsal wedge osteotomy of the proximal phalanx. An articulated external fixator was used to maintain the diastasis of the joint. Barca retrospectively reviewed a series of 12 patients over a period of 21 months. All patients reported good or excellent results, and dorsiflexion was improved by an average of 44 degrees. Coughlin and Shurnas[15] used a gracilis tendon as a graft and retrospectively reviewed seven patients over an average of 42 months of follow-up. All seven patients rated their result as good or excellent with a mean increase in AOFAS scores from 46 to 86. Mean dorsiflexion improved from 9 to 34 degrees and all demonstrated good to excellent plantarflexion strength. Four patients did report mild metatarsalgia. The authors conclude that this technique gave excellent pain relief and reliable function of the hallux.[15]

Arthrodesis. Arthrodesis of the first MTP joint has been one of the mainstays of surgical treatment of severe hallux rigidus, particularly in the younger, more active population. This procedure eliminates the painful movement of the joint and provides a stable medial column for ambulation. However, it has not been without controversy. An arthrodesis has a prolonged recovery course compared with other procedures, and there are complications such as nonunion, progressive arthrosis of the interphalangeal joint, and lateral metatarsalgia.[16] The long-term success and the impact on the gait cycle have also been a concern.

Joint Preparation and Fixation Technique. Authors have debated on the methods to prepare the joint surfaces and stabilize the arthrodesis site. There are two popular methods to prepare the fusion site. The first method is using a cone reamer system where one reamer is used to create a convex surface at the base of the proximal phalanx whereas a reciprocal reamer leads to a concave surface on the metatarsal head. The second method of planar excision is simpler, where an oscillating saw can be used to create flat cancellous surfaces on either side of the joint that are then brought together. Various fixation techniques have been described; older studies have used wire suture, K-wires, or Steinmann pins, whereas more recent authors have used a dorsal plate, interfragmentary screws, or Herbert screws. Several biomechanical studies have compared both different methods of joint preparation and fixation techniques. Curtis and researchers[17] compared four fixation techniques: (1) planar excision with K-wire fixation, (2) planar excision and fixation with dorsal plate and screws, (3) planar excision and fixation with a single interfragmentary screw, and (4) cup and cone preparation and fixation with an interfragmentary screw. Their results revealed that the cup and cone group had greater stiffness and load to failure compared with all other groups. It was concluded that the cup and cone method of fusion provided the majority of the stability, whereas the method of fixation was secondary.[17] Politi and coauthors[18] compared the strength of five techniques of first MTP arthrodesis: (1) surface excision with a machined reaming and fixation with a 3.5-mm cortical interfragmentary lag screw, (2) surface excision with machined conical reaming and fixation with crossed K-wires, (3) surface excision with machined conical reaming and fixation with a 3.5-mm cortical lag screw and a four-hole dorsal miniplate, (4) surface excision with machined conical reaming and fixation with a four-hole dorsal miniplate and no lag screw, and (5) planar surface excision and fixation with a single oblique 3.5-mm interfragmentary cortical lag screw. The most stable technique found was the combination of the machined conical reaming and an oblique interfragmentary lag screw and dorsal plate, whereas the dorsal plate and K-wire fixation alone were the weakest.[18]

Clinical Outcomes. Clinical studies have shown high success rates with fusion using a variety of techniques. Goucher and Coughlin[19] prospectively evaluated 50 patients who underwent first MTP arthrodesis using dome-shaped reamers and a dorsal plate and crossed screws. Diagnoses included hallux rigidus, hallux valgus, rheumatoid arthritis, failure of prior first MTP procedures, hallux varus, and neuromuscular disorders. They achieved a 96% satisfaction rate and 92% union rate at an average of 16 months of follow-up. A significant improvement was found in AOFAS scores.[19] Flavin and colleagues[20] in a prospective study had similar results. Twelve first MTP arthrodeses were performed using cone reaming preparation and fixation with a dorsal plate with an average follow-up period of 18 months. Diagnoses included hallux valgus, hallux rigidus, and nonunion of a previous first MTP fusion. All patients showed evidence of radiographic union at 6 weeks and had significant increases in both AOFAS hallux and SF-36 (36-Item Short Form Health Survey) scores.[20] The literature has limitations because most series include a number of preoperative diagnoses besides hallux rigidus, mainly hallux valgus.

The absence of any prospective comparative clinical trials evaluating the different techniques of first MTP arthrodesis for the treatment of advanced hallux rigidus leads to uncertainty of ideal technique of first MTP arthrodesis (grade I recommendation for arthrodesis of the treatment of advanced or end-stage hallux).

Prosthetic Replacement Arthroplasty. Over the past several decades, prosthetic replacement arthroplasties have been developed for the treatment of severe hallux rigidus with the anticipation of not only pain relief but restoration of joint stability and motion.

Silastic Implants. Because of the success of silastic implants in the hand, they were adapted for the first MTP joint. This led to the development of a double-stemmed implant, which allowed the implant to act as a dynamic spacer and, as a result, maintain joint space and motion. Although clinical studies showed good clinical satisfaction, there was concern about the longevity of the prosthesis. In a prospective study, Cracchiolo and coworkers[21] observed 66 patients over an average of 5.8 years. Subjectively, 83% of the patients were satisfied while the average range of motion was 42 degrees. However, radiographically, the implant did not fare as well. Osteophyte formation was present in 23 patients, and of those, 12 had nearly 50% articular space encroachment. Radiographic cysts were noted in 35% of the patients, and eight implant fractures were identified.[21] The area of concern for implant failure was at the hinged portion of the prosthesis, which was subjected to high shear forces at the joint. Titanium grommets were added to protect this area and increase durability of the implants. In a retrospective review, Swanson and de Groot[22] retrospectively report on 90 implants; all patients were clinically improved, and no implant fractures were identified. Sebold and Cracchiolo[23] also retrospectively reviewed a series of 47 feet that received a silicone implant with titanium grommets over an average follow-up period of 51 months. Thirty of 47 patients were completely satisfied with no radiographic evidence of implant fracture, although 5 feet had radiolucencies around the implant, and subsidence was noted in 15 feet. This was compared with a similar group of patients who had been treated with hinged implants, and it was noted that 30 of 41 feet had evidence of radiolucencies around the implant with two implant fractures. It was concluded that the titanium grommets appeared to protect the silicone implant and may help improve its longevity.[23] Despite the modification with titanium grommets, the use of silicone implants remains controversial, in particular, with the potential complications of silicone debris. The silicone particles can cause a foreign body reaction that leads to synovitis and potential bone erosion. Systemic effects are also a concern because silicone microfragments invade the lymphoreticular system, and the long-term complications of this process have yet to be identified.[24]

Metallic Implants. With the success of the metallic hip and knee arthroplasty, similar implants were designed for the hallux. In a prospective trial, Pulavarti and colleagues[25] prospectively reviewed the results of 36 Bio-Action prostheses (Osteomed, Addison, Texas) a nonconstrained, uncemented implant, with a minimum follow-up period of 3 years. Diagnoses included hallux rigidus, hallux valgus with degenerative changes, failed hallux surgery, gouty arthritis, and rheumatoid arthritis. Results showed a significant improvement in dorsiflexion, MTP arc of motion, and Hallux MTP scale after surgery. Subjective satisfaction was rated as either excellent or good in 77.5% of patients. Two patients required revision surgery (resection arthroplasty and arthrodesis) after poor outcomes; however, the authors did not identify any obvious cause for the failures. Radiographic studies did reveal periprosthetic radiolucency and subsidence in 33% of the implants, although this did not affect functional outcome.[25] Fuhrmann and coauthors[26] prospectively reviewed the results of 43 ReFlexion (Osteomed, Addison, Texas) MTP endoprostheses with an average follow-up period of 3 years. The ReFlexion endoprosthesis is a modular, nonconstrained, porous-coated implant that allows for either cementless or cemented fixation. Thirty-two patients had painful end-stage hallux rigidus, whereas other diagnoses included failed resection arthroplasty, cheilectomy, and silicone implants. Because of poor bone stock, cement was used in 20 phalangeal components and 5 metatarsal components. Results revealed all patients reported significant reduction in pain levels with a visual analogue scale pain. AOFAS scores and passive dorsiflexion significantly improved after surgery. However, the main area of concern was a reduction of MTP joint stability. About 28% of patients had an increased dorsoplantar drawer test, and 16% had medial instability (2+) with the toe in a slight valgus position. Radiographically, 30% of patients had mild hallux valgus deformities, 9% had slight varus deformities, and 21% showed plantar subluxation of the phalangeal component. Radiolucent lines were evident in 23% of phalangeal components (35% cemented vs. 13% cemented) and 9% of metatarsal components (equal cemented vs. uncemented percentages).[26]

Hemiarthroplasty. Although hemiarthroplasties of the proximal phalanx for the treatment of hallux rigidus have been available in the past half century, they have not gained much popularity compared with other forms of surgical treatment. Correspondingly, the literature reveals few published studies on their outcomes. Advocates of metallic hemiarthroplasties believe that it avoids the high dorsal shear forces associated with arthroplasties involving the metatarsal heads and does not possess the inherent structural flaws of a silastic implant.[27,28]

Townley and Taranow[27] performed a long retrospective review of 279 patients treated with a metallic hemiarthroplasty of the proximal phalanx with a follow-up range from 8 months to 33 years. Indications for treatment included hallux rigidus ($n = 171$), rheumatoid arthritis ($n = 29$), and varying degrees of osteoarthritis associated with hallux valgus ($n = 79$). The authors report good or excellent results in 95% of patients. Only two patients with hallux rigidus were unsatisfied: one was complicated by an infection, whereas the other received an oversized implant. The remainder of failures occurred in eight of the patients with hallux valgus and three with rheumatoid arthritis. Only one case of clinical or radiographic evidence of loosening was reported, which

occurred in a patient with rheumatoid arthritis with poor bone quality.[27] Taranow and coworkers[28] retrospectively reviewed 28 patients who received metallic hemiarthroplasties for severe hallux rigidus over an average follow-up period of 33 months. Twenty-three of 28 patients were completely satisfied, 3 were satisfied with reservations, and 2 were dissatisfied. Radiographically, four implants were inserted in a dorsiflexed position, which was demonstrated on postoperative radiographs, and three of these showed evidence of subsidence and loosening. No other cases of loosening or progressive deformities were reported. Two patients demonstrated mild recurrence of osteophytes, but this did not correlate with patient satisfaction. The authors conclude that technical errors likely contributed to radiographic loosening.[28] However, not all results have been positive. Kondel and Menger[29] retrospectively reviewed 10 patients (13 feet) who underwent a titanium hemiarthroplasty for grade II or III hallux rigidus. Follow-up ranged from 37 to 105 months. Eleven of 13 toes had absent or mild pain. However, all implants had evidence of varying degrees of radiolucencies and subsidence. One implant was removed and underwent interpositional arthroplasty after fracture and painful nonunion.[29]

Comparative Studies

Keller Arthroplasty versus Arthrodesis. O'Doherty and coauthors[30] report a prospective randomized trial comparing Keller's arthroplasty and arthrodesis of the first MTP joint for the treatment of both hallux valgus and rigidus in 110 feet with a minimum follow-up period of 2 years. The inclusion criteria were age older than 45 years, with a mean of 60.5 years. They report similar results among the two groups with a satisfactory or excellent result in 98% who underwent a Keller arthroplasty compared with 95% in the arthrodesis group. No significant difference was found between the groups in the incidence of postoperative transfer metatarsalgia or cock-up deformity. However, the incidence rate of nonunion in the arthrodesis group was extremely high at 44%. The majority of patients were asymptomatic, with only 4 of 22 requiring revision. The authors attributed this to the wire suture and K-wire fixation technique, which was a poor biomechanical construct.[30]

Arthrodesis versus Total Joint Replacement. Gibson and Thomson[31] performed a prospective, randomized, controlled trial comparing arthrodesis versus total replacement arthroplasty for hallux rigidus. Sixty-three patients (77 feet) were randomized to either arthrodesis (22 patients, 38 toes) or a BioMet, uncemented total joint arthroplasty (27 patients, 39 toes). Patient mean age was 55 (range, 34–77) years. Arthrodesis was performed using planar excision preparation and metal cerclage wire and K-wire for fixation; all arthroplasties were uncemented. Results revealed that all 38 arthrodeses united, although 7 acquired minor wound infections and 2 required extraction of the K-wire. In contrast, 6 of 39 arthroplasties required removal because of loosening of the phalangeal components. At 2 years, final range of active joint dorsiflexion was no greater than preoperative movement. Visual analogue pain scores revealed significant reduction in both groups. However, those who had an arthrodesis improved more than those in the arthroplasty group. More patients in the arthrodesis group preferred both their function result and the appearance of their toe after arthrodesis. At 2 years, only 3% of patients in the arthrodesis group would not have undergone the same surgery again compared with 40% in the arthroplasty group. The authors conclude that outcomes after arthrodesis were better than those after arthroplasty, and arthrodesis was clearly preferred by most patients.[31]

Arthrodesis versus Hemiarthroplasty. Raikin and coworkers[32] retrospectively reviewed a series of patients with severe hallux rigidus who were treated with either a metallic hemiarthroplasty or an arthrodesis. Twenty-one hemiarthroplasties with a mean follow-up period of 79 months were compared with 27 arthrodeses with a mean follow-up period of 30 months. The Biopro implant (Biopro, Port Huron, Michigan) was utilized for the hemiarthroplasties, whereas the arthrodesis technique involved planar excision with two obliquely oriented screws for fixation. Results revealed that all arthrodesis went on to unite within 12 weeks, and no revisions were required. Only two patients required screw removal for prominent hardware. Of the 21 hemiarthroplasties, 5 required revision surgery (1 was revised, 4 were converted to an arthrodesis), whereas eight that had survived showed evidence of plantar cutout of the prosthetic stem. Patients who underwent arthrodesis had significantly greater satisfaction rates, greater AOFAS hallux scores, and lower visual analogue pain scores compared with the hemiarthroplasty group. The authors conclude that arthrodesis was more predictable than hemiarthroplasty for alleviating symptoms and restoring function in patients with severe hallux rigidus.[32]

RECOMMENDATIONS

The best treatment for end-stage hallux rigidus remains controversial. The quality of the literature is poor because there are few prospective comparative studies, a lack of standardized outcome measures, few long-term studies, and most studies include other diagnoses beyond hallux rigidus.

Initial treatment of hallux rigidus should be nonoperative. Arthrodesis is the mainstay operative treatment for end-stage hallux rigidus. Conical reaming and fixation with a dorsal plate and interfragmentary screw is the strongest construct. A Keller resection arthroplasty is a viable option in older or lower demand patients; however, the complications of cock-up toe deformity and transfer metatarsalgia must be taken into consideration.

Cheilectomy cannot be recommended for treatment of end-stage hallux rigidus. Current total joint replacements have shown a high incidence of radiographic evidence of early loosening and wear. Because their longevity has not yet been established, it cannot be recommended at this time.

Hemiarthroplasty has shown some promise in long-term survivorship, but results overall have been variable. Biologic interpositional arthroplasty has not shown consistent, reliable results. There is insufficient evidence to allow for a recommendation for or against this treatment of end-stage hallux rigidus. Table 72–1 provides a summary of recommendations for the treatment of end-stage hallux rigidus.

TABLE 72–1. Summary of Recommendations

STATEMENT	GRADE OF RECOMMENDATION	LEVEL OF EVIDENCE	REFERENCES
1. Arthrodesis is the mainstay operative treatment for end-stage hallux rigidus.	B	II	19, 20, 30–32
2. Conical reaming and fixation with a dorsal plate and interfragmentary screw is the strongest construct for an arthrodesis.	B	II	17, 18
3. Keller resection arthroplasty is a viable option for older or lower demand patients.	B	II	10, 30
4. Cheilectomy cannot be recommended for treatment of end-stage hallux rigidus.	C	IV	5, 6
5. Total joint replacements have shown a high incidence of radiographic evidence of early loosening and wear cannot be recommended.	B	II	25, 26, 31
6. Hemiarthroplasty has shown inconsistent results.	I	IV	27–29, 32
7. Biologic interpositional arthroplasty has shown inconsistent results.	I	IV	1, 12–16

REFERENCES

1. Lau JT, Daniels TR: Outcomes following cheilectomy and interpositional arthroplasty in hallux rigidus. Foot Ankle Int 22:462–470, 2001.
2. Gould N, Schneider W, Ashikaga T: Epidemiological survey of foot problems in the continental United States: 1978-1979. Foot Ankle Int 1:8–10, 1980.
3. Coughlin MJ, Shurnas PS: Hallux Rigidus: Demographics, etiology, and radiographic assessment. Foot Ankle Int 24:731–743, 2003.
4. Hattrup SJ, Johnson KA: Subjective results of hallux rigidus following treatment with cheilectomy. Clin Orthop Related Res 226:182–191, 1988.
5. Mann RA, Clanton TO: Hallux rigidus: Treatment by cheilectomy. J Bone Joint Surg Am 70:400–406, 1988.
6. Feltham GT, Hanks SE, Marcus RE: Age-based outcomes of cheilectomy for the treatment of hallux rigidus. Foot Ankle Int 22:192–197, 2001.
7. Coughlin MJ, Shurnas PS: Hallux rigidus. Grading and long-term results of operative treatment. J Bone Joint Surg Am 85-A:2072–2088, 2003.
8. Easley ME, Davis WH, Anderson RB: Intermediate to long-term follow-up of medial-approach dorsal cheilectomy for hallux rigidus. Foot Ankle Int 20:147–152, 1999.
9. Henry AP, Waugh W, Wood H: The use of footprints in assessing the results of operations for hallux valgus: A comparison of Keller's operation and arthrodesis. J Bone Joint Surg Br 57:478–481, 1975.
10. Love TR, Whynot AS, Farine I, Lavoie M, Hunt L, Gross A: Keller arthroplasty: A prospective review. Foot Ankle 8:46–54, 1987.
11. Keiserman LS, Sammarco VJ, Sammarco GJ: Surgical treatment of hallux rigidus. Foot Ankle Clin N Am 10:75–96, 2005.
12. Hamilton W, O'Malley MJ, Thompson FM, Kovatis PE: Capsular interpositional arthroplasty for severe hallux rigidus. Foot Ankle Int 18:68–70, 1997.
13. Kennedy JG, Chow FY, Dines J, Gardner M, Bohne WH: Outcomes after interposition arthroplasty for treatment of hallux rigidus. Clin Orthop Relat Res 445:210–215, 2006.
14. Barca F: Tendon arthroplasty of the first metatarsophalangeal joint in hallux rigidus: Preliminary communication. Foot Ankle Int 18:222–228, 1997.
15. Coughlin MJ, Shurnas PS: Soft-tissue arthroplasty for hallux rigidus. Foot Ankle Int 24:661–672, 2003.
16. Brage ME, Ball ST: Surgical options for salvage of end-stage hallux rigidus. Foot Ankle Clin N Am 7:49–73, 2002.
17. Curtis MJ, Myerson M, Jinnah RH, Cox QG, Alexander I: Arthrodesis of the first metatarsophalangeal joint: A biomechanical study of internal fixation techniques. Foot Ankle 14:395–399, 1993.
18. Politi J, John H, Njus G, Bennett GL, Kay DB: First metatarsal-phalangeal joint arthrodesis: A biomechanical assessment of stability. Foot Ankle Int 24:332–337, 2003.
19. Goucher NR, Coughlin MJ: Hallux metatarsophalangeal joint arthrodesis using dome-shaped reamers and dorsal plate fixation: A prospective study. Foot Ankle Int 27:869–876, 2006.
20. Flavin R, Stephens MM: Arthrodesis of the first metatarsophalangeal joint using a dorsal titanium contoured plate. Foot Ankle Int 25:783–787, 2004.
21. Cracchiolo A 3rd, Weltmer JB Jr, Lian G, Dalseth T, Dorey F: Arthroplasty of the first metatarsophalangeal joint with a double-stem silicone implant. Results in patients who have degenerative joint disease, failure of previous operations, or rheumatoid arthritis. J Bone Joint Surg Am 74:552–563, 1992.
22. Swanson AB, de Groot SG: Use of grommets for flexible hinge implant arthroplasty of the great toe. Clin Orthop Relat Res 340:87–94, 1997.
23. Sebold EJ, Cracchiolo 3rd A: Use of titanium grommets in silicone implant arthroplasty of the hallux metatarsophalangeal joint. Foot Ankle Int 17:145–151, 1996.
24. Esway J, Conti SF: Joint replacement in the hallux metatarsophalangeal joint. Foot Ankle Clin N Am 10:97–115, 2005.
25. Pulavarti RS, McVie JL, Tulloch CJ: First metatarsophalangeal joint replacement using the Bio-Action great toe implant: Intermediate results. Foot Ankle Int 26:1033–1037, 2005.
26. Fuhrmann RA, Wagner A, Anders JO: First metatarsophalangeal joint replacement: The method of choice for end-stage hallux rigidus? Foot Ankle Clin N Am 8:711–721, 2003.
27. Townley CO, Taranow WS: A metallic hemiarthroplasty resurfacing prosthesis for the hallux metatarsophalangeal joint. Foot Ankle Int 15:575–580, 1994.
28. Taranow WS, Moutsatson MJ, Cooper JM: Contemporary approaches to Stage II and III hallux rigidus: The role of metallic hemiarthroplasty of the proximal phalanx. Foot Ankle Clin N Am 10:713–728, 2005.
29. Konkel KF, Menger AG: Mid-term results of titanium hemi-great toe implants. Foot Ankle Int 27:922–929, 2006.
30. O'Doherty DP, Lowrie IG, Magnussen PA, Gregg PJ: The management of the painful first metatarsophalangeal joint in the older patient. J Bone Joint Surg Br 72-B:839–842, 1990.
31. Gibson A, Thomson CE: Arthrodesis or total replacement arthroplasty for hallux rigidus. Foot Ankle Int 26:680–690, 2005.
32. Raikin SM, Ahmad J, Pour AE, Abidi N: Comparison of arthrodesis and metallic hemiarthroplasty of the hallux metatarsophalangeal joint. J Bone Joint Surg Am 89:1979–1985, 2007.

Chapter 73

What Is the Best Treatment for Hallux Valgus?

Mark E. Easley, MD, John S. Reach, Jr, MD, MSc, and Hans-Joerg Trnka, MD

Theories on the pathology and appropriate treatment of hallux valgus have been extensively described in the orthopedic literature. The wealth of information on the surgical management of hallux valgus has been molded into frequently taught treatment algorithms and principles. Although these algorithms and principles aim to provide consistency in treating symptomatic hallux valgus, the wide variety of approaches to treating hallux valgus suggests that they are far from commonly accepted. The purpose of this current concept review is to provide a balanced representation of current thinking on the pathomechanics, assessment, and treatment of hallux valgus. Orthopedic management of hallux valgus remains challenging. Despite the appeal of establishing universally accepted treatment protocols and algorithms, a critical review of the literature suggests that the surgeon treating hallux valgus deformity should individualize management to the particular patient.

HISTORY OF THE CONDITION AND OVERVIEW OF CAUSATIVE FACTORS

Bunion, a term evolving from the Latin word bunio, meaning "turnip," poorly defines the condition hallux valgus. To our knowledge, the first published reference to hallux valgus is by Carl Hueter in 1870.[1] Hallux valgus is commonly thought to develop because of unaccommodative shoe wear. Some support this conclusion,[2,3] but consistently sufficient evidence does not exist to confirm unaccommodative shoe wear as a causative factor in the development of hallux valgus. Conversely, the observation that many individuals do not experience development of hallux valgus despite wearing nonphysiologic shoe wear for many years implies that some individuals may have an incompletely defined predisposition to hallux valgus. Other studies report that hallux valgus develops in some unshod individuals, implying a congenital predisposition.[4–10] Hallux valgus in juveniles, adolescents, or male individuals whose feet have not been sub-

jected to shoes with narrow toe boxes supports a congenital predisposition. An association between hallux valgus and female sex is also suggested.[11,12] It has also been proposed that there is a familial predisposition to development of hallux valgus.[6,13–15] The exact cause leading to the development of a hallux valgus deformity remains unclear and may be multifactorial. However, as the bunion deformity tends to develop over time, it seems reasonable to conclude that repetitive forces applied to the first metatarsal phalangeal joint leads to hallux valgus.

CAUSATIVE FACTORS AND PATHOMECHANICS (PROPOSED THEORIES)

Anatomic Considerations

Patients without hallux valgus maintain physiologic alignment of the hallux metatarsophalangeal (MTP) joint with the following anatomic conditions: (1) congruent/symmetric alignment of the articular surfaces of the first proximal phalanx and the first metatarsal head during the repetitive joint loading associated with gait, (2) physiologic relation of the distal first metatarsal articular surface and the first metatarsal shaft axis, (3) stable balance of soft tissues about the first MTP joint, and (4) stable first tarsometatarsal (TMT) joint. Given that there is no muscular/tendinous attachment to the metatarsal head, any divergence from these physiologic factors predisposes a patient to hallux valgus.

Repetitively forcing the hallux into a valgus position, particularly with weight bearing and ambulation, is believed to eventually result in a valgus deformity at the first MTP joint. The summation of ground reactive forces and dynamic muscular forces eventually leads to attenuation of the medial joint capsule, contractures of the lateral joint capsule and adductor tendons, with a resultant medial deviation of the first metatarsal head ("bunion deformity").

Ground reactive forces may play a role in the gradual development of a hallux valgus deformity. The forefoot is subject to ground reactive forces equal to more than body weight with each step. If these forces are channeled through the plantar pulp of the hallux, the first MTP joint will move through a physiologic range of motion. However, if these forces are channeled through the plantar medial aspect of the hallux, then the structures restraining the medial

Much of this text, by the same authors, has been published in Foot and Ankle International as a two-part Current Concepts Review of hallux valgus (Easley ME, Trnka HJ: Current concepts review: Hallux valgus. Part 1: Pathomechanics, clinical assessment, and nonoperative management. Foot Ankle Int 28:654–659, 2007; and Easley ME, Trnka HJ: Current concepts review: Hallux valgus. Part II: Operative treatment. Foot Ankle Int 28:748–758, 2007). Reprinted with permission of Data Trace Publishing Company.

aspect of the first MTP joint will tend to become attenuated over time. In this model, anything that leads the hallux to accept weight bearing asymmetrically on the medial aspect of the hallux can predispose to hallux valgus. Restrictive shoe wear and hypermobility of the first ray are examples that may produce this situation.

Dynamic muscular forces across the first MTP joint may also contribute to the development of the hallux valgus deformity. If the medial dynamic structures, particularly the abductor hallucis, have their pull redirected plantarward, the force opposing the adductor hallucis is forfeited. The extensor hallucis longus and flexor hallucis longus gradually create a more lateral force across the joint, the plantar aponeurosis (windlass mechanism) is directed more laterally, and the flexor hallucis brevis forces also shift slightly more laterally. With these eccentric forces, the crista under the first metatarsal head fails to maintain proper tracking of the sesamoids. The resulting muscular forces across the first MTP joint function to deviate the hallux laterally.

Several factors have been reputed to be associated with the development of hallux valgus. These include: (1) pes planus, (2) hypermobility of the first TMT joint, (3) the relation and characteristics of the first metatarsal head and proximal phalanx, and (4) the condition of the medial capsule.

Pes Planus and Hallux Valgus

Pes planus may lead to hallux valgus because of increased forefoot abduction that creates a nonphysiologic load on the plantarmedial aspect of the great toe during heel rise. The association between pes planus and hallux valgus is controversial. Although some authors suggest that patients with pes planus have a greater tendency to experience development of hallux valgus than patients with maintained arches,[16–23] others fail to support this association.[14,24–26] The combination of conflicting reports and consistently Level III-V evidence provide insufficient evidence (grade I) to prove or disprove an association between pes planus and hallux valgus.

Hypermobility of the First Tarsometatarsal Joint

Mobility of the first TMT joint is observed in the sagittal and transverse plane.[27] The actual prevalence of medial column hypermobility continues to be controversial. It is theorized that hypermobility could lead to the development of hallux valgus in two ways. First, greater than physiologic dorsal subluxation of the first metatarsal could result in pes planus alignment, increased forefoot abduction, and a nonphysiologic load on the plantarmedial aspect of the great toe during heel rise. Second, greater than physiologic medial subluxation of the first metatarsal could result in increasing the 1-2 intermetatarsal angle (IMA), promoting metatarsus

primus varus. Some foot and ankle surgeons maintain that hypermobility of the first TMT joint or lack of stability of the foot's medial column contributes to the development of hallux valgus[28–32] and resultant pain,[33] a theory popularized by Morton.[9,34–37] Lapidus[38–40] supports this theory and suggests surgical correction with a first TMT joint arthrodesis. Although a convincing argument in theory, no evidence exists to support such a correlation, and in fact, other investigators have demonstrated that hypermobility of the first TMT joint is not directly associated with hallux valgus.[37,41–45] Insufficient evidence (Level III-V) exists to support or disprove the contribution of first TMT joint hypermobility to the development of hallux valgus (grade I).

Shape of the First Metatarsal Head

A "square" or flattened configuration of the MTP joint may resist valgus forces and limit development of hallux valgus; in contrast, a rounded, concentric relation of the MTP joint may predispose to hallux valgus if a valgus stress is consistently maintained on the hallux. To our knowledge, the contribution of metatarsal head configuration to the development of hallux valgus remains an observation; no evidence supports the association of metatarsal head configuration to hallux valgus.

Distal Metatarsal Articular Angle

Hallux valgus may exist with a congruent/symmetric relation between the first proximal phalanx and the first metatarsal head, suggesting a congenital predisposition in select patients with an increased distal metatarsal articular angle (DMAA).[46–48] Richardson and colleagues[49] note that the DMAA ranged from 6.3 to 18 degrees; as the angle increases, so does the propensity for hallux valgus, albeit congruent/symmetric. Coughlin[14] adds that the DMAA tends to be greater in patients with juvenile hallux valgus younger than 10 years when compared with those older than 10. Although Richardson and colleagues[49] suggest that the DMAA can be reliably determined radiographically, others have reported poor interobserver reliability.[50–52]

Medial Capsular Integrity

Uchiyama and investigators[53] demonstrate, in a cadaveric model, that feet with hallux valgus have a different organization of collagen fibrils than that observed in normal feet. These findings may be in response to abnormal stress repetitively applied to this part of the joint capsule. Alternatively, abnormal mechanical properties of the medial capsule such as those seen in patients with conditions such as rheumatoid arthritis may increase the propensity to develop hallux valgus.

CLINICAL MANIFESTATION/TYPICAL PRESENTATION

History Taking

Not all patients with hallux valgus are symptomatic. Besides an obvious cosmetic deformity, patients with symptomatic hallux valgus generally report pain exacerbated by shoe wear, particularly shoe wear with a narrow toe box. Frequently reported complaints include pain over the medial eminence and pain with first MTP joint motion. Pain may also be reported at the second MTP joint, under the second metatarsal head, and occasionally with impingement of the first toe on the second. In addition to identifying pain related to hallux valgus, the physician should determine limitations in shoe wear and activity level resulting from the deformity.

Physical Examination

The severity of hallux valgus deformity and pes planus are assessed with the patient weight bearing. To illustrate appropriateness of shoe wear, the physician may wish to contrast an outline of the patient's foot with nonphysiologic shoe wear. Medial eminence tenderness, first MTP joint range of motion, and first TMT hypermobility may be evaluated with the patient seated.[43] Limited first MTP joint range of motion with or without crepitance should alert the physician to potential first MTP joint degenerative changes.

Because physiologically normal values of first TMT joint mobility have not been defined, first ray hypermobility remains a controversial finding and a diagnostic challenge, despite some authors providing methods to objectively quantitate first TMT joint motion.[54] Even though a validated Klaue device exists to measure first ray mobility,[55,56] it is not particularly practical in the clinical setting. Moreover, first TMT joint hypermobility may not only occur in the sagittal plane but also in the transverse plane.[27] Clinical evaluation may not be adequately specific to isolate the first TMT joint, and therefore may assess only medial column mobility. Physical examination should also include the evaluation of the second MTP joint for presence of synovitis, metatarsal head overload, and/or second toe deformity, all of which are often associated with hallux valgus.

Imaging Studies

Proper evaluation of a hallux valgus deformity necessitates weight-bearing anteroposterior (AP) and lateral radiographs of the entire foot. From these radiographs, the angular relations that identify the presence and determine magnitude of the deformities of the bones and the joints associated with hallux valgus are measured. Other conditions, such as instability, arthrosis, and malalignment of joints elsewhere in the foot or the manifestations of vascular, neurogenic, or systemic disorders that affect the function of the foot may also be appreciated. Oblique views of the foot may facilitate the recognition of these associated problems; however, they are not used to measure any of conventional parameters of pedal alignment, and are therefore often unnecessary.

Radiographic Measurements Pertinent to Hallux Valgus. Several parameters measured from AP radiographs aid in the basic characterization of a hallux valgus deformity. The hallux valgus angle (HVA), defined as the angle formed by the intersection of longitudinal axes of the diaphyses of the first metatarsal and the proximal phalanx, quantifies the malalignment of the first MTP joint. Several authors have suggested that the upper limit of normal for this measurement is 15 degrees.[6,57–59] The IMA represents the angle formed between the diaphyses of the first and second metatarsals. This measurement quantifies the extent of metatarsus primus varus. The upper limit of normal for the IMA is 9 degrees.[6,57–59] The interphalangeal angle, which measures the angle between the metaphysis and diaphysis of the proximal phalanx, determines the amount of hallux valgus interphalangeus (HVI). The physiologic upper limit of normal for this parameter is 10 degrees.[51,58,59] The DMAA assesses the angular relation between the articular surface of the head and diaphysis of the first metatarsal. The upper limit of normal DMAA is 10 degrees.[37,49,51] The literature suggests that, although preoperative intraobserver and interobserver reliability for the HVA and IMA is excellent (<5 degrees, 95% confidence interval),[51,59–61] assessment of the DMAA remains a diagnostic challenge, with poor intraobserver and interobserver reliability.[47,49–52]

Radiographic Measurements Purported to Suggest Hypermobility. Second metatarsal diaphyseal hypertrophy, a medially oriented first TMT joint, and first TMT joint obliquity have been suggested to indirectly determine hypermobility of the first ray. Diaphyseal hypertrophy of the second metatarsal, particularly the medial cortex, has been suggested as a sign of hypermobility of the first ray.[28,29,31,62,63] No investigation has demonstrated a correlation between radiographic changes in the second metatarsal and hypermobility.[37,44,64] However, one study demonstrated a marginal correlation between the IMA and dorsal mobility of the TMT joint in patients with hallux valgus.[65] A medially oriented obliquity of the first TMT joint has proposed as an associated sign of a hypermobility, but Brage and colleagues[66] demonstrated that changing the inclination of the x-ray beam relative to the floor created wide variation in the measurement of the first TMT joint obliquity. Based on these findings, Brage and colleagues[66] concluded that first TMT joint obliquity was not a reliable indication for first TMT arthrodesis in the management of hallux valgus. An investigation observed significant dorsal translation and dorsiflexion of this joint in a series of patients with moderate-to-severe hallux valgus compared with normal control subjects.[67] The appearance of plantar gapping at the TMT joint has been attributed to radiographic projection and discounted as an indication of hypermobility.[33,71] Currently, no investigation has correlated these presumed radiographic abnormalities of the TMT joint with clinical hypermobility.

Correlating Physical and Radiographic Findings. Thordarson and coworkers[68] evaluated 285 women, with an average age of 49 years, scheduled for corrective surgery for hallux valgus. Validated AAOS foot-specific outcomes data collection questionnaires were used. Preoperative radiographic data (HVA and IMA) were stratified into degree of deformity. The data were stratified into age groups consistent with those reported for the 36-Item Short Form Health Survey (SF-36), and the results were compared with the SF-36 for the general population. The global foot and ankle score and the shoe comfort score were compared with the general population, and the severity of the preoperative deformity was correlated with the baseline scores. Bodily pain scores were uniformly worse for hallux valgus patients compared with the general population, with significantly lower global foot and ankle and shoe comfort scores, a finding that suggests that the bodily pain score from the SF-36 represents a sensitive measure of the difficulties experienced by patients undergoing corrective hallux valgus surgery. The preoperative radiographically determined severity of deformity failed to correlate with any scores measured.

CLASSIFICATION

Classification of deformity, based on radiographic parameters, may serve to formulate a surgical plan in the management of hallux valgus deformity. Although algorithms exist, the authors caution that hallux valgus surgery may need to be individualized. The following classification provides general guidelines:

Hallux Valgus

Step 1: Rule out degenerative joint disease of the first MTP joint

Step 2: Congruent versus incongruent joint (i.e., increased DMAA or not)

Step 3: Degree of severity

Mild deformity (IMA < 13 degrees; HVA < 30 degrees)

stable first TMT joint

Moderate-to-severe deformity (IMA > 13 degrees; HVA > 30 degrees)

stable first TMT joint

Severe deformity (IMA > 20 degrees; HVA > 40 degrees)

stable first TMT joint

Step 4: Hypermobility of the first TMT joint

Step 5: Evaluate for increased HVI angle

NONOPERATIVE TREATMENT

Nonoperative management of hallux valgus can improve a patient's symptoms and avoids the complications that may be associated with hallux valgus

surgery. To ensure appropriate nonsurgical treatment of hallux valgus, the treating surgeon should focus on identifying the patient's specific complaints. Pain may not be a major component of the patient's symptoms. Cosmetic concerns and difficulty using restrictive shoe wear are often common complaints. Because of the recovery time associated with bunion surgery and the potential for complications, surgical correction of hallux valgus for cosmesis is not indicated.

Symptoms of pain are best treated with shoe wear and activity modification. Shoes with a wider toe box and a comfortable upper are often helpful. Padding over the medial eminence or adjustments to the shoe to create more space medially can be helpful. However, nonoperative management cannot reverse hallux valgus deformity, and successful surgery may lead to an improved functional outcome. A randomized, controlled trial in 209 consecutive patients with symptomatic hallux valgus treated in four Finnish general community hospitals demonstrated that, although orthoses provided short-term symptomatic relief, surgical management of hallux valgus led to superior functional outcome and patient satisfaction as compared with orthotic management at a minimum follow-up of 12 months.[69] Surgical correction also led to better functional outcome and patient satisfaction than observation ("watchful waiting"), suggesting that the natural history of symptomatic hallux valgus deformity, at 12 months, is not one of improvement (Level I evidence). Although this prospective, randomized study demonstrates benefits of surgical correction of hallux valgus when compared with nonoperative treatment, insufficient evidence exists to support that corrective bunion surgery should be favored over nonoperative management (grade I).

OVERVIEW OF OPERATIVE TREATMENT

More than 100 different operative treatments have been proposed for hallux valgus. As a general principle, the severity of the deformity dictates treatment options. Although mild-to-moderate deformities often can be corrected with a more distal procedure such as a chevron osteotomy, more severe deformities typically are managed with a more proximal procedure such as a proximal metatarsal osteotomy or Lapidus procedure. A first MTP joint arthrodesis generally is reserved for hallux valgus associated with first MTP joint arthrosis, severe deformities, or salvage of failed previous hallux valgus procedures.

MILD-TO-MODERATE DEFORMITY

Distal Procedures

Incongruent Hallux Valgus.

Simple Bunionectomy. Few recent orthopedic articles report on simple bunionectomy (medial eminence resection with medial capsular plication). In a retrospective review of simple bunionectomy, Kitaoka and coauthors[70] note high recurrence and high patient dissatisfaction rates. Given the limited Level IV evidence for simple bunionectomy, no specific recommendation (grade I) can be made for medial eminence resection in hallux valgus correction.

Modified McBride Procedure (Distal Soft-Tissue Procedure). The McBride distal soft-tissue procedure, although common as an adjunct procedure in many hallux valgus corrective surgeries, has also been described as an isolated procedure for hallux valgus correction. In 1923, Silver[22] reported the combination of medial eminence resection, lateral capsular release, adductor hallucis tendon release, and medial capsular plication for the treatment of hallux valgus deformity. The modified McBride procedure includes medial capsulotomy (and subsequent plication), division of the ligament between the lateral capsule and fibular sesamoid, adductor hallucis release, lateral capsular fenestration, and a controlled varus stress to the first MTP joint.[71-73] A concern about hallux varus after the original McBride procedure[74] prompted the preservation of the fibular sesamoid in the modification.

Few recent orthopedic articles report on isolated modified McBride procedures for the correction of hallux valgus deformity. In a retrospective review, Mann and Pfeffinger[72] note acceptable patient satisfaction rates and improvement in hallux alignment (Level IV evidence). However, a selection bias to patients with mild and flexible deformities was suggested.[75] Johnson and coworkers[71] retrospectively compared the modified McBride procedure and distal chevron osteotomy, with the two groups matched for age, severity of deformity, and length of follow-up (Level III evidence). Although postoperative satisfaction rates were not significantly different, the distal chevron group exhibited significantly better correction of alignment. Given the limited Level III and IV evidence for the modified McBride procedure, no specific recommendation (grade I) can be made for the McBride distal soft-tissue procedure when used in isolation for hallux valgus correction.

Distal Chevron Osteotomy. The distal chevron osteotomy is a V-shaped osteotomy of the first metatarsal, described by Corless,[76] Johnson and coworkers,[77] and Austin and Leventen.[78] The capital fragment is shifted laterally to narrow the forefoot. An anatomic study suggested that the capital fragment can be safely shifted laterally 6.0 mm in men and 5.0 mm in women, and still maintain greater than 50% bony apposition of the fragments.[79] The procedure has been performed with or without fixation of the shifted capital fragment.[80-85] The symmetric orientation of the distal chevron osteotomy[78] has undergone several modifications to accommodate fixation.[77,80] The combination of a medial closing wedge osteotomy of the first proximal phalanx (Akin) and a distal chevron osteotomy has been described when hallux valgus with metatarsus primus varus is associated with HVI.[86,87] The distal chevron osteotomy also has been combined with a lateral capsular or adductor tendon release, or both.[83,85,88-90]

For mild-to-moderate hallux valgus correction, the effectiveness of the distal chevron osteotomy in providing favorable outcomes and patient satisfaction, regardless of fixation method, addition of lateral soft-tissue release, length of follow-up, or patient age, is supported by numerous retrospective reviews (Level IV evidence).[80-85,90-97] The average preoperative IMA was less than 15 degrees in all studies. DeOrio and Ware[81] report satisfactory outcomes and patient satisfaction with a low complication rate with bioabsorbable fixation (Level IV evidence). Crosby and Bozarth[93] and Gill and colleagues[82] note no significant differences in favorable outcomes or patient satisfaction and minimal complications in case series comparisons of screw, Kirschner wire, and no fixation and Kirschner wires versus bioabsorbable fixation, respectively (Level IV evidence).

Although the addition of a lateral release to a distal chevron osteotomy may improve global correction of hallux alignment, patient satisfaction is similar in patients who have distal chevron osteotomies with or without lateral release. Resch and investigators'[89] Level I evidence investigation compares distal chevron osteotomy with and without adductor tenotomy. Although the clinical appearance and radiographic alignment were significantly improved in the group with adductor release, patient satisfaction was not. Mann and Donatto,[80] in a small case series (Level IV evidence), note satisfactory outcome for distal chevron osteotomy without lateral release: similar to results of Level IV evidence studies of distal chevron osteotomies with lateral release.[92,95,97]

Two recently published Level IV case series of distal chevron osteotomies with lateral release[83,85] note that the results were maintained with longer follow-up: Trnka and coworkers'[83] follow-up period was 2 to 5 years, and Schneider and colleagues'[85] follow-up period was 5.6 to 12.7 years. Furthermore, both studies suggest that results were equal for patients older and younger than the arbitrarily chosen age of 50 years.

Congruent Hallux Valgus. Although subject to poor interobserver reliability,[47,50-52] the DMAA[47,49] can be decreased by combining the distal chevron osteotomy with Akin osteotomy[80] or by making a biplanar distal chevron osteotomy in mild hallux valgus deformity[46,98] (Level IV evidence). Whereas the goal of a combination of distal chevron and Akin osteotomies is to improve clinical alignment through extra-articular correction, the biplanar distal chevron osteotomy aims to simultaneously correct hallux valgus and decrease the DMAA. In the biplanar distal chevron procedure, two different osteotomy configurations can be used. With the conventional, symmetric pattern of two osteotomy limbs of equal length, a second oblique wedge resection for each cut allows a reduction in the DMAA in combination with the lateral shift of the metatarsal head[46] (Level IV evidence). With a short, relatively vertical dorsal limb and long, horizontal plantar limb, a second wedge resection dorsally permits redirection of the metatarsal head simultaneous with the lateral shift[98] (Level IV evidence).

Risk for Osteonecrosis of the First Metatarsal Head with Distal Chevron Osteotomy. Adding a lateral capsular release to a chevron osteotomy may improve deformity correction,[84,88,95,96,99,100] but this type of release may increase the risk for osteonecrosis of the first metatarsal head[90] (Level IV evidence). A distal chevron osteotomy disrupts the intraosseous blood supply to the metatarsal head, and the medial capsular release eliminates a substantial portion of the blood supply to the metatarsal head.[88] Retrospective reviews[83–85,94–96] (Level IV evidence) suggest that a lateral capsular release or adductor tenotomy can be safely combined with a distal chevron osteotomy. Moreover, in a prospective, randomized study (Level I evidence), Resch and investigators[99] used scintigraphy to demonstrate that an adductor hallucis tenotomy performed with a distal chevron osteotomy did not lead to an increased circulatory disturbance to the first metatarsal head compared with distal chevron osteotomies performed without a lateral soft-tissue procedure. Kuhn and colleagues[88] prospectively (Level III evidence) utilized an intraoperative laser Doppler probe to demonstrate that the combination of chevron osteotomy, medial capsular release, and lateral release plus adductor tenotomy resulted in a cumulative decrease in blood flow to the metatarsal head of 71%, with the greatest insult being attributed to the medial capsular release (45%). None of the 20 metatarsal heads analyzed in Kuhn and colleagues'[88] study experienced development of osteonecrosis. Some investigations have noted initial radiographic findings suggestive of avascular change in the first metatarsal head, but with further follow-up these changes resolved in most patients.[80,96,99] Even after chevron osteotomy without lateral release, subtle findings suggestive of osteonecrosis may be identified, but these rarely have long-term sequelae[80,99] (Level I and IV evidence). Jones and coauthors[100] propose an overpenetration with the saw blade through the lateral first metatarsal cortex and the lateral capsule as the technical error potentially leading to osteonecrosis.

Levels of Evidence for Distal Chevron Osteotomy. Given the numerous positive Level IV evidence investigations and one Level I evidence study in the orthopedic literature, a grade B treatment recommendation can be made to support the use of a distal chevron osteotomy for correction of mild-to-moderate hallux valgus deformity. One Level I evidence study and multiple Level IV evidence investigations that provide grade B evidence that hallux alignment and functional outcome may be better after a distal chevron osteotomy with a lateral soft-tissue procedure than without suggest that patient satisfaction is no different in these two groups. Moreover, consistently positive Level IV evidence and one Level I evidence investigation allow a grade B recommendation that a lateral capsular or adductor hallucis tendon release can be done with a distal chevron osteotomy without increased risk for first metatarsal head osteonecrosis. Two relatively recent Level IV evidence stud-

ies exist for the distal chevron and Akin osteotomies and the biplanar distal chevron osteotomy to correct mild-to-moderate hallux valgus associated with an increased DMAA.[46,86,87,98] Although functional outcomes and patient satisfaction for these case series are favorable, only grade C evidence supports their use in the management of mild-to-moderate hallux valgus with an increased DMAA.

Keller Resection Arthroplasty. Several Level IV retrospective case series have been published on the Keller resection arthroplasty.[21,101–107] The Keller resection arthroplasty is the resection of the first proximal phalanx base to correct hallux valgus deformity. In a prospective comparison, Turnbull and Grange[101] demonstrate better HVA and IMA correction, hallux MTP joint motion, and metatarsal head relation with the sesamoid complex for the distal chevron osteotomy compared with the Keller procedure (Level II evidence). Although some authors have reported satisfactory results with the Keller resection arthroplasty, these authors note that acceptable results were achieved because of ancillary procedures. Specifically, Donley and researchers[108] note acceptable postoperative alignment when the resection arthroplasty is combined with a fibular sesamoidectomy (Level IV). Likewise, several authors[105,106,109–111] attribute improved outcome applying a *cerclage fibreux* (described by LeLievre and LeLievre[112]) distal soft-tissue procedure or tendon transfer in conjunction with the resection (Level IV). Zembsch and investigators,[102] in a retrospective, uncontrolled comparative case series, demonstrate worse results with the Keller procedure than with proximal metatarsal closing wedge osteotomy, with significantly better correction of hallux valgus deformity in the proximal osteotomy group. Both groups had high rates of transfer metatarsalgia (Level IV evidence). Anecdotally, most authors suggest that the Keller procedure be used only in older patients with limited functional expectations who may be at risk if subjected to corrective surgery. Given that no more than Level IV evidence exists in the orthopedic literature, only grade C evidence exists for recommending the Keller procedure in the management of hallux valgus deformity.

MODERATE-TO-SEVERE DEFORMITY

Incongruent Hallux Valgus Deformity

Proximal Procedures and First Metatarsophalangeal Joint Arthrodesis. For a moderate-to-severe hallux valgus deformity associated with metatarsus primus varus, a more powerful deformity correction generally is required. A wide variety of approaches have been described for correction of severe hallux valgus deformity, including various proximal first metatarsal osteotomies, corrective first TMT joint arthrodesis (Lapidus), or first MTP joint arthrodesis. Typically, a distal soft-tissue procedure is performed in conjunction with a proximal osteotomy or a Lapidus procedure.

Whereas crescentic[113–117] and closing wedge osteotomies are done through a dorsal approach, proximal chevron, opening wedge Ludloff, and scarf osteotomies are done from the medial aspect of the proximal first metatarsal.[118–121] Several authors suggest that dorsiflexion malunion is less likely to occur with proximal osteotomies done from the medial aspect of the first metatarsal than from the dorsal aspect.[115,118,121] Most proximal first metatarsal osteotomies require full transection of the first metatarsal; the opening and closing wedge procedures maintain lateral and medial cortical hinges, respectively. For all proximal osteotomies combined with a distal soft-tissue procedure, potential complications include recurrence, hallux varus, first MTP joint stiffness, malunion, nonunion, and infection.

Proximal Crescentic Osteotomy. The proximal crescentic osteotomy for correction of hallux valgus associated with metatarsus primus varus has been popularized by Mann and colleagues.[122] Unique to the proximal crescentic osteotomy is the use of a crescentic saw blade. A commonly cited potential complication of the proximal crescentic osteotomy is dorsiflexion malunion.[115,116,122,123] Jones and coauthors[124] describe a technique to aid surgeons in properly orienting the crescentic saw blade in the coronal plane to minimize the risk for initial dorsiflexion malpositioning.

Several case series (Level IV evidence) reported satisfactory radiographic correction, high rates of satisfaction, and significant improvement in functional outcomes with the proximal crescentic osteotomy at intermediate- to long-term follow-up periods.[113,114,116,117,122,123,125,126] A prospective, randomized comparison[115] (Level II evidence) of the proximal crescentic and proximal chevron osteotomies suggested favorable radiographic correction and clinical outcomes for both procedures, with American Orthopaedic Foot and Ankle Society (AOFAS) outcome scores and radiographic correction of HVA and IMA improving significantly at an average follow-up of 24 (proximal crescentic) and 20 months (proximal chevron). Dorsiflexion malunion was observed in 17% of the proximal crescentic cohort. Mann and colleagues,[122] in one of the original articles describing this procedure, note dorsiflexion malunions in 28% of cases. The consistently favorable results from several case series and one Level II evidence study impart a grade B recommendation for the use of the proximal crescentic osteotomy in the surgical management of hallux valgus.

Proximal Chevron Osteotomy. The proximal chevron osteotomy, first reported by Sammarco and researchers,[118] relies not simply on lateral translation of the distal fragment, as with the distal chevron procedure, but concomitantly incorporates an opening wedge principle.[115,118–120] The large contact area is relatively stable, and recommended fixation is with a combination of a screw and a Kirschner wire, two screws, or a plate.[115,118–120,127,128] The procedure has been described using a single-[119,120] or two-incision[115,118] technique.

Three case series[118,120] (Level IV evidence) and one prospective, randomized comparative study[115] (Level II evidence) reported favorable radiographic correction, high rates of satisfaction, and significant improvements in the functional outcomes with the proximal chevron osteotomy at intermediate follow-up. In the Level II investigation comparing the proximal chevron and crescentic osteotomies, healing time was shorter and the tendency for first metatarsal shortening was less for the proximal chevron cohort. Dorsiflexion malunion was observed in 0% and 17% for the proximal chevron and crescentic cohorts, respectively. Taking the limited (but favorable) Level IV evidence and the positive Level II evidence into consideration, a grade B recommendation for the use of the proximal chevron osteotomy in the operative management of hallux valgus can be made.

Opening Wedge Proximal First Metatarsal Osteotomy. The opening wedge proximal first metatarsal osteotomy was described by Trethowen in 1923[129] but was largely abandoned because of concerns of stability and nonunion. With improved fixation techniques, including fixed-angle plating, the opening wedge has regained acceptance in some centers. It probably is inaccurate to state that an opening wedge proximal first metatarsal osteotomy lengthens the metatarsal, but it may maintain length, a feature that may be beneficial when the first metatarsal is relatively short compared with the second metatarsal. Healing rarely is problematic despite the gap that is created; minimal periosteal stripping and an intact lateral cortex allow relatively rapid incorporation of local autograft, allograft, or bone graft substitutes.

Despite the attention given this technique in recent years, to our knowledge, no investigations have been published that report the results of hallux valgus correction using an opening wedge proximal first metatarsal osteotomy. Thus, insufficient (grade I) evidence exits to make a recommendation.

Proximal Oblique ("Ludloff") Osteotomy. The proximal oblique first metatarsal osteotomy was introduced in 1918 by Ludloff,[130] but it failed to gain acceptance because the original description did not include fixation. More recently, a modified technique included fixation with two screws.[121] The first screw is placed before the osteotomy is completed, allowing the surgeon to maintain full control of the osteotomy throughout the procedure.[121] Beischer and coauthors[131] report the optimal geometric parameters of the modified Ludloff osteotomy in a three-dimensional computer analysis. Specifically, they determined that first metatarsal shortening and rotational malalignment can be controlled if the osteotomy is started dorsally at the first TMT joint and extended distally to the plantar first metatarsal, just proximal to the sesamoid complex. They also explain that first metatarsal elevation is avoided by tilting the osteotomy 10 degrees plantarward, thereby directing the distal fragment plantarward during correction.

A few orthopedic clinical series (Level IV evidence) have analyzed the modified Ludloff osteotomy combined with a distal soft-tissue procedure.[121,132,133] At intermediate follow-up, in prospective case series (Level IV evidence), Hofstaetter and colleagues,[132] Petroutsas and Trnka,[133] and Chiodo and coworkers[121] report significant improvement in the AOFAS Hallux-IP joint score, favorable patient satisfaction, and significant correction of radiographic hallux alignment. Based on the limited clinical series of Level IV articles, a grade B recommendation exists for the modified Ludloff osteotomy and distal soft-tissue procedure in the operative management of moderate-to-severe hallux valgus deformity.

Closing Wedge Proximal First Metatarsal Osteotomy. A proximal closing wedge osteotomy perpendicular to the first metatarsal longitudinal axis is not universally accepted by orthopedic foot and ankle surgeons because of concerns regarding complications, including shortening and dorsiflexion malunion.[102,134,135] Perhaps by utilizing an oblique wedge orientation (as has been espoused at various meetings), these risks might be diminished. To date, however, no peer-reviewed published data exist in support of this in the orthopedic literature. The proximal closing wedge first metatarsal osteotomy is done through a dorsal approach, with the base of the resected segment directed laterally. Despite a medial hinge being maintained, most published series acknowledge a risk for dorsiflexion malunion. Given the natural propensity for the wedge osteotomy to shorten the ray, theoretically, this osteotomy may be uniquely suitable for patients with a relatively long first metatarsal.

Several retrospective case series (Level IV evidence) of proximal first metatarsal closing wedge osteotomies and distal soft-tissue procedures with intermediate- to long-term follow-up periods have been reported in the orthopedic literature.[102,134–136] Trnka and researchers[135] report long-term retrospective results (follow-up range, 10–22 years) of basal metatarsal closing wedge osteotomies. Despite good-to-excellent results in 85% of patients who returned for follow-up, a considerable number of complications occurred, including dorsiflexion malunion, first metatarsal shortening (mean, 5 mm), transfer metatarsalgia, and hallux varus. In an uncontrolled comparative study (Level IV evidence), the same authors report that a subset of the same patients compared favorably with a group of similar patients undergoing Keller resection arthroplasties.[102] Although the incidence of transfer metatarsalgia was equal in the two groups, the basal closing wedge osteotomy had significantly better AOFAS Hallux-IP joint scores and radiographic outcomes. Again, the frequency of dorsiflexion malunion and hallux varus was high. In an intermediate follow-up case series, Resch and investigators[134] cite a long average time to healing of the osteotomy and a 20% incidence rate of dorsiflexion malunion associated with transfer metatarsalgia.

Granberry and Hickey[136] report a retrospective, uncontrolled comparative study (Level III evidence) of proximal first metatarsal closing wedge and Akin osteotomies with or without a distal soft-tissue procedure. Although the same combination of osteotomies was done in the two groups, only one group had release of the lateral joint capsule from the sesamoid and transfer of the adductor tendon into the first metatarsal neck. The significantly better radiographic

correction of hallux valgus in those with a distal soft-tissue procedure was accompanied by significantly less first MTP joint motion. Several dorsiflexion malunions were observed in the entire group of patients. With the Level III and IV evidence, a grade B recommendation can be made for the closing wedge proximal first metatarsal osteotomy in the correction of hallux valgus, with the observation that dorsiflexion malunion and considerable shortening of the first metatarsal are frequent.

Scarf Osteotomy. The scarf osteotomy is not a proximal first metatarsal osteotomy per se but is commonly used outside of the United States for moderate-to-severe hallux valgus deformity.[137–141] The configuration of the osteotomy with a distal dorsal limb (virtually identical to that of a traditional distal chevron osteotomy), a long transverse cut, and a proximal limb (similar to the distal extension of the Ludloff osteotomy) confers stability and permits fixation with two screws. It is designed primarily as an osteotomy that laterally translates the distal fragment, but with slight modification of the bone cuts, rotation also can be imparted to the distal fragment to further correct the IMA increased DMAA. A potential complication unique to the scarf osteotomy is "troughing" (i.e., an impaction of the two osteotomy fragments, resulting in loss of metatarsal height).

Several prospective and retrospective case series (Level IV evidence) have reported favorable radiographic correction, high rates of patient satisfaction, and significant improvements in the functional outcomes and pedobaric foot pressure analyses with the scarf osteotomy.[137–145] Aminian and coauthors,[142] in their retrospective review, note no transfer metatarsalgia pattern in foot pressure analysis. Prospectively, Lorei and coworkers[141] observed a redistribution from the lateral forefoot to the first ray after scarf osteotomies in their case series using pedobarographic analysis (Level IV evidence). Jones and coauthors,[139] prospectively, and Crevoisier and investigators,[137] retrospectively, reported favorable outcomes and radiographic correction using a combination of scarf and Akin osteotomies (Level IV evidence).

In contrast, Coetzee[146] reports poor AOFAS outcome scores and an alarming complication rate in a prospective case series of scarf osteotomies (Level IV evidence). Complications included "troughing" (35%), rotational malunion (30%), metatarsal fracture (10%), and early recurrence of deformity (25%). Although many authors have acknowledged the complexity of this osteotomy, several have provided technique tips and experience to accelerate the learning curve in mastering the procedure.[138,143,145,147–149]

Despite one Level IV evidence case series condemning the procedure, the favorable results from numerous case series support a grade B recommendation for the use of the scarf osteotomy in the treatment of primary hallux valgus.

First Tarsometatarsal Joint Arthrodesis (Modified Lapidus Procedure). Lapidus[38] originally described an arthrodesis between the bases of the first and second metatarsals and the first intercuneiform joint to correct metatarsus primus varus in patients with hallux valgus. Currently, the modified Lapidus procedure incorporates an isolated arthrodesis of the first TMT joint with a lateral and plantar based closing wedge osteotomy of the medial cuneiform.[31,138,150–152] This procedure has been indicated for the correction of metatarsus primus varus in patients with moderate-to-severe hallux valgus and hypermobility of the first ray. First ray hypermobility has been controversial and often is questioned.[37,42,45,152]

Several retrospective case series (Level IV evidence) have collectively reported excellent radiographic correction, high rates of satisfaction, and significant improvements in functional outcomes with the modified Lapidus procedure.[28–30,32,153,154] Faber and coauthors,[152] in a prospective, randomized study comparing the Hohmann procedure (distal first metatarsal osteotomy) with the modified Lapidus procedure in 101 feet (Level I evidence), found no significant differences in clinical outcomes, radiographic correction, or patient satisfaction. Feet with preoperatively identified hypermobility had equally favorable outcomes with either procedure when compared with feet without hypermobility. A prospective study (Level II evidence) evaluated the efficacy of the modified Lapidus procedure in the treatment of recurrent hallux valgus. Significant decreases in the pain score, IMAs, and HVAs, and increases in the AOFAS clinical ratings score were associated with an 81% satisfaction rate at 2 years after surgery.[155]

Early reports identified nonunion rates of 10% to 12% with the modified Lapidus procedure.[29,31,156] However, a more recent large clinical series reported a 4% nonunion rate and a 2% revision rate in feet treated with the Lapidus procedure.[32] The authors reported that five of the eight patients with nonunions had previous bunion surgery, and two patients smoked. Another study reported no nonunions with the use of the modified Lapidus procedure for the primary correction of hallux valgus.[157] The uniformly successful results from numerous case series, supported by one Level I evidence study, justify a grade B recommendation for the use of the modified Lapidus procedure in the treatment of primary hallux valgus. Although the results of Coetzee and co-workers[155,158] suggest that the modified Lapidus procedure also is an effective salvage procedure for recurrent hallux valgus, this evidence from a single Level II study is insufficient (grade I) to make a recommendation.

Congruent Hallux Valgus Deformity

Double/Triple Osteotomies for Hallux Valgus Correction. A large IMA in combination with an increased DMAA cannot be corrected with a proximal osteotomy alone; reducing the IMA will effectively increase the DMAA. In hallux valgus with a large IMA and increased DMAA, a double osteotomy, with a proximal first

metatarsal osteotomy or medial opening wedge osteotomy of the first cuneiform (Cotton procedure) to correct the increased IMA and a distal medial closing wedge osteotomy of the metatarsal head (Reverdin osteotomy) to reduce the DMAA, may be considered. With severe deformity, an opening wedge medial cuneiform osteotomy (Cotton procedure) can be added to proximal MT osteotomy and Reverdin to further correct the IMA, creating a triple osteotomy. When associated with HVI, an Akin osteotomy also should be added because none of the aforementioned osteotomies directly corrects angulation in the hallux proximal phalanx.[159] One Level IV evidence investigation suggested favorable outcomes in a limited number of patients undergoing multiple osteotomies for a more comprehensive hallux valgus correction.[159] Several case series (Level IV evidence) have reported favorable outcomes with Akin osteotomies added to distal chevron osteotomies[86,87] and more proximal osteotomies.[137,139] The limited published Level IV evidence available for double and triple osteotomies is insufficient (grade I) to make a recommendation for their use in the management of hallux valgus deformity.

First Metatarsophalangeal Joint Arthrodesis. Arthrodesis of the first MTP joint generally is reserved for patients with severe hallux valgus deformity, or patients in whom hallux valgus is associated with arthrosis of the joint, failed prior surgical correction, or a neuromuscular disorder; it also is used as part of the reconstruction of a rheumatoid forefoot. Coughlin and coauthors[160] (Level IV evidence) report significant decreases in pain after fusion for moderate-to-severe hallux valgus. There were no dissatisfied patients, and most patients were able to wear conventional or comfort shoe wear at an average of 8 years after surgery. However, radiographic progression of arthritis was evident at the interphalangeal joint in 7 of the 21 feet in their series.[160] Grimes and Coughlin[151] report satisfactory outcomes at an average follow-up period of 8 years in a retrospective case series of first MTP joint arthrodeses performed for failed hallux valgus procedures. When fusion was compared with resection of the first MTP joint for reconstruction of the rheumatoid forefoot (Level II evidence), no differences were detected other than a significant increase in the duration of the procedure for the group undergoing arthrodesis.[161] Salvage of a failed Keller procedure with fusion was associated with a greater rate of satisfaction and AOFAS clinical rating score, and avoided the onset of postoperative valgus or cock-up deformity when compared with isolated soft-tissue release (Level III evidence).[162] A case series (Level IV evidence) evaluating the results of arthrodesis for hallux valgus in children with cerebral palsy reported high rates of fusion and satisfaction with the procedure. Together, these investigations favor a grade B recommendation for the use of arthrodesis in the management of a wide spectrum of hallux valgus deformities.

RECOMMENDATIONS

Our evidence-based recommendations for the treatment of hallux valgus are as follows (Table 73–1):

- Nonoperative treatment for hallux valgus can mitigate patient symptoms but does not alter the natural history of the deformity.
- A distal chevron osteotomy appears to be a predictable treatment for mild and some moderate hallux valgus deformities.
- The addition of a limited lateral capsular release, adductor hallucis tenotomy, or both to a distal chevron osteotomy does not seem to increase the risk for first metatarsal osteonecrosis.

- Multiple proximal first metatarsal procedures, when combined with a distal soft-tissue procedure, appear to provide satisfactory treatment for moderate-to-severe hallux valgus deformity (hallux valgus associated with metatarsus primus varus). These include proximal crescentic, proximal chevron, proximal oblique (Ludloff), proximal closing wedge, and scarf osteotomies and the Lapidus procedure.
- First MTP joint arthrodesis appears to offer satisfactory outcome in patients with severe hallux valgus.

TABLE 73–1. Summary of Recommendations

STATEMENT	LEVEL OF EVIDENCE/GRADE OF RECOMMENDATIONS	REFERENCE
1. A distal chevron osteotomy apears to be a predictable treatment for mild and some moderate hallux valgus deformities.	Level IV/Grade B	80–85, 90–97
2. The addition of a limited lateral capsular release or adductor hallucis tenotomy or both to a distal chevron ostetomy does not seem to increase the risk of first metatarsal head osteonecrosis.	Level I, IV/Grade B	83–85, 88, 94–96, 99, 100
3. Multiple proximal first metatarsal procedures, when combined with a distal soft-tissue procedure, appear to provide satisfactory treatment for moderate-to-severe hallux valgus deformity (hallux valgus associated with metatarsus primus varus). These include proximal crescentic, proximal chevron, proximal oblique (Ludloff), proximal closing wedge, and Scarf osteotomies and the Lapidus procedure.	Level II, IV/Grade B	113, 114, 116, 117, 122, 123, 125, 126, 118, 119, 120, 115, 121, 132, 133, 136, 137–145, 28–30, 32, 153, 154
4. First metatarsophalangeal joint arthrodesis appears to offer satisfactory outcome in patients with severe hallux valgus.	Level II, III, IV/Grade B	151, 160, 161

REFERENCES

1. Hueter C: [Klinik der Gelenkkrankungen mit Einschluss der Orthopaedie]. Leipzig, Vogel, 1870.
2. Kato TWS: The etiology of hallux valgus in Japan. Clin Orthop Relat Res 158:78, 1981.
3. Lam SL, Hodgson AR: A comparison of foot forms among the non-shoe and shoe-wearing Chinese population. J Bone Joint Surg 40:1058, 1958.
4. MacLennan R: Prevalence of hallux valgus in a neolithic New Guinea population. Lancet 1:1398, 1966.
5. Creer W: The feet of the industrial worker: Clinical aspect; relation to footwear. Lancet 2:1482, 1938.
6. Hardy RH, Clapham JC: Observations on hallux valgus; based on a controlled series. J Bone Joint Surg Br 33-B:376–391, 1951.
7. Barnicot NA, Hardy RH: The position of the hallux in West Africans. J Anat 89:355, 1955.
8. James CS: Footprints and feet of natives of Soloman Islands. Lancet (2):1390, 1939.
9. Engle ET, Morton DJ. Notes on foot disorders among natives of the Belgian Congo. J Bone Joint Surg 13:311, 1931.
10. Wells LE: The foot of the south African native. Am J Phys Anthropol 15:185, 1931.
11. Wilkins E: Feet with particular reference to school children. Med Officer 66:5,13,21,9, 1941.
12. Hewitt DS, Stewart AM, Webb JW: The prevalence of foot defects among wartime recruits. Br Med J 2:745, 1953.
13. Glynn MK, Dunlop JB, Fitzpatrick D: The Mitchell distal metatarsal osteotomy for hallux valgus. J Bone Joint Surg Br 62-B:188–191, 1980.
14. Coughlin M: Juvenile hallux valgus: Etiology and treatment. Foot Ankle 16:682–697, 1995.
15. Johnson O: Further studies of the inheritance of hand and foot anomalies. Clin Orthop Relat Res 8:146–160, 1956.
16. Hohmann G: Der hallux valgus und die uebrigen Zehenverkruemmungen. Ergeb Chir Orthop 18:308–348, 1925.
17. Anderson RL: Hallux valgus: report of end results. South Med Surg 91:74–78, 1929.
18. Craigmile D: Incidence, origin, and prevention of certain foot defects. Br Med J 2:749, 1953.
19. Galland WI, Jordan H: Hallux valgus. Surg Gunecol Obstet 66:95, 1938.
20. Joplin RJ: Sling procedure for correction of splayfoot, metatarsus primus varus, and hallux valgus. J Bone Joint Surg 32:779, 1950.
21. Rogers WAJ, Joplin RJ: Hallux valgus, weak foot, and the Keller operations: An end-result study. Surg Clin North Am 1947;27:1295–1302.
22. Silver D: The operative treatment of hallux valgus. J Bone Joint Surg 5:225, 1923.
23. Stein HC: Hallux valgus. Surg Gunecol Obstet 66:889–898, 1938.
24. Mann RA, Coughlin MJ: Hallux valgus: Etiology, anatomy, treatment and surgical considerations. Clin Orthop Relat Res 157:31, 1981.
25. Kilmartin TE, Wallace WA: The significance of pes planus in juvenile hallux valgus. Foot Ankle 13:53–56, 1992.
26. Canale PB, Aronsson DD, Lamont RL, Manoli A 2nd: The Mitchell procedure for the treatment of adolescent hallux valgus. A long-term study. J Bone Joint Surg Am 75:1610–1618, 1993.

27. Faber FW, Kleinrensink GJ, Verhoog MW, et al: Mobility of the first tarsometatarsal joint in relation to hallux valgus deformity: Anatomical and biomechanical aspects. Foot Ankle Int 20:651–656, 1999.
28. Bednarz PA, Manoli A 2nd: Modified lapidus procedure for the treatment of hypermobile hallux valgus. Foot Ankle Int 21:816–821, 2000.
29. Sangeorzan BJ, Hansen ST Jr: Modified Lapidus procedure for hallux valgus. Foot Ankle 9:262–266, 1989.
30. Kopp FJ, Patel MM, Levine DS, Deland JT: The modified Lapidus procedure for hallux valgus: A clinical and radiographic analysis. Foot Ankle Int 26:913–917, 2005.
31. Myerson M: Metatarsocuneiform arthrodesis for treatment of hallux valgus and metatarsus primus varus. Orthopedics 13:1025–1031, 1990.
32. Thompson IM, Bohay DR, Anderson JG: Fusion rate of first tarsometatarsal arthrodesis in the modified Lapidus procedure and flatfoot reconstruction. Foot Ankle Int 26:698–703, 2005.
33. Ito H, Shimizu A, Miyamoto T, et al: Clinical significance of increased mobility in the sagittal plane in patients with hallux valgus. Foot Ankle Int 20:29–32, 1999.
34. Morton D: Hypermobility of the first metatarsal bone: The interlinking factor between metatarsalgia and longitudinal arch strains. J Bone Joint Surg Am 10:187–196, 1928.
35. Morton D: Significant characteristics of the Neanderthal foot. Natural History 26:310–314, 1926.
36. Morton D: The human foot: Its evolution, physiology and functional disorders. New York, Columbia University Press, 1935.
37. Grebing BR, Coughlin MJ: Evaluation of Morton's theory of second metatarsal hypertrophy. J Bone Joint Surg Am 86-A:1375–1386, 2004.
38. Lapidus PW: Operative correction of the metatarsus varus primus in hallux valgus. Surg Gynecol Obstet 58:183–191, 1934.
39. Lapidus PW: A quarter of a century experience with the operative correction of the metatarsus varus primus in hallux valgus. Bull Hosp Joint Dis 17:404–421, 1956.
40. Lapidus PW: The author's bunion operation from 1931 to 1959. Clin Orthop Relat Res 16:119–135, 1960.
41. Coughlin MJ, Jones CP, Viladot R, et al: Hallux valgus and first ray mobility: A cadaveric study. Foot Ankle Int 25:537–544, 2004.
42. Coughlin MJ, Shurnas PS: Hallux valgus in men. Part II: First ray mobility after bunionectomy and factors associated with hallux valgus deformity. Foot Ankle Int 24:73–78, 2003.
43. Grebing BR, Coughlin MJ: The effect of ankle position on the exam for first ray mobility. Foot Ankle Int 25:467–475, 2004.
44. Prieskorn DW, Mann RA, Fritz G: Radiographic assessment of the second metatarsal: Measure of first ray hypermobility. Foot Ankle Int 17:331–333, 1996.
45. Glasoe WM, Coughlin MJ: A critical analysis of Dudley Morton's concept of disordered foot function. J Foot Ankle Surg 45:147–155, 2006.
46. Chou LB, Mann RA, Casillas MM: Biplanar chevron osteotomy. Foot Ankle Int 19:579–584, 1998.
47. Coughlin MJ: Hallux valgus in men: Effect of the distal metatarsal articular angle on hallux valgus correction. Foot Ankle Int 18:463–470, 1997.
48. Coughlin MJ: Roger A. Mann Award. Juvenile hallux valgus: Etiology and treatment. Foot Ankle Int 16:682–697, 1995.
49. Richardson EG, Graves SC, McClure JT, Boone RT: First metatarsal head-shaft angle: A method of determination. Foot Ankle 14:181–185, 1993.
50. Chi TD, Davitt J, Younger A, et al: Intra- and inter-observer reliability of the distal metatarsal articular angle in adult hallux valgus. Foot Ankle Int 23:722–726, 2002.
51. Coughlin MJ, Freund E: Roger A. Mann Award. The reliability of angular measurements in hallux valgus deformities. Foot Ankle Int 22:369–379, 2001.
52. Vittetoe DA, Saltzman CL, Krieg JC, Brown TD: Validity and reliability of the first distal metatarsal articular angle. Foot Ankle Int 15:541–547, 1994.
53. Uchiyama E, Kitaoka HB, Luo ZP, et al: Pathomechanics of hallux valgus: Biomechanical and immunohistochemical study. Foot Ankle Int 26:732–738, 2005.
54. Voellmicke KV, Deland JT: Manual examination technique to assess dorsal instability of the first ray. Foot Ankle Int 23:1040–1041, 2002.
55. Jones CP, Coughlin MJ, Pierce-Villadot R, et al: The validity and reliability of the Klaue device. Foot Ankle Int 26:951–956, 2005.
56. Glasoe WM, Grebing BR, Beck S, et al: A comparison of device measures of dorsal first ray mobility. Foot Ankle Int 26:957–961, 2005.
57. Steel MW 3rd, Johnson KA, DeWitz MA, Ilstrup DM: Radiographic measurements of the normal adult foot. Foot Ankle 1:151–158, 1980.
58. Mann RA: Bunion surgery: Decision making. Orthopedics 13:951–957, 1990.
59. Saltzman CL, Brandser EA, Berbaum KS, et al: Reliability of standard foot radiographic measurements. Foot Ankle Int 15:661–665, 1994.
60. Schneider W, Csepan R, Knahr K: Reproducibility of the radiographic metatarsophalangeal angle in hallux surgery. J Bone Joint Surg Am 85-A:494–499, 2003.
61. Smith RM, Reynolds JC, Stewart MJ: Hallux valgus assessment: Report of research committee of American Orthopaedic Foot and Ankle Society. Foot Ankle 5:92–103, 1984.
62. Hansen ST Jr: Functional reconstruction of the foot and ankle. Philadelphia, Lippincott Williams & Wilkins, 2000.
63. Myerson MS, Badekas A: Hypermobility of the first ray. Foot Ankle Clin 5:469–484, 2000.
64. Faber FW, Kleinrensink GJ, Mulder PG, Verhaar JA: Mobility of the first tarsometatarsal joint in hallux valgus patients: A radiographic analysis. Foot Ankle Int 22:965–969, 2001.
65. Glasoe WM, Allen MK, Saltzman CL: First ray dorsal mobility in relation to hallux valgus deformity and first intermetatarsal angle. Foot Ankle Int 22:98–101, 2001.
66. Brage ME, Holmes JR, Sangeorzan BJ: The influence of x-ray orientation on the first metatarsocuneiform joint angle. Foot Ankle Int 15:495–497, 1994.
67. King DM, Toolan BC: Associated deformities and hypermobility in hallux valgus: An investigation with weightbearing radiographs. Foot Ankle Int 25:251–255, 2004.
68. Thordarson DB, Ebramzadeh E, Rudicel SA, Baxter A: Age-adjusted baseline data for women with hallux valgus undergoing corrective surgery. J Bone Joint Surg Am 87:66–75, 2005.
69. Torkki M, Malmivaara A, Seitsalo S, et al: Surgery vs orthosis vs watchful waiting for hallux valgus: A randomized controlled trial. Jama 285:2474–2480, 2001.
70. Kitaoka HB, Franco MG, Weaver AL, Ilstrup DM: Simple bunionectomy with medial capsulorrhaphy. Foot Ankle 12:86–91, 1991.
71. Johnson JE, Clanton TO, Baxter DE, Gottlieb MS: Comparison of Chevron osteotomy and modified McBride bunionectomy for correction of mild to moderate hallux valgus deformity. Foot Ankle 12:61–68, 1991.
72. Mann RA, Pfeffinger L: Hallux valgus repair. DuVries modified McBride procedure. Clin Orthop Relat Res (272):213–218, 1991.
73. Pfeffinger LL: The modified McBride procedure. Orthopedics 13:979–984, 1990.
74. McBride ED: The conservative operation for bunions. J Bone Joint Surg 10:735, 1928.
75. Mann R, Coughlin MJ: Adult hallux valgus. In Coughlin M, Mann RA (eds): Surgery of the Foot and Ankle. Philadelphia, Mosby, 1999, pp 150–269.
76. Corless JR: A modification of the Mitchell procedure. J Bone Joint Surg 55:138, 1976.
77. Johnson KA, Cofield RH, Morrey BF: Chevron osteotomy for hallux valgus. Clin Orthop Relat Res (142):44–47, 1979.
78. Austin DW, Leventen EO: A new osteotomy for hallux valgus: A horizontally directed "V" displacement osteotomy of the metatarsal head for hallux valgus and primus varus. Clin Orthop Relat Res (157):25–30, 1981.
79. Badwey TM, Dutkowsky JP, Graves SC, Richardson EG: An anatomical basis for the degree of displacement of the distal chevron osteotomy in the treatment of hallux valgus. Foot Ankle Int 18:213–215, 1997.

80. Mann RA, Donatto KC: The chevron osteotomy: A clinical and radiographic analysis. Foot Ankle Int 18:255–261, 1997.

81. Deorio JK, Ware AW: Single absorbable polydioxanone pin fixation for distal chevron bunion osteotomies. Foot Ankle Int 22:832–835, 2001.

82. Gill LH, Martin DF, Coumas JM, Kiebzak GM: Fixation with bioabsorbable pins in chevron bunionectomy. J Bone Joint Surg Am 79:1510–1518, 1997.

83. Trnka HJ, Zembsch A, Easley ME, et al: The chevron osteotomy for correction of hallux valgus. Comparison of findings after two and five years of follow-up. J Bone Joint Surg Am 82-A:1373–1378, 2000.

84. Trnka HJ, Zembsch A, Wiesauer H, et al: Modified Austin procedure for correction of hallux valgus. Foot Ankle Int 18:119–127, 1997.

85. Schneider W, Aigner N, Pinggera O, Knahr K: Chevron osteotomy in hallux valgus. Ten-year results of 112 cases. J Bone Joint Surg Br 86:1016–1020, 2004.

86. Mitchell LA, Baxter DE: A Chevron-Akin double osteotomy for correction of hallux valgus. Foot Ankle 12:7–14, 1991.

87. Tollison ME, Baxter DE: Combination chevron plus Akin osteotomy for hallux valgus: Should age be a limiting factor? Foot Ankle Int 18:477–481, 1997.

88. Kuhn MA, Lippert FG 3rd, Phipps MJ, Williams C: Blood flow to the metatarsal head after chevron bunionectomy. Foot Ankle Int 26:526–529, 2005.

89. Resch S, Stenstrom A, Reynisson K, Jonsson K: Chevron osteotomy for hallux valgus not improved by additional adductor tenotomy. A prospective, randomized study of 84 patients. Acta Orthop Scand 65:541–544, 1994.

90. Meier PJ, Kenzora JE: The risks and benefits of distal first metatarsal osteotomies. Foot Ankle 6:7–11, 1985.

91. Caminear DS, Pavlovich R Jr, Pietrzak WS: Fixation of the chevron osteotomy with an absorbable copolymer pin for treatment of hallux valgus deformity. J Foot Ankle Surg 44:203–210, 2005.

92. Chen YJ, Hsu RW, Shih HN, et al: Distal chevron osteotomy with intra-articular lateral soft-tissue release for treatment of moderate to severe hallux valgus deformity. J Formos Med Assoc 95:776–781, 1996.

93. Crosby LA, Bozarth GR: Fixation comparison for chevron osteotomies. Foot Ankle Int 19:41–43, 1998.

94. Peterson DA, Zilberfarb JL, Greene MA, Colgrove RC: Avascular necrosis of the first metatarsal head: Incidence in distal osteotomy combined with lateral soft tissue release. Foot Ankle Int 15:59–63, 1994.

95. Pochatko DJ, Schlehr FJ, Murphey MD, Hamilton JJ: Distal chevron osteotomy with lateral release for treatment of hallux valgus deformity. Foot Ankle Int 15:457–461, 1994.

96. Thomas RL, Espinosa FJ, Richardson EG: Radiographic changes in the first metatarsal head after distal chevron osteotomy combined with lateral release through a plantar approach. Foot Ankle Int 15:285–292, 1994.

97. Trnka HJ, Hofmann S, Salzer M, Ritschl P: Clinical and radiological results after Austin bunionectomy for treatment of hallux valgus. Arch Orthop Trauma Surg 115(3-4):171–175, 1996.

98. Nery C, Barroco R, Ressio C: Biplanar chevron osteotomy. Foot Ankle Int 23:792–798, 2002.

99. Resch S, Stenstrom A, Gustafson T: Circulatory disturbance of the first metatarsal head after Chevron osteotomy as shown by bone scintigraphy. Foot Ankle 13:137–142, 1992.

100. Jones KJ, Feiwell LA, Freedman EL, Cracchiolo A 3rd: The effect of chevron osteotomy with lateral capsular release on the blood supply to the first metatarsal head. J Bone Joint Surg Am 77:197–204, 1995.

101. Turnbull T, Grange W: A comparison of Keller's arthroplasty and distal metatarsal osteotomy in the treatment of adult hallux valgus. J Bone Joint Surg Br 68:132–137, 1986.

102. Zembsch A, Trnka HJ, Ritschl P: Correction of hallux valgus. Metatarsal osteotomy versus excision arthroplasty. Clin Orthop Relat Res (376):183–194, 2000.

103. Jordan HH, Brodsky AE: Keller operation for hallux valgus and hallux rigidus. Arch Surg 62:586–596, 1951.

104. Richardson EG: Keller resection arthroplasty. Orthopedics 13:1049–1053, 1990.

105. Sarda G, Bertini G, Celenza M, et al: [Review of 64 cases of hallux valgus surgically treated with the Keller-Leviere technique]. Minerva Med 81(7-8 suppl):121–122, 1990.

106. Schneider W, Knahr K: Keller procedure and chevron osteotomy in hallux valgus: Five-year results of different surgical philosophies in comparable collectives. Foot Ankle Int 23:321–329, 2002.

107. Viladot R, Rochera R, Alvarez F, Pasarin A: [Resection arthroplasty in the treatment of hallux valgus]. Orthopade 25:324–331, 1996.

108. Donley BG, Vaughn RA, Stephenson KA, Richardson EG: Keller resection arthroplasty for treatment of hallux valgus deformity: Increased correction with fibular sesamoidectomy. Foot Ankle Int 23:699–703, 2002.

109. Bardelli M, Gusso MI, Allegra M: [Hallux valgus treated by the Keller-Lelievre-Viladot technic: indications and results]. Arch Putti Chir Organi Mov 33:201–211, 1983.

110. Grandi A, Neri M: [Critical review of cases operated for hallux valgus using the Keller-Lelievre-Viladot method]. Chir Organi Mov 71:115–117, 1986.

111. Capasso G, Testa V, Maffulli N, Barletta L: Molded arthroplasty and transfer of the extensor hallucis brevis tendon. A modification of the Keller-Lelievre operation. Clin Orthop Relat Res (308):43–49, 1994.

112. LeLievre J, LeLievre J-F: [Technique chirurgicale de l'avant pied]. In LeLievre J (ed): Pathologie due Pied. Paris, Masson et Cie, 1967, pp 809–812.

113. Mann RA: Distal soft tissue procedure and proximal metatarsal osteotomy for correction of hallux valgus deformity. Orthopedics 13:1013–1018, 1990.

114. Dreeben S, Mann RA: Advanced hallux valgus deformity: Long-term results utilizing the distal soft tissue procedure and proximal metatarsal osteotomy. Foot Ankle Int 17:142–144, 1996.

115. Easley ME, Kiebzak GM, Davis WH, Anderson RB: Prospective, randomized comparison of proximal crescentic and proximal chevron osteotomies for correction of hallux valgus deformity. Foot Ankle Int 17:307–316, 1996.

116. Markbreiter LA, Thompson FM: Proximal metatarsal osteotomy in hallux valgus correction: A comparison of crescentic and chevron procedures. Foot Ankle Int 18:71–76, 1997.

117. Veri JP, Pirani SP, Claridge R: Crescentic proximal metatarsal osteotomy for moderate to severe hallux valgus: A mean 12.2 year follow-up study. Foot Ankle Int 22:817–822, 2001.

118. Sammarco GJ, Brainard BJ, Sammarco VJ: Bunion correction using proximal Chevron osteotomy. Foot Ankle 14:8–14, 1993.

119. Sammarco GJ, Conti SF: Proximal Chevron metatarsal osteotomy: Single incision technique. Foot Ankle 14:44–47, 1993.

120. Sammarco GJ, Russo-Alesi FG: Bunion correction using proximal chevron osteotomy: A single-incision technique. Foot Ankle Int 19:430–437, 1998.

121. Chiodo CP, Schon LC, Myerson MS: Clinical results with the Ludloff osteotomy for correction of adult hallux valgus. Foot Ankle Int 25:532–536, 2004.

122. Mann RA, Rudicel S, Graves SC: Repair of hallux valgus with a distal soft-tissue procedure and proximal metatarsal osteotomy. A long-term follow-up. J Bone Joint Surg Am 74:124–129, 1992.

123. Zettl R, Trnka HJ, Easley M, et al: Moderate to severe hallux valgus deformity: Correction with proximal crescentic osteotomy and distal soft-tissue release. Arch Orthop Trauma Surg 120(7-8):397–402, 2000.

124. Jones C, Coughlin M, Villadot R, Golano P: Proximal crescentic metatarsal osteotomy: The effect of saw blade orientation on first ray elevation. Foot Ankle Int 26:152–157, 2005.

125. Okuda R, Kinoshita M, Morikawa J, et al: Surgical treatment for hallux valgus with painful plantar callosities. Foot Ankle Int 22:203–208, 2001.

126. Thordarson DB, Leventen EO: Hallux valgus correction with proximal metatarsal osteotomy: Two-year follow-up. Foot Ankle 13:321–326, 1992.

127. Anderson RB, Davis WH: Internal fixation of the proximal chevron osteotomy. Foot Ankle Int 18:371–372, 1997.

128. Gallentine JW DJ, DeOrio MJ: Bunion surgery using locking-plate fixation of proximal metatarsal chevron osteotomies. Foot Ankle Int 28:361–368, 2007.

129. Trnka HJ: Osteotomies for hallux valgus correction. Foot and Ankle Clinics of North America 10(1):15–33, 2005.

130. Ludloff K: Die Beseitigung des Hallux Valgus durch die schraege planta-dorsale Osteotomie des Metatarsus. I Arch Klin Chir 110:364–387, 1918.

131. Beischer AD, Ammon P, Corniou A, Myerson M: Three-dimensional computer analysis of the modified Ludloff osteotomy. Foot Ankle Int 26:627–632, 2005.

132. Hofstaetter SG, Gruber F, Ritschl P, Trnka HJ: [The modified Ludloff osteotomy for correction of severe metatarsus primus varus with hallux valgus deformity]. Z Orthop Ihre Grenzgeb 144:141–147, 2006.

133. Petroutsas J, Trnka HJ: The Ludloff osteotomy for correction of hallux valgus. Oper Orthop Traumatol 17:102–117, 2005.

134. Resch S, Stenstrom A, Egund N: Proximal closing wedge osteotomy and adductor tenotomy for treatment of hallux valgus. Foot Ankle 9:272–280, 1989.

135. Trnka HJ, Muhlbauer M, Zembsch A, et al: Basal closing wedge osteotomy for correction of hallux valgus and metatarsus primus varus: 10- to 22-year follow-up. Foot Ankle Int 20:171–177, 1999.

136. Granberry WM, Hickey CH: Hallux valgus correction with metatarsal osteotomy: Effect of a lateral distal soft tissue procedure. Foot Ankle Int 16:132–138, 1995.

137. Crevoisier X, Mouhsine E, Ortolano V, et al: The scarf osteotomy for the treatment of hallux valgus deformity: A review of 84 cases. Foot Ankle Int 22:970–976, 2001.

138. Barouk LS: Scarf osteotomy for hallux valgus correction. Local anatomy, surgical technique, and combination with other forefoot procedures. Foot Ankle Clin 5:525–558, 2000.

139. Jones S, Al Hussainy HA, Ali F, et al: Scarf osteotomy for hallux valgus. A prospective clinical and pedobarographic study. J Bone Joint Surg Br 86:830–836, 2004.

140. Kristen KH, Berger C, Stelzig S, et al: The SCARF osteotomy for the correction of hallux valgus deformities. Foot Ankle Int 23:221–229, 2002.

141. Lorei TJ, Kinast C, Klarner H, Rosenbaum D: Pedographic, clinical, and functional outcome after scarf osteotomy. Clin Orthop Relat Res 2006;451:161–166.

142. Aminian A, Kelikian A, Moen T: Scarf osteotomy for hallux valgus deformity: An intermediate followup of clinical and radiographic outcomes. Foot Ankle Int 27:883–886, 2006.

143. Dereymaeker G: Scarf osteotomy for correction of hallux valgus. Surgical technique and results as compared to distal chevron osteotomy. Foot Ankle Clin 5:513–524, 2000.

144. Perugia D, Basile A, Gensini A, et al: The scarf osteotomy for severe hallux valgus. Int Orthop 27:103–106, 2003.

145. Smith AM, Alwan T, Davies MS: Perioperative complications of the scarf osteotomy. Foot Ankle Int 24:222–227, 2003.

146. Coetzee JC: Scarf osteotomy for hallux valgus repair: The dark side. Foot Ankle Int 24:29–33, 2003.

147. Weil LS: Scarf osteotomy for correction of hallux valgus. Historical perspective, surgical technique, and results. Foot Ankle Clin 5:559–580, 2000.

148. Madhav R, Singh D: Re: Scarf osteotomy for hallux valgus repair: The dark side, Coetzee, JC, Foot Ankle Int 24(1):29-33, 2003.

149. Saragas NP: Technique tip: Preventing "troughing" with the scarf osteotomy. Foot Ankle Int 26:779–780, 2005.

150. Capasso G, Testa V, Maffulli N, Barletta L: Molded arthroplasty and transfer of the extensor hallucis brevis tendon. A modification of the Keller-Lelievre operation. Clin Orthop Relat Res (308):43–49, 1994.

151. Grimes JS, Coughlin MJL: First metatarsophalangeal joint arthrodesis as a treatment for failed hallux valgus surgery. Foot Ankle Int 27:887–893, 2006.

152. Faber FW, Mulder PG, Verhaar JA: Role of first ray hypermobility in the outcome of the Hohmann and the Lapidus procedure. A prospective, randomized trial involving one hundred and one feet. J Bone Joint Surg Am 86-A:486–495, 2004.

153. Coetzee JC, Wickum D: The Lapidus procedure: A prospective cohort outcome study. Foot Ankle Int 25:526–531, 2004.

154. Johnson KA, Kile TA: Hallux valgus due to cuneiform-metatarsal instability. J South Orthop Assoc 3:273–282, 1994.

155. Coetzee JC, Resig SG, Kuskowski M, Saleh KJ: The Lapidus procedure as salvage after failed surgical treatment of hallux valgus: A prospective cohort study. J Bone Joint Surg Am 85-A:60–65, 2003.

156. Myerson M, Allon S, McGarvey W: Metatarsocuneiform arthrodesis for management of hallux valgus and metatarsus primus varus. Foot Ankle 13:107–115, 1992.

157. Okuda R, Kinoshita M, Morikawa J, et al: Distal soft tissue procedure and proximal metatarsal osteotomy in hallux valgus. Clin Orthop Relat Res (379):209–217, 2000.

158. Coetzee JC, Resig SG, Kuskowski M, Saleh KJ: The Lapidus procedure as salvage after failed surgical treatment of hallux valgus. Surgical technique. J Bone Joint Surg Am 86-A(suppl 1):30–36, 2004.

159. Coughlin MJ, Carlson RE: Treatment of hallux valgus with an increased distal metatarsal articular angle: Evaluation of double and triple first ray osteotomies. Foot Ankle Int 20:762–770, 1999.

160. Coughlin MJ, Grebing BR, Jones CP: Arthrodesis of the first metatarsophalangeal joint for idiopathic hallux valgus: Intermediate results. Foot Ankle Int 26:783–792, 2005.

161. Grondal L, Hedstrom M, Stark A: Arthrodesis compared to Mayo resection of the first metatarsophalangeal joint in total rheumatoid forefoot reconstruction. Foot Ankle Int 26:135–139, 2005.

162. Machacek F Jr, Easley ME, Gruber F, et al: Salvage of a failed Keller resection arthroplasty. J Bone Joint Surg Am 86-A:1131–1138, 2004.

What Is the Best Treatment for a Charcot Foot and Ankle?

LEW SCHON, MD AND MEENA SHATBY, MD

Charcot, or neuropathic arthropathy, of the lower extremity is a destructive disease in which patients present with swelling, erythema, and progressive deformity of their feet. Despite diabetes becoming the most common causative agent, the incidence of Charcot neuropathy is quite low in the diabetic population. In a radiographic study,[1] the incidence was noted to be less than 1%, with similar incidence in retrospective clinical studies.[2] Other studies have reported the presence of Charcot radiographic bony changes in almost 16% of patients with diabetes.[3] This large variability may be attributed to difference in definition, alternate diagnosis, and lack of clinical signs despite radiographic changes.

The cause of Charcot disease is related to presence of peripheral neuropathy. Two theories currently exist regarding the pathophysiology of the disease. One theory considers neurotraumatic destruction of the joint, in which multiple trauma to the insensate joint results in microfractures, which over time result in macrofractures and progressive deformity. This concept also includes major fractures that progress to clinical deformity and is similar to the pathway by which arthritic joints in neuropathic patients become Charcot joints with advanced bony changes. The second theory relies on neurosympathetic destruction in which vascular and absorptive changes occur secondary to abnormal neural function, leading to autonomic sympathectomy and vascular alterations, which eventually progresses to gross deformity.[4] It is thought that a combination of both pathologies contributes to the disease process. A common finding that is not as frequently evaluated is that peripheral perfusion is maintained in this group of patients.

Biologically, the progressive bone resorption seen in Charcot joints is associated with a large number of osteoclasts lining resorptive bone lacunae. The osteoclasts outnumber osteoblasts and demonstrate immunoreactivity to cytokines: interleukin (IL)-1, IL-6, and tumor necrosis factor-α (TNF-α). One study concludes that alteration in the synthesis, secretion, or activity of these regulatory molecules may alter bone remodeling and lead to healing without collapse or malalignment.[5]

CLASSIFICATION

The disease process has been divided into stages as described by Eichenholtz.[6] Stage I is characterized by significant inflammatory response with hyperemia, erythema, swelling, and warmth. Radiographically,

this is associated with bony fragmentation. Stage II, known as coalescence, involves decreasing inflammation and edema, with bony coalescence noted radiographically. In Stage III, the bones are consolidated with an absence of inflammatory signs leading to the presence of fixed deformity.[4] A prodromal stage 0 ("pre-stage I") category has been described in patients with neuropathy with an acute sprain or fracture that places them at risk for the development of full-blown Charcot arthropathy.[7] Other classification systems have been developed since then that are based on anatomic location and type of deformity.[8,9] The only classification system tested to be reliable and reproducible involved the midtarsus.[9,10] In this radiographic classification, Charcot anatomic variants of midtarsus deformities are identified by Roman numerals (I-IV) beginning from the Lisfranc joints (I) and extending proximally to the transverse tarsal joints (IV). A severity stage (α [low risk] or β [high risk]) is assigned depending on radiographic features. If one of the following criteria is met, the foot is considered at high risk (β):

1. A dislocation is present
2. The lateral talar-first metatarsal angle is ≥ 30 degrees
3. The lateral calcaneal-fifth metatarsal angle ≥ 0 degrees
4. The anteroposterior talar-first metatarsal angle is ≥ 35 degrees

An α stage can be assigned when all four features are absent. By testing the system on 75 orthopedic surgeons, reliability and reproducibility were found to be high. It was believed to be useful as a tool for diagnosis, planning treatment, and assessing the prognosis.[10]

MANAGEMENT

Goals of treatment include the creation and maintenance of a stable plantigrade foot, wound and bone healing, elimination of infection, and prevention of deformity. Current treatment recommendations are based on the stage of disease presentation. Pinzur[11] had reported that reviewing current orthopaedic textbooks reveals almost universal agreement that acute Charcot foot arthropathy, Stage I Eichenholtz, should be treated conservatively, and surgery has only been advised when accommodative treatment has failed.[12,13] Despite this general consensus, significant lack of evidence-based studies exist to support this recommendation, with a majority of current data from Level III and IV studies.[11] Therefore, a grade C recommendation exists regarding the use of total contact cast (TCC) for the initial management of Charcot arthropathy.

The American Orthopaedic Foot and Ankle Society (AOFAS) has taken an initiative to develop objective data for basing diagnostic and therapeutic guidelines for this disease. A two-part survey was done. Whereas the first part surveyed treatment patterns for 94 patients, the second part consisted of a questionnaire of the clinical preferences completed by 37 AOFAS members with special interest in the disease process.[14] The AOFAS notes from their results that management of the Charcot foot in the community is inconsistent, and significant variability occurs from the current guidelines by both physicians in the community and the specialists.[14]

Adjuvant Medical Treatment

In addition to better diabetic control, a number of studies have looked at adjuvant medications during the acute phase to relieve the symptoms.[15] A Level I, randomized, controlled, therapeutic trial of 39 patients with active Charcot neuroarthropathy randomly assigned patients to treatment with 90 mg pamidronate or placebo.[16] The authors report the treatment group had statistically significant reduction of symptoms and warmth; there was also significant reduction in bone turnover markers, bone-specific alkaline phosphate and dehydroxypyridinoline, from 4 to 24 weeks. The authors conclude that pamidronate had a substantial effect on reducing symptoms and bone turnover markers in patients with active Charcot arthropathy.[16] They also suggest that further studies may be necessary to evaluate dosing regimen and frequency of pamidronate administration. Therefore, a grade B recommendation exists for the use of pamidronate in reducing symptoms of active Charcot arthropathy.

Nonsurgical Management

Traditionally, acute Charcot arthropathy, or Eichenholtz Stage I, has been treated with non–weight bearing and TCC. In healthy subjects, plantar peak pressure was shown to be significantly less, and contact duration greater, under the metatarsal heads and heel during gait in a TCC than in a standard shoe.[17] A general belief exists that the healing time for diabetic Charcot fractures may be twice as long as nondiabetic fractures[15,18]; nevertheless, Boddenberg's[19] literature review found no conclusive evidence to support that assumption.[19] His experience with 28 patients with diabetes compared with 17 patients in a control group found a healing rate of 3.5 versus 3 months in the control group.[19] Another study noted differences in healing based on the location of pathology at an average of 86 ± 45 days, with hindfoot and midfoot Charcot taking longer than forefoot disease to complete healing.[20] Thus, grade B level of recommendation exists that the

length of treatment of fractures in patients with Charcot arthropathy is similar or only slightly larger in nondiabetic fractures.

In a study of 55 patients with acute Charcot arthropathy who were treated with serial TCC for an average of 18.5 ± 10.6 weeks, all patients returned to permanent footwear over a period of 28.3 ± 14.5 weeks after casting.[21] The authors note that the casting time to return to footwear was independent of anatomic site of involvement.[21] However, patients with bilateral involvement required a longer duration of TCC treatment (28 ± 15 weeks) and a longer subsequent period for return to permanent footwear (48 ± 18 weeks; $P <$ 0.02).[21] A retrospective review of 237 patients showed successful nonoperative management with non–weight-bearing TTC in 115 (48.5%) patients. The cast was changed weekly and discontinued after dissipation of swelling and warmth.[13] Another study involving 147 patients noted that 87 patients (59.2%) were successfully managed conservatively.[11] An additional retrospective study of 221 neuropathic fractures or Charcot joints identified 136 that were managed without surgical reconstruction.[22]

However, compliance with non–weight-bearing status is variable and can be limited by physical or medical conditions, or both.[15] Pinzur and colleagues[15,23] managed 9 patients treated with TTC who were allowed to bear full weight on their casts. At 5 months, all patients progressed to consolidation without any complications or wound problems. In another case series, the authors used a well-padded bivalved cast (moldable, removable to check skin and padding) in 25 (51%) acute Charcot feet with good success.[24] Another study by Conti and coauthors[25,26] compared plantar pressure measurements between short leg casts (SLCs) and TTC in 10 healthy subjects. They identified no significant difference between SLC and TTC, although there were marginal decreased hindfoot pressures in TTC.[25]

In subacute (stage II) midfoot Charcot arthropathy, Myerson and coauthors[27] note that TTC was successful in 70% of patients. As the stages evolved, weight bearing was advanced to full weight bearing, and patients were then placed in protective bracing to decrease the risk for flare-up or displacement.[15,27]

From these studies, one may summarize a grade B recommendation exists to support the concept "short leg cast is equivalent to TCC in dissipating pressure and grade C recommendations exist that 'weightbearing is permissible in cast, in allowing significant proportional of Charcot patients to successfully follow a nonoperative protocol.'"

Complications of Casting

Casting is not risk free, and contraindications to total contact casting include deep infection, osteomyelitis, extensive drainage, poor skin quality, severe arterial insufficiency, and poor patient compliance.[28] Guyton's[29] retrospective review of 71 patients was performed to evaluate iatrogenic complications of TCCs. The average cast was changed every 7.69 days. Complications occurred in 22 casts (5.52% per cast). These included six new pretibial ulcers, six new midfoot ulcers, four forefoot or toe ulcers, five hindfoot ulcers, and one malleolar ulcer. He notes that all the iatrogenic ulcers, except for one, healed within 3 weeks, and there was no worsening of the original wound or ulcer.[29]

No studies exist that have compared alternative forms of protective immobilization. It appears that a significant number of methods have been used including well-padded bivalved casts, Unna boots, compression hoses, molded splints, braces, bivalved ankle-foot orthosis (AFO), and SLCs.[12,14,15,30–32] Therefore, a grade I recommendation exists for these alternative forms of protective immobilization of Charcot arthropathy.

Surgical Treatment

Indications for surgery in the Charcot foot include acute fracture or dislocation, severe or progressive deformity, and recurrent ulceration, secondary to either instability or bony prominence.[22,31,33] Surgical procedures include debridement, exostectomy of bony prominences, osteotomies with realignment, and fusion. In a Level IV series by Myerson and coauthors,[27] a cohort of 41 feet with chronic Charcot, stage III, underwent total contact casting initially. Subsequent surgery in this group included arthrodesis in nine (22%) feet, exostectomy in six (14%) feet, drainage of an abscess in two (5%) feet, and amputation in two (5%) feet.[27] In stage II midfoot neuroarthropathy, 3 (10%) of 30 feet were treated surgically (two arthrodeses and one exostectomy) after reaching the chronic stage, stage III.[27] In another level IV study, 29 (17%) of 168 patients with Charcot arthropathy were treated surgically in either stages II or III.[34] Saltzman and colleagues[35] (Level IV) performed 53 procedures on 115 patients (49%), excluding amputations. Another group of 122 of 237 patients (51.5%) required surgical intervention that included bony stabilization, debridement, and partial limb amputations.[13] Another group had a surgical rate of 40.8%.[11]

Exostectomies. Exostectomies are indicated for stable Charcot deformities and are supported by Level IV studies, in which there are bony prominences that are promoting recurrent ulceration or hindering healing of a chronic ulcer.[4,11,36,37] A retrospective review (Level IV) of 20 patients who underwent 27 ostectomy procedures evaluated medial and lateral column ulcerations.[38] There were 18 medial and 9 lateral ulcers. After surgery, 20 wounds had resolved, resulting in a 74% healing rate. The majority of failed procedures involved lateral column wounds (six of seven). Revision surgery was required in five of the nine lateral column wounds for limb salvage. The authors warn that ostectomy for ulcers that involve the lateral column was less predictable and may require further surgery.[38] Therefore, a grade C recommendation exists for exostectomy for stable Charcot arthropathy in which there are bony prominences that are promoting recurrent ulceration or hindering healing of a chronic ulcer.

Internal Fixation. Traditionally, elective operative fusion of Charcot joints had been performed in Eichenholtz stage III or after. This protocol is followed to avoid the poorer bone quality and increased technical difficulties associated with stages I and II.[15,33] Currently, no studies in the literature support that theory, however, and surgery may be indicated in stage I disease if there is gross instability, dislocation, or deformity.[7] Simon and coworkers[39] published the results of 14 of 43 patients with stage I disease who underwent acute extensive debridement, open reduction, and internal fixation of the tarsal-metatarsal region with autologous bone graft. They note successful union in all patients. The mean time to assisted weight bearing was 10 ± 3.3 weeks, the mean time to unassisted weight bearing was 15 ± 8.8 weeks, and the mean time to return to the use of regular shoes was 27 ± 14.4 weeks.[39]

Associated procedures may include Achilles tendon lengthening[21,22,33,40] if there is associated equines contracture, bone grafting with internal or external fixation[40] for defects, or increased risk for nonunion.[22]

Methods of Fixation. Despite many case series recommending open reduction and internal fixation.[11,12,33,34] No studies have looked at comparing different modalities of fixations. A variety of midfoot arthrodesis techniques has been described. Despite Charcot arthropathy being a major cause of multiple midfoot joint arthroses, most of these studies did not focus solely on the disease. Internal fixation techniques included staples, Steinmann pins, tension band wires, screws, dowels, and medial or plantar plates.[41–46] A biomechanical study comparing multiscrew fixation with a plate applied to the plantar (tension) side of the medial midfoot demonstrated that the latter was stronger.[47]

Traditionally, fixation plates have been placed medial and plantar, areas thought to be of greatest stress.[29,34,35,39] However, a retrospective review of nine patients undergoing fusion through a dorsally placed plate (four were secondary to Charcot arthropathy) had a 95% success rate.[45] Another retrospective review of 10 patients treated with open reduction and internal fixation with iliac crest bone grafting resulted in 90% union rate.[48] This included five osseous and four fibrous unions.[48]

For hindfoot fixation, plantar or medial plates, and screws have been utilized. A biomechanical study assessing the calcaneocuboid (CC) screw placement found that a screw placed axially from posterior to anterior starting at the calcaneal tuberosity and crossing the CC joint perpendicularly was superior to an obliquely placed screw.[49]

Caravaggi and researchers[50] evaluated ankle arthrodesis with a compressive intramedullary nail in 14 patients. Patients had severe ankle instability with previous recommendation of undergoing below-knee amputation (BKA). After a mean follow-up of 18 months, 10 patients (71.4%) achieved a solid arthrodesis, 3 patients (21.4%) experienced development of fibrous union, after hardware failure, and 1 patient went on to a BKA.[50] Another study by Pinzur and colleagues[51] evaluated 21 attempted ankle fusion with a retrograde nail, of which 11 limbs had the talus absent or required complete talectomy for realignment. A significantly increased complication rate was present in this subgroup of patients compared with the group with preserved talus.[51]

External fixation may be used as an alternative form of fixation and deformity correction. This may be especially useful in patients with extensive open wounds and recurrent or persistent ulcerations.[34] A retrospective review reported on 11 patients with significant ulcerations who underwent wound debridement, ostectomy, corrective osteotomies, and external fixation. Average time of fixator placement was 57 days, after which all patients were placed in TCC for an average of 131 days. All patients progressed to full healing, with four osseous and five fibrous unions.[52] Another report by Pinzur[53] advocates the use of ring external fixators for patients with high risks for wound complications for internal fixation. Based on the wide variety of surgical techniques and method of fixation, the absence of studies comparing different modality of fixation leads to a grade I recommendation.

Complications of Arthrodesis with Internal Fixation

In a series of 29 operative patients, 10 (34%) patients experienced development of pseudarthroses.[34] Other complications in 19 of the 29 patients included malunion, superficial wound infection, early or late fatigue failure of screw fixation, wound slough, skin irritation and ulceration, distal tibia fracture, osteomyelitis, and BKA. However, 7 (70%) of the pseudarthroses were stable, and limb salvage was achieved in 27 (93%) patients.[34] Papa and coauthors[34] report a complication rate of 65% in their study of 29 patients. These included nine pseudarthroses (six tibiocalcaneal, one tibiotalar, and two talonavicular). In another series, the complication rate was 53%.[54]

COMPLICATIONS OF CHARCOT ARTHROPATHY

Saltzman and colleagues'[35] retrospective review of 115 patients demonstrated an approximately 2.7% annual rate of amputation, a 23% risk for requiring bracing for more than 18 months, and a 49% risk for recurrent ulceration. Limbs with open ulcers at initial presentation or chronically recurrent ulcers had increased risk for amputation.[35] Pinzur[13] reports an overall lower extremity amputation rate of 9% (of 237 patients) during a 10-year period.

In a meta-analysis of 15 studies, the death rate was 4% (11 deaths in 301 patients) within 2.5 years after treatment for Charcot arthropathy.[55] Partial or complete foot amputation had been done in 20 (7%) of 301 patients in the follow-up period. A total of 83 (28%) of 301 patients required an AFO, permanent bracing, or assistive devices.[55]

PREVENTION

Charcot arthropathy may occur after acute trauma in the patient with neuropathy.[37] Therefore, it is prudent to treat this population group with extra caution including immobilization and protective bracing after injury. In patients with diabetes with decreased sensation, preventive patient education may include frequent inspection, extra protection against traumatic events, and low tolerance in seeking medical evaluation.[37] A single-blinded, randomized, clinical trial study was conducted to evaluate the effectiveness of at-home infrared temperature monitoring for preventing the development of ulceration and wound complications in patients with diabetes at high risk.[56] The authors divided 85 patients into 2 groups, with the first group undergoing standard foot care and evaluation, and the second group adding home infrared thermometer to monitor skin temperature, and reducing their activity with any detectable increase in temperature. The authors used a temperature differential of 4 degrees between corresponding sites of opposite feet to trigger the subsequent decreased activity level and to contact a healthcare worker. They note that patients in the standard management group were 10.3 times more likely to experience development of foot ulcerations than the group monitoring skin temperature changes and adjusting their activity level accordingly. Two cases of Charcot arthropathy were observed in the standard treatment group, and none was observed in the second group. Their recommendation was to use home infrared thermometry as an adjunct tool for diabetic foot care and monitoring.[56]

Although this one Level I study possibly supports a grade A recommendation, this is only one study, and this diagnostic modality needs to be substantiated in further studies. Table 74–1 provides a summary of recommendations for the treatment of Charcot foot and ankle.

TABLE 74–1. Summary of Recommendations

RECOMMENDATIONS	LEVEL OF EVIDENCE/GRADE OF RECOMMENDATION
1. Home monitoring of foot skin temperatures is successful in preventing ulceration.	A
2. Short leg cast is equivalent to total contact casting in dissipating pressure.	B
3. Length of treatment of fractures in patients with Charcot arthropathy is similar to or slightly longer than with nondiabetic fractures.	B
4. Total contact cast should be used for initial management of Charcot arthropathy.	C
5. Weight bearing is permissible during the initial phase of total contact cast treatment.	C
6. Exostectomy is appropriate for bony prominences.	C
7. Internal fixation is necessary for gross deformity.	C
8. There is no difference between early and late operative arthrodesis.	C
9. External fixation is a valid treatment in high-risk or infected feet.	C
10. Use of pamidronate for treatment of active Charcot arthropathy is effective in reducing symptoms.	C

REFERENCES

1. Smith, DG, Barnes BC, Sands AK, et al: Prevalence of radiographic foot abnormalities in patients with diabetes. Foot Ankle Int 18:342–346, 1997.
2. Fabrin J, Larsen K, Holstein PE: Long-term follow-up in diabetic Charcot feet with spontaneous onset. Diabetes Care 23:796–800, 2000.
3. Cavanagh PR, Young MJ, Adams JE, et al: Radiographic abnormalities in the feet of patients with diabetic neuropathy. Diabetes Care 17:201–209, 1994.
4. Brodsky JW: Charcot's joints. In Mann RA, Coughlin MJ (eds): Surgery of the Foot and Ankle, 8th ed. St. Louis, Mosby, 2006, pp 1281–1368.
5. Baumhauer JF, O'Keefe RJ, Schon LC, et al: Cytokine-induced osteoclastic bone resorption in Charcot arthropathy: An immunohistochemical study. Foot Ankle Int 27:797–800, 2006.
6. Eichenholtz SN: Charcot Joints. Springfield, IL, Charles C Thomas, 1966.
7. Schon LC, Marks RM: The management of neuroarthropathic fracture-dislocations in the diabetic patient. Orthop Clin North Am 26:375–392, 1995.
8. Brodsky JW: The diabetic foot. In: Mann RA, Coughlin MJ (eds): Surgery of the Foot and Ankle. St. Louis, Mosby-Year Book, 1993, pp 877–958.
9. Schon LC, Weinfeld SB, Horton GA, et al: Radiographic and clinical classification of acquired midtarsus deformities. Foot Ankle Int 19:394–404, 1998.
10. Schon LC, Easley ME, Cohen I, et al: The acquired midtarsus deformity classification system—interobserver reliability and intraobserver reproducibility. Foot Ankle Int 23:30–36, 2002.
11. Pinzur M: Surgical versus accommodative treatment for Charcot arthropathy of the midfoot. Foot Ankle Int 25:545–549, 2004.
12. Pinzur MS, Sage R, Stuck R, et al: Treatment algorithm for neuropathic (Charcot) midfoot deformity. Foot Ankle Int 14:189–197, 1993.
13. Pinzur MS: Benchmark analysis of diabetic patients with neuropathic (Charcot) foot deformity. Foot Ankle Int 20:564–567, 1999.
14. Pinzur MS, Shields N, Trepman E, et al: Current practice patterns in the treatment of Charcot foot. Foot Ankle Int 21:916–920, 2000.
15. Trepman E, Nihal A, Pinzur MS: Current topics review: Charcot neuroarthropathy of the foot and ankle. Foot Ankle Int 26:46–63, 2005.
16. Jude EB, Selby PL, Burgess J, et al: Bisphosphonates in the treatment of Charcot neuroarthropathy: A double-blind randomised controlled trial. Diabetologia 44:2032–2037, 2001.
17. Baumhauer JF, Wervey R, McWilliams J, et al: A comparison study of plantar foot pressure in a standardized shoe, total contact cast, and prefabricated pneumatic walking brace. Foot Ankle Int 18:26–33, 1997.
18. Schwarz RJ, Macdonald MRC, Van der Pas M: Results of arthrodesis in neuropathic feet. J Bone Joint Surg Br 88:747–750, 2006.
19. Boddenberg U: Healing time of foot and ankle fractures in patients with diabetes mellitus: Literature review and report on own cases. Zentralbl Chir 129:453–459, 2004.
20. Sinacore DR: Acute Charcot arthropathy in patients with diabetes mellitus: Healing times by foot location. J Diabetes Complications 12:287–293, 1998.
21. Armstrong DG, Todd WF, Lavery LA, et al: The natural history of acute Charcot's arthropathy in a diabetic foot specialty clinic. Diabet Med 14:357–363, 1997.
22. Schon LC, Easley ME, Weinfeld SB: Charcot neuroarthropathy of the foot and ankle. Clin Orthop 349:116–131, 1998.
23. Pinzur MS, Lio T, Posner M: Treatment of Eichenholtz stage I Charcot foot arthropathy with a weightbearing total contact cast. Foot Ankle Int 27:324–329, 2006.
24. Pinzur MS, Sage R, Stuck R, et al: A treatment algorithm for neuropathic (Charcot) midfoot deformity. Foot Ankle 14:189–197, 1993.
25. Conti SF, Martin RL, Chaytor ER, et al: Plantar pressure measurements during ambulation in weightbearing conventional short leg casts and total contact casts. Foot Ankle Int 17:464–469, 1996.
26. Martin RL, Conti SF: Plantar pressure analysis of diabetic rockerbottom deformity in total contact casts. Foot Ankle Int 17:470–472, 1996.
27. Myerson MS, Henderson MR, Saxby T, et al: Management of midfoot diabetic neuroarthropathy. Foot Ankle Int 15:233–241, 1994.
28. Conti SF: Total contact casting. AAOS Instr Course Lect 48:305–315, 1999.
29. Guyton GP: An analysis of iatrogenic complications from the total contact cast. Foot Ankle Int 26:903–907, 2005.
30. Harrelson JM: The diabetic foot: Charcot arthropathy. Instr Course Lect 42:141–146, 1993.
31. Lesko P, Maurer RC: Talonavicular dislocations and midfoot arthropathy in neuropathic diabetic feet. Clin Orthop 240:226–231, 1989.
32. Boninger ML, Leonard JA: Use of bivalved ankle-foot orthosis in neuropathic foot and ankle lesions. J Rehabil Res Dev 33:16–22, 1996.
33. Johnson JE: Surgical treatment for neuropathic arthropathy of the foot and ankle. Instr Course Lect 48:269–277, 1999.
34. Papa J, Myerson M, Girard P: Salvage, with arthrodesis, in intractable diabetic neuropathic arthropathy of the foot and ankle. J Bone Joint Surg Am 75-A:1056–1066, 1993.
35. Saltzman CL, Hagy ML, Zimmerman B, et al: How effective is intensive nonoperative initial treatment of patients with diabetes and Charcot arthropathy of the feet? Clin Orthop Relat Res 435:185–190, 2005.
36. Bono JV, Roger DJ, Jacobs RL: Surgical arthrodesis of the neuropathic foot. A salvage procedure. Clin Orthop Relat Res 14–20, 1993.
37. Johnson JE: Operative treatment of neuropathic arthropathy of the foot and ankle. J Bone Joint Surg 80-A:1700–1709, 1998.
38. Catanzariti AR, Mendicino R, Haverstock B: Ostectomy for diabetic neuroarthropathy involving the midfoot. J Foot Ankle Surg 39:291–300, 2000.
39. Simon SR, Tejwani SG, Wilson DL, et al: Arthrodesis as an early alternative to nonoperative management of Charcot arthropathy of the diabetic foot. J Bone Joint Surg Am 82-A:939–950, 2000.
40. Deresh GM, Cohen M: Reconstruction of the diabetic Charcot foot incorporating bone grafts. J Foot Ankle Surg 35:474–488, 1996.
41. Horton GA, Olney BW: Deformity correction and arthrodesis of the midfoot with a medial plate. Foot Ankle Int 14:493–499, 1993.
42. Johnson JE, Johnson KA: Dowel arthrodesis for degenerative arthritis of the tarsometatarsal (Lisfranc) joints. Foot Ankle Int 6:243–253, 1986.
43. Kupcha PC, Fitzpatrick MJ: Application of the tension band technique for arthrodesis of the forefoot and midfoot. Foot Ankle Int 12:784, 1996.
44. Treadwell JR, Kahn MD: Lisfranc arthrodesis for chronic pain: A cannulated screw technique. J Foot Ankle Surg 37:28–36, 1998.
45. Suh J-S, Amendola A, Lee K-B, et al: Dorsal modified calcaneal plate for extensive midfoot arthrodesis. Foot Ankle Int 26:503–509, 2005.
46. Sticha RS, Frascone ST, Wertheimer SJ: Major arthrodeses in patients with neuropathic arthropathy. J Foot Ankle Surg 35:560–566, 1996.
47. Marks RM, Parks B, Schon LC: Midfoot fusion technique for neuropathic feet: Biomechanical analysis and rationale. Foot Ankle Int 19:507–510, 1998.
48. Craig Stone N, Daniels TR: Midfoot and hindfoot arthrodeses in diabetic Charcot arthropathy. Can J Surg 43:449–455, 2000.
49. Kann JN, Parks BG, Schon LC: Biomechanical evaluation of two different screw positions for fusion of the calcaneocuboid joint. Foot Ankle Int 20:33–36, 1999.
50. Caravaggi C, Cimmino M, Caruso S, et al: Intramedullary compressive nail fixation for the treatment of severe Charcot deformity of the ankle and rear foot. J Foot Ankle Surg 45:20–24, 2006.

51. Pinzur MS, Kelikian A: Charcot ankle fusion with a retrograde locked intramedullary nail. Foot Ankle Int 18:699–704, 1997.
52. Farber DC, Juliano PJ, Cavanagh PR, et al: Single stage correction with external fixation of the ulcerated foot in individuals with Charcot neuroarthropathy. Foot Ankle Int 23:130–134, 2002.
53. Pinzur MS: The role of ring external fixation in Charcot foot arthropathy. Foot Ankle Clin 11:837–847, 2006.
54. Early JS, Hansen ST: Surgical reconstruction of the diabetic foot: A salvage approach for midfoot collapse. Foot Ankle Int 17:325–330, 1996.
55. Sinacore DR, Withrington NC: Recognition and management of acute neuropathic (Charcot) arthropathies of the foot and ankle. J Orthop Sports Phys Ther 29:736–746, 1999.
56. Lavery LA, Higgins KR, Lanctot DR, et al: Home monitoring of foot skin temperatures to prevent ulceration. Diabetes Care 27:2642–2647, 2004.

Chapter 75

What Is the Best Treatment for Displaced Intra-Articular Calcaneal Fractures?

Richard E. Buckley, MD, FRCSC

All patients who present with a displaced intra-articular calcaneal fracture should be treated initially with rest, ice, compression, and elevation. After initial assessment of the injured patient, decision making becomes much more difficult. Certain factors in patients with displaced intra-articular calcaneal fractures are critically important in deciding whether to operate.[1]

An early (1976) Level II study[2] demonstrated that more patients in the group who had a surgical reduction of their subtalar joint had resumed heavy work. Other studies, reviews, and meta-analyses have shown consistent direction that surgical treatment provides slight advantages in certain circumstances for individual patients with defined patient and fracture factors.[3–9]

TREATMENT OPTIONS

Nonoperative Treatment

A common theme among prospective trials of operative versus nonoperative treatment for displaced intra-articular calcaneal fractures is that the hindfoot becomes stiff when immobilized. Because of this, nonoperative care was thought best without immobilization.[2,6,7] One small, randomized, controlled trial was quick to dismiss nonoperative care because operative care was much better in their Level II trial.[9] However, nonoperative care has withstood the test of time in certain patient populations, especially those patients who are elderly, presenting with multiple medical problems, distal vascular insufficiency, or incorrigible smoking habits. This means ice, elevation, tensoring, and early range of motion establishing full weight bearing by 6 weeks. These patients, especially sedentary patients,[1,6] have reasonable long-term results with nonoperative care.

Percutaneous Fixation

No Level I or II trials exist showing efficacy for percutaneous fixation versus operative care in those patients where surgery has been chosen as the best option for treatment. In situations where the medical circumstance dictates that less surgery may be a better option for an individual patient, percutaneous fixation done with the aid of fluoroscopy, usually from the lateral or medial side, may result in rational care for an individual patient.

Operative Reduction

The debate has raged over whether operative care is better than nonoperative care in many randomized clinical trials.[2,6,7,9] However, one thing becomes clear with careful review of well-performed Level II studies with good follow-up and computerized tomography. Those cases where an operative reduction has been done perfectly end in a better result.[6,10] Nonoperative care, when compared with operative care, has consistently less successful results. Interestingly, the worst outcomes appear to be in those patients who have had operative reduction and internal fixation with a less than optimal anatomic reduction proved by computerized tomography.[6,10] This is also reinforced by a study[11] in which all prospective randomized trials were reviewed to judge operative reduction. This study suggests that there was only weak evidence to support open reduction and internal fixation versus nonoperative care. There was weak evidence to show an improved plain radiographic anatomic alignment in this group of radiographic studies.[7,9,12]

A common theme with these studies and the earlier-mentioned randomized, controlled trials is that patient selection is important. Simple, displaced fractures that can be easily reduced (Sanders type II)[12] are best reduced surgically. Sanders type III and IV fractures (comminuted) are more difficult to reduce accurately and to maintain reduction.[13]

Another article has stated the significance of avoiding complications.[14] Complications will often result in a less than optimal long-term result with problems such as pain, stiffness, or infection lessening the long-term outcome.[1,6,14] It is clear that complications occur regardless of management strategy (even by experienced surgeons). Complications are a cause of significant morbidity, especially failure to obtain and maintain a reduction, infection, and late and long-term stiffness.[14] Surgeon decision making was thought to be crucial for patient outcome. The right patient must receive surgery to minimize possible complications (long-term problems from nonoperative care). The right patient should also be treated without surgery (to minimize operative complications in that patient deemed more suitably treated without surgery).[1,14] The patient and fracture factors thought to be important include age, sex, smoking history, compensation claim information, workload on foot, fracture classification, bilaterality, and description of whether the calcaneus is an open or closed fracture.

EVIDENCE

Nonoperative Treatment

No Level I evidence provides guidance for treatment of displaced intra-articular calcaneal fractures. There are combinations of demographic groups or types of patients who are best treated by nonoperative care.[1,6] Older patients (>60 years), medically unwell patients or unrepentant smokers, sedentary workers, or those with simple fractures patterns such as extra-articular type can be treated without surgery.[1,6] The nonoperative protocol for these patients includes early range of motion, ice, elevation, and good follow-up. These decisions are based on the proviso that a computerized tomographic calcaneal scan demonstrates that the foot does not have any deformity. One of the features that was important from Howard and coauthors'[14] article was that foot deformity treated without surgery will respond poorly, but given the fact that no gross foot deformity (marked varus or valgus) exists, this patient should have little in the way of complications and may be a candidate for nonoperative care.

Percutaneous Fixation

For those displaced fractures where full surgical approaches are not advisable (skin or soft-tissue concerns, elderly patients with vascular problems, or patients with diabetes), percutaneous fixation may be used. Essex-Lopresti[15] introduced the use of the reduction technique with a posterior joystick elevating the depressed posterior facet. Tornetta[16] reintroduced the percutaneous techniques for posterior facet percutaneous reduction more recently with a Level IV study. No Level I or II studies suggest that percutaneous reduction provides better long-term results for displaced intra-articular calcaneal fractures.

Operative Reduction

Once soft tissues have settled (7–10 days), operative treatment is suggested by a number of Level II studies.[2-6,8-10] Young patients are found to respond better

than older adult patients.[6] Female patients may respond better than male patients with displaced intra-articular calcaneal fractures.[6] Open fractures, because of the amount of energy and violence imparted with the foot injury, will have marked foot deformities and have better outcomes with operative care. If a patient presents with a Böhler's angle of greater than 15 degrees, then operative care may be suggested because these patients will do better with operative strategies.[6] Those with a Böhler's angle of less than 0 degrees show equivocal results with operative care, although at least one study by Thordarson and Krieger[9] suggests much better results with operative care. Simple fracture patterns, such as Sanders fracture types II and III, respond better with operative care.[4,6] Fractures that are severely comminuted provide treatment dilemmas. Fractures with Sanders type IV characteristics can be treated with primary operative repair or primary fusion treatment. One study demonstrated that the amount of initial injury involved with the displaced intra-articular calcaneal fracture was a primary prognostic determinant of long-term patient outcome.[17] Patients with Böhler's angle presentation of less than 0 degrees were 10 times more likely to require late subtalar fusion than a Böhler's angle presentation of greater than 15 degrees, whereas a Sanders type IV presentation was 5.5 times more likely to be fused than a simple Sanders type II fracture. Workers with insurance claims were three times more likely to need fusion than those without an insurance claim, whereas nonoperative care resulted in fusion six times more likely than in those patients treated with initial open reduction and internal fixation.[17]

AREAS OF UNCERTAINTY

Age

Ceccarelli and colleagues[18] provided long-term follow-up care on calcaneal fractures in children. Children were defined as younger than 17 years. Those patients who presented with fractures when they were younger than 14 years responded well regardless of nonoperative or operative care. Those patients who were 15 to 17 years old responded better with operative care. This Level II study also showed that extra-articular fractures could be treated without surgery.

Workers' Compensation (Insurance Claims)

Buckley and colleagues[6] determined that results were equivocal with their Level II study when these patients suffered displaced intra-articular calcaneal fractures. Any patient without workers' compensation insurance claim did better with operative care, whereas those patients with an insurance claim did not score as well on the standard scoring scales (scored 20 points less on a 100-point scoring scale).[6]

Bilateral

Patients with bilateral calcaneal injuries seem to have less successful outcomes than patients with one fracture.[6] Gait and occupation are compromised. Treatment strategies are unclear.

Subtalar Fusion

Patients with severe fractures (Sanders type IV) on initial presentation may be treated operatively with primary reconstruction or fusion. No evidence has been reported that one is better than the other in the literature. However, late subtalar fusion is predicted by a number of presenting patient features.[17] Importantly, those patients who were fused late (>6 months after injury) demonstrated outcome scores similar to those treated with surgery early.[17] Level II evidence suggests that if someone is treated without surgery initially because of ongoing medical circumstance, but they require a late subtalar fusion for pain, then their outcome will be similar to patients who had early operative care.

GUIDELINES

The spectrum of care for displaced intra-articular calcaneal fractures is dependent on patient factors and fracture factors. Level II evidence suggests that young patients, any patient without a worker compensation insurance claim, and simple fracture types with good soft tissue will have optimal results with operative care.[1,6,10] Importantly, a surgeon must be wary of patient complications during surgery.[14] Should complications occur, the outcome for the patient significantly lessens because of further surgical needs. The surgical team must be adept at provision of an accurate reduction. Level II evidence[6,10] suggests that if the operative reduction is not well achieved and the surgical team is able only to achieve a partial reduction, then long-term outcome for the patient is compromised. Lastly, for patients who are medically unwell, older, have extra-articular fractures, or perform light or sedentary work, Level II evidence suggests nonoperative care may be the best choice.

RECOMMENDATIONS

Patient must be carefully assessed to ensure they are good operative candidates. Smoking cessation attempts and good soft-tissue care are

---

mandated. Investigation with plain radiograph and computed tomographic scanning can quantify and qualify the type of fracture present. When nonsurgical management is chosen, functional care is preferable to casting with early motion, non–weight bearing, and stretching. At 6 weeks, progressive weight bearing can be started with the use of custom orthoses and good footwear.[1]

Percutaneous operative treatment is best utilized in patients who are medically unwell or who have simple fracture patterns. With careful use of small incisions and intraoperative fluoroscopy, posterior facet reduction is accomplished and maintained with limited internal fixation. Knowing that an anatomic reduction provides the best result, this particular technique should be saved for those patients who, for medical reasons, should not have a large incision for open reduction internal fixation.

Surgery is the standard of care for most displaced intra-articular fractures of the calcaneus. Skeletally mature patients,[18] young adult patients,[6] and any patient without an insurance claim[6] should have operative reduction internal fixation with an experienced surgical team. Simple fracture types are more easily reduced and the fracture reductions maintained. Difficult reductions occur in the Sanders type III and IV fractures, and the surgeon must always be aware that "the achievement of a reduction and the maintenance of a reduction" determines whether a patient will have a good result.[6,10] If the result is compromised with a less than adequate surgical procedure, then the patient will probably have results that are equal to or no better than nonoperative care.[6] Complications must be avoided because patients with complications will have less successful results and long-term outcome.[1,14] Subtalar arthritis, if it does occur, may be treated with late subtalar fusion[17] with good results.

In conclusion, this clinical scenario has proved to be a clinical conundrum. Unfortunately, the surgical team may focus on the fracture and may overlook significant patient characteristics that could help in guiding optimal patient care. Operative management is the treatment of choice as long as complications can be minimized. Nonoperative care can lead to successful results in select patients in a high percentage of cases. Table 75–1 provides a summary of recommendations for the treatment of displaced intra-articular calcaneal fractures.

TABLE 75–1. Summary of Recommendations

FACTORS	LEVEL OF EVIDENCE/ GRADE OF RECOMMENDATION	SURGERY RECOMMENDED	RESULTS EQUIVOCAL	NONOPERATIVE CARE
Patient Factor				
Age[1,3,6]	B	Adolescent; adult	Middle age (50 yr)	>60 yr
Sex[1,3,6]	B	Female patients; young male patients	Middle-aged male patients	Older patients
Smoking history[14]	C	–	–	Recommended
Chronic medical illness[6]	C	–	–	Recommended
Insurance claim[6]	B	–	+	–
Workload[6]	B	Any patient without insurance claim	Insurance claim pending	Light or sedentary work
Fracture Factor				
Bilateral injury[6]	B	–	+	–
Open fracture[1,4]	C	Recommended	–	–
Böhler's angle[6]	B	>0°	<0°	–
Fracture classification[6]	B	Sanders types II, III, and IV	Type IV fractures ORIF or primary fusion	Extra-articular type (percutaneous ORIF?)
Surgical team probability of achieving surgical goal[6]	B	Excellent chance of achieving reduction	Equivocal reduction	Little chance of achieving operative reduction or maintenance of reduction

ORIF, open reduction and internal fixation.

REFERENCES

1. Buckley R, Tough S: Displaced intra-articular calcaneal fractures. J Am Acad Orthop Surg 12:172–178, 2004.
2. Aaron D, Howat T: Intra-articular fractures of the calcaneum. Injury 7:205–211, 1976.
3. Bajammal S, Tornetta IP, Sanders D, et al: Displaced intra-articular calcaneal fractures. J Orthop Trauma 19:360–364, 2005.
4. Bridgman S, Dunn K, McBride D, et al: Interventions for treating calcaneal fractures. Cochrane Database Syst Rev CD001161, 2000.
5. Bridgeman S, Dunn K, McBride D, et al: Interventions for treating calcaneal fractures. Foot 12:47–61, 2002.
6. Buckley R, Tough S, McCormack R, et al: Operative compared with non-operative treatment of displaced intra-articular calcaneal fractures: A prospective randomized controlled multicentre trial. J Bone Joint Surg Am 84:1733–1744, 2002.
7. Parmar H, Triffitt P, Gregg P: Intra-articular fractures of the calcaneum treated operatively or conservatively, a prospective study. J Bone Joint Surg Br 75:932–937, 1993.
8. Randle J, Kreder H, Stephen D, et al: Should calcaneal fractures be treated surgically? Meta-analysis. Clin Orthop Relat Res 217–227, 2000.
9. Thordarson D, Krieger L: Operative vs. non-operative treatment of intra-articular fractures of the calcaneus: A prospective randomized trial. Foot Ankle Int 17:2–9, 1996.
10. Richards P, Bridgman S: Review of the radiology in randomized controlled trials in open reduction and internal fixation (ORIF) of displaced intra-articular calcaneal fractures. Injury 32:633–636, 2001.
11. O'Farrell D, O'Byrne J, McCabe J, et al: Fractures of the os calcis: improved results with internal fixation. Injury 24:263–265, 1993.
12. Sanders R: Intra-articular fractures of the calcaneus: Present state of the art. J Orthop Trauma 6:252–265, 1992.
13. Longino D, Buckley R: Bone graft in the operative treatment of displaced intra-articular calcaneal fractures: Is it helpful? J Orthop Trauma 15:280–286, 2001.
14. Howard J, Buckley R, McCormack R, et al: Complications following management of displaced intra-articular calcaneal fractures: A prospective randomized trial comparing open reduction internal fixation with non-operative management. J Orthop Trauma 17:241–249, 2003.
15. Essex-Lopresti P: The mechanism, reduction technique and results in fractures of the os calcis. Br J Surg 39:395–419, 1952.
16. Tornetta P: The Essex-Lopresti reduction for calcaneal fractures revisited. J Orthop Trauma 12:469–473, 1998.
17. Csizy M, Buckley R, Tough S, et al: Displaced intra-articular calcaneal fractures: Variables predicting late subtalar fusion. J Orthop Trauma 17:106–112, 2003.
18. Ceccarelli F, Faldini C, Piras F, et al: Surgical vs. non-surgical treatment of calcaneal fractures in children: A long term results comparative study. Foot Ankle Int 21:825–832, 2000.

Chapter 76

What Is the Best Treatment of Displaced Talar Neck Fractures?

NICOLE L. FETTER, MD AND CHRISTOPHER P. CHIODO, MD

Talus fractures have been recognized in the scientific literature for centuries, with Fabricus' 1608 description often cited as the first reference.[1] Fractures of the talar neck comprise 3% of all foot fractures, but 50% of all talus fractures. They are usually high-energy injuries, and as such, often are associated with poor outcomes. Certain aspects of the talar anatomy further exacerbate this. For instance, the talus has no muscular attachments, with approximately 70% of its surface covered by articular cartilage. The talar neck itself has fewer trabeculae compared with the head or body, and these trabeculae have a different orientation.[2] The precarious blood supply of the talus has been studied extensively, and it is vulnerable to disruption with fractures of the talar neck. This puts patients with displaced talar neck fracture at risk for the development of avascular necrosis (AVN).

Historical treatment options described for displaced talar neck fractures have ranged from closed reduction and casting to open reduction with and without internal fixation. More recent studies have investigated the timing of surgery and the optimal method of fixation. When faced with a displaced talar neck fracture, the treating orthopedist is faced by three main questions. First, is surgery necessary, or can the fracture be treated without surgery? Second, if open management is indicated, is it necessary to perform surgery on an emergent basis? Third, what is the best method of fixing these fractures? This chapter attempts to answer these questions using an evidenced-based review of the pertinent literature on displaced talar neck fractures.

CLASSIFICATION

Hawkins[3] introduced the popular classification system of talar neck fractures that remains commonly used today. This system is based on the degree of fracture fragment displacement and divides talar neck fractures into three groups. Type I fractures are nondisplaced. Type II fractures are displaced with subtalar subluxation or dislocation. Type III talar neck fractures are displaced with dislocation of the subtalar and tibiotalar joints. This classification system was modified by Canale and Kelly[4] in 1978 to include type IV fractures that involve not only dislocation of the subtalar and tibiotalar joints but also

dislocation of the talar head from the talonavicular joint.

CLOSED VERSUS OPEN MANAGEMENT

The first question that must answered when taking care of a patient with a displaced talar neck fracture is whether open reduction and internal fixation (ORIF) is indicated. Traditionally, concerns regarding the development of AVN and post-traumatic arthritis have led to the general consensus that displaced talar neck fractures require ORIF.

In the twentieth century, before Hawkins's work, several clinical series on talus fractures were reported.[5-8] In 1919, Anderson coined the term *aviator's astragalus* after observing this injury in downed pilots.[5] In 1952, Coltart[6] reported a large Level IV clinical series examining this injury in British Air Force pilots during World War II. In this series, a poor outcome was associated with inadequate reduction of the subtalar joint, leading the author to advocate anatomic reduction with or without internal fixation.

Subsequently, Kenwright and Taylor[7] examined 58 talus fractures in civilians. In 14 patients with talar neck fractures and subtalar subluxation, closed reduction and cast immobilization was attempted; however, in 10 patients (71%), satisfactory reduction could not be obtained or maintained, and open reduction was necessary. In some instances (the authors did not specify how many), the reduction was held with a Kirschner wire. Similar results were noted for talar neck fractures with tibiotalar dislocation. As such, the authors conclude that "a good result occurs only if accurate reduction is effected and maintained."[7]

If these studies are considered to be Level II prognostic studies (i.e., investigating the outcome of the injury with and without reduction), they constitute fair evidence (grade B) that for displaced talar neck fractures, some form of reduction is necessary. The question then remains, is ORIF necessary?

In 1970, Hawkins'[3] landmark review and classification system of talar neck fractures was published. In this retrospective review (Level IV therapeutic study, Level II prognostic study), he drew attention to the incidence of AVN after talar neck fractures and emphasized the importance of open reduction.

Nevertheless, in this series, Hawkins only peripherally mentions internal fixation in two patients but does not give details regarding fracture type or method of fixation. Of the 24 type II fractures in this series, 10 were treated with closed reduction and cast immobilization, whereas 14 were treated with open reduction.[3] The overall incidence of AVN for type II fractures was 42%.[3] For type III fractures, 2 of these injuries were treated with closed reduction and 20 with some form of open reduction for an overall AVN rate of 91%.[3]

Meanwhile, Canale and Kelly[4] used closed reduction, as well as open reduction with and without internal fixation, in their historical series. Closed reduction was limited to those fractures in which adequate alignment (defined as less than 5 mm of displacement and less than 5 degrees of angular deformity) could be obtained. Of the 30 cases of type II fractures in this series, 19 were treated with closed reduction and casting, 1 presented late and was treated with only non–weight bearing, and 10 underwent open reduction with internal fixation. The overall AVN rate for type II fractures was 50%. Meanwhile, for type III fractures, 5 underwent closed reduction and 15 had open reduction (only 11 of which had internal fixation). The AVN rate in this group was 84%.[4]

Unfortunately, in both Hawkins'[3] and Canale and Kelly's[4] series, the incidence and rate of AVN were not stratified by treatment type. Therefore, it is difficult to draw from these two studies any conclusions as to whether open treatment provides a lower AVN rate than closed reduction.

Other studies have reported varied rates of AVN. In a large Level IV review of 123 talar neck fractures, Lorentzen and colleagues[9] found the overall incidence rate of AVN to be 21%. The majority of the fractures in this series were treated with cast immobilization. Among the 53 type II fractures, only 4 underwent open reduction. Thirty fractures were treated with closed reduction and casting, whereas 19 were treated with no reduction and casting only. Notably, although Lorentzen and colleagues report a 21% incidence rate of AVN, 44% of the fractures in their series were nondisplaced. The incidence rate of AVN was 35% when only the displaced talar neck fractures are considered.[9]

In those studies that examine the results of ORIF, the type of fixation often varies dramatically within the study. In a Level IV retrospective review, Grob and coworkers[10] report the results of ORIF in 41 displaced talar neck fractures treated with malleolar screws, Kirschner wires, or cancellous screws. In this series, the incidence rate of AVN was only 16%.[10] These encouraging data would seem to indicate that ORIF does reduce the incidence of AVN when compared with previous series in which patients were more commonly treated with closed techniques. However, in Vallier and colleagues'[11] retrospective review (Level II prognostic study) of 102 displaced talar neck fractures in which all patients were treated with ORIF, the incidence of AVN was 39% for Hawkins group II fractures and 64% for Hawkins group III fractures.[11]

In addition to AVN, the development of malunion and post-traumatic osteoarthritis are two other clinical concerns associated with displaced talar neck fractures. Canale and Kelly[4] report that subtalar degenerative changes occurred in approximately 50% of their patients, of which one third was said to have a malunion. Notably, in this series, 18 of 71 patients (25%) experienced development of a malunion. Because 11 of these 18 were initially treated with only closed reduction and casting, Canale and Kelly[4] attributed subtalar arthritis to inadequate reduction or fixation. Comfort and colleagues'[12] work supports the hypothesis that the incidence of malunion can be reduced with internal fixation. In this retrospective review of 28 patients with displaced talar neck fractures all treated with ORIF, there were no malunions and no nonunions. Radiographic evidence of ankle arthritis was noted in eight patients.[12] Similarly, in the series reported by Vallier and coworkers,[11] all 102 fractures were treated with ORIF. No patients experienced development of a malunion or nonunion. Although 54% of patients had *radiographic* evidence of arthritis, this was more common after comminuted and open fractures.[11] Finally, Fleuriau Chateau and colleagues[13] report a clinical series of displaced and highly comminuted talar neck fractures treated with open reduction and plate fixation. These authors note no varus malunions despite the fact that the fractures in this series were characterized by substantial comminution.

Although the aforementioned studies offer evidence that ORIF reduces the incidence of malunion, Sanders and colleagues'[14] series does have a high malunion rate despite the use of internal fixation. In this series, 70 displaced talar neck fractures were treated with open reduction and screw fixation. Signs of radiographic arthritis were present in 40% of affected ankles and 78% of subtalar joints. The authors acknowledge malunion as "an important clinical problem" and note hindfoot malalignment in 30% of patients. When interpreting the results of this study, it is important to note that, in this series, surgery was performed or "directly supervised" by a consultant orthopedic trauma surgeon, and that eight fractures were treated by "other orthopedic surgeons at the trauma center."[14] In addition, malunion was seemingly not assessed by radiographs but rather hindfoot alignment alone.

Beyond these series, Grob and coauthors[10] report osteoarthritis of the ankle joint in 32% of cases and of the subtalar joint in 37% of cases. All fractures in this series were treated with some form of ORIF. Unfortunately, data stratification with regard to post-traumatic arthritis and fracture type was not provided. No mention was made to malunion or nonunion. Pajenda and researchers[15] reviewed 50 fractures of the talar neck and body (Level IV evidence), and reported osteoarthritis in 48% of the fractures. Severe ankle arthritis was noted in 11 of 30 displaced talar fractures (types II, III, and IV), but the form of fixation varied greatly including open reduction and internal with screws, external fixation, percutaneous screws, and closed reduction with percutaneous pinning using Kirschner wires.[15]

Collectively, these results justify a grade C recommendation that patients with displaced talar neck fractures should undergo ORIF of their displaced fractures.

TIMING OF SURGERY

When faced with a displaced talus fracture, the next issue to be decided is the timing of surgery. Specifically, the surgeon must decide whether this is an operation that must be performed on an emergent or an urgent basis. Traditionally, concern regarding the development of AVN has led many to advocate emergent ORIF of these fractures.

At least three studies, two clinical series and one survey, have addressed this issue. In a recent clinical investigation, Vallier and colleagues[11] performed a Level II retrospective review of 100 patients with 102 fractures of the talar neck. The average time to fixation was 3.4 days for patients who experienced development of AVN compared with 5.0 days for patients who did not. Rather than the timing of surgery, AVN was associated with talar neck comminution and the presence of an open injury. No correlation between surgical delay and the development of AVN could be identified.

These results are similar to those that Comfort and colleagues[12] reported. In this retrospective review, the results of 28 patients who underwent ORIF of displaced talar neck fractures were reported and analyzed.[12] Time to surgery was less than 12 hours for 18 patients, 1 to 7 days in 9, and 17 days in 1. Twelve of the 28 patients (43%) experienced development of AVN. Like Vallier and colleagues,[11] the authors report that there was no trend between delay in operation and the degree of necrosis, and that the presence of necrosis correlated with the degree of displacement.

Recently, 89 expert orthopedic surgeons working at Level 1 trauma centers were surveyed regarding the current state of practice for the treatment of displaced talar neck fractures (Level V evidence).[16] In this survey, 60% of respondents stated that, for displaced talar neck fractures, treatment after 8 hours is acceptable. Forty-six percent of respondents stated that treatment at or after 24 hours is acceptable. The authors of this study conclude that "most expert orthopedic trauma surgeons do not believe that an immediate operation is necessary to adequately treat a displaced talar neck fracture."[16]

These studies, especially the work of Vallier and colleagues,[11] offer fair (grade B) evidence that displaced talar neck fractures do not need to undergo ORIF on an urgent or emergent basis. Nevertheless, it should be noted that Vallier's group did advocate emergent reduction of dislocations through either closed or percutaneous manipulation. Meanwhile, Comfort's group[12] recommends that ORIF "should be performed early," although they did not expand on the definition of "early."

METHOD OF FIXATION

The third question that must be answered in the treatment of displaced talar neck fractures is what form of surgical fixation should be used. Traditionally, surgical fixation of talar neck fractures has been achieved with Kirschner wires or screws placed in an anterior-to-posterior direction. Only a few clinical studies have examined other fixation constructs. Lemaire and Bustin[17] analyzed their results using closed reduction followed by placement of a lag screw via the posterior tubercle. These authors suggest that the posterior approach allowed them to place the screw perpendicular to the fracture line. They also postulate that the posterior approach would have less effect on blood supply compared with an anterior approach. They report three excellent results and four good results, with AVN developing in two of the seven cases.[17]

Fayazi and coauthors[18] describe a technique in which they closed reduced talar neck fractures and then performed percutaneous fixation using fluoroscopy and two partially threaded cannulated screws placed in opposite directions and parallel to each other. In this Level V technique article, the authors emphasize that if an anatomic reduction could not be obtained by closed methods, then open reduction was required. They state that their percutaneous approach resulted in shorter surgery, less pain, and minimal soft-tissue manipulation. Unfortunately, they report only on their technique and do not offer any results.[18]

Finally, Fleuriau Chateau and coworkers[13] studied the effects of fixation of talar neck fractures using mini-fragment plates. In this retrospective review, 23 talar neck fractures were stabilized with a combination of mini-fragment plates augmented with lag screws if required. These fractures included type II, III, and IV injuries, and all were characterized by substantial comminution. The plates were placed on the more comminuted side of the fracture (either medial or lateral). With an average follow-up period of 20 months, the authors report no wound complications, a 100% union rate, and no evidence of varus malunion. Radiographically, there were two cases of tibiotalar arthritis and one case of subtalar arthritis. These patients were clinically asymptomatic. The authors argue that plate fixation minimizes varus malunion in highly comminuted fractures by avoiding excessive compression of the comminuted neck with lag screws.[13]

Although biomechanical studies do not provide direct clinical evidence, they are helpful in providing surgeons with basic principles that may provide guidance in the clinical setting. Several biomechanical studies have examined various methods of surgical fixation for talar neck fractures. Swanson and coworkers[19] created a fracture model with cadaveric tali and compared four different fixation constructs: (1) Kirschner wires alone, (2) 4.0-mm cancellous screws placed from anterior to posterior, (3) 4.0-mm cancellous screws placed from posterior to anterior, and (4) a 6.5-mm cancellous screw placed from posterior to anterior combined with a Kirschner wire.[19] Results showed that screw fixation was superior to Kirschner-wire fixation. Furthermore, screws placed in a posterior-to-anterior direction were found to provide stronger fixation than those placed in an anterior-to-posterior direction.[19] More recently, Charlson and colleagues[20] created a comminuted talar neck fracture model fixed with either two 4.0-mm cancellous screws placed in a posterior-to-anterior direction or a lateral mini-fragment plate augmented with a medial 2.7-mm lag screw.[20] Their results showed superior fixation with the two-screw technique compared with plate fixation. Also, their results demonstrated failure at a load significantly below that shown by Swanson and coworkers.[19] They attribute this to the comminuted component of the fracture model.[20] Attiah and coauthors[21] compared fixation among 3 3.5-mm cortical and 4.0-mm cancellous screws placed in an anterior-to-posterior direction, 2 4.0-mm cancellous screws placed in posterior-to-anterior direction, and a 2.7-mm blade plate placed on the medial aspect with a 4.0-mm cancellous screw placed laterally.[21] Unlike Charlson and colleagues,[20] these authors report no significant difference in the failure load between screw and plate fixation, but they did note that the screws failed by bending or pulling out, whereas the blade plate model failed by fracture of the talar head around the plate.[21]

Taken together, the combination of clinical evidence and biomechanical studies for fixation of talar neck fractures suggest the following: Screws placed in a posterior-to-anterior direction provide stronger fixation than those placed in the traditional anterior-to-posterior direction. Biomechanical studies have conflicting results whether screw fixation is equal to or superior to plate fixation. However, Fleuriau Chateau and colleagues[13] offer limited Level IV clinical evidence that plate fixation may minimize varus malunion in highly comminuted fractures.

CONCLUSION

In conclusion, displaced talar neck fractures continue to pose a clinical challenge with an uncertain prognosis and potentially poor long-term morbidity. An evidenced-based review of the scientific literature regarding the optimal treatment of these injuries allows for several recommendations. First, such fractures should be treated with ORIF, rather than cast immobilization alone or open reduction without internal fixation. Second, surgery does not have to be performed on an emergent basis. Third, various fixation constructs are biomechanically advantageous, especially screws placed in a posterior-to-anterior direction and plate fixation for highly comminuted fractures. Table 76–1 provides a summary of recommendations for the treatment of displaced talar neck fractures.

TABLE 76–1. Summary of Recommendations for the Treatment of Displaced Talar Neck Fractures

RECOMMENDATIONS	LEVEL OF EVIDENCE/ GRADE OF RECOMMENDATION
1. Some form of reduction is necessary in treatment of displaced talar neck fractures.	B
2. Patients with displaced talar neck fractures should undergo open reduction and internal fixation.	B
3. Displaced talar neck fractures do not need open reduction and internal fixation on an urgent or emergent basis.	C
4. Plate fixation minimizes malunion in highly comminuted fractures.	C

REFERENCES

1. Adelaar RS: Complex fractures of the talus. Instr Course Lect 46:323–338, 1997.
2. Ebraheim NA, Sabry FF, Nadim Y: Internal architecture of the talus: Implication for talar fracture. Foot Ankle Int 20:794–796, 1999.
3. Hawkins LG: Fractures of the neck of the talus. J Bone Joint Surg Am 52:991–1002, 1970.
4. Canale ST, Kelly FB Jr: Fractures of the neck of the talus. Long-term evaluation of seventy-one cases. J Bone Joint Surg Am 60:143–156, 1978.
5. Anderson HG, FM, Gotch OH (eds): The Medical and Surgical Aspects of Aviation. London, H Frowde, 1919.
6. Coltart WD: Aviator's astragalus. J Bone Joint Surg Br 34-B:545–566, 1952.
7. Kenwright J, Taylor RG: Major injuries of the talus. J Bone Joint Surg Br 52:36–48, 1970.
8. Kleiger B: Fractures of the talus. J Bone Joint Surg 30A:735–744, 1948.
9. Lorentzen JE, Christensen SB, Krogsoe O, Sneppen O: Fractures of the neck of the talus. Acta Orthop Scand 48:115–120, 1977.
10. Grob D, Simpson LA, Weber BG, Bray T: Operative treatment of displaced talus fractures. Clin Orthop Relat Res (199):88–96, 1985.
11. Vallier HA, Nork SE, Barei DP, et al: Talar neck fractures: Results and outcomes. J Bone Joint Surg Am 86-A:1616–1624, 2004.
12. Comfort TH, Behrens F, Gaither DW, et al: Long-term results of displaced talar neck fractures. Clin Orthop Relat Res (199):81–87, 1985.
13. Fleuriau Chateau PB, Brokaw DS, Jelen BA, et al: Plate fixation of talar neck fractures: Preliminary review of a new technique in twenty-three patients. J Orthop Trauma 16:213–219, 2002.
14. Sanders DW, Busam M, Hattwick E, et al: Functional outcomes following displaced talar neck fractures. J Orthop Trauma 18:265–270, 2004.
15. Pajenda G, Vecsei V, Reddy B, Heinz T: Treatment of talar neck fractures: Clinical results of 50 patients. J Foot Ankle Surg 39:365–375, 2000.
16. Patel R, Van Bergeyk A, Pinney S: Are displaced talar neck fractures surgical emergencies? A survey of orthopaedic trauma experts. Foot Ankle Int 26:378–381, 2005.
17. Lemaire RG, Bustin W: Screw fixation of fractures of the neck of the talus using a posterior approach. J Trauma 20:669–673, 1980.
18. Fayazi AH, Reid JS, Juliano PJ: Percutaneous pinning of talar neck fractures. Am J Orthop 31:76–78, 2002.
19. Swanson TV, Bray TJ, Holmes GB Jr: Fractures of the talar neck. A mechanical study of fixation. J Bone Joint Surg Am 74:544–551, 1992.
20. Charlson MD, Parks BG, Weber TG, Guyton GP: Comparison of plate and screw fixation and screw fixation alone in a comminuted talar neck fracture model. Foot Ankle Int 27:340–343, 2006.
21. Attiah M, Sanders DW, Valdivia G, et al: Comminuted talar neck fractures: A mechanical comparison of fixation techniques. J Orthop Trauma 21:47–51, 2007.

Chapter 77

What Is the Best Treatment for Injury to the Tarsometatarsal Joint Complex?

Dominic Carreira, MD and Mark S. Myerson, MD

The tarsometatarsal joints, commonly but incorrectly called the *tarsometatarsal joint,* divides the midfoot from the forefoot, and injuries to this joint complex continue to be both a diagnostic and a treatment challenge. The term *tarsometatarsal joint complex* was introduced by Myerson and colleagues[1] to highlight the more extensive nature of this injury to include not only the joints between the metatarsals and cuneiforms or cuboid, but also the intercuneiform and the naviculocuneiform joints. The presentation of this injury is quite varied and may take the form of a joint subluxation, dislocation with or without fracture. Although the reported occurrence is 1 per 55,000 fractures per year,[2] these injuries seem to be increasing in frequency since the late 1990s, particularly in certain sports.

Diagnosis is made based on a high index of suspicion with tenderness about the midfoot. Radiographs must be taken while bearing weight, and if equivocal, a fluoroscopic stress test with forefoot abduction and pronation is performed. Various treatment modalities have been utilized, including closed treatment with immobilization, closed reduction and percutaneous pinning, open reduction and internal fixation (ORIF), and primary arthrodesis. The best approach to achieve and maintain an anatomic reduction must be balanced with the risks for operative intervention and the possible development of arthritis and the need for future surgery.

Treatment of these injuries does not have uniformly excellent outcomes, even with anatomic reduction and stable internal fixation. Arthritis and hence disability may result even with surgical treatment,[3] and the reported prevalence of painful arthrosis with these injuries has ranged from 0 of 9 patients[4] to 15 (58%) of 26 patients.[5] In a series of 69 patients, degenerative joint disease developed in 21 (30%).[6] Regardless of the incidence of posttraumatic arthritis, it is now well accepted that an anatomic reduction is critical to a successful outcome. One such study by Arntz and Hansen[7] demonstrated an overall good or excellent functional result in 95% of patients in whom an anatomic reduction was obtained. In contrast, a satisfactory result was obtained in only one of five patients in whom congruity of the joint was not accurately restored.

Multiple confounding factors make it difficult to make treatment recommendations, few Level I studies exist to support any single approach, and the best treatment approach is unclear if not controversial. This chapter initially reviews treatment recommendations based on levels of evidence followed by specific issues associated with this topic.

LEVEL I STUDY

Only a single Level I study has been published on clinical outcomes of surgical treatment of the tarsometatarsal joint. Ly and Coetzee[8] compared ORIF versus primary arthrodesis in a study of 41 patients with isolated acute and subacute primarily ligamentous injuries. The average follow-up was 42 months with a minimum of 2 years after treatment. The primary arthrodesis group included a fusion of the first two or three rays, but never included the lateral rays. The mean American Orthopaedic Foot and Ankle Society (AOFAS) midfoot score was 68.6 for the open reduction group and was 88 in the arthrodesis group. In the open reduction group, five patients who had persistent midfoot pain with or without the development of deformity eventually underwent arthrodesis. Patients treated with a primary arthrodesis estimated achievement of postoperative level of activity was 92% of their preinjury level, whereas the open reduction group estimated that the postoperative level was only 65% of their preoperative level ($P < 0.005$). Multiple criticisms have been made for this Level I study. The medium-to long-term results of primary arthrodesis and the risk for arthritis in adjacent joints over the long term remain unknown. Furthermore, significant bony injuries were not addressed in this study because this treatment was based on ligamentous injuries (subluxation and dislocation). Lastly, the inclusion and exclusion criteria are not clear, given that no high-performance athlete was treated in this manner, and no massive and complete high-energy dislocations were treated.

LEVEL II STUDY

Only a single Level II study has been published on tarsometatarsal injuries. In a surgeon randomized study, Mulier and colleagues[9] analyzed patients with severe tarsometatarsal injuries who were treated by surgical intervention, with one surgeon always performing an arthrodesis and the other surgeon always performing ORIF. ORIF (16 patients) and partial arthrodesis (6 patients) was recommended over complete arthrodesis of all 5 tarsometatarsal joints (6 patients). The subgroups were identical in age, follow-up, type of fracture, type of injury, and time to intervention. Anatomic reduction was achieved in 8 of the 12 patients in the arthrodesis group and in 12 of the 16 patients in the ORIF group. The Baltimore painful foot score was greater in the ORIF group than in the complete arthrodesis group, meaning the ORIF group had less pain. Stiffness of the forefoot, loss of the metatarsal arch, and sympathetic dystrophy occurred more frequently in the complete arthrodesis group. However, it is noted that 94% of the open-reduction group had signs of radiographic degeneration at the average final follow-up of 30 months.

LEVEL III AND IV STUDIES

Several Level III and IV studies also have been published that provide guidance in decision making. Closed treatment with plaster immobilization has resulted in poor results.[10–12] Wilson[13] reports that only 1 of 14 patients undergoing closed reduction and cast immobilization had an anatomic reduction, and 7 of the 14 patients were noted to have residual displacement of 5 mm or more. These studies consist of limited small numbers, and their poor results are of historic interest only. The demographics of tarsometatarsal injury have changed markedly, and with closer attention to diagnosis, subtle injuries have been diagnosed with increased frequency. Although closed reduction or closed reduction and percutaneous screw fixation does not allow for assessment under direct visualization of the reduction or for removal of osteocartilaginous debris, percutaneous screw fixation has gained popularity.

Based on these reports, and because the potential for long-term morbidity after tarsometatarsal injuries, any patient with a displaced fracture-dislocation or with any degree of instability of the tarsometatarsal joint should be treated with surgery. The question remains, however, as to what is the ideal method of surgical treatment (Level IV).

Open Reduction and Internal Fixation

Multiple authors have correlated outcomes with the accuracy of surgical reduction. Arntz and Hansen[7] retrospectively reviewed 34 tarsometatarsal fracture-dislocations treated with open reduction and temporary internal fixation with AO screws (Level IV). They emphasize the importance of screw fixation, given the previous problems that they had experienced with percutaneous pin fixation, including pin infection, migration of pins, and loss of reduction. Of the patients with an anatomic reduction, a good or excellent result was obtained in all but two patients at an average follow-up of 3.4 years. An analysis of the six patients who had a fair or poor result showed the following: two patients had an anatomic reduction, two patients had a fair reduction, and two a nonanatomic reduction; five had an associated grade II or III open injury.

Kuo and coworkers[14] performed a retrospective study of patients who underwent an open reduction and screw fixation of a tarsometatarsal injury (Level IV). Forty-eight patients were observed for an average of 52 months (range, 13–114 months). Twelve patients (25%) had post-traumatic osteoarthritis of the tarsometatarsal joints, and six of them required arthrodesis. The average AOFAS midfoot score was 77 (out of 100). No significant difference in outcome scores could be detected when purely ligamentous injuries were compared with combined ligamentous and osseous injuries, open wounds were compared with closed wounds, involvement of five tarsometatarsal joints was compared with involvement of fewer than five, the presence of associated cuneiform and/or cuboid injury was compared with the absence of either injury, isolated injury was compared with multiple injuries, multiple trauma was compared with the absence of multiple trauma, the presence of associated injury of the ipsilateral lower limb was compared with the absence of such injury, acute diagnosis was compared with delayed diagnosis, and work-related injury was compared with nonwork-related injury. Based on these studies and their levels, grade C recommendation exists for ORIF and screw fixation of tarsometatarsal fracture dislocation.

Late Treatment with Arthrodesis

Delayed treatment of injuries beyond 6 weeks has been associated with poorer outcomes.[15] This, however, depends on the magnitude of the deformity. For those injuries associated with complete subluxation of all the joints, then, indeed, delayed treatment is more complicated because the realignment and arthrodesis required is more complex. However, this does not apply to more minor injuries where limited subluxation and dislocation is present. These luxations can be treated months after injury with either closed reduction and percutaneous fixation or ORIF without resorting to arthrodesis. Sangeorzan and Hansen's[19] study of salvage of tarsometatarsal injuries yielded significant results based on different statistical analyses. By Pearson coefficient, they found several significant factors: less time to treatment was more likely to result in a good or excellent result; adequate reduction was correlated with better outcome;

and work-related injuries were more likely to have a bad outcome. No correlation was found between the age of the patient and result of treatment. By multiple regression analysis, reduction was the only factor found to be predictive of result.[16] Komenda and Myerson[17] retrospectively reviewed 32 patients who underwent an arthrodesis of the midfoot after a traumatic injury. The arthrodesis was performed at a mean of 35 months (range, 6–108 months) after the injury. All of the patients were treated with rigid internal fixation, and autogenous bone graft was used in 24 patients in whom a defect had been created after preparation of the bone surfaces. At an average of 50 months after the arthrodesis, the mean AOFAS midfoot postoperative score was 78 points (vs. 44 before surgery). Given the number of patients in this study, it was not possible to determine whether the extent of arthrodesis, the involvement of other joints in the hindfoot or forefoot, or the involvement of workers' compensation affected outcome.

Primary Arthrodesis

Several Level III and IV studies have analyzed the role of primary arthrodesis for tarsometatarsal dislocation in addition to the Level I study by Ly and Coetzee[8] described earlier in this chapter. Granberry and Lipscomb[18] recommend primary fusion in any unstable injury requiring open reduction because of the high incidence (11/25) of these injuries subsequently being treated with arthrodesis. However, no information was provided on the type and magnitude of either the injury or the type of treatments available that might have predisposed the patients to development of posttraumatic arthritis. Furthermore, no outcome data were provided subsequently for those 11 patients who underwent arthrodesis. Kuo and coworkers[14] suggest that there may be a subset of patients with purely ligamentous injuries who would benefit from primary arthrodesis, given that 6 of 15 of their patients with purely ligamentous injuries experienced development of painful osteoarthrosis.

Because of the limited number of grade I/and multiple Level III/IV studies, a Grade C recommendation exists for primary arthrodesis. As noted in the treatment algorithm (Fig. 77–1), we recommend primary arthrodesis in a subset of patients with Lis Franc injuries.

Extent of Arthrodesis

In the setting of arthrosis, the extent of fusion has been an area of controversy, particularly the inclusion versus exclusion of the lateral column. Interestingly, the middle column (second and third metatarsocuneiform joints) has the least motion, and yet

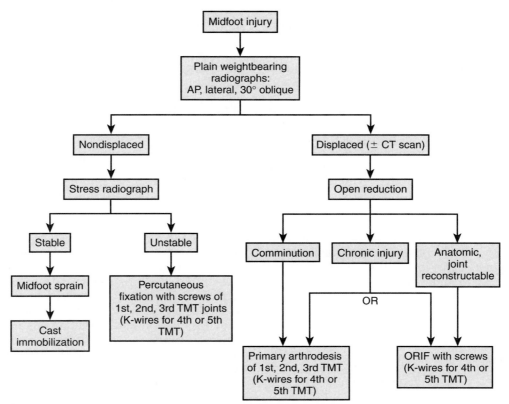

FIGURE 77–1. Recommended treatment algorithm for Lis Franc injuries.

are the joints most likely to develop post-traumatic arthritis and require an arthrodesis. The contrary applies to the lateral column (the fourth and fifth metatarsocuboid joints), which is mobile but is rarely symptomatic. The sagittal plane movements of the tarsometatarsal joints, as determined by cadaveric study, are significantly greater for the fourth (9.6 mm) and fifth (10.2 mm), as compared with the first (3.5 mm), second (0.6 mm), and third (1.6 mm) joints.[16] Given this increased physiologic motion across the lateral column, the benefit of arthrodesis across these joints has been called into question. In the setting of chronic degenerative changes, Sangeorzan and coauthors[19] and Komenda and Myerson[17] have recommended that only the medial and/or middle column should be fused. The only two patients who underwent arthrodesis of all three columns in Komenda and Myerson's study subsequently required a revision procedure with metatarsal osteotomies because of metatarsalgia. Furthermore, a third patient who underwent fusion with an interposition bone block arthrodesis of the calcaneocuboid joint for a traumatic abduction deformity also experienced intractable pain at the metatarsocuboid joints and subsequently underwent metatarsocuboid fusions. Raikin and Schon[20] presented a report of 28 feet that were treated with arthrodesis of the fourth

and fifth tarsometatarsal joints at a 2-year minimum follow-up, but most of these arthrodeses (22/28) were performed for neurarthopathic rocker-bottom deformity and have no relevance in this type of discussion pertaining to a neurologic intact person with post-traumatic arthritis. Based on current evidence, we recommend limiting fusions to the medial and middle columns.

UTILITY OF BONE SCAN FOR LATE TREATMENT

No studies exist that specifically address the ideal diagnostic modalities for determining the extent of arthrodesis. In addition to plain radiographs, Level IV evidence alone supports the use of nuclear bone scans and selective anesthetic injections. Komenda and Myerson[17] did not find bone scan to be useful because it tended to show uptake in areas that were painless. They did not recommend any additional imaging studies, given that clinical examination and plain radiographs were useful in determining which joints should be fused. However, Mann and Sobel[21] used a bone scan to determine the extent of arthrodesis in 8 of 40 patients in their series. The majority of patients in this latter series, however, were treated for idiopathic osteoarthritis and not post-traumatic deformity.

RECOMMENDATIONS

After diagnosis with either weight-bearing radiographs or fluoroscopic stress manipulation of the foot, anatomic restoration of the tarsometatarsal joint complex should be obtained either by closed or open means. If closed, percutaneous screw fixation is an acceptable method of restoring joint alignment, and open reduction with either fixation or primary arthrodesis used where comminution or failure to obtain an anatomic reduction is noted. The dilemma remains with respect to

primary arthrodesis. If comminuted, this is the procedure of choice, but it is technically difficult to perform because of lack of joint congruity and bone support. Based on Ly and Coetzee's[8] work, primary arthrodesis should, however, be part of the current treatment regimen used by orthopedic surgeons in the management of tarsometatarsal joint injury. Table 77–1 provides a summary of recommendations for the treatment for injury to the tarsometatarsal joint complex.

TABLE 77–1. Summary of Recommendations

STATEMENT	LEVEL OF EVIDENCE/GRADE OF RECOMMENDATION	REFERENCES
1. LisFranc injuries that are fracture dislocations or that are unstable should be treated surgically	Level I/III/IV Grade B	7, 8, 10-12, 14, 18
2. Tarsometatarsal fracture dislocations should be treated with anatomic reduction and screw fixation	Level III/IV Grade C	7, 14
3. Tarsometatarsal fracture dislocations and unstable injuries should be treated with arthrodesis	Level I/III/IV Grade C	8, 14, 17-19
4. Arthrodesis of the LisFranc joints should be limited to the medial and middle column in the neurologically intact patient	Level III/IV Grade B	9, 17, 19
5. Bone scan should be used to determine the extent of arthrodesis	Level IV Grade I	17, 21

REFERENCES

1. Myerson MS, Fisher RT, Burgess AR, Kenzora JE: Fracture dislocations of the tarsometatarsal joints: End results correlated with pathology and treatment. Foot Ankle 6:225–242, 1986.
2. Hardcastle P: Injury to tarsometatarsal joint. J Bone Joint Surg Br 64-B:349–356, 1982.
3. Buzzard BM, Briggs PJ: Surgical management of acute tarsometatarsal dislocation in the adult. Clin Orthop Relat Res 353:125–133, 1998.
4. Aitken AP, Poulson D: Dislocations of the tarsometatarsal joint. J Bone Joint Surg 45-A:246–260, 1963.
5. Wilppula E: Tarsometatarsal fracture-dislocation. Late results in 26 patients. Acta Orthop Scand 44:335–345, 1973.
6. Hardcastle PH, Reschauer R, Kutscha-Lissberg E, Schoffmann W: Injuries to the tarsometatarsal joint. Incidence, classification, and treatment. J Bone Joint Surg Br 64-B:349–356, 1982.
7. Arntz CT, Veith RG, Hansen ST: Fractures and fracture-dislocations of the tarsometatarsal joint. J Bone Joint Surg Am 70:173–181, 1988.
8. Ly TV, Coetzee JC: Treatment of primarily ligamentous tarsometatarsal joint injuries: Primary Arthrodesis compared with open reduction and internal fixation. J Bone Joint Surg Am 88-A:514–520, 2006.
9. Mulier T, Reynders P, Dereymaeker G, Broos P: Severe tarsometatarsal injuries: Primary arthrodesis or ORIF? Foot Ankle Int 23:902–905, 2002.
10. Goosens M, DeStoop N: Tarsometatarsal's fracture dislocation: Etiology, readiology, and results of treatment. Clin Orthop 176:154–162, 1983.
11. Willpula E: Tarsometatarsal fracture-dislocation. Acta Orthop Scand 44:335–345, 1973.
12. Myerson M: The diagnosis and treatment of injuries of the tarsometatarsal joint complex. Orthop Clin North Am 20:655–664, 1989.
13. Wilson DW: Injuries of the tarso-metatarsal joints: Etiology, classification and results of treatment. J Bone Joint Surg Br 54:677–686, 1972.
14. Kuo RS, Tejwani NC, DiGiovanni CW, et al: Outcome after open reduction and internal fixation of tarsometatarsal joint injuries. J Bone Joint Surg Am 82-A:1609–1618, 2000.
15. Myerson MS, Fisher RT, Burgess AR, et al: Fracture dislocations of the tarsometatarsal joints: End results correlated with pathology and treatment. Foot Ankle 6:225–242, 1986.
16. Ozononian T, Shereff M: In vitro determinant of midfoot motion. Foot Ankle Int 10:140–146, 1989.
17. Komenda GA, Myerson MS, Biddinger KR: Results of arthrodesis of the tarsometatarsal joints after traumatic injury. J Bone Joint Surg Am 78:1665–1676, 1996.
18. Granberry W, Lipscomb P: Dislocation of the tarsometatarsal joints. Surg Gynecol Obstet 114:467–469, 1962.
19. Sangeorzan BJ, Veith RG, Hansen ST Jr: Salvage of tarsometatarsal joint by arthrodesis. Foot Ankle 193–200, 1990.
20. Raikin SM, Schon LC: Arthodesis of the fourth and fifth metatarsal joints of the midfoot. Foot Ankle Int 24:584–590, 2003.
21. Mann RA, Prieskorn D, Sobel M: Mid-tarsal and tarsometatarsal arthrodesis for primary degenerative osteoarthrosis or osteoarthrosis after trauma. J Bone Joint Surg Am 78:1376–1385, 1996.

What Is the Best Treatment for Recurrent Ankle Instability?

Alastair Younger, MB, ChB, FRCSC, Msc, ChM

Incidence of Recurrent Ankle Instability

Most acute injuries are treated by a rehabilitation program. The remaining 15% to 20% who remain symptomatic may require surgical intervention.[1] In the United Kingdom, 302,000 sprains are treated per year.[2] Recurrent sprains may result in more lost days of sport than the initial injury.[3]

Anatomy of the Lateral Collateral Ligaments

The lateral collateral ligaments stabilize the ankle joint to episodes of inversion sprains. The anterior talofibular ligament runs from the anterior aspect of the fibula to the neck of the talus laterally at its junction to the body of the talus.[4] The calcaneofibular ligament starts just inferior and posterior to the origin of the talofibular ligament, and inserts into the lateral border of the calcaneus running posteriorly.[5] The talofibular ligament therefore stabilizes the ankle by preventing the talus from subluxing anteriorly in the ankle mortise, whereas the calcaneofibular ligament prevents inversion of both the talus and calcaneus at the ankle joint and subtalar joint, respectively.

Pathoanatomy

Rupture of the lateral ligaments may cause instability in the ankle, in the subtalar joint, or both. During an acute episode of instability, the talus will rotate within the ankle mortise and can subject a shear load onto the cartilage on the dome of the talus. The medial dome may impinge on the medial side of the distal tibia causing a central to posteromedial chondral injury. Alternatively, the lateral dome may impinge on the fibula causing a posterolateral injury. Ongoing instability and the chondral injury can cause further cartilaginous degeneration, allowing the ankle joint to become inflamed with associated synovitis. If long-term instability is persistent, significant ankle degeneration occurs with osteophytes formation, both of which may cause symptomatic impingement. Inversion sprains may also overload the peroneal tendon complex, causing stretching or incompetency of SPR, peroneal subluxation/injury, and synovitis.

The anatomy of the hindfoot has a critical effect on the loading of the lateral ligament complex. A cavus foot position may cause medial displacement of the joint reaction force in the ankle, increasing strain on the lateral collateral ligaments.[6] Posterior displacement of the tip of the fibula has been hypothesized as being the cause of recurrent instability. These anatomic variations may, however, represent part of a constellation of cavus foot deformity.[7] Symptomatic chronic instability may be caused by the combination of foot shape and an acute injury. A study of patients with ankle instability awaiting surgery compared with normal control subjects showed that those with instability had a more varus heel.[6]

PREVENTION OF ANKLE INSTABILITY

Theoretically, bracing may prevent recurrent ankle instability. The application of a brace may assist in prevention of instability by mechanical support and by improved proprioception. Bracing has also been used to prevent ankle instability; this is supported through reviews in the Cochrane database but is beyond the scope of this chapter.

TREATMENT OF THE ACUTE INJURY

The general consensus of the literature is that the results of early surgical repair do not result in better outcomes than nonoperative treatment.[8-11] Two Cochrane database reviews showed insufficient evidence to recommend surgical intervention. The most recent is based on the review of 20 articles. A trend existed toward worse outcome in the surgical group for longer recovery times, stiffness, and surgical complications {Kerkhoffs, 2007 #585} (grade B). Repair and reconstruction is therefore recommended only for patients with chronic symptoms of ankle instability.

Limitations of Outcomes Studies

In the Cochrane database review, no evidence was found to support acute lateral ligament reconstruction compared with conservative treatment. However, the studies analyzed were not designed well enough to definitively answer the question.[9] The obvious limitations of articles on recurrent lateral ankle instability include retrospective design with nonvalidated outcome scores without control groups. Less obvious may be the presence or absence of copathologies with ankle instability. Hintermann and colleagues[12] report on 148 patients with medial or lateral instability. Cartilage injury was found in 66% of patients with lateral instability, and 98% of patients with medial instability. Another study showed a 98% rate of intra-articular pathology is associated with lateral ankle instability. The author notes the most common finding was synovitis with a 25% rate of chondral injuries in the ankle.[13] Other authors have documented similar findings.[13-15] Injury to the peroneal tendons and tendonitis are associated with recurrent lateral ankle instability[16,17] with 25% of patients having a peroneal tendon injury.

In summary, older studies do not address the copathologies, nor do they discuss or outline their concomitant treatment protocol on finding these associated issues. For this reason alone, the outcomes for ankle ligament stabilization may be improved in recent articles with the advent of routine magnetic resonance imaging (MRI) and ankle arthroscopy, and treatment of osteochondral defects. Based on the Level IV studies, a grade I recommendation exists for the routine use of advanced diagnostic testing, such as MRI. The diagnostic role of routine arthroscopic debridement at the time of lateral ligament reconstruction has not been determined; however, its use is now recommended by some authors[15,18] (grade I). More studies are required in regard to this specific issue.

Nonoperative Treatment of Recurrent Ankle Instability

Nonoperative treatment of recurrent ankle instability may include casting, bracing, anti-inflammatory medication, taping, and physiotherapy. A review of the literature showed a number of studies related physiotherapy, cast, and brace treatment. Most of these modalities are used in combination. Physiotherapy seems to be better studied and the outcomes outlined better than brace treatment.

Brace Treatment. Overall bracing may be more effective than no treatment with Level C evidence: poor-quality evidence (Level IV or V with consistent findings) for or against recommending intervention, with most studies being of Level IV quality. Although bracing may be effective, the literature is too inconsistent to recommend bracing over taping or to recommend one brace over another.

Strengths of these brace studies in general are that the majority are prospective and do contain a control group. One criticism is that they do not have clinical results as an end point, but instead use indirect measures such as dynamometer testing or peroneal reaction times. This weakness makes many of the articles, which otherwise have good study design, hard to place in the context of outcome research.

The obvious study, comparison of brace versus no brace treatment on the midterm outcome of ankle instability or symptoms reported by the patient, has not been done. The articles written on bracing for chronic instability are summarized in Table 78–1. Future research should ideally be prospective, randomized, and based on patient-reported outcomes.

Physiotherapy. Three studies of Level II quality exist supporting the use of physiotherapy for recurrent instability. Four studies are Level II and IV quality, and three cannot be rated because they report outcomes that were not clinical and focused on indirect evidence such as peroneal reaction times. Based on these studies, a grade B recommendation exists for treatment of ankle instability with physiotherapy. One study used an unusual treatment regimen[28] that is an unconventional form of physiotherapy—a bidirectional bicycle pedal that is not available to most patients (Table 78–2).

Surgical Treatment of Recurrent Ankle Instability

After failed nonoperative treatment of ankle instability, patients may opt for surgical stabilization. The ligaments may be repaired or reconstructed. In the Broström repair, the torn ligaments are imbricated and may be augmented by the extensor retinaculum (Gould modification). Karlson modified the Broström technique by recommending repair through drill holes in bone.

Alternatively, the ligaments can be reconstructed. The reconstruction can be either anatomic or nonanatomic. Nonanatomic reconstructions include the Evans procedure (rerouting of the peroneus brevis through the fibula) or the Watson–Jones procedure (peroneal tendon weave). These reconstructions as a result sacrifice the active evertors of the ankle for a static restraint. Because the reconstruction is nonanatomic, joint motion may be restricted, so that the Evans procedure, for example, restricts subtalar joint motion.[37,38] In one retrospective case–control study with long-term follow-up, the rate of arthritis, ongoing instability, and reoperation rate all favored anatomic repair over Evans tenodesis.[39] Nine studies recommend against the use of nonanatomic reconstructions.[39-47] Another study showed impaired kinematics after Evans tenodesis and recommended against its use.[42] In a review of patients undergoing the Broström procedure compared with the Christman–Snook nonanatomic reconstruction, patients with the reconstruction complained of the ankle feeling "too tight."[48] Current opinion supports the use of an anatomic reconstruction or repair without sacrifice of the active evertors of the ankle.

Anatomic Repair. Anatomic repair (Broström repair, with or without modifications) remains one of the mainstays of surgical treatment of recurrent ankle instability.[49] Broström[50] described the imbrication of the lateral collateral ligaments. Karlsson and coworkers[51] modified the Broström repair by bringing the distal segments of the ligaments through drill holes and

TABLE 78–1. Brace Treatment for Ankle Instability

AUTHOR	YEAR	PATIENTS (N)	PROCEDURE	OUTCOME	COMMENTS	LEVEL
De Simoni et al.[19]	1996	30	Functional brace	93% better	Recommend prospective	IV
Eils et al.[20]	2002	24	10 brace types	Tilting platform		UR
Jerosch and Schoppe[21]	2000	21	Ankle support	Sport specific activities	Improved with brace	IV
Hals et al.[22]	2000	25	Rigid brace	Shuttle run times	Better with brace	III/UR
Baier and Hopf[23]	1998	22	Rigid vs. flexible brace	Reduced mediolaterals way	Both flexible and rigid braces work	III/UR
Jerosch et al.[24]	1997	23 ankles 18 control subjects	Various braces	Jumping performance	Braces better than no brace—aircast best	III/UR
Jerosch et al.[24]	1997	23 ankles 18 control subjects	Various braces	Time for ankle stabilization	Braces better than no brace	III
Els et al.[25]	1996	89 patients 0 control subjects	Lace brace	Acute injury—recurrent instability	Braces beneficial	IV
Regis et al.[26]	1995	20 dynamic 10 cast	Dynamic brace versus cast	Clinical outcome and Cybex	Dynamic brace better	III
Jerosch and Bischof[27]	1994	16 athletes 14 healthy volunteers	Brace vs. taping	Dynamic reaction time	Brace and tape better than nothing	UR IV

Grade of recommendation C: Poor-quality evidence (Level IV or V with consistent findings) for or against recommending intervention.

TABLE 78–2. Treatment of Ankle Instability with Physiotherapy

AUTHOR	YEAR	PATIENTS (N)	INTERVENTION	OUTCOME	COMMENTS	LEVEL
Kaminski et al.[29]	2003	30	Proprioception; strength training;	Peak torque Kin-Com	No difference	11
Hoiness et al.[28]	2003	19	Bidirectional pedal	Increased peak eversion torque + clinical review	Prospective randomized	11
Matsusaka et al.[30]	2001	22	Tape and disc	Proprioception	Tape improved proprioception	11
Eils and Rosenbaum[31]	2001	48	Multistation proprioception	Joint position sense and proprioception	Exercise better	111
Rozzi et al.[32]	1999	13	Balance training	Stability test	Improved	III
Wester et al.[33]	1998	48	Wobble board	Recurrent instability—control group	Wobble board beneficial	II
Wester et al.[34]	1996	48	Wobble board—acute injury	Clinical assessment	Wobble board beneficial	II
Regis et al.[26]	1995	20	20 dynamic brace vs. 10 cast	Clinical outcome and Cybex	Dynamic brace better	III
Karlsson et al.[35]	1991	100	Functional rehabilitation	49 good or excellent	Recommend physiotherapy as initial treatment	IV
Linde et al.[36]	1986	150	Functional rehabilitation	8% significantly impaired at 1 year	Physiotherapy recommended as initial treatment	IV

oversewing the repair to reinforce it. Gould and investigators[52] modified the Broström repair by oversewing the extensor retinaculum over the top of the repaired ligaments. I prefer to use both the Karlsson and Gould modifications.[53] Three studies are prospective, although one study compares two postoperative regimens for one type of reconstruction.[54] The strongest study was performed by Pijnenburg and researchers,[55] a Level I, randomized, prospective study. The remainder of the studies is Level IV quality. Overall, the grade of re-commendation is B for anatomic repair of the lateral ligaments for recurrent instability. All of the studies support the anatomic reconstruction, as opposed to the significant number of studies failing to support nonanatomic reconstruction. Notably, the majority of ideal studies have been done within the anatomic repair group, with consistent results. The anatomic repair should therefore be considered the standard of care for surgical intervention of recurrent lateral ankle instability, based on the level of evidence with the current studies and outcomes available (Table 78–3).

Instability in Children. Children and teenagers have weaker bones than adults; as a result, they are at risk for avulsing the tip of the fibula with an inversion sprain. In this case, the unstable ankle joint is associated with a fracture, providing a different pathology and a different reconstruction. The outcome of removal of the bone fragment and repair of the ligament to bone has been studied previously. The outcome studies on this procedure are summarized later in this chapter. As a subgroup of patients with ankle instabilities, they represent a small percentage of all patients with ankle instability. Notably, few patients have been studied in retrospective reviews, but all reporting good outcomes. Therefore, with a limited number of patients studied, a level C grade of recommendation exists for this procedure in children with ankle instability (see Table 78–4).

Nonanatomic Reconstruction. Nonanatomic reconstructions are more historical interest at this time. A number of repairs have been described. The Evans repair sacrifices the peroneus brevis muscle and uses it as a static restraint on the lateral ankle by repairing the proximal end to the fibula. It is the least anatomic of the nonanatomic reconstructions. It does not reconstruct the calcaneofibular ligament and runs perpendicular to the native ligament. Patients, therefore, may describe loss of inversion range, and loss of active eversion may cause greater feeling of instability beyond the instability being treated.

The Watson–Jones reconstruction uses peroneus brevis in a similar manner to the Evans repair, but brings the tendon through the front of the fibula and also reconstructs the talofibular ligament. The Christman–Snook repair reconstructs both ligaments with peroneus brevis by bringing the tendon from front to back and making a more anatomic reconstruction of the calcaneofibular ligament.

Grade of recommendation I exists for the nonanatomic reconstructions in view of the conflicting evidence for reconstruction. A large number of articles advocate against nonanatomic reconstruction and that these procedures should not be performed, and anatomic reconstruction or repair used instead. The articles on poor outcomes of nonanatomic reconstructions support the abandonment of the procedure (Table 78–5 and 78–6).

Anatomic Reconstruction with Use of Allograft or Autograft Tendon Augmentation. Anatomic reconstruction uses allograft or autograft to reconstruct the lateral collateral ligaments of the ankle in a manner that as closely as possible resembles the normal anatomy. Anatomic reconstructions preserve the function of the peroneus brevis. Like an anterior cruciate reconstruction of the knee, the anatomy cannot be completely reproduced, but the technique is designed within the limits of the surgery to resemble the normal anatomy.

Segesser[79] and Anderson[84] have used the plantaris tendon to reconstruct the lateral collateral ligaments.

TABLE 78–3. Surgical Treatment of Ankle Instability Using an Anatomic Lateral Ligament Repair Such as a Broström Procedure

AUTHOR	YEAR	PATIENTS (N)	PROCEDURE	OUTCOME	COMMENTS	LEVEL
Pijnenburg et al.[55]	2003	370	Repair vs. nonoperative treatment	Surgery better	Randomized prospective	II
Jarde et al.[56]	2002	43	Repair?	Surgery better	Retrospective	IV
Karlsson et al.[57]	1998	22	Repair	Surgery improved outcomes	Retrospective	IV
Rudert et al.[58]	1997	94	Repair with periosteal flap	81% good to excellent	Retrospective	IV
Liu and Jacobson[59]	1995	39	Repair with capsule	92% satisfied	Retrospective review	IV
Karlsson et al.[54]	1995	40	Repair: early ROM vs. cast	80% satisfaction—cast 91% satisfaction— early ROM	Prospective randomized	II
Karlsson et al.[51]	1988	148	Repair and imbrication	86% satisfied	Retrospective	IV
Duquennoy et al.[60]	1989	50	Repair	32 good or excellent	Retrospective	IV
Duquennoy et al.[61]	1980	22	Repair anterior TFL	21 good and excellent		IV
Hennrikus et al.[48]	1996	80	Repair vs. Christman–Snook	Repair better	Randomized prospective	II
Krips et al.[39]	2002	54	Repair vs. Evans	Repair better	Retrospective case–control	IV
Messer et al.[62]	2000	22	Broström	91% good or excellent	Retrospective review	IV
Hamilton et al.[63]	1993	27	Broström	26 of 27 did well	Retrospective review	IV

Grade of recommendation: B.
ROM, range of motion; TFL, talofibular ligament.

TABLE 78–4. Results for Surgery for Ankle Instability in Children

AUTHOR	YEAR	PATIENTS (N)	PROCEDURE	OUTCOME	COMMENTS	LEVEL
Busconi and Pappas[64]	1996	10	Excision of fibular fragment	All "better"	In favor	IV
Danielsson[65]	1980	5	Excision fibular fragment	All better	In favor	IV
Letts et al.[66]	2003	12	Nonanatomic reconstruction	"Better"	In favor	IV

TABLE 78–5. Outcomes of Surgery for Nonanatomic Reconstructions: Articles in Favor of the Technique

AUTHOR	YEAR	PATIENTS (N)	PROCEDURE	OUTCOME	COMMENTS	LEVEL
Cheng and Tho[67]	2002	15	Christman–Snook	14 excellent and good	Retrospective study nonvalidated outcome	IV
Colombet et al.[68]	1999	32	Christman–Snook	Karlson score and Telos	6 bad 24 return to sport	IV
Eskander and Macdonald[69]	1993	23	Watson–Jones	Not stated		IV
van der Rijt and Evans[47]	1984	9	Watson–Jones	22-year follow-up: only 3 asymptomatic	Recommends against	IV
Lauttamus et al.[70]	1982	33	Evans	32 good	? Quality	IV
Kristiansen[71]	1982	18	Evans	67% stable; 33% return to full activity	? Quality	IV
Kristiansen[72]	1981	24	Evans	73% stable postoperative		IV
Horstman et al.[41]	1981		Evans, Watson–Jones, Elmslie		Believed these ORs were inappropriate	IV
Baltopoulos et al.[37]	2004	27	Evans	92 average AOFAS points	Retrospective study	IV
Smith et al.[73]	1995	18	Christman–Snook		Retrospective study	IV
Marsh et al.[74]	2006	44	Christman–Snook	Good outcomes—children	Retrospective study	IV
Rosenbaum et al.[75]	1999	10	Evans	Equal results to periosteal repair		

AOFAS, American Orthopaedic Foot and Ankle Society.

TABLE 78–6. Nonanatomic Reconstruction: The 11 Articles Reporting Poor Outcomes

AUTHOR	YEAR	PATIENTS (N)	PROCEDURE	OUTCOME	COMMENTS	LEVEL
Juliano et al.[40]	2000	10	Christman–Snook	Revision surgery	Poor outcomes	IV
Boszotta and Sauer[46]	1989	44	Watson–Jones	61% arthrosis	Recommends against	IV
van der Rijt and Evans[47]	1984	9	Watson–Jones	22-year follow-up: only 3 asymptomatic	Recommends against	IV
Horstman et al.[41]	1981		Evans, Watson–Jones, Elmslie		Believed these ORs were inappropriate	IV
Hedeboe and Johannsen[76]	1979	21	Watson–Jones	80% good and excellent but not better than repair		IV
Krips et al.[39]	2002	45	Evans	Compared with Broström—higher reoperation rate in Evans	Retrospective case–control review	IV
Labs et al.[42]	2001	79	Evans	Recommended against Evans	Retrospective review	IV
Nimon et al.[43]	2001	89	Modified Evans	Recommended against 65% good or excellent	Retrospective review	IV
Becker et al.[44]	1994	38	Evans	40% reported ongoing pain: restricted motion	Retrospective review	IV
Orava et al.[45]	1983	42	Evans	6 poor results—radiographic subluxation Recommend against	Retrospective review	IV
Karlsson et al.[77]	1988	42	Evans	Only 50% satisfied—against Evans	Retrospective review	IV

Grade of recommendation I: The nonanatomic reconstructions have conflicting evidence for reconstruction. In view of the large number of articles advocating against nonanatomic reconstruction, these procedures should be not be performed, and anatomic reconstruction or repair used instead.

A drill hole is made through the calcaneus to deliver the tendon at the insertion of the calcaneofibular ligament. The tendon is then brought up through drill holes in the fibula and back onto the insertion of the anterior talofibular ligament, repairing to the talus with drill holes. Colville[80] repaired the lateral ligaments using half of peroneus brevis, thus preserving the function of the brevis muscle as an evertor. Coughlin[83] uses a free gracilis graft through drill holes. A modification of the Anderson technique using a free gracilis autograft is our preferred technique for lateral ligament reconstruction. No outcome review has been performed to date.[78]

All articles to date support the concept of an anatomic reconstruction. Some surgeons select the anatomic reconstruction for patients with more attenuated tissue. Because these tendon autograft or allograft lateral ligament reconstruction are newer techniques, limited outcome data are available. However, all articles support of anatomic reconstruction with a grade C recommendation (see Table 78–7).

Revision Lateral Ligament Reconstruction. Only two articles identified the outcome of lateral ligament reconstruction for revision of a previous failed repair. As would be expected, few articles have been published in this area. Those two articles support the principle with a grade C recommendation, with the caution that few patients have been studied. Table 78–9 provides a summary of recommendations for the treatment of recurrent ankle instability.

TABLE 78–7. Outcomes of Anatomic Reconstruction with Autograft or Allograft Tendon

AUTHOR	YEAR	PATIENTS (N)	PROCEDURE	OUTCOME	COMMENTS	LEVEL
Segesser and Goesele[79]	1996	443	Reconstruction with plantaris	88% good/excellent	Supports repair	IV
Colville and Grondel[80]	1995	12	Reconstruction half peroneal brevis		Supports repair ? Anatomic	IV
Solheim et al.[81]	1980	30	Medial third Achilles	All except 1 asymptomatic		IV
Sugimoto et al.[82]	2002	13	Repair with bone patella bone	All		IV
Coughlin et al.[83]	2004	28	Gracilis free graft	All good outcome		IV
Anderson[84]	1985	9	Plantaris	All good outcome		IV

Grade of recommendation C: One article has a large series; however, the number of articles currently supporting anatomic reconstruction with a free tendon graft is few.

TABLE 78–8. Outcomes of Revision Lateral Ligament Reconstruction

AUTHOR	YEAR	PATIENTS (N)	PROCEDURE	OUTCOME	COMMENT	LEVEL
Kuhn and Lippert[85]	2006	15	Revision lateral ligament with Broström	12/15 good	Favorable	IV
Sammarco and Carrasquillo[86]	1995	10	Elmslie with tendon graft	9/10 good		IV

Grade of recommendation C or I: There are only 25 patients in total studied in these series. However, it is not surprising that this is a limited area of publication.

TABLE 78–9. Summary of Recommendations

STATEMENT	LEVEL OF EVIDENCE/ GRADE OF RECOMMENDATION	REFERENCES
1. Acute ankle sprains should be treated non operatively.	B	8-11, [1]
2. Brace treatment may be effective for non operative treatment of ankle instability.	C	19-27
3. Physiotherapy is beneficial for patients with recurrent ankle instability.	B	26,28-36
4. For failed non operative treatment a Brostrom repair of the ligaments is effective, including Karlsson and Gould Modifications.	B	55-63
5. There is insufficient research to determine the best treatment for ankle instability in children, although studies to date show benefit.	C	64-66
6. Non anatomic reconstructions of the ankle are not recommended due to the large number of papers documenting poor outcomes with Evans and Watson Jones Procedures.	C	39-47,76,77
7. There is insufficient evidence to support non anatomic reconstructions.	C	37, 47, 68-75
8. Anatomic reconstruction should be used if a repair cannot be performed because of poor or insufficient residual ligaments.	C	79-84
9. There is insufficient evidence for the use of anatomic reconstruction as a primary procedure.	C	79-84

REFERENCES

1. Baumhauer JF, O'Brien T: Surgical considerations in the treatment of ankle instability. J Athl Train 37:458–462, 2002.
2. Van Bergeyk AB, Younger A, Carson B: CT analysis of hindfoot alignment in chronic lateral ankle instability. Foot Ankle Int 23:37–42, 2002.
3. Berkowitz MJ, Kim DH: Fibular position in relation to lateral ankle instability. Foot Ankle Int 25:318–321, 2004.
4. Ferran NA, Maffulli N: Epidemiology of sprains of the lateral ankle ligament complex. Foot Ankle Clin 11:659–662, 2006.
5. Brooks JH, Fuller CW, Kemp SP, et al: Epidemiology of injuries in English professional rugby union: Part 2 training injuries. Br J Sports Med 39:767–775, 2005.
6. Colville MR: Surgical treatment of the unstable ankle. J Am Acad Orthop Surg 6:368–377, 1998.
7. Burks RT, Morgan J: Anatomy of the lateral ankle ligaments. Am J Sports Med 22:72–77, 1994.
8. Karlsson J, Eriksson BI, Sward L: Early functional treatment for acute ligament injuries of the ankle joint. Scand J Med Sci Sports 6:341–345, 1996.
9. Kerkhoffs GM, Handoll HH, de Bie R, et al: Surgical versus conservative treatment for acute injuries of the lateral ligament complex of the ankle in adults. Cochrane Database Syst Rev (3):CD000380, 2002.
10. Kerkhoffs GM, Rowe BH, Assendelft WJ, et al: Immobilisation for acute ankle sprain. A systematic review. Arch Orthop Trauma Surg 121:462–471, 2001.
11. Karlsson J, Lansinger O: Lateral instability of the ankle joint. Clin Orthop Relat Res (276):253–261, 1992.
12. Hintermann B, Boss A, Schafer D: Arthroscopic findings in patients with chronic ankle instability. Am J Sports Med 30:402–409, 2002.
13. Komenda GA, Ferkel RD: Arthroscopic findings associated with the unstable ankle. Foot Ankle Int 20:708–713, 1999.
14. Taga I, Shino K, Inoue M, et al: Articular cartilage lesions in ankles with lateral ligament injury. An arthroscopic study. Am J Sports Med 21:120–127, 1993.
15. Ferkel RD, Chams RN: Chronic lateral instability: Arthroscopic findings and long-term results. Foot Ankle Int 28:24–31, 2007.
16. Takao M, Komatsu F, Naito K, et al: Reconstruction of lateral ligament with arthroscopic drilling for treatment of early-stage osteoarthritis in unstable ankles. Arthroscopy 22:1119–1125, 2006.
17. DIGiovanni BF, Fraga CJ, Cohen BE, Shereff MJ: Associated injuries found in chronic lateral ankle instability. Foot Ankle Int 21:809–815, 2000.
18. Bonnin M, Tavernier T, Bouysset M: Split lesions of the peroneus brevis tendon in chronic ankle laxity. Am J Sports Med 25:699–703, 1997.
19. De Simoni C, Wetz HH, Zanetti M, et al: Clinical examination and magnetic resonance imaging in the assessment of ankle sprains treated with an orthosis. Foot Ankle Int 17:177–182, 1996.
20. Eils E, Demming C, Kollmeier G, et al: Comprehensive testing of 10 different ankle braces. Evaluation of passive and rapidly induced stability in subjects with chronic ankle instability. Clin Biomech (Bristol, Avon) 17:526–535, 2002.
21. Jerosch J, Schoppe R: Midterm effects of ankle joint supports on sensomotor and sport-specific capabilities. Knee Surg Sports Traumatol Arthrosc 8:252–259, 2000.
22. Hals TM, Sitler MR, Mattacola CG: Effect of a semi-rigid ankle stabilizer on performance in persons with functional ankle instability. J Orthop Sports Phys Ther 30:552–556, 2000.
23. Baier M, Hopf T: Ankle orthoses effect on single-limb standing balance in athletes with functional ankle instability. Arch Phys Med Rehabil 79:939–944, 1998.
24. Jerosch J, Thorwesten L, Frebel T, et al: Influence of external stabilizing devices of the ankle on sport-specific capabilities. Knee Surg Sports Traumatol Arthrosc 5:50–57, 1997.
25. Els M, Niggli A, Ochsner PE: [Functional therapy using a laced ankle brace in supination trauma of the ankle joint with lesions of the capsule-ligament apparatus]. Swiss Surg 2:280–283, 1996.
26. Regis D, Montanari M, Magnan B, et al: Dynamic orthopaedic brace in the treatment of ankle sprains. Foot Ankle Int 16:422–426, 1995.
27. Jerosch J, Bischof M: [The effect of proprioception on functional stability of the upper ankle joint with special reference to stabilizing aids]. Sportverletz Sportschaden 8:111–121, 1994.
28. Hoiness P, Glott T, Ingjer F: High-intensity training with a bi-directional bicycle pedal improves performance in mechanically unstable ankles—a prospective randomized study of 19 subjects. Scand J Med Sci Sports 13:266–271, 2003.
29. Kaminski TW, Buckley BD, Powers ME, et al: Effect of strength and proprioception training on eversion to inversion strength ratios in subjects with unilateral functional ankle instability. Br J Sports Med 37:410–415, 2003.
30. Matsusaka N, Yokoyama S, Tsurusaki T, et al: Effect of ankle disk training combined with tactile stimulation to the leg and foot on functional instability of the ankle. Am J Sports Med 29:25–30, 2001.
31. Eils E, Rosenbaum D: A multi-station proprioceptive exercise program in patients with ankle instability. Med Sci Sports Exerc 33:1991–1998, 2001.
32. Rozzi SL, Lephart SM, Sterner R, et al: Balance training for persons with functionally unstable ankles. J Orthop Sports Phys Ther 29:478–486, 1999.
33. Wester JU, Jespersen SM, Nielsen KD, et al: [Training on a wobble board following lateral ankle joint sprains]. Ugeskr Laeger 160:632–634, 1998.
34. Wester JU, Jespersen SM, Nielsen KD, et al: Wobble board training after partial sprains of the lateral ligaments of the ankle: A prospective randomized study. J Orthop Sports Phys Ther 23:332–336, 1996.
35. Karlsson J, Lansinger O, Faxen E: [Lateral instability of the ankle joint (2). Active training programs can prevent surgery]. Lakartidningen 88:1404–1407, 1991.
36. Linde F, Hvass I, Jurgensen U, et al: Early mobilizing treatment in lateral ankle sprains. Course and risk factors for chronic painful or function-limiting ankle. Scand J Rehabil Med 18:17–21, 1986.
37. Baltopoulos P, Tzagarakis GP, Kaseta MA: Midterm results of a modified evans repair for chronic lateral ankle instability. Clin Orthop Relat Res (422):180–185, 2004.
38. Fujii T, Kitaoka HB, Watanabe K, et al: Comparison of modified Brostrom and Evans procedures in simulated lateral ankle injury. Med Sci Sports Exerc 38:1025–1031, 2006.
39. Krips R, Brandsson S, Swensson C, et al: Anatomical reconstruction and Evans tenodesis of the lateral ligaments of the ankle. Clinical and radiological findings after follow-up for 15 to 30 years. J Bone Joint Surg Br 84:232–236, 2002.
40. Juliano PJ, Jordan JD, Lippert FG, et al: Persistent postoperative pain after the Chrisman-Snook ankle reconstruction. Am J Orthop 29:449–452, 2000.
41. Horstman JK, Kantor GS, Samuelson KM: Investigation of lateral ankle ligament reconstruction. Foot Ankle 1:338–342, 1981.
42. Labs K, Perka C, Lang T: Clinical and gait-analytical results of the modified Evans tenodesis in chronic fibulotalar ligament instability. Knee Surg Sports Traumatol Arthrosc 9:116–122, 2001.
43. Nimon GA, Dobson PJ, Angel KR, et al: A long-term review of a modified Evans procedure. J Bone Joint Surg Br 83:14–18, 2001.
44. Becker HP, Rosenbaum D, Zeithammer G, et al: Gait pattern analysis after ankle ligament reconstruction (modified Evans procedure). Foot Ankle Int 15:477–482, 1994.
45. Orava S, Jaroma H, Weitz H, et al: Radiographic instability of the ankle joint after Evans' repair. Acta Orthop Scand 54:734–738, 1983.
46. Boszotta H, Sauer G: [Chronic fibular ligament insufficiency at the upper ankle joint. Late results after modified Watson-Jones plastic surgery]. Unfallchirurg 92:11–16, 1989.
47. van der Rijt AJ, Evans GA: The long-term results of Watson-Jones tenodesis. J Bone Joint Surg Br 66:371–375, 1984.

48. Hennrikus WL, Mapes RC, Lyons PM, et al: Outcomes of the Chrisman-Snook and modified-Broström procedures for chronic lateral ankle instability. A prospective, randomized comparison. Am J Sports Med 24:400–404, 1996.

49. Harper MC: Modification of the Gould modification of the Broström ankle repair. Foot Ankle Int 19:788, 1998.

50. Broström L: Sprained ankles. VI. Surgical treatment of "chronic" ligament ruptures. Acta Chir Scand 132:551–565, 1966.

51. Karlsson J, Bergsten T, Lansinger O, et al: Reconstruction of the lateral ligaments of the ankle for chronic lateral instability. J Bone Joint Surg Am 70:581–588, 1988.

52. Gould N, Seligson D, Gassman J: Early and late repair of lateral ligament of the ankle. Foot Ankle 1:84–89, 1980.

53. Ajis A, Younger AS, Maffulli N: Anatomic repair for chronic lateral ankle instability. Foot Ankle Clin 11:539–545, 2006.

54. Karlsson J, Rudholm O, Bergsten T, et al: Early range of motion training after ligament reconstruction of the ankle joint. Knee Surg Sports Traumatol Arthrosc 3:173–177, 1995.

55. Pijnenburg AC, Bogaard K, Krips R, et al: Operative and functional treatment of rupture of the lateral ligament of the ankle. A randomised, prospective trial. J Bone Joint Surg Br 85:525–530, 2003.

56. Jarde O, Duboille G, Abi-Raad G, et al: [Ankle instability with involvement of the subtalar joint demonstrated by MRI. Results with the Castaing procedure in 45 cases.] Acta Orthop Belg 68:515–528, 2002.

57. Karlsson J, Eriksson BI, Renstrom P: Subtalar instability of the foot. A review and results after surgical treatment. Scand J Med Sci Sports 8:191–197, 1998.

58. Rudert M, Wulker N, Wirth CJ: Reconstruction of the lateral ligaments of the ankle using a regional periosteal flap. J Bone Joint Surg Br 79:446–451, 1997.

59. Liu SH, Jacobson KE: A new operation for chronic lateral ankle instability. J Bone Joint Surg Br 77:55–59, 1995.

60. Duquennoy A, Fontaine C, Martinot JC, et al: [Surgical reduction of the external ligament for chronic instability of the tibio-tarsal joint. Apropos of 58 reviewed cases]. Rev Chir Orthop Reparatrice Appar Mot 75:387–393, 1989.

61. Duquennoy A, Letendard J, Loock P: [Chronic instability of the ankle treated by reefing of the lateral ligament (author's transl)]. Rev Chir Orthop Reparatrice Appar Mot 66:311–316, 1980.

62. Messer TM, Cummins CA, Ahn J, et al: Outcome of the modified Broström procedure for chronic lateral ankle instability using suture anchors. Foot Ankle Int 21:996–1003, 2000.

63. Hamilton WG, Thompson FM, Snow SW: The modified Broström procedure for lateral ankle instability. Foot Ankle 14:1–7, 1993.

64. Busconi BD, Pappas AM: Chronic, painful ankle instability in skeletally immature athletes. Ununited osteochondral fractures of the distal fibula. Am J Sports Med 24:647–651, 1996.

65. Danielsson LG: Avulsion fracture of the lateral malleolus in children. Injury 12:165–167, 1980.

66. Letts M, Davidson D, Mukhtar I: Surgical management of chronic lateral ankle instability in adolescents. J Pediatr Orthop 23:392–397, 2003.

67. Cheng M, Tho KS: Chrisman-Snook ankle ligament reconstruction outcomes—a local experience. Singapore Med J 43:605–609, 2002.

68. Colombet P, Bousquet V, Allard M, et al: [Treatment of chronic ankle instability with the Chrisman-Snook's technique]. Rev Chir Orthop Reparatrice Appar Mot 85:722–726, 1999.

69. Eskander M, Macdonald R: Watson-Jones tenodesis for chronic ankle joint instability. J R Army Med Corps 139:115–116, 1993.

70. Lauttamus L, Korkala O, Tanskanen P: Lateral ligament injuries of the ankle. Surgical treatment of late cases. Ann Chir Gynaecol 71:164–167, 1982.

71. Kristiansen B: Surgical treatment of ankle instability in athletes. Br J Sports Med 16:40–45, 1982.

72. Kristiansen B: Evans' repair of lateral instability of the ankle joint. Acta Orthop Scand 52:679–682, 1981.

73. Smith PA, Miller SJ, Berni AJ: A modified Chrisman-Snook procedure for reconstruction of the lateral ligaments of the ankle: Review of 18 cases. Foot Ankle Int 16:259–266, 1995.

74. Marsh JS, Daigneault JP, Polzhofer GK: Treatment of ankle instability in children and adolescents with a modified Chrisman-Snook repair: A clinical and patient-based outcome study. J Pediatr Orthop 26:94–99, 2006.

75. Rosenbaum D, Engelhardt M, Becker HP, et al: Clinical and functional outcome after anatomic and nonanatomic ankle ligament reconstruction: Evans tenodesis versus periosteal flap. Foot Ankle Int 20:636–639, 1999.

76. Hedeboe J, Johannsen A: Recurrent instability of the ankle joint. Surgical repair by the Watson-Jones method. Acta Orthop Scand 50:337–340, 1979.

77. Karlsson J, Bergsten T, Lansinger O, et al: Lateral instability of the ankle treated by the Evans procedure. A long-term clinical and radiological follow-up. J Bone Joint Surg Br 70:476–480, 1988.

78. Boyer DS, Younger AS: Anatomic reconstruction of the lateral ligament complex of the ankle using a gracilis autograft. Foot Ankle Clin 11:585–595, 2006.

79. Segesser B, Goesele A: [Weber fibular ligament-plasty with plantar tendon with Segesser modification]. Sportverletz Sportschaden 10:88–93, 1996.

80. Colville MR, Grondel RJ: Anatomic reconstruction of the lateral ankle ligaments using a split peroneus brevis tendon graft. Am J Sports Med 23:210–213, 1995.

81. Solheim LF, Denstad TF, Roaas A: Chronic lateral instability of the ankle. A method of reconstruction using the Achilles tendon. Acta Orthop Scand 51:193–196, 1980.

82. Sugimoto K, Takakura Y, Kumai T, et al: Reconstruction of the lateral ankle ligaments with bone-patellar tendon graft in patients with chronic ankle instability: A preliminary report. Am J Sports Med 30:340–346, 2002.

83. Coughlin MJ, Schenck RC Jr, Grebing BR, et al: Comprehensive reconstruction of the lateral ankle for chronic instability using a free gracilis graft. Foot Ankle Int 25:231–241, 2004.

84. Anderson ME: Reconstruction of the lateral ligaments of the ankle using the plantaris tendon. J Bone Joint Surg Am 67:930–934, 1985.

85. Kuhn MA, Lippert FG: Revision lateral ankle reconstruction. Foot Ankle Int 27:77–81, 2006.

86. Sammarco GJ, Carrasquillo HA: Surgical revision after failed lateral ankle reconstruction. Foot Ankle Int 16:748–753, 1995.

87. Kerkhoffs GM, Handoll HH, de Bie R, et al.: Surgical versus conservative treatment for acute injuries of the lateral ligament complex of the ankle in adults. Cochrane Database Syst Rev 2007(2):CD000380.

ARTHROPLASTY TOPICS

Regional Anesthesia for Total Hip and Knee Arthroplasty:
Is It Worth the Effort?

Richard Brull, MD, FRCPC, G Arun Prasad, MBBS, DA, FRCA, and Vincent W. S. Chan, MD, FRCPC

Regional anesthesia (RA) for total hip arthroplasty (THA) and total knee arthroplasty (TKA) has been associated with numerous benefits compared with general anesthesia (GA). Regional anesthesia can afford both dense surgical anesthesia and long-lasting, opioid-sparing, postoperative analgesia with a low rate of serious complications.[1-7] Regional anesthesia techniques for THA and TKA include, either alone or in combination, central neuraxial blockade (CNB) (i.e., epidural and spinal anesthesia) and peripheral nerve blockade (PNB). For example, combined spinal-epidural is an excellent technique for THA or TKA because it combines the benefits of spinal and epidural blockade, that is, reliable rapid-onset dense surgical anesthesia provided by the intrathecal dose of local anesthetic and the flexibility to administer supplemental local anesthetic as necessary via the epidural catheter for prolonged intraoperative anesthesia or postoperative analgesia, or both. Alternatively, PNB avoids many of the unwanted adverse effects of both GA and CNB, such as hypotension, nausea and vomiting, and pruritus, and allows for targeted unilateral blockade of the operative limb providing excellent analgesia.[8,9] Continuous PNB (CPNB) for TKA has gained tremendous popularity in recent years[10,11] because continuous perineural infusions of dilute, long-acting local anesthetic solution via an indwelling catheter can significantly prolong postoperative analgesia compared with single-injection techniques[12,13] and, importantly, can facilitate rehabilitation[14-17] because opioid-related adverse effects are spared.[9,18,19]

Despite the benefits of regional anesthesia for THA and TKA, many orthopedic surgeons have been reluctant to embrace regional anesthesia because of concerns of operating room delay and block failure.[20] Indeed, GA affords a near 100% success rate in comparison with regional anesthesia, which carries an inherent failure rate even in experienced hands.[21] GA can often be performed faster than regional anesthesia, and the technical skills needed to administer GA are easier to acquire than regional anesthesia. Furthermore, the choice of anesthetic technique—regional anesthesia versus GA—is oftentimes influenced by time constraints, the availability of a "block room,"[22] skilled anesthetic personnel, and perceived

liability risk.[23] These obstacles have prompted many orthopedic surgeons (and anesthesiologists alike) to ask: "Is regional anesthesia worth the effort?"

Numerous recent meta-analyses have addressed the question of regional anesthesia versus GA for major orthopedic surgery with conflicting results.[24-29] Much of the source data for these meta-analyses are dated because databases such as MEDLINE capture indexed articles published as early as 1950. These older studies do not reflect advances in training, anesthetic techniques, and perioperative surgical practices, such as routine low-molecular-weight heparin thromboprophylaxis and standardized clinical pathways. Moreover, meta-analyses are notoriously limited by the inclusion of studies with small sample sizes, heterogeneity between source studies, publication bias, informed censoring, and meta-analyst bias.[30,31] Accordingly, results of meta-analyses oftentimes do not reflect those of corresponding large, randomized, controlled trials (RCTs).[32] In this chapter, we review and summarize (Tables 79–1 and 79–2) the best contemporary data available regarding the effects of anesthetic technique, either regional anesthesia or GA, on important perioperative outcomes for patients undergoing THA or TKA. We included RCTs of adult patients who underwent regional anesthesia or GA for THA or TKA that were published in English from 1990 to July 2007. We included trials that compared a regional anesthesia technique for primary surgical anesthesia or postoperative analgesia, or both, with conventional GA for surgery and/or systemic analgesia for postoperative pain control.

MORTALITY

No contemporary RCTs are designed primarily to assess differences in mortality after regional anesthesia versus GA for THA or TKA. Because death is such a rare occurrence in modern anesthetic practice, prohibitively large numbers of patients would be required for study to determine the effects of anesthetic technique on patient mortality. In a widely cited meta-analysis of 141 clinical trials (almost 10,000 patients in total) comparing CNB or GA for a variety of surgery types (mostly orthopedic),

TABLE 79–1. Perioperative Outcomes after Regional Anesthesia versus General Anesthesia for Total Hip Arthroplasty

AUTHOR (YEAR OF PUBLICATION)	N	ANESTHESIA	ANALGESIA	RESULTS	P	OUTCOME*	REMARKS
Mortality							
Wulf et al. (1999)[54]	43 45	EA GA	CEA IV PCA	No deaths reported in the course of the study	NS	2°	
Planes et al. (1991)[61]	65 60 62	SA[I] SA[II] GA[III]	Paracetamol Paracetamol Paracetamol	No difference in postoperative mortality	NS	2°	I. No additional enoxaparin II. 20 mg enoxaparin 1 hour after SA III. 40 mg enoxaparin 12 hours before GA Enoxaparin 12 hours after surgery and daily thereafter
Cardiovascular Morbidity							
Borghi et al. (2002)[62]	70 70 70	EA EA+GA GA	Undisclosed Undisclosed Undisclosed	Incremental increase in incidence of clinically significant hypotension EA+GA vs. GA vs. EA alone	<0.05	1°	
Wulf et al. (1999)[54]	43 45	EA GA	CEA IV PCA	1. Increased incidence of hypotension in EA (4%) vs. GA (11%) 2. Increased incidence of bradycardia in EA (2%) vs. GA (14%)	1. <0.05 2. <0.05	2°	
Dauphin et al. (1997)[63]	20 17	EA+GA GA	IV/IM opioid IV/IM opioid	No difference in perioperative dysrhythmias or ischemic episodes	NS	2°	Perioperative (48-hour) Holter monitoring
Deep Venous Thrombosis							
Brueckner et al. (2003)[64]	16 10	SA GA	Undisclosed Undisclosed	1. No cases of clinically evident DVT 2. No difference in hemostatic molecular markers	1. NS 2. NS	1°	Daily nadroparin thromboprophylaxis and compression stockings
Dauphin et al. (1997)[63]	20 17	EA+GA GA	IV/IM opioid IV/IM opioid	No difference in DVT	NS	2°	Daily warfarin thromboprophylaxis
Planes et al. (1991)[61]	65 60 62	SA[I] SA[II] GA[III]	Paracetamol Paracetamol Paracetamol	1. No difference in total and proximal DVT 2. Incremental reduction in distal DVT in group I (11%) vs. group II (5%) vs. group III (0%)	1. NS 2. <0.01	1°	I. No additional enoxaparin II. 20 mg enoxaparin 1 hour after SA III. 40 mg enoxaparin 12 hours before GA Enoxaparin 12 hours after surgery and daily thereafter Venography on POD 13
Pulmonary Embolism							
Brueckner et al. (2003)[64]	16 10	SA GA	Undisclosed Undisclosed	No cases of clinically evident PE	NS	1°	Daily nadroparin thromboprophylaxis and compression stockings
Planes et al. (1991)[61]	65 60 62	SA[I] SA[II] GA[III]	Paracetamol Paracetamol Paracetamol	No cases of PE	NS	1°	I. No additional enoxaparin II. 20 mg enoxaparin 1 hour after SA III. 40 mg enoxaparin 12 hours before GA Enoxaparin 12 hours after surgery and daily thereafter Venography on POD 13
Blood Loss							
Borghi et al. (2005)[65]	70 70 70	EA EA+GA GA	Undisclosed Undisclosed Undisclosed	1. No difference in intraoperative or postoperative blood loss 2. Faster recovery of circulating RBC mass in EA vs. EA+GA or GA	1. NS 2. <0.05	1°	Nitrous oxide in GA can inhibit erythropoiesis by altering vitamin B_{12}
Brueckner et al. (2003)[64]	16 10	SA GA	Undisclosed Undisclosed	Reduced intraoperative bleeding in SA (572 mL) vs. GA (750 mL)	<0.05	2°	No difference in Hb and Hct up to POD 6

TABLE 79–1. Perioperative Outcomes after Regional Anesthesia versus General Anesthesia for Total Hip Arthroplasty—cont'd

AUTHOR (YEAR OF PUBLICATION)	N	ANESTHESIA	ANALGESIA	RESULTS	P	OUTCOME*	REMARKS
Borghi et al. (2002)[62]	70	EA	Undisclosed	No difference in intraoperative or postoperative blood loss or transfusion requirements	NS	2°	
	70	EA+GA	Undisclosed				
	70	GA	Undisclosed				
Stevens et al. (2000)[66]	28	GA	LPB	1. Reduced intraoperative blood loss in LPB (420 mL) vs. IV PCA (538 mL) 2. Reduced postoperative blood loss in LPB (170 mL) vs. IV PCA (310 mL)	1. <0.05 2. <0.05	2°	LPB performed before surgery
	29	GA	IV PCA				
D'Ambrosio et al. (1999)[67]	15	EA+GA[I]	CEA	Increased perioperative blood loss and transfusion requirements in GA[IV] vs. all other groups	<0.001	1°	I. Aprotinin 500,000 KIU before surgery and 500,000 KIU/hr intraoperatively II. No aprotinin (placebo) III. Aprotinin 500,000 KIU before surgery and 500,000 KIU/h intraoperatively IV. No aprotinin (placebo) Daily naproparin thromboprophylaxis
	15	EA+GA[II]	CEA				
	15	GA[III]	IV opioid				
	15	GA[IV]	IV opioid				
Dauphin et al. (1997)[63]	20	EA+GA	IV/IM opioid	1. Reduced intraoperative blood loss in EA+GA (664 mL) vs. GA (1259 mL) 2. Reduced transfusion requirements in EA+GA (35%) vs. GA (88%) 3. No difference in postoperative Hb	1. <0.01 2. <0.01 3. NS	1°	Reduced average intraoperative MAP in EA+GA (80 mm Hg) vs. GA (88 mm Hg) (*P* < 0.05)
	17	GA	IV/IM opioid				
Planes et al. (1991)[61]	65	SA[I]	Paracetamol	No difference in intraoperative blood loss, postoperative blood drainage, or transfusion requirements	NS	2°	I. No additional enoxaparin II. 20 mg enoxaparin 1 hour after SA III. 40 mg enoxaparin 12 hours before surgery All patients received 40 mg enoxaparin 12 hours after surgery and daily thereafter
	60	SA[II]	Paracetamol				
	62	GA[III]	Paracetamol				
Salo and Nissila (1990)[68]	11	SA	IM opioid	No difference in surgical blood loss	NS	2°	
	11	GA	IM opioid				
Jones et al. (1990)[69]	43	SA	IM morphine	1. Reduced transfusion requirements in SA (50%) vs. GA (72%) 2. No difference in postoperative Hb	1. <0.05 2. NS	2°	
	46	GA	IM morphine				
Surgical Time							
Borghi et al. (2005)[65]	70	EA	Undisclosed	No difference in surgical duration	NS	2°	
	70	EA+GA	Undisclosed				
	70	GA	Undisclosed				
Biboulet et al. (2004)[70]	15	GA	FNB	No difference in surgical duration	NS	2°	
	15	GA	LPB				
	15	GA	IV PCA				
Brueckner et al. (2003)[64]	16	SA	Undisclosed	No difference in surgical duration	NS	2°	
	10	GA	Undisclosed				
Borghi et al. (2002)[62]	70	EA	Undisclosed	No difference in surgical duration	NS	2°	
	70	EA+GA	Undisclosed				
	70	GA	Undisclosed				
Stevens et al. (2000)[66]	29	GA	LPB	No difference in surgical duration	NS	2°	LPB performed before surgery
	30	GA	IV PCA				
D'Ambrosio et al. (1999)[67]	15	EA+GA[I]	CEA	No difference in surgical duration	NS	2°	See above for explanation of groups
	15	EA+GA[II]	CEA				
	15	GA[III]	IV opioid				
	15	GA[IV]	IV opioid				
Dauphin et al. (1997)[63]	20	EA+GA	IV/IM opioid	No difference in surgical duration	NS	2°	
	17	GA	IV/IM opioid				

Continued

TABLE 79–1. Perioperative Outcomes after Regional Anesthesia versus General Anesthesia for Total Hip Arthroplasty—cont'd

AUTHOR (YEAR OF PUBLICATION)	N	ANESTHESIA	ANALGESIA	RESULTS	P	OUTCOME*	REMARKS
Moiniche et al. (1994)[71]	11	EA	CEA	No difference in surgical duration	NS	2°	
	11	GA	IM morphine		NS	2°	
Planes et al. (1991)[61]	65	SA[I]	Paracetamol	No difference in surgical duration	NS	2°	See above for explanation of groups
	60	SA[II]	Paracetamol				
	62	GA[III]	Paracetamol				
Pain							
Biboulet et al. (2004)[70]	15	GA	FNB	Reduced pain scores and morphine consumption up to 4 hours in LPB vs. FNB or IV PCA	<0.05	1°	No difference in pain scores or morphine consumption at rest or during mobilization beyond 4 hours
	15	GA	LPB				
	15	GA	IV PCA				
Stevens et al. (2000)[66]	28	GA	LPB	Reduced pain scores and morphine consumption up to 6 hours in LPB vs. IV PCA	<0.01	1°	LPB performed before surgery
	29	GA	IV PCA				No difference in pain scores or morphine consumption beyond 6 hours
Wulf et al. (1999)[54]	43	EA	CEA	Reduced pain scores at rest up to 24 hours in EA vs. GA	<0.01	1°	No difference in pain scores after mobilization
	45	GA	IV PCA				
Moiniche et al. (1994)[71]	11	EA	CEA	Reduced pain scores at (1) rest, (2) flexion, and (3) walk up to 48 hours in EA vs. GA	1. <0.01 2. <0.01 3. 0.01	1°	No difference in pain scores beyond 48 hours
	11	GA	IM morphine				
Adverse Effects							
Biboulet et al. (2004)[70]	15	GA	FNB	No difference in PONV, pruritus, or sedation	NS	2°	No difference in patient satisfaction
	15	GA	LPB				
	15	GA	IV PCA				
Stevens et al. (2000)[66]	28	GA	LPB	No difference in PONV symptoms	NS	2°	LPB performed before surgery
	29	GA	IV PCA				
Wulf et al. (1999)[54]	43	EA	CEA	1. Reduced incidence of nausea in EA (16%) vs. GA (28%) 2. Reduced incidence of vomiting in EA (11%) vs. GA (22%) 3. Earlier return of bowel motility in EA (26 hours) vs. GA (47 hours)	1. <0.05 2. <0.05 3. <0.05	2°	
	45	GA	IV PCA				
Cognitive Deficit							
Wulf et al. (1999)[54]	43	EA	CEA	Earlier mental clarity and cooperativeness in EA vs. GA	<0.05	2°	
	45	GA	IV PCA				
Rehabilitation							
Biboulet et al. (2004)[70]	15	GA	FNB	1. No difference in articular mobility on admission to rehabilitation center 2. No difference in duration of stay at rehabilitation center	1. NS 2. NS	2°	
	15	GA	LPB				
	15	GA	IV PCA				
Moiniche et al. (1994)[71]	11	EA	CEA	No difference in postoperative activity	NS	2°	
	11	GA	IM morphine				
Length of Stay							
Wulf et al. (1999)[54]	43	EA	CEA	No difference in LOS	NS	2°	Earlier discharge readiness from PACU in EA vs. GA (P < 0.05)
	45	GA	IV PCA				
Moiniche et al. (1994)[71]	11	EA	CEA	No difference in LOS	NS	2°	
	11	GA	IM morphine				

*1° denotes primary outcome measure of parent study; 2° denotes secondary outcome measure of parent study.
CEA, continuous epidural analgesia; EA, epidural anesthesia; FNB, femoral nerve block; GA, general anesthesia; Hb, hemoglobin; Hct, hematocrit; IM, intramuscular; IV, intravenous; LOS, length of stay; LPB, lumbar plexus block; MAP, mean arterial pressure; NS, not significant; PACU, postanesthesia care unit; PCA, patient-controlled analgesia; PE, pulmonary embolism; POD, postoperative day; PONV, postoperative nausea and vomiting; SA, spinal anesthesia.

TABLE 79–2. Perioperative Outcomes after Regional Anesthesia versus General Anesthesia for Total Knee Arthroplasty

AUTHOR (YEAR OF PUBLICATION)	N	ANESTHESIA	ANALGESIA	RESULTS	P	OUTCOME*	REMARKS
Mortality							
Williams-Russo et al. (1996)[15]	134	EA	CEA	No difference in postoperative mortality	NS	2°	
Williams-Russo et al. (1995)[56]	128	GA	IV opioid				
Cardiovascular Morbidity							
Chelly et al. (2001)[60]	29 30 33	GA EA GA	CFNB+SNB CEA IV PCA	1. Decreased incidence of hypotension in GA+CFNB+SNB (66% RRR) vs. GA alone 2. Decreased incidence of bradycardia in GA+CFNB+SNB (77% RRR) vs. GA alone 3. Decreased incidence of hypotension in GA+CFNB+SNB (69% RRR) vs. EA 4. Decreased incidence of bradycardia in GA+CFNB+SNB (81% RRR) vs. EA 5. No difference in postoperative MI or CVA	1. <0.05 2. <0.05 3. <0.05 4. <0.05 5. NS	2°	CFNB+SNB placed before surgery
Williams-Russo et al. (1996)[15]	134	EA	CEA	No difference in adverse cardiovascular outcomes	NS	2°	
Williams-Russo et al. (1995)[56]	128	GA	IV analgesia				
Deep Venous Thrombosis							
Chelly et al. (2001)[60]	29 30 33	GA EA GA	CFNB+SNB CEA IV PCA	No difference in DVT	NS	2°	Daily warfarin thromboprophylaxis
Kohro et al. (1998)[72]	11 11	EA GA	Undisclosed Undisclosed	Reduced blood coagulability (mean maximum amplitude) in EA vs. GA	<0.05	1°	Study limited to intraoperative period No thromboprophylaxis disclosed
Sharrock et al. (1997)[73]	15 16	EA GA	Undisclosed Undisclosed	No difference in thrombin generation or fibrinolytic activity	NS	1°	Study limited to intraoperative period Daily ASA thromboprophylaxis
Williams-Russo et al. (1996)[15]	97 81	EA GA	CEA IV opioid	No difference in DVT	NS	2°	Daily ASA thromboprophylaxis, graded elastic stockings, and early mobilization Postoperative venography
Sharrock and Go (1992)[74]	11 10	EA GA	Undisclosed Undisclosed	No difference in clot formation or fibrinolytic activity	NS	1°	Postoperative venography
Jorgensen et al. (1991)[34]	17 22	EA GA	CEA IM opioid	1. Reduced overall incidence of DVT in EA (15%) vs. GA (59%) 2. Reduced incidence of calf vein thrombosis in EA (12%) vs. GA (45%)	1. 0.02 2. 0.05	1°	Compression stockings
Mitchell et al. (1991)[75]	34 38	EA GA	Undisclosed Undisclosed	No difference in DVT or PE (combined incidence)	NS	1°	Daily ASA thromboprophylaxis (males) or low-dose warfarin (females) Postoperative venography Reduced incidence of proximal vein clots in EA vs. GA

Continued

TABLE 79–2. Perioperative Outcomes after Regional Anesthesia versus General Anesthesia for Total Knee Arthroplasty—cont'd

AUTHOR (YEAR OF PUBLICATION)	N	ANESTHESIA	ANALGESIA	RESULTS	P	OUTCOME*	REMARKS
Pulmonary Embolism							
Williams-Russo et al. (1996)[15]	86 67	EA GA	PCEA IV PCA	No difference in PE	NS	2°	Daily ASA thromboprophylaxis, graded elastic stockings, and early mobilization Postoperative lung perfusion scans
Jorgensen et al. (1991)[34]	17 22	EA GA	CEA IM opioid	No difference in PE	NS	2°	Compression stockings. One case of nonfatal PE in GA
Mitchell et al. (1991)[75]	34 38	EA GA	Undisclosed Undisclosed	No difference in DVT or PE (combined incidence)	NS	1°	Daily ASA thromboprophylaxis (males) or low-dose warfarin (females) Postoperative lung perfusion scans
Blood Loss							
Chelly et al. (2001)[60]	29 30 33	GA EA GA	CFNB+SNB CEA IV PCA	1. Reduced postoperative bleeding and transfusion requirements in CFNB+SNB (72% and 68% RRR) vs. IV PCA 2. Reduced postoperative bleeding and transfusion requirements in CEA (64% and 50% RRR) vs. IV PCA	1. <0.05 2. <0.05	2°	
Kohro et al. (1998)[72]	11 11	EA GA	Undisclosed Undisclosed	No difference in postoperative blood loss	NS	2°	
Jorgensen et al. (1991)[34]	17 22	EA GA	CEA IM opioid	No difference in postoperative blood drainage or transfusion requirements	NS	2°	
Mitchell et al. (1991)[75]	34 38	EA GA	Undisclosed Undisclosed	No difference in blood loss or number of units transfused	NS	2°	
Nielson et al. (1990)[55]	25 39	SA GA	Opioid Opioid	No difference in transfusion requirements	NS	2°	
Surgical Time							
Capdevila et al. (1999)[14]	20 17 19	GA GA	CFNB CEA IV PCA	No difference in duration of surgery	NS	2°	
Ganapathy et al. (1999)[76]	20 20 22	GA GA GA	CFNB 0.2% B CFNB 0.1% B Placebo	No difference in duration of surgery	NS	2°	
Sharrock et al. (1997)[73]	15 16	EA GA	Undisclosed Undisclosed	No difference in duration of surgery	NS	2°	
Williams-Russo et al. (1996)[15] Williams-Russo et al. (1995)[56]	134 128	EA GA	CEA IV opioid	No difference in duration of surgery	NS	2°	
Mitchell et al. (1991)[75]	34 38	EA GA	Undisclosed Undisclosed	No difference in duration of surgery	NS	2°	
Nielson et al. (1990)[55]	25 39	SA GA	Opioid Opioid	No difference in duration of surgery	NS	2°	
Serpell et al. (1991)[41]	13 16	SA SA	CFNB IV PCA	No difference in duration of surgery	NS	2°	
Pain							
Seet et al. (2006)[45]	17 18 20	SA SA SA	CFNB 0.15% R CFNB 0.2% R IV PCA	1. No difference in pain scores 2. Reduced morphine consumption in CFNB 0.15% R and 0.2% R vs. IV PCA	1. NS 2. <0.05	1°	

TABLE 79–2. Perioperative Outcomes after Regional Anesthesia versus General Anesthesia for Total Knee Arthroplasty—cont'd

AUTHOR (YEAR OF PUBLICATION)	N	ANESTHESIA	ANALGESIA	RESULTS	P	OUTCOME*	REMARKS
Wang et al. (2002)[44]	15 15	GA GA	FNB Placebo	1. Reduced pain scores at rest and during rehabilitation up to POD 1 in FNB vs. placebo 2. Reduced total postoperative morphine consumption in FNB (0.7 mg/kg) vs. placebo (2.5 mg/kg)	1. <0.05 2. <0.05	1°	No difference in pain scores on POD 2 and 3
Chelly et al. (2001)[60]	29 30 33	GA EA GA	CFNB+SNB CEA IV PCA	1. Reduced morphine consumption up to POD 3 in CFNB+SNB (59% RRR) vs. CEA 2. Reduced morphine consumption up to POD 3 in CFNB+SNB (74% RRR) vs. IV PCA	1. <0.05 2. <0.05	2°	
Capdevila et al. (1999)[14]	20 17 19	GA GA GA	CFNB CEA IV PCA	Reduced pain scores at rest and during CPM up to 48 hours in CFNB and CEA vs. IV PCA	<0.05	1°	No difference in pain scores or morphine requirements between CFNB and CEA
Ganapathy et al. (1999)[76]	20 20 22	SA SA SA	CFNB 0.2% B CFNB 0.1% B Placebo	Reduced pain scores during activity on DOS only in CFNB 0.2% B and 0.1% B vs. placebo	<0.05	1°	No difference in pain scores during activity from POD 1 up to day of discharge Inconsistent reduction in morphine consumption in CFNB groups vs. placebo
Allen et al. (1998)[43]	12 12 12	SA SA SA	FNB FNB+SNB Placebo	1. Reduced pain scores at rest up to 8 hours in FNB and FNB+SNB vs. placebo 2. Reduced morphine consumption up to POD 2 in FNB and FNB+SNB vs. placebo	1. <0.05 2. <0.02	1°	Incomplete data beyond 8 hours SNB did not improve analgesia compared with FNB alone
Singelyn et al. (1998)[16]	15 15 15	GA GA GA	CFNB CEA IV PCA	Reduced pain scores at rest and with movement up to 48 hours in CFNB and CEA vs. IV PCA	<0.05	1°	
Hirst et al. (1996)[39]	11 11 11	GA GA GA	FNB CFNB IV PCA	Reduced pain scores with motion in PACU in FNB and CFNB vs. IV PCA	<0.05	1°	No difference in pain scores or morphine requirements beyond PACU
Moiniche et al. (1994)[71]	10 10	EA GA	CEA IM morphine	Reduced pain scores at rest, flexion, and walk in CEA vs. IM morphine	<0.05	1°	
Edwards and Wright (1992)[38]	19 18	GA GA	CFNB IM opioid	1. Reduced pain scores up to 24 hours in CFNB vs. IM opioid 2. Reduced morphine consumption up to 24 hours in CFNB vs. IM opioid	1. <0.01 2. <0.01	1°	No data beyond 24 hours
Nielson et al. (1990)[55]	25 39	SA GA	Opioid Opioid	No difference in the amount or choice of postoperative opioid use	NS	2°	
Serpell et al. (1991)[41]	13 16	SA SA	CFNB IV PCA	1. No difference in pain scores at 24 and 48 hours 2. Reduced total morphine consumption at 48 hours in CFNB (60 mg) vs. IV PCA (91 mg)	1. NS 2. <0.05	1°	Intermittent boluses via CFNB for 48 hours

Continued

TABLE 79–2. Perioperative Outcomes after Regional Anesthesia versus General Anesthesia for Total Knee Arthroplasty—cont'd

AUTHOR (YEAR OF PUBLICATION)	N	ANESTHESIA	ANALGESIA	RESULTS	P	OUTCOME*	REMARKS
Adverse Effects							
Seet et al. (2006)[45]	17	SA	CFNB 0.15% R	No difference in PONV, urinary retention, and sedation between the groups	NS	2°	Superior patient satisfaction in both CFNB groups vs. IV PCA
	18	SA	CFNB 0.2% R				
	20	SA	IV PCA				
Wang et al. (2002)[44]	15	GA	FNB	Reduced incidence of opioid-related adverse effects in FNB (5%) vs. placebo (54%)	<0.05	2°	
	15	GA	Placebo				
Chelly et al. (2001)[60]	29	GA	CFNB+SNB	1. Reduced PONV in CFNB+SNB (63% RRR) vs. IV PCA	1. <0.05	2°	
	30	EA	CEA	2. Reduced pruritus in CFNB+SNB and CEA (73% RRR) vs. IV PCA	2. <0.05		
	33	GA	IV PCA	3. Reduced constipation in CFNB+SNB (88% RRR) vs. IV PCA	3. <0.05		
				4. Reduced constipation in CFNB+SNB (66% RRR) vs. CEA	4. <0.05		
Capdevila et al. (1999)[14]	20	GA	CFNB	1. Reduced urinary retention in PACU in CFNB (0%) and IV PCA (21%) vs. CEA (53%).	1. <0.05	2°	
	17	GA	CEA	2. Reduced nausea at 24 hours in CFNB (5%) vs. IV PCA (21%)	2. <0.05		
	19	GA	IV PCA	3. Incremental reduction in hypotension at 24 hours in IV PCA (26%) vs. CFNB (50%) vs. CEA (76%)	3. <0.05		
Ganapathy et al. (1999)[76]	20	GA	CFNB 0.2% B	No difference in PONV symptoms	NS	2°	
	20	GA	CFNB 0.1% B				
	22	GA	Placebo				
Allen et al. (1998)[43]	12	SA	FNB	No difference in pruritus, nausea, or sedation	NS	2°	No difference in patient satisfaction
	12	SA	FNB+SNB				
	12	SA	Placebo				
Singelyn et al. (1998)[16]	15	GA	CFNB	1. No difference in PONV symptoms	1. NS	2°	
	15	GA	CEA	2. Increased urinary retention in CEA (40%) vs. CFNB (0%)	2. <0.05		
	15	GA	IV PCA				
Hirst et al. (1996)[39]	11	GA	FNB	Reduced PONV in FNB and CFNB vs. IV PCA	<0.05	2°	No difference in patient satisfaction
	11	GA	CFNB				
	11	GA	IV PCA				
Serpell et al. (1991)[41]	13	SA	CFNB	No difference in PONV symptoms	NS	2°	
	16	SA	IV PCA				
Cognitive Deficit							
Williams-Russo et al. (1995)[56]	134	EA	CEA	No difference in cognitive function tests 1 week or 6 months after surgery	NS	1°	Midazolam and fentanyl for intraoperative sedation in EA group
	128	GA	IV opioid				
Nielson et al. (1990)[55]	25	SA	Opioid	No difference in cognitive or psychosocial function tests up to 3 months after surgery	NS	1°	All patients undergoing SA received intraoperative sedation with diazepam or lorazepam
	39	GA	Opioid				
Rehabilitation							
Seet et al. (2006)[45]	17	SA	CFNB 0.15% R	No difference in the median day of first ambulation	NS	2°	
	18	SA	CFNB 0.2% R				
	20	SA	IV PCA				

TABLE 79–2. Perioperative Outcomes after Regional Anesthesia versus General Anesthesia for Total Knee Arthroplasty—cont'd

AUTHOR (YEAR OF PUBLICATION)	N	ANESTHESIA	ANALGESIA	RESULTS	P	OUTCOME*	REMARKS
Wang et al. (2002)[44]	15 15	GA GA	FNB Placebo	1. Superior ambulation from POD 1 up to discharge in FNB vs. placebo 2. Greater knee flexion on POD 2 in FNB (70 degrees) vs. placebo (60 degrees)	1. <0.05 2. <0.05	2°	No difference in knee flexion at time of discharge
Chelly et al. (2001)[60]	29 30 33	GA EA GA	CFNB+SNB CEA IV PCA	1. Increased ROM on CPM up to POD 3 in CFNB+SNB and CEA vs. IV PCA 2. Earlier mobilization in CFNB+SNB vs. IV PCA	1. <0.05 2. <0.05	2°	
Capdevila et al. (1999)[14]	20 17 19	GA GA GA	CFNB CEA IV PCA	1. Earlier achievement of rehabilitation goals in CFNB and CEA vs. IV PCA 2. Greater maximal knee flexion on POD 5 in CEA (85 degrees) and CFNB (80 degrees) vs. IV PCA (60 degrees) 3. Shorter stay in rehabilitation facility in CEA (37 days) and CFNB (40 days) vs. IV PCA (50 days)	1. <0.05 2. <0.05 3. <0.05	2°	No difference in knee flexion at 1 and 3 months
Ganapathy et al. (1999)[76]	20 20 22	GA GA GA	CFNB 0.2% B CFNB 0.1% B Placebo	Improved ROM on POD 1 in CFNB 0.2% B vs. CFNB 0.1% B and placebo	<0.05	2°	No difference in ROM after POD 1
Singelyn et al. (1998)[16]	15 15 15	GA GA GA	CFNB CEA IV PCA	1. Superior knee flexion up to 6 weeks discharge in CFNB and CEA vs. IV PCA 2. Earlier walking in CFNB (3.5 days) and CEA (3.5 days) vs. IV PCA (4.3 days)	1. <0.05 2. 0.02	2°	No difference in knee flexion between CFNB and CEA at any time No difference in knee flexion at 3 months
Williams-Russo et al. (1996)[15]	134 128	EA GA	CEA IV opioid	1. Earlier achievement of 90-degrees flexion in EA (6.9 days) vs. GA (7.8 days) 2. Earlier achievement of assisted stair climbing in EA (7.9 days) vs. GA (9.5 days)	1. <0.03 2. <0.01	1°	No difference in all other functional milestones
Moiniche et al. (1994)[71]	10 10	EA GA	CEA IM morphine	No difference in postoperative activity	NS	2°	
Length of Stay							
Seet et al. (2006)[45]	17 18 20	SA SA SA	CFNB 0.15% R CFNB 0.2% R IV PCA	No difference in LOS	NS	2°	
Wang et al. (2002)[44]	15 15	GA GA	FNB Placebo	Shorter LOS in FNB (3 days) vs. placebo (4 days)	<0.05	2°	
Chelly et al. (2001)[60]	29 30 33	GA EA GA	CFNB+SNB CEA IV PCA	Shorter LOS in CFNB+SNB (20% RRR) vs. IV PCA	<0.05	2°	
Singelyn et al. (1998)[16]	15 15 15	GA GA GA	CFNB CEA IV PCA	Shorter LOS in CFNB (17 days) and CEA (16 days) vs. IV PCA (21 days)	<0.001	2°	Duration of hospital stay included rehabilitation phases of recovery

Continued

TABLE 79–2. Perioperative Outcomes after Regional Anesthesia versus General Anesthesia for Total Knee Arthroplasty—cont'd

AUTHOR (YEAR OF PUBLICATION)	N	ANESTHESIA	ANALGESIA	RESULTS	P	OUTCOME*	REMARKS
Williams-Russo et al. (1995)[56]	134	EA	CEA	No difference in LOS	NS	2°	
	128	GA	IV opioid				
Moiniche et al. (1994)[71]	10	EA	CEA	No difference in LOS	NS	2°	
	10	GA	IM morphine				
Mitchell et al. (1991)[75]	34	EA	Undisclosed	No difference in LOS	NS	2°	
	38	GA	Undisclosed				

Numeric data are presented for significant differences between groups wherever possible. Pain scores are presented out of 10 (maximum) on a verbal rating scale.
*1° denotes primary outcome measure of parent study; 2° denotes secondary outcome measure of parent study.
ASA, acetylsalicylic acid; B, bupivacaine; CEA, continuous epidural analgesia; CFNB, continuous femoral nerve block; CPM, continuous passive motion; CVA, cerebrovascular accident; DOS, day of surgery; DVT, deep vein thrombosis; EA, epidural anesthesia; FNB, femoral nerve block; GA, general anesthesia; IM, intramuscular; IV, intravenous; LOS, length of stay; LPB, lumbar plexus block; MI, myocardial infarction, NS, not significant; PACU, postanesthesia care unit; PCA, patient-controlled analgesia; PCEA, patient-controlled epidural analgesia; PE, pulmonary embolism; POD, postoperative day; PONV, postoperative nausea and vomiting; R, ropivacaine; ROM, range of motion; RRR, relative risk reduction; SA, spinal anesthesia; SNB, sciatic nerve block.

Rodgers and colleagues[25] found that overall mortality was reduced by one third (odds ratio [OR], 0.70; 95% confidence interval [CI], 0.54–0.90) in patients allocated to CNB. Furthermore, Rodgers and colleagues[25] demonstrated that overall mortality was reduced regardless of whether neuraxial blockade was continued after surgery.[25] For epidural analgesia after THA, Wu and colleagues[26] similarly found no reduction in mortality compared with systemic analgesia after reviewing a random sample of 23,136 patients from a national Medicare claims database between 1994 and 1999. It may be that any observed reduction in mortality conferred by regional anesthesia is due to the surgical anesthetic rather than postoperative analgesia.

DEEP VENOUS THROMBOSIS AND PULMONARY EMBOLISM

It has long been thought that CNB can decrease the incidence of deep venous thrombosis (DVT) rates by enhancing lower extremity venous blood flow,[33] and perhaps "washing out" the thrombogenic load accumulated during surgery. In addition, epidural analgesia and CPNB each facilitate postoperative rehabilitation after THA and TKA,[14–16] which may indirectly prevent DVT formation. Mauermann and colleagues[28] reported a meta-analysis of 10 studies examining the incidences of DVT and pulmonary embolism (PE) in patients randomized to CNB or GA for THA. The pooled data revealed a significantly lower risk for DVT (OR, 0.27; 95% CI, 0.17–0.42) and PE (OR, 0.26; 95% CI, 0.12–0.56) for patients who received CNB in comparison with those who received GA.

Importantly, among the 10 RCTs included in Mauermann and colleagues'[28] meta-analysis, 8 were carried out before 1990 when routine thromboprophylaxis was not commonplace. In only 1 of these 10 trials did patients receive heparin thromboprophylaxis. However, after the introduction of routine thromboprophylaxis, there appears to be no significant difference in the incidence of DVT and PE for patients undergoing THA (see Table 79–1). For TKA, only two studies[21,34] currently reviewed showed a decreased incidence of DVT in favor of regional anesthesia, and these without chemical thromboprophylaxis. Furthermore, none of the TKA studies indicated that the incidence of PE is affected by anesthetic technique (see Table 79–2). It therefore remains questionable whether regional anesthesia offers any additive effect in reducing DVT and PE when used in combination with modern routine thromboprophylaxis.

BLOOD LOSS

In a meta-analysis investigating the effects of CNB on surgical blood loss, Joanne Guay[35] found that CNB for THA significantly reduced the likelihood of transfusion by three fourths (OR, 0.25; 95% CI, 0.11–0.53). Peripheral vasodilation most likely accounts for any observed blood-sparing effects of CNB for THA. By contrast, however, we found conflicting results in the contemporary literature for intraoperative bleeding and transfusion requirements in patients receiving regional anesthesia either alone or in combination with GA for THA (see Table 79–1). For TKA, the contemporary literature demonstrates no significant difference in intraoperative blood loss with regional anesthesia compared with GA, and this lack of effect is most likely due to the use of an intraoperative tourniquet.

DURATION OF SURGERY

Mauermann and colleagues'[28] meta-analysis demonstrated a modest, but significant, decrease in surgical time with CNB compared with GA for THA. This difference may be a reflection of the reduction in bleeding afforded by CNB and, by extension, a "drier" operative field. Among the studies currently reviewed, the duration of surgery was not influenced by the type of anesthetic for THA or TKA (see Tables 79–1 and 79–2). However, none of these studies considered the total operating room time that includes anesthetic intervention. Endless efforts to improve operating room efficiency have spawned modifications of how anesthetic services are delivered, such as the introduction of a "block room" or anesthesia induction room where regional techniques are performed before operating room entry. These models have been shown to reduce the anesthesia-related operating room time when compared with GA[22,36] and may prove cost-saving in the future.[37]

PAIN

Choi and colleagues'[24] meta-analysis examines the efficacy of postoperative lumbar epidural analgesia compared with systemic analgesia after THA or TKA. These authors hesitantly conclude that epidural analgesia affords superior pain relief for up to 6 hours after surgery compared with conventional systemic analgesia. One important limitation of this meta-analysis is that all patients, whether THA or TKA, were analyzed in aggregate despite important differences between these surgical procedures, especially concerning the severity of postoperative pain.

Our review identified only four recently published RCTs that investigated regional anesthesia versus systemic analgesia for THA (see Table 79–1). It appears that the analgesic benefit of regional anesthesia is short-lived and does not confer extended benefit once the local anesthetic recedes or the infusion ceased. However, in one THA study, there was a significant reduction in morphine consumption beyond the expected duration of action of the local anesthetic, possibly suggesting a pre-emptive analgesic effect of regional anesthesia. For TKA, epidural analgesia, single-injection femoral nerve block (FNB), and continuous catheter-based FNB can each improve postoperative pain control compared with systemic analgesia (see Table 79–2).[14,15,38–45] Only one study included a comparison of single-injection FNB with continuous catheter-based FNB (CFNB) for postoperative analgesia after TKA and showed little additional benefit by the placement of a catheter as opposed to the single-injection technique,[39] but this finding has since been countered.[13,17] Furthermore, a study comparing CFNB with intravenous (IV) patient-controlled analgesia (PCA) for TKA revealed an opioid-sparing effect, which is a surrogate marker of pain relief, and better patient satisfaction scores favoring CFNB to IV PCA, despite no significant differences in reported pain scores between the groups.[45] Lastly, whether sciatic afferents (i.e., posterior aspect of the knee) contribute significantly to pain after TKA remains a subject of controversy.[43,46–48]

ADVERSE EFFECTS

Opioid-related adverse effects, especially nausea and vomiting, are of primary concern to patients[49] and can delay discharge from hospital.[50] In many published studies examining regional anesthesia versus GA, including most examined herein, significant differences in opioid-related adverse effects were observed in favor of regional anesthesia. Unfortunately, however, opioid-related adverse effects are almost never designated as primary outcome measures. Reported "significant" differences in secondary outcomes must be interpreted with caution because the parent studies are often inadequately powered to detect such differences.[51] For example, in Seet and colleagues'[45] RCT, there was a significant opioid-sparing effect in patients receiving regional anesthesia compared with IV PCA, but no significant difference in opioid-related adverse effects such as PONV and sedation.[45] For this reason, each listed outcome in Tables 79–1 and 79–2 is identified as the primary or secondary outcome measure of the corresponding parent study.

COGNITIVE DEFICIT

It has long been suggested that regional anesthesia allows for rapid recovery of cognitive function after surgery compared with GA.[52,53] In our review of the contemporary literature, we found only one recent RCT that reported cognitive performance after regional anesthesia versus GA for THA with results in favor of regional anesthesia (see Table 79–1).[54] By contrast, two robust studies demonstrated no difference in short- and long-term cognitive function between regional anesthesia and GA for patients with TKA (see Table 79–2), but IV sedation was administered to the regional anesthesia groups, which can introduce bias.[55,56]

REHABILITATION AND LENGTH OF STAY

Regional anesthesia can significantly hasten postoperative rehabilitation and shorten length of stay in hospital after TKA, but not after THA (see Tables 79–1 and 79–2). This difference is likely because the severity of pain decreases rapidly after THA in comparison with TKA, where pain can often be severe, and exacerbates with physical therapy. Epidural analgesia and CFNB for TKA can each significantly improve rehabilitation and help to attain milestones earlier than IV PCA.[8] CFNB is generally preferred over epidural analgesia because important unwanted effects such as bilateral blockade, hypotension, bradycardia, and nausea and vomiting are avoided,[14,16,57] whereas the patient's anticoagulation status is less of a concern.[58,59] A shorter length of stay in hospital has consistently been demonstrated in patients receiving CFNB or FNB for pain relief after TKA.[16,44,60] Remarkably, the early rehabilitation achievements facilitated by regional anesthesia for TKA can translate into shorter patient stays in rehabilitation centers after discharge from hospital.[14]

SUMMARY

In modern anesthetic practice, both GA and regional anesthesia can be reliably performed for THA and TKA with high success and few major complications. Contemporary evidence strongly suggests that regional anesthesia techniques, especially PNB, can provide superior early postoperative analgesia and decrease opioid consumption compared with traditional systemic analgesia after THA or TKA. Accordingly, fair evidence has been reported to suggest that regional anesthesia minimizes opioid-related adverse effects. For TKA, the analgesic benefits of regional anesthesia can afford superior rehabilitation or earlier hospital discharge, but the same is not true for THA. By contrast, regional anesthesia techniques may reduce blood loss and transfusion requirements after THA, but not TKA. Finally, in the current environment of routine thromboprophylaxis and standardized clinical pathways, regional anesthesia techniques do not appear to decrease the incidence of DVT and PE, preserve cognitive function, or reduce the duration of surgery compared with GA for THA or TKA. Table 79–3 provides a summary of recommendations based on levels of evidence for primary outcome measures.[77,78]

TABLE 79–3. Summary of Recommendations

STATEMENT	LEVEL OF EVIDENCE/ GRADE OF RECOMMENDATION	
When compared with GA:	THA	TKA
1. RA decreases postoperative pain scores.	A[54,66,70,71]	A[14,16,38,39,43, 44,60, 71,76]
2. RA reduces postoperative morphine consumption.	A[66,70]	A[38,41,43–45]
3. RA does not decrease incidence of DVT or PE in the presence of thromboprophylaxis.	A[61,64]	A[72,73]
4. RA reduces perioperative bleeding.	A[63,67]	No primary outcome studies
5. RA does not affect postoperative cognitive function.	No primary outcome studies	A[55,56]

DVT, deep vein thrombosis; GA, general anesthesia; PE, pulmonary embolism; RA, regional anesthesia; THA, total hip arthroplasty; TKA, total knee arthroplasty.

REFERENCES

1. Aromaa U, Lahdensuu M, Cozanitis DA: Severe complications associated with epidural and spinal anaesthesias in Finland 1987-1993. A study based on patient insurance claims. Acta Anaesthesiol Scand 41:445–452, 1997.
2. Auroy Y, Narchi P, Messiah A, et al: Serious complications related to regional anesthesia: Results of a prospective survey in France. Anesthesiology 87:479–486, 1997.
3. Borgeat A, Ekatodramis G, Kalberer F, Benz C: Acute and nonacute complications associated with interscalene block and shoulder surgery: A prospective study. Anesthesiology 95:875–880, 2001.
4. Fanelli G, Casati A, Garancini P, Torri G: Nerve stimulator and multiple injection technique for upper and lower limb blockade: Failure rate, patient acceptance, and neurologic complications. Study Group on Regional Anesthesia. Anesth Analg 88:847–852, 1999.
5. Moen V, Dahlgren N, Irestedt L: Severe neurological complications after central neuraxial blockades in Sweden 1990-1999. Anesthesiology 101:950–959, 2004.
6. Auroy Y, Benhamou D, Bargues L, et al: Major complications of regional anesthesia in France: The SOS Regional Anesthesia Hotline Service. Anesthesiology 97:1274–1280, 2002.
7. Brull R, McCartney CJ, Chan VW, El Beheiry H: Neurological complications after regional anesthesia: Contemporary estimates of risk. Anesth Analg 104:965–974, 2007.
8. Davies AF, Segar EP, Murdoch J, et al: Epidural infusion or combined femoral and sciatic nerve blocks as perioperative analgesia for knee arthroplasty. Br J Anaesth 93:368–374, 2004.
9. Zaric D, Boysen K, Christiansen C, et al: A comparison of epidural analgesia with combined continuous femoral-sciatic nerve blocks after total knee replacement. Anesth Analg 102:1240–1246, 2006.
10. Hebl JR, Kopp SL, Ali MH, et al: A comprehensive anesthesia protocol that emphasizes peripheral nerve blockade for total knee and total hip arthroplasty. J Bone Joint Surg Am 87(suppl 2):63–70, 2005.
11. Pagnano MW, Hebl J, Horlocker T: Assuring a painless total hip arthroplasty: A multimodal approach emphasizing peripheral nerve blocks. J Arthroplasty 21:80–84, 2006.
12. Boezaart AP: Perineural infusion of local anesthetics. Anesthesiology 104:872–880, 2006.
13. Salinas FV, Liu SS, Mulroy MF: The effect of single-injection femoral nerve block versus continuous femoral nerve block after total knee arthroplasty on hospital length of stay and long-term functional recovery within an established clinical pathway. Anesth Analg 102:1234–1239, 2006.
14. Capdevila X, Barthelet Y, Biboulet P, et al: Effects of perioperative analgesic technique on the surgical outcome and duration of rehabilitation after major knee surgery. Anesthesiology 91:8–15, 1999.
15. Williams-Russo P, Sharrock NE, Haas SB, et al: Randomized trial of epidural versus general anesthesia: Outcomes after primary total knee replacement. Clin Orthop Relat Res 199–208, 1996.
16. Singelyn FJ, Deyaert M, Joris D, et al: Effects of intravenous patient-controlled analgesia with morphine, continuous epidural analgesia, and continuous three-in-one block on postoperative pain and knee rehabilitation after unilateral total knee arthroplasty. Anesth Analg 87:88–92, 1998.
17. Watson MW, Mitra D, McLintock TC, Grant SA: Continuous versus single-injection lumbar plexus blocks: Comparison of the effects on morphine use and early recovery after total knee arthroplasty. Reg Anesth Pain Med 30:541–547, 2005.
18. Richman JM, Liu SS, Courpas G, et al: Does continuous peripheral nerve block provide superior pain control to opioids? A meta-analysis. Anesth Analg 102:248–257, 2006.
19. Brull R, Sharrock NE: Anesthesia for knee surgery. In Insall JN, Scott WN (eds): Surgery of the Knee, 4th ed. New York, Churchill Livingstone, 2006, pp 1064–1073.
20. Oldman M, McCartney CJ, Leung A, et al: A survey of orthopedic surgeons' attitudes and knowledge regarding regional anesthesia. Anesth Analg 98:1486–1490, 2004.
21. Nielsen KC, Steele SM: Outcome after regional anaesthesia in the ambulatory setting—is it really worth it? Best Pract Res Clin Anaesthesiol 16:145–157, 2002.
22. Armstrong KP, Cherry RA: Brachial plexus anesthesia compared to general anesthesia when a block room is available. Can J Anaesth 51:41–44, 2004.
23. Katz J: A survey of anesthetic choice among anesthesiologists. Anesth Analg 52:373–375, 1973.
24. Choi PT, Bhandari M, Scott J, Douketis J: Epidural analgesia for pain relief following hip or knee replacement. Cochrane Database Syst Rev CD003071, 2003.

25. Rodgers A, Walker N, Schug S, et al: Reduction of postoperative mortality and morbidity with epidural or spinal anaesthesia: Results from overview of randomised trials. BMJ 321:1493, 2000.

26. Wu CL, Hurley RW, Anderson GF, et al: Effect of postoperative epidural analgesia on morbidity and mortality following surgery in medicare patients. Reg Anesth Pain Med 29:525–533, 2004.

27. Block BM, Liu SS, Rowlingson AJ, et al: Efficacy of postoperative epidural analgesia: A meta-analysis. JAMA 290:2455–2463, 2003.

28. Mauermann WJ, Shilling AM, Zuo Z: A comparison of neuraxial block versus general anesthesia for elective total hip replacement: A meta-analysis. Anesth Analg 103:1018–1025, 2006.

29. Urwin SC, Parker MJ, Griffiths R: General versus regional anaesthesia for hip fracture surgery: A meta-analysis of randomized trials. Br J Anaesth 84:450–455, 2000.

30. Higgins MS, Stiff JL: Pitfalls in performing meta-analysis: I. Anesthesiology 79:405, 1993.

31. McKenzie PJ: Pitfalls in performing meta-analysis: II. Anesthesiology 79:406–408, 1993.

32. LeLorier J, Gregoire G, Benhaddad A, et al: Discrepancies between meta-analyses and subsequent large randomized, controlled trials. N Engl J Med 337:536–542, 1997.

33. Modig J, Malmberg P, Karlstrom G: Effect of epidural versus general anaesthesia on calf blood flow. Acta Anaesthesiol Scand 24:305–309, 1980.

34. Jorgensen LN, Rasmussen LS, Nielsen PT, et al: Antithrombotic efficacy of continuous extradural analgesia after knee replacement. Br J Anaesth 66:8–12, 1991.

35. Guay J: The effect of neuraxial blocks on surgical blood loss and blood transfusion requirements: A meta-analysis. J Clin Anesth 18:124–128, 2006.

36. Williams BA, Kentor ML, Williams JP, et al: Process analysis in outpatient knee surgery: Effects of regional and general anesthesia on anesthesia-controlled time. Anesthesiology 93:529–538, 2000.

37. Williams BA, Kentor ML, Vogt MT, et al: Economics of nerve block pain management after anterior cruciate ligament reconstruction: Potential hospital cost savings via associated postanesthesia care unit bypass and same-day discharge. Anesthesiology 100:697–706, 2004.

38. Edwards ND, Wright EM: Continuous low-dose 3-in-1 nerve blockade for postoperative pain relief after total knee replacement. Anesth Analg 75:265–267, 1992.

39. Hirst GC, Lang SA, Dust WN, et al: Femoral nerve block. Single injection versus continuous infusion for total knee arthroplasty. Reg Anesth 21:292–297, 1996.

40. Raj PP, Knarr DC, Vigdorth E, et al: Comparison of continuous epidural infusion of a local anesthetic and administration of systemic narcotics in the management of pain after total knee replacement surgery. Anesth Analg 66:401–406, 1987.

41. Serpell MG, Millar FA, Thomson MF: Comparison of lumbar plexus block versus conventional opioid analgesia after total knee replacement. Anaesthesia 46:275–277, 1991.

42. Weller R, Rosenblum M, Conard P, Gross JB: Comparison of epidural and patient-controlled intravenous morphine following joint replacement surgery. Can J Anaesth 38:582–586, 1991.

43. Allen HW, Liu SS, Ware PD, et al: Peripheral nerve blocks improve analgesia after total knee replacement surgery. Anesth Analg 87:93–97, 1998.

44. Wang H, Boctor B, Verner J: The effect of single-injection femoral nerve block on rehabilitation and length of hospital stay after total knee replacement. Reg Anesth Pain Med 27:139–144, 2002.

45. Seet E, Leong WL, Yeo AS, Fook-Chong S: Effectiveness of 3-in-1 continuous femoral block of differing concentrations compared to patient controlled intravenous morphine for post total knee arthroplasty analgesia and knee rehabilitation. Anaesth Intensive Care 34:25–30, 2006.

46. Pham DC, Gautheron E, Guilley J, et al: The value of adding sciatic block to continuous femoral block for analgesia after total knee replacement. Reg Anesth Pain Med 30:128–133, 2005.

47. Cook P, Stevens J, Gaudron C: Comparing the effects of femoral nerve block versus femoral and sciatic nerve block on pain and opiate consumption after total knee arthroplasty. J Arthroplasty 18:583–586, 2003.

48. Morin AM, Kratz CD, Eberhart LH, et al: Postoperative analgesia and functional recovery after total-knee replacement: Comparison of a continuous posterior lumbar plexus (psoas compartment) block, a continuous femoral nerve block, and the combination of a continuous femoral and sciatic nerve block. Reg Anesth Pain Med 30:434–445, 2005.

49. Macario A, Weinger M, Carney S, Kim A: Which clinical anesthesia outcomes are important to avoid? The perspective of patients. Anesth Analg 89:652–658, 1999.

50. Pavlin DJ, Rapp SE, Polissar NL, et al: Factors affecting discharge time in adult outpatients. Anesth Analg 87:816–826, 1998.

51. Mariano ER, Ilfeld BM, Neal JM: "Going fishing"-the practice of reporting secondary outcomes as separate studies. Reg Anesth Pain Med 32:183–185, 2007.

52. Sharrock NE, Fischer G, Goss S, et al: The early recovery of cognitive function after total-hip replacement under hypotensive epidural anesthesia. Reg Anesth Pain Med 30:123–127, 2005.

53. Tzabar Y, Asbury AJ, Millar K: Cognitive failures after general anaesthesia for day-case surgery. Br J Anaesth 76:194–197, 1996.

54. Wulf H, Biscoping J, Beland B, et al: Ropivacaine epidural anesthesia and analgesia versus general anesthesia and intravenous patient-controlled analgesia with morphine in the perioperative management of hip replacement. Ropivacaine Hip Replacement Multicenter Study Group. Anesth Analg 89:111–116, 1999.

55. Nielson WR, Gelb AW, Casey JE, et al: Long-term cognitive and social sequelae of general versus regional anesthesia during arthroplasty in the elderly. Anesthesiology 73:1103–1109, 1990.

56. Williams-Russo P, Sharrock NE, Mattis S, et al: Cognitive effects after epidural vs general anesthesia in older adults. A randomized trial. JAMA 274:44–50, 1995.

57. Barrington MJ, Olive D, Low K, et al: Continuous femoral nerve blockade or epidural analgesia after total knee replacement: A prospective randomized controlled trial. Anesth Analg 101:1824–1829, 2005.

58. Hantler C, Despotis GJ, Sinha R, Chelly JE: Guidelines and alternatives for neuraxial anesthesia and venous thromboembolism prophylaxis in major orthopedic surgery. J Arthroplasty 19:1004–1016, 2004.

59. Horlocker TT, Wedel DJ, Benzon H, et al: Regional anesthesia in the anticoagulated patient: Defining the risks (the second ASRA Consensus Conference on Neuraxial Anesthesia and Anticoagulation). Reg Anesth Pain Med 28:172–197, 2003.

60. Chelly JE, Greger J, Gebhard R, et al: Continuous femoral blocks improve recovery and outcome of patients undergoing total knee arthroplasty. J Arthroplasty 16:436–445, 2001.

61. Planes A, Vochelle N, Fagola M, et al: Prevention of deep vein thrombosis after total hip replacement. The effect of low-molecular-weight heparin with spinal and general anaesthesia. J Bone Joint Surg Br 73:418–422, 1991.

62. Borghi B, Casati A, Iuorio S, et al: Frequency of hypotension and bradycardia during general anesthesia, epidural anesthesia, or integrated epidural-general anesthesia for total hip replacement. J Clin Anesth 14:102–106, 2002.

63. Dauphin A, Raymer KE, Stanton EB, Fuller HD: Comparison of general anesthesia with and without lumbar epidural for total hip arthroplasty: Effects of epidural block on hip arthroplasty. J Clin Anesth 9:200–203, 1997.

64. Brueckner S, Reinke U, Roth-Isigkeit A, et al: Comparison of general and spinal anesthesia and their influence on hemostatic markers in patients undergoing total hip arthroplasty. J Clin Anesth 15:433–440, 2003.

65. Borghi B, Casati A, Iuorio S, et al: Effect of different anesthesia techniques on red blood cell endogenous recovery in hip arthroplasty. J Clin Anesth 17:96–101, 2005.

66. Stevens RD, Van Gessel E, Flory N, et al: Lumbar plexus block reduces pain and blood loss associated with total hip arthroplasty. Anesthesiology 93:115–121, 2000.

67. D'Ambrosio A, Borghi B, Damato A, et al: Reducing perioperative blood loss in patients undergoing total hip arthroplasty. Int J Artif Organs 22:47–51, 1999.

68. Salo M, Nissila M: Cell-mediated and humoral immune responses to total hip replacement under spinal or general anaesthesia. Acta Anaesthesiol Scand 34:241–248, 1990.

69. Jones MJ, Piggott SE, Vaughan RS, et al: Cognitive and functional competence after anaesthesia in patients aged over 60: Controlled trial of general and regional anaesthesia for elective hip or knee replacement. BMJ 300:1683–1687, 1990.

70. Biboulet P, Morau D, Aubas P, et al: Postoperative analgesia after total-hip arthroplasty: Comparison of intravenous patient-controlled analgesia with morphine and single injection of femoral nerve or psoas compartment block. A prospective, randomized, double-blind study. Reg Anesth Pain Med 29:102–109, 2004.

71. Moiniche S, Hjortso NC, Hansen BL, et al: The effect of balanced analgesia on early convalescence after major orthopaedic surgery. Acta Anaesthesiol Scand 38:328–335, 1994.

72. Kohro S, Yamakage M, Arakawa J, et al: Surgical/tourniquet pain accelerates blood coagulability but not fibrinolysis. Br J Anaesth 80:460–463, 1998.

73. Sharrock NE, Go G, Williams-Russo P, et al: Comparison of extradural and general anaesthesia on the fibrinolytic response to total knee arthroplasty. Br J Anaesth 79:29–34, 1997.

74. Sharrock NE, Go G: Fibrinolytic activity following total knee arthroplasty under epidural or general anesthesia. Reg Anesth 17:94, 1992.

75. Mitchell D, Friedman RJ, Baker JD III, et al: Prevention of thromboembolic disease following total knee arthroplasty. Epidural versus general anesthesia. Clin Orthop Relat Res 109–112, 1991.

76. Ganapathy S, Wasserman RA, Watson JT, et al: Modified continuous femoral three-in-one block for postoperative pain after total knee arthroplasty. Anesth Analg 89:1197–1202, 1999.

77. Wright JG, Swiontkowski MF, Heckman JD: Introducing levels of evidence to the journal. J Bone Joint Surg Am 85:1–3, 2003.

78. Wright JG: A practical guide to assigning levels of evidence J Bone Joint Surg Am 89:1128–1130, 2007.

Chapter 80

Should Thromboprophylaxis Be Used for Lower Limb Joint Replacement Surgery?

ERIK L. YEO, MD, FRCPC

THROMBOEMBOLIC DISEASE IN JOINT REPLACEMENT SURGERY

Venous thromboembolic events (VTEs) are among the most feared complication of total hip replacement (THR) and total knee replacement (TKR) surgeries, and these patients are in the greatest surgical risk group for this complication. The development of deep venous thrombosis (DVT) with the potential to propagate a potentially lethal pulmonary embolus (PE) is the complication that presents the greatest risk for perioperative mortality after lower limb joint replacement. This has led to the adoption of routine thromboprophylaxis as a standard of care in joint replacement surgery since the late 1980s.[1,2]

The natural history of VTE disease, after joint replacement surgery, has been well characterized. Based on data before 1980 and from trials with placebo patients, the incidence of lower extremity DVT without thromboprophylaxis in THR and total knee arthroplasty (TKA) has been reported as 40% to 60% and 41% to 85%, respectively (Table 80–1).[3–9] Many of these statistics are based on venography end points. At least 50% of these patients had either asymptomatic or distal DVTs that resolved spontaneously without clinical sequelae.[10,11] In the absence of thromboprophylaxis, clinically more important proximal DVTs occurred in THR and TKA at 18% to 36% and 5% to 22%, respectively, but again many were asymptomatic. With prophylaxis, symptomatic VTE was seen in 2.4% and 1.7%, respectively, of patients within 3 months of THR or TKA in studies done between 1992 and 1996.[12] Many of these thrombotic events occur after hospital discharge, and the VTE risk remains increased for at least 8 weeks after surgery.

The incidence of PEs is less certain. The incidence of asymptomatic PE ranges from 3% to 20% and symptomatic PE from 0.5% to 3%,[13,14] and with the current routine use of thromboprophylaxis, fatal PE is uncommon.[15] Without thromboprophylaxis, perioperative mortality in THR and TKA from PE was reported from 0.1% to 2%.[5,16,17] With thromboprophylaxis for 7 to 10 days, there is a 0.1% rate of postdischarge fatal PE at 90 days after surgery in THR.[18]

Although there have been great strides in identifying genetic and biochemical thrombophilic abnormalities and acquired medical risk factors to help stratify patient risk for VTE, there remains no robust way of identifying and separating out individuals who will go on to experience development of symptomatic VTE. This has led to prevention strategies as the key to minimizing the risk for VTE and the recommendation of thromboprophylaxis for all patients undergoing major joint replacement surgery. Numerous means, including compression stockings, mechanical compression devices, early mobilization, anesthetic or analgesic techniques, and anticoagulant drugs are utilized to decrease the risk for VTE, and their study remains a major focus in the field.

The ideal VTE prophylaxis includes clear effectiveness compared with placebo or other active interventions; good risk/benefit profile; good compliance by patients, nurses, and physicians; easy administration or intervention; and requiring no need for monitoring whereas being cost effective.[19] The best means to attain this goal remains an evolving science.

VENOUS THROMBOEMOBLIC EVENT RISKS

Understanding VTE risk factors is key in helping to further risk stratify individual patients for selection of best thromboprophylaxis, including length of duration of intervention. Multiple risk factors are common, and the overall risk for postsurgical VTE increases with each additional risk factor identified.

The interaction of age, genetic factors, and secondary, acquired persistent or transient environment or local factors is the accepted model for the pathogenesis of venous thrombotic disease. VTE risk has a direct and major relation to age.[19] At ages 20, 50, and 80 years, the prevalence of VTE is 1 in 10,000, 1 in 1000, and 1 in 100 individuals per year, respectively, with a lifetime risk of 10%.[20] Ethnicity is a risk factor.[21,22] VTE is more common among blacks compared with whites and Asians by 1.4- and 7-fold, respectively.

Up to 15% to 20% of the general population has demonstrable endogenous biochemical hypercoagulable states.[23,24] These defects may be on a genetic or acquired basis and include defects or deficiencies in anticoagulant proteins (protein S or C, antithrombin [AT]), altered procoagulant proteins (factor V and prothrombin), or fibrinolytic processes.[25] Genetic hypercoagulable states include factor V Leiden (2–4% of the white population) and prothrombin 20210 defect (2–4% of the white population), AT deficiency (1/1000), protein C deficiency (1/2000), and protein S deficiency (1/2000).[26] Acquired defects include anti-phospholipid

TABLE 80–1. Venous Thromboembolic Event Frequency after Orthopedic Joint Replacement Surgery

	DVT		PE	
	TOTAL	PROXIMAL	TOTAL	PROXIMAL
THR	42–57%[1,5,13]	18–36%[1,5,13]	0.9–28%[1,4,13]	0.1–2.0%[5,6,16]
TKA	41–85%[8,14,15]	5–22%[8,14,15]	1.5–10%[8,14,15]	0.1–1.7%[6,14]

DVT, venous thromboembolic event; PE, pulmonary embolism; THR, total hip replacement; TKA, total knee arthroscopy.

antibodies (2–5%) that can be found in up to 25% of population by age 75.[23] Increased factor VIII, found in up to 10% of the well population, has a dose-related relation to VTE and is one of the more recently identified common risk factors.[27] Factor V Leiden is the most common cause of inherited thrombophilia, found in up to 20% of VTE cases. In addition, local factors play a key role in thrombosis related to lower limb joint surgery and include vascular injury and thrombotic repair response, as well as venous stasis caused by prolonged immobility.

Independent VTE risk factors identified in studies of surgical populations for VTE included age older than 50 years, varicose veins, prior myocardial infarction, cancer, atrial fibrillation, ischemic stroke, diabetes mellitus, current use of estrogen-containing compounds, and chronic and acute inflammatory states including infections.[28] Additional risk factors that increase the risk for surgery-related VTE include previous VTE, obesity, heart failure, and paralysis.[29]

VTE risk is increased, in a stepwise and fairly linear manner, with multiple risk factors. One surgical study noted a 10% to 15% increased risk for VTE with each additional risk factor identified.[30] Multiple risk factors in orthopedic patients should be expected given the age, increasing numbers of patients undergoing joint replacement, and frequency of underlying VTE predispositions.

Medical and surgical patients have been risk stratified into low, intermediate, high, and highest VTE risk groups, to assist in creating robust clinical recommendation for best thromboprophylaxis practice.[2,31] Patients undergoing elective joint replacement surgery fall into the highest risk category of this well-accepted clinical model. Patients at highest risk for VTE include surgical patients older than 40 years with multiple risk factors, those with THR or TKA, patients undergoing hip fracture surgery, or patients with major trauma and spinal cord injury. Risk for VTE in this aggregate group include calf DVT (40–80%), proximal DVT (10–20%), clinical PE (4–10%), and fatal PE (0.2–5%).

Prevention of Venous Thromboembolic Events: Introduction

Two approaches, primary and secondary, are used to prevent fatal PE. Primary VTE prophylaxis, the accepted current standard of care using drugs and physical methods, is cost-effective and supported by evidence-based medicine. Secondary prevention approaches are strongly discouraged in other than extenuating clinical circumstances. Secondary approaches include the use of sensitive VTE screening methods, such as Doppler ultrasound (DUS), for postoperative VTE detection followed by treatment of subclinical venous thrombosis to prevent PE. Secondary prevention should never replace primary prophylaxis and is reserved for patients in whom primary prophylaxis is either contraindicated or ineffective.

Features of the ideal VTE prophylaxis include clearly demonstrated effectiveness in evidence-based trials compared with placebo or active approaches, good risk/benefit profiles with low bleeding risk and high degree of prevention, excellent compliance because of ease of us and simplicity of the intervention, lack of need for laboratory monitoring, and cost-effectiveness compared with other interventions.

The prophylactic measures most commonly used in surgery include low-dose unfractionated heparin (LDUFH), low-molecular-weight heparin (LMWH), the substituted pentasaccharide, fondaparinux, oral adjusted-dose vitamin K antagonists (VKAs) (international normalized ratio [INR], 2.0–3.0), and lower limb mechanical compression approaches. For joint replacement surgery, LDUFH is not an acceptable option in normal circumstances.[2]

A large and strong body of evidence-based studies, from randomized trials and meta-analysis, in thromboprophylaxis makes current prophylaxis recommendations robust for most common procedures including joint replacement surgery. A primary reference that is increasingly seen as the authoritative reference body that sets the North American standard of care in thromboprophylaxis is the periodic report on the "Prevention of Venous Thrombosis" for the American College of Chest Physicians Conference on Antithrombotic and Thrombolytic Therapy.[2] It is strongly recommended that individual hospitals, as well as subspecialty and physician groups, should develop, adopt, and evolve formal strategies for the prevention of VTE disease for all risk categories for surgical and medical patients.

Drugs Used in Venous Thromboembolic Event Prevention

Low-Dose Unfractionated Heparin. Although UFH is not considered an acceptable prophylactic drug for lower limb joint replacement surgery because of its lack of efficacy compared with other pharmacologic intervention, it is the parent compound from which the current recommended agents, LMWH and fondaparinux, were developed, and the mechanisms of action are closely related.

UFH is a heterogeneous glycosaminoglycan (5000–30,000 molecular weight [MW]) that binds to AT, altering AT so that AT then binds to and inactivates circulating factor Xa and factor IIa (thrombin). UFH then dissociates from these inactive, AT-serpin complexes that are then cleared. This anti–factor Xa and anti–factor IIa activity accounts for UFH anticoagulant activity. UFH inactivates free but not clot-bound factors IIa and Xa in a 1:1 ratio and, to a lesser extent, the other serine proteases.[32]

Clearance of UFH is dose dependent, with an approximate half-life of 30 to 60 minutes. This short half-life explains the need for two or three times daily dosing when prophylaxis is used. One major biophysical drawback with UFH, but not with LMWH or fondaparinux, is that UFH binds to and is made unavailable by a large number of endogenous, intravascular heparin-binding proteins (von Willebrand factor, fibronectin, platelet factor 4) that reduce its anticoagulant activity, because only free UFH is active.[33] This may in part explain LMWH superiority to UFH in high-risk prothrombotic situations such as joint surgery. LDUFH has the advantage that it is relatively inexpensive compared with LMWH and fondaparinux, and is easily administered. Anticoagulant monitoring is not required for prophylaxis.

Limitations of UFH include the pharmacokinetic, biophysical properties and risk for heparin-induced thrombocytopenia (HIT).[34] HIT is an immunologic disorder in which antibodies form against heparin-PF4 complex bound to the platelet and endothelial cell surface, and result in vascular cell (platelet and endothelial cell) activation, thrombocytopenia, and arterial and venous thrombosis. These pathologic antibodies form in 1% to 3% of patients receiving UFH, and although more common with full-dose UFH, the syndrome is well described with LDUFH. HIT is associated with significant morbidity (stroke, coronary events, peripheral arterial occlusions) in 10% to 15% of HIT cases. All patients receiving UFH must be followed with regular platelet counts while remaining on UFH, and any unexplained thrombocytopenia (decline in platelets of >50% from baseline or platelet count < 100,000/μL) during UFH use requires investigation and elucidation of its cause. If HIT is suspected, UFH must be stopped and replaced by an alternative anticoagulant not associated with HIT (hirudin, argatroban, or danaparoid) until the diagnosis is established.[35] HIT antibodies cross-react with LMWH. Patients diagnosed with HIT should never be exposed to either UFH or LMWH.

Low-Molecular-Weight Heparins. LMWH is a thromboprophylactic drug of choice for joint replacement surgery. LMWHs are fractionated, low-molecular-weight moieties (3000–5000 MW) of UFH, produced by chemical and physical methods, that are approximately one-third as long as native UFH.[32] LMWHs when compared with UFH have a number of desirable pharmacologic and clinical properties that include: (1) superior and predictable pharmacokinetics that allow once or twice daily subcutaneous (SC) dosing based on body weight, (2) no laboratory monitoring, (3) more favorable benefit/risk ratio, and (4) less anti–factor IIa and more anti–factor Xa activity. Because of these properties and its demonstrated improved clinical efficacy in preventing VTE disease, LMWH has replaced UFH for many clinical indications including joint replacement surgery thromboprophylaxis.[36]

Like UFH, LMWH induces its anticoagulant effect through complex formation with AT and factor Xa, and to a lesser extent, thrombin. The anti–factor IIa/anti–factor Xa ratio is 1:1 for UFH, but 1:2 to 1:5 for different LMWHs. A number of pharmaceutical formulations are available in North America, including nadroparin, enoxaparin, dalteparin, and tinzaparin. They are prepared by different methods resulting in slightly different pharmacokinetic and anticoagulant properties, although clinical efficacy is similar for all indications other than acute coronary syndromes.[37] Bleeding risk is similar or slightly lower with LMWH compared with UFH, and there is no true antidote for its anticoagulant action, unlike UFH.

Biophysical properties of LMWH are its major advantage. Because LMWH does not bind to intravascular proteins or cells, they have predictable pharmacokinetics including dose–response relations and an increased plasma half-life. Peak anticoagulant effect is seen at 4 to 8 hours after SC injection. Half-life of this renally cleared agent is much longer than UFH at 3 to 6 hours, and any measurable anticoagulant effect of LMWH is gone in 24 hours in the absence of kidney dysfunction. Depending on the formulation and supporting clinical evidence, LMWHs are administered either once or twice a day for thromboprophylaxis.[37]

HIT is much less common with LMWH use than UFH, although the precise incidence is not clear. As an example, one randomized, double-blind study of patients after hip surgery found that thrombocytopenia occurred in 9 of 332 patients (2%) receiving UFH compared with none receiving LMWH.[38] Because of LMWH cross-reactivity with HIT antibodies, patients with a history of HIT should never be exposed to either LMWH.

Pentasaccharide. Fondaparinux (Arixtra), a synthetic heparin analog, is a highly sulfated, pentasaccharide sequence, derived from the AT binding region of UFH. It is the newest, currently available anticoagulant for joint surgery thromboprophylaxis and has demonstrated improved efficacy compared with LMWH.[39,40] The anticoagulant action of fondaparinux is via a mechanism similar to LMWH in which the drug binds to AT and causes AT to bind to and inactivate factor Xa, but not thrombin. Its action is directed against factor Xa only. Fondaparinux, like LMWH, does not bind to or interact with other plasma proteins or cells resulting in predictable and stable pharmacokinetics. Its half-life at 17 hours is much longer than UFH (0.5–1 hour) or LMWH (4–6 hours), and prophylactic doses (2.5 mg SC) are given daily. Although clinical HIT has not been described with fondaparinux, HIT antibodies do develop with it use.[41] Bleeding with prophylactic fondaparinux is slightly more common than with LMWH or VKA, and like LMWH, this agent is not reversible.[15,42]

Oral Anticoagulants. VKA has been available in clinical practice since the 1950s and is commonly used for VTE prophylaxis in lower limb joint replacement surgery. Certain anticoagulant properties including long half-life, delayed onset of action, and reversibility have made it a favored drug for joint replacement thromboprophylaxis in North America.[43] The VKA warfarin induces an anticoagulant state by interfering with the vitamin K–dependent, post-translational modification of hepatically synthesized blood clotting factors II, VII, IX, and X. This results in near-normal circulating levels of hypofunctional clotting factors II, VII, IX, and X.

These factors have markedly different half-lives, from 6 to 60 hours. It is the half-lives of these factors that dictate the anticoagulant effect of VKA. The anticoagulant efficacy of VKA most closely correlates with the functional level of factor II (prothrombin) that has the longest half-life (60 hours).[44]

VKA is rapidly absorbed from the gut and is 90% albumin bound in circulation. Only free, unbound VKA is biologically active. The half-life of VKA is 36 to 48 hours, and it is the hepatic metabolism by microsomal enzymes, including cytochrome P450 variants, that explains, in part, the marked interindividual variation in dosage required for drug effect. Numerous factors affect the biologic activity of VKA, including patient age, activity level, diet, drug absorption, albumin level, vitamin K intake, general state of health, and interfering drugs. The list of drugs known to interact by either potentiating or attenuating the VKA effect is lengthy, and knowledge of their identity and expected interactions is important given its narrow therapeutic index.[45] Diet can also impact warfarin effect because ingestion of foodstuffs high in vitamin K will counteract the effects of warfarin within 6 to 12 hours.[46]

The average oral dosage of VKA is 5 mg/day, and for patients older than 70 years is 4 mg/day. The use of VKA dosing nomograms should be adopted and have been convincingly demonstrated to accelerate the attainment of a target INR whereas simplifying management for healthcare providers.[47] The optimal INR target for treatment and prophylaxis of VTE indications is 2.5 (2.0–3.0). For any given indication, there is a trend to lower bleeding risk with no loss in clinical efficacy the lower the INR is kept within the therapeutic range. Target INR should be 2.0 to 3.0 as per published trials as opposed to lower targets. There is no rationale to use a loading dose for the initiation of VKA therapy.[43] Given the long half-lives of both VKA (36 hours) and factor II (60 hours), this means that to attain full anticoagulant effect, the INR must be within the therapeutic range for at least 4 to 6 days for all of the vitamin K–dependent proteins to decrease to 20% to 30% of normal.

Unlike LMWH and fondaparinux, frequent PT/INR blood testing is required with VKA thromboprophylaxis, making infrastructure support necessary for adequate posthospital anticoagulation control. Point of care testing (POCT) of INR, analogous to POCT glucose monitoring, has been developed for VKA therapy. A number of small handheld home models are available, and results obtained with them correlate reasonably well with reference laboratory results in the range of an INR of 1.0 to 3.5.

VKA is generally well tolerated, with few side effects other than the bleeding risk. Gastrointestinal (GI) upset and hair thinning may be seen in 10% to 15% of cases. An outpatient bleeding risk index has been developed that includes independent risk factors: age older than 65, history of GI bleeding, history of stroke.[48] Low-, intermediate-, and high-risk patients had, respectively, 3%, 12%, and 53% probability of bleeding. The bleeding risk is directly correlated with INR; it begins to increase quite markedly when the INR increases to more than 3.5, and an INR greater than 5 requires active intervention (hold drug, oral or SC vitamin K_1, fresh-frozen plasma) to reverse the drug effect.

Aspirin. Although aspirin decreases the frequency of VTE after orthopedic surgery when analyzed in meta-analysis, this efficacy is significantly less than that obtained using other anticoagulant agents.[49] A large randomized trial involving 4088 patients undergoing THR and TKR received placebo or 160 mg/day aspirin for 35 days, in addition to other thromboprophylactic measures prescribed at the discretion of the treating physician.[50] Fatal PE and DVT were both significantly decreased by aspirin: relative risk reduction (RRR) of 40% and absolute risk reduction of 4 fatal PEs per 1000 patients. Wound-related bleeding, GI bleeding, and the need for transfusion were significantly more common in the aspirin-treated group. Thus, although aspirin may have some activity in preventing VTE, its efficacy and safety profile are markedly inferior to other available measures, precluding its use as monotherapy.[51] Aspirin cannot currently be recommended for the prophylaxis of VTE.[2]

New Anticoagulant Agents. Further improvements in thromboprophylaxis are going to come from the evolution of better pharmacologic agents with not only an increased efficacy in VTE prevention but a lower bleeding risk and improved biologic properties including reversibility and longer half-lives. The quest for this holy grail in anticoagulant therapy among pharmaceutical companies is ongoing. Examples of agents that have demonstrable efficacy with similar benefit/risk profiles when compared with LMWH and have been studied in THR and TKA include the direct thrombin inhibitors parenteral recombinant hirudin, parenteral melagatran, and oral ximelagatran and the new oral direct anti Xa inhibitor rivaroxaban.[2,52,53,145,146] Emerging drugs include idraparinux, a long-acting pentasaccharide congener to fondaparinux, currently in trials, that can be given once a week and the biotinylation of pentasaccharides so that their anticoagulant action can be reversed with an infusion of avidin.[39] None of these agents has been approved for thromboprophylaxis use in North America.

Mechanical Approaches to Venous Thromboembolic Event Prevention

Compared with drug interventions for thromboprophylaxis, mechanical devices have been studied in fewer patients. Thus, the confidence around the recommendation for their use is weaker. A major practical issue related to using this approach is patient and health provider compliance.[54] Intermittent pneumatic leg compression (IPC), graduated compression stockings (GCS), and venous foot pump (VFP) mechanically prevent venous thrombosis by augmenting blood flow and theoretically decreasing venous stasis in the deep veins of the legs. Pneumatic compression has an added biochemical anticoagulant effect by reducing plasminogen activator inhibitor-1 levels, resulting in increased endogenous fibrinolytic activity.[55] Thus, mechanical leg compression approaches have both local and systemic effects.

These devices are generally free of clinically important side effects and offer a valuable alternative or adjunct in patients who have a high risk for bleeding. They must be used continuously until the patient is fully ambulatory and removal can be only temporary to be fully effective. They produce discomfort in some patients, which impacts compliance, and should be used with caution in patients with peripheral vascular disease. They are contraindicated in patients at bed rest or immobilized for more than 72 hours without other active prophylaxis, because there use may cause a newly formed clot to dislodge.

Although IPC[56–59] has been demonstrated to reduce the incidence of DVT in moderate-risk surgical patients,[60] it is less effective in patients undergoing hip surgery or knee replacement, and although it reduces RRR of total DVTs and prevents calf vein thrombosis, it is not clinically effective for more important proximal DVTs.[56,59] IPC use has decreased with decreasing length of hospital stay and rapid ambulation in patients undergoing orthopedic surgery.[61] In a review, the duration, degree of compression, and overall compliance were significantly less than expected, even with a concerted education program, in patients undergoing THR when IPC was the only form of prophylaxis.[62]

GCS[16,63–65] reduce venous stasis in the limb by applying decreasing degrees of compression moving proximally from the ankle to calf, but reduce the incidence of postoperative VTE only in low-risk surgical patients.[66] In a meta-analysis, GCS in combination with other forms of prophylaxis does not result in any further risk reduction in VTE.[67]

Evidence of efficacy with VFP[65,68] is less developed than the other mechanical methods, and although it does appear to reduce overall rates of DVT, it is inferior to current anticoagulant approaches.[9,69] Mechanical devices are not recommended as a sole therapy for thromboprophylaxis in joint replacement surgery, and good comparative studies with these devices as part of multimodal approaches are lacking, making it difficult to make any firm recommendations despite their attractiveness because of their biomechanical action.

TOTAL HIP REPLACEMENT

Thromboprophylaxis has been recommended in all patients undergoing THR for at least 20 years. This recommendation is supported by many randomized, clinical trials between active interventions with and without placebo groups, and guidelines have been well refined. Three pharmacologic approaches have been demonstrated to be effective and safe. LMWH (SC once or twice daily), fondaparinux (SC once daily), or adjusted-dose VKA (target INR, 2.5).[2,15,70–76]

Mechanical prophylaxes GCS,[16,63–65] IPC,[56–59] and VFP[65,68] have all been studied in THR. Each of these methods provides some level of protection compared with placebo with a RRR of DVT of 20% to 70%. However, this RRR is inferior compared with current pharmacologic interventions in preventing VTE, especially proximal DVTs.[2,59,63] Mechanical, lower limb methods are not recommended as a primary prophylactic modality.[2]

Multimodal prophylaxis, although frequently adopted in orthopedic surgery, is less well studied using accepted randomized, clinical trials approaches versus other active intervention and in large enough patient populations, making it difficult to make any firm recommendations.

In THR, both aspirin[51] and fixed-dose LDUH[77] are superior to placebo in meta-analyses for the prevention of VTE. However, neither of these modalities is recommended as monotherapy because of inferior efficacy when compared with LMWH or VKA.[3,53,78–80]

In North America, as opposed to the European Union, thromboprophylaxis utilizing adjusted-dose VKA (target INR, 2.5) continues to the most common pharmacologic intervention used in THR.[81–86] In the European Union, LMWH has largely replaced VKA because of the lower comparative efficacy of VKA. Advantages of VKA include its later onset of action, physicians' comfort and familiarity with the drug and its actions, the ability to reverse anticoagulant effect, lower cost compared with fondaparinux and LMWH, and more acceptable bleeding risk. Disadvantages of VKA include the need for frequent blood testing, necessity of complex ongoing infrastructure for monitoring and dose adjustment, wide patient intervariability in drug dosage, variable patient response, narrow therapeutic index, and significant drug and food interactions. There is a delay in full anticoagulant action with VKA,[87] for at least 3 to 5 days, that may explain VKA bleeding risk advantage compared with fondaparinux and LMWH.[2]

Different LMWHs have been studied extensively and demonstrated to be safe and highly efficacious in the thromboprophylaxis of THR.[70–73,75,76,88–92] A meta-analysis of 13 studies comparing LMWH with placebo demonstrated that LMWH significantly reduced the risk for asymptomatic DVT (RR, 0.51) without significantly increasing the risk for major bleeding, and indicated that the different LMWH regimens studied and currently recommended are similarly effective and safe.[93] Pooled results of a number of large clinical trials[75,76,91,94] of adjusted-dose VKA versus LMWH in THR reveal that LMWH is more effective, but at the cost of increased bleeding risk. Overall pooled DVT rates were 20.7% versus 13.7% ($P = 0.0002$), and proximal DVT was 4.8% versus 3.4% ($P = 0.08$) in the VKA and LMWH groups, respectively. In a trial of greater than 3000 patients with THR treated with LMWH twice daily versus VKA, there was a threefold reduction in in-hospital, symptomatic VTE (0.3% vs. 1.1%), and major bleeding was 1.2% versus 0.5%, respectively, whereas the 3-month overall VTE rates, between treatments, were no different.[95] In another major randomized clinical trial, LMWH, started either 2 hours before or 4 hours after surgery, versus adjusted-dose VKA demonstrated a significant reduction in total and proximal DVT, and significant reduction in symptomatic DVT (2.2% vs. 4.4%).[76] A meta-analyses of up to 10,000 patients undergoing lower limb orthopedic surgery compared the benefit/risk ratio of VKA versus LMWHs and concluded that VKAs were less effective than LMWH in preventing total and proximal DVTs, and that differences between VKA and LMWH in major hemorrhage and wound hematoma were not significant.[96] Thus, LMWHs are more efficacious than VKA in prevention of VTE, but this efficacy comes at a cost of a slightly increased bleeding risk.

The pentasaccharide fondaparinux is the most recently available anticoagulant with indications for thromboprophylaxis with apparent improved efficacy in THR. In the initial European Union study comparing fondaparinux and enoxaparin, in which fondaparinux (2.5 mg SC daily) was started 4 to 8 hours after surgery and LMWH 12 hours before surgery, demonstrated a 50% decrease in overall VTE rates (4% vs. 9%) in favor of fondaparinux.[42] In the North American study with LMWH starting 12 to 24 hours after surgery, there was no statistical difference between overall and proximal VTE rates (6% vs. 8% and 2% vs. 1%, respectively).[92] There was a nonsignificant trend to more bleeding with fondaparinux versus all LMWH.[42,92,97,98] Studies directly comparing fondaparinux and VKA have not been performed. A meta-analysis of four multicenter, randomized, double-blind trials for the prevention of VTE after major orthopedic surgery, in which fondaparinux (2.5 mg/day) begun 4 to 8 hours after surgery was compared with enoxaparin, demonstrated a significantly reduced risk for all VTEs by day 11 (6.8% vs. 13.7%; $P < 0.001$) but at an increased bleeding risk.[15]

Comparison of bleeding risks across trials of thromboprophylaxis drugs in THR is difficult, because the agents, dosing schedules, dosage, and definition of major and minor bleeding often vary from one trial to another. General conclusion can be inferred that the bleeding risk increases from VKA to LMWH and fondaparinux. First, surgery-related bleeding risk must be put in context by the observation that in the placebo groups of pooled, randomized, clinical trials of THR, the aggregate major bleeding rate was 2% to 4%.[99,100] One meta-analysis concluded that there was no significant difference in bleeding risk between VKA and LMWH.[96] In four major trials pooled, significant bleeding in VKA and LMWH groups was 3.3% versus 5.3%, respectively,[75,76,91,94] whereas the rates of major bleeding ranged from 1.8% to 4.1% for fondaparinux and 1.0% to 3.5% for LMWH. A nonsignificant trend to more bleeding with fondaparinux versus all LMWHs was reported.[42,92,97,98]

In conclusion, LMWH, and by indirect comparison fondaparinux, is more effective than VKA in preventing

symptomatic and asymptomatic VTE in THR at a slightly increased risk for surgical-site bleeding. Increased bleeding and improved VTE efficacy is likely on the basis of earlier proximity to surgery of anticoagulant activity of LMWH and fondaparinux.

TOTAL KNEE REPLACEMENT

TKA differs from THR in a number of important ways. The total VTE rate is greater in TKA, whereas more important proximal and symptomatic DVTs are less common. The efficacy of LMWH versus VKA is more pronounced in TKA, and major bleeding is less common but clinically more worrisome. After elective TKR, LMWH, fondaparinux, or adjusted VKA (target INR, 2.5) can be used.[2,75,89,91,97,101] Finally, although the number of patients undergoing TKR now equals the number undergoing THR in North America, there have been fewer trials in patients undergoing knee replacement.

Like THR studies of IPC[102,103] and VFP,[104] but not GCS,[66] mechanical devices show some efficacy. However, issues of compliance and inability to maintain usage limit this efficacy. The relatively smaller number of patients enrolled in mechanical device, randomized, clinical trials compared with pharmacologic studies results in weak confidence around recommendations related to their use. Although IPC may have some adjunctive role in in-hospital prophylaxis, its combined use has not been studied in randomized, controlled studies. Both LDUH[99,105] and aspirin[7,78,103] have been studied in TKA and have been shown to be much less efficacious than LMWH, fondaparinux, or adjusted-dose VKA; they are not recommended.

Numerous randomized trials of VKA in TKA have been reported, and confidence around VKA recommendations is high.[7,75,91,101,102,106–109] Despite adjusted-dose VKA, thromboprophylaxis total, venographic, DVT rates remain high (25–50%), with treatment out to 2 weeks. However, unlike THR, symptomatic VTE rates are low (1–2%) when assessed at up to 3 months after surgery.[86,110] A 2004 meta-analysis of VKA trials in orthopedic surgery demonstrated that VKAs were less effective than LMWH in preventing total and proximal DVTs (9822 patients; RR, 1.51; $P < 0.001$; and 6131 patients; RR, 1.51; $P = 0.028$, respectively), whereas the differences between VKA and LMWH in major hemorrhage and wound hematoma were not significant. The authors conclude that VKAs are less effective than LMWH, without any significant difference in the bleeding risk in lower limb orthopedic procedures including TKR and THR.[96] When compared with LMWH in patients with TKA, VKA is less efficacious with a similar or slightly lower bleeding risk.

LMWH in TKA is well-studied, and is a safe and effective prophylactic measure with clear superior efficacy compared with VKA. Pooled clinical trials directly comparing VKA and LMWH demonstrate overall DVT rates of 48% versus 33% and proximal DVT rates of 10.4% versus 7.1%, respectively.[75,91,101,107,111,112] A 2001 meta-analysis of thromboprophylaxis studies in

TKA evaluated 14 studies (3482 patients) and reported that for proximal DVT rates, LMWH was significantly better than warfarin ($P = 0.0002$), whereas there was no significant difference for symptomatic PE, fatal PE, major hemorrhage, or total mortality.[113] Another meta-analysis confirmed the superior efficacy of LMWH over VKA without increased bleeding.[114]

Large-scale clinical trials have shown that fondaparinux further reduces the likelihood of VTE complications after major orthopedic surgery.[115] Fondaparinux was shown to be superior to LMWH in reduction of total VTE events after TKA in a large, randomized trial of more than 1000 patients.[97,115] Fondaparinux (2.5 mg SC daily) started 6 hours after surgery versus LMWH started 12 to 24 hours after surgery resulted in a halving of total VTE (12.5% vs. 27.8%; $P < 0.001$) and proximal DVT rates (2.4% vs. 5.4%; $P = 0.06$) respectively. This improved efficacy came at a cost of increased major bleeding (2.1% vs. 0.2%; $P = 0.006$). In a systematic review of the four thromboprophylaxis studies in major orthopedic surgery, fondaparinux was 50% more effective in reducing VTE than LMWH (enoxaparin), with an overall 1% increased rate of major bleeding, whereas the incidence of fatal bleeding, critical organ bleeding, or bleeding leading to reoperation did not differ between the two treatment groups.[39,115]

VTE after TKR results in a significant cost burden because of rehospitalization, prolonged stay, morbidity, mortality, and long-term postphlebitic syndrome. Both LMWH and fondaparinux are significantly more costly on a daily basis than VKA for thromboprophylaxis. When cost-effectiveness, comparing VKA and LMWH, has been studied, conflicting conclusions using slightly different methodologies have been drawn, suggesting that there may be little difference in cost-effectiveness of VKA versus LMWH.[116–118] A review of the pharmacoeconomic evaluations of fondaparinux leads to the conclusion that fondaparinux is a cost-effective alternative to LMWHs in VTE prophylaxis.[119]

In conclusion, LMWH, and by indirect comparison fondaparinux, is more effective than VKA in preventing symptomatic and asymptomatic VTE. The bleeding risk is similar for VKA and LMWH but increased for fondaparinux. Increased bleeding and improved VTE efficacy is likely on the basis of earlier proximity to surgery of anticoagulant activity of these two former drugs.

OTHER ISSUES

Timing of Prophylaxis

Prophylaxis should ideally be started in close proximity to surgery, either before or after, and continued until the patient is fully ambulatory and VTE risk begins to approach baseline. In North America, prophylaxis has routinely started 12 to 24 hours after surgery because of a greater concern for bleeding complications and to facilitate same-day admissions.

VKA prophylaxis can be commenced at any convenient time perioperatively, usually the night before or 12 to 24 hours after surgery. The onset of anticoagulant effect is delayed until the third or fourth postoperative day.[87]

There is likely little difference in efficacy in preoperative or postoperative commencement of LMWH.[76,88] LMWH at a first injection, 50% dose reduction, started immediately before or early after (<7 hours) surgery in patients undergoing THR, resulted in similar VTE rates of both total and proximal DVT but significantly lower VTE rates when compared with warfarin.[120] No difference was found between the preoperative and postoperative LMWH arms with respect to efficacy, but there was more major bleeding in the preoperative LMWH group when compared with warfarin and the postoperative arm. In a meta-analysis comparing preoperative with postoperative initiation of LMWH for prophylaxis of DVT after THR, it was shown that total DVT rates (but not proximal DVT rates) and major bleeding occurred significantly less frequently in the preoperative group compared with those who received postoperative prophylaxis.[121] The timing of the first dose of LMWH after THR was further assessed in a meta-analysis of four trials of LMWH given at half the regular dose within 6 to 8 hours compared with full dose at 12 to 24 hours, VKA was associated with a large risk reduction, and major bleeding occurred significantly less frequently in the preoperative group compared with those who received postoperative prophylaxis.[121] This study concluded that the timing of initiating LMWH significantly impacts efficacy, and delaying initiation of LMWH prophylaxis results in loss of efficacy without an enhanced safety advantage. The closer to surgery prophylaxis is initiated the better the efficacy, but this is offset by an increased risk for major bleeding.[122,123]

Findings are similar with fondaparinux with respect to perioperative timing of prophylactic dose.[15,39,122,124] In a benefit/risk analysis, the incidence of major bleeding was significantly less (2.1% vs. 3.2%) in those patients receiving fondaparinux 6 versus less than 6 hours after surgery, whereas there was no significant difference in efficacy (7.0% vs. 6%, respectively).[124] This finding resulted in a regulatory agency recommending fondaparinux initiation at 6 to 8 hours after surgery rather than the timing used in the trials (4–8 hours).

Duration of Prophylaxis

For a patient undergoing THR or TKR, the minimum duration of pharmaco-thromboprophylaxis for all patients should be 7 to 10 days.[2] Extending prophylaxis with VKA, LMWH, or fondaparinux beyond this time appears to have greatest efficacy in THR as opposed to TKR. VKA use extended for 4 weeks in THR compared with in-hospital use was associated with a 5- to 10-fold decrease in VTE rates as assessed by DUS at little increased bleeding risk.[125] Multiple reports and two meta-analyses clearly support continued prophylaxis with LMWH for 28 to 42 days after THR.[70–72,74,126,127] The meta-analyses, when compared with placebo, showed a significant decrease in total DVT and PE without a significant increased risk for major bleeding but increased minor bleeding.[121,126,127] There is less of a need for extended prophylaxis beyond 10 days for patients undergoing TKR because prolonging therapy for an additional 3 to 6 weeks in TKR does not appear to provide significant further benefit.[74,75,126]

The benefit of thromboprophylaxis in THR with fondaparinux (2.5 mg/day) for 1 month, rather than 6 to 8 days, was studied in a double-blind, multicenter trial and summarized in two other reviews of all fondaparinux-related joint surgery randomized studies.[39,115,128] Compared with 1 week of fondaparinux followed by 3 weeks of placebo in the PENTHIFRA-PLUS trial, extended fondaparinux resulted in a significant reduction in total VTE from 35.0% to 1.4%, as well as an 87% reduction in symptomatic VTE. However, a nonsignificant trend toward more major bleeding in the 1-month group was found.

Recommendations include prophylaxis for 7 to 10 days in all patients undergoing THR and TKA. Extended prophylaxis up to 42 days is recommended in patients with THR and in at-risk but not in routine-risk patients with TKR.

SCREENING

It has been clearly demonstrated with numerous studies that postoperative screening for VTE using noninvasive methods is an unacceptable and costly alternative to primary prophylaxis.[129] Noninvasive screening methods, such as the DUS, have been demonstrated as having low sensitivity and specificity, after THR, for both distal and proximal DVT.[130–132] This has been shown in studies of both TKR and THR.[110,133,134] A meta-analysis demonstrated that venous ultrasound imaging has moderate sensitivity and moderate positive predictive value when used to screen for DVT after orthopedic surgery; thus, ultrasound imaging is not a reliable approach for DVT screening.[135] Consequently, DVT screening as secondary prophylaxis is not recommended for patients with lower limb joint replacement.[2]

NEURAXIAL ANESTHESIA

Lower limb arthroplasty surgery that involves spinal or epidural invasive procedures for regional anesthesia or continued analgesia in conjunction with prophylactic anticoagulants must be used with extreme caution, and current and evolving recommendations of the American Association for Regional Anesthesia should be consulted for evolving recommendations. Spinal hematoma, although a serious concern, is rare.[136] Bleeding risk concerns should not outweigh the anticipated benefits of regional anesthesia in joint arthroplasty or its efficacy in thromboprophylaxis, which are much more common complications of lower limb arthroplasty.[2,137,138] A recent meta-analysis of 10 trials showed that compared with general anesthesia (GA), neuraxial block reduced many serious complications in all patients. Pooled results from five trials showed that neuraxial block significantly decreased the incidence of all radiologic DVT or PE in THR. The odds ratio for DVT and PE was 0.27 (confidence interval [CI], 0.17–0.42) and 0.26 (CI, 0.12–0.56), respectively, and the authors concluded that patients undergoing THR with neuraxial anesthesia have better outcomes than those under GA and less frequent VTE events.[139] Second, as the 2003 ASRA Consensus Conference statement makes clear, regional anesthesia may be used safely with LMWH prophylaxis[136] as long as key factors including timing issues in relation to the regional anesthetic procedure are considered.

COST-EFFECTIVENESS

VTE represents a huge health economic burden of nearly $500 million per year in the United States, and patients undergoing major lower limb surgery are at high risk for development of VTE. Prophylaxis with warfarin substantially reduces the risk for VTE after lower limb arthroplasty and is more cost-effective than no prophylaxis.[119] Although LMWHs are more expensive than VKA, they are superior to warfarin in VTE prevention and are cost-effective.[140,141] A review of the pharmacoeconomic evaluations of fondaparinux leads to the conclusion that fondaparinux is a cost-effective alternative to LMWHs in lower limb joint surgery.[119] Fondaparinux, LMWH, and VKA in extended prophylaxis for 28 days all appear to be cost-effective.[142–144]

RECOMMENDATIONS

In making overall recommendations for thromboprophylaxis, an increased weight/value is placed on the risks (bleeding) of thromboprophylaxis given the relative low incidence of symptomatic VTE, proximal DVT, and PE with current pharmacologic interventions. VKA, fondaparinux, and LMWH are all efficacious in the prevention of VTE in lower limb joint replacement surgery. This improved efficacy, moving progressively from VKA to LMWH to fondaparinux, is offset by a similar trend toward increasing bleeding rates. This risk/benefit ratio for each intervention needs to be weighed on an individual patient basis. Patients who, on clinical analysis, are at greater risk for bleeding or clotting should be considered for prophylaxis with an approach that carries a lower risk for these respective deleterious complications.[2]

Specific decisions of thromboprophylaxis approach for THR and TKA should be made at a hospital level, ideally both through a professional consensus approach and at an individual patient level. Decision should be based on issues of local cost, infrastructure support for monitoring of VKA if being considered, patient compliance, and duration of prophylaxis. Table 80–2 provides a summary of recommendations.

TABLE 80–2. Summary of Recommendations

RECOMMENDATIONS	LEVEL OF EVIDENCE/GRADE OF RECOMMENDATION
Elective THR	
The routine use of one of the following is recommended for all patients undergoing elective THR: (1) LMWH, at standard high-risk prophylactic dosage, started either 12 hours before or 12 to 24 hours after surgery, or a 50% dose reduction at 4 to 6 hours after surgery escalating to full-dose prophylaxis at 24 hours and daily thereafter; (2) VKA, dose adjusted with INR-warfarin nomogram to a target INR of 2.5, started before surgery or the evening after surgery; or (3) fondaparinux (2.5 mg) started 6 to 8 hours after surgery and daily thereafter.	A
The use of aspirin, LDUFH, GCS, IPC, or VFP as monotherapy for thromboprophylaxis is *not* recommended.	A
Elective TKR	
The routine use of one of the following is recommended for all patients undergoing elective TKR: (1) LMWH, at standard high-risk prophylactic dosage, started either 12 hours before or 12 to 24 hours after surgery, or a 50% dose reduction at 4 to 6 hours after surgery escalating to full-dose prophylaxis at 24 hours and daily thereafter; (2) VKA, dose adjusted with INR-warfarin nomogram to a target INR of 2.5, started before surgery or the evening after surgery; or (3) fondaparinux (2.5 mg) started 6 to 8 hours after surgery and daily thereafter.	A
The use of aspirin, LDUFH, GCS, IPC, or VFP as monotherapy for thromboprophylaxis is *not* recommended.	A
Timing	
The efficacy-to-bleeding risk needs to be individualized for all patients at increased risk to bleed or clot based on clinical assessment and on the bases of each agent. Preoperative or postoperative initiation off all three agents (fondaparinux, LMWH, or VKA) is acceptable.	A
Screening	
The routine use of postoperative VTE screening in asymptomatic patients is *not* recommended.	A
Length of Prophylaxis	
In elective THR and TKA, thromboprophylaxis with LMWH, VKA, or fondaparinux should be continued for a minimum of 7 to 10 days for patients. Patients undergoing THR and patients at high risk for thrombosis undergoing TKA should be given extended prophylaxis for up to 28 to 42 days after surgery.	A
Neuraxial Anesthesia/Analgesia	
Special caution should be used with concurrent use of anticoagulant prophylaxis.	B

DVT, venous thromboembolic event; GCS, graduated compression stockings; INR, international normalized ratio; IPC, intermittent pneumatic leg compression; LDUFH, low-dose unfractionated heparin; LMWH, low-molecular-weight heparin; PE, pulmonary embolism; THR, total hip replacement; TKA, total knee arthroscopy; TKR, total knee replacement; VFP, venous foot pump; VKA, vitamin K antagonist.

REFERENCES

1. NIH Consensus Conference: Prevention of venous thrombosis and pulmonary embolism. JAMA 256:744–749, 1986.
2. Geerts W, Pineo GF, Heit JA, et al: Prevention of venous thrombosis: The Seventh ACCP Conference on Antithrombotic and Thrombolytic Therapy. Chest 126:338S–400S, 2004.
3. Freedman KB, Brookenthal KR, Fitzgerald RH Jr, Williams S, Lonner JH: A meta-analysis of thromboembolic prophylaxis following elective total hip arthroplasty. J Bone Joint Surg Am 82-A:929–938, 2000.
4. Beisaw NE, Groth HE, Merli GJ, Weitz HH, et al: Dihydroergotamine/heparin in the prevention of deep-vein thrombosis after total hip replacement. A controlled, prospective, randomized multicenter trial. J Bone Joint Surg Am 70:2–10, 1988.
5. Haake DA, Berkman SA: Venous thromboembolic disease after hip surgery. Risk factors, prophylaxis, and diagnosis. Clin Orthop Relat Res (242):212–231, 1989.
6. Mohr DN, Silverstein MD, Ilstrup DM, Heit JA, Morrey BF: Venous thromboembolism associated with hip and knee arthroplasty: Current prophylactic practices and outcomes. Mayo Clin Proc 67:861–870, 1992.
7. Lotke PA, Palevsky H, Keenan AM, et al: Aspirin and warfarin for thromboembolic disease after total joint arthroplasty. Clin Orthop Relat Res (324):251–258, 1996.
8. Stulberg BN, Insall JN, Williams GW, Ghelman B: Deep-vein thrombosis following total knee replacement. An analysis of six hundred and thirty-eight arthroplasties. J Bone Joint Surg Am 66:194–201, 1984.
9. Warwick D, Harrison J, Whitehouse S, Mitchelmore A, Thornton M: A randomised comparison of a foot pump and low-molecular-weight heparin in the prevention of deep-vein thrombosis after total knee replacement. J Bone Joint Surg Br 84:344–350, 2002.
10. Ginsberg JS, Turkstra F, Buller HR, MacKinnon B, Magier D, et al: Postthrombotic syndrome after hip or knee arthroplasty: A cross-sectional study. Arch Intern Med 160:669–672, 2000.
11. Kim YH, Oh SH, Kim JS: Incidence and natural history of deep-vein thrombosis after total hip arthroplasty. A prospective and randomised clinical study. J Bone Joint Surg Br 85:661–665, 2003.
12. White RH, Romano PS, Zhou H, Rodrigo J, Bargar W: Incidence and time course of thromboembolic outcomes following total hip or knee arthroplasty. Arch Intern Med 158:1525–1531, 1998.
13. Eriksson BI, Kälebo P, Anthymyr BA, Wadenvik H, Tengborn L: Prevention of deep-vein thrombosis and pulmonary embolism after total hip replacement: Comparison of low-molecular-weight heparin and unfractionated heparin. J Bone Joint Surg Am 73:484–493, 1991.
14. Khaw FM, Moran CG, Pinder IM, Smith SR: The incidence of fatal pulmonary embolism after knee replacement with no prophylactic anticoagulation. J Bone Joint Surg Br 75:940–941, 1993.
15. Turpie AGG, Bauer KA, Eriksson BI, Lassen MR: Fondaparinux vs enoxaparin for the prevention of venous thromboembolism in major orthopedic surgery: A meta-analysis of 4 randomized double-blind studies. Arch Intern Med 162:1833–1840, 2002.
16. Warwick D, Bannister GC, Glew D, Mitchelmore A, Thornton M, et al: Perioperative low-molecular-weight heparin. Is it effective and safe. J Bone Joint Surg Br 77:715–719, 1995.
17. Fender D, Harper WM, Thompson JR, Gregg PJ: Mortality and fatal pulmonary embolism after primary total hip replacement. Results from a regional hip register. J Bone Joint Surg Br 79:896–899, 1997.

18. Paiement G: Prevention and treatment of venous thromboembolic disease complications in primary hip arthroplasty patients. Instr Course Lect 47:331–335, 1998.

19. Montgomery KD, Geerts WH, Potter HG, Helfet DL: Practical management of venous thromboembolism following pelvic fractures. Orthop Clin North Am 28:397, 1997.

20. Langlois NJ, Wells PS: Risk of venous thromboembolism in relatives of symptomatic probands with thrombophilia: A systematic review. Thromb Haemost 90:17–26, 2003.

21. Moores L, Bilello KL, Murin S: Sex and gender issues and venous thromboembolism. Clin Chest Med 25:281–297, 2004.

22. White RH, Zhou H, Murin S, Harvey D: Effect of ethnicity and gender on the incidence of venous thromboembolism in a diverse population in California in 1996. Thromb Haemost 93:298–305, 2005.

23. Mateo J, Oliver A, Borrell M, Sala N, Fontcuberta J: Laboratory evaluation and clinical characteristics of 2,132 consecutive unselected patients with venous thromboembolism—results of the Spanish Multicentric Study on Thrombophilia (EMET-Study). Thromb Haemost 77:444–451, 1997.

24. Crowther MA, Kelton JG: Congenital thrombophilic states associated with venous thrombosis: A qualitative overview and proposed classification system. Ann Intern Med 138:128–134, 2003.

25. Kearon C, Crowther M, Hirsh J: Management of patients with hereditary hypercoagulable disorders. Annu Rev Med 51:169–185, 2000.

26. Emmerich J, Rosendaal FR, Cattaneo M, Margaglione M, De Stefano V, et al: Combined effect of factor V Leiden and prothrombin 20210A on the risk of venous thromboembolism—pooled analysis of 8 case-control studies including 2310 cases and 3204 controls. Study Group for Pooled-Analysis in Venous Thromboembolism. Thromb Haemost 86:809–816, 2001.

27. Kyrle PA, Minar E, Hirschl M, Bialonczyk C, Stain M, et al: High plasma levels of factor VIII and the risk of recurrent venous thromboembolism. N Engl J Med 343:457–462, 2000.

28. Zaw HM, Osborne IC, Pettit PN, Cohen AT: Risk factors for venous thromboembolism in orthopedic surgery. Isr Med Assoc J 4:1040–1042, 2002.

29. Vaughan P, Gardner J, Peters F, Wilmott R: Risk factors for venous thromboembolism in general surgical patients. Isr Med Assoc J 4:1037–1039, 2002.

30. Spencer FA, Emery C, Lessard D, Anderson F, Emani S, et al: The Worcester Venous Thromboembolism study: A population-based study of the clinical epidemiology of venous thromboembolism. J Gen Intern Med 21:722–727, 2006.

31. Caprini JA, Arcelus JI, Reyna JJ: Effective risk stratification of surgical and nonsurgical patients for venous thromboembolic disease. Semin Hematol 38(2 suppl 5):12–19, 2001.

32. Hirsh J, Raschke R: Heparin and low-molecular-weight heparin: The Seventh ACCP Conference on Antithrombotic and Thrombolytic Therapy. Chest 126(3 suppl):188S–203S, 2004.

33. Turpie AG: Pharmacology of the low-molecular-weight heparins. Am Heart J 135(6 pt 3 suppl):S329–S335, 1998.

34. Warkentin TE, Greinacher A: Heparin-induced thrombocytopenia: recognition, treatment, and prevention: The Seventh ACCP Conference on Antithrombotic and Thrombolytic Therapy. Chest 126(3 suppl):311S–337S, 2004.

35. Greinacher A, Warkentin TE: Recognition, treatment, and prevention of heparin-induced thrombocytopenia: Review and update. Thromb Res 118:165–176, 2006.

36. Prandoni P: Heparins and venous thromboembolism: Current practice and future directions. Thromb Haemost 86:488–498, 2001.

37. White RH, Ginsberg JS: Low-molecular-weight heparins: Are they all the same? Br J Haematol 121:12–20, 2003.

38. Warkentin TE, Roberts RS, Hirsh J, Kelton JG: An improved definition of immune heparin-induced thrombocytopenia in postoperative orthopedic patients. Arch Intern Med 163:2518–2524, 2003.

39. Nijkeuter M, Huisman MV: Pentasaccharides in the prophylaxis and treatment of venous thromboembolism: A systematic review. Curr Opin Pulm Med 10:338–344, 2004.

40. Turpie AG, Gallus AS, Hoek JA; Pentasaccharide Investigators: A synthetic pentasaccharide for the prevention of deep-vein thrombosis after total hip replacement. N Engl J Med 344:619–625, 2001.

41. Warkentin TE, Cook RJ, Marder VJ, Sheppard JA, Moore JC, et al: Anti-platelet factor 4/heparin antibodies in orthopedic surgery patients receiving antithrombotic prophylaxis with fondaparinux or enoxaparin. Blood 106:3791–3796, 2005.

42. Lassen MR, Bauer KA, Eriksson BI, Turpie AG; European Pentasaccharide Elective Surgery Study (EPHESUS) Steering Committee: Postoperative fondaparinux versus preoperative enoxaparin for prevention of venous thromboembolism in elective hip-replacement surgery: A randomised double-blind comparison. Lancet 359:1715–1720, 2002.

43. Ansell J, Hirsh J, Poller L, Bussey H, Jacobson A, Hylek E: The pharmacology and management of the vitamin K antagonists: the Seventh ACCP Conference on Antithrombotic and Thrombolytic Therapy. Chest 126(3 suppl):204S–233S, 2004.

44. Freedman MD: Oral anticoagulants: Pharmacodynamics, clinical indications and adverse effects. J Clin Pharmacol 32:196–209, 1992.

45. Juurlink D: Drug interactions with warfarin: What clinicians need to know. CMAJ 177:369–371, 2007.

46. Schurgers LJ, Shearer MJ, Hamulyák K, Stöcklin E, Vermeer C: Effect of vitamin K intake on the stability of oral anticoagulant treatment: Dose-response relationships in healthy subjects. Blood 104:2682–2689, 2004.

47. Ebell MH: Evidence-based initiation of warfarin (Coumadin). Am Fam Physician 71:763–765, 2005.

48. Aspinall SL, DeSanzo BE, Trilli LE, Good CB: Bleeding Risk Index in an anticoagulation clinic. Assessment by indication and implications for care. J Gen Intern Med 20:1008–1013, 2005.

49. Collaborative overview of randomised trials of antiplatelet therapy—I: Prevention of death, myocardial infarction, and stroke by prolonged antiplatelet therapy in various categories of patients. Antiplatelet Trialists' Collaboration. BMJ 308:81–106, 1994.

50. Prevention of pulmonary embolism and deep vein thrombosis with low dose aspirin: Pulmonary Embolism Prevention (PEP) trial. Lancet 355:1295–1302, 2000.

51. Hovens MM, Snoep JD, Tamsma JT, Huisman MV: Aspirin in the prevention and treatment of venous thromboembolism. J Thromb Haemost 4:1470–1475, 2006.

52. Eriksson BI, Kälebo P, Ekman S, Lindbratt S, Kerry R, et al: Direct thrombin inhibitor melagatran followed by oral ximelagatran in comparison with enoxaparin for prevention of venous thromboembolism after total hip or knee replacement. Thromb Haemost 89:288–296, 2003.

53. Eriksson BI, Ekman S, Kalebo P, Zachrisson B, Bach D, et al: Prevention of deep-vein thrombosis after total hip replacement: Direct thrombin inhibition with recombinant hirudin, CGP 39393. Lancet 347:635–639, 1996.

54. Westrich GH, Specht LM, Sharrock NE, Sculco TP, Salvati EA, et al: Pneumatic compression hemodynamics in total hip arthroplasty. Clin Orthop Relat Res (372):180–191, 2000.

55. Comerota AJ, Chouhan V, Harada RN, Sun L, Hosking J, Veermansunemi R, et al: The fibrinolytic effects of intermittent pneumatic compression: Mechanism of enhanced fibrinolysis. Ann Surg 226:306–314, 1997.

56. Hull RD, Raskob GE, Gent M, McLoughlin D, Julian D, et al: Effectiveness of intermittent pneumatic leg compression for preventing deep vein thrombosis after total hip replacement. Jama 263:2313–2317, 1990.

57. Paiement G, Wessinger SJ, Waltman AC, Harris WH: Low-dose warfarin versus external pneumatic compression for prophylaxis against venous thromboembolism following total hip replacement. J Arthroplasty 2:23–26, 1987.

58. Norgren L, et al: Low incidence of deep vein thrombosis after total hip replacement: An interim analysis of patients on low molecular weight heparin vs sequential gradient compression prophylaxis. Int Angiol 15(3 suppl 1):11–14, 1996.

59. Francis CW, Pellegrini VD Jr, Marder VJ, Totterman S, Harris CM, et al: Comparison of warfarin and external pneumatic compression in prevention of venous thrombosis after total hip replacement. Jama 267:2911–2915, 1992.

60. Ramos R, Salem BI, De Pawlikowski MP, Coordes C, Eisenberg S, et al: The efficacy of pneumatic compression stockings in the prevention of pulmonary embolism after cardiac surgery. Chest 109:82–85, 1996.

61. White RH, Gettner S, Newman JM, Trauner KB, Romano PS: Predictors of rehospitalization for symptomatic venous thromboembolism after total hip arthroplasty. N Engl J Med 343:1758–1764, 2000.

62. Haddad FS, Kerry RM, McEwen JA, Appleton L, Garbuz DS, et al: Unanticipated variations between expected and delivered pneumatic compression therapy after elective hip surgery: A possible source of variation in reported patient outcomes. J Arthroplasty 16:37–46, 2001.

63. Samama CM, Clergue F, Barre J, Montefiore A, Ill P, Samii K: Low molecular weight heparin associated with spinal anaesthesia and gradual compression stockings in total hip replacement surgery. Br J Anaesth 78:660–665, 1997.

64. Barnes RW, Brand RA, Clarke W, Hartley N, Hoak JC: Efficacy of graded-compression antiembolism stockings in patients undergoing total hip arthroplasty. Clin Orthop Relat Res (132):61–67, 1978.

65. Fordyce MJ, Ling RS: A venous foot pump reduces thrombosis after total hip replacement. J Bone Joint Surg Br 74:45–49, 1992.

66. Hui ACW, Heras-Palou C, Dunn I, Triffitt PD, Crozier A, Imeson J, et al: Graded compression stockings for prevention of deep-vein thrombosis after hip and knee replacement. J Bone Joint Surg Br 78:550–554, 1996.

67. Wells PS, Lensing AW, Hirsh J: Graduated compression stockings in the prevention of postoperative venous thromboembolism. A meta-analysis. Arch Intern Med 154:67–72, 1994.

68. Warwick D, Harrison J, Glew D, Mitchelmore A, Peters TJ, Donovan J: Comparison of the use of a foot pump with the use of low-molecular-weight heparin for the prevention of deep-vein thrombosis after total hip replacement. A prospective, randomized trial. J Bone Joint Surg Am 80:1158–1166, 1998.

69. Pitto RP, Hamer H, Heiss-Dunlop W, Kuehle J: Mechanical prophylaxis of deep-vein thrombosis after total hip replacement a randomised clinical trial. J Bone Joint Surg Br 86:639–642, 2004.

70. Lassen MR, Borris LC, Anderson BS, Jensen HP, Skejø Bro HP, et al: Efficacy and safety of prolonged thromboprophylaxis with a low molecular weight heparin (dalteparin) after total hip arthroplasty—the Danish Prolonged Prophylaxis (DaPP) Study. Thromb Res 89:281–287, 1998.

71. Dahl OE, Andreassen G, Aspelin T, Müller C, Mathiesen P, et al: Prolonged thromboprophylaxis following hip replacement surgery: Results of a double-blind, prospective, randomised, placebo-controlled study with dalteparin (Fragmin(TM)). Thromb Haemost 77:26–31, 1997.

72. Planes A, Vochelle N, Darmon JY, Fagola M, Bellaud M, et al: Risk of deep-venous thrombosis after hospital discharge in patients having undergone total hip replacement: Double-blind randomised comparison of enoxaparin versus placebo. Lancet 348:224–228, 1996.

73. Bergqvist D, Benoni G, Björgell O, Fredin H, Hedlundh U, et al: Low-molecular-weight heparin (enoxaparin) as prophylaxis against venous thromboembolism after total hip replacement. N Engl J Med 335:696–700, 1996.

74. Comp PC, et al: Prolonged enoxaparin therapy to prevent venous thromboembolism after primary hip or knee replacement. Enoxaparin Clinical Trial Group. J Bone Joint Surg Am 83-A:336–345, 2001.

75. Hull R, et al: A comparison of subcutaneous low-molecular-weight heparin with warfarin sodium for prophylaxis against deep-vein thrombosis after hip or knee implantation. N Engl J Med 329:1370–1376, 1993.

76. Hull RD, Pineo GF, Francis C, Bergqvist D, Fellenius C, et al: Low-molecular-weight heparin prophylaxis using dalteparin in close proximity to surgery vs warfarin in hip arthroplasty patients: A double-blind, randomized comparison. The North American Fragmin Trial Investigators. Arch Intern Med 160:2199–2207, 2000.

77. Collins R, Scrimgeour A, Yusuf S, Peto R: Reduction in fatal pulmonary embolism and venous thrombosis by perioperative administration of subcutaneous heparin. Overview of results of randomized trials in general, orthopedic, and urologic surgery. N Engl J Med 318:1162–1173, 1988.

78. Anonymous: Prevention of pulmonary embolism and deep vein thrombosis with low dose aspirin: Pulmonary Embolism Prevention (PEP) trial. Lancet 355:1295–1302, 2000.

79. Anderson DR, O'Brien BJ, Levine MN, Roberts R, Wells PS, et al: Efficacy and cost of low-molecular-weight heparin compared with standard heparin for the prevention of deep vein thrombosis after total hip arthroplasty. Ann Intern Med 119:1105–1112, 1993.

80. Kakkar VV, Howes J, Sharma V, Kadziola Z: A comparative double-blind, randomised trial of a new second generation LMWH (bemiparin) and UFH in the prevention of post-operative venous thromboembolism. The Bemiparin Assessment group. Thromb Haemost 83:523–529, 2000.

81. Paiement GD, Wessinger SJ, Hughes R, Harris WH: Routine use of adjusted low-dose warfarin to prevent venous thromboembolism after total hip replacement. J Bone Joint Surg Am 75:893–898, 1993.

82. Mesko JW, Brand RA, Iorio R, Gradisar I, Heekin R, et al: Venous thromboembolic disease management patterns in total hip arthroplasty and total knee arthroplasty patients: A survey of the AAHKS membership. J Arthroplasty 16:679–688, 2001.

83. Gross M, Anderson DR, Nagpal S, O'Brien B: Venous thromboembolism prophylaxis after total hip or knee arthroplasty: A survey of Canadian orthopedic surgeons. Can J Surg 42:457–461, 1999.

84. Amstutz HC, Friscia DA, Dorey F, Carney BT: Warfarin prophylaxis to prevent mortality from pulmonary embolism after total hip replacement. J Bone Joint Surg Am 71:321–326, 1989.

85. Janku GV, Paiement GD, Green HD: Prevention of venous thromboembolism in orthopaedics in the United States. Clin Orthop Relat Res (325):313–321, 1996.

86. Lieberman JR, Wollaeger J, Dorey F, Thomas BJ, Kilgus DJ et al: The efficacy of prophylaxis with low-dose warfarin for prevention of pulmonary embolism following total hip arthroplasty. J Bone Joint Surg Am 79:319–325, 1997.

87. Brotman DJ, Jaffer AK, Hurbanek JG, Morra N: Warfarin prophylaxis and venous thromboembolism in the first 5 days following hip and knee arthroplasty. Thromb Haemost 92:1012–1017, 2004.

88. Hull RD, Pineo GF, Francis C, Bergqvist D, Fellenius C, et al: Low-molecular-weight heparin prophylaxis using dalteparin extended out-of-hospital vs in-hospital warfarin/out-of-hospital placebo in hip arthroplasty patients: A double-blind, randomized comparison. North American Fragmin Trial Investigators. Arch Intern Med 160:2208–2215, 2000.

89. Comp PC, et al: Prolonged enoxaparin therapy to prevent venous thromboembolism after primary hip or knee replacement. Enoxaparin Clinical Trial Group. J Bone Joint Surg Am 83-A:336–345, 2001.

90. Samama CM, Vray M, Barré J, Fiessinger JN, Rosencher N, et al: Extended venous thromboembolism prophylaxis after total hip replacement: A comparison of low-molecular-weight heparin with oral anticoagulant. Arch Intern Med 162:2191–2196, 2002.

91. Hamulyak K, Lensing AW, van der Meer J, Smid WM, van Ooy A, et al: Subcutaneous low-molecular weight heparin or oral anticoagulants for the prevention of deep-vein thrombosis in elective hip and knee replacement? Thromb Haemost 74:1428–1431, 1995.

92. Turpie AGG, Bauer KA, Eriksson BI, Lassen MR; PENTATHALON 2000 Study Steering Committee: Postoperative fondaparinux versus postoperative enoxaparin for prevention of venous thromboembolism after elective hip-replacement surgery: A randomised double-blind trial [erratum appears in Lancet 2002 Oct 5;360(9339):1102]. Lancet 359:1721–1726, 2002.

93. Zufferey P, Laporte S, Quenet S, Molliex S, Auboyer C, Decousus H, et al: Optimal low-molecular-weight heparin regimen in major orthopaedic surgery: A meta-analysis of randomised trials. Thromb Haemost 90:654–661, 2003.

94. Francis CW, Pellegrini VD Jr, Totterman S, Boyd AD Jr, Marder VJ, et al: Prevention of deep-vein thrombosis after total hip arthroplasty: Comparison of warfarin and dalteparin. J Bone Joint Surg Am 79:1365–1372, 1997.

95. Colwell CW Jr, Collis DK, Paulson R, McCutchen JW, Bigler GT, et al: Comparison of enoxaparin and warfarin for the prevention of venous thromboembolic disease after total hip arthroplasty. Evaluation during hospitalization three months after discharge. J Bone Joint Surg Am 81:932–940, 1999.

96. Mismetti P, Laporte S, Zufferey P, Epinat M, Decousus H, Cucherat M: Prevention of venous thromboembolism in orthopedic surgery with vitamin K antagonists: A meta-analysis. J Thromb Haemost 2:1058–1070, 2004.

97. Bauer KA, Eriksson BI, Lassen MR, Turpie AG; Steering Committee of the Pentasaccharide in Major Knee Surgery Study: Fondaparinux compared with enoxaparin for the prevention of venous thromboembolism after elective major knee surgery. N Engl J Med 345:1305–1310, 2001.

98. Eriksson BI, Bauer KA, Lassen MR, Turpie AG; Steering Committee of the Pentasaccharide in Hip-Fracture Surgery Study: Fondaparinux compared with enoxaparin for the prevention of venous thromboembolism after hip-fracture surgery. N Engl J Med 345:1298–1304, 2001.

99. Colwell CW Jr, Spiro TE, Trowbridge AA, et al: Efficacy and safety of enoxaparin versus unfractionated heparin for prevention of deep venous thrombosis after elective knee arthroplasty. Clin Orthop Relat Res 321:19–27, 1995.

100. Turpie AG, Levine MN, Hirsh J, Carter CJ, Jay RM, Powers PJ, et al: A randomized controlled trial of a low-molecular-weight heparin (enoxaparin) to prevent deep-vein thrombosis in patients undergoing elective hip surgery. N Engl J Med 315:925–929, 1986.

101. Fitzgerald RH Jr, Spiro TE, Trowbridge AA, Gardiner GA Jr, Whitsett TL, et al: J Bone Joint Surg Am 83-A:900–906, 2001.

102. Kaempffe FA, Lifeso RM, Meinking C: Intermittent pneumatic compression versus coumadin: Prevention of deep vein thrombosis in lower-extremity total joint arthroplasty. Clin Orthop Relat Res (269):89–97, 1991.

103. Haas SB, Insall JN, Scuderi GR, Windsor RE, Ghelman B: Pneumatic sequential-compression boots compared with aspirin prophylaxis of deep-vein thrombosis after total knee arthroplasty. J Bone Joint Surg Am 72:27–31, 1990.

104. Westrich GH, Specht LM, Sharrock NE, Windsor RE, Sculco TP, et al: Venous haemodynamics after total knee arthroplasty: Evaluation of active dorsal to plantar flexion and several mechanical compression devices. J Bone Joint Surg Br 80:1057–1066, 1998.

105. Fauno P, Suomalainen O, Rehnberg V, Hansen TB, Krøner K, et al: Prophylaxis for the prevention of venous thromboembolism after total knee arthroplasty. A comparison between unfractionated and low-molecular-weight heparin. J Bone Joint Surg Am 76:1814–1818, 1994.

106. Francis CW, Pellegrini VD Jr, Leibert KM, Totterman S, Azodo MV, et al: Comparison of two warfarin regimens in the prevention of venous thrombosis following total knee replacement. Thromb Haemost 75:706–711, 1996.

107. Leclerc JR, Geerts WH, Desjardins L, Laflamme GH, L'Espérance B, et al: Prevention of venous thromboembolism after knee arthroplasty. A randomized, double-blind trial comparing enoxaparin with warfarin. Ann Intern Med 124:619–626, 1996.

108. Francis CW, Davidson BL, Berkowitz SD, Lotke PA, Ginsberg JS, et al: Ximelagatran versus warfarin for the prevention of venous thromboembolism after total knee arthroplasty. A randomized, double-blind trial. Ann Intern Med 137:648–655, 2002.

109. Francis CW, Berkowitz SD, Comp PC, Lieberman JR, Ginsberg JS, et al: Comparison of ximelagatran with warfarin for the prevention of venous thromboembolism after total knee replacement. N Engl J Med 349:1703–1712, 2003.

110. Robinson KS, Anderson DR, Gross M, Petrie D, Leighton R, et al: Ultrasonographic screening before hospital discharge for deep venous thrombosis after arthroplasty: The post-arthroplasty screening study. A randomized, controlled trial. Ann Intern Med 127:439–445, 1997.

111. RD Heparin Arthroplasty Group. RD heparin compared with warfarin for prevention of venous thromboembolic disease following total hip or knee arthroplasty. J Bone Joint Surg Am 76:1174–1185, 1994.

112. Heit JA, Berkowitz SD, Bona R, Cabanas V, Corson JD, et al: Efficacy and safety of low molecular weight heparin (ardeparin sodium) compared to warfarin for the prevention of venous thromboembolism after total knee replacement surgery: A double-blind, dose-ranging study. Thromb Haemost 77:32–38, 1997.

113. Brookenthal KR, et al: A meta-analysis of thromboembolic prophylaxis in total knee arthroplasty. J Arthroplasty 16:293–300, 2001.

114. Howard AW, Aaron SD: Low molecular weight heparin decreases proximal and distal deep venous thrombosis following total knee arthroplasty. A meta-analysis of randomized trials. Thromb Haemost 79:902–906, 1998.

115. Turpie AGG: Venous thromboembolism prophylaxis: Role of factor Xa inhibition by fondaparinux. Surg Technol Int 13:261–267, 2004.

116. Menzin J, Colditz GA, Regan MM, Richner RE, Oster G et al: Cost-effectiveness of enoxaparin vs low-dose warfarin in the prevention of deep-vein thrombosis after total hip replacement surgery. Arch Intern Med 155:757–764, 1995.

117. Hull RD, Raskob GE, Pineo GF, Feldstein W, Rosenbloom D, et al: Subcutaneous low-molecular-weight heparin vs warfarin for prophylaxis of deep vein thrombosis after hip or knee implantation. An economic perspective. Arch Intern Med 157:298–303, 1997.

118. Friedman RJ, Dunsworth GA: Cost analyses of extended prophylaxis with enoxaparin after hip arthroplasty. Clin Orthop Relat Res (370):171–182, 2000.

119. Hawkins D: Pharmacoeconomics of thrombosis management. Pharmacotherapy 24(7 Pt 2):95S–99S, 2004.

120. Hull RD, Brant RF, Pineo GF, Stein PD, Raskob GE, Valentine KA: Preoperative vs postoperative initiation of low-molecular-weight heparin prophylaxis against venous thromboembolism in patients undergoing elective hip replacement. Arch Intern Med 159:137–141, 1999.

121. Hull RD, Pineo GF, Stein PD, Mah AF, MacIsaac SM, et al: Timing of initial administration of low-molecular-weight heparin prophylaxis against deep vein thrombosis in patients following elective hip arthroplasty: A systematic review. Arch Intern Med 161:1952–1960, 2001.

122. Raskob GE, Hirsh J: Controversies in timing of the first dose of anticoagulant prophylaxis against venous thromboembolism after major orthopedic surgery. Chest 124(6 suppl):379S–385S, 2003.

123. Strebel N, Prins M, Agnelli G, Büller HR: Preoperative or postoperative start of prophylaxis for venous thromboembolism with low-molecular-weight heparin in elective hip surgery? Arch Intern Med 162:1451–1456, 2002.

124. Turpie A, Bauer K, Eriksson B, Lassen M; Steering Committees of the Pentasaccharide Orthopedic Prophylaxis Studies: Efficacy and safety of fondaparinux in major orthopedic surgery according to the timing of its first administration. Thromb Haemost 90:364–366, 2003.

125. Prandoni P, Bruchi O, Sabbion P, Tanduo C, Scudeller A, et al: Prolonged thromboprophylaxis with oral anticoagulants after total hip arthroplasty: A prospective controlled randomized study. Arch Intern Med 162:1966–1971, 2002.

126. Eikelboom JW, Quinlan DJ, Douketis JD: Extended-duration prophylaxis against venous thromboembolism after total hip or knee replacement: A meta-analysis of the randomised trials. Lancet 358:9–15, 2001.

127. Hull RD, Pineo GF, Stein PD, Mah AF, MacIsaac SM, et al: Extended out-of-hospital low-molecular-weight heparin prophylaxis against deep venous thrombosis in patients after elective hip arthroplasty: A systematic review. Intern Med 135:858–869, 2001.

128. Turpie AGG, Eriksson BI, Bauer KA, Lassen MR: New pentasaccharides for the prophylaxis of venous thromboembolism: Clinical studies. Chest 124(6 suppl):371S–378S, 2003.

129. Kearon C: Noninvasive diagnosis of deep vein thrombosis in postoperative patients. Semin Thromb Hemost 27:3–8, 2001.

130. Agnelli G, Cosmi B, Ranucci V, Renga C, Mosca S, et al: Impedance plethysmography in the diagnosis of asymptomatic deep vein thrombosis in hip surgery. A venography-controlled study. Arch Intern Med 151:2167–2171, 1991.

131. Ciccone WJ 2nd, Fox PS, Neumyer M, Rubens D, Parrish WM, Pellegrini VD Jr: Ultrasound surveillance for asymptomatic deep venous thrombosis after total joint replacement. J Bone Joint Surg Am 80:1167–1174, 1998.

132. Magnusson M, Eriksson BI, Kälebo P, Sivertsson R: Is colour Doppler ultrasound a sensitive screening method in diagnosing deep vein thrombosis after hip surgery? Thromb Haemost 75:242–245, 1996.

133. Schmidt B, et al: Ultrasound screening for distal vein thrombosis is not beneficial after major orthopedic surgery. A randomized controlled trial. Thromb Haemost 90:949–954, 2003.

134. Leclerc JR, et al: The incidence of symptomatic venous thromboembolism during and after prophylaxis with enoxaparin: A multi-institutional cohort study of patients who underwent hip or knee arthroplasty. Canadian Collaborative Group. Arch Intern Med 158:873–878, 1998.

135. Wells PS, Lensing AW, Davidson BL, Prins MH, Hirsh J: Accuracy of ultrasound for the diagnosis of deep venous thrombosis in asymptomatic patients after orthopedic surgery. A meta-analysis. Ann Intern Med 122:47–53, 1995.

136. Horlocker TT, Wedel DJ, Benzon H, Brown DL, Enneking FK, et al: Regional anesthesia in the anticoagulated patient: Defining the risks (the second ASRA Consensus Conference on Neuraxial Anesthesia and Anticoagulation). Reg Anesth Pain Med 28:172–197, 2003.

137. Modig J: The role of lumbar epidural anaesthesia as antithrombotic prophylaxis in total hip replacement. Acta Chir Scand 151:589–594, 1985.

138. Capdevila X, Barthelet Y, Biboulet P, Ryckwaert Y, Rubenovitch J, d'Athis F: Effects of perioperative analgesic technique on the surgical outcome and duration of rehabilitation after major knee surgery. Anesthesiology 91:8–15, 1999.

139. Mauermann WJ, Shilling AM, Zuo Z: A comparison of neuraxial block versus general anesthesia for elective total hip replacement: A meta-analysis. Anesth Analg 103:1018–1025, 2006.

140. Botteman MF, Caprini J, Stephens JM, Nadipelli V, Bell CF, et al: Results of an economic model to assess the cost-effectiveness of enoxaparin, a low-molecular-weight heparin, versus warfarin for the prophylaxis of deep vein thrombosis and associated long-term complications in total hip replacement surgery in the United States. Clin Ther 24:1960–1986; discussion 1938, 2002.

141. Matzsch T: Thromboprophylaxis with low-molecular-weight heparin: Economic considerations. Haemostasis 30(suppl 2):141–145; discussion 128–129, 2000.

142. Tran AH, Lee G: Fondaparinux for prevention of venous thromboembolism in major orthopedic surgery. Ann Pharmacother 37:1632–1643, 2003.

143. Skedgel C, Goeree R, Pleasance S, Thompson K, O'Brien B, Anderson D: The cost-effectiveness of extended-duration antithrombotic prophylaxis after total hip arthroplasty. J Bone Joint Surg Am 89:819–828, 2007.

144. Dahl OE, Pleil AM: Investment in prolonged thromboprophylaxis with dalteparin improves clinical outcomes after hip replacement. J Thromb Haemost 1:896–906, 2003.

145. Eriksson BI, Borris LC, Friedman RJ, et al: Rivaroxaban versus enoxaparin for thromboprophylaxis after hip arthroplasty. N Engl J Med 26;358(26):2765–2775, 2008.

146. Lassen MR, Ageno W, Borris LC et al: Rivaroxaban verus enoxaparin for thromboprophylaxis after total knee arthroplasty. N Engl J Med Jun 26;358(26):2776–2786, 2008.

What Blood Conservation Techniques for Total Joint Arthroplasty Work?

STUART A. MCCLUSKEY, MD, PhD, FRCPC AND ATUL PRABHU, MD

In 1997, after the tainted blood issues of the 1980s, the Canadian Commission of Inquiry on the Blood Supply (The Krever Commission; more information is available online at: http://www.hc-sc.gc.ca/ahc-asc/activit/com/krever_e.html) recommended the promotion of the "appropriate use of, and alternatives to, blood components and blood products." Therefore, it is not a question of whether blood conservation should be considered, but rather which of the available modalities of blood conservation is effective, and moreover cost-effective, in joint arthroplasty.

The primary focus of blood conservation in joint arthroplasty, as well as the focus of this chapter, is on limiting the perioperative need for 1 or 2 units of allogeneic red blood cells (RBCs). Although, reducing the amount of blood lost and maintaining a higher hemoglobin concentration peri-operatively are similar objectives to avoiding an allogeneic blood transfusion, there is no clear evidence that there will be any effect on measurable patient outcomes.

It should be stressed that blood conservation is not limited to avoiding allogeneic blood utilization but also includes the appropriate utilization of blood and blood products. Simple rules to ordering and administering blood products should be established, published, and reinforced at every institution carrying out joint arthroplasty: (1) A transfusion guideline should be established (Table 81–1); (2) ordering of blood product should include the indication for its administration (e.g., transfuse 1 unit of RBCs for a hemoglobin concentration of 70 g/L), and (3) RBC units should be administered one unit at a time with the patient reassessed before a second unit is administered. Following these simple guidelines will improve the utilization of blood products and reduce unnecessary transfusions.

OPTIONS

Blood conservation includes preoperative, intraoperative and postoperative modalities. Preoperative modalities focus on the expansion of the RBC mass either ex vivo using preoperative autologous blood donation (PAD) or in vivo using iron supplementation and erythrocyte-stimulating agents (ESA) (e.g., Eprex, Ortho Biotech, Toronto, Ontario, Canada). Intraopera-

tive techniques focus on reducing the loss of RBCs or the reclamation of shed blood. Surgical technique and the strict attention to hemostasis is the single-most important factor for which there is no alternative. Other methods purported to reduce blood loss include controlled hypotension, acute normovolemic hemodilution (ANH), antifibrinolytic agents, and cell salvage. Postoperative blood conservation modalities include cell salvage, continued adherence to a transfusion guideline, and the careful management of hemostasis, keeping in mind the need for postoperative deep vein thrombosis prophylaxis (see Chapter 2).

EVIDENCE

Preoperative Autologous Donation

PAD is a method of expanding the RBC mass by removing blood for storage in the blood bank and allowing the patient to replace the sequestered RBCs before surgery. Although some protocols allow for blood collection from patients with anemia (hemoglobin concentration <130 g/L) and allow for blood collection up to 48 hours before surgery, this practice should be avoided because the patient is unlikely to replace the sequestered RBCs before surgery, and the risk for an allogeneic blood transfusion will be unchanged at best.

The efficacy of PAD in reducing patient exposure to allogeneic blood has been demonstrated in numerous randomized clinical trials in several operative settings.[1] This evidence is supported by controlled observational trials, but the overall level of evidence remains poor because there are no blinded trials.[1]

In joint arthroplasty, the evidence in support of PAD is less convincing (Figs. 81–1[2–4] and 81–2[5–11]). Some authors have concluded that there is no role for PAD in joint arthroplasty, and if the entire surgical population were considered candidates for PAD, then the evidence would support this contention.[1] However, for patients who are at increased risk for a blood transfusion (e.g., revision surgery, small body habitus [<70 kg]) and are not anemic (i.e., patient capable of regenerating RBC mass after donation), PAD may be a viable blood conservation modality. It should be the role of a perioperative blood conservation program to identify appropriate patients for PAD using an up-to-date database to evaluate its use.

TABLE 81–1. Guideline for Red Blood Cell Transfusion Based on Hemoglobin Concentration

HEMOGLOBIN CONCENTRATION (G/L)	TRANSFUSION RECOMMENDATION
>100	Transfusion required only in exceptional circumstances
70–100	Transfusion required only if there are signs and symptoms of impaired oxygen delivery or if patient is at high risk*
<70	Likely be appropriate
<60	Transfusion highly recommended

Level III evidence.

*Patients at high risk include those with known coronary artery or valvular hearts disease, previous cerebral vascular event, or poor oxygenation.

Preoperative Iron and Erythropoietin Therapy

The incidence of preoperative anemia in patients scheduled for the total arthroplasty is between 20% and 35%.[12,13] The causative factor of this anemia is multifactorial, but the two most common causes are iron deficiency anemia and anemia of chronic disease. Importantly, preoperative anemia is the single-most treatable risk factor for a blood transfusion associated with joint arthroplasty surgery.[12] Iron supplementation and the use of erythropoietin (Epo) are the primary modes of therapy of preoperative anemia.

The incidence of preoperative iron deficiency anemia is unknown, but elderly patients have a number of risk factors for iron deficiency including use of nonsteroidal anti-inflammatory drugs and poor diet. Iron deficiency anemia is a hypochromic, microcytic anemia, and the RBC mean cell volume (MCV) is a good predictor for response to iron supplementation.[14] For anemia (hemoglobin concentration <120 g/L) and MCV less than 80 fL, a 4-week course of supplemental iron results in an 11- to 12-g/L increase in hemoglobin concentration.[14] In contrast, anemia with an MCV greater than 90 fL does not respond to iron supplementation alone.[14]

The routine use of perioperative supplemental iron therapy is controversial in that it has little effect on blood transfusion.[15,16] However, in patients in whom erythropoiesis is either stimulated by PAD or recombinant Epo, iron supplementation is recommended. The source of iron is arguably unimportant as long as the goal is to add approximately 100 mg elemental iron to the daily diet. In fact, dietary heme-iron in red meat, poultry, and fish is more readily absorbed than formulated dietary supplements. Other sources of iron include plant food such as lentils and beans. If, however, oral iron absorption is poor and iron supplementation is still required, intravenous iron sucrose is a safe and effective alternative.[17,18] Iron sucrose is no more effective than oral iron preparations in increasing the RBC mass.[19,20]

Epo is a naturally-occurring hormone secreted by the kidneys in response to low partial pressure of oxygen. Epo stimulates effective erythropoiesis only if there are adequate iron stores, and the use of Epo should be combined with supplemental iron. The efficacy of preoperative Epo in total joint arthroplasty (TJA) has been demonstrated in double-blind, randomized, controlled trials, increasing preoperative hemoglobin concentration by 15 g/L whereas reducing the frequency of RBC transfusion by 50%.[21] In a systematic review of the literature, Laupacis and colleagues[22] found that the overall odds ratio of RBC transfusion in patients who received Epo was 0.36 (95% confidence interval [CI], 0.24–0.56).[22]

In addition, several studies have evaluated the use of Epo in the clinical setting and confirmed it effectiveness in reducing the exposure of patient to allogeneic

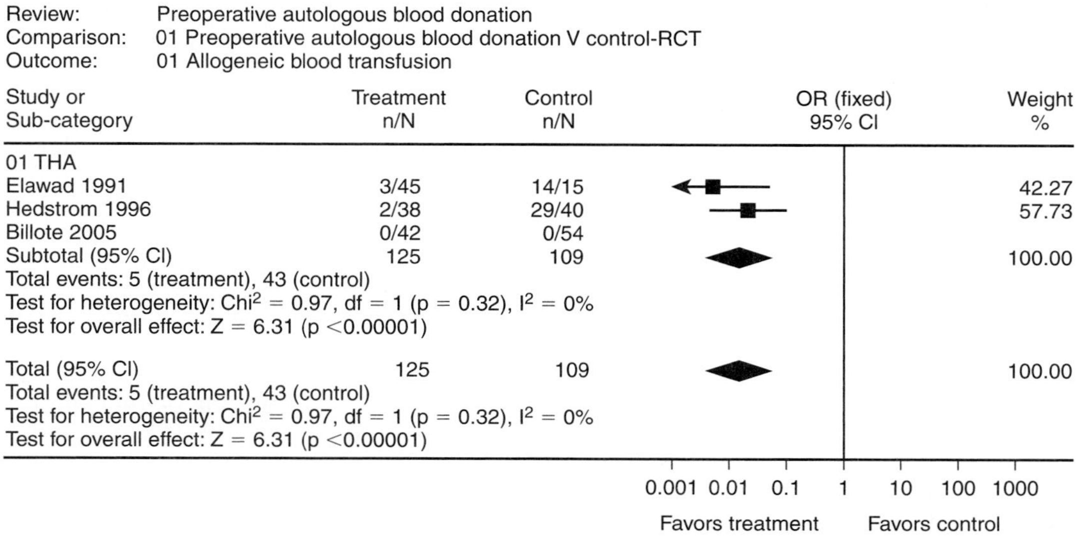

Review: Preoperative autologous blood donation
Comparison: 01 Preoperative autologous blood donation V control-RCT
Outcome: 01 Allogeneic blood transfusion

Study or Sub-category	Treatment n/N	Control n/N	OR (fixed) 95% CI	Weight %
01 THA				
Elawad 1991	3/45	14/15		42.27
Hedstrom 1996	2/38	29/40		57.73
Billote 2005	0/42	0/54		
Subtotal (95% CI)	125	109		100.00
Total events: 5 (treatment), 43 (control)				
Test for heterogeneity: Chi² = 0.97, df = 1 (p = 0.32), I² = 0%				
Test for overall effect: Z = 6.31 (p <0.00001)				
Total (95% CI)	125	109		100.00
Total events: 5 (treatment), 43 (control)				
Test for heterogeneity: Chi² = 0.97, df = 1 (p = 0.32), I² = 0%				
Test for overall effect: Z = 6.31 (p <0.00001)				

0.001   0.01   0.1   1   10   100   1000

Favors treatment   Favors control

FIGURE 81–1. Randomized, controlled trials of preoperative autologous blood donation (PAD) in joint arthroplasty. Exposure to allogeneic red blood cell transfusion. CI, confidence interval; OR, odds ratio; THA, total hip arthroplasty.

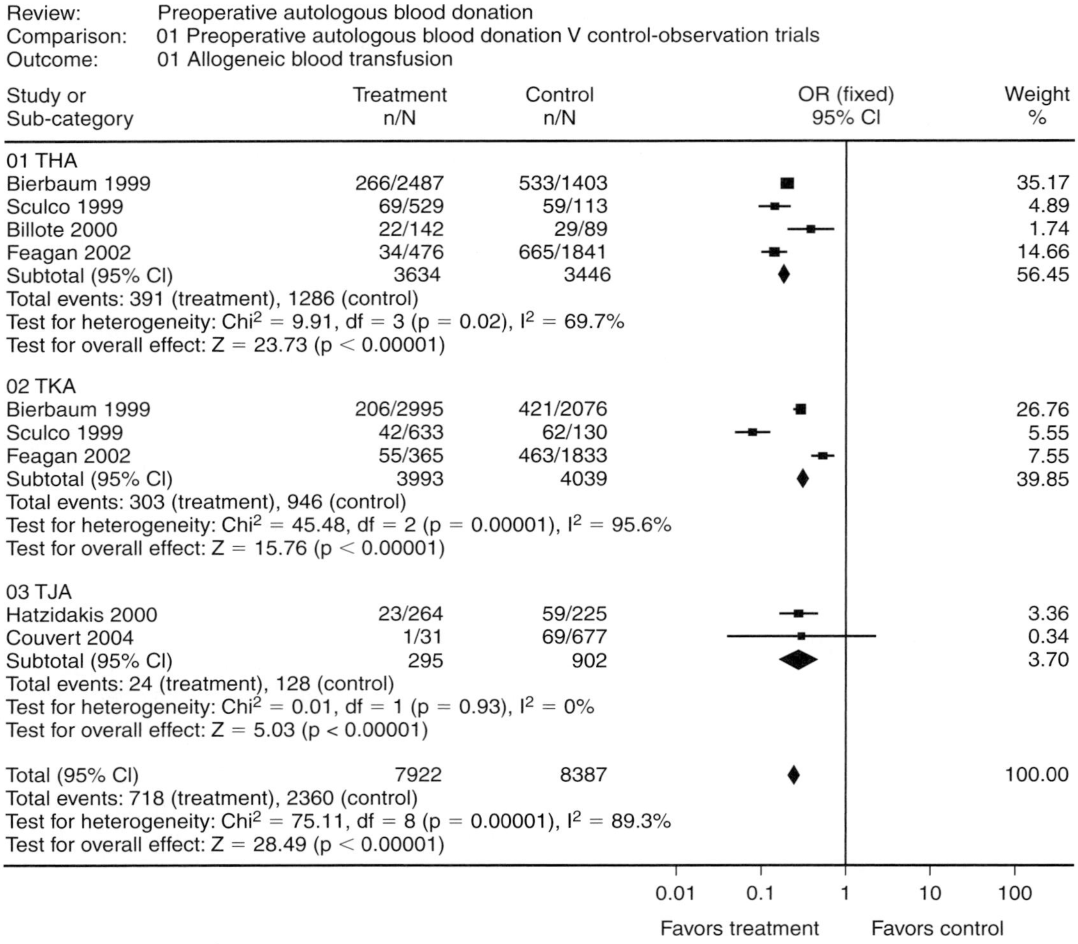

Review: Preoperative autologous blood donation
Comparison: 01 Preoperative autologous blood donation V control-observation trials
Outcome: 01 Allogeneic blood transfusion

Study or Sub-category	Treatment n/N	Control n/N	OR (fixed) 95% CI	Weight %
01 THA				
Bierbaum 1999	266/2487	533/1403		35.17
Sculco 1999	69/529	59/113		4.89
Billote 2000	22/142	29/89		1.74
Feagan 2002	34/476	665/1841		14.66
Subtotal (95% CI)	3634	3446		56.45

Total events: 391 (treatment), 1286 (control)
Test for heterogeneity: Chi^2 = 9.91, df = 3 (p = 0.02), I^2 = 69.7%
Test for overall effect: Z = 23.73 (p < 0.00001)

02 TKA				
Bierbaum 1999	206/2995	421/2076		26.76
Sculco 1999	42/633	62/130		5.55
Feagan 2002	55/365	463/1833		7.55
Subtotal (95% CI)	3993	4039		39.85

Total events: 303 (treatment), 946 (control)
Test for heterogeneity: Chi^2 = 45.48, df = 2 (p = 0.00001), I^2 = 95.6%
Test for overall effect: Z = 15.76 (p < 0.00001)

03 TJA				
Hatzidakis 2000	23/264	59/225		3.36
Couvert 2004	1/31	69/677		0.34
Subtotal (95% CI)	295	902		3.70

Total events: 24 (treatment), 128 (control)
Test for heterogeneity: Chi^2 = 0.01, df = 1 (p = 0.93), I^2 = 0%
Test for overall effect: Z = 5.03 (p < 0.00001)

Total (95% CI)	7922	8387		100.00

Total events: 718 (treatment), 2360 (control)
Test for heterogeneity: Chi^2 = 75.11, df = 8 (p = 0.00001), I^2 = 89.3%
Test for overall effect: Z = 28.49 (p < 0.00001)

```
        0.01   0.1    1    10   100
     Favors treatment   Favors control
```

FIGURE 81–2. Observational trials of preoperative autologous blood donation (PAD) in joint arthroplasty. Exposure to allogeneic red blood cell transfusion. CI, confidence interval; OR, odds ratio; THA, total hip arthroplasty; TJA, total joint arthroplasty; TKA, total knee arthroplasty.

blood transfusions.[13,23,24] In a clinical observation trial, Karkouti and colleagues[13] demonstrated a reduction in transfusion rates for patients with anemia undergoing TJA from 56.1% to 16.4% when treated before surgery with Epo, and the adjusted odds ratio of RBC transfusion in the Epo group was 0.33 (95% CI, 0.21–0.49).[13]

Although Epo is undeniably an effective therapy in reducing the risk for an allogeneic blood transfusion, particularly for the patient with anemia, there are two caveats to its routine use that should be considered. First, it remains an expensive therapy ($500 [Canadian currency] per injection), and second, concerns about the safety of Epo have been identified. The first safety concern is that the use of an ESA can increased the risk for thromboembolic events. In a large ($N = 681$), randomized, control trial, patients with anemia who received Eprex before spinal surgery had a significantly greater rate of thromboembolic events compared with patients given placebo (8.2% vs. 4.1%; more information is available online at: http://download.veritas-medicine.com/PDF/CR004621_CSR.pdf). The second and perhaps more worrisome safety concern is the increased risk for serious adverse events and death when they are used to treat anemia in patients with

cancer.[25] These concerns led the U.S. Food and Drug Administration (FDA) to enhance its safety warnings for Epo and other ESAs (more information is available online at: http://www.fda.gov/cder/drug/infopage/RHE/default.htm). Patients should be informed of these newly recognized safety concerns, and the cautious use of ESA should be recommended. It will likely be some time before the importance of these safety concerns for patients with TJA can be clarified.

Intraoperative Acute Normovolemic Hemodilution

For ANH, autologous whole blood is sequestered in the operating room, and the intravascular volume is replaced with crystalloid or colloid to maintain normovolemia. As a result, the blood lost during surgery is diluted, and the amount of hemoglobin or number of RBCs lost is reduced. The sequestered whole blood is retransfused if a transfusion trigger is met or the case is completed.

Several meta-analyses have considered the efficacy of ANH, including trials from various surgical procedures.[1,26,27] Conclusions from these reviews are as follows: (1) The effectiveness of ANH is dependent of the number of units sequestered and the degree of hemodilution tolerated; (2) the trials included in the review were not blinded, resulting in an overestimated effect size; and (3) when the outcome decision (i.e., allogeneic blood transfusion) was considered under a transfusion protocol, the effect size was reduced.

Randomized, controlled trials conducted in the joint arthroplasty are presented in Figure 81–3.[28–32] Oishi and colleagues[30] utilized ANH and intraoperative cell salvage, and compared the rate of any transfusion, allogeneic or autologous. ANH is of minimal benefit in total knee arthroplasty (TKA) when a tourniquet is used because most blood loss occurs after the tourniquet is deflated at a time when the sequestered blood is retransfused. For total hip arthroplasty (THA), a prolonged severe anemia would be required to accomplish sufficient hemodilution to reduce the risk for an allogeneic blood transfusion, and this has perioperative risk in and of itself. Therefore, the evidence does not support the routine use of ANH because it offers only limited benefit in terms of blood conservation and has an unproven safety profile.

Intraoperative Antifibrinolytics

Surgical stress, limb trauma, and the application of a tourniquet can activate fibrinolysis and increase blood loss. Several systematic reviews and meta-analyses have focused on the use of antifibrinolytics in joint arthroplasty (Table 81–2).[33–36] While these reviews conclude that antifibrinolytics reduce blood loss and allogeneic blood transfusion, there are caveats that should not be overlooked before tranexamic acid or aprotinin are used in clinical practice. The first consideration relates to the law of diminishing returns. Zufferey and coworkers[36] point to a direct relation between transfusion rate and effect size such that the number needed to treat to avoid an allogeneic blood transfusion decreases as baseline transfusion rate increases.[36] Therefore, the benefit of antifibrinolytics will be reduced as transfusion rates are reduced, and many of the studies had greater transfusion rates than are found currently.

The second caveat has to do with the different dosing regimens used in the trials included in these systematic reviews. Although the high-dose aprotinin and tranexamic acid (Cyklokapron) treatments would seem to be effective, the optimal dose has not been established. In addition, several observational studies and a meta-analysis of randomized, controlled trials have shown that aprotinin is associated with increased risk for renal dysfunction.[37–39] These findings led the FDA to restrict the indications for aprotinin to high-risk coronary artery bypass surgery (more information is available at: http://www.fda.gov/bbs/topics/NEWS/2006/NEW01529.html). Tranexamic acid has been shown to significantly reduce allogeneic blood exposure in joint arthroplasty, but its benefit may be limited to settings associated with high blood loss.[33–36] Importantly, the adverse-effect profile or risks for these drugs has not been established, making it difficult to establish a risk/benefit estimate.

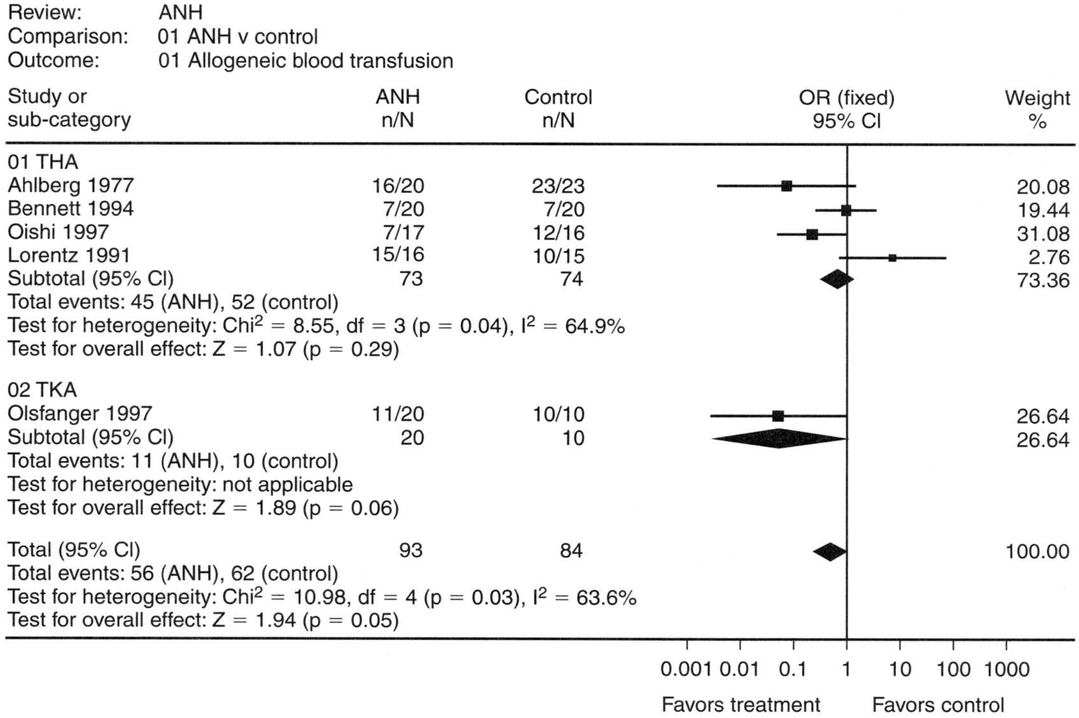

Review: ANH
Comparison: 01 ANH v control
Outcome: 01 Allogeneic blood transfusion

Study or sub-category	ANH n/N	Control n/N	OR (fixed) 95% CI	Weight %
01 THA				
Ahlberg 1977	16/20	23/23		20.08
Bennett 1994	7/20	7/20		19.44
Oishi 1997	7/17	12/16		31.08
Lorentz 1991	15/16	10/15		2.76
Subtotal (95% CI)	73	74		73.36
Total events: 45 (ANH), 52 (control)				
Test for heterogeneity: Chi² = 8.55, df = 3 (p = 0.04), I² = 64.9%				
Test for overall effect: Z = 1.07 (p = 0.29)				
02 TKA				
Olsfanger 1997	11/20	10/10		26.64
Subtotal (95% CI)	20	10		26.64
Total events: 11 (ANH), 10 (control)				
Test for heterogeneity: not applicable				
Test for overall effect: Z = 1.89 (p = 0.06)				
Total (95% CI)	93	84		100.00
Total events: 56 (ANH), 62 (control)				
Test for heterogeneity: Chi² = 10.98, df = 4 (p = 0.03), I² = 63.6%				
Test for overall effect: Z = 1.94 (p = 0.05)				

0.001 0.01 0.1 1 10 100 1000

Favors treatment   Favors control

FIGURE 81–3. Randomized trials of acute normovolemic hemodilution (ANH) in joint arthroplasty. Exposure to allogeneic red blood cell transfusion. CI, confidence interval; OR, odds ratio; THA, total hip arthroplasty; TKA, total knee arthroplasty.

TABLE 81–2. Meta-analytic Results for the Allogeneic Transfusion Rates for Patient Undergoing Joint Arthroplasty Surgery Comparing the Effects of Antifibrinolytic with Placebo

REVIEW (YEAR OF PUBLICATION)	SURGERY	TREATMENT (n/N)	PLACEBO (n/N)	OR (95% CI)
Ho and Ismail (2003)[33]	TKA, THA	TA/AP: 99/286	145/237	0.16 (0.09–0.26)
Cid and Lozano (2005)[34]	TKA	TA: 88/255	135/202	0.10 (0.06–0.18)
Gill and Rosenstein (2006)[35]	THA	TA/AP		Reduces
Zufferey et al. (2006)[36]	THA/THA	AP: 83/375	87/196	0.42 (0.27–0.66)
		TA: 112/357	185/305	0.18 (0.09–0.26)

AP, aprotinin; CI, confidence interval; OR, odds ratio; TA, tranexamic acid; THA, total hip arthroplasty; TKA, total knee arthroplasty.

INTRAOPERATIVE AND POSTOPERATIVE CELL SALVAGE

Cell salvage can be accomplished producing either a washed or filtered RBC product and can continue into the postoperative period for up to 6 hours by reclaiming shed blood from surgical drains. The inflammatory response to retransfusion of filtered blood has been found to be greater than the response to a washed RBC product, but the consequence of this difference has not been identified.[40–42]

Although not supported by clinical evidence, drains are used in joint arthroplasty surgery to reduce hematoma formation and the incidence of wound infection. Some evidence would suggest that these benefits are not realized, and that drain placement may increase postoperative blood loss.[43,44] If a drain is placed, there is evidence from randomized, controlled trails, particularly in TKA, that cell salvage can effectively reduce the need for an allogeneic blood transfusion (Fig. 81–4).[2,45–49]

Intraoperative cell salvage can be utilized in THA; however, there are no randomized, control trials to support its general use. In revision THA, the use of cell salvage is reported in retrospective cohort studies to reduce both net perioperative blood loss[50] and number of allogeneic blood transfusions.[51] This Level III evidence is not sufficient to recommend the routine use of cell salvage in THA.

AREAS OF UNCERTAINTY

Levels of Evidence

PAD, ANH, and cell salvage have never been compared using blinded, randomized, controlled trials, and we must rely on open-labeled trails, which can

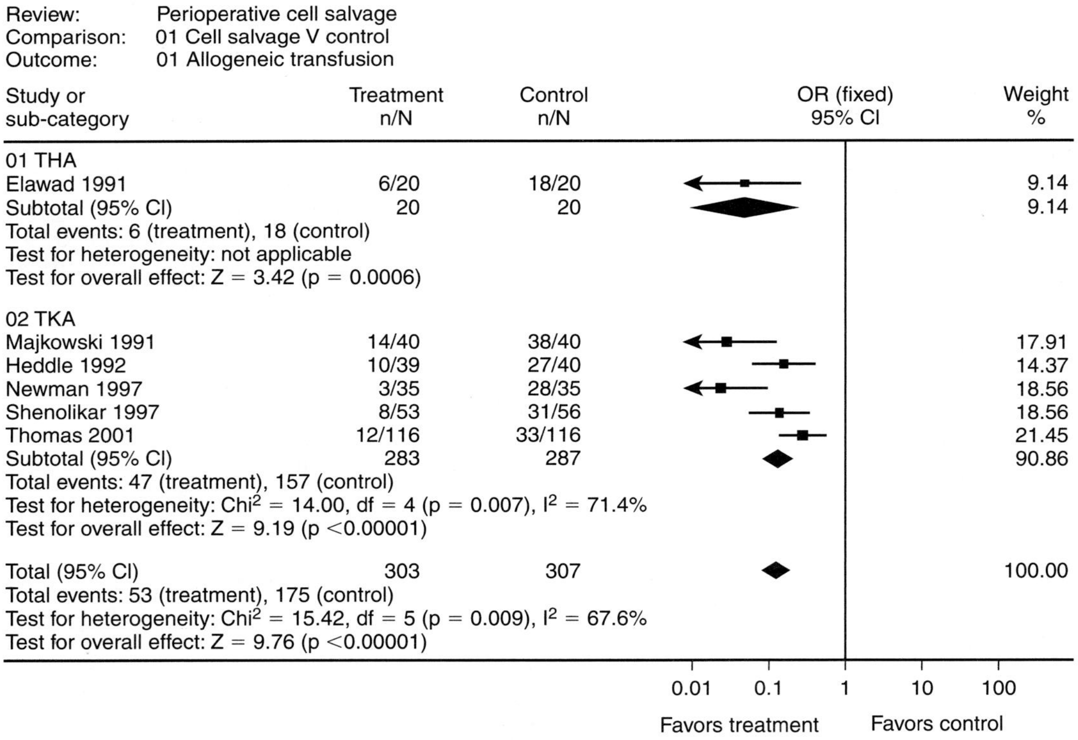

Review: Perioperative cell salvage
Comparison: 01 Cell salvage V control
Outcome: 01 Allogeneic transfusion

Study or sub-category	Treatment n/N	Control n/N	OR (fixed) 95% CI	Weight %
01 THA				
Elawad 1991	6/20	18/20		9.14
Subtotal (95% CI)	20	20		9.14
Total events: 6 (treatment), 18 (control)				
Test for heterogeneity: not applicable				
Test for overall effect: Z = 3.42 (p = 0.0006)				
02 TKA				
Majkowski 1991	14/40	38/40		17.91
Heddle 1992	10/39	27/40		14.37
Newman 1997	3/35	28/35		18.56
Shenolikar 1997	8/53	31/56		18.56
Thomas 2001	12/116	33/116		21.45
Subtotal (95% CI)	283	287		90.86
Total events: 47 (treatment), 157 (control)				
Test for heterogeneity: Chi² = 14.00, df = 4 (p = 0.007), I² = 71.4%				
Test for overall effect: Z = 9.19 (p <0.00001)				
Total (95% CI)	303	307		100.00
Total events: 53 (treatment), 175 (control)				
Test for heterogeneity: Chi² = 15.42, df = 5 (p = 0.009), I² = 67.6%				
Test for overall effect: Z = 9.76 (p <0.00001)				

0.01   0.1   1   10   100

Favors treatment   Favors control

FIGURE 81–4. Randomized, control trials of postoperative cell salvage in joint arthroplasty surgery. Exposure to allogeneic red blood cell transfusion. CI, confidence interval; OR, odds ratio; THA, total hip arthroplasty; TKA, total knee arthroplasty.

overestimate the effect size. Some studies are in the planning stage to overcome this shortfall, but in the meantime, the use of these modalities should be limited to patients at high risk for a blood transfusion with surgery.

Comparison of Blood Conservation Modalities

Numerous trials compare the efficacy of one blood conservation modality with another (e.g., PAD compared with ANH[52] or PAD with perioperative cell salvage).[53,54] These comparisons would be valuable if the efficacy of at least one modality was well established, but as described earlier, this is not the case. Trials comparing different as yet unproven modalities were not considered in this chapter unless a placebo group was included.

Combining Blood Conservation

It would seem logical that if one modality of blood conservation was effective, then adding a second modality would be more effective. However, this should be done with caution because there would be an obvious reduction in cost-effectiveness and a potential increase in risk for adverse effects without known benefit.

Cost Benefit

One of the limitations of any cost-effective analysis is the ability to include all the relevant costs and similarly all the potential cost savings. For some

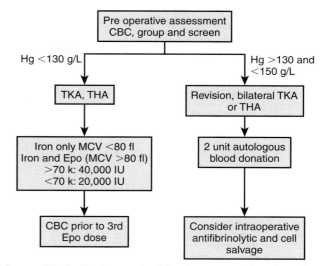

FIGURE 81–5. Perioperative blood conservation algorithm for patients undergoing joint arthroplasty. CBC, complete blood count; Epo, erythropoietin; Hb, hemoglobin concentration; MCV, mean cell volume; THA, total hip arthroplasty; TKA, total knee arthroplasty.

patients, avoiding a blood transfusion is an important objective, but one that is usually superseded by the surgical outcome. Clear evidence that avoiding a blood transfusion or avoiding moderate anemia (hemoglobin concentration, 70–90 g/L) improves patient outcome has yet to be definitively demonstrated in joint arthroplasty surgery.

RECOMMENDATIONS

Effective perioperative blood conservation is a multidisciplinary perioperative management concern. It requires the cooperation of orthopedic surgery with transfusion medicine, the providers of blood products, anesthesiology, the managers of perioperative hemodynamics, fluid resuscitation and hemostasis, and perioperative nursing to identify patients at risk for a blood transfusion. Patients need to be informed of the perioperative risk for a blood transfusion and the strategies available to reduce this risk. If the cost-effectiveness of blood conservation is to be assessed, efforts for blood conservation need to look beyond the number of units of blood transfused to the perioperative patient outcome.

Until evidence supports more aggressive perioperative blood conservation management, we recommend the restricted management outline in Figure 81–5 and Table 81–3. Iron and Epo therapy for moderate preoperative anemia and PAD for patients at high risk for an allogeneic blood transfusion with hemoglobin concentration in the reference range are recommended. Evidence from observational[11,13] and randomized[21,22] trials support a program approach to perioperative blood conservation, but each program should be tailored to its institution using site-specific data to guide the utilization of specific interventions.

TABLE 81–3. Summary of Recommendations

STRATEGY	RECOMMENDATIONS	LEVEL OF EVIDENCE/GRADE OF RECOMMENDATION	REFERENCES
Preoperative autologous blood donation	Not routinely recommended	B	1–11
Acute normovolemic hemodilution	Not recommended	B	28–32
Cell salvage	Notrecommended	B	2, 43–49
Preoperative iron	Recommended	B	15–19
Preoperativeerythropoietin	Recommended	A	13, 22–24, 36
Tranexamic acid	Not routinely recommended	B	33–36
Aprotinin	Not recommended	B	33, 35, 36

REFERENCES

1. Carless P, Moxey A, O'Connell D, et al: Autologous transfusion techniques: A systematic review of their efficacy. Transfus Med 14:123–144, 2004.
2. Elawad AA, Ohlin AK, Berntorp E, et al: Intraoperative autotransfusion in primary hip arthroplasty. A randomized comparison with homologous blood. Acta Orthop Scand 62:557–562, 1991.
3. Hedstrom M, Flordal PA, Ahl T, et al: Autologous blood transfusion in hip replacement. No effect on blood loss but less increase of plasminogen activator inhibitor in a randomized series of 80 patients. Acta Orthop Scand 67:317–320, 1996.
4. Billote DB, Glisson SN, Green D, et al: A prospective, randomized study of preoperative autologous donation for hip replacement surgery. J Bone Joint Surg Am 84-A:1299–1304, 2002.
5. Bierbaum BE, Callaghan JJ, Galante JO, et al: An analysis of blood management in patients having a total hip or knee arthroplasty. J Bone Joint Surg Am 81:2–10, 1999.
6. Sculco TP, Gallina J: Blood management experience: Relationship between autologous blood donation and transfusion in orthopedic surgery. Orthopedics 22(suppl):S129–S134, 1999.
7. Billote DB, Glisson SN, Green D, et al: Efficacy of preoperative autologous blood donation: Analysis of blood loss and transfusion practice in total hip replacement. J Clin Anesth 12:537–542, 2000.
8. Feagan BG, Wong CJ, Johnston WC, et al: Transfusion practices for elective orthopedic surgery. CMAJ 166:310–314, 2002.
9. Woolson ST, Pottorff G: Use of preoperatively deposited autologous blood for total knee replacement. Orthopedics 16:137–141, 1993.
10. Hatzidakis AM, Mendlick RM, Mckillip T, et al: Preoperative autologous donation for total joint arthroplasty: An analysis of risk factors for allogenic transfusion. J Bone Joint Surg Am 82:89–100, 2000.
11. Couvret C, Laffon M, Baud A, et al: A restrictive use of both autologous donation and recombinant human erythropoietin is an efficient policy for primary total hip or knee arthroplasty. Anesth Analg 99:262–271, 2004.
12. Shander A, Knight K, Thurer R, et al: Prevalence and outcomes of anemia in surgery: A systematic review of the literature. Am J Med 116(suppl 7A):58S–69S, 2004.
13. Karkouti K, Mccluskey SA, Evans L, et al: Erythropoietin is an effective clinical modality for reducing RBC transfusion in joint surgery. Can J Anaesth 52:362–368, 2005.
14. Andrews CM, Lane DW, Bradley JG: Iron pre-load for major joint replacement. Transfus Med 7:281–286, 1997.
15. Kasper SM, Ellering J, Stachwitz P, et al: All adverse events in autologous blood donors with cardiac disease are not necessarily caused by blood donation. Transfusion 38:669–673, 1998.
16. Sutton PM, Cresswell T, Livesey JP, et al: Treatment of anaemia after joint replacement. a double-blind, randomised, controlled trial of ferrous sulphate versus placebo. J Bone Joint Surg Br 86:31–33, 2004.
17. Faich G, Strobos J: Sodium ferric gluconate complex in sucrose: Safer intravenous iron therapy than iron dextrans. Am J Kidney Dis 33:464–470, 1999.
18. Reed J, Charytan C, Yee J: The safety of intravenous iron sucrose use in the elderly patient. Consult Pharm 22:230–238, 2007.
19. Miller HJ, Hu J, Valentine JK, et al: Efficacy and tolerability of intravenous ferric gluconate in the treatment of iron deficiency anemia in patients without kidney disease. Arch Intern Med 167:1327–1328, 2007.
20. Weisbach V, Skoda P, Rippel R, et al: Oral or intravenous iron as an adjuvant to autologous blood donation in elective surgery: A randomized controlled study. Transfusion 39:465–472, 1999.
21. Feagan BG, Wong CJ, Kirkley A, et al: Erythropoietin with iron supplementation to prevent allogeneic blood transfusion in total hip arthroplasty. A randomized, controlled trial. Ann Intern Med 133:845–854, 2000.
22. Laupacis A, Feagan B, Wong C: Effectiveness of perioperative recombinant human erythropoietin in elective hip replacement. COPES Study Group. Lancet 342:378, 1993.
23. Rosencher N, Poisson D, Albi A, et al: Two injections of erythropoietin correct moderate anemia in most patients awaiting orthopedic surgery. Can J Anaesth 52:160–165, 2005.
24. Wong CJ, Vandervoort MK, Vandervoort SL, et al: A cluster-randomized controlled trial of a blood conservation algorithm in patients undergoing total hip arthroplasty. Transfusion 47:832–841, 2007.
25. Burton A: Is it all over for erythropoietin? Lancet Oncol 8:285, 2007.
26. Bryson GL, Laupacis A, Wells GA: Does acute normovolemic hemodilution reduce perioperative allogeneic transfusion? A meta-analysis. The International Study of Perioperative Transfusion. Anesth Analg 86:9–15, 1998.
27. Segal JB, Blasco-Colmenares E, Norris EJ, et al: Preoperative acute normovolemic hemodilution: A meta-analysis. Transfusion 44:632–644, 2004.
28. Ahlberg A, Nillius A, Rosberg B, et al: Preoperative normovolemic hemodilution in total hip arthroplasty. A clinical study. Acta Chir Scand 143:407–411, 1977.
29. Bennett SR: Perioperative autologous blood transfusion in elective total hip prosthesis operations. Ann R Coll Surg Engl 76:95–98, 1994.
30. Oishi CS, D'Lima DD, Morris BA, et al: Hemodilution with other blood reinfusion techniques in total hip arthroplasty. Clin Orthop Relat Res 132–139, 1997.
31. Lorentz A, Osswald PM, Schilling M, et al: [A comparison of autologous transfusion procedures in hip surgery]. Anaesthesist 40:205–213, 1991.
32. Olsfanger D, Fredman B, Goldstein B, et al: Acute normovolaemic haemodilution decreases postoperative allogeneic blood transfusion after total knee replacement. Br J Anaesth 79:317–321, 1997.
33. Ho KM, Ismail H: Use of intravenous tranexamic acid to reduce allogeneic blood transfusion in total hip and knee arthroplasty: A meta-analysis. Anaesth Intensive Care 31:529–537, 2003.

34. Cid J, Lozano M: Tranexamic acid reduces allogeneic red cell transfusions in patients undergoing total knee arthroplasty: Results of a meta-analysis of randomized controlled trials. Transfusion 45:1302–1307, 2005.

35. Gill JB, Rosenstein A: The use of antifibrinolytic agents in total hip arthroplasty: A meta-analysis. J Arthroplasty 21:869–873, 2006.

36. Zufferey P, Merquiol F, Laporte S, et al: Do antifibrinolytics reduce allogeneic blood transfusion in orthopedic surgery? Anesthesiology 105:1034–1046, 2006.

37. Karkouti K, Beattie WS, Dattilo KM, et al: A propensity score case-control comparison of aprotinin and tranexamic acid in high-transfusion-risk cardiac surgery. Transfusion 46:327–338, 2006.

38. Mangano DT, Tudor IC, Dietzel C: The risk associated with aprotinin in cardiac surgery. N Engl J Med 354:353–365, 2006.

39. Brown JR, Birkmeyer NJ, O'Connor GT: Meta-analysis comparing the effectiveness and adverse outcomes of antifibrinolytic agents in cardiac surgery. Circulation 115:2801–2813, 2007.

40. Tylman M, Bengtson JP, Avall A, et al: Release of interleukin-10 by reinfusion of salvaged blood after knee arthroplasty. Intensive Care Med 27:1379–1384, 2001.

41. Bottner F, Sheth N, Chimento GF, et al: Cytokine levels after transfusion of washed wound drainage in total knee arthroplasty: A randomized trial comparing autologous blood and washed wound drainage. J Knee Surg 16:93–97, 2003.

42. Cheng SC, Hung TSL, Tse PYT: Investigation of the use of drained blood reinfusion after total knee arthroplasty: A prospective randomised controlled study. J Orthop Surg (Hong Kong) 13:120–124, 2005.

43. Esler CNA, Blakeway C, Fiddian NJ: The use of a closed-suction drain in total knee arthroplasty. A prospective, randomised study. J Bone Joint Surg Br 85:215–217, 2003.

44. Tsumara N, Yoshiya S, Chin T, et al: A prospective comparison of clamping the drain or post-operative salvage of blood in reducing blood loss after total knee arthroplasty. J Bone Joint Surg Br 88:49–53, 2006.

45. Majkowski RS, Currie IC, Newman JH: Postoperative collection and reinfusion of autologous blood in total knee arthroplasty. Ann R Coll Surg Engl 73:381–384, 1991.

46. Heddle NM, Brox WT, Klama LN, et al: A randomized trial on the efficacy of an autologous blood drainage and transfusion device in patients undergoing elective knee arthroplasty. Transfusion 32:742–746, 1992.

47. Newman JH, Bowers M, Murphy J: The clinical advantages of autologous transfusion. A randomized, controlled study after knee replacement. J Bone Joint Surg Br 79:630–632, 1997.

48. Shenolikar A, Wareham K, Newington D, et al: Cell salvage auto transfusion in total knee replacement surgery. Transfus Med 7:277–280, 1997.

49. Thomas D, Wareham K, Cohen D, et al: Autologous blood transfusion in total knee replacement surgery. Br J Anaesth 86:669–673, 2001.

50. Zarin J, Grosvenor D, Schurman D, et al: Efficacy of intraoperative blood collection and reinfusion in revision total hip arthroplasty. J Bone Joint Surg Am 85-A:2147–2151, 2003.

51. Bridgens JP, Evans CR, Dobson PM, et al: Intraoperative red blood-cell salvage in revision hip surgery. A case-matched study. J Bone Joint Surg Am 89:270–275, 2007.

52. Goodnough LT, Despotis GJ, Merkel K, et al: A randomized trial comparing acute normovolemic hemodilution and preoperative autologous blood donation in total hip arthroplasty. Transfusion 40:1054–1057, 2000.

53. Goodnough LT, Monk TG, Despotis GJ, et al: A randomized trial of acute normovolemic hemodilution compared to preoperative autologous blood donation in total knee arthroplasty. Vox Sang 77:11–16, 1999.

54. Woolson ST, Wall WW: Autologous blood transfusion after total knee arthroplasty: A randomized, prospective study comparing predonated and postoperative salvage blood. J Arthroplasty 18:243–249, 2003.

What Is the Role of Antibiotic Cement in Total Joint Replacement?

J. Roderick Davey, MD, FRCSC and Rajiv Gandhi, MD, FRCSC

Deep wound infection after total joint arthroplasty can be a devastating complication for the patient. Data from the Swedish Knee Registry demonstrates a deep infection rate after total knee arthroplasty (TKA) of 1.7% in patients with osteoarthrosis and 4.4% in patients with rheumatoid arthritis.[1] Data from other large series of patients have shown infection rates to be between 0.2% to 1%.[2–4] Antibiotic-loaded bone cement (ALBC) is a well-accepted adjunct in the treatment of an established infection. However, its role in the prevention of infection remains controversial because of issues regarding drug resistance, sensitivity, efficacy, and cost.

When considering whether to use ALBC during joint arthroplasty, it is important to define whether the intended use is for prophylaxis or treatment of infection, primary or revision joint arthroplasty, and whether there are specific high-risk patients for whom ALBC would be beneficial.

BACKGROUND

For an antibiotic to be effective when mixed with methylmethacrylate, the preparation must be thermally stable to withstand the heat of polymerization. The antibiotic must be water soluble so that it can diffuse into surrounding tissues and have a bactericidal effect at the tissue levels attained. In addition, it must be released gradually over time.

The course and amount of antibiotic that is released from the cement depends on the porosity and the overall surface area of the bone cement exposed. Antibiotic is released from the surface of the cement, and also from cracks and voids in the cement.[5,6]

Palacos (Zimmer, Warsaw, IN, USA) bone cement has been shown to have greater elution levels than other types of bone cement.[7,8] This difference is attributed to the increased porosity of Palacos cement. Although the majority of the antibiotic release occurs in the first 9 weeks, late fracture of the cement mantle can liberate substantial levels of antibiotic many years after implantation.[9,10]

Commercially prepared antibiotic cement may be superior to cement in which antibiotics are mixed intraoperatively. Elution of gentamicin and tobramycin from surgeon-mixed Simplex (Stryker, Mahwah, NJ, USA) or Palacos beads compared with elution from commercially prepared gentamicin-PMMA (Septopal,

Biomet, Warsaw, IN, USA) beads showed that more total antibiotic was released from the latter and was maintained at greater concentrations than it was in the cement to which antibiotics were mixed by hand.[11]

Some antibiotics elute better from bone cement than others.[12] A study of antibiotic elution from Simplex bone cement examined cefazolin (4.5 g per 40 g cement powder), ciprofloxacin (6 g per 40 g powder), clindamycin (6 g per 40 g powder), ticarcillin (12 g per 40 g powder), tobramycin (9.8 g per 40 g powder), and vancomycin (4 g per 40 g powder). The authors conclude that clindamycin, vancomycin, and tobramycin displayed the best elution characteristics into bone and granulation tissue.[13]

The use of local antibiotic delivery from ALBC in the treatment of musculoskeletal infection is well established.[14–17] It has been shown that at least 3.6 g antibiotic per 40 g cement is optimal for the best elution kinetics and sustained therapeutic levels.[18] Doses as high as 6 to 8 g antibiotic per 40 g bone cement have been shown to be safe clinically.[17] The use of these high doses is important for the sustained release of antibiotics at levels that are bacteriocidal for the organisms being treated.

PROPHYLAXIS

Total Knee Arthroplasty

The use of ALBC for treating active infections in joint arthroplasty has been well established. The basis for the use of ALBC as a prophylactic measure is to reduce the prevalence of deep joint infection. Gentamicin, cefuroxime, and tobramycin are the antibiotics most commonly used in bone cement in clinical studies worldwide.[19–22] Of the three antibiotics, gentamicin has been used most frequently and studied most extensively.[23] We are not aware of any clinical studies comparing the efficacy of one antibiotic over another as a prophylaxis in cement.

In a randomized clinical trial of 340 primary TKAs, Chiu and colleagues[19] evaluated the deep infection rates for patients with cefuroxime bone cement as compared with standard bone cement. No deep infections occurred in the study group, whereas a deep infection developed in 5 of the 162 knees (3.1%) in the control group ($P = 0.02$). Even with the small sample size, a significant reduction in deep infections was noted with the use of antibiotic bone cement.

The same authors then performed a second prospective randomized trial on just 78 patients with diabetes undergoing primary TKA.[20] Once again, cefuroxime bone cement was used in one group and standard bone cement in the other. The authors note a significant reduction in deep infection rate in this high-risk patient population with the use of antibiotic bone cement ($P < 0.02$). The reported a deep infection rate of 13.5% (5/37) in the control group and no infections in the ALBC group. This overall infection rate for patients with diabetes is greater than that reported in the literature of 3.1% to 7%.[24-26]

In another randomized trial, McQueen and coworkers[27] found that, in 295 patients undergoing primary hip or knee replacement, there was no difference in infection rates between the use of cefuroxime-impregnated bone cement or administration of the cefuroxime intravenously. They report an overall infection rate of 6.8%.

Prophylaxis: Total Hip Arthroplasty

Josefsson and Kolmert[28] performed a large randomized trial of 1688 patients undergoing hip replacement and found that at 2 years, the group treated with intravenous antibiotics had a deep infection rate of 1.6% (13/835) versus 0.4% (3/853) in the group treated with gentamycin-impregnated bone cement ($P < 0.05$).

Espehaug and coauthors[21] report on 10,905 primary cemented total hip replacements from the Norwegian Arthroplasty Registry. There were four treatment groups: (1) systemic antibiotics and antibiotic-impregnated bone cement, (2) systemic antibiotics only, (3) antibiotic-impregnated bone cement only, and (4) no antibiotic prophylaxis. The overall infection rate was 0.4%. The use of antibiotic bone cement and systemic antibiotics was found to be significantly more effective in preventing deep infection than using either systemic antibiotics or antibiotic bone cement alone ($P < 0.001$). The adjusted failure rate ratios in the remaining groups were 4.3 (systemic antibiotics only), 6.3 (antibiotic-impregnated cement only), and 11.5 (no antibiotic prophylaxis). The authors conclude that the best prophylaxis against infection was a combination of systemic antibiotics and antibiotic-impregnated cement.

The Swedish Hip Registry data consisted of 92,675 primary and revision total hip replacements performed between 1978 and 1990. Malchau and researchers[22] found that the quality of the operating room ventilation and the use of gentamycin-impregnated antibiotic bone cement were the only significant factors in reducing deep infection ($P < 0.001$). Also, the benefit was greater for revision surgery than for primary hip replacements. Interestingly, the data showed a decrease in deep infection rates from 1979 to 1991 in all patients, regardless of the use of ALBC, because of other measures of infection control introduced over this period.

A large retrospective study of 22,170 primary total hip replacements from the Norwegian Arthroplasty Register during the period of 1987 to 2001 was reported by Engesaeter and investigators.[29] Patients who received only systemic antibiotic prophylaxis (5960 patients) had a 1.8 times greater rate of infection than patients who received systemic antibiotic prophylaxis combined with gentamicin-loaded bone cement (15,676 patients) ($P = 0.01$).

In another retrospective review of 1542 total hip replacements, no difference was found in infection rate between primary total hip replacements performed with (1.65%) compared with those performed without gentamicin-loaded bone cement (1.72%).[30] However, with revision surgery, gentamicin-loaded bone cement provided significantly better results, with a 0.81% infection rate, as compared with a rate of 3.46% after those done with plain cement.[30]

Tunney and colleagues'[31] in vitro study examined the efficacy of gentamicin-impregnated bone cement and preoperative and postoperative administration of cefuroxime in the prevention of biofilm formation. The authors conclude that with a low bacterial inoculum, the combination of gentamicin and cefuroxime was effective in preventing biofilm formation but had no effect in an environment of high bacterial concentrations (Table 82–1).

STUDY LIMITATIONS

In the literature, the event rate for deep infection has been reported at about 1% in many large series.[1-4] Taking a 50% reduction in infection rate as significant and assuming a power of 0.8, a well-powered, randomized, controlled study would need approximately 5000 patients to adequately document a difference between groups.

The randomization process in the two studies by Chiu and colleagues[19,20] used a system based on even and odd medical record numbers as opposed to a formal, computer-generated randomization schedule.

TABLE 82–1. Summary of Level I Evidence for Prophylactic Antibiotic-Loaded Bone Cement in Joint Arthroplasty

AUTHOR	JOINTS STUDIED	DEEP INFECTION RATES	CONTROL TREATMENT
Chiu et al.[19] (N = 340)	Primary knees	5/162 (3.1%)	0/178 (0%)
Chiu et al.[20] (N = 78)	Primary knees	5/37 (13.5%)	0/41 (0%)
McQueen et al.[27] (N = 295)	Primary hips and knees	2/149 (1.3%)	1/146 (0.7%)
Josefsson and Kolmert[28] (N = 1688)	Primary hips	13/835 (1.6%)	(3/853) (0.4%)

Potential Disadvantages of Routine Use of Antibiotic-Loaded Bone Cement

The unanswered question remains whether the benefits of prophylaxis with ALBC in the current era of joint arthroplasty with an extremely low rate of infection are outweighed by the potential disadvantages associated with its routine use. The issues of toxicity and detrimental effects to the mechanical properties of bone cement are inconsequential when using low-dose ALBC (0.5–1.0 g antibiotic per 40 g cement). Biomechanical testing has shown that, in contrast with the use of high-dose antibiotics, which can weaken bone cement, the low-dose, antibiotic-impregnated bone cements that are used in practice have negligible reductions in fatigue strength, and fixation is not compromised.[32–34]

Two reports showed that the addition of gentamicin powder into Palacos R bone cement (Zimmer) or either erythromycin plus colistin or tobramycin powder into Simplex P (Stryker) bone cement did not decrease the fatigue strength compared with that of the respective plain-cement controls.[35,36] In contrast, DeLuise and Scott[6] showed that hand-mixing tobramycin into Simplex P bone cement results in a 36% decrease in the strength of the cement compared with the strength of commercially prepared, tobramycin-loaded bone cement (Simplex T) and that of plain Simplex P cement. Radiosterometric analysis studies have revealed comparable fixation of cemented implants with and without commercially prepared antibiotic-impregnated bone cement.[34]

Other concerns are the potential for an allergic reaction to the antibiotic being used and the potential development of drug-resistant organisms. No reports have been made of allergic reactions in more than 100,000 cases of ALBC thus far in the literature.[37] Some authors have described gentamycin-resistant organisms and have suggested the use of other antibiotics such as the cephalosporins ciprofloxacin, erythromycin, or vancomycin as alternative choices.[31,38,39]

The cost of commercially available ALBC products is considerable. Compared with the cost of plain bone cement, the cost of equivalent ALBC is increased from $284 to $349 (U.S currency) per 40-g package.[40] This increased cost needs to be balanced against the potential cost savings from avoiding a deep prosthetic joint infection.

Potentially High-Risk Populations

Patients with the following characteristics are at potentially high risk for infection:
1. *Prolonged operating time:* Smabrekke et al.[41] evaluated 31,745 total hip replacements in Norway and found that an operating time of more than 150 minutes was associated with a greater infection rate.
2. *Revision surgery:* Blom and researchers[42] examined the results of 931 primary and

69 revision total knee replacements, and found the prevalence of deep infection to be 1% after primary total knee replacement compared with 5.8% after revision total knee replacement.
3. *Inflammatory arthritis:* Infection rates in rheumatoid arthritis have been reported to be between 2% and 4% in various studies.[36,40,41]
4. *Diabetes mellitus:* Various authors have reported infection rates between 3.1% and 7% in patients with diabetes undergoing primary total joint arthroplasty.[20,24–26]

RECOMMENDATIONS

The use of ALBC in prophylaxis in primary total joint arthroplasty remains controversial. ALBC should be considered as a defense against direct contamination at the time of surgery or during the early postoperative period as the wound seals. In a survey of 1015 American adult arthroplasty surgeons, only 56% routinely use ALBC in their practice.[43]

Kurtz and colleagues[44] have projected that between the years of 2005 and 2030, the revision burden in the United States for hip and knee surgery will increase by 137% and 601%, respectively. The healthcare costs for treating joint sepsis after arthroplasty has been estimated at $40 to $80 million annually in the United States.[45] Sculco[46] estimates the direct costs of revision surgery for deep infection at more than $55,000.

In the literature there exist four prospective, randomized trials in which three have demonstrated a decreased rate of deep infection with ALBC prophylaxis for primary joint arthroplasty at short-term follow-up. Dividing the patients by hip and knee surgery, there are insufficient numbers in these studies to adequately conclude a definite benefit in the use of ALBC for routine primary joint arthroplasty.

Many unanswered questions remain such as which is the best antibiotic for use in prophylaxis in bone cement, whether commercially available ALBC is mechanically superior to less expensive hand-mixed ALBC in the clinical setting, and whether an increased use of low-dose ALBC will result in an increased prevalence of drug-resistant organisms.

With concerns of cost and antibiotic-resistant organisms, the use of ALBC in all routine primary hip and knee replacements cannot be recommended based on the current evidence. Antibiotics in bone cement has a more definitive role in those populations at high risk described earlier and in revision joint arthroplasty. Table 82–2 provides a summary of recommendations.

TABLE 82–2. Summary of Recommendations

RECOMMENDATIONS	LEVEL OF EVIDENCE/GRADE OF RECOMMENDATION	REFERENCES
1. ALBC is indicated in the treatment of active bone/joint infections.	A	14–17
2. ALBC decreases the early deep infection rates after primary THA/TKA.	B	19, 20, 28, 29
3. ALBC leads to increased complications such as allergic reaction and drug-resistantorganisms.	I	31, 37–39

ALBC, antibiotic-loaded bone cement; THA, total hip arthroplasty; TKA, total knee arthroplasty.

REFERENCES

1. Robertsson O, Knutson K, Lewold S, et al: The Swedish knee arthroplasty register 1975–1997: An update with special emphasis of 41,223 knees operated on in 1988–1997. Acta Orthop Scand 72:603, 2001.
2. Blom AW, Brown J, Taylor AH, et al: Infection after total knee arthroplasty. J Bone Joint Surg Br 86:688–691, 2004.
3. Mahomed NN, Barrett J, Katz JN, et al: Epidemiology of total knee replacement in the United States Medicare population. J Bone Joint Surg Am 87:1222–1228, 2005.
4. Phillips CB, Barrett JA, Losina E, et al: Incidence rates of dislocation, pulmonary embolism, and deep infection during the first six months after elective total hip replacement. J Bone Joint Surg Am 85:20–26, 2003.
5. Neut D, van de Belt H, van Horn JR, et al: The effect of mixing on gentamicin release from polymethylmethacrylate bone cements. Acta Orthop Scand 74:670–676, 2003.
6. DeLuise M, Scott CP: Addition of hand-blended generic tobramycin in bone cement: Effect on mechanical strength. Orthopedics 27:1289–1291, 2004.
7. Penner MJ, Duncan CP, Masri BA: The in vitro elution characteristics of antibiotic-loaded CMW and Palacos-R bone cements. J Arthroplasty 14:209–214, 1999.
8. Baker AS, Greenham LW: Release of gentamicin from acrylic bone cement. Elution and diffusion studies. J Bone Joint Surg Am 70:1551–1557, 1988.
9. Powles JW, Spencer RF, Lovering AM: Gentamicin release from old cement during revision hip arthroplasty. J Bone Joint Surg Br 80:607–610, 1998.
10. Fletcher MD, Spencer RF, Langkamer VG, Lovering AM: Gentamicin concentrations in diagnostic aspirates from 25 patients with hip and knee arthroplasties. Acta Orthop Scand 75:173–176, 2004.
11. Nelson CL, Griffin FM, Harrison BH, Cooper RE: In vitro elution characteristics of commercially and noncommercially prepared antibiotic PMMA beads. Clin Orthop 284:303–309, 1992.
12. Lawson KJ, Marks KE, Brems J, Rehm S: Vancomycin vs tobramycin elution from polymethylmethacrylate: An in vitro study. Orthopedics 13:521–524, 1990.
13. Adams K, Couch L, Cierny G, et al: In vitro and in vivo evaluation of antibiotic diffusion from antibiotic-impregnated polymethylmethacrylate beads. Clin Orthop Relat Res (278):244–252, 1992.
14. Buchholz HW, Elson RA, Engelbrecht E, et al: Management of deep infection of total hip replacement. J Bone Joint Surg Br 63:342–353, 1981.
15. Duncan CP, Masri BA: The role of antibiotic-loaded cement in the treatment of an infection after a hip replacement. Instr Course Lect 44:305–313, 1995.
16. Hanssen AD, Rand JA, Osmon DR: Treatment of the infected total knee arthroplasty with insertion of another prosthesis. The effect of antibiotic-impregnated bone cement. Clin Orthop Relat Res (309):44–55, 1994.
17. Springer BD, Lee GC, Osmon D, et al: Systemic safety of high-dose antibiotic-loaded cement spacers after resection of an infected total knee arthroplasty. Clin Orthop Relat Res (427):47–51, 2004.
18. Penner MJ, Duncan CP, Masri BA: The in vitro elution characteristics of antibiotic-loaded CMW and Palacos-R bone cements. J Arthroplasty 14:209, 1999.

19. Chiu FY, Chen CM, Lin CFJ, et al: Cefuroxime impregnated cement in primary total knee arthroplasty. J Bone Joint Surg Am 84:759, 2002.
20. Chiu FY, Lin CF, Chen CM, et al: Cefuroxime-impregnated cement at primary total knee arthroplasty in diabetes mellitus. A prospective, randomized study. J Bone Joint Surg Br 83:691, 2001.
21. Espehaug B, Engesaeter LB, Vollset SE, et al: Antibiotic prophylaxis in total hip arthroplasty: Review of 10,905 primary cemented total hip replacements reported to the Norwegian arthroplasty register, 1987 to 1995. J Bone Joint Surg Br 79:590, 1997.
22. Malchau H, Herberts P, Ahngelt L: Prognosis of total hip replacement in Sweden. Follow-up of 92,675 operations performed 1978-1990. Acta Orthop Scand 64:497–506, 1993.
23. Hanssen AD: Prophylactic use of antibiotic bone cement: An emerging standard—in opposition. J Arthroplasty 19(4 suppl 1):73–77, 2004.
24. Yang K, Yeo SJ, Lee BP, Lo NN: Total knee arthroplasty in diabetic patients: A study of 109 consecutive cases. J Arthroplasty 16:102–106, 2001.
25. England SP, Stern SH, Insall JN, Windsor RE: Total knee arthroplasty in diabetes mellitus. Clin Orthop Relat Res (260):130–134, 1990.
26. Meding JB, Reddleman K, Keating ME, et al: Total knee replacement in patients with diabetes mellitus. Clin Orthop Relat Res (416):208–216, 2003.
27. McQueen M, Littlejohn A, Hughes SP: A comparison of systemic cefuroxime and cefuroxime loaded bone cement in the prevention of early infection after total joint replacement. Int Orthop 11:241–243, 1987.
28. Josefsson G, Kolmert L: Prophylaxis with systematic antibiotics versus gentamicin bone cement in total hip arthroplasty. A ten-year survey of 1,688 hips. Clin Orthop Relat Res (292):210–214, 1993.
29. Engesaeter LB, Lie SA, Espehaug B, et al: Antibiotic prophylaxis in total hip arthroplasty: Effects of antibiotic prophylaxis systemically and in bone cement on the revision rate of 22,170 primary hip replacements followed 0-14 years in the Norwegian Arthroplasty Register. Acta Orthop Scand 74:644–651, 2003.
30. Lynch M, Esser MP, Shelley P, Wroblewski BM: Deep infection in Charnley low friction arthroplasty. Comparison of plain and gentamicin-loaded cement. J Bone Joint Surg Br 69:355–360, 1987.
31. Tunney MM, Ramage G, Patrick S, et al: Antimicrobial susceptibility of bacteria isolated from orthopedic implants following revision hip surgery. Antimicrob Agents Chemother 42:3002, 1998.
32. Davies JP, Harris WH: Effect of hand mixing tobramycin on the fatigue strength of Simplex P. J Biomed Mater Res 25:1409, 1991.
33. Masari BA, Duncan CP, Beauchamp CP: Long-term elution of antibiotics from bone cement: An in vivo study using the prosthesis of antibiotic-loaded acrylic cement (PROSTALAC) system. J Arthroplasty 13:331, 1998.
34. Adelberth G, Nilsson KG, Karrholm J, et al: Fixation of the tibial component using CMW-1 or Palacos bone cement with gentamicin: Similar outcome in a randomized radiostereometric study of 51 total knee arthroplasties. Acta Orthop Scand 73:531, 2002.

35. Davies JP, Harris WH: Effect of hand mixing tobramycin on the fatigue strength of Simplex P. J Biomed Mater Res 25:1409–1414, 1991.
36. Davies JP, O'Connor DO, Burke DW, Harris WH: Influence of antibiotic impregnation on the fatigue life of Simplex P and Palacos R acrylic bone cements, with and without centrifugation. J Biomed Mater Res 23:379–397, 1989.
37. Bourne R: Prophylactic use of antibiotic bone cement an emerging standard—in the affirmative. J Arthroplasty 19:69–72, 2004.
38. Sanzen L, Walder M: Antibiotic resistance of coagulase-negative staphylococci in an orthopaedic department. J Hosp Infect 12:103, 1988.
39. Taggart T, Kerry RM, Norman P, et al: The use of vancomycin-impregnated cement beads in the management of infection of prosthetic joints. J Bone Joint Surg Br 84:70, 2002.
40. Jiranek W, Hanssen AB, Greenwalk AS: Antibiotic-loaded bone cement for infection prophylaxis in total joint replacement. J Bone Joint Surg Am 88:2487–2500, 2006.
41. Lentino JR: Prosthetic joint infections: Bane of orthopedists, challenge for infectious disease specialists. Clin Infect Dis 36:1157–1161, 2003.
42. Blom AW, Brown J, Taylor AH, et al: Infection after total knee arthroplasty. J Bone Joint Surg Br 86:688–691, 2004.
43. Heck D, Rosenberg A, Schink-Ascani M, et al: Use of antibiotic impregnated cement during hip and knee arthroplasty in the United States. J Arthroplasty 10:470–475, 1995.
44. Smabrekke A, Espehaug B, Havelin LI, Fumes O: Operating time and survival of primary total hip replacements: an analysis of 31,745 primary cemented and uncemented total hip replacements from local hospitals reported to the Norwegian Arthroplasty Register 1987-2001. Acta Orthop Scand 75:524-32, 2004.
45. Brause BD: Infections with prostheses in bones and joints. In Mandell GL, Bennett Je, Dolin R (eds): Principles and Practice of Infectious Diseases, 4th ed. New York, Churchill Livingstone Inc, 1995, pp 1051–1055.
46. Sculco TP: The economic impact of infected total joint arthroplasty. Instr Course Lect 42:349–351, 1993.

Total Hip Replacement:
Hybrid versus Uncemented: Which Is Better?

Khaled Saleh, MD, MSc, FRCSC, FACS, Mark McCarthy, MSI, William Mihalko, MD, PhD, Quanjun Qui, MD, MS, and Thomas E. Brown, MD

Chapter 83

Total hip replacement (THR) is one of the most common procedures performed in orthopedic surgery. With an ever-aging population and increasing levels of obesity, arthritic joints are becoming more prevalent. Furthermore, arthroplasty is being performed in younger and younger patients. Although THR results in substantial improvement in quality of life, it is not without intraoperative and postoperative risks, including fat embolism, deep venous thrombosis (DVT), pulmonary embolism, and ultimately failed prosthesis, necessitating another, more significant revision surgery. This chapter examines the decision to cement the femoral component.

Surgical technique is paramount to a successful THR outcome. Currently, much research is being dedicated to evaluate the potential merits and downfalls of minimally invasive surgery (MIS). With regards to total hip arthroplasty, this option remains in its infancy of evaluation. With consumer interest in this cosmetically pleasing, smaller scar, further studies are warranted to ensure minimally invasive THR is a safe and reproducible surgery that parallels the traditional approach and its historically sound results.

The first issue is the risk of intraoperative fat emboli. Fat emboli presents a potential intraoperative adverse event, including the rare but critical bone cement implantation syndrome (BCIS), which leads to death in 0.6% to 1% of patients.[1] BCIS is characterized by hypoxemia, hypotension, cardiac arrhythmias, and cardiac arrest in any or all combinations. Transesophageal echocardiography (TEE) has been used in many studies to evaluate the size and magnitude of embolic cascade during the reaming of the femoral canal. Here, we compare different techniques in hip arthroplasty and show examples of measures taken to reduce the risk for complications from fat emboli in cemented and uncemented arthroplasty.

In one study, the incidence of bone marrow and fat emboli among cemented and uncemented THR was similar[2] (Level of Evidence II). Here, 50 consecutive bilateral hip replacements and 106 unilateral hip replacements were enrolled in this study, for a total of 206 hip arthroplasties. One hundred of the hips were treated with cemented stems, whereas 106 of the hips were replaced with uncemented stems. Arterial and right atrial blood samples were obtained before implantation, at 1-, 3-, 4-, and 10-minute intervals after implantation, and at 24 and 48 hours after the surgery. This study found no difference between the prevalence of fat embolism in cemented and uncemented stems, regardless of patients receiving bilateral or unilateral arthroplasties.

Christie and colleagues[3] found that cemented compared with uncemented hemiarthroplasty in the treatment of femoral neck fractures caused greater and more prolonged embolic cascades (Level II). A subsequent study evaluated minimal versus thorough lavage of the femoral canal and found a statistically significant reduction in duration of the embolic responses and number of large emboli, together with less pulmonary function disturbance[4] (Level II). Although these studies were not done in the context of hip arthroplasty for arthritic joints, it speaks to the importance of thorough femoral canal lavage before cementation.

A modified cementing technique using vacuum drainage into the proximal femur has been successful in reducing intramedullary pressure and the incidence of embolism[5] (Level II). Koessler and coworkers[5] studied the effects of placing vacuum drainage in the proximal femur to reduce the increase in intramedullary pressure during prosthesis insertion. To perform this study, 2 groups of 120 patients were randomized. One group received a total hip arthroplasty using a conventional cementing technique, and the other group used the modified technique described earlier. Perioperative monitoring of embolic events was done by continuous TEE, hemodynamic monitoring, and blood gas analysis. The results in this study show that 93.3% of patients receiving the conventional cementation experienced embolism contrasted with 13.3% occurrence rate in patients undergoing total hip arthroplasty using the modified technique ($P < 0.05$). Intraoperative shunt values increased from 8.2% to 10.3% during femoral component insertion in the conventional cementation group ($P < 0.05$). No significant changes were found during femoral stem insertion in the modified group. No patients in either group sustained fat embolism syndrome. These results show that the embolic events seen under TEE can lead to increased pulmonary shunt values during THR, most notably in those patients with systemic disease. The modified technique, designed to reduce increases in intramedullary pressure, reduced the incidence of embolism.

Pitto and investigators[6] performed a similar study, utilizing a bone-vacuum technique in the experimental group (Level II). Here, 130 patients were randomized to receive a standard cemented hip without the use of a bone vacuum or to have the arthroplasty performed with the use of a bone vacuum (65 patients in each study). This study examined the incidence of embolic events via TEE as well. However, serial duplex ultrasonography was used to assess the occurrence of DVT in each of the groups. This was done the day before surgery and on postoperative days 4, 14, and 45. The control, standard cementation group had significantly more embolic particles and masses (in 59 patients, or 91%) versus the group that underwent femoral component implantation with the concurrent use of a bone vacuum (10 patients, or 15%). Furthermore, ultrasonography on postoperative day 4 found DVT in 12 of the patients in the control group (18%) compared with a DVT rate of 3% (2 patients) on postoperative day 4 in the experimental group ($P < 0.05$).

Pitto and investigators[7] also examined the incidence of fat embolism in uncemented versus cemented hip arthroplasty in the following study. To assess this, they randomized 60 patients to 1 of 3 groups of 20 patients each. Group 1 received uncemented femoral stems, group 2 received femoral stems with conventional cementation, and group 3 stems with modified cementation technique. Again, TEE, hemodynamic, and blood-gas analyses were performed intraoperatively to assess for embolic events. Severe embolic events, defined as a cascade of fine echogenic particles less than 5 mm in diameter, were observed in 17 of 20 patients in group 2 (85%). Group 1, the uncemented group, has no patients with this occurrence. Group 3, with stems implanted using modified cementation technique, had one patient with severe embolic events (5%)[7] (Level II). Group 1 had an average increase in intrapulmonary shunt values of 24% ($P < 0.05$), whereas the other two groups did not have a significant change detected. Thus, this study showed it is imperative to consider the overall health of the patient with THR in preoperative planning, most notably in their ability to cope with embolic events or intraoperative pulmonary impairment if a conventional cementation is to be performed. This is less of an issue if bone-vacuum cementation is performed or an uncemented stem is implanted. This study shows that the defined severe embolic events, together with intraoperative pulmonary impairment, are quite common (85%) in the setting of conventional cementation of the femoral component. It also revealed that modified cementation using the bone-vacuum technique significantly reduces the risk for these embolic events.

Other issues in deciding to cement the femoral component in THR includes incidence of postoperative thigh pain, periprosthetic proximal femur fractures, and rate of femoral revision. Several studies have directly compared cemented versus uncemented femoral stems. In a study that compared titanium-cemented and uncemented stems, it was found that cementless stems had better 10-year survival rates (100%) than the cemented counterparts (84%), in which survivorship was defined by femoral revision[8] (Level II). The authors compare two similar stems, one randomized to be cemented ($n = 102$ hips) whereas the other was uncemented ($n = 78$ hips). Radiographic analysis was performed, with an average follow-up period of 6.7 and 7.0 years for the cemented and cementless groups, respectively. In this analysis, osteolysis below the joint line, in zones 2 through 6, occurred in 12.7% (13/102) of hips in the cemented group and in 0% of the uncemented hips ($P < 0.001$). Although each study group had the same number of acetabular revisions (17 in each), the uncemented stem group had zero femoral stem revisions. Nine of the 17 acetabular revisions from the cemented group underwent concurrent femoral revision.

In a double-blinded study that assessed mortality, revision rate, and health-related quality of life, 250 patients with diagnoses of osteoarthritis of the hip were randomized to receive the same femoral, titanium-alloy prosthesis, one implanted with cement and the other without. Of the 250 patients, 124 of them received cemented femoral stems and 126 uncemented. The mean age was 64 years, and average follow-up was 6.3 years. The results showed that 13 revisions were required in the cemented stem group versus 6 in the uncemented group ($P = 0.11$). However, of the 13 revisions in the cemented group, 12 of them required femoral revisions versus 1 in 6 from the uncemented group ($P = 0.002$)[9] (Level II). In this study, the authors conclude that one type of cemented prosthesis required more femoral revisions than uncemented femoral stems.

Osteoarthritis of the hip in a younger population presents a particular problem in planning for a revision arthroplasty at a later point in time. With this foresight in mind, uncemented stems have been utilized often in younger populations. One study compared cemented and uncemented stems in a younger population (<65 years; average age, 54 years) with hip osteoarthritis.[10] Forty-five patients who met the above criteria were randomized to receive an uncemented or cemented stem, then observed for a period of 2 years (Level II). Outcomes were measured via Merle d'Aubigne score, conventional radiography, and repeated radiostereometric analysis. Furthermore, the authors managed 81 of the uncemented stems for an average of 8 years (range, 7–12 years) with revision as their end point. The results showed the cemented stems remained stable throughout the follow-up period. The uncemented stems subsided and rotated into retroversion in the first three postoperative months, then remained stable radiographically thereafter. Postoperative thigh pain, traditionally a problem in uncemented hip prostheses, was not observed in any patient from this study. The authors conclude both cemented and uncemented femoral Cone stems give stable results younger patients with osteoarthritis. However, longer-term studies are warranted to assess long-term viability.

DVT and pulmonary embolism are great concerns after surgery in total hip arthroplasty. Laupacis and coauthors[11] directly assess this issue in a randomized study of 250 patients undergoing unilateral THR. The patients were randomized to receive the same prosthesis: one group to be cemented, and the other uncemented. Both groups received prophylaxis against DVT, with aspirin being used in the first half of the study and warfarin in the second. Of the 250 patients, 80% agreed to undergo postoperative bilateral venography. All of them were clinically evaluated for pulmonary embolus. The results of this study showed that the frequency of DVT was not statistically significant (50% in the cemented patient group and 47% from the uncemented group; $P = 0.73$).

Heterotopic ossification (HO) can be a debilitating aftereffect of THR, leading to increased pain, decreased mobility, and potentially necessitating a challenging revision arthroplasty. In a prospective, randomized, controlled trial, HO was compared between cemented and uncemented hip arthroplasties, with 112 patients receiving uncemented implants and 114 receiving cemented implants.[12] The Brooker classification was used to assess heterotopic bone formation from postoperative radiographs. Overall, 148 of the hips (66%) did not develop HO: 76 from the uncemented group (68%) and 72 from the cemented group (63%). Of the HO cases that did develop in the remainder, neither of the groups progressed to Brooker class IV. Rates of Brooker classes I, II, and III were approximately the same between the two groups. This study showed that there is no significant difference in the formation of HO between cemented and uncemented THR.

To further protect from the formation of heterotopic bone formation, some have advocated the use of nonsteroidal anti-inflammatory drugs (NSAIDs) as a postoperative prophylactic measure. Regardless of cemented or uncemented prosthesis, evidence shows that the use of these medications can reduce the amount and severity of heterotopic bone formation. In a study of the use of NSAIDs after cementless hip arthroplasty, patients were randomized to receive a 4- or an 8-day course of indomethacin, 50 mg three times daily. The longer course group of patients, it was discovered, had less severe HO formation than the shorter course group ($P = 0.003$).[13]

Another study examined the use of naproxen, 500 mg twice daily, for the first 7 postoperative days. The control group consisted of 23 patients from a previous study, none of which received any NSAID. HO was measured radiographically, with the radiographs mixed randomly. One year after the operation, 4 of the 27 patients (17%) in the naproxen group experienced development of HO versus 12 (52%) in the untreated group of 23 patients ($P < 0.05$).[14]

THR remains a highly successful procedure that greatly improves quality of life in those stricken with degenerative arthritis. When considering whether to cement the femoral component, many considerations must be taken, including age of the patient and overall health status. Cementation can increase the risk for embolic events, especially when used without thorough or vacuum-assisted lavage of the femoral canal. Furthermore, revision rates of the femoral component are found to be greater in cemented THRs. DVT rates were found to be similar in either cemented or uncemented hip replacements, provided the femoral canal is appropriately prepared via lavage before cementation.

If patients are older and in good health overall, it would seem appropriate to utilize uncemented femoral stems if their bone has a high enough quality. In the setting of poor bone quality, utilizing a modified cementation technique to minimize the ill effects of embolic cascade is the most appropriate course. If younger patients are in need of hip replacement, uncemented stems are appropriate in planning for possible revision surgery in the future. If cementation of the femoral component is performed, thorough lavage or vacuum-assisted lavage of the femoral canal before femoral component insertion decreases embolic problems. After surgery, other than greater rates of revision in cemented THR, there does not seem to be any difference in cemented or uncemented hip replacements in many important parameters. The incidence rates of DVT and pulmonary embolism are similar. Quality of life and overall improvement scores studied are similar among the cemented and uncemented THR. Table 83–1 provides a summary of recommendations for the treatment of THR.

TABLE 83–1. Summary of Recommendations for the Treatment of Total Hip Replacement

STATEMENT	LEVEL OF EVIDENCE/ GRADE OF RECOMMENDATION	REFERENCES
1. Vacuum-assisted drainage in cementation of femoral components reduces fat embolism events and incidence of deep vein thrombosis to levels comparable with uncemented femoral stem procedures.	B	7, 8
2. Uncemented femoral stems have prolonged survivorship versus cemented femoral stems when femoral revision is the end point.	B	10, 11
3. No difference exists in the prevalence or severity of heterotopic bone formation when cemented and uncemented femoral stems are compared.	A	14

REFERENCES

1. Lamade WR, Friedl W, Schmid B, Meeder PJ: Bone cement implantation syndrome. A prospective randomised trial for use of antihistamine blockade. Arch Orthop Trauma Surg 114:335–339, 1995.
2. Kim Y-H, Oh SW, Kim JS: Prevalence of fat embolism following bilateral simultaneous and unilateral total hip arthroplasty performed with or without cement: A prospective, randomized clinical study. J Bone Joint Surg Am 84-A:1372–1379, 2002.
3. Christie J, Burnett R, Potts HR, Pell ACH: Echocardiography of transatrial embolism during cemented and uncemented hemiarthroplasty of the hip. J Bone Joint Surg Br 76:409–412, 1994.
4. Christie J, Robinson CM, Singer B, Ray DC: Medullary lavage reduces embolic phenomena and cardiopulmonary changes during cemented hemiarthroplasty. J Bone Joint Surg Br 77:456–459, 1995.
5. Koessler MJ, Fabiani R, Hamer H, Pitto RP: The clinical relevance of embolic events detected by transesophageal echocardiography during cemented total hip arthroplasty: A randomized clinical trial. Anesth Analg 92:49–55, 2001.
6. Pitto RP, Hamer H, Fabiani R, et al: Prophylaxis against fat and bone-marrow embolism during total hip arthroplasty reduces the incidence of postoperative deep-vein thrombosis: A controlled, randomized clinical trial. J Bone Joint Surg Am 84-A:39–48, 2002.
7. Pitto RP, Koessler M, Kuehle JW: Comparison of fixation of the femoral component without cement and fixation with use of a bone-vacuum cementing technique for the prevention of fat embolism during total hip arthroplasty. A prospective, randomized clinical trial. J Bone Joint Surg Am 81:831–843, 1999.
8. Emerson Jr RH, Head WC, Emerson CB, et al: A comparison of cemented and cementless titanium femoral components used for primary total hip arthroplasty: A radiographic and survivorship study. J Arthroplasty 17:584–591, 2002.
9. Laupacis A, Bourne R, Rorabeck C, et al: Comparison of total hip arthroplasty performed with and without cement: A randomized trial. J Bone Joint Surg Am 84-A:1823–1828, 2002.
10. Strom H, Kolstad K, Mallmin H, et al: Comparison of the uncemented Cone and the cemented Bimetric hip prosthesis in young patients with osteoarthritis: An RSA, clinical and radiographic study. Acta Orthopaedica 77:71–78, 2006.
11. Laupacis A, Rorabeck C, Bourne R, et al: The frequency of venous thrombosis in cemented and non-cemented hip arthroplasty. J Bone Joint Surg Br 78:210–212, 1996.
12. Nayak KN, Mulliken B, Rorabeck CH, et al: Prevalence of heterotopic ossification in cemented versus noncemented total hip joint replacement in patients with osteoarthrosis: A randomized clinical trial. Can J Surg 40:368–374, 1997.
13. Dorn U, Grethen C, Effenberger H, et al: Indomethacin for prevention of heterotopic ossification after hip arthroplasty. A randomized comparison between 4 and 8 days of treatment. Acta Orthop Scand 69:107–110, 1998.
14. Gebuhr P, Wilbek H, Soelberg M: Naproxen for 8 days can prevent heterotopic ossification after hip arthroplasty. Clin Orthop Relat Res (314):166–169, 1995.

Chapter 84

Which Bearing Surface Should Be Used: Highly Cross-Linked Polyethylene versus Metal or Metal versus Ceramic on Ceramic?

RICHARD A. HOCKING, BSc (MED), MBBS (HONS), FRACS (ORTH)
AND STEVEN J. MACDONALD, MD, FRCSC

Total hip replacement changes the lives of more than one million patients worldwide each year. In well-selected patients, the success of the implant has historically meant that for nearly 90% of patients, their primary hip replacement is their only hip replacement.[1] This level of success has been reached with multiple implants including cemented mono-block femoral stems with conventional cemented, all-polyethylene, acetabular components of several different designs. If this is the case, why are we looking for alternative bearings?

First, the levels of success in historical data were achieved only in select groups of patients. Many historical studies had an inbuilt selection bias. Surgeons were aware that there were certain diagnoses that fared poorly with the implants and techniques available to them, and in particular, younger patients did not respond as well in terms of survivorship of the implant. As such, patients who were perceived to be at high risk for unsuccessful results were not offered a total hip replacement. National registries are probably the best tool for observing the effect that age and diagnosis have on the revision rate. The Swedish registry has been collecting data relating age and diagnosis to the success of hip arthroplasty since 1979. Over this period, they have observed an overall diminishing revision burden, which they speculate may be caused by better surgical training, an improvement in the performance of modern implants compared with their historical counterparts, and surgeons modifying their practice to use combinations of implants that have performed well in the registry.[2] Despite these favorable conditions for hip arthroplasty, there has been a relative increase in the revision rate of total hip replacements performed for inflammatory arthropathies, childhood hip disorders, and post-traumatic arthritis[2]—all diagnoses found predominantly in young people having total hip arthroplasties.

Second, patient demands have significantly changed since the introduction of total hip arthroplasty. Today's patients and surgeons are unlikely to proceed with operations such as arthrodesis and resection arthroplasty. Patients perceive that total hip replacement is almost universally successful and offers a return to near-normal function. This perception has contributed to the fact that greater numbers of younger patients are seeking total hip arthroplasty than ever before; in addition, the activity level and expectations of all patients undergoing total hip replacement has significantly increased.

Therefore, patients not only expect to be more active than their historical counterparts, data demonstrate that these patients will live longer. All of this leads to greater tribological loads on the bearing surface; hence, there have been concerted efforts by the orthopedic scientific community to develop new bearing surfaces that will meet the demands of the patients who are currently seeking total hip replacement. To this end, advances have been made with polyethylene-bearing surfaces with the development of highly cross-linked polyethylene, and there has been renewed interest and advances in both engineering and the understanding of metal on metal in both total hip and resurfacings and ceramic-on-ceramic bearings.

WHAT ARE THE TRIBOLOGICAL DEMANDS ON TOTAL HIP ARTHROPLASTY ARTICULATIONS?

Historically, wear particles from conventional polyethylene gamma irradiated in air, coupled with small-diameter metal or ceramic heads, has led to osteolysis and failure of the components after 5 to 15 years of use.[3,4] In a study of Charnley hips retrieved at time of revision for aseptic loosening,[5] the mean time to revision was 12 years, and the mean volumetric wear at failure was 785 mm.[4] The same polyethylene had been tested in another study using a hip simulator, and this degree of volumetric wear was obtained after 12 years of wear when it was assumed that 1.5 million steps were taken in a year.[6,7] Assuming 1.5 million steps per year as average use of the joint replacement, conventional articulations should have a total lifetime of between 10 and 20 million cycles before failure.

Young people have higher levels of activity than older patients by up to an additional million steps per year.[8] They should also expect to live 20 to 40 years longer than the conventional recipients of total hip replacements. Younger patients are also planning to return to more vigorous activities with their hip replacements, and as such, we would expect that they would be at a greater risk for polyethylene failure and osteolysis, as well as an increased risk for dislocation than their historical counterparts. To improve both range of motion and stability, larger and larger diameter femoral heads have been developed.[9] A progression has occurred from the 22.25-mm to the 26-, 28-, 32-, and now 36- and 38-mm metal heads for use in metal/poly articulations. These larger heads have increased wear associated with the increased surface area of the articulation.[4,10] In hip simulator data, this is seen with conventional polyethylene and significantly reduced with highly cross-linked polyethylene. Even with the biggest heads, the wear of the highly cross-linked polyethylene is still significantly less than the historical wear rates of smaller heads against conventional polyethylene. Metal-on-metal articulations have even greater available bearing diameters and are now up to 44 mm with conventional stems and shells, and anatomic head sizes with surface replacement components.

Thus, the lifetime tribological demand that young people place on their hip replacements may have increased to between 100 and 200 million cycles. If a single implanted articulation is to cope with the expected increase in demand of the younger or more active patient, there would need to be at least a 10-fold improvement in the wear characteristics of the alternative bearing couple compared with conventional polyethylene for the bearing couple to survive without need for revision. This is the driving force behind the development of alternative bearing surfaces.[11]

Evidence

Hip simulator studies have been used extensively since the late 1990s to support the research and development of new bearing systems for hip prostheses.[12–15] Total hip replacements often fail because of polyethylene wear debris-induced osteolysis.[16] Most studies comparing cross-linked polyethylene and conventional polyethylene have concentrated only on volumetric wear. Osteolysis is, however, dependent on the size, shape, and chemical activity of the wear debris generated.[17] To compare alternative bearing surfaces, one must determine the relative biological activity of the debris generated and then relate it to the volumetric wear of the articulation. This then gives a means of directly comparing the tribological and biological performances of different alternative bearings.[5,17–25]

CROSS-LINKED POLYETHYLENE

Ultra-high-molecular-weight polyethylene comprises long chains of polyethylene molecules, some in parallel and others in random orientation. When the polyethylene molecules are exposed to gamma irradiation, free radicals are released. With the release of free radicals from adjacent polyethylene molecules, two chains may link at the site from which the free radicals were released. The amount of cross linking is determined by the type of irradiation the polyethylene is exposed to, the dosage of radiation applied, the atmosphere in which the polyethylene is exposed to the radiation, and the postradiation treatment of the polyethylene.[26] Cross linking improves the resistance of the polyethylene to adhesive and abrasive wear. This should result in decreased linear and volumetric wear in cross-linked polyethylene articulations compared with conventional polyethylene.

In hip simulator studies, there is an eightfold reduction in volumetric wear of cross-linked polyethylene compared with conventional polyethylene.[19,24] Improvements in wear rate by an additional 40% are seen when ceramic heads are used against the cross-linked polyethylene.[19,24] In clinical studies, a reduction in linear and volumetric wear has been seen using cross-linked polyethylene ranging from 28% to 95%.[26–30] These observations would suggest that if volumetric wear alone determined osteolysis potential, cross-linked polyethylene should be a much better articulation than conventional polyethylene.

Unfortunately, cross-linked polyethylene produces wear debris that theoretically may have a specific biological activity double that of conventional polyethylene.[19,24] Thus, even though there is an eightfold reduction in volumetric wear, there is only a fourfold improvement in the functional biological activity of the bearing couple. Thus, in vitro, cross-linked polyethylene articulations do not reach the 10-fold improvement in wear characteristics that are estimated to be required by younger patients having total hip replacement. In vitro experiments thus predict a reduction in osteolysis when highly cross-linked polyethylene is used; however, the reduction may not be proportionate to the observed reduction in the volumetric wear.

In a randomized, prospective study with minimum 4-year radiographic follow-up, the incidence of osteolysis was significantly less in the cross-linked arm of the study.[27] This observation was more pronounced on the femoral side where the difference between the cross-linked and noncross-linked group was highly significant ($P = 0.001$). However, when the volume of the osteolytic area was examined, one finds that although the total volume of osteolysis was less in the cross-linked group, the difference was not significant ($P = 0.4$). In another 5-year retrospective study comparing cross-linked and conventional polyethylenes, there were no osteolytic lesions observed around the femoral components in the cross-linked group[28] (Level of Evidence IV).

Thus far we have concentrated on the improved material property of wear resistance that cross-linked polyethylene has compared with conventional polyethylene. There are, however, downsides to cross-linking polyethylene, namely, the physical properties of yield strength, overall tensile strength, and resistance to elongation or crack propagation are all reduced.[31] These physical properties are important to the overall survival of the implant because they each represent a mode through which the implant may fail. One needs to remember that wear-related osteolysis and aseptic loosening are not the only reasons that an implant may fail. Impingement of the neck of the femoral component on the polyethylene insert may result in catastrophic failure caused by fracture of the polyethylene. Fatigue failure of the locking mechanism may lead to loosening of the insert within the modular shell again, causing catastrophic failure.[31] These failure mechanisms are rarely seen with conventional polyethylene; however, the diminished mechanical properties of cross-linked polyethylene raise concerns that failures because of these mechanisms may become more frequent.[32] A balance therefore needs to be reached between the improved wear properties and the reduced physical properties of cross-linked polyethylene. To date, this balance has not been determined.

METAL ON METAL

Of all the alternative bearings, metal on metal has data with the longest follow-up period, with clinical data available on the McKee–Farrar prosthesis for nearly 30 years of follow-up.[33] Currently, there are two main iterations of the metal-on-metal articulation in North America: a modular metal insert that fits into a traditional press-fit shell, or a surface replacement metal head that articulates against nonmodular acetabular components.

Metal-on-metal articulations have the most complex tribology of the alternative bearings. The wear properties are dependent on the exact composition of the alloy used, the size of the articulation, the time after implantation, and the clearance between the components. In simulator studies, high-carbon alloys have been compared with low-carbon alloys with the findings that low-carbon alloys had a six times greater volumetric wear rate than high-carbon alloys.[33] From this observation, the investigators recommend that low-carbon alloys should not be used in metal-on-metal articulations. This has been supported by other authors.[34] Metal-on-metal articulations feature a significant running in phenomenon. In the first million cycles, the articulation has a significantly increased wear rate compared with the steady-state wear rate observed after this.[35] Paradoxically, articulations of larger diameters have less volumetric wear than smaller articulations. This applies both to the wearing in and the steady-state wear rates.[36] Lubrication analysis revealed that as the head size increased, the fluid film also increased, hence reducing wear.[37]

Radial clearance has also been examined as a contributor to volumetric wear rate. As the radial clearance increases between 20 and 150 μm and beyond, the volumetric wear in both the running-in and the steady-state phase increases. Lubrication analysis revealed that as radial clearance increased, fluid film decreased, which explains the worsening wear rates for increased radial clearance.[37]

In summary, metal-on-metal articulations have the advantages that they produce low volumetric wear rates, that increasing the diameter of the articulation improves the volumetric wear rates, and that metal-on-metal articulations can be manufactured in a large variety of sizes as either conventional total hip replacements or surface replacements. Is this then the ideal bearing surface for the young adult who intends to be active with his or her total hip replacement? What are the disadvantages of metal-on-metal articulations?

The single greatest concern with the use of metal-on-metal bearings continues to be the increased levels of metal ions measurable in patients' blood and urine after implantation. Many studies have evaluated the circulating heavy metal ions (Table 84–1).[38] There are, however, multiple complex issues associated with the analysis of metal ions, including collection techniques, analysis, statistical methodologies, and reporting of results. To date, the literature on this topic has been characterized by significant variability in all of these factors. Attempts have been made to standardize these methods.[39] What then are the observed biological effects of the wear debris?

Wear debris from metal-on-metal articulations is in the nanometer size range, and these particles have been found to be cytotoxic to cells at volumes of $5 \ \mu m^3$/cell and greater.[40] Necrosis has been observed histologically around retrieved implants of both historical and modern design.[41] This cytotoxic effect of the wear debris to the local tissue remains of concern to users of metal-on-metal articulations. Concerns are also raised about the effect of elevated heavy metal ions in remote tissues to the hip replacement. Both chromium and cobalt levels are increased above baseline with metal-on-metal articulations.[35,42] Concerns have also been expressed about potential metal ion carcinogenicity. More than 700,000 metal-on-metal total hip arthroplasties have been performed globally with no causal links to cancer.[43,44] Metal wear debris also may cause inflammatory or allergic local tissue reactions in some individuals. This may lead to pain at the site of implantation from synovitis or implant loosening.[45]

These potential adverse biological effects of metal-on-metal articulations are the rationale behind ongoing research into novel hard-bearing articulations. For example, currently under investigation are a delta ceramic head on metal insert bearing, and the use of metal components coated with a thick layer of chromium cyanide (CrCN). Both ceramic-on-metal and the CrCN-coated metal-on-metal articulations have volumetric wear rates 10 to 100 times less than metal-on-metal articulations of the same diameter head size.[46–48] The improvement observed with the ceramic-on-metal articulation is thought to be because of the differential hardness of the metal and the ceramic, and the smoother surface and improved lubrication that ceramics offer. The wear debris from the CrCN-coated bearings was also found to be more biocompatible and less cytotoxic than the metallic debris.[49]

TABLE 84–1. Cobalt and Chromium Levels of Metal-on-Metal Implants

IMPLANT	ANALYTIC TECHNIQUE	SAMPLE	NO. OF IMPLANTS	TIME IN VIVO (YR)	COBALT LEVELS (PARTS PER BILLION)	CHROMIUM LEVELS (PARTS PER BILLION)	REFERENCE
Metasul*	AAS	Serum	27	1	1.1	—	57
Metasul	AAS	Serum	36	5	0.7	—	58
Metasul	AAS	Serum	15	2	0.88	—	59
Metasul	AAS	Serum	15	4.3	0.81	—	59
Metasul	AAS	Serum	60	2	1.70	4.28	60
Metasul	AAS	Serum	42	4	1.57	2.10	61
Metasul average					1.13	3.19	
M²a†	ICP-MS	Erythrocytes	22	2	1.10	2.50	62
M²a	AAS	Serum	10	6	1.55	0.84	63
M²a average					1.33	1.67	
BHR‡	ICP-MS	Serum	16	1	2.10		64
BHR	AAS	Serum	111	2	4.28	5.12	60
BHR	AAS	Serum	16	2	1.88	3.53	65
BHR	ICP-MS	Whole blood	26	4	1.20	1.10	66
BHR average					2.37	3.25	

*Metasul (Zimmer Inc., Winterthur, Switzerland).
†M²a (Biomet, Warsaw, IN).
‡Birmingham Hip Resurfacing (BHR; Midland Medical Technologies, Birmingham, United Kingdom).
AAS, atomic absorption spectrophotometry; ICP-MS, inductively coupled plasma mass spectrometry.

CERAMIC ON CERAMIC

Ceramic-on-ceramic articulations in simulated wear testing outperform other articulations. Volumetric wear rates for ceramic-on-ceramic articulations using traditional hip simulators have been as low as 0.1 mm³/million cycles.[37] To put this in perspective, this is about 350 times lower than the volumetric wear rates of metal on conventional polyethylene and 50 times less than the volumetric wear rate of metal on cross-linked polyethylene. Unfortunately, these wear rates have not been observed in clinical retrieval studies of worn ceramic on ceramic articulations. As the hip moves in vivo, the femoral head does not stay in the exact center of the joint at all times through the gait cycle, and at times may come in contact with the rim of the cup. Standard hip simulators have not been able to replicate the stripe wear that is seen on retrieved femoral heads.[50] Thus, a microseparation hip simulator has been developed that replicates the stripe wear seen on retrieved femoral heads. Volumetric wear rates of 1.4 mm³/million cycles have been observed using this simulator.[51] These observations are consistent with retrieval studies of ceramic-on-ceramic articulations.[37] Comparing these results with other bearings, the ceramic-on-ceramic articulation produces 25 times less debris than conventional polyethylene and 4 times less debris than highly cross-linked polyethylene.[37] In vivo, ceramic-on-ceramic bearings produce similar volumetric wear to metal-on-metal bearings when the metal-on-metal bearing has finished running in and is within its steady-state wear.

When examining the functional biological activity of the debris from the microseparation hip simulator in the same way that the debris of polyethylene articulations was analyzed, there was a bimodal distribution of particle size in the ceramic debris: nanometer-sized debris from the normal articulation surfaces and micron-sized debris from grain boundary failure and pull out from the regions of stripe wear.[52] When this debris was cultured with human macrophages, measured tumor necrosis factor-α production produced a specific biological activity of 0.18. When combined with volumetric wear, substantially lower functional biological activity is derived for ceramic-on-ceramic articulations than either conventional polyethylene (80 times lower) or cross-linked polyethylene (20 times lower).[37] This lower functional biological activity is reflected in retrieval studies where there has been a low incidence of osteolysis.[53]

Ceramics are brittle materials. A real risk exists for fracturing one of the components if the component dislocates or if the neck of the femoral component impinges on the rim of the acetabular insert.[54] There have also been reports of spontaneous fracture of ceramic femoral heads (zirconia heads).[54] Modern ceramics have a fracture risk rate of 0.004%[54] (Level of Evidence III). One of the theoretical concerns that this raises is that when there is a ceramic fracture, the bearing used for the revision should also be ceramic because the hardness of the residual fragments after revision will cause accelerated wear because of third body wear in either a metal-on-metal or a metal-on-polyethylene articulation. When the ceramic fractures, damage may also occur to the femoral trunnion, which then may necessitate removal of a well-fixed femoral stem because the morse taper may be too damaged for another modular head to be implanted on it.[54]

Another complication that occurs uniquely with ceramic-on-ceramic bearings is squeaking. For reasons yet to be determined, a small percentage of patients (0.5–7%)[55,56] (Level of Evidence IV) experience a positional- or activity-related squeaking noise arising from their articulation. This can be unsettling for the patient and rarely may necessitate a revision. Squeaking does not appear to be a problem with metal-on-metal articulations because when squeaking does occur, it is usually only a temporary phenomenon during the metal-on-metal bearing run-in period. More information, however, is needed to understand more fully the squeaking phenomenon in both ceramic-on-ceramic and metal-on-metal bearing couples.

RECOMMENDATIONS

Thus far, only the tribological and biological effects of the alternative bearings have been considered. What is important to remember is that these articulations are being used for total hip replacement, and as such, other considerations need to be met when considering what would be the best articulation for an individual patient. All of these articulations are used in our institution in variable clinical scenarios.

Highly cross-linked polyethylene is an extremely versatile articular bearing surface with a variety of options available to the reconstructive surgeon. Fully cemented components can be manufactured, acetabular inserts can be designed with hoods of various degrees, extra offset can be built into the liner, the liner may have an angled offset opening (a face-changing liner), or the liner may be incorporated into a bipolar or tripolar head. This versatility cannot be achieved with other alternative bearings. Highly cross-linked polyethylene thus gives the surgeon flexibility in obtaining stability in a total hip replacement. This may be even more critical in revision total hip replacements where the increased options available to the surgeon make this an ideal alternate bearing surface.

Ceramic-on-ceramic articulations have as their strengths the lowest volumetric wear rates and the fact that they produce the least biologically active wear debris. Their weakness is that they have limited sizing options, the rare flaw of catastrophic failure, and the clinical issue of a squeaking bearing. We see the role of ceramic-on-ceramic articulations to be the articulation of choice for young and active patients for whom you have concerns that the increased metal ions associated with metal-on-metal articulations may prove problematic—for example, the young female individual of child-bearing years, the young patient with a history of cardiac or renal disease, or the young patient with a history of metal hypersensitivity. (Level of Evidence V).

A significant renewal in interest in metal-on-metal articulations has occurred. Metal heads are able to be manufactured in a greater range of sizes and neck lengths than ceramic heads. Metal acetabular articulations can also be made in a variety of sizes in both modular and nonmodular

forms. This gives the surgeon greater flexibility in terms of improving the stability at time of surgery. Currently, acetabular components can be manufactured only with neutral openings, and as such, the range of options as with polyethylene liners is not available. Large-head, conventional metal-on-metal articulations have the advantage of modularity on both the femoral and acetabular side, and offer the ability to use screws to obtain primary stability of the acetabular shell. In the future, modified metal articulations—ceramic on metal or metal coated with CrCN—may offer the solution to the adverse biological properties of current metal-on-metal articulations (Level of Evidence V).

The 2000s has seen a significant improvement in the materials and options that are available for use as articulating surfaces in total hip arthroplasty. Currently, most of the commercially available bearings have only short- to mid-term follow-up, but results to date are encouraging. Long-term follow-up is, however, required to confirm in vivo results will replicate in vitro data. There continues to be much ongoing work in the improvement of current bearing materials, as well as the evaluation of potential newer bearing couples. Table 84–2 summarizes the levels of evidence for bearing surfaces.

TABLE 84–2. Bearing Surfaces: Levels of Evidence

STATEMENT	LEVEL OF EVIDENCE/ GRADE OF RECOMMENDATION	REFERENCES
1. In hip simulator studies, there is an eightfold reduction in volumetric wear of cross-linked polyethylene compared with conventional polyethylene.	Basic science article	19, 24
2. Metal against cross-linked UHMWPE produces less osteolysis than against non–cross-linked UHMWPE	B B	27 28, 29
3. Low-carbon alloys should not be used in metal-on-metal articulations.	Basic science article	33
4. In metal-on-metal articulations, the larger the diameter of the articulation, the lower the wear.	Basic science article	37
5. In vitro, ceramic-on-ceramic articulations have about 350 times lower the volumetric wear rates of metal on conventional polyethylene and 50 times less than the volumetric wear rate of metal on cross-linked polyethylene.	Basic science article	37
6. Osteolysis is infrequent with ceramic-on-ceramic articulations.	B	53, 54

UHMWPE, ultra-high-molecular-weight polyethylene.

REFERENCES

1. Callaghan JJ, Templeton JE, Liu SS, et al: Results of Charnley total hip arthroplasty at a minimum of thirty years. A concise follow-up of a previous report. J Bone Joint Surg Am 86:690–695, 2004.

2. Malchau H, Garellick G, Eisler T, et al: Presidential Guest Address. The Swedish Hip Registry. Clin Orthop 441:19–29.

3. Ingham E, Fisher J: Biological reactions to wear debris in total joint replacement. Proc Inst Mech Eng 214:21–37, 2000.

4. Livermore J, Ilstrup D, Murray B: Effect of head size on the wear of the polyethylene acetabular component. J Bone Joint Surg Am 72:518–528, 1990.

5. Tipper JL, Ingham E, Hailey JL, et al: Quantitative analysis of polyethylene wear debris, wear rate and head damage in retrieved Charnley hip prostheses. J Mater Sci Mater Med 11:117–124, 2000.

6. Barbour PS, Stone MH, Fisher J: A hip joint simulator study using simplified loading and motion cycles generating physiological wear paths and rates. Proc Inst Mech Eng 213:455–467, 1999.

7. Barbour PS, Stone MH, Fisher J: A hip joint simulator study using new and physiologically scratched femoral heads with ultra-high molecular weight polyethylene acetabular cups. Proc Inst Mech Eng 214:569–576, 2000.

8. Schmalzried TP, Szuszczewicz ES, Northfield MR, et al: Quantitative assessment of walking activity after total hip and total knee replacement. J Bone Joint Surg Am 80:54–58, 1998.

9. Crowninshield RD, Maloney WJ, Wentz DH, et al: Biomechanics of large diameter heads. Clin Orthop Relat Res (429):102–107, 2004.

10. Fisher J: Wear of joint replacements. In Shanbhag A, Rubash HE, Jacobs JJ (eds): Joint Replacement and Bone Resorption—Pathology, Biomaterials and Clinical Practice. New York, Taylor and Francis, 2006, pp 145–169.

11. Heisel C, Silva M, Schmalzried TP: Bearing surface options for total hip replacements in young patients. Instr Course Lect 53:49–65, 2004.

12. Chan FW, Bobyn JD, Medley JB: Engineering issues and wear performance of metal on metal hip implants. Clin Orthop Relat Res (333):96–107, 1996.

13. D'Lima DD, Hermida JC, Chen PC, Colwell CW Jr: Polyethylene cross-linking by two different methods reduces acetabular liner wear in a hip joint wear simulator. J Orthop Res 21:761–766, 2003.

14. Jin ZM, Dowson D, Fisher J: Analysis of fluid film lubrication in artificial hip joint replacements with surfaces of high elastic modulus. Proc Inst Mech Eng [H] 211:247–256, 1997.

15. Wang A, Essner A, Schmidig G: The effects of lubricant composition on in vitro wear testing of polymeric acetabular components. J Biomed Mater Res B Appl Biomater 68:45–52, 2004.

16. Willert HG, Semliitsch M: Reactions of the articular capsule to wear products of artificial joint prostheses. J Biomed Mater Res 11:157–164, 1977.

17. Ingram JH, Stone M, Fisher J, Ingham E: The influence of molecular weight, crosslinking and counterface roughness on TNF-alpha production by macrophages in response to ultra high molecular weight polyethylene particles. Biomaterials 25:3511–3522, 2004.

18. Tipper JL, Firkins PJ, Besong AA, et al: Characterisation of wear debris from UHMWPE on zirconia ceramic, metal-on-metal and alumina ceramic-on-ceramic hip prostheses generated in a physiological anatomical hip joint simulator. Wear 250:120–128, 2001.

19. Galvin AL, Tipper JL, Ingham E, Fisher J: Nanometre size wear debris generated from crosslinked and non-crosslinked ultra high molecular weight polyethylene in artificial joints. Wear 259:977–983, 2005.

20. Hatton A, Nevelos JE, Nevelos AA, et al: Alumina-alumina artificial hip joints. Part I: A histological analysis and characterisation of wear debris by laser capture microdissection of tissues retrieved at revision. Biomaterials 23:3429–3440, 2002.

21. Tipper JL, Hatton A, Nevelos JE, et al: Alumina-alumina artificial hip joints: Part II: Characterisation of the wear debris from in vitro hip joints simulations. Biomaterials 23:3441–3448, 2002.

22. Firkins PJ, Tipper JL, Saadatzadeh MR, et al: Quantitative analysis of wear and wear debris from metal-on-metal hip prostheses tested in a physiological hip joint simulator. Biomed Mater Eng 11:143–157, 2001.

23. Green TR, Fisher J, Stone M, et al: Polyethylene particles of a "critical size" are necessary for the induction of cytokines by macrophages in vitro. Biomaterials 19:2297–2302, 1998.

24. Endo M, Tipper JL, Barton DC, et al: Comparison of wear, wear debris and functional biological activity of moderately crosslinked and non-crosslinked polyethylene in hip prostheses. Proc Inst Mech Eng [H] 216:111–122, 2002.

25. Fisher J, Bell J, Barbour PS, et al: A novel method for the prediction of functional biological activity of polyethylene wear debris. Proc Inst Mech Eng [H] 215:127–132, 2001.

26. Geerdink CH, Grimm B, Ramakrishnan R, et al: Crosslinked polyethylene compared to conventional polyethylene in total hip replacement: Pre-clinical evaluation, in-vitro testing and prospective clinical followup study. Acta Orthopaedica 77:719–725, 2006.

27. Engh CA Jr, Stepniewski AS, Ginn SD, et al: A randomized prospective evaluation of outcomes after total hip arthroplasty using cross-linked marathon and non–cross-linked enduron polyethylene liners. J Arthoplasty 21(suppl 2):17–25, 2006.

28. D'Antonio JA, Manley MT, Capello WN, et al: Five-year experience with crossfire highly cross-linked polyethylene. Clin Orthop Relat Res (441):143–150.

29. Manning DW, Chiang PP, Martell JM, et al: In vivo comparative wear study of traditional and highly cross-linked polyethylene in total hip arthroplasty. J Arthroplasty 20:880–886, 2005.

30. Digas G, Kärrholm J, Thanner J, et al: Highly cross-linked polyethylene in total hip arthroplasty. Clin Orthop Relat Res 429:6–16, 2004.

31. Bradford L, Baker D, Ries MD, Pruitt LA: Fatigue crack propagation resistance of highly crosslinked polyethylene. Clin Orthop Relat Res (429):68–72.

32. Birman MV, Noble PC, Conditt MA, et al: Cracking and impingement in ultra–high-molecular-weight polyethylene acetabular liners. J Arthroplasty 20(suppl 3):87–92.

33. Brown SR, Davies WA, DeHeer DH, Swanson AB: Long-term survival of McKee-Farrar total hip prostheses. Clin Orthop Relat Res (402):157, 2002.

34. Chan FW, Bobyn JD, Medley JB, et al: The Otto Aufranc Award: Wear and lubrication of metal-on metal hip implants. Clin Orthop Relat Res (369):10, 1999.

35. Lhotka C, Szekeres T, Steffan I, et al: Four-year study of cobalt and chromium blood levels in patients managed with two different metal-on-metal total hip replacements. J Orthop Res 21:189–195, 2003.

36. Hu XQ, Isaac GH, Fisher J: Changes in contact area during the bedding-in of different sizes of metal on metal hip prostheses. Biomed Mater Eng 14:145–149, 2004.

37. Fisher J, Jin Z, Tipper J, et al: Tribology of alternative bearings. Clin Orthop 453:25–34, 2006.

38. MacDonald SJ: Can a safe level for metal ions in patients with metal-on-metal total hip arthroplasties be determined? J Arthroplasty 19(suppl 3):71–77, 2004.

39. MacDonald, SJ, Brodner W, Jacobs JJ: A consensus paper on metal ions in metal-on-metal hip arthroplasties. J Arthroplasty 19:12–16, 2004.

40. Germain MA, Hatton A, Williams S, et al: Comparison of the cytotoxicity of clinically relevant cobalt-chromium and alumina ceramic wear particles in vitro. Biomaterials 24:469–479, 2003.

41. Doorn PE, Mirra JM, Campbell PA, Amstutz HC: Tissue reaction to metal on metal total hip prostheses. Clin Orthop Relat Res 329S:S187–S205.

42. Daniel J, Ziaee H, Pradhan C, et al: Blood and urine metal ion levels in young and active patients after Birmingham hip resurfacing arthroplasty. J Bone Joint Surg Br 89-B:169–173, 2007.

43. Visuri TI, Pulkkinen P, Paavolainen P: Malignant tumors at the site of total hip prosthesis. Analytic review of 46 cases. J Arthroplasty 21:311–323, 2006.

44. Visuri TI, Pukkala E, Pulkkinen P, Paavolainen P: Cancer incidence and causes of death among total hip replacement patients: A review based on Nordic cohorts with a special

emphasis on metal-on-metal bearings. Proc Inst Mech Eng [H] 220:399–407, 2006.

45. Jacobs JJ, Hallab J: Loosening and osteolysis associated with metal-on-metal bearings: A local effect of metal hypersensitivity? J Bone Joint Surg Am 88:1171–1172, 2006.

46. Firkins PJ, Tipper JL, Ingham E, et al: A novel low wearing differential hardness, ceramic-on-metal hip joint prostheses. J Biomech 34:1291–1298, 2001.

47. Fisher J, Hu XQ, Stewart TD, et al: Wear of surface engineered metal-on-metal hip prostheses. J Mater Sci Mater Med 15:225–235, 2004.

48. Fisher J, Hu XQ, Tipper JL, et al: An in vitro study of the reduction in wear of metal on metal hip prostheses using surface-engineered femoral heads. Proc Inst Mech Eng [H] 216:219–230, 2002.

49. Williams S, Tipper JL, Ingham E, et al: In vitro analysis of the wear, wear debris and biological activity of surface-engineered coatings for use in metal-on-metal total hip replacements. Proc Inst Mech Eng [H] 217:155–163, 2003.

50. Walter WL, Insley GM, Walter WK, Tuke MA: Edge loading in third generation alumina ceramic-on-ceramic bearings. J Arthroplasty 19:402–413, 2004.

51. Stewart T, Tipper JL, Streicher R, et al: Long-term wear or HIPed alumina on alumina bearings for THR under microseparation conditions. J Mater Sci Mater Med 12:1053–1056, 2001.

52. Tipper JL, Hatton A, Nevelos JE, et al: Alumina-alumina artificial hip joints: Part II: Characterisation of the wear debris from in vitro hip joints simulations. Biomaterials 23:3441–3448, 2002.

53. Hamadouche M, Boutin P, Daussange J, et al: Alumina-on-alumina total hip arthroplasty: A minimum 18.5-year follow-up study. J Bone Joint Surg Am 84:69–77, 2002.

54. Bierbaum BJ, Nairus J, Kuesis D, et al: Ceramic-on-ceramic bearings in total hip arthroplasty. Clin Orthop Relat Res 405:158–163, 2002.

55. Walter WL, O'Toole GC, Walter WK, et al: Squeaking in ceramic on ceramic hips. J Arthroplasty 22:496–503, 2007.

56. Jarrett C, Ranawat AS, Bruzzone M, et al: "The squeaking hip" An under reported phenomenon of ceramic on ceramic total hip arthroplasty. Presented at the Hip Society Summer Meeting; Iowa City, IA, 2006.

57. Brodner W, Bitzan P, Meisinger V, et al: Elevated serum cobalt with metal on metal articulating surfaces. J Bone Joint Surg Br 79:316, 1997.

58. Brodner W, Bitzan P, Meisinger V, et al: Serum cobalt levels after metal-on-metal total hip arthroplasty. J Bone Joint Surg Am 85:2168, 2003.

59. Savarino L, Granchi D, Ciapetti G, et al: Ion release in stable hip arthroplasties using metal-on-metal articulating surfaces: A comparison between short- and medium-term results. J Biomed Mater Res 66A:450, 2003.

60. Witzleb WC, Ziegler J, Krummenauer F, et al: Exposure to chromium, cobalt and molybdenum from metal-on-metal total hip replacement and hip resurfacing arthroplasty. Acta Orthop 77:697–705, 2006.

61. Savarino L, Greco M, Cenni E, et al: Differences in ion release after ceramic-on-ceramic and metal-on-metal total hip replacement. Medium-term follow-up. J Bone Joint Surg Br 88:472–476, 2006.

62. MacDonald SJ, McCalden RW, Chess DG, et al: Metal-on-metal versus polyethylene in hip arthroplasty: A randomized clinical trial. Clin Orthop Relat Res (406):282, 2003.

63. Rasquinha VJ, Ranawat CS, Weiskopf J, et al: Serum metal levels and bearing surfaces in total hip arthroplasty. J Arthroplasty 21(6 suppl 2):47–52, 2006.

64. Clarke MT, Lee PTH, Arora A, Villar RN: Levels of metal ions after small and large diameter metal-on-metal hip arthroplasty. J Bone Joint Surg Br 85:913, 2003.

65. Back DL, Young DA, Shimmin AJ: How do serum cobalt and chromium levels change after metal-on-metal hip resurfacing? Clin Orthop Relat Res (438):177–181, 2005.

66. Daniel J, Ziaee H, Pradham C, et al: Blood and urine metal ion levels in young and active patients after Birmingham hip resurfacing arthroplasty. Four-year results of a prospective longitudinal study. J Bone Joint Surg Br 89:169–173, 2006.

Chapter 85

What Are the Facts and Fiction of Minimally Invasive Hip and Knee Arthroplasty Surgery?

David Backstein, MD, Med, FRCSC

Although minimally invasive surgical (MIS) techniques such as laparoscopic cholecystectomy and arthroscopic anterior cruciate ligament reconstruction have gained widespread acceptance in the surgical community, reduced invasiveness in total joint replacement has stirred much controversy and debate. The concept of minimizing iatrogenic trauma has always been a fundamental surgical principle. However, it is only recently that the concept of small-incision surgery and minimal musculotendinous disturbance has come to the forefront in the total hip and total knee arthroplasty (THA and TKA) literature, the lay press, and commercial advertising.

There are several key characteristics of what is generally considered MIS joint replacement including reduced skin incision length, mobile windows of exposure, reduced muscle and tendon damage, avoidance of extreme maneuvers such as patellar eversion, and utilization of low-profile instrumentation. Any discussion of this topic must distinguish between those techniques that involve surgical approaches through smaller skin incisions and lessened muscle dissection from those procedures that describe truly novel and potentially technically challenging approaches to the hip and knee. In addition, it is important to recognize that any MIS joint replacement protocol also incorporates specialized preoperative and postoperative patient education, anesthesia routines, as well as nursing and rehabilitation programs.

Advocates for MIS joint replacement proclaim the benefits of less blood loss, less postoperative pain, reduced length of hospital stay, more rapid recovery of function, and better cosmesis without increased risk for complication or diminished duration of implant survivorship.[1-11] However, other investigators have failed to find significant benefit from MIS joint replacement and have encountered steep and difficult learning curves.[10,12-18] Some investigators have discovered concerning rates of serious complications such as implant malposition, intraoperative fracture, skin complications, and prolonged operative durations.[18-24] These data combined with the well-documented and highly favorable long-term results of traditional-incision joint replacement have resulted in some vocal opposition to the placement

of excessive emphasis on incision length.[25-27] Some authors have questioned the ethics of the broad application of such techniques without proven benefit, as well as the role that direct-to-consumer advertising and commercial interests have played before thorough study.[28-30]

The purpose of this chapter is to review the available evidence in the literature that is capable of directing potential incorporation of novel MIS techniques into the already successful practice regimens of hip and knee arthroplasty, which have been developed over more than three decades. Techniques that involve smaller and modified implant plant components such as unicompartmental knee arthroplasty or resurfacing of the hip are not considered here. Although the overwhelming majority of data on this topic is derived from retrospective cohort studies and case–control series, there is a modest amount of Level I and II evidence available to draw some conclusions and make practice recommendations (Tables 85–1 and 85–2).

OPTIONS

Hip

In MIS hip surgery, the dominant approaches have been modifications of standard anterior, posterior, and lateral surgical exposures, as well as a combined anterior and posterior approach commonly called the "two-incision" technique. This has led to the development of surgical instrument systems that are smaller and of lower profile, but the actual implants themselves have not changed in any significant way. The posterior technique of mini-incision THA has been described by authors such as Chimento and coworkers.[31] This approach involves an incision of 6 to 10 cm in length without disruption of the gluteus maximus tendon or the quadratus femoris muscle. Berger[1] has described an anterolateral approach that transects less gluteus medius and minimus through an 8- to 10-cm incision. Toms and Duncan[32] have published a description of a single incision intermuscular anterolateral approach that they claim has advantages of standard lateral patient positioning, simple conversion to an extensile approach, no need for fluoroscopy, and a short learning curve for surgeons.

TABLE 85–1. Summary of Level I and II Evidence

STUDY	LEVEL OF EVIDENCE	DESIGN	APPROACH	CASES (N)	FINDINGS
Level I and II Studies of MIS THA					
Chimento et al.[31]	II	Prospective, randomized	8 vs. 16 cm posterolateral	28 MIS vs. 32 standard	Less intraoperative and total blood loss in MIS, but no difference in transfusion requirements Less limp at 6 weeks No difference in complication rate
Mardones et al.[40]	II	Randomized, controlled	Two-incision vs. miniposterior, cadaveric	10 two-incision vs. 10 miniposterior	Two-incision group had greater damage to abductor muscles
Bennett et al.[12]	II	Prospective, blinded cohort	10 vs. 16 cm posterior	17	Standard group achieved more normal hip joint kinematics after surgery compared with MIS MIS group showed no early benefit (postoperative day 2) in any kinematic of temporospatial measures compared with standard
Mow et al.[5]	II	Blinded scar comparison	<10 vs. >15 cm	31	Cosmesis of mini-incision THA scars may be inferior to standard-incision scars
Hart et al.[6]	II	Prospective, randomized	<10 vs. >10 cm posterior	120	Less blood loss in MIS group; trend toward better clinical scores for MIS at 6 weeks after surgery; no clinical difference by 6 months; no difference in complications
Ogonda et al.[13]	I	Prospective, randomized	<10 vs. 16 cm posterior	219	Mini-incision safe but of no benefit in the early postoperative phase; more investigation required for lower volume, less experienced surgeons
Level I and II Studies of MIS TKA					
Kolisek et al.[50]	II	Prospective, randomized	MIS midvastus with skin incision <13 cm vs. >13-cm incision with midvastus or medial parapatellar	80	No differences in functional or radiographic results; no differences in adverse outcomes
Aglietti et al.[45]	I	Prospective, randomized	Mini-subvastus vs. "quadriceps sparing"	60	No significant differences between groups at 3 months after surgery Quadriceps sparing technically more challenging
Boerger et al.[44]	II	Prospective	10-cm mini-subvastus vs. standard medial parapatellar	120	Early, short-lived functional benefit in MIS, but with greater significant complication rate; no radiographic differences; MIS more technically challenging

TABLE 85–2. Summary of Recommendations

RECOMMENDATIONS	LEVEL OF EVIDENCE/GRADE OF RECOMMENDATION
1. Short incision approaches to the hip utilizing less invasive modifications of traditional posterior, lateral, and anterior approaches are a viable option in nonobese patients without prior hip surgery or major alterations to normal anatomy (such as protrusion or developmental dysplasia of the hip).	A
2. Minimally invasive hip approaches utilizing novel surgical approach (two-incision approach) are not recommended because of lack of evidence of any benefit and unacceptable complication rates.	B
3. Short-incision approaches to the knee utilizing less invasive modifications of traditional medial parapatellar, subvastus, or midvastus approaches are a viable option in nonobese patients without prior knee surgery or major alterations to normal anatomy.	A
4. Minimally invasive knee approaches utilizing novel surgical approach (quadriceps-sparing approach) is not recommended because of lack of evidence of clinical benefit and concerns about technical difficulty.	B

Among the most controversial novel hip approaches has been the two-incision method written about extensively by Berger.[33] It has been claimed that this technique is completely intermuscular and "avoids the transection of any muscle or tendon."[1] The two-incision technique utilizes an anterior, Smith–Peterson interval for the acetabular exposure, and a posterior incision between the abductors and the external rotators for stem insertion. The described technique requires intraoperative fluoroscopic imaging.

Knee

Three modifications of standard techniques have gained wider utilization in the knee, as well as one novel approach, which has much less general acceptance. All four techniques have in common abandonment of the formerly common practice of patellar eversion and tibiofemoral dislocation for exposure purposes.[34] They also make use of the concept of "mobile windows" of exposure that utilize varying degrees of flexion and extension throughout the procedure to allow visualization of the femur or the tibia, but not both simultaneously.

Scuderi and coworkers[35] use a 10- to 14-cm skin incision and a medial parapatellar arthrotomy that differs from a standard approach in that the quadriceps tendon is incised only 2 to 4 cm above the superior pole of the patella. The subvastus approach that Hofmann[36] described has been modified to make it less invasive. A shortened anterior, midline skin incision is made, and a medial parapatellar arthrotomy follows. The attachment of the vastus medialis obliquus (VMO) muscle to the quadriceps tendon and upper patellar pole is left intact. The VMO muscle belly is then retracted so that limited dissection can occur posterior to the muscle belly, anterior to the intermuscular septum. Synovial release of the suprapatellar pouch is required, and the patella is subluxed laterally.[35] The standard midvastus approach that Engh and colleagues[37] described has been modified to lessen its damage to the VMO. A shortened midline anterior skin incision is utilized. A medial arthrotomy is made and the incision is extended proximally into the full thickness of the vastus medialis, in-line with its muscle fibers for a

length or 4 to 5 cm starting at the superior-medial pole of the patella. The patella is then lateralized but not dislocated.[35]

The technique that deviates to the greatest degree from traditional techniques and has gained the least general acceptance has been described by Tria and Coon[38] and is commonly referred to as the "quadriceps-sparing" technique. This technique uses a curved medial incision from the superior pole of the patella to the tibial joint line. An arthrotomy is then made in line with the skin incision. Bony cuts are made using instruments and guides that fixate and cut from the medial side of the knee rather than the standard anterior location. The quadriceps tendon and VMO are theoretically left completely intact.

EVIDENCE

Hip

Because of the earlier interest and development of MIS applications to THA, the hip literature is more robust than that of the knee. The earliest work in this realm consisted almost exclusively of case series and expert opinions. Despite the absence of high-quality research, many orthopedic surgeons have determined the degree to which they would incorporate MIS concepts into their practice based on the recommendation of opinion leaders, as well as their own personal experience. Fortunately, sufficient time has now elapsed to allow several Level I and II studies to be published.

In 2005, Ogonda and coauthors[13] reported on a prospective, randomized, controlled trial of 219 patients with 219 THAs studied over a period of 6 months. Patients were blinded to length of incision, and all surgery was performed by a single surgeon using a posterior approach. Of critical importance, and one of the strengths of this study, was the fact that the treating surgeon had already become adept at MIS techniques by previously performing 300 short-incision THAs. In the standard-incision group, the subcutaneous tissues and fascia lata were divided in line with the skin incision, which was 16 cm long. In the MIS group, only the proximal 1 cm of the fascia lata was incised. The distal fibers of the gluteus maximus were split by blunt dissection, and the short external rotators were detached close to their insertion into the greater trochanter. These authors found no difference in component position and wound complications, and no evidence of lessened inflammation in the MIS group based on C-reactive protein measurements at 48 hours after surgery. Most remarkably, there were no differences in function immediately after surgery or at 6 weeks, based on Harris hip scores, Oxford hip scores, WOMAC Index of Osteoarthritis and SF-12 general health questionnaire. There was also no benefit for the MIS group in terms of length of hospital stay. These authors conclude that MIS incision surgery performed by an experienced surgeon through a posterior approach is safe but of no benefit in the early postoperative phase. They also caution that more investigation is required to determine the appropriateness of this technique for lower volume and less experienced surgeons.[13]

Chimento and investigators[5] conducted a prospective, randomized comparison of a group of 60 patients with THA through a 15-cm incision with a group that had a modified posterolateral approach and an 8-cm incision. Only patients with a body mass index of less than 30 and no previous hip surgery were included. All procedures involved a single surgeon and anesthetist. After surgery, all patients were supervised by a single physiotherapist. The MIS group was found to have significantly less intraoperative and total blood loss. At 6 weeks after surgery, significantly fewer MIS patients had a residual limp (21.4% vs. 46.8%). No differences were found in any other parameter including length of hospital stay, number of units transfused, postoperative interleukin-6 levels, volume of narcotic used, or utilization of a cane at 6 weeks. There were also no differences between the groups in terms of the position of components or incidence of complications. This well-designed study did indicate that the MIS group may benefit in terms of reduced blood loss; however, the lack of any difference in transfused units and the possibility that there was inadequate numbers to detect differences in complication rates results in no definitive evidence in favor of the MIS approach.

Lawlor and researchers[39] have conducted a prospective study of 219 THA replacements that were randomized into either an MIS group (<10 cm) or standard incision (16 cm), performed by a single surgeon with a standardized analgesia and physiotherapy regimen. No significant improvement was noted in the MIS group in terms of ability to transfer, mobilize weight bearing, or walking velocity at 2 days after surgery. No statistically significant difference was found in the length of hospital stay. No significant differences between groups were found at the 6-week mark after surgery. These authors conclude that the MIS approach offered no benefit over the 16-cm incision. It is clear that a posterior approach was used for all hips in this study; however, there is no indication that deep soft-tissue management differed between the two groups. Therefore, this study cannot have implication beyond the impact of a smaller skin incision.

Another study, conducted by Bennett and coworkers,[12] also failed to show any significant benefit of MIS THA techniques. These authors compared objective postoperative gait mechanics data by means of a prospective, blinded cohort study of 25 randomly selected patients evaluated on postoperative days 1, 2, and 42 (6 weeks). Nine patients with MIS and eight with standard incision were available for a full set of gait analyses. The standard group experienced greater improvement in sagittal plane hip joint movement between day 2 and week 6 compared with the MIS group. Measurements also suggested that the standard group achieved more normal hip joint kinematics after surgery than did the MIS group. The MIS group demonstrated no early benefit (at day 2) in any kinematic or temporospatial measures. Even at 6 weeks, the temporospatial variables and kinematic ranges of motion were reduced compared with the traditional group. The lack of any significant difference in velocity, step length of the affected or unaffected leg, or stride length or stance phase duration between groups failed to lend support to the MIS technique.

Hart and coworkers[6] conducted a prospective study comparing 60 patients randomly selected to have a posterior approach THA with an incision 10 cm or less to a second group of 60 with a standard posterolateral approach. Mean follow-up period was 39 months, and no patients were lost to follow-up. No statistically significant differences were observed between the two groups including pain, motion, and function. There were also no differences in component positioning or complication rates. These authors caution that the MIS approach has a greater requirement for assistants and should not be attempted in patients with protrusio deformity, fibrous or osseus ankylosis, hips scarred by previous surgery, or obese patients.

The two-incision approach to THA has been among the most controversial of MIS techniques. The developers of this operation have published several technical and experiential reports that were largely favorable and described rapid recovery of function.[1,2,7] However, several studies by other authors have since revealed a difficult learning curve and a complication rate that is of significant concern. Archibeck and White[19] examined data provided by the implant manufacturer that played a role in the development of this procedure, which was collected to track the early experiences of surgeons trained in the technique. These authors discovered that the learning curve was likely longer than initially expected based on the 851 cases they reviewed. The rates of femoral fractures (6.5%) and nerve injuries (3.2%) were also found to be much greater than traditional THA. Bal and coauthors[20] have also raised concern as they compared the results of the two-incision technique as described by initial innovators[1,2,7] with an MIS approach, which used a single incision. In the two-incision group, 10% of patients required repeat surgery because of a femoral fracture identified after surgery (two hips), dislocation (one hip), a wound complication (two hips), or subsidence and loosening of the femoral implant (four hips). Twenty-five percent of patients suffered an injury of the lateral femoral cutaneous nerve, and one patient (one hip) had a neuropraxia of the femoral nerve. In comparison, of the 96 THAs that had been performed with use of a single MIS direct lateral exposure of the hip joint, the overall complication rate was 6% and the reoperation rate was 3%. Although the rate of complications with the two-incision technique decreased significantly as the surgeon gained experience, this study raises concern about highly consequential complications early in the learning curve, particularly because these authors are experienced hip surgeons who took the necessary training before initiating the two-incision technique.

Further evidence questioning the value and utility of the two-incision technique was reported by Mardones and coworkers.[40] These authors elegantly quantified the extent and location of damage to the abductor and external rotator muscles and tendons after 10 two-incision and 10 miniposterior THAs were conducted on contralateral sides of 10 fresh-frozen cadavers. A surgeon experienced with such procedures performed each approach. A third surgeon assessed the degree of muscle damage using a standardized, published technique,[41] and found damage to gluteus medius and gluteus minimus from the two-incision technique was greater than the miniposterior approach. Every two-incision procedure had damage to abductors, external rotators, or both. The mean amount of damage to the gluteus medius muscle for the two-incision technique was 15.14% of its muscular area, whereas the miniposterior technique had a mean of only 4.73%. The damage to the gluteus minimus muscle was similarly greater in the two-incision technique as compared with the miniposterior group. Six of 10 two-incision THAs had complete detachment of the external rotators. Although this was a cadaveric study, and therefore not precisely comparable with living patients, the indications for the two-incision procedure were further eroded because there was absolutely no evidence of lessened muscle or tendon damage. In fact, the extent of abductor damage was actually greater in the two-incision group than in the matched miniposterior group.

Knee

Although a review of the literature reveals fewer data of high quality in the area of MIS TKA than that of THA, adequate information is available to draw some conclusions. Haas and colleagues[42] compared 40 consecutive MIS midvastus TKAs without patellar eversion with an age- and sex-matched cohort of TKAs done with a standard technique. Patients achieved motion faster in the MIS group. Mean flexion for minimally invasive total knee replacement at 6 and 12 weeks was 114 (range, 90–132) and 122 (range, 103–135) degrees, respectively, compared with 95 (range, 65–125) and 110 (range, 80–125) degrees for the standard group. The average range of motion at 1 year after surgery in the MIS group was

125 (range, 110–135) degrees compared with 116 (range, 95–130) degrees in the standard group. Postoperative Knee Society scores were greater in the MIS group, and there was no difference in radiographic alignment, infections, extensor mechanism complications, or neurovascular injury. The authors conclude that mini-midvastus approach without patella eversion combined with a small incision was associated with a more rapid functional recovery and improved range of motion without compromise of implant position.[42] Laskin and colleagues'[43] retrospective mini-midvastus study has also shown improved early range of motion and greater Knee Society functional outcome scores without compromise in radiographic alignment.

In a prospective, observer-blinded study, Boerger and researchers[44] studied 120 consecutive patients with TKAs performed by a single surgeon using either the MIS subvastus approach without patella eversion or the standard parapatellar approach with patella eversion. Patients were matched by age, sex, body mass index, knee flexion, deformity, and preexisting high tibial osteotomy. The authors found that the MIS approach was technically more demanding, and inferior visibility prolonged the tourniquet time by an average of 15 minutes. They attributed two intraoperative complications to the poorer exposure. Patients in the MIS subvastus group lost, on average, 100 mL less blood and had better pain scores on day 1 (mean visual analogue scale score: 2.4 vs. 3.89). The MIS group reached 90 degrees of knee flexion earlier (2.8 vs. 4.5 days), and an active straight-leg raise earlier (3.2 vs. 4.1 days). Although the MIS group average flexion at 30, 60, and 90 days was statistically better (100 vs. 94, 110 vs. 106, and 112 vs. 109 degrees), the benefits diminished with time, and the authors doubted the clinical relevance. All patients including those with complications had good results with good component and leg alignment. The authors conclude that the MIS subvastus approach offers early but short-lived benefits for patients at the expense of a longer operation and a greater risk for complications.

A prospective, randomized, double-blind study was conducted by Aglietti and researchers[45] to compare the postoperative recovery and early results "quadriceps-sparing" technique with the MIS subvastus approach.[45] Thirty patients in each group received the same anesthesia protocol and had surgery performed by the same surgeon using the same TKA implants. Evaluation was performed before surgery, in the first week after surgery, and at 1 and 3 months. The authors questioned the feasibility of the quadriceps-sparing technique because these highly experienced knee surgeons required extension of the incision in five cases in the "quadriceps-sparing" group for exposure. Active straight leg raising was achieved half a day earlier, on average, in the MIS subvastus group (1.9 vs. 1.4 days). No further difference was found between the two approaches in relation to short-term recovery or early results; thus, the utility of the technically more challenging quadriceps-sparing technique was questioned. Further evidence by Pagnano and researchers[49] used a cadaveric study that reported that any medial arthrotomy that extends more proximal than the midpole of the patella detaches a portion of the quadriceps tendon; thus, the term *quadriceps-sparing TKA* may be inaccurate.

Nuelle and Mann[46] examined 2 groups of 25 patients in a single surgeon's practice who underwent THA and TKA with standard incisions. The only difference between groups was the anesthesia, pain management, and physical therapy protocols. One group received the protocols described for MIS surgery, whereas the second group had protocols for standard procedures. The surgical technique itself was identical between the two groups. A dramatic reduction in the time it took to achieve the goals for discharge was observed in the MIS protocol group. The MIS protocol group benefited in terms of time to straight leg raise, time to walk 100 m, time to get in and out of bed without assistance, and length of stay. Most patients with the MIS protocols were ready for discharge within 24 hours. The implications of these results are that the benefits of MIS surgery may be unrelated to the surgical procedure itself but rather directly a result of perioperative protocols. If true, this would make the reduction in exposure and the potential inherent risks of MIS surgery of no particular value.

Dalury and Dennis[47] have raised concerns about component malposition and potential long-term compromise when MIS TKA techniques are used. In this retrospective, comparative study, the authors compared a group of 30 patients who had MIS TKA with a similar group of 30 patients who had a standard-incision TKA. Exposure in both groups was primarily through a midvastus approach, although a medial parapatellar was used in 7 of 30 of the MIS and 9 of 30 standard patients. The MIS group had some minor early advantages in terms of pain medication use and earlier improvement in range of motion; however, by 3 months, the groups were equivalent. Radiographic evaluation revealed that 4 of 30 patients with MIS exposures had tibial component varus (<87 degrees) and none of the standard group had such malalignment.

GUIDELINES

In 2004, the American Association of Hip and Knee Surgeons (AAHKS) published an advisory statement on the topic of MIS.[48] At the time of this statement's publication, the AAHKS was of the opinion that the potential of MIS surgery for better long-term results, with shorter and less painful recovery, had yet to be scientifically proven. The AAHKS states that is the responsibility of the surgeon to be competent at these techniques and obtain informed consent before performing them.[49]

The American Academy of Orthopaedic Surgeons (AAOS; http://www.aaos.org/home.asp) similarly recognizes the importance of studying and validating these procedures but considers MIS surgery to be an "evolving" technique.

CONCLUSIONS

Review of the orthopedic literature indicates that total hip and knee replacement through smaller incisions utilizing traditional approaches that minimize soft-tissue damage can be performed without unacceptable complications rates. However, only minimal benefit has been demonstrated in terms of recovery, and without a doubt, modern perioperative anesthesia and physiotherapy regimens play a contributing role.

In contrast, techniques that involve major deviations from the traditional surgical approaches have yet to be proven beneficial and likely have unacceptable complication rates when performed by surgeons other than the designers and innovators themselves. These procedures cannot be recommended at this time.

RECOMMENDATIONS

Review of the available literature allows for certain recommendations regarding the applicability of minimally invasive approaches to hip and knee replacement in the broader orthopedic community. The published literature naturally divides itself into two categories. One category involves procedures that utilized smaller incisions in combination with modifications of standard approaches to minimize muscle and tendon damage. The second category of procedure includes those that are distinctly different from traditional both in terms of the location of skin incisions and the nature of the deeper surgical approach (two-incision THA and "quadriceps-sparing" TKA).

At this time, a definitive recommendation in favor of smaller incisions with modifications of standard approaches cannot be made because the published evidence has failed to reveal any significant and clinically relevant difference between the early outcomes of any MIS technique when contrasted with the comparable traditional approach. Longer-term studies have also found no advantages of MIS procedures. Several retrospective, case-controlled, and case series studies have shown moderate early advantages of MIS surgery in terms of blood loss and early functional outcome. These studies have also generally demonstrated an absence of adverse outcomes with respect to component positioning, fixation, or postoperative complications. Thus, these "small-incision" procedures can be acceptable when adequate training and consent is obtained.

In distinct contrast, however, techniques such as "two-incision" approach to THA and the

Continued

REFERENCES

1. Berger R: Mini-incision total hip replacement using an anterolateral approach: Technique and results. Orthop Clin North Am 35:143–145, 2004.
2. Berger RA, Jacobs JJ, Meneghini RM, et al: Rapid rehabilitation and recovery with minimally invasive total hip arthroplasty. Clin Orthop Relat Res (429):239–247, 2004.
3. Chung WK, Liu D, Foo LS: Mini-incision total hip replacement—surgical technique and early results. J Orthop Surg 12:19–24, 2004.
4. Wenz JF, Gurkan I, Jibodh SR: Mini-incision total hip arthroplasty: A comparative assessment of perioperative outcomes. Orthopedics 25:1031–1043, 2002.
5. Mow CS, Woolson ST, Ngarmukos SG, Park EH, Lorenz HP: Comparison of scars from total hip replacements done with a standard or a mini-incision. Clin Orthop Relat Res (441):80–5, 2005.
6. Hart R, Stipak V, Janecek M, et al: Component position following total hip arthroplasty through miniinvasive posterolateral approach. Acta Orthop Belg 71:60–64, 2005.
7. Duwelius PJ, Burkhart RL, Hayhurst JO, et al: Comparison of the 2-incision and mini incision posterior total hip arthroplasty technique: A retrospective match-pair controlled study. J Arthroplasty 22:48–56, 2007.
8. Floren M, Lester DK: Durability of implant fixation after less-invasive total hip arthroplasty. J Arthroplasty 21:783–790, 2006.
9. O'Brien DA, Rorabeck CH: The mini-incision direct lateral approach in primary total hip arthroplasty. Clin Orthop Relat Res 441:99–103, 2005.
10. Wright JM, Crockett HC, Delgado S, et al: Mini-incision for total hip arthroplasty: A prospective, controlled investigation with 5-year follow-up evaluation. J Arthroplasty 19:538–545, 2004.
11. DiGioia AM 3rd, Blendea S, Jaramaz B: Computer-assisted orthopaedic surgery: Minimally invasive hip and knee reconstruction. Orthop Clin North Am 35:183–189, 2004.
12. Bennett D, Ogonda L, Elliott D, et al: Comparison of gait kinematics in patients receiving minimally invasive and traditional hip replacement surgery: A prospective blinded study. Gait Posture 23:374–382, 2006.
13. Ogonda L, Wilson R, Archbold P, et al: A minimal-incision technique in total hip arthroplasty does not improve early postoperative outcomes. A prospective, randomized, controlled trial. J Bone Joint Surg Am 87:701–710, 2005.
14. Ciminiello M, Parvizi J, Sharkey PF, et al: Total hip arthroplasty: Is small incision better? J Arthroplasty 21:484–488, 2006.
15. de Beer J, Petruccelli D, Zalzal P, et al: Single-incision, minimally invasive total hip arthroplasty: Length doesn't matter. J Arthroplasty 19:945–950, 2004.
16. Rosenberg AG: A two-incision approach: Promises and pitfalls. Orthopedics 28:935–936, 2005.
17. Weng HH, Fitzgerald J: Current issues in joint replacement surgery. Curr Opin Rheumatol 18:163–169, 2006.
18. Woolson ST, Mow CS, Syquia JF, et al: Comparison of primary total hip replacements performed with a standard incision or a mini-incision. J Bone Joint Surg Am 86-A:1353–1358, 2004.
19. Archibeck MJ, White RE Jr: Learning curve for the two-incision total hip replacement. Clin Orthop Relat Res (429):232–238, 2004.
20. Bal BS, Haltom D, Aleto T, et al: Early complications of primary total hip replacement performed with a two-incision minimally invasive technique. J Bone Joint Surg Am 87:2432–2438, 2005.
21. Bottner F, Delgado S, Sculco TP: Minimally invasive total hip replacement: The posterolateral approach. Am J Orthop 35:218–224, 2006.
22. Howell JR, Masri BA, Duncan CP: Minimally invasive versus standard incision anterolateral hip replacement: A comparative study. Orthop Clin North Am 35:153–156, 2004.
23. Parvizi J, Sharkey PF, Pour AE, et al: Hip arthroplasty with minimally invasive surgery: A survey comparing the opinion of highly qualified experts vs patients. J Arthroplasty 21(6 suppl 2):38–46, 2006.
24. Teet JS, Skinner HB, Khoury L: The effect of the "mini" incision in total hip arthroplasty on component position. J Arthroplasty 21:503–507, 2006.
25. Berry DJ, Berger RA, Callaghan JJ, et al: Minimally invasive total hip arthroplasty. Development, early results, and a critical analysis. Presented at the Annual Meeting of the American Orthopaedic Association, Charleston, South Carolina, USA, June 14, 2003. J Bone Joint Surg Am 85-A:2235–2246, 2003.
26. Hungerford DS: Minimally invasive total hip arthroplasty: In opposition. J Arthroplasty 19(4 suppl 1):81–82, 2004.
27. Woolson ST: In the absence of evidence—why bother? A literature review of minimally invasive total hip replacement surgery. Instr Course Lect 55:189–193, 2006.
28. Holt G, Wheelan K, Gregori A: The ethical implications of recent innovations in knee arthroplasty. J Bone Joint Surg Am 88-A:226–229, 2006.
29. Ranawat CS, Ranawat AS: A common sense approach to minimally invasive total hip replacement. Orthopedics 28:937–938, 2005.
30. American Association of Hip and Knee Surgeons Advisory Statement: Minimally Invasive and Small Incision Joint Replacement Surgery: What Surgeons Should Consider. American Association of Hip and Knee Surgeons online. http://www.aahks.org/pdf/MIS_position_statement.pdf. Accessed August 2007.
31. Chimento GF, Pavone V, Sharrock N: Minimally invasive total hip arthroplasty: A prospective randomized study. J Arthroplasty 20:139–144, 2005.
32. Toms A, Duncan CP: The limited incision, anterolateral, intermuscular technique for total hip arthroplasty. Instr Course Lect 55:199–203, 2006.
33. Berger RA: The technique of minimally invasive total hip arthroplasty using the two-incision approach. Instr Course Lect 53:149–155, 2004.
34. Bonutti PM, Mont MA: Minimally invasive total knee arthroplasty. J Bone Joint Surg Am 86-A(suppl 2):26–32, 2004.
35. Scuderi GR, Tenholder M, Capeci C: Surgical approaches in mini-incision total knee arthroplasty. Clin Orthop Relat Res (428):61–67, 2004.
36. Hofmann AA, Plaster RL, Murdock LE: Subvastus (Southern) approach for primary total knee arthroplasty. Clin Orthop Relat Res (269):70–77, 1991.
37. Engh GA, Holt BT, Parks NL: A midvastus muscle-splitting approach for total knee arthroplasty. J Arthroplasty 12:322–331, 1997.
38. Tria AJ Jr, Coon TM: Minimal incision total knee arthroplasty: Early experience. Clin Orthop Relat Res (416):185–190, 2003.
39. Lawlor M, Humphreys P, Morrow E, et al: Comparison of early postoperative functional levels following total hip replacement using minimally invasive versus standard incisions. A prospective randomized blinded trial. Clin Rehabil 19:465–474, 2005.
40. Mardones R, Pagnano MW, Nemanich JP: The Frank Stinchfield Award: Muscle damage after total hip arthroplasty done with the two-incision and mini-posterior techniques. Clin Orthop Relat Res (441):63–67, 2005.

41. McConnell T, Tornetta P 3rd, Benson E: Gluteus medius tendon injury during reaming for gamma nail insertion. Clin Orthop Relat Res (407):199–202, 2003.

42. Haas SB, Cook S, Beksac B: Minimally invasive total knee replacement through a mini midvastus approach: A comparative study. Clin Orthop Relat Res (428):68–73, 2004.

43. Laskin RS, Beksac B, Phongjunakorn A: Minimally invasive total knee replacement through a mini-midvastus incision: An outcome study. Clin Orthop Relat Res (428):74–81, 2004.

44. Boerger TO, Aglietti P, Mondanelli N: Mini-subvastus versus medial parapatellar approach in total knee arthroplasty. Clin Orthop Relat Res (440):82–87, 2005.

45. Aglietti P, Baldini A, Sensi L: Quadriceps-sparing versus mini-subvastus approach in total knee arthroplasty. Clin Orthop Relat Res (452):106–111, 2006.

46. Nuelle DG, Mann K: Minimal incision protocols for anesthesia, pain management, and physical therapy with standard incisions in hip and knee arthroplasties: The effect on early outcomes. J Arthroplasty 22:20–25, 2007.

47. Dalury DF, Dennis DA: Mini-incision total knee arthroplasty can increase risk of component malalignment. Clin Orthop Relat Res 440:77–81, 2005.

48. American Academy of Orthopaedic Surgeons: Advisory Statement: Minimally Invasive and Small Incision Joint Replacement Surgery. Available at: http://www.aaos.org/home.asp. Accessed August 2007.

49. Pagnano MW, Meneghini RM, Trousdale RT: Anatomy of the extensor mechanism in reference to quadriceps-sparing TKA. Clin Orthop Relat Res (452):102–105, 2006.

50. Kolisek FR, Bonutti FM, Hozack WJ et al: Clinical experience using a minimally invasive surgical approach for total knee arthroplasty: early results of a prospective randomized study compared to a standard approach. J Arthroplasty 22:8–13, 2007.

Chapter 86

What Is the Role for Hip Resurfacing Arthroplasty?

A. Kursat Barin, MSc, Peter Faris, PhD, and James Powell, MD, FRCSC

Hip resurfacing is a technique that has re-emerged since the late 1990s. Hip resurfacing using different methods of fixation and different bearing surfaces have previously been unsuccessful. The experience with the Wagner resurfacing in the early 1980s was reported by Bell and coauthors[1] in their study of implant failures with the Wagner resurfacing. They note that loosening was associated with the development of a membrane at the bone-cement interface. This histologic examination of the membrane demonstrated foreign body response to wear products from the arthroplasty. This suggested that the bearing materials used in this second generation of resurfacing devices was a major factor in the high early failure rate.[2]

The high volumetric of polyethylene of the earlier designs led several investigators to simultaneously and independently investigate in the early 1990s the use of metal-on-metal (MOM) bearing surfaces.[3,4] The bearings designed during the 1990s have proved more durable and are the subject of this review.

Hip resurfacing arthroplasty is an increasingly popular hip arthroplasty option for young, active patients who will likely loosen a conventional total hip replacement (THR) prosthesis. THR has proved to be highly effective in elderly and less active patients, who can expect an implant failure rate less than 10% at 10 years after surgery.[5] These excellent results, however, are not observed in younger, more active recipients of THR, who routinely put significant strain on their hip prosthesis during work and recreational pursuits. In these patients, implant failure rates of 25% to 30% have been reported at 15 years.[6] This is likely caused by an active lifestyle that contributes to excessive wear, osteolysis, and loosening of the implant.[7,8]

Modern hip resurfacing offers a more conservative approach to hip arthroplasty in terms of bone stock. With this arthroplasty, MOM bearings are used to resurface the worn surfaces of the hip joint. A femoral component is cemented in the majority of systems in current usage onto the proximal femur, and an uncemented acetabular cup is press-fit into the pelvis. This technique minimizes femoral bone resection and potentially restores normal biomechanics. It is generally believed that, compared with THR, MOM hip resurfacing offers the following advantages:

- Maintenance of normal hip biomechanics
- Better proprioceptive feedback

- Improved wear characteristics with no polyethylene-induced osteolysis
- Reduced risk for dislocation because of a larger femoral head
- Greater levels of postsurgical activity
- The possibility for ease of conversion to THR should the resurfacing implant fail

Despite the promising advantages of hip resurfacing, long-term clinical outcomes and safety profiles are not well understood. This chapter presents a summary of the evidence on the clinical effectiveness and safety of hip resurfacing arthroplasty.

EVIDENCE

Systematic Reviews

At this time, there are two Level IV systematic reviews available on the outcomes of hip resurfacing arthroplasty. The systematic review by Vale and colleagues[9] compared the reported outcomes of hip resurfacing with other treatments including THR. This review included 20 articles (1990–2001) that met the inclusion criteria, which included study patients who were active and younger than 65 years, and who would likely outlive a THR. Hip resurfacing revision rates were found to range from 0% to 14% over a 3-year follow-up period compared with THR revision rates of 10% or less over a 10-year period. Furthermore, 91% of patients with hip resurfacing were reported to be pain free at 4-year follow-up evaluation, compared with 84% at 11 years for patients with THRs. Unfortunately, that review was limited to eight case series reports of hip resurfacing outcomes. Hence, no comparative studies were available that directly compared hip resurfacing with THR.

Wyness and researchers[10] provide a follow-up systematic review on the effectiveness of hip resurfacing based on studies published before 2002 (Level IV). This review includes data from four hip resurfacing studies, four THR studies, and one watchful waiting study. In addition, the authors include three unpublished hip resurfacing studies supplied from manufacturers for analysis. Unfortunately, similar to Vale and colleagues'[9] review, no comparative studies were available to this systematic review. The studies included in this review rate poorly for study description and for controlling bias. Of the hip resurfacing reports, revision rates were between 0% and 14.3% over a follow-up range of 8.3 to 48 months.

Prospective, Randomized Studies

One prospective, randomized, controlled trial (RCT)[11] has assessed outcomes after modern hip resurfacing with THR. Howie and coauthors[12] also report a hip resurfacing RCT that featured 24 patients 55 years or younger. That study compared the outcomes of 11 patients who randomly received McMinn resurfacing devices with 13 patients with THR. The surgeries were performed between 1993 and 1995, and unlike current hip resurfacing techniques, cement fixation of the acetabular component was used. An extremely high revision rate of 73% was observed in the resurfacing group, which contributed to the abandonment of cement fixation for the acetabular component.

Vendittoli and coworkers'[11] RCT compares the clinical outcomes of patients with hip resurfacing (107 hips) with THR (103 hips) over a study period from 2003 to 2006. The average age of the hip resurfacing group (49.1 years; range, 23–64 years) was similar to that of the THR group (50.6 years; range, 24–65 years), although the hip resurfacing group had a lower body mass index (27.2 vs. 29.6) than the THR group. Osteoarthritis was the primary diagnosis for all patients, and outcome measures included the, Western Ontario and McMaster Universities (WOMAC) index, Postel-Merle-d'Aubigne (PMA) functional assessment, and the UCLA activity score. This RCT found that hip resurfacing, compared with THR, took longer operating time (101 vs. 85 min) and resulted in shorter length of hospital stay (5.0 days vs. 6.1 days). At 1-year follow-up examination, WOMAC and PMA scores were similar for both groups, although patients with hip resurfacing had greater average UCLA activity scores. Vendittoli and coworkers[11] also note that more resurfacing patients returned to work and resumed heavy or moderate activities at 1-year follow-up compared with the THR group. No dislocations or femoral neck fractures were observed in the resurfacing group, although two cases of femoral aseptic loosening led to revision surgery (one at 6 months and the other at 9 months after surgery). In the THR group, one revision was performed for recurrent dislocation. Those authors conclude that hip resurfacing and THR result in similar satisfaction rates in young patients, but hip resurfacing may give better functional performance in terms of activity level and capacity to return to work. Although this RCT is the best experimental study conducted to date on hip resurfacing, it is limited by its short-term follow-up period.

Comparative and Case Series Studies

Numerous comparative and case series studies have been published since the late 1990s on patient clinical outcomes after hip resurfacing. An overview of these studies is provided in Table 86–1.

HIP RESURFACING OUTCOMES

Implant Survival Rates

The most important outcome after hip resurfacing is the rate of surgical revision, which is the primary indicator of implant failure. Although a revision of a resurfaced hip to a THR is relatively straightforward, it is inconvenient to the patient, costly, and associated with the risks of revision surgery.

Currently, there are no long-term outcomes on revision rates for the current generation of hip resurfacings. Reported short-term outcomes of up to 5 years after surgery have indicated various rates of revision (see Table 86–1). We summarized the revision rates for these studies as the overall revision rates per 100 hip-years of follow-up. We used a Poisson distribution to determine the rates after first testing for overdispersion of study rates using a negative binomial distribution. We used hip-time of follow-up as an offset in estimating the failure rate. At the 5% level of significance, there was no evidence of overdispersion among the rates. The overall rate per 100 hip-years of follow-up was 0.99 (95% confidence interval, 0.83–1.17).

Table 86–2 provides a summary of the revision rates and study duration reported in comparative and case series hip resurfacing studies. In addition, it includes the 3-year revision rates for each study based on an exponential failure distribution. Numerous factors contribute to the variance in revision rates reported in the literature. These include surgeon experience[13,14] and appropriate patient selection.

Adverse Events

The major complication after MOM hip resurfacing is femoral neck fracture. This contributes to the earlier revision rate noted with hip resurfacing when compared with total hip arthroplasty. The overall incidence rate of femoral neck fracture as reported by Shimmin and Back[15] is 1.46%. The incidence rate for women is 1.91% and for men is 0.98%. The mean time to fracture was 15.4 weeks. Significant varus placement of the femoral component and intraoperative notching of the femoral neck were predisposing factors in 85% of cases.

Implant Wear and Metal Ion Effects

The advent of MOM arthroplasty has led to an increased concern about the consequence of metal ion debris with respect to both toxicity and carcogenicity. Keegan and coauthors'[16] review article outlines the potential toxicities of metal ions. Visuri and investigators'[17] work shows no increase in the cancer rate on long-term follow-up of patients with MOM total joint arthroplasty. However, because the event rate is low, the literature must be considered inconclusive on this issue. No evidence exists for an increased risk for cancer with the ion levels that are currently seen in clinical practice. Further surveillance is required.

TABLE 86–1. Comparative and Case Series Studies on Patient Clinical Outcomes after Hip Resurfacing

AUTHOR (YEAR OF PUBLICATION)	DESIGN	LEVEL OF EVIDENCE	NO. OF HIPS (NO. OF PATIENTS)	AGE (RANGE), YR	STUDY NOTES AND FINDINGS
Amstutz et al. (2004)[24]	Prospective case series	IV	400 (355)	48.2 (15–77)	400 Conserve Plus MOM hip resurfacings (355 patients) performed between 1996 and 2000. Average patients was 48 (range, 15–77), with OA being the primary diagnosis for surgery. Average follow-up examination was at 3.5 years (range, 2.2–6.2), and 3 patients were lost to follow-up. Significant improvements in clinical outcomes and quality of life were found. Revision rate at follow-up was 3%. Reasons for revision were femoral component loosening (7 hips), femoral neck fracture (3 hips), recurrent dislocation (1 hip), and a deep infection (1 hip).
Amstutz et al. (2007)[20]	Prospective case series	IV	600 (519)	48.9 (15–78)	Outcomes of 600 Conserve Plus MOM hip resurfacings in 519 patients were assessed. Surgeries were performed between 1996 and 2003. Average patient age was 49 years. This study assessed surgeon experience with outcomes. Modifications to technique were introduced after the first 300 hips. The mean follow-up time was 5.9 years for the first 300 hips and 3.5 years for the second 300. Significant improvement was noted for the second 300 hips over the first half. 94.4% (17 hips) of all the revised hips (18) occurred in the first 300 hips.
Back et al. (2005)[22]	Prospective case series	IV	230	52.1 (18–82)	The clinical and radiological outcomes of 230 consecutive patients with Birmingham hip resurfacing (average age, 52) who underwent surgery between 1999 and 2001 were studied. Follow-up was at an average of 3 years. Survivorship rate at follow-up was 99.14% (1 patient suffered a femoral neck fracture that required revision). 97% of patients reported their outcome as good or excellent. Study authors suggest that results from hip resurfacing are superior to the earlier generation of hip resurfacing devices that used cement and metal-on-polyethylene bearings.
Beaule et al. (2004)[25]	Retrospective case series	IV	42 (39)	47.5 (22–69)	39 patients received 42 McMinn MOM hip resurfacings between 1993 and 1996. Average patient age was 48 years (range, 22–69), and OA was the primary reason for surgery. Mean follow-up period was at 8.7 years (range, 7.2–10.0), and 1 patient was lost to follow-up due to death. This study reported a poor survival rate of 79% at 7-year follow-up. Considering aseptic-only failures, the femoral and acetabular component survivorship at 7 years was 93% and 80%, respectively. Cement fixation was used for the acetabular component, resulting in acetabular loosening. The current generation of hip resurfacings uses cementless acetabular components.
Beaule et al. (2004)[26]	Retrospective case series	IV	94 (83)	34.2 (15–40)	Outcomes of 94 Conserve Plus MOM hip resurfacings in a group of 83 young patients (average age, 34 years; range, 15–40) was studied. The mean follow-up period was 3 years (range, 2.0–5.6), and 2 patients (2 hips) were lost to follow-up. Significant improvements in clinical outcomes and quality of life were found at follow-up. The survival rate was 96.8% at follow-up. Three revisions were performed at a mean of 27 months. The survivorship of the hip resurfacings was superior to the published results of THR devices for this younger patient population.
Daniel et al. (2004)[23]	Retrospective case series	IV	446 (384)	48.3 (26.8–54.9)	446 hip resurfacings (403 Birmingham and 43 McMinn devices) were performed between 1994 and 2001. OA was the primary diagnoses, and the average patient age was 48 years old (range, 27–55 years). Follow-up occurred at an average of 3.3 years (range, 1.1–8.2 years), and no patient was lost to follow-up. Six patients died of unrelated causes, whereas 1 suffered a femoral neck fracture. The survival rate was 99.8% (1 revision was required). The results suggest that MOM hip resurfacing offers superior results over THR for younger patients with degenerative joint disease.

TABLE 86–1. Comparative and Case Series Studies on Patient Clinical Outcomes after Hip Resurfacing—cont'd

AUTHOR (YEAR OF PUBLICATION)	DESIGN	LEVEL OF EVIDENCE	NO. OF HIPS (NO. OF PATIENTS)	AGE (RANGE), YR	STUDY NOTES AND FINDINGS
De Smet (2005)[27]	Prospective case series	IV	268 (252)	49.7 (16–75)	Study assessed outcomes of 268 consecutive Birmingham hip resurfacings performed on 252 patients from 1998 to 2004. Average patient age was 50 years (range, 16–75), and the primary diagnosis was OA. Follow-up occurred at an average of 2.8 years (range, 2–5), and 3 patients (4 prostheses) were lost to follow-up because of death. At follow-up, 97.8% of patients had no pain, total Harris Hip Score averaged 97.2, 61% engaged in strenuous activities, hip flexion averaged 123 degrees, 19.4% experienced temporary clicking in the prosthesis within the first 6 months after surgery, and 2.8% had a persistent slight groin pain. Prosthesis survival rate was 98.8%. Reasons for revision were a femoral neck fracture, a low-grade infection, and avascular necrosis in the femoral head. This study shows promising short-term results with hip resurfacing for young, active patients.
Falez et al. (2008)[28]	Prospective case series	IV	60 (58)	46.82 (30–60)	60 hips (58 patients) resurfaced between 2001 and 2005. Mean follow-up period was 2.7 years, and average patient age was 47 (range, 30–60). Postoperative complication rate was 11.7%, with 8.3% (5 cases) requiring revision. The authors conclude that short-term hip resurfacing outcomes are strongly correlated with surgical approach and between prosthesis design and fixation technique.
Grigoris et al. (2005)[29]	Retrospective case Series	IV	200 (186)	48 (22–72)	186 consecutive patients (200 hips) received Durom hip resurfacings between 2001 and 2003. Average patient age was 48 years (range, 22–72), and the primary preoperative diagnosis was OA. Average follow-up was at 2.2 years (range, 1.0–3.4), and no patients were lost to follow-up. Early results had 100% prosthesis survivorship, with no indications of impending device failure in any patient.
Lilikakis et al. (2005)[30]	Retrospective case series	IV	70 (66)	51.5 (23.3–72.7)	Outcomes of 70 MOM Cormet 2000 hip resurfacings in 66 patients (average age, 52 years) were assessed. Surgeries were performed from 2001 to 2002. Unique to this study was the use of hydroxyapatite coating on the femoral component rather than cement fixation. The mean follow-up period was 2.4 years (range, 2.0–3.2). The survival rate was 97.1%, with 2 revisions (one because of infection and the other aseptic loosening of the acetabular component).
McAndrew et al. (2007)[31]	Prospective case series	IV	180 (155)	56 (25–75)	180 consecutive hip resurfacing procedures (150 patients) were performed between 2000 and 2004 with a mean follow-up of 2.6 years. Average age was 56 (range, 25–75), and OA was the primary diagnosis. Nine complications in 7 patients were reported: 3 femoral neck fractures, 2 superficial wound infections, 2 cases of deep vein thrombosis, 2 cases of pulmonary embolism, and 1 femoral nerve palsy. Implant survival rate was 98.3% at follow-up. Study outcomes are comparable with others. Authors recommend that hip resurfacing is suitable for younger, active patients who present with degenerative joint disease.
Mont et al. (2006)[13]	Retrospective comparative study	III	1016 (906)	50 (15–80)	1016 MOM total hip resurfacings were performed in 906 patients from 2000 to 2006. The average follow-up period was 2.6 years. Mean patient age was 50 (range, 15–80). Over the course of this study, surgical technique was modified to adjust for femoral cysts and prosthesis sizes. The impact of these modifications on outcomes was studied. The overall complication rate declined from 13.4% to 2.1%, and femoral neck fracture rates declined from 7.2% to 0.8% after the modifications. This study indicates the importance of patient selection and optimized surgical technique in the reduction of complications.

Continued

TABLE 86–1. Comparative and Case Series Studies on Patient Clinical Outcomes after Hip Resurfacing—cont'd

AUTHOR (YEAR OF PUBLICATION)	DESIGN	LEVEL OF EVIDENCE	NO. OF HIPS (NO. OF PATIENTS)	AGE (RANGE), YR	STUDY NOTES AND FINDINGS
Pollard et al. (2006)[32]	Retrospective comparative study	III	54 (53)	49.8 (18–67)	Results of 54 Birmingham hip resurfacings performed from 1999 to 2001 were compared with those of 54 hybrid THRs performed from 1996 to 2001 by the same surgeon. OA was the primary diagnoses in both groups. Outcomes comparisons included radiologic, clinical, and quality-of-life measures. Patients in both groups were matched before surgery for gender, age, surgery, BMI, and preoperative activity levels before disease limitations. Average follow-up time was 5.1 years for the resurfacing group and 6.7 for the THR. Postoperative function was excellent in both groups, but resurfacing patients had higher postoperative activity and quality-of-life scores. The revision or intent-to-revise rates were 6% for the resurfacing group and 8% for the hybrid THR group. The 6% revision rate of the resurfacing group was likely because of the surgeon's inexperience. Study suggests hip resurfacing provides better outcomes to younger patients compared with THR.
Schmalzried et al. (2005)[33]	Retrospective case series	IV	91 (79)	48 (30–67)	91 Conserve Plus MOM hip resurfacings in 79 patients performed between 2000 and 2004. Average age was 48 years (range, 30–67), and OA was the primary diagnosis for surgery. 70 patients (81 hips) were managed up at 2.6 years (range, 2.0–4.0). Significant clinical improvements were observed with no implant failures. Hips with least OA degeneration had best outcomes. The authors advocate strict patient selection criteria for optimal resurfacing outcomes. Limitations of study include the use of multiple femoral component fixation techniques.
Siebel et al. (2006)[14]	Prospective case series	IV	300 (300)	56.8 (18–76)	Clinical outcomes of 300 consecutive ASR MOM hip resurfacings in 300 patients (average age, 57 years) performed between 2003 and 2005. OA was the primary diagnosis, and 15 patients had previous surgery of the affected hip. Average follow-up time was 202 days (0.6 year). Implant survival rate was 97.3%. Reasons for revision were 5 femoral neck fractures and 3 acetabular component revisions. Revision rates were predominately in the early group of hips, indicating a steep learning curve in hip resurfacing arthroplasty. Of the first 150 patients, 7 revisions were performed later, whereas only 1 was required in the next 150 patients.
Treacy et al. (2005)[21]	Retrospective case series	IV	144 (130)	52.1 (17–76)	144 consecutive Birmingham hip resurfacings in 130 patients performed between 1997 and 1998. Average patient age was 52 years (range, 17–76), and the primary diagnosis was OA. The survival rate at 5 years after surgery was 98% overall and 99% for asepticive revisions only. Authors note that hip resurfacing offers medium-term solution for younger, more active adults who need surgical intervention for hip disease.
Vail et al. (2006)[34]	Retrospective comparative study	III	57 (52)	47 (22–64)	Comparison of outcomes of 57 patients with Conserve Plus hip resurfacing with 47 matched patients with THR. The study follow-up period was 3 years (range, 2–4). At follow-up, the patients with hip resurfacing had better clinical outcomes and lower patient-reported limitations compared with the THR group. Survival rates were similar between the hip resurfacing (96.5%) and THR (95.7%) groups.

BMI, body mass index; MOM, metal on metal; OA, osteoarthritis; THR, total hip replacement.

TABLE 86–2. Summary of Revision Rates Reported in Comparative and Case Series Studies

STUDY	STUDY PERIOD	NO. OF HIPS (NO. OF PATIENTS)	PROSTHESIS	MEAN FOLLOW-UP (RANGE), YR	REVISION RATE	3-YEAR REVISION RATE*
Beaule et al. (2004)[25]	1993–1996	42 (39)	McMinn	8.7 (7.2–10.0)	35.9%	14.2%
Beaule et al. (2004)[26]	NR	94 (83)	Conserve Plus	3 (2.0–5.6)	3.6%	3.6%
Treacy et al. (2005)[21]	1997–1998	144 (130)	BHR	5	2.3%	1.4%
Amstutz et al. (2004)[24]	1996–2000	400 (355)	Conserve Plus	3.5 (2.2–6.2	3.4%	2.9%
Pollard et al. (2006)[32]	1999–2001	54 (53)	BHR	5.1 (4.3–5.9)	6%	3.6%
Back et al. (2005)[22]	1999–2001	230	BHR	3 (2.1–4.3)	0.4%	0.4%
Daniel et al. (2004)[23]	1994–2001†	446 (384)	BHR: 403 hips McMinn: 43 hips	3.3 (1.1–8.2)	0.3%	0.3%
Lilikakis et al. (2005)[30]	2001–2002	70 (66)	Cormet 2000	2.4 (2.0–3.2)	2.9%	3.6%
Amstutz et al. (2007)[20]	1996–2003	600 (519)	Conserve Plus	4.7 (2.8–9.1)	3%	1.9%
Vail et al. (2006)[34]	2000–2003	57 (52)	Conserve Plus	3.0 (2.0–4.0)	3.5%	3.5%
Grigoris et al. (2005)[29]	2001–2003	200 (186)	Durom System	2.2 (1.0–3.4)	0%	0.0%
De Smet (2005)[27]	1998–2004	268 (252)	BHR	2.8 (2–5)	1.2%	1.3%
Schmalzried et al. (2005)[33]	2000–2004	91 (79)	Conserve Plus	2.6 (2.0–4.0)	0%	0.0%
McAndrew et al. (2007)[31]	2000–2004	180 (155)	MMT BHR	2.6 (NR)	2%	2.3%
Falez et al. (2008)[28]	2001–2005	60 (58)	BHR, ASR, MRS, RECAP	2.7 (0.2–3.7)	8%	8.8%
Siebel et al. (2006)[14]	2003–2005	300 (300)	ASR	0.6 (NR)	2.7%	12.8%
Mont et al. (2006)[13]	2000–2006	1016 (906)	Conserve Plus	2.8 (2–5)	5%	5.3%

*Three-year revision rate assumes exponential failure distribution.
†1996 data excluded because of prosthesis production problems.
BHR, Birmingham hip resurfacing; NR, not reported

RECOMMENDATIONS

A major drawback with metal-on-polyethylene hip arthroplasty devices is their wear profile and subsequent release of polyethylene particles into the joint. This wear debris is believed to be a significant cause of osteolysis and long-term implant failure.[18,19]

MOM bearings for THR and hip resurfacing are becoming increasingly popular because of their improved wear characteristics. The literature shows considerable variation in revision rates for MOM resurfacing. Much of this is due to variation in study durations, and when we interpolated 3-year rates using an exponential failure distribution, the rates ranged from 0% to 14.2%. Early articles reported greater revision rates than typically seen with THRs because of the early occurrence of femoral neck fractures leading to conversion to total hip arthroplasty. Reports by experienced surgeons[20–23] (Level IV) showed excellent midterm results with lower projected revision rates than that for THR as reported by the Swedish Joint Replacement Registry.

Reported results from the Australian registry show an acceptable midterm survivorship of several of the resurfacing systems, surpassing the reports of a high failure rate for the Wagner resurfacing system by midterm assessment. The greater earlier failure rate is largely a consequence of femoral neck fracture. Based on Shimmin and Back's[15] analysis, many of the fractures were as a consequence of technical error. Appropriate physician training, attention to intraoperative detail, and careful patient selection to avoid patients with poor bone quality should lead to a reduction in the postoperative rate of femoral neck fracture. The authors recommend continued study of the outcome of resurfacing and surveillance for possible adverse consequences of increased metal ion levels. Resurfacing arthroplasty shows great promise in young adults with osteoarthritis who have a high functional demand and when performed by an experienced surgeon. Table 86–3 provides a summary of recommendations.

TABLE 86–3. Summary of Recommendation

STATEMENT	LEVEL OF EVIDENCE/GRADE OF RECOMMENDATIONS
Resurfacing arthroplasty may have a role in young adults.	I

REFERENCES

1. Bell RS, Schatzker J, Fornasier VL, et al: A study of implant failure in the Wagner resurfacing arthroplasty. J Bone Joint Surg Am 67:1165–1175, 1985.
2. Howie DW, Campbell D, McGee M, et al: Wagner resurfacing hip arthroplasty. The results of one hundred consecutive arthroplasties after eight to ten years. J Bone Joint Surg Am 72:708–714, 1990.
3. Schmalzried TP, Fowble VA, Ure KJ, et al: Metal on metal surface replacement of the hip. Technique, fixation, and early results. Clin Orthop Relat Res (329 suppl):S106–S114, 1996.
4. McMinn D, Daniel J: History and modern concepts in surface replacement. Proc Inst Mech Eng [H] 220:239–251, 2006.
5. Malchau H, Herberts P, Eisler T, et al: The Swedish Total Hip Replacement Register. J Bone Joint Surg Am 84-A (suppl 2):2–20, 2002.
6. Northmore-Ball MD: Young adults with arthritic hips. BMJ 315:265–266, 1997.
7. Crowther JD, Lachiewicz PF: Survival and polyethylene wear of porous-coated acetabular components in patients less than fifty years old: Results at nine to fourteen years. J Bone Joint Surg Am 84-A:729–735, 2002.
8. Duffy GP, Berry DJ, Rowland C, et al: Primary uncemented total hip arthroplasty in patients <40 years old: 10- to 14-year results using first-generation proximally porous-coated implants. J Arthroplasty 16:140–144, 2001.
9. Vale L, Wyness L, McCormack K, et al: A systematic review of the effectiveness and cost-effectiveness of metal-on-metal hip resurfacing arthroplasty for treatment of hip disease. Health Technol Assess 6:1–109, 2002.
10. Wyness L, Vale L, McCormack K, et al: The effectiveness of metal on metal hip resurfacing: A systematic review of the available evidence published before 2002. BMC Health Serv Res 4:39, 2004.
11. Vendittoli PA, Lavigne M, Roy AG, et al: A prospective randomized clinical trial comparing metal-on-metal total hip arthroplasty and metal-on-metal total hip resurfacing in patients less than 65 years old. Hip International 16:S73–S81, 2006.
12. Howie DW, McGee MA, Costi K, et al: Metal-on-metal resurfacing versus total hip replacement: The value of a randomized clinical trial. Orthop Clin North Am 36:195–201, ix, 2005.
13. Mont MA, Ragland PS, Etienne G, et al: Hip resurfacing arthroplasty. J Am Acad Orthop Surg 14:454–463, 2006.
14. Siebel T, Maubach S, Morlock MM: Lessons learned from early clinical experience and results of 300 ASR hip resurfacing implantations. Proc Inst Mech Eng [H] 220:345–353, 2006.
15. Shimmin AJ, Back D: Femoral neck fractures following Birmingham hip resurfacing: A national review of 50 cases. J Bone Joint Surg Br 87:463–464, 2005.
16. Keegan GM, Learmonth ID, Case CP: Orthopaedic metals and their potential toxicity in the arthroplasty patient: A review of current knowledge and future strategies. J Bone Joint Surg Br 89:567–573, 2007.
17. Visuri T, Pukkala E, Paavolainen P, et al: Cancer risk after metal on metal and polyethylene on metal total hip arthroplasty. Clin Orthop Relat Res (329 suppl):S280–S289, 1996.
18. Schmalzried TP, Jasty M, Harris WH: Periprosthetic bone loss in total hip arthroplasty. Polyethylene wear debris and the concept of the effective joint space. J Bone Joint Surg Am 74:849–863, 1992.
19. Schmalzried TP, Kwong LM, Jasty M, et al: The mechanism of loosening of cemented acetabular components in total hip arthroplasty. Analysis of specimens retrieved at autopsy. Clin Orthop Relat Res 60–78, 1992.
20. Amstutz HC, Le Duff MJ, Campbell PA, et al: The effects of technique changes on aseptic loosening of the femoral component in hip resurfacing. Results of 600 Conserve Plus with a 3 to 9 year follow-up. J Arthroplasty 22:481–489, 2007.
21. Treacy RB, McBryde CW, Pynsent PB: Birmingham hip resurfacing arthroplasty. A minimum follow-up of five years. J Bone Joint Surg Br 87:167–170, 2005.
22. Back DL, Dalziel R, Young D, et al: Early results of primary Birmingham hip resurfacings. An independent prospective study of the first 230 hips. J Bone Joint Surg Br 87:324–329, 2005.
23. Daniel J, Pynsent PB, McMinn DJ: Metal-on-metal resurfacing of the hip in patients under the age of 55 years with osteoarthritis. J Bone Joint Surg Br 86:177–184, 2004.
24. Amstutz HC, Beaule PE, Dorey FJ, et al: Metal-on-metal hybrid surface arthroplasty: Two to six-year follow-up study. J Bone Joint Surg Am 86-A:28–39, 2004.
25. Beaule PE, Le DM, Campbell P, et al: Metal-on-metal surface arthroplasty with a cemented femoral component: A 7-10 year follow-up study. J Arthroplasty 19:17–22, 2004.
26. Beaule PE, Dorey FJ, Leduff M, et al: Risk factors affecting outcome of metal-on-metal surface arthroplasty of the hip. Clin Orthop Relat Res 87–93, 2004.
27. De Smet KA: Belgium experience with metal-on-metal surface arthroplasty. Orthop Clin North Am 36:203–213, ix, 2005.
28. Falez F, Favetti F, Casella F, et al: Hip resurfacing: Why does it fail? Early results and critical analysis of our first 60 cases. Int Orthop 32:209–216, 2007.
29. Grigoris P, Roberts P, Panousis K, et al: The evolution of hip resurfacing arthroplasty. Orthop Clin North Am 36:125–134, vii, 2005.
30. Lilikakis AK, Vowler SL, Villar RN: Hydroxyapatite-coated femoral implant in metal-on-metal resurfacing hip arthroplasty: Minimum of two years follow-up. Orthop Clin North Am 36:215–222, ix, 2005.
31. McAndrew AR, Khaleel A, Bloomfield MD, Aweid A: A District General Hospital's Experience of hip resurfacing. Hip International 17:1–3, 2007.
32. Pollard TC, Baker RP, Eastaugh-Waring SJ, et al: Treatment of the young active patient with osteoarthritis of the hip. A five- to seven-year comparison of hybrid total hip arthroplasty and metal-on-metal resurfacing. J Bone Joint Surg Br 88:592–600, 2006.
33. Schmalzried TP, Silva M, de la Rosa MA, et al: Optimizing patient selection and outcomes with total hip resurfacing. Clin Orthop Relat Res 441:200–204, 2005.
34. Vail TP, Mina CA, Yergler JD, et al: Metal-on-metal hip resurfacing compares favorably with THA at 2 years followup. Clin Orthop Relat Res 453:123–131, 2006.

Chapter 87

When Should a Unicompartmental Knee Arthroplasty Be Considered?

Michael J. Dunbar, MD, FRCSC, PhD

The first unicompartmental knee arthroplasty (UKA), the Polycentric, was released in 1968 by Gunston,[1] after which UKA became a viable treatment option for selected patients with unicompartmental osteoarthritis. Initial results for UKA in the 1970s were somewhat unimpressive, perhaps suggestive of the learning curve associated with the introduction of a novel technology.[2] After publication of improved UKA results in the 1980s and continued refinement of patient selection, technology, and surgical procedure, Kozinn and Scott[3] published what have now become referred to as the "classic" indications for UKA.[4] These inclusion and exclusion criteria were selected for an elderly, nonobese patient with noninflammatory medial compartment arthritis and intact ligaments. Although an important and widely quoted publication, the development of the classic indications for UKA was largely based on observational series often using survivorship as the sole outcome metric. Survivorship of UKA demonstrated equivalent survivorship in the first decade between UKA and total knee arthroplasty (TKA), but worse survivorship for UKA in the second decade. Thus, UKA was initially seen as a definitive procedure that would not need to be revised in an elderly patient.

Interest in UKA has been renewed since the 1990s associated with newer designs and minimally invasive surgery (MIS).[5] This renewed interest may also be associated with the unmet burden of middle-aged patients with unicompartmental osteoarthritis of the knee.[6] Without the underpinnings of strong evidenced-based indications, UKA is increasingly being recommended as a bridging procedure for younger patients with isolated osteoarthritis of the medial or lateral compartment,[7] in addition to a definitive procedure in the older patient. Furthermore, some authors have expanded the indications to include patients with anterior cruciate ligament (ACL) deficiency and patients with significant patella-femoral arthritis. The variability and lack of consensus of indications for UKA have led to a reported range of potential candidates for UKA in a knee arthroplasty population of between 5% and 30%.[8] Despite the fact that UKA preceded TKA and the renewed interest in UKA, the cumulative revision rates for UKA have not improved in Sweden since the 1970s. This is in distinction to TKA, which has seen a significant reduction in cumulative revision rate (CRR) over the same period.

OPTIONS

Surgical options for patients with unicompartmental osteoarthritis of the knee include proximal tibial osteotomy, TKA, chondral transplant with or without corrective osteotomy, and arthroscopic debridement.

Proximal tibial osteotomy has similar indications for a UKA, including lack of significant flexion contracture with intact range of motion. The results generally demonstrate 80% survivorship at 5 years and 60% survivorship at 10 years.[10] The result, however, is often cosmetically unsatisfying and questions remain regarding the results of salvage procedures after UKA, such as TKA.[11] The traditional method, and that with the most evidence, is the closing wedge osteotomy, as described by Coventry.[12] Opening wedge osteotomy and opening wedge hemicallostosis osteotomy have become increasing popular.[13,14] Although long-term data are lacking, the techniques are appealing in that they tend to be more "physiologic" with respect to joint biomechanics because the osteotomy is usually performed below the tubercle, and they have been suggested to be more reproducible and reduce the incidence of adverse effects such as reversed tibial slope, intra-articular fracture, patellar baja, and medial proximal tibial overhang with metaphyseal-diaphyseal mismatch[11,15] (Level of Evidence IV). Proximal tibial osteotomy is generally reserved for younger patients with higher levels of demand (Level of Evidence V).

TKA has similar or better survivorship to UKA in the first decade and better survivorship in the second decade.[16,17] As such, TKA is more reliable and is appropriate for older patients who may outlive their UKA. TKA has similar satisfaction rates to medial UKA (82%).[18] TKA has the major advantage over UKA of being able to accommodate major ligament releases and resections, including the ACL and PCL, as well as significant bone resection to address deformity. The survivorship of TKA is adversely affected by younger age and obesity.[19–22]

Fresh osteochondral allografting has been recommended for the treatment of large focal defects. Matched osteochondral surfaces are transplanted from the donor to the recipient host, often with an unloading osteotomy. Reasonable success rates have been reported, but this technique has limitations in that it requires immunosuppressive drugs, carries the risk for disease transfer, and requires a large catchment area to find suitable donors.[23,24] This technique has had limited success at a few centers around the world. Chondral transplant has been advocated for focal defects in one of the femoral condyles.[25–27] Although it has been possible to grow chondrocytes in vitro, results of transplanted chondrocytes have been mixed because of the large biomechanical forces to which the immature chondral cells are exposed.

Arthroscopic debridement of the knee for unicompartmental arthroplasty has been shown in general to be ineffective[28] (Level of Evidence I). However, evidence suggests that arthroscopic debridement can relieve symptoms temporarily for patients with mechanical symptoms, such as catching or locking, associated with arthritis[28] (Level of Evidence I).

EVIDENCE

Unfortunately, UKA studies in the literature with high levels of evidence are limited (Table 87–1). In a randomized trial, Newman and colleagues[29] compared 52 TKAs with 50 fixed-bearing UKAs. All patients were selected for surgery as candidates for UKA using the classic indications of intact cruciate ligaments: "normal" other compartments, flexion deformity less than 15 degrees, and varus/valgus less than 15 degrees. The mean age at surgery was 69 years. Patients in the UKA group had less morbidity, shorter length of stays, and better range of motion both in the short and the long term (109.3 vs. 102.6 degrees). Two failures occurred in the UKA group and one in the TKA group, with an additional pending failure. The number of knees able to flex greater than 120 degrees was proportionally greater in the UKA group. Pain relief was similar in both groups using the Bristol Knee Score. The authors conclude that UKA gives better results than TKA at 5 years in patients who meet the conservative criteria for UKA (Level of Evidence I).

Amin and coworkers[16] report on a matched study of 54 consecutive UKAs compared with 54 consecutive TKAs. The two groups of patients were matched for age, sex, body mass index, preoperative range of movement, and preoperative Knee Society scores. The mean follow-up period was 59 months in both groups. Classic selection criteria were used for the UKA group. The UKA was mobile bearing. The survivorship for the UKA group at 5 years was 88% compared with 100% for the TKA group. Subjective outcomes were similar for both groups. The range of motion was greater for the UKA group. This study differed from Newman and colleagues'[29] work in that the patients with TKA were not candidates for UKA, and the UKA was mobile bearing (Level of Evidence III).

Stukenborg-Colsman and investigators[30] completed a prospective, randomized trial comparing UKA with proximal tibial osteotomy. The selection criteria for the patients were medial unicompartmental osteoarthritis, varus malalignment less than 10, flexion contraction less than 15 degrees, minimal ligament instability, and age older than 60 years. The osteotomies were performed according to Coventry's[12] technique and the UKAs were fixed bearing. Thirty-two patients received osteotomies and 28 received UKAs with mean follow-up period of 7.5 years. The UKA group had fewer intraoperative and postoperative complications, had a greater percentage of patients with good or excellent results on the Knee Society Score, and had a better 7- to 10-year survivorship rate of 77% compared with 60%. The authors conclude that UKA offered better long-term results compared with Coventry-type proximal tibial osteotomy in patients older than 60 years (Level of Evidence I).

UKA has experienced a resurgence in interest since the last 1990s partly because of its adaptability to MIS. Despite the popularity of MIS, most data to support its use are anecdotal or of a low quality of evidence. Furthermore, reported MIS results are most often associated with a specific implant of interest, hence the results may not be generalizable to all implant/instrument

TABLE 87–1. Summary of Studies with Levels of Evidence Greater Than II for Unicompartmental Knee Arthroplasty

STUDY	DESIGN	DESCRIPTION	UKA DESIGN	RESULT	LEVEL OF EVIDENCE	CASES (N)	AVERAGE PATIENT AGE (YR)	FOLLOW-UP (YR)
Newman et al.[29]	Prospective randomized	UKA vs. TKA	Fixed bearing	Favors UKA	I	102	69	5
Amin et al.[16]	Matched prospective	UKA vs. TKA	Mobile bearing	UKA = better range of motion UKA = worse survivorship	II	54	68	5
Stukenborg-Colsman et al.[30]	Prospective randomized	UKA vs. HTO	Fixed bearing	Favors UKA	I	60	67	7.5
Carlsson et al.[31]	Prospective randomized	MIS vs. conventional UKA	Fixed bearing	Favors MIS	I	41	65	2

HTO, high tibial osteotomy; MIS, minimally invasive surgery; TKA, total knee arthroplasty; UKA, unicompartmental knee arthroplasty.

types. Carlsson and coauthors[31] have reported on the only randomized trial comparing a conventional approach in 20 patients with MIS in 21 patients, using a fixed-bearing UKA. Patients were selected for the study who had intact ligaments and unicompartmental disease; however, moderate patella-femoral arthritis was accepted. Average patient age was 64 years, and the length of follow-up was 2 years. Patients receiving the MIS approach had significantly shorter hospital stays (3 vs. 6 days). However, the subjective outcomes (Hospital for Special Surgery Score) were the same for both groups, as were the clinical outcomes such as alignment and range of motion. Precise and accurate radiostereometric analysis (RSA) data demonstrated similar migration patterns in both patients, suggesting that the long-term survivorship should be the same for both groups (Level of Evidence I).

AREAS OF UNCERTAINTY

Acceptable Degree of Patella-Femoral Joint Arthritis

Classic indications for UKA suggest that rest pain in the patella-femoral joint is a relative contraindication to UKA, whereas asymptomatic patella-femoral arthritis is not. However, full-thickness cartilage lesions in the patella-femoral groove have been suggested to be a contraindication to surgery.[3] Some authors more recently have suggested that significant patella-femoral arthritis, including that associated with pain, is not a contraindication.[32] No randomized trials published to date address this issue.

Obesity

Previous literature suggests that UKA should be avoided in obese patients.[3] More recent articles have refuted this notion, which appears to be based on anecdote and the expectation that increased body mass index will lead to increased load on a small area of tibia. Tabor and coauthors[33] report that on a 20-year follow-up of UKA, the survivorship of the UKAs in the obese group was actually better than the nonobese group, whereas Berend and Lombardi[32] report increased failures in a retrospective review (Level of Evidence II). Few data address differences in functional outcome between the two groups.

Mobile versus Fixed Bearing

Early failure patterns in UKA treatment included delamination and failure of the polyethylene bearing. Partly in an effort to address this, a more congruent but mobile-bearing polyethylene was developed. In a small, randomized trial to look at this issue, Li and researchers[34] randomized 56 UKAs to a fixed-bearing versus a mobile-bearing device. In their study, the mobile-bearing knees had better kinematics, a lower incidence of radiolucency, but no difference in multiple subjective outcome questionnaires at 2 years[34]

(Level of Evidence II). The increased incidence of radiolucent lines is significant but difficult to interpret because radiolucent lines do not necessarily correlate with failure. Also, other that one being mobile bearing and the other fixed, the two designs of knees studied were quite disparate, and these differences in design may just as easily account for the improved kinematics. Emerson and coauthors[35] report on 50 matched mobile-bearing UKAs with 51 fixed-bearing UKAs with 7.7 years of follow-up. The mobile-bearing group demonstrated a survivorship rate of 99% at 11 years, whereas the fixed-bearing group had a rate of 93%. However, the two groups had significantly different postoperative alignment, forcing the authors to conclude that the results could be attributable to surgical technique and prosthesis design (Level of Evidence III). Gleeson[9] reports on the early results of a prospective study comparing 47 mobile-bearing UKAs with 57 fixed bearings. At 2 years, the mobile-bearing group had a greater failure rate, mostly because of polyethylene dislocation, and better subjective pain scores (Level of Evidence II). According to the Swedish Knee Registry,[20] mobile-bearing UKAs have a greater rate of mechanical failures but a lower rate of failure for polyethylene wear than do fixed-bearing designs[36] (Level of Evidence III).

Lateral Compartment Unicompartmental Knee Arthroplasty

Considerable debate is included in the literature regarding UKA of the lateral compartment. Initially, before tricondylar knee systems, it was not uncommon to use a UKA for lateral joint disease.[37] In a nonrandomized, consecutive series comparing lateral with medial UKAs in 159 knees, the authors conclude that lateral UKA is a viable alternative to TKA (Level of Evidence III). However, in a large series investigating satisfaction after UKA and TKA in more than 29,000 patients from the Swedish Knee Registry, satisfaction rates after lateral UKA were significantly lower than for medial UKA[18] (Level of Evidence III). Because of significant differences in the kinematics between the medial and lateral compartments, some authors have recommended caution when using meniscal bearings in the lateral compartment[38,39] (Level of Evidence V).

Anterior Cruciate Ligament Deficiency

ACL deficiency has been defined in the early literature as a contraindication for UKA[3] (Level of Evidence V). The concern has been that ACL laxity can ultimately culminate in increased polyethylene wear because of the altered joint kinematics, particularly with anteroposterior translation.[40,41] Both favorable and unfavorable results have been reported with UKA in patients with ACL deficiency.[41] ACL reconstruction at the same time as UKA has been reported in a matched series of 15 patients receiving UKA with

ACL reconstruction and 15 patients receiving UKA with an intact ACL. Similar excellent short-term outcomes were reported for both groups[42] (Level of Evidence III).

GUIDELINES

No published guidelines are specific to patient selection for UKA from any of the major international orthopedic or arthritis care organizations. The "classic" indications for UKA have been described by Kozinn and Scott,[3] and have generally been accepted by the orthopedic community as such. However, the "classic" indications are not necessarily believed to be the contemporary indications.

RECOMMENDATIONS

UKA is a technical operation, made more complex when associated with MIS, with significant controversy regarding patient selection, including age, body mass index, extent of patella-femoral arthritis, and condition of the ACL. UKA is no longer seen as exclusively a definitive procedure in the elderly but rather increasingly as a bridging procedure in the younger patient. A paucity of appropriate randomized trials exists to address many of the controversial aspects of patient selection. Subsequently, UKA is difficult in the sense of both the "incision" and the "decision."

The greatest preponderance and length of follow-up in the literature still suggest that the ideal patient for UKA is an older, nonobese patient with medial compartment osteoarthritis, intact ligaments, a correctable deformity, small or no flexion contracture, good range of motion, and no significant arthritis in the lateral or patella-femoral joint (grade B). It appears that, with a fixed bearing at least, there are advantages of the MIS approach without significant disadvantages in the short- and long-term clinical outcome (grade I). This may be prosthesis and instrument specific, however.

UKA in younger patients has shown favorable outcomes in selected series. These series are usually from high-volume UKA knee surgeons, often with advanced knowledge of the prosthesis in question. As such, it is difficult to extrapolate the results to the larger surgical community. The Swedish Knee Arthroplasty Registry has reported that in the experience of all surgeons living in one nation using multiple prostheses design and techniques, the survivorship of UKA in patients younger than 60 years is worse than in those older than 60[19] (Level of Evidence III). UKA eventually will fail in the younger patient population, and it is unclear as to the survivorship of revised UKA relative to TKA. Based on the available evidence, UKA should be used judiciously in obese and highly active patients (grade C). Reports of good outcomes in UKA with ACL reconstruction and significant arthritic changes in the patella-femoral joint tend to be prosthetic specific from expert UKA surgeons. I do not recommend the routine use of UKA in these circumstances (grade C).

Given that a volume effect has been reported on more technically demanding implants, such as mobile-bearing designs,[43] the casual UKA surgeon should strongly consider simpler designs with larger incisions, if necessary (grade C). Ideally, potential UKA patients would be referred to a small enough number of surgeons with a particular interest in UKA to take maximum advantage of the surgical learning curve, and ensure greater consistency and reproducibility in patient selection.

A significant need exists for appropriate studies with high levels of evidence to address the areas of controversy and to further define who are the best candidates for UKA. Table 87–2 provides a summary of recommendations.

TABLE 87–2. Summary of Recommendations

STATEMENT	LEVEL OF EVIDENCE/GRADE OF RECOMMENDATION	REFERENCES
1. Older patients with classic* indications for UKA do as well or better with a UKA than with TKA.	A	29
2. Patients aged 60 years or older with classic indications for UKA do better with UKA than with high tibial osteotomy.	A	30
3. Lateral UKA has significantly lower satisfaction rates than medial UKA.	B	18
4. The survivorship of UKA in patients less than 60 years of age is worse than in patients older than 60.	B	19

*Classic indications: isolated medial compartment osteoarthritis, flexion deformity less than 15 degrees, varus/valgus less than 15 degress, intact anterior cruciate ligament

REFERENCES

1. Gunston FH: Polycentric knee arthroplasty. Prosthetic simulation of normal knee movement. J Bone Joint Surg 53:272–277, 1971.
2. Scott RD: Unicondylar arthroplasty: Redefining itself. Orthopedics 26:951–952, 2003.
3. Kozinn SC, Scott R: Unicondylar knee arthroplasty. J Bone Joint Surg Am 71:145–150, 1989.

4. Scott RD, Santore RF: Unicondylar unicompartmental replacement for osteoarthritis of the knee. J Bone Joint Surg Am 63:536–544, 1981.
5. Meek RM, Masri BA, Duncan CP: Minimally invasive unicompartmental knee replacement: Rationale and correct indications. Orthop Clin N Am 35:191–200, 2004.
6. Canadian Institute for Health Information: Canadian Joint Replacement Registry (CJRR) 2006 Report—Hip and Total Knee Replacements in Canada. Canadian Institute for Health Information, Toronto Ontario, 2006.
7. Price AJ, Dodd CA, Svard UG, Murray DW: Oxford medial unicompartmental knee arthroplasty in patients younger and older than 60 years of age. J Bone Joint Surg Br 87:1488–1492, 2005.
8. Mont MA, Stuchin SA, Paley D, Sharkey PF, Parvisi J, et al: Different surgical options for monocompartmental osteoarthritis of the knee: High tibial osteotomy versus unicompartmental knee arthroplasty versus total knee arthroplasty: Indications, techniques, results, and controversies. Instruc Course Lect 53:265–283, 2004.
9. Gleeson RE, Evans R, Ackroyd CE, Webb J, and Newman JH: Fixed or mobile bearing unicompartmental knee replacement? A comparative cohort study. Knee 11(5):379-384, 2004.
10. Naudie D, Bourne RB, Rorabeck CH, Bourne TJ: The Install Award. Survivorship of the high tibial valgus osteotomy. A 10- to 22-year follow-up study. Clin Orthop Relat Res (367):18–27, 1999.
11. Windsor RE, Insall JN, Vince KG: Technical considerations of total knee arthroplasty after proximal tibial osteotomy. J Bone Joint Surg Am 70:547–555, 1988.
12. Coventry MB: Osteotomy of the upper portion of the tibia for degenerative arthritis of the knee. A preliminary report. J Bone Joint Surg Am 47:984–990, 1965.
13. Amendola A, Fowler PJ, Litchfield R, Kirkley S, Clatworthy M: Opening wedge high tibial osteotomy using a novel technique: Early results and complications. J Knee Surg 17:164–169, 2004.
14. Weale AE, Lee AS, MacEachern AG: High tibial osteotomy using a dynamic axial external fixator. Clin Orthop Relat Res (382):154–167, 2001.
15. Insall J, Salvati E: Patella position in the normal knee joint. Radiology 101:101–104, 1971.
16. Amin AK, et al: Unicompartmental or total knee arthroplasty? Results from a matched study. Clin Orthop Relat Res 451:101–106, 2006.
17. Scott RD, Cobb AG, McQueary FG, Thornhill TS: Unicompartmental knee arthroplasty. Eight- to 12-year follow-up evaluation with survivorship analysis. Clin Orthop Relat Res (271):96–100, 1991.
18. Robertsson O, Dunbar M, Pehrsson T, Knutson K, Lidgren L: Patient satisfaction after knee arthroplasty: A report on 27,372 knees operated on between 1981 and 1995 in Sweden. Acta Orthop Scand 71:262–267, 2000.
19. Harrysson OL, Robertsson O, Nayfeh JF: Higher cumulative revision rate of knee arthroplasties in younger patients with osteoarthritis. Clin Orthop Relat Res (421):162–168, 2004.
20. Swedish Knee Arthroplasty Register, Annual Report 2006— The Swedish Knee Arthroplasty Register 2006. Department of Orthopedics, Lund University Hospital, Lund, Sweden, 2006.
21. Gillespie GN, Porteous AJ: Obesity and knee arthroplasty. Knee 14:81–86, 2007.
22. Amin AK, Clayton RA, Patton JT, Gaston M, Cook RE, Brenkel IJ: Total knee replacement in morbidly obese patients. Results of a prospective, matched study. J Bone Joint Surg Br 88:1321–1326, 2006.
23. Gross AE, Shasha N, Aubin P: Long-term followup of the use of fresh osteochondral allografts for posttraumatic knee defects. Clin Orthop Relat Res (435):79–87, 2005.
24. Maury AC, Safir O, Heras FL, Pritzker KP, Gross AE: Twenty-five-year chondrocyte viability in fresh osteochondral allograft. A case report. J Bone Joint Surg Am 89:159–165, 2007.
25. Gillogly SD, Myers TH, Reinold MM: Treatment of full-thickness chondral defects in the knee with autologous chondrocyte implantation. J Orthop Sports Phys Ther 36:751–764, 2006.
26. Lahav A, Burks RT, Greis PE, Chapman AW, Ford GM, Fink BP: Clinical outcomes following osteochondral autologous transplantation (OATS). J Knee Surg 19:169–173, 2006.
27. Steinwachs M, Kreuz PC: Autologous chondrocyte implantation in chondral defects of the knee with a type I/III collagen membrane: A prospective study with a 3-year follow-up. Arthroscopy 23:381–387, 2007.
28. Bradley JD, Heilman DK, Katz BP, Gsell P, Wallick JE, Brandt KD: Tidal irrigation as treatment for knee osteoarthritis: A sham-controlled, randomized, double-blinded evaluation. Arthritis Rheum 46:100–108, 2002.
29. Newman JH, Ackroyd CE, Shah NA: Unicompartmental or total knee replacement? Five-year results of a prospective, randomised trial of 102 osteoarthritic knees with unicompartmental arthritis. J Bone Joint Surg Br 80:862–865, 1998.
30. Stukenborg-Colsman C, Wirth CJ, Lazovic D, Wefer A: High tibial osteotomy versus unicompartmental joint replacement in unicompartmental knee joint osteoarthritis: 7-10-year follow-up prospective randomised study. Knee 8:187–194, 2001.
31. Carlsson LV, Albrektsson BE, Regner LR: Minimally invasive surgery vs conventional exposure using the Miller-Galante unicompartmental knee arthroplasty: A randomized radiostereometric study. J Arthroplasty 21:151–156, 2006.
32. Berend KR, Lombardi AV Jr: Liberal indications for minimally invasive oxford unicondylar arthroplasty provide rapid functional recovery and pain relief. Surg Technol Int 16:193–197, 2007.
33. Tabor OB Jr, Tabor OB, Bernard M, Wan JY: Unicompartmental knee arthroplasty: Long-term success in middle-age and obese patients. J Surg Orthop Adv 14:59–63, 2005.
34. Li MG, Yao F, Joss B, Ioppolo J, Nivbrant B, Wood D: Mobile vs. fixed bearing unicondylar knee arthroplasty: A randomized study on short term clinical outcomes and knee kinematics. Knee 13:365–370, 2006.
35. Emerson RH Jr, Hansborough T, Reitman RD, Rosenfeldt W, Higgins LL: Comparison of a mobile with a fixed-bearing unicompartmental knee implant. Clin Orthop Relat Res (404):62–70, 2002.
36. Lewold S, Goodman S, Knutson K, Robertsson O, Lidgren L: Oxford meniscal bearing knee versus the Marmor knee in unicompartmental arthroplasty for arthrosis. A Swedish multicenter survival study. J Arthroplasty 10:722–731, 1995.
37. Lewold S, Robertsson O, Knutson K, Lidgren L: Revision of unicompartmental knee arthroplasty: Outcome in 1,135 cases from the Swedish Knee Arthroplasty study. Acta Orthop Scand 69:469–474, 1998.
38. Robinson BJ, Rees JL, Price AJ, Beard DJ, Murray DM; OHKG. Oxford Hip and Knee Group: A kinematic study of lateral unicompartmental arthroplasty. Knee 9:237–240, 2002.
39. Robinson BJ, Rees JL, Price AJ, Beard DJ, Murray DW, McLardy Smith P, Dodd CA: Dislocation of the bearing of the Oxford lateral unicompartmental arthroplasty. A radiological assessment. J Bone Joint Surg Br 84:653–657, 2002.
40. Suggs JF, Li G, Park SE, Steffensmeier S, Rubash HE, Freiberg AA: Function of the anterior cruciate ligament after unicompartmental knee arthroplasty: An in vitro robotic study. J Arthroplasty 19:224–229, 2004.
41. Engh GA, Ammeen D: Is an intact anterior cruciate ligament needed in order to have a well-functioning unicondylar knee replacement? Clin Orthop Relat Res (428):170–173, 2004.
42. Pandit H, Beard DJ, Jenkins C, Kimstra Y, Thomas NP, Dodd CA, Murray DW: Combined anterior cruciate reconstruction and Oxford unicompartmental knee arthroplasty. J Bone Joint Surg Br 88:887–892, 2006.
43. Robertsson O, Knutson K, Lewold S, Lidgren L: The routine of surgical management reduces failure after unicompartmental knee arthroplasty. J Bone Joint Surg Br 83:45–49, 2001.

Chapter 88

Should You Save or Substitute the Posterior Cruciate Ligament in Total Knee Replacement?

Paul R. T. Kuzyk, BSc, MASc, MD, FRCS(C) and Emil H. Schemitsch, MD, FRCS(C)

The posterior cruciate ligament (PCL) serves several important functions in the native knee joint. The PCL is the strongest ligament in the knee and runs from the posteromedial portion of the medial femoral condyle to the posterior aspect of the tibia.[1] Because of its direction of attachment, it is the primary ligament resisting posterior subluxation of the tibia on the femur. During flexion, the PCL ensures that the femoral condyles are positioned appropriately on the tibial plateau. The ligament also contains receptors that are sensitive to stretch and allow for normal knee joint proprioception.

The PCL is present and functional in almost all patients who present for total knee arthroplasty. Furthermore, it is possible to retain this ligament without significantly increasing surgical time or expense. Sacrifice of the PCL, however, may facilitate ligament balancing and enhance correction of deformity. This has sparked debate concerning how the PCL should be treated during total knee arthroplasty. Orthopedic surgeons follow one of two differing philosophies: save the PCL or sacrifice the PCL.

OPTIONS

Arguments for Sparing the Posterior Cruciate Ligament in Total Knee Arthroplasty

Advocates for PCL sparing total knee arthroplasty generally cite five theoretical advantages: (1) increases passive range of motion, (2) preserves the quadriceps lever arm, (3) enhances joint stability, (4) reduces bone-implant interfacial stress on the tibial component, and (5) improves joint proprioception. A review of the normal function of the PCL in the knee is required to understand these arguments.

As the knee is flexed, the PCL tethers the femur to the posterior tibia. This causes the femoral condyles to roll backward on the tibial plateau. The resulting anterior-to-posterior translation of the femur on the tibia has been termed *femoral roll back*.[2] The medial femoral condyle is more constrained than the lateral femoral condyle and, therefore, undergoes less roll back. This causes internal rotation of the tibia on the femur with knee flexion.

Preservation of normal femoral roll back is suggested as the mechanism for increased passive range of motion. Because of roll back, the femur moves backward on the tibia by 10 mm from full extension to full flexion. This posterior translation of the femur prevents it from impinging on the posterior portion of the tibial plateau during flexion. Posterior translation of the femur by 10 mm also increases the quadriceps lever arm by approximately 40% (Fig. 88–1).[1] This improves quadriceps power for knee extension from a flexed position. Proponents of PCL sparing have argued that this leads to improved stair climbing. They have suggested that patients without normal femoral roll back need to lean forward while climbing stairs so that their center of gravity falls anterior to the knee (counteracting the reduced quadriceps lever arm).[1]

The PCL is the primary stabilizer for posteriorly directed forces on the tibia. These forces may be quite high during normal activities (e.g., approaching body weight during walking).[1] Without the native PCL, these forces may be transferred to the bone-implant interface. Two types of PCL-sacrificing implants recreate the posterior stabilizing effect of the PCL using different designs: (1) posterior stabilized (PS) implants have a post on the tibial component and a cam on the femoral component, and (2) ultra-congruent (UC) implants have deep troughs in the tibial component to accommodate the femoral condyles. In these PCL-sacrificing implants, a posterior-directed force on the tibia will pass through the tibial component and result in a shear force at the bone-implant interface. This may accelerate loosening of the tibial component.

Because of its location in the middle of the knee, the PCL is also a secondary stabilizer for both varus and valgus forces placed on the tibia.[1] The typical varus thrust that occurs with walking on level ground results in an adduction moment about the knee joint. This is resisted by the PCL through a relatively short lever arm (Fig. 88–2). This function of the PCL may not be fully replicated by PS and UC implants. As a result, there may be greater forces through the medial compartment than the lateral compartment when the PCL is sacrificed.

The PCL, like the anterior cruciate ligament (ACL), contains mechanoreceptors that detect knee joint position (i.e., proprioception). These mecha-

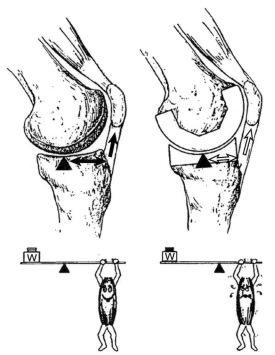

FIGURE 88–1. An illustration of increased quadriceps lever arm due to femoral roll back. (From Andriacchi TP, Galante JO: Retention of the posterior cruciate in total knee arthroplasty. J Arthroplasty 3(Suppl): 13-19, 1988, p.S17.)

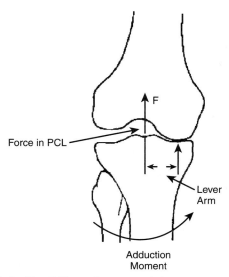

FIGURE 88–2. The PCL produces a stabilizing moment (force in PCL) that acts at a distance (lever arm) from the medial compartment. The PCL is therefore a secondary stabilizer acting against the normal adduction moment (or varus thrust) that occurs with walking. (From Andriacchi TP, Galante JO: Retention of the posterior cruciate in total knee arthroplasty. J Arthroplasty 3(Suppl): 13-19, 1988, p.S17.)

noreceptors sense stress placed on the ligaments and act through a reflex arc to stimulate the dynamic stabilizers of the knee (i.e., muscles that cross the knee joint). Proprioceptive deficiency in the knee may lead to knee instability, gait abnor-

malities, and difficulties with balance.[3] Improved knee joint proprioception through retention of the PCL may result in better patient function after total knee arthroplasty.[4]

Arguments for Sacrificing the Posterior Cruciate Ligament in Total Knee Arthroplasty

Advocates for PCL-sacrificing total knee arthroplasty generally cite three possible advantages: (1) it facilitates correction of deformity, (2) it enhances range of passive motion, and (3) it decreases stress at the bone-implant interface. Several authors suggest that release of the PCL allows for improved correction in knees with more than 15 degrees of varus or valgus deformity and knees with more than 15 degrees of fixed flexion deformity.[5,6] Matsueda and colleagues[7] showed in a cadaver study that release of the PCL led to the ability to achieve significantly greater tibiofemoral coronal angles during both medial and lateral releases. They also found that release of the PCL produced extension gaps of 10.9 mm and flexion gaps of 6.6 mm. This would allow for correction of significant flexion deformities.

The PS implant recreates the femoral roll back through the articulation between the cam on the femoral component and the post on the tibial component. Femoral roll back, as stated earlier, allows for increased passive range of motion and quadriceps mechanical function. Through fluoroscopic analysis, femoral roll back has been shown to be more consistent with PS implants than cruciate-sparing implants.[8] Some cruciate-sparing implants exhibited paradoxical anterior femoral translation. The UC implant has an anterior lip and tibial surface that conforms to the femoral condyles to substitute for the PCL. This does not recreate femoral roll back; however, the axis of rotation of the femur on the tibia is placed posterior on the tibial plateau. This allows for improved range of motion and quadriceps mechanical function in the absence of femoral roll back.[2]

The PCL is thought to impart posterior stability to the flexed knee through two mechanisms. First, it is taut in flexion and orientated somewhat horizontal to the tibia, so that it may directly resist posterior displacement of the tibia on the femur.[2] Second, the PCL holds the femoral condyles down on the tibial surface. The tibial surface slopes upward anteriorly, and this is further enhanced by the menisci.[2] With the PCL securing the femoral condyles to the tibial surface, the condyles will impinge on the anterior sloping tibial surface if the tibia experiences a posterior-directed force. For the PCL to provide posterior stability through these mechanisms, it must have the appropriate tension in flexion. This is achieved by varying bone cuts on the superior tibia and posterior femur (i.e., varying the flexion gap).

The success of total knee arthroplasty with retention of the PCL is highly dependent on proper tensioning of the PCL. If the flexion gap is "overstuffed" (i.e., too large of a femoral component or too thick of a polyethylene spacer), the PCL will be under too much tension with flexion. This causes a large compressive force between the femoral condyles and the posterior aspect of the tibial surface. Unbalanced force on the tibial surface causes the tibial component to "book open" (i.e., the anterior portion of the tibial component lifts off the tibia). This must be recognized intraoperatively and the appropriate measures taken (recessing the PCL, reducing thickness of the spacer, or decreasing size of the femoral component). Otherwise, this unbalanced force on the tibial component will place undue stress on the bone-implant interface. Overtensioning the PCL has also been reported to increase the rate of polyethylene wear and may result in posterior femoral subluxation.[9,10] On the other hand, leaving the flexion space too lax or over-recessing the PCL will lead to a slack PCL and subsequent flexion instability.

Differences in passive range of motion, tibial component loosening, proprioception, and patient function (i.e., quadriceps strength and knee stability) are cited for choosing PCL retention over sacrifice and vice versa. Therefore, studies should incorporate outcome measures that address these variables.

Evidence

A Cochrane meta-analysis was performed recently to identify differences in functional, clinical, and radiological outcomes for patients receiving either a cruciate retaining or sacrificing total knee arthroplasty.[11] Eight randomized, controlled trials were identified in the literature. These consisted of four level I studies and four level II studies (Table 88–1).[3,12–18] Two treatment options were compared to PCL retention: PCL sacrifice with use of a PCL-retaining (CR) implant, and PCL sacrifice with use of a PS implant. The group receiving PCL sacrifice with a PS implant were found to have a significantly greater (8.1 degrees; $P = 0.01$) range of motion after surgery as compared with the

TABLE 88–1. Studies Reporting Outcomes for Posterior Cruciate Ligament–Retaining Implants, Posterior Cruciate Ligament–Substituting Implants and Posterior Cruciate Ligament Sacrifice with Use of a Posterior Cruciate Ligament–Retaining Implant

STUDY	LEVEL OF EVIDENCE	DESIGN	RATE OF FOLLOW-UP	MEAN DURATION OF FOLLOW-UP (YR)	N	MEAN AGE (YR)	TYPE OF IMPLANT
Catani et al. (2004)[12]	I	Prospective RCT	100%	2	A: 20 B: 20	70	A: CR B: PS
Maruyama et al. (2004)[13]	I	Prospective RCT	100%	2.64 (2–4.42)	20	74.3	A: CR B: PS
Swanik et al. (2004)[3]	I	Prospective RCT	100%	0.63	A: 10 B: 10	A: 71.1 B: 69.4	A: CR B: PS
Tanzer et al. (2002)[14]	I	Prospective RCT	100%	2	A: 20 B: 20	A: 68 B: 66	A: CR B: PS
Misra et al. (2003)[15]	II	Prospective RCT	77%	>5	A: 51 B: 54	A: 66.8 B: 67.2	A: CR B: CR (PCL resected)
Straw et al. (2003)[16]	II	Prospective RCT	56%	3.5	A: 66 B: 59 C: 42	73.2	A: CR B: CR (PCL resected) C: PS
Clark et al. (2001)[17]	II	Prospective RCT	51%	3	A: 67 B: 76	A: 72 B: 71	A: CR B: PS
Shoji et al. (1994)[18]	II	Prospective RCT	51%	3.2 (2.5–4.5)	28	60.2	A: CR B: CR (PCL resected)

* Bilateral total knee arthroplasty studies with the PCL spared in one knee and resected in the contralateral knee.
CR, posterior cruciate ligament retaining; HSS, Hospital for Special Surgery; KS, Knee Society; PCL, posterior cruciate ligament; PS, posterior stabilized; RCT, randomized, controlled trial; ROM, range of motion.

CR group. There was no significant difference in range of motion in patients receiving CR implants with either PCL retention or sacrifice. The Hospital for Special Surgery score was significantly better for PCL sacrifice (CR and PS implants together) than PCL retention. This outcome measure evaluates overall patient function and specific clinical variables (e.g., knee range of motion and radiographic appearance). All other variables did not reveal any significant difference between treatment groups. The authors of the Cochrane analysis were reluctant to make conclusions because the methodologic quality of the studies, as determined by the van Tulder score, was quite variable.[11] For future studies, they suggest more information on the patient population, more information on the type of treatment and intraoperative findings, and better outcome measures (e.g., range of motion, contact position of the femur on the tibia, and knee stability). Despite their hesitation to make a conclusion, these authors state that there is "strong" evidence that there is no difference be-

tween PCL retention and sacrifice using the same prosthesis.[11]

Long-term case series (Level IV) are available for similarly designed CR and PS implants. The Press-Fit Condylar prosthesis (PFC; Johnson and Johnson, Raynham, MA) has been used since 1984, and survival data have been published for both CR and PS designs.[19] Survival of the CR design has been reported at 91.5% at a mean of 15.8 years, and survival of the PS design has been reported at 94.6% at 12 years.[19,20] The similar longevity of these implant designs suggests that the PCL may be substituted without increasing revision rates. Therefore, rates of aseptic loosening, knee instability, and component wear may be unaffected by PCL substitution.

Authors have suggested sacrifice of the PCL and use of a PS implant for certain clinical scenarios: severe deformity (varus/valgus > 15 degrees and fixed flexion deformity > 15 degrees), previous patellectomy, and inflammatory arthritis.[6] Laskin[21] has reported a retrospective case series (Level IV) showing poor results in

RANGE OF MOTION (BEFORE SURGERY)	RANGE OF MOTION (AFTER SURGERY)	KS KNEE SCORE	HSS SCORE	X-RAY SCORE	PROPRIOCEPTION	COMMENTS
A: 106 ± 12 degrees B: 106 ± 21 degrees	A: 97 ± 15 degrees B: 114 ± 21 degrees	No difference	No difference	No difference	Not reported	PS showed significantly increased ROM at 2 years after surgery.
A: 120 ± 8 degrees B: 120 ± 18 degrees	A: 122 ± 15 degrees B: 131 ± 13 degrees	No difference	No difference	No difference	Not reported	PS showed significantly increased ROM at more than 2 years after surgery.
Not reported	Not reported	Not reported	Not reported	Not reported	Significantly better in PS group	Proprioception improves after surgery with both CR and PS arthroplasty.
A: 110 ± 12 degrees B: 101 ± 23 degrees	A: 112 ± 13 degrees B: 111 ± 17 degrees	No difference	Not reported	No difference	Not reported	No difference in results for CR or PS implants.
Not reported	Not reported	Not reported	No difference	No difference	Not reported	PCL not useful when retained. PS knee implant may not be required for PCL-deficient knees.
Not reported	A: 100 degrees B: 110 degrees C: 110 degrees	No difference	Not reported	No difference	Not reported	No significant difference between CR, CR (PCL released), and PS groups.
A: 110.6 degrees B: 111.6 degrees	A: 108.5 degrees B: 108.3 degrees	No difference	Not reported	No difference	Not reported	No difference in results for CR or PS implants.
A: 95.4 degrees B: 94.3 degrees	A: 114.2 degrees B: 117.4 degrees	Not reported	No difference	No difference	Not reported	No difference between retention and sacrifice of PCL.

patients with a fixed varus deformity treated with a CR prosthesis. Laskin and others[5,21] suggest PCL sacrifice and use of a PS implant for varus or valgus deformity greater than 15 degrees (Level V). Lombardi and colleagues[6,22] originally believed that a fixed flexion contracture of greater than 15 degrees required PCL sacrifice; however, based on a recent retrospective comparative study (Level III), these authors now recommend an intraoperative algorithm to determine whether the PCL should be sacrificed for flexion deformity. Sacrifice of the PCL is recommended if full extension cannot be achieved with CR trial, or more than 2 mm (beyond the amount required using a measured resection technique) of distal femur must be resected to achieve full extension. Paletta and Laskin[23] published a retrospective, comparative trial (Level III) on total knee arthroplasty after a patellectomy that showed superior results for a PS implant as compared with a CR implant. In a case series of CR implants used to treat patients with rheumatoid arthritis compared with a case series of CR implants used to treat patients with osteoarthritis, Laskin and O'Flynn[24] found an increased incidence of posterior instability and recurvatum deformity in the patients with rheumatoid arthritis. They recommend use of a PS implant in patients with inflammatory arthritis (Level IV).

AREAS OF UNCERTAINTY

Does Sacrifice of the Posterior Cruciate Ligament Lead to Changes in Knee Joint Proprioception?

The neurosensory function of the PCL is often used as an argument to retain this ligament during knee arthroplasty.[4] Proprioception is used to regulate motor control, coordination, and stability of a joint. An association between reduced proprioception and function has been reported in patients with osteoarthritis.[3] Given the importance of joint stability and coordination in an elderly population (i.e., prevention of falls), every effort should be made to preserve knee joint proprioception. However, many other structures other than the PCL contribute to proprioception (e.g., ACL, collateral ligaments, and joint capsule). Should the PCL be retained to allow for improved proprioception?

Swanik and colleagues[3] conducted a prospective, randomized, controlled trial to investigate the effect of PCL sacrifice on proprioception (Level I evidence). They assessed joint position sense, threshold to detect joint motion, and ability to balance on an unstable platform both before surgery and over 6 months after surgery. Ten patients were randomized to the CR group, and 10 to the PCL-sacrificing group with use of a PS implant group. Joint position sense and balance were significantly better after surgery as compared with before surgery for both treatment groups. The only significant difference between treatment groups was an improvement in joint sensation (sensing extension from a flexed position) for the PS implant group. The authors conclude that arthroplasty improves knee joint proprioception, and sacrifice of the PCL has no significant effect on proprioception. This agrees with two other retrospective comparative studies (Level III) that showed no difference in proprioception with PCL sacrifice.[25,26]

Is a Posterior Stabilized Implant Required When the Posterior Cruciate Ligament Is Sacrificed?

The PS implant reproduces the stability of the PCL through a post and cam mechanism. Articulation of the tibial post within the femoral cam during flexion also simulates physiologic femoral roll back. However, the cam-post articulation can be an additional source of polyethylene wear debris and may dislocate (i.e., the cam may jump anteriorly over the post) if collateral ligament laxity is present.[27] Therefore, UC implants have been proposed as an alternative to PS implants.

Parsley and coworkers[28] conducted a retrospective comparative study (Level III) with 121 patients in the PS treatment group and 89 patients in the UC treatment group.[28] They found no significant difference between groups for terminal flexion, range of motion, and functional scores at the time of follow-up (the time of follow-up was undefined). The authors conclude that there was no clinical difference between implant designs.

Is it possible to use a CR implant with sacrifice of the PCL? Three Level II studies were identified that compared PS implants with CR implants used without retention of the PCL (see Table 88–1).[15,16,18] These studies did not show any significant difference in range of motion, functional score, or radiographic assessment between the two treatment groups. This led the authors to conclude that a PS implant is not required when the PCL is sacrificed. However, follow-up periods for the studies were relatively short (i.e., only one study had a follow-up period of at least 5 years). Instability and polyethylene wear may become apparent beyond this follow-up time.

RECOMMENDATIONS

The literature contains significant debate regarding the fate of the PCL during total knee arthroplasty. However, both long- and short-term studies suggest little difference between PCL retention and sacrifice. Based on our examination of the literature, we make the following recommendations (Table 88–2):

- Primary total knee replacements with PCL sacrifice exhibit slightly greater early range of motion (approximately 8 degrees difference). Otherwise, there is no significant difference in clinical outcomes (functional measures, radiographic measures, and revision rates) between retention and sacrifice of the PCL during routine primary total knee arthroplasty (grade A).
- The PCL should be sacrificed and a PS implant used for patients with severe varus or valgus deformity (>15 degrees, grade C), severe fixed flexion deformity (unable to obtain

intraoperative correction with a CR implant, grade B), previous patellectomy (grade B), and inflammatory arthritis (grade C).
- Sacrifice of the PCL during total knee arthroplasty does not decrease joint proprioception (grade A).
- Insufficient evidence exists that a PS implant is required when the PCL is sacrificed during routine primary total knee arthroplasty.

TABLE 88–2. Grades of Evidence for Recommendations Regarding Posterior Cruciate Ligament in Total Knee Arthroplasty

RECOMMENDATIONS	LEVEL OF EVIDENCE/ GRADE OF RECOMMENDATION
1. No significant difference was found in clinical outcomes between retention and sacrifice of the PCL during routine primary total knee arthroplasty.	A
2. The PCL should be sacrificed and a PS implant used for patients with previous patellectomy.	B
3. The PCL should be sacrificed and a PS implant used for patients with severe fixed flexion deformity (unable to obtain intraoperative correction with a CR implant).	B
4. The PCL should be sacrificed and a PS implant used for patients with severe varus or valgus deformity (>15 degrees).	C
5. The PCL should be sacrificed and a PS implant used for patients with inflammatory arthritis.	C
6. Sacrifice of the PCL during total knee arthroplasty does not decrease knee joint proprioception.	A
7. A PS implant is required when the PCL is sacrificed during routine primary total knee arthroplasty.	I

CR, posterior cruciate ligament retaining; PCL, posterior cruciate ligament; PS, posterior stabilized.

REFERENCES

1. Andriacchi TP, Galante JO: Retention of the posterior cruciate in total knee arthroplasty. J Arthroplasty 3(suppl):13–19, 1988.
2. Freeman MA, Railton GT: Should the posterior cruciate ligament be retained or resected in condylar nonmeniscal knee arthroplasty? The case for resection. J Arthroplasty 3(Suppl): 3–12, 1988.
3. Swanik CB, Lephart SM, Rubash HE: Proprioception, kinesthesia, and balance after total knee arthroplasty with cruciate-retaining and posterior stabilized prostheses. J Bone Joint Surg 86-A:328–334, 2004.
4. Simmons S, Lephart S, Rubash H, et al: Proprioception following total knee arthroplasty with and without the posterior cruciate ligament. J Arthroplasty 11:763–768, 1996.
5. Laskin RS, Rieger M, Schob C, et al: The posteriorstabilized total knee prosthesis in the knee with a severe fixed deformity. Am J Knee Surg 1:199–203, 1988.
6. Lombardi AV Jr, Mallory TH, Fada RA, et al: An algorithm for the posterior cruciate ligament in total knee arthroplasty. Clin Orthop Relat Res 392:75–87, 2001.
7. Matsueda M, Gengerke TR, Murphy M, et al: Soft tissue release in total knee arthroplasty. Cadaver study using knees without deformities. Clin Orthop Relat Res (366):264–273, 1999.
8. Dennis DA, Komistek RD, Mahfouz MR, et al: Multicenter determination of in vivo kinematics after total knee arthroplasty. Clin Orthop Relat Res (416):37–57, 2003.
9. Yamakado K, Worland RL, Jessup DE, et al: Tight posterior cruciate ligament in posterior cruciate-retaining total knee arthroplasty: A cause of posteromedial subluxation of the femur. J Arthroplasty 18:570–574, 2003.
10. Swany MR, Scott RD: Posterior polyethylene wear in posterior cruciate ligament-retaining total knee arthroplasty. A case study. J Arthroplasty 8:439–446, 1993.
11. Jacobs WC, Clement DJ, Wymenga AB: Retention versus sacrifice of the posterior cruciate ligament in total knee replacement for treatment of osteoarthritis and rheumatoid arthritis. Cochrane Database Syst Rev 4:CD004803, 2005.
12. Catani F, Leardini A, Ensini A, et al: The stability of the cemented tibial component of total knee arthroplasty: Posterior cruciate-retaining versus posterior-stabilized design. J Arthroplasty 19:775–782, 2004.
13. Maruyama S, Yoshiya S, Matsui N, et al: Functional comparison of posterior cruciate-retaining versus posterior stabilized total knee arthroplasty. J Arthroplasty 19:349–353, 2004.
14. Tanzer M, Smith K, Burnett S: Posterior-stabilized versus cruciate-retaining total knee arthroplasty: Balancing the gap. J Arthroplasty 17:813–819, 2002.
15. Misra AN, Hussain MR, Fiddian NJ, et al: The role of the posterior cruciate ligament in total knee replacement. J Bone Joint Surg 85-B:389–392, 2003.
16. Straw R, Kulkarni S, Attfield S, et al: Posterior cruciate ligament at total knee replacement. Essential, beneficial or a hindrance? J Bone Joint Surg 85-B:671–674, 2003.
17. Clark CR, Rorabeck CH, MacDonald S, et al: Posterior-stabilized and cruciate-retaining total knee replacement: A randomized study. Clin Orthop Relat Res (392):208–212, 2001.
18. Shoji H, Wolf A, Packard S, et al: Cruciate retained and excised total knee arthroplasty. A comparative study in patients with bilateral total knee arthroplasty. Clin Orthop Relat Res (305):218–222, 1994.
19. Rodricks DJ, Patil S, Pulido P, et al: Press-fit condylar design total knee arthroplasty. Fourteen to seventeen-year follow-up. J Bone Joint Surg Am 89-A:89–95, 2007.
20. Rasquinha VJ, Ranawat CS, Cervieri CL, et al: The press-fit condylar modular total knee system with a posterior cruciate-substituting design. A concise follow-up of a previous report. J Bone Joint Surg Am 88-A:1006–1010, 2006.
21. Laskin RS: Total knee replacement with posterior cruciate ligament retention in patients with a fixed varus deformity. Clin Orthop Relat Res (331):29–34, 1996.
22. Berend KR, Lombardi AV Jr, Adams JB: Total knee arthroplasty in patients with greater than 20 degrees flexion contracture. Clin Orthop Relat Res (452):83–87, 2006.
23. Paletta GA, Laskin RS: Total knee arthroplasty after a previous patellectomy. J Bone Joint Surg Am 77-A:1708–1712, 1995.
24. Laskin RS, O'Flynn HM: The Insall Award. Total knee replacement with posterior cruciate ligament retention in rheumatoid arthritis. Problems and complications. Clin Orthop Relat Res (345):24–28, 1997.
25. Cash RM, Gonzalez MH, Garst J, et al: Proprioception after arthroplasty: Role of the posterior cruciate ligament. Clin Orthop Relat Res (331):172–178, 1996.
26. Lattanzio PJ, Chess DG, MacDermid JC: Effect of the posterior cruciate ligament in knee-joint proprioception in total knee arthroplasty. J Arthroplasty 13:580–585, 1998.
27. Puloski SK, McCalden RW, MacDonald SJ, et al: Tibial post wear in posterior stabilized total knee arthroplasty. An unrecognized source of polyethylene debris. J Bone Joint Surg Am 83-A:390–397, 2001.
28. Parsley BS, Conditt MA, Bertolusso R, et al: Posterior cruciate ligament substitution is not essential for excellent postoperative outcomes in total knee arthroplasty. J Arthroplasty 21(suppl 2):127–131, 2006.

Chapter 89

Should the Patella Be Resurfaced in Total Knee Replacement?

Raphael C. Y. Hau, MBBS, FRACS, Bassam A. Masri, MD, FRCSC, and Donald S. Garbuz, MD, MHSc, FRCSC

The issue of whether the patella should be replaced during total knee replacement (TKR) for osteoarthritis is controversial. Three options are available to the surgeon, namely, always resurface, never resurface, or selectively resurface. This chapter examines the available evidence in the literature to help make a supported decision.

The specific questions examined in this chapter are as follows:

1. What is the evidence for or against routine resurfacing of the patella during TKR for osteoarthritis?
2. What is the evidence for the reliability of the factors used to predict postoperative anterior knee pain?
3. What is the evidence for or against selective resurfacing of the patella during TKR for osteoarthritis?

RESURFACING VERSUS NONRESURFACING

Thirteen Level I-II studies and four meta-analyses found in the English literature examine the role of routine resurfacing of the patella. All of these studies compared two groups of patients with one group having routine resurfacing of their patellae and the other group routine retention of their patellae. These studies are examined paying specific attention to statistically significant differences in the incidence of patellofemoral complications or revisions, the incidence of anterior knee pain, and clinical or functional scores in these studies. There are a further 13 Level III-IV studies on the subject. However, this chapter examines only the Level I-II evidence available to make a recommendation.

Among the 13 Level I/II studies, only one found an inferior result in the resurfaced group favoring nonresurfacing as the preferred management. Eight studies found conflicting results within the same cohort over time or statistically nonsignificant results. Four studies found superior results in the resurfaced group (Table 89–1).

Evidence Favoring Nonresurfacing

Feller and coauthors[1] report a prospective randomized, control trial (RCT) of 40 patients who had unilateral TKR by a single surgeon. Patients with se-

verely deformed patellae were excluded. Removal of osteophytes was performed on the nonresurfaced group, and cemented, all-polyethylene components were inserted in patients in the resurfaced group. One patient in each group had died on follow-up. Thirty-eight knees were reviewed at 3 years after surgery. There were no patellar complications or revisions in either group. No statistically significant difference was found in Hospital for Special Surgery (HSS) and specific Patellar scores between the resurfaced and nonresurfaced groups. Women and heavier patients were found to have significantly lower HSS and Patellar scores. Significantly worse scores were reported for stair climbing in the resurfaced group. The authors conclude that there were no significant benefits to resurfacing the patella if it was not severely deformed.

EVIDENCE FAVORING NEITHER ROUTINE RESURFACING NOR NONRESURFACING

Bourne and colleagues[2] report a series of 90 patients in a RCT with 50 knees in each group. At a minimum of 2 years, two nonresurfaced patellae had subsequent resurfacing for intractable knee pain. They found no statistically significant difference in Knee Society functional score, 30-second stair climbing, and the knee extension torque. The nonresurfaced patients had significantly less pain and better clinical rating. At the 8- to 10-year follow-up examination, Mayman and coauthors[3] report results on the same group of patients. Twenty-nine patients had died leaving 71 patients to follow-up. One patient in the resurfaced group fell and fractured the patella, requiring a patellectomy. The clinical results had changed since the last report in favor of resurfacing. The incidence of anterior knee pain with walking and stair climbing was significantly less in the resurfaced group. More patients were either satisfied or extremely satisfied in the resurfaced group. At the minimum of 10 years review, Burnett and researchers[4] report on 50 knees. From the original 90 patients, 7 refused to participate after enrollment in the study, 36 patients had died, and 2 patients could not attend the follow-up because of dementia and a stroke. Consequently, 45 patients and 50 knees remained to review. One more patient in the nonresurfaced group had had a subsequent resurfacing for anterior knee pain since the last review. No statistically significant difference was found between the groups regarding revision rates, Knee Society clinical rating and functional scores, patient satisfaction, anterior knee pain, and patellofemoral radiographic outcomes. The authors recommend a selective resurfacing approach.

Keblish and colleagues[5] report on a quasi-randomized, prospective, control trial of 52 patients who had bilateral TKR. Forty-four patients had osteoarthritis, six had rheumatoid arthritis, and two had post-traumatic osteoarthritis. All patients had a resurfacing on one side and nonresurfacing on the other. Fifty-one of the 52 had a metal-backed uncemented mobile-bearing patella, and 1 had a cemented all-polyethylene component. Only 58% (30/52) of patients were available for review. At a mean follow-up examination of 5.24 years, no statistically significant difference was found in subjective preference, performance on ascending and descending stairs, or the incidence of anterior knee pain. The authors conclude that nonresurfaced patellae could perform as well as resurfaced patellae.

Barrack and coauthors[6] report on 118 knees in 86 patients at 2.5 years in a RCT. 10% of those in the non-resurfaced group had subsequent resurfacing because of pain. No patient in the resurfaced group had another operation. The statistical significance of this apparent difference in the incidence of reoperation was not reported. No statistically significant difference was found in regarding overall score, pain score, functional score, patient satisfaction, or the incidence of anterior knee pain. At the 5- to 7-year follow-up examination, Barrack and coauthors[6a] report on 88 knees in 64 patients in the same cohort. One more patient in the nonresurfaced group had had a subsequent patellar resurfacing for anterior knee pain. Again, the statistical significance of the apparent difference in the incidence of reoperation was not reported. No statistically significant difference was found in any of the parameters previously examined. The conclusion of the authors was that the occurrence of anterior knee pain was unlikely to be related to whether the patella was resurfaced.

Peng and investigators[7] report on 35 patients having bilateral TKR by a single surgeon in a quasi-randomized prospective study. A variety of implants was used: 30 NexGen (Zimmer, Warsaw, Indiana), 36 Miller-Galante II (Zimmer, Warsaw, Indiana), 2 PFC (Johnson & Johnson, Langhorne, Philadelphia), 2 Genesis (Smith & Nephew, Memphis, Tennessee). One patient in the nonresurfaced group had a patellar realignment for lateral subluxation after a fall. No statistically significant difference was found in Knee Society overall, clinical or function scores, incidence of anterior knee pain or reoperation, and no patient preference for either knee. No recommendation was made by the authors.

Campbell and researchers[8] report on 100 TKRs in a RCT. At 10-year follow-up examination, 22 patients had died, 7 had dementia, 10 were lost to follow-up, and 3 had refused to participate because of poor health. Fifty-eight knees were therefore available to

be reviewed. Two patients in the nonresurfaced group had undergone subsequent resurfacing for anterior knee pain. One patient in the resurfaced group had an arthroscopic lateral release for lateral tilting and anterior knee pain. No statistically significant difference was found in Knee Society score, Western Ontario and McMaster University Osteoarthritis Index, and specific patellofemoral-related questions. The authors conclude that they were not able to recommend routine resurfacing of the patella.

In all the articles previously mentioned in this section, no mention in any of the studies is made of a power analysis. Indeed, in each study, multiple outcomes are mentioned and no primary outcome is identified. Given that these trials were all negative, it is imperative that the reader know what the primary outcome of interest was and the sample size needed to achieve adequate power. Without this information, these negative trials give limited information to the reader. Given the numbers in these studies, it is most likely they were underpowered, rendering their conclusions that there is no difference between the treatment options open to question.

Evidence Favoring Routine Resurfacing

Schroeder-Boersch and investigators[9] report on 40 patients in a RCT. One patient in the nonresurfaced group had a lateral release for subluxation. Better functional and clinical Knee Society scores, as well as better stair-climbing score, were found in the resurfaced group. The authors recommend routine resurfacing, especially in those with severe osteoarthritis. One major deficiency in this article is that there were no preoperative scores on the patients. Because this is known to be the single strongest predictor of postoperative scores, the lack of these scores is a major concern. In addition, the method of randomization was not described.

Newman and colleagues[10] reported on a well-designed RCT involving 125 knees. Forty-two knees were in each of the resurfaced and nonresurfaced groups. Twenty patients had died at the last follow-up; therefore, 105 knees were available for review. No patient in the resurfaced group required a reoperation. Six knees in the nonresurfaced group had a subsequent resurfacing for anterior knee pain. The difference in the incidence of reoperation was statistically significant. No statistically significant difference was found in Bristol Knee score. The authors recommend routine patellar resurfacing.

Wood and coworkers[11] report on a well-designed RCT involving 201 patients. Nine had died and 12 had withdrawn from the study. A total of 198 knees in 180 patients were therefore available for review. Fifteen of 128 nonresurfaced knees required a reoperation because of patellofemoral problems. Eleven of these were secondary patellar resurfacing, one had an arthroscopy for anterior knee pain, two had surgeries for mal-tracking, and one had tibial tubercle transfer after a traumatic patellar dislocation. Nine of

TABLE 89–1. Resurfacing versus Nonresurfacing

AUTHOR (YEAR OF PUBLICATION)	LOE	DX	NO. OF KNEES (RS/NR)	IMPLANT	MEAN FOLLOW-UP (YR)	REOPERATIONS RS	REOPERATIONS NR	AKP RS	AKP NR	KNEE SCORES	OTHER FINDINGS
Feller et al. (1996)[1]	I	OA	40 (20/20) recruited 38 (19/19) reviewed	PCA	3	0	0			Better stair-climbing score in nonresurfaced patients*	
Bourne et al. (1995)[2]†	I	OA	100 (50/50)	AMK	2	0/50, significance not stated	2/50, significance not stated			Less pain and better clinical score in nonresurfaced patients*	Better flexion torque in nonresurfaced knees*
Mayman et al. (2003)[3]†	I	OA	71 reviewed	AMK	8–10	1/50, NS	2/50, NS	10% on stairs* 0% on walking*	47% on stairs* 33% on walking*	NS	More resurfaced patients were either satisfied or extremely satisfied*
Burnett et al. (2004)[4]†	I	OA	50 reviewed	AMK	>10	1/42, NS	3/48, NS	7/19, NS	5/20, NS	NS	
Keblish et al. (1994)[5]	II	OA/RA/post-traumatic	104 (52/52) recruited 60 (30/30) reviewed	Low contact stress	5.2	0	0	3/30, significance not stated	3/30, significance not stated	NS	NS in patient satisfaction
Barrack et al. (1997)[6‡]	I	OA	118 (58/60)	Miller-Galante II	2.5	0%, significance not stated	10%, significance not stated	7%, NS	13%, NS	NS	NS in patient satisfaction
Barrack (2001)[6a]	I	OA	88 (44/44)	Miller-Galante II	5–7	0%, significance not stated	12%, significance not stated	19% NS	17% NS	NS	NS in patient satisfaction
Peng et al. (2003)[7]	II	OA	70 (35/35)	NexGen, Miller-Galante II, Genesis, PFC	3.2	0/35, significance not stated	1/35, significance not stated	20%, NS	20%, NS	NS	NS in patient satisfaction

Study	LOE	Dx	No. of Knees	Implant	Follow-up (y)					Outcome	Outcome
Campbell et al. (2006)[8]	I	OA	100 (46/54) recruited 58 (30/28) Reviewed	Miller-Galante II	10	1/30, significance not stated	2/28, significance not stated	47% NS	43% NS	NS on WOMAC or AKS	Better score on climbing stairs subitem in resurfaced patients*
Schroeder-Boersch et al. (1998)[9]	II	OA	40 (20/20)	Duracon	2	0/20, significance not stated	1/20, significance not stated	NS	NS	Better overall and functional knee scores in the resurfaced group*	
Newman et al. (2000)[10]	I	OA	125 (42/42), 41 selectively resurfaced, 105 reviewed	Kinematic	>5	0/42*	6/42*			NS	
Wood et al. (2002)[11]	I	OA	220 (92/128), 198 reviewed	Miller-Galante II	2	10% NS	12% NS	16%*	31%*	NS in Knee Society scores; Greater overall score in resurfaced knees*	NS on stair descent or ascent; Higher patient satisfaction in resurfaced patients*
Waters and Bentley (2003)[12]	I	403 OA, 71 RA	514 recruited 474 (243/231) reviewed	PFC	5.3	3/243*	11/231*	5.3%*	25.1%*		
Forster (2004)[13]	I§	OA	3 RCTs, 235 knees	Kinematic, Miller-Galante II, AMK	5–10	0.7%*	11%*				
Pakos et al. (2005)[14]	I§	OA/RA	10 RCTs, 1223 knees		1–10	1.9%*	7.3%*	6.4%*	21.2%*	NS	
Nizard et al. (2005)[15]	II§	OA/RA	12 RCTs, 1490 knees		1–10	2.3%*	6.5%*	7.6%*	22.3%*		Less pain during stair climbing in resurfaced patients*; NS in patient satisfaction
Parvizi et al. (2005)[16]	II§	OA/RA	14 RCTs, 1519 knees			NS	NS	15.5%*	30.3%*	NS	Higher patient satisfaction in those resurfaced*

*Statistically significant difference found.
†Same cohort.
‡Same cohort.
§Meta-analysis.

AKP, rate of anterior knee pain; AKS, American Knee Society score; AMK, anatomic medullary knee; Dx, diagnosis; LOE, level of evidence; NR, nonresurfaced; NS, no statistically significant difference; OA, osteoarthritis; PCA, porous coated anatomic, PFC, press-fit condylar; RA, rheumatoid arthritis; reoperations, rate of reoperations for patellofemoral problems; RCT, prospective, randomized, control trials; RS, resurfaced; WOMAC, Western Ontario and McMaster University Arthritis Index.

the 92 resurfaced knees required reoperations. There were five patellar revisions; three of these were done for loosening. One patient had a patellectomy for a comminuted patellar fracture, one had a lateral release, and two had arthroscopies. A significantly lower incidence of anterior knee pain was found in the resurfaced group. There was no statistically significant difference in Knee Society score. Better ability with borderline statistical significance was found in stair descent in the resurfaced group. The authors note that the results of their study are specific to the Miller-Galante type II knee.

Waters and Bentley[12] report on 474 knees in 390 patients in a RCT. Eleven of 231 knees had to have a secondary resurfacing in the nonresurfaced group. This was a well-designed RCT looking at the Press Fit Condylar Knee from Johnson & Johnson. In the resurfaced group, one loose patellar component was removed, and two knees had lateral releases. There was a significantly lower incidence of reoperation, lower incidence of anterior knee pain, greater Knee Society score, and higher patient satisfaction in the resurfaced group. The authors recommend routine patellar resurfacing.

Even though a few well-designed, prospective, randomized trials with adequate follow-up have shown results in favor of routine resurfacing, the majority of the Level I/II studies yielded equivocal results. The potential problems such as small patient numbers, lost to follow-up, and inadequate power may increase the chance of a type II error. A number of meta-analyses have been performed to minimize this chance.

Meta-analyses

Forster[13] examined three prospective, randomized trials with a minimum of 5-year follow-up and strict inclusion criteria. A 78% follow-up rate was reported with a total of 235 knees. The resurfaced patients had a significantly lower incidence of reoperation. Anterior knee pain could not be analyzed because of study heterogeneity. The authors conclude that there was no mid- to long-term benefit to leaving the patella nonresurfaced.

Pakos and colleagues[14] examined 10 prospective, randomized trials with a total of 1223 knees. The range of follow-up was between 1 and 10 years. There was a well-designed meta-analysis with strict inclusion criteria. A significantly lower risk for having a reoperation or anterior knee pain was found in the resurfaced patients. No statistically significant difference was found in terms of knee scores. The authors conclude that routine resurfacing was a marginally superior strategy.

Nizard and coworkers[15] examined 12 prospective trials with a total of 1490 knees. Randomized and quasi-randomized trials were included. A significantly lower risk for having a reoperation, anterior knee pain, or pain during stair climbing was found in the resurfaced patients. No statistically significant difference was found in terms of patient satisfaction. The authors conclude that there seemed to be an advantage in routine resurfacing the patella.

Parvizi and investigators[16] examined 14 prospective trials with a total of 1519 knees. Randomized and quasi-randomized trials were included. A significantly lower risk for having anterior knee pain and a higher patient satisfaction rate was found in the resurfaced patient. No statistically significant difference was found in the incidence of reoperation, complications, or knee scores. The authors did not make a recommendation.

Summary

Most of the Level I/II studies have shown either no difference in results or have shown advantages of routine resurfacing over nonresurfacing. Notably, of the 13 studies mentioned, only three of the RCTs and two of the meta-analyses were of a high-quality design, and all of these studies support routine patellar resurfacing. In conclusion, there is good evidence to support routine resurfacing of the patella over nonresurfacing in the treatment of osteoarthritis with total knee arthroplasty. However, this evidence is specific to certain total knee designs. Clearly, there is a need for further RCTs on this subject. However, for these to be successful, a well-designed scoring system needs to be defined that will answer this important question.

SELECTIVE RESURFACING

Selective resurfacing has been advocated by some to reduce the incidence of postoperative anterior knee pain whereas minimizing the complications such as patellar fractures and component loosening associated with resurfacing. In this approach, the surgeon has to make an assessment before and during surgery as to which patients are likely to experience postoperative anterior knee pain. The patients who are deemed at high risk for having postoperative knee pain will then be selected to have a patella resurfacing at the time of their TKR. This section examines the evidence for the *validity* of factors used to predict the occurrence of postoperative anterior knee pain.

Evidence for and against the Reliability of Predictors for Postoperative Anterior Knee Pain

Four Level I studies and four Level IV studies have presented data on the validity of different predictive factors for postoperative anterior knee pain. These factors include age, sex, weight, height, body mass index, preoperative anterior knee pain, preoperative Knee Society score, preoperative range of movement, degree of osteophytes, grading of the articular surface of the patellofemoral joint, and the need for a lateral release. No Level I/II data are available on the diagnosis of inflammatory arthritis as a predictor of postoperative anterior knee pain. Only the Level I evidence is considered here (Table 89–2).

TABLE 89–2. Predictors for Postoperative Anterior Knee Pain

AUTHOR (YEAR OF PUBLICATION)	LOE	NO. OF KNEES	FINDINGS
Newman et al. (2000)[10]	I	125 recruited, 105 reviewed	Grading of articular cartilage was found not to be a predictor.
Wood et al. (2002)[11]	I	220 recruited, 198 reviewed	Age, sex, weight, body mass index, preoperative anterior knee pain, preoperative Knee Society score, preoperative range of movement, grading of patellar articular cartilage, degree of osteophytes formation, and lateral release were not significant predictors of postoperative anterior knee pain. The weight of the patient was a significant predictor of anterior knee pain in those without patellar resurfacing.*
Waters and Bentley (2003)[12]	I	514 recruited 474 reviewed	Age, sex, weight, preoperative radiographic appearance, lateral release, or whether the posterior cruciate ligament was sacrificed were not found to be predictors.
Campbell et al. (2006)[8]	I	100 recruited, 58 reviewed	Grading of the articular surfaces of either the patella or the trochlea was not found to be a predictor.

*Statistically significant difference found.
LOE, level of evidence.

TABLE 89–3. Resurfaced versus Selectively Resurfaced

AUTHOR (YEAR OF PUBLICATION)	LOE	DX	NO. OF KNEES (RS/SR)	IMPLANT	MEAN FOLLOW-UP (YR)	REOPERATIONS RS	REOPERATIONS SR	AKP RS	AKP SR	KNEE SCORES	RECOMMENDATIONS
Newman et al. (2000)[10]	I	OA	125 (42/41), 42 non-resurfaced	Kinematic (Stryker, Mahwah, New Jersey)	>5	0/42, NS	1/41, NS			NS	Recommended routine resurfacing
Tabutin et al. (2005)[17]	III	OA	5915 (487/5428)	NexGen (Zimmer, Warsaw, Indiana)	2			0.7%*	6.3%*		

*Statistically significant difference found.
AKP, rate of anterior knee pain; Dx, diagnosis; LOE, level of evidence; NS, no statistically significant difference; reoperations, rate of reoperations for patellofemoral problems; RS, resurfaced; SR, selectively resurfaced.

TABLE 89–4. Selective Resurfacing Case Series

AUTHOR (YEAR OF PUBLICATION)	LOE	DX	NO. OF KNEES (RS/NR)	IMPLANT	MEAN FOLLOW-UP (YR)	REOPERATIONS/COMPLICATIONS		AKP		OTHER FINDINGS	RECOMMENDATION BY AUTHORS
						RS	NR	RS	NR		
Boyd et al. (1993)[18]	IV	OA/RA	891 (396/495)	Johnson & Johnson (Langhorne, Pennsylvania)	6.5	4%*	12%*		RA 13%* OA 6%*		Routine resurfacing
Ewald et al. (1999)[19]	IV	OA/RA	306 (242/64)	Kinematic (Stryker, Mahwah, New Jersey)	10–14	11/242, significance not stated	1/64, significance not stated	11.2%*	21.8%*	Better stair-climbing abilities in nonresurfaced group*	Resurfacing not appropriate for this prosthesis RCTs needed
Misra et al. (2003)[20]	IV	OA	129 recruited, 105 (48/57) reviewed	PFC (Johnson and Johnson, Langhorne, Pennsylvania)	4.75	0/48	0/57	4.2%	3.5%	NS in HSS score Greater rate of lateral release in nonresurfaced group*	RCTs needed
Arbuthnot et al. (2004)[21]	IV	OA/RA	378 (236/142)	Insall–Berstein II				38/236, significance not stated	40/142, significance not stated	Better Knee Society score in resurfaced group*	RCTs needed

*Statistically significant difference found.

AKP, rate of anterior knee pain; Dx, diagnosis; HSS, Hospital for Special Surgery; LOE, level of evidence; NR, nonresurfaced; NS, no statistically significant difference; OA, osteoarthritis; PFC, press-fit condylar; RA, rheumatoid arthritis; RCT, prospective, randomized, control trials; reoperations, rate of reoperations for patellofemoral problems; RS, resurfaced.

Newman and colleagues[10] found in their RCT that the intraoperative grade of the articular cartilage of the patellofemoral joint did not correlate with the occurrence of postoperative knee pain. Wood and coworkers[11] found that age, sex, weight, body mass index, preoperative anterior knee pain, preoperative Knee Society score, preoperative range of movement, grading of patellar articular cartilage, degree of osteophytes formation, and lateral release did not correlate with the incidence of postoperative anterior knee pain. However, when the nonresurfaced group was considered in isolation, the weight of the patient was found to be a significant predictor of anterior knee pain. Waters and Bentley[12] found that age, sex, weight, preoperative radiographic appearance, lateral release, and whether the posterior cruciate ligament was sacrificed were not to predictive of postoperative anterior knee pain. Campbell and researchers[8] found that the grading of the articular surfaces of either the patella or of the trochlea was not predictive of postoperative anterior knee pain.

Therefore, a lack of consistent evidence exists to support any of the factors mentioned earlier as valid predictors of postoperative knee pain after a TKR without patellar resurfacing. Without reliable predictors of anterior knee pain, the criteria for selective resurfacing, therefore, are subjective and do not confer any prognostic value. The whole basis of selective resurfacing should therefore be questioned.

Data on Selective Resurfacing

In contrast with routine resurfacing, there are few direct comparative studies on selective resurfacing against other treatment options in the literature. Most of the evidence on this subject is of low quality. In the English literature, there is one RCT (Level I) comparing routine resurfacing, nonresurfacing and selective resurfacing. There is one case–control study (Level III) and four case series (Level IV). Because of the paucity of Level I-II evidence, studies of all levels of evidence are considered (Tables 89–3 and 89–4).

Selective Resurfacing versus Routine Resurfacing

Newman and colleagues[10] compared 42 patients who had their patellae resurfaced and 41 patients who had selective resurfacing of their patellae in an RCT. One patella had to be revised in the selective group for loosening. None of the patients in the resurfaced group had a reoperation. No statistically significant difference was found in terms of incidence of reoperations, Bristol knee score, and clinical Patellar score. However, although not significantly different, the nonresurfaced group and nonresurfaced knees in the selected group scored worse than the knees that were resurfaced, either selectively or by random allocation. The authors recommend routine patellar resurfacing.

Tabutin and coauthors[17] report on the incidence of anterior knee pain as a part of a multicenter 5-year clinical and radiologic study on 5915 Nex Gen TKRs. Only osteoarthritic knees with no previous osteotomies or replacements were included. The 2-year results of French (487 knees) and the international (5428 knees) groups were reported. A significantly greater incidence of preoperative anterior knee pain was found in the French group (85.1% vs. 66.6%). The percentage of patellar resurfacing was also found to be significantly different between the two groups with the French resurfacing 98.8% and the international group resurfacing 35.7% of the knees. The main finding in this report was the significant difference in postoperative anterior knee pain with 0.7% in the French group and 6.3% in the international group. The incidence of patellofemoral complication or reoperations was not reported. It must be pointed out that this is not a true comparison between routine resurfacing and selective resurfacing. Not the entire French cohort was resurfaced, and the criteria for resurfacing in the international group were not reported. The authors conclude with caution that resurfacing was a better option with this prosthesis.

Selective Resurfacing Case Series

Boyd and coworkers[18] retrospectively evaluated a group of 891 selectively resurfaced knees. A total of 396 knees were selectively resurfaced based on the gross appearance of the patellofemoral joint and on the patellar tracking intraoperatively. A posterior cruciate–retaining prosthesis was used. Thirty percent of resurfaced knees and 37% of the knees that were not resurfaced had osteoarthritis. The incidence of reoperations was significantly lower in the resurfaced group compared with the nonresurfaced group. The incidence of anterior knee pain was significantly lower in patients with osteoarthritis as compared with those with inflammatory arthropathy in the nonresurfaced group. The authors recommend routine resurfacing when a cruciate-retaining prosthesis was used.

Ewald and colleagues[19] reported on a prospective case series of 306 knees. Approximately 45.5% of the patients had osteoarthritis, 49.5% had rheumatoid arthritis, and 5% had post-traumatic arthritis. About 79% of the patellae were resurfaced. The indications included rheumatoid arthritis, eburnated patellofemoral joint, and patellar deformity. Ten of the 242 resurfaced patellae became loose and were revised. One resurfaced patella had to be realigned for recurrent dislocation. One nonresurfaced patella was resurfaced for recurrent dislocation. A significantly greater incidence of anterior knee pain was found in the nonresurfaced group, but significantly better stair-climbing abilities were found in the nonresurfaced group. The authors conclude that routine resurfacing may not be the most effective strategy with that prosthesis.

Misra and coauthors[20] report a case series on 105 TKRs that were treated with selective resurfacing. The criteria for resurfacing included preoperative patellofemoral symptoms, patellar instability/malalignment, and grade III-IV articular changes. Forty-eight knees were resurfaced according to these criteria. A significantly greater incidence of lateral release was found in the nonresurfaced group. No statistically significant difference was found in the incidence of anterior knee pain or in the HSS score. No revisions were required in any knees. The authors conclude that an RCT was needed.

Arbuthnot and investigators[21] report on a prospective case series of 378 TKRs. All of these knees had preoperative patellofemoral pain. A total of 236 knees were resurfaced at the surgeons' discretion. The criteria for resurfacing were not described. A significantly better Knee Society score was found in the resurfaced group. No statistically significant difference was found in the incidence of postoperative anterior knee pain, reoperations, or complications. The authors were unable to make a recommendation.

CONCLUSION

The literature on patellar resurfacing has been reviewed in an attempt answer whether we should always resurface, never resurface, or selectively resurface the patella in TKR. For selective resurfacing, there is insufficient evidence to support the use of any factors as *valid* predictors of postoperative anterior knee pain. Therefore, there is a great deal of difficulty in designing high-quality RCTs to answer this question. The evidence available is insufficient to support the management option of selective resurfacing at the time of TKR for osteoarthritis.

To date, the best evidence available supports routine resurfacing of the patella. This is based on three well-designed RCTs and two meta-analyses. However, the conclusions of these studies are specific to the prosthesis used. Meta-analysis, although providing some insight, again is limited because of many factors including limited number of high-quality RCTs, multiple prosthetic designs, multiple surgeries, and ill-defined primary outcomes. Given that this is an important question to be answered, future high-quality RCTs are of value. However, equally important is the clinician's decision on what primary outcome would be of utmost importance for him/her and his/her patients. In this way, RCTs can be appropriately powered to show a difference in important clinical outcome if the difference truly exists. Until further evidence becomes available, routine resurfacing of the patella is recommended. Table 89–5 provides a summary of recommendations.

TABLE 89–5. Summary of Recommendations

STATEMENT	LEVEL OF EVIDENCE/GRADE OF RECOMMENDATION	REFERENCES
1. The patella should be routinely resurfaced in total knee replacement	I	10, 11, 12, 13, 14

REFERENCES

1. Feller JA, Bartlett RJ, Lang DM: Patellar resurfacing versus retention in total knee arthroplasty. J Bone Joint Surg Br 2:226, 1996.
2. Bourne RB, Rorabeck CH, Vaz M, et al.: Resurfacing versus not resurfacing the patella during total knee replacement. Clin Orthop Relat Res (321):156, 1995.
3. Mayman D, Bourne RB, Rorabeck CH, et al: Resurfacing versus not resurfacing the patella in total knee arthroplasty: 8- to 10-year results. J Arthroplasty 5:541, 2003.
4. Burnett RS, Haydon CM, Rorabeck CH, et al: Patella resurfacing versus nonresurfacing in total knee arthroplasty: Results of a randomized controlled clinical trial at a minimum of 10 years' followup. Clin Orthop Relat Res (428):12, 2004.
5. Keblish PA, Varma AK, Greenwald AS: Patellar resurfacing or retention in total knee arthroplasty. A prospective study of patients with bilateral replacements. J Bone Joint Surg Br 6:930, 1994.
6. Barrack RL, Wolfe MW, Waldman DA, et al: Resurfacing of the patella in total knee arthroplasty. A prospective, randomized, double-blind study. J Bone Joint Surg Am 8:1121, 1997.
6a. Barrack RL, Bertot AJ, Wolfe MW, et al: Patellar resurfacing in total knee arthroplasty. A prospective, randomized, double-blind study with five to seven years of follow-up. J Bone Joint Surg Am 9:1376–1381, 2001.
7. Peng CW, Tay BK, Lee BP: Prospective trial of resurfaced patella versus non-resurfaced patella in simultaneous bilateral total knee replacement. Singapore Med J 7:347, 2003.
8. Campbell DG, Duncan WW, Ashworth M, et al.: Patellar resurfacing in total knee replacement: A ten-year randomised prospective trial. J Bone Joint Surg Br 6:734, 2006.
9. Schroeder-Boersch H, Scheller G, Fischer J, et al.: Advantages of patellar resurfacing in total knee arthroplasty. Two-year results of a prospective randomized study. Arch Orthop Trauma Surg 1-2:73, 1998.
10. Newman JH, Ackroyd CE, Shah NA, et al: Should the patella be resurfaced during total knee replacement? Knee 1:17, 2000.
11. Wood DJ, Smith AJ, Collopy D, et al: Patellar resurfacing in total knee arthroplasty: A prospective, randomized trial. J Bone Joint Surg Am 2:187, 2002.
12. Waters TS, Bentley G: Patellar resurfacing in total knee arthroplasty. A prospective, randomized study. J Bone Joint Surg Am 2:212, 2003.
13. Forster MC: Patellar resurfacing in total knee arthroplasty for osteoarthritis: A systematic review. Knee 6:427, 2004.
14. Pakos EE, Ntzani EE, Trikalinos TA: Patellar resurfacing in total knee arthroplasty. A meta-analysis. J Bone Joint Surg Am 7:1438, 2005.
15. Nizard RS, Biau D, Porcher R, et al: A meta-analysis of patellar replacement in total knee arthroplasty. Clin Orthop Relat Res 432:196, 2005.
16. Parvizi J, Rapuri VR, Saleh KJ, et al: Failure to resurface the patella during total knee arthroplasty may result in more knee pain and secondary surgery. Clin Orthop Relat Res (438):191–196, 2005.
17. Tabutin J, Banon F, Catonne Y, et al: Should we resurface the patella in total knee replacement? Experience with the Nex Gen prothesis. Knee Surg Sports Traumatol Arthrosc 7:534, 2005.

18. Boyd AD Jr, Ewald FC, Thomas WH, et al: Long-term complications after total knee arthroplasty with or without resurfacing of the patella. J Bone Joint Surg Am 5:674, 1993.
19. Ewald FC, Wright RJ, Poss R, et al: Kinematic total knee arthroplasty: A 10- to 14-year prospective follow-up review. J Arthroplasty 4:473, 1999.
20. Misra AN, Smith RB, Fiddian NJ: Five year results of selective patellar resurfacing in cruciate sparing total knee replacements. Knee 2:199, 2003.
21. Arbuthnot JE, McNicholas MJ, McGurty DW, et al: Total knee replacement and patellofemoral pain. Surgeon 4:230, 2004.

Chapter 90

What Is the Role of Computer Navigation in Hip and Knee Arthroplasty?

RAJIV GANDHI, MD, FRCSC AND NIZAR N. MAHOMED, MD, SCD, FRCSC

Achieving the correct rotation and alignment of the implant components is critical for the short- and long-term survival of hip and knee arthroplasty. In total hip arthroplasty (THA), wear,[1,2] range of motion,[3] and stability[4] are all affected by component orientation. In total knee arthroplasty (TKA), authors have shown that knee implants malpositioned by more than 3 degrees had a 24% loosening rate by 3 years after surgery as compared with 3% for correctly aligned implants.[5,6]

The correct placement of implants is guided by preoperative radiographs and templating, intraoperative anatomic landmarks, and mechanical alignment guides on the instrumentation sets. However, patient positioning on the table is variable, anatomic landmarks are often difficult to reliably identify in arthritic joints, and mechanical alignment guides have not improved accuracy of acetabular positioning.[7,8]

Computer-assisted surgery (CAS) has the potential to improve surgical accuracy through less invasive techniques and to improve clinical outcomes for patients. Computer-based tools allow for preoperative templating with three-dimensional imaging and intraoperative real-time positional information on tracking tools and bony structures. The clinical utility of these tools as compared with conventional techniques is being investigated in total joint arthroplasty.

BACKGROUND

Picard and colleagues[9] have classified CAS into active robotic systems, semiactive robotic systems, and passive systems. Active robotic systems are those in which a robot performs some surgical tasks such as drilling and reaming without the direct intervention of the surgeon. Many systems use a preoperative computed tomographic (CT) scan to plan the surgery. These systems are costly and involve complex equipment in the operating room, and thus have not been widely used.

Semiactive robots do not perform surgical tasks directly but rather direct placement of surgical tools in space. With this system, the surgeon first indicates the desired position and orientation of the implant on a three-dimensional template. The robot then positions the saw and drill guides so that the surgeon can make the necessary cuts. Passive systems include CT-based, fluoroscopy-based, or imageless navigation.

CT-based systems require a preoperative CT scan that is used to construct a three-dimensional model of the joint including the mechanical, transepicondylar, and tibial rotation axis. Surface landmarks of the joint are then acquired intraoperatively by touching the bony points with a tracking probe. Fluoroscopy-based navigation uses two or more intraoperative fluoroscopic views that are entered into the computer, thereby calculating the required anatomic references. A third method requires no images be obtained before or during surgery, but rather relies on the computer system having a database of prescanned CT images to calculate reference axes. The surgeon inputs multiple bony reference points into the computer that are compared with the database to define a three-dimensional model of the patient's anatomy.

Regardless of the type of computerized navigation system, the main goal is to increase surgical accuracy and reduce the chance of malposition of the implants. The potential downsides of navigation are the increased cost, exposure to radiation, and increased surgical time.

CLINICAL RESULTS

Total Hip Arthroplasty

Achieving the correct abduction and anteversion of the acetabular component could potentially improve the longevity of a THR, improve the range of motion,[3] and decrease the dislocation rate.[10–12] Lewinnek and coauthors[13] recommend an abduction angle of 40 ± 10 degrees and an anteversion angle of 15 ± 10 degrees as the safe zone for cup orientation. Many studies have investigated whether CAS can help improve accuracy in cup placement.

Kalteis and investigators,[14] in a prospective, randomized trial, examined CT-based navigation versus imageless navigation versus conventional techniques for positioning of the acetabulum. The data showed that the incidence of component malposition was 53% in the freehand group, 17% in the CT-based group, and 7% with imageless navigation. The authors conclude that navigation significantly improved component alignment ($P = 0.003$), and there was no difference between CT-based and imageless navigation ($P = 0.23$). In comparing the mean abduction and anteversion angles between the groups, navigation was significantly better than conventional techniques with no difference between the CT-based versus imageless navigation. Surgical time was increased 8 minutes with imageless navigation and 17 minutes with CT-based navigation with no difference in blood loss among the three groups.

Parratte and Argenson[15] compared image-free navigation and freehand techniques for cup placement in a prospective randomized study of 60 patients. They found that 57% of the cups in the freehand group were malpositioned outside the acceptable range as compared with 20% in the navigation group ($P = 0.002$). When they compared the mean cup angles for both abduction and anteversion between the two groups, there was no significant difference. The mean surgical time was 12 minutes greater for the navigation group.

Leenders and researchers[16] undertook a prospective, randomized trial comparing CT-based navigation and freehand techniques for positioning of the acetabular component. CAS surgery led to a significantly improved accuracy for placing the cup within the safe zone of 45 to 55 degrees as compared with traditional methods ($P < 0.001$). The authors found that only 2 of the 50 patients in the CAS group had abduction angles of cup outside the safe zone.

Other authors have concluded similar findings that navigation helped improve alignment in cup position and reduce the number of outliers from the acceptable range.[17,18] Many of these studies are short-term follow-up, and it would be prudent to follow these patients long term to see whether the improved component alignment leads to an improved outcome and survival of the implant. Overall, there is no reported increase in complication rate associated with CAS.

A further advancement has been the use of active systems and a robot that serves as a delivery tool for a surgical procedure planned before surgery on a computer. The surgeon positions a robot by means of a referencing procedure and then can supervise the robot throughout the process.

A prospective, randomized study from Germany by Schwieger and colleagues[19] compared robotic insertion (ROBODOC) and conventional techniques for total hip replacement. After 24 months of follow-up,

the authors conclude that limb-length equality and varus/valgus alignment of the femoral component was improved with the robot ($P < 0.001$). Recurrent dislocations and subsequently the revision rate was greater in the robotic group ($P < 0.001$), and the duration of surgery was increased in the robotic group ($P < 0.001$). No difference was found at 2 years in the Harris hip, Merle d'Aubigné, and the Mayo clinical scores between the two groups. The authors conclude that the 18% dislocation rate in the robot group was due to the abductor muscle deficiencies either from the wide surgical approach needed for the robot or the damage it caused to the tendon during the reaming process, but not from malposition of the components. Furthermore, the authors suggest this technology needs some further development before it can be considered for routine use in THA.

The stability of the femoral implant inserted with ROBODOC was evaluated by Nogler and researchers[20] in a prospective, randomized cadaveric study. The authors conclude that there was no difference in femoral component micromotion at the time of insertion; therefore, the robot system did not enhance stability as compared with manual insertion techniques (Table 90–1 and Fig. 90–1).

Total Knee Arthroplasty

Minor implant malpositioning can lead to early wear and loosening, and poorer clinical results. Ritter and coworkers[21] have proposed that implants should be aligned in a neutral mechanical axis ±3 degrees varus or valgus for better survivorship. Ten percent of knees lie outside of this range using standard instrumentation. Rotational malpositioning can affect patellar tracking and cause subluxation.[22] Traditional techniques for determining femoral component alignment include the epicondylar axis, posterior femoral condyles, and Whiteside's line.[23] Studies have shown that the intraobserver and interobserver reproducibility of these techniques in arthritic knees is poor[24–26] Computer navigation has the potential to improve component alignment and also to record information on intraoperative knee kinematics, joint range of motion, and soft-tissue balance.[27]

Chin and investigators[28] performed a prospective, randomized trial to compare postoperative radiographic alignment of TKA using standard alignment techniques, both intramedullary (IM) and extramedullary, with CAS. The authors found that CAS was

TABLE 90–1. Summary of Best Evidence for Navigation and Hip Arthroplasty

AUTHOR	PARAMETER	CONTROL	STUDY GROUP	
			IMAGE-FREE NAVIGATION	COMPUTED TOMOGRAPHIC NAVIGATION
Kalteis et al.[14] ($N = 90$)	Outliers from accepted range	16/30 (53%)	2/30 (7%)	5/30 (17%)
Parratte and Argenson[15] ($N = 60$)	Outliers from accepted range	17/30 (57%)	6/30 (20%)	
Leenders et al.[16] ($N = 60$)	Outliers from accepted range	8/30 (27%)		2/30 (7%)

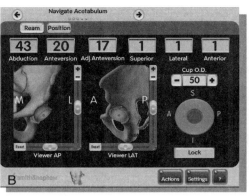

FIGURE 90–1. Navigation in total hip replacement. *A,* Intraoperative tracking of landmarks. *B,* Real-time feedback on acetabular positioning. (Courtesy Smith & Nephew, Memphis, TN)

more accurate and consistent with placement of the components in both the sagittal and coronal planes as compared with conventional techniques ($P < 0.05$). When the overall mechanical axes of the limbs were compared, there was no difference among the three groups ($P = 0.274$). The authors conclude that there are fewer outliers from the acceptable alignment of ±3 degrees with computer navigation. Operative time was significantly greater in the CAS group by 30 minutes ($P < 0.001$). The volume of drainage in the drains was less in the computer navigation group ($P = 0.046$); however, the decline in hemoglobin was no different ($P = 0.176$).

In a randomized prospective trial by Chauhan and coworkers,[29] 70 patients were randomized to jig-based TKA versus computer-assisted TKA. They found that computer-navigated knees scored significantly better in terms of femoral coronal plane alignment ($P = 0.032$), femoral rotation ($P = 0.001$), and tibial alignment ($P = 0.047$). Overall, blood loss was less with CAS ($P = 0.0001$), and the duration of surgery was greater by an average of 13 minutes ($P = 0.0001$).

Matziolis and investigators[30] performed a prospective, randomized study comparing CAS and conventional techniques in TKA. They conclude that computer guidance led to a smaller range of deviation from a neutral mechanical axis as compared with conventional techniques ($P < 0.004$). Rotational alignment of the tibial and femoral components showed no difference between the two groups. Other authors have reported similar results whereby computer navigation decreases the number of outliers from the acceptable range of alignment.[31,32]

Another potential benefit to CAS is avoid having to cannulate the IM canals of the femur and tibia, which can potentially lead to decreased blood loss and less systemic fat embolus load. Kalairajah and colleagues[33] investigated the incidence of cranial emboli in a prospective, randomized study of 24 patients undergoing either CAS or traditional TKA using intramedullary femoral and tibial guides. In the computer-assisted group, there were, on average, 0.64 emboli detected versus 10.7 in the conventional total knee group ($P = 0.003$). However, this study did not determine the size of these emboli or the nature of the emboli being fat, air, platelets, or bone. No difference was reported in

mean mental scores conducted on the patients on postoperative days 1 or 3.

The issue of blood loss was addressed by Kalairajah and colleagues[34] in a prospective, randomized study of 60 patients undergoing TKA with either computer-based navigation or by conventional methods. The mean blood loss in the CAS group was 1183 versus 1747 mL in the conventional group. This difference was statistically significant ($P = 0.001$). The authors conclude that despite an increase in mean surgical time in the CAS group, 89 versus 74 minutes ($P = 0.002$), CAS surgery can potentially lead to a decrease in need for blood transfusions.

Keene and investigators[35] randomized patients undergoing bilateral medial unicompartmental arthroplasty into two groups, one side with computer navigation and the other with traditional techniques. Preoperative valgus stress view radiographs and clinical assessments were used to determine the desired postoperative coronal alignment. The results demonstrated that the mean variation between the desired alignment and the achieved correction was significantly improved in the navigation group, 0.9 versus 2.8 degrees ($P < 0.001$). The mean tourniquet time for the navigated knees was 70 minutes as compared with 53 minutes in the non-navigated knees.

A meta-analysis taking restoration of the mechanical axis as an end point was reported by Bauwens and coauthors.[36] They included 33 studies, 11 of which were randomized studies for a total of 3423 patients. They conclude that mean values for alignment were no different between the computer navigation group of patients and the conventional technique group. Computer navigation did, however, decrease the risk for malalignment beyond the critical threshold of 3 degrees. Mean surgical time was 23% greater in the navigation group.

The benefits of computer navigation in revision surgery have not been well described in the literature. Sikorski[37] reported on 14 knees revised for aseptic failure and concluded that no component was perfectly aligned after surgery and the most difficulty came in femoral rotation. Overall, the author believes that the alignment obtained in computer-assisted revision knee surgery is not as accurate as computer-assisted primary knee arthroplasty (Table 90–2 and Fig. 90–2).

TABLE 90–2. Summary of Best Evidence for Navigation and Knee Arthroplasty

AUTHOR	PARAMETER	CONTROL	STUDY GROUP	
			IMAGE-FREE NAVIGATIOIN	COMPUTED TOMOGRAPHIC NAVIGATION
Matziolis et al.[30] (N = 60)	Outliers from ±3-degree mechanical axis	7/28 (25%)	1/32 (3%)	
Chauhan et al.[29] (N = 70)	Outliers from ±3-degree mechanical axis	8/35 (23%)	5/35 (14%)	
Chin et al.[28] (N = 90)	Outliers from ±3-degree mechanical axis	22/60 (37%)		6/30 (20%)
Decking et al.[38] (N = 52)	Outliers from ±5-degree mechanical axis	8/25 (32%)	1/27 (4%)	
Bathis et al.[39] (N = 160)	Outliers from ±3-degree mechanical axis	18/80 (22%)	3/80 (4%)	

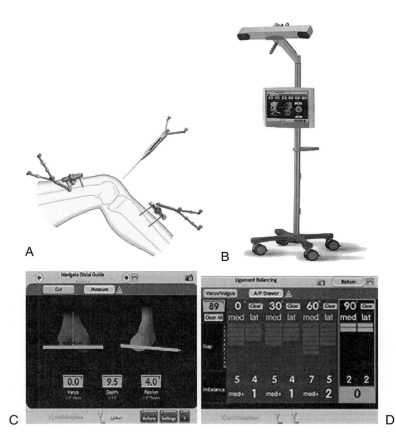

FIGURE 90–2. Navigation in total knee replacement. *A–B,* Diagram of patient setup with tracker pins in femur and tibia, and computer base with infrared sensors. *C,* Distal femoral alignment. *D,* Soft-tissue balancing. (Courtesy Smith & Nephew, Memphis, TN)

STUDY LIMITATIONS

Many of the studies in the hip and knee literature around CAS have reported the overall mean alignment for the study groups. We suggest that this measure may not be an accurate comparison for reporting the data. For example, two cups in one study group aligned at 50 and 30 degrees of abduction will present the same mean as two cups aligned in 40 degrees of abduction; however, they represent different surgical precision.

Computer navigation is an emerging technology whereby the software and hardware components are all continuing to evolve. There is a significant learning curve with computer navigation.[17] Potential improvements may be a pinless system to avoid stress risers in the tibia and femur, as well as a computer base with a sterile handle such that it can be adjusted by the surgeon. New systems are using electromagnetic pulses rather than line-of-sight infrared determination of implant position, which may help reduce some of

Continued

RECOMMENDATIONS—CONT'D

the clutter of the crowded operating room.

At the time of this publication, there are few randomized controlled trials to clearly document an advantage to CAS. From both the hip and knee literature, it appears clear that navigation does decrease the number of outliers from the desired component alignment. Long-term studies to document an overall clinical benefit in component survival with CAS are yet to be published.

The computer software systems provide the surgeon with much data on soft-tissue stability and ligament balance to which no standard and accepted values are known. How much laxity is acceptable at full extension, midflexion, or 90 degrees of flexion is yet to be determined and remains an area in need of further study.

Navigation systems generally do not provide any information about either patellofemoral kinematics or placement of the patellar component. With improved software, computer navigation may prove to become a valuable tool to assess patellofemoral kinematics in osteoarthritic knees and reduce patellofemoral complications.

At the current costs of the equipment, the use of navigation may be limited to higher volume arthroplasty centers. However, its greatest benefit may be in the hands of the low-volume arthroplasty surgeon who is not as comfortable with the traditional alignment guides. Whether these systems prove to be cost-effective in the long term by reducing the revision burden remains to be seen.

The role of computer navigation may be limited to difficult cases with altered anatomy or in association with small incision techniques to improve component alignment. Its consistent use in every primary total joint replacement would likely require a reduction in costs to the hospital, a decrease in added surgical time to the case, and an alternate funding model for the surgeon. Table 90–3 provides a summary of recommendations.

TABLE 90–3. Summary of Recommendations

RECOMMENDATIONS	LEVEL OF EVIDENCE/GRADE OF RECOMMENDATION	REFERENCES
1. CAS improves precision in component alignment in THA/TKA.	A	3, 14–16, 28, 29
2. CAS increases mean surgical time versus conventional techniques.	A	14, 15, 28, 29
3. CAS decreases blood loss in THA/TKA.	I	3, 14, 28, 29, 34, 40
4. CAS leads to an improved long-term clinical outcome in THA/TKA.	I	

CAS, computer-assisted surgery; THA, total hip arthroplasty; TKA, total knee arthroplasty.

REFERENCES

1. Schmalzried TP, Guttman D, Grecula M, Amstutz HC: The relationship between design, position and articular wear of acetabular components inserted without cement and the development of pelvic osteolysis. J Bone Joint Surg Am 76:677–688, 1994.
2. Kennedy JG, Rogers WB, Soffe KE, et al: Effect of acetabular component orientation on recurrent dislocation, pelvic osteolysis, polyethylene wear, and component migration. J Arthroplasty 13:530–534, 1998.
3. Kummer FJ, Shah S, Iyer S, DiCesare PE: The effect of acetabular cup orientations on limiting hip rotation. J Arthroplasty 14:509–513, 1999.
4. Jolles BM, Zangger P, Leyvraz PF: Factors predisposing to dislocation after primary total hip arthroplasty. J Arthroplasty 17:282, 2002.
5. Fehring TK, Odum S, Griffin WL, et al: Early failures in total knee arthroplasty. Clin Orthop Relat Res 392:315–318, 2001.
6. Jeffery RS, Morris RW, Denham RA: Coronal alignment after total knee replacement. J Bone Joint Surg Br 73:709–714, 1995.
7. Siston RA, Patel JJ, Goodman SB, et al: The variability of femoral rotational alignment in total knee arthroplasty. J Bone Joint Surg Am 87:2276–2280, 2005.
8. DiGioia AM, Jaramaz B, Plakseychuk Ay, et al: Comparison of a mechanical acetabular alignment guide with computer placement of the socket. J Arthroplasty 17:359–364, 2002.
9. Picard F, Moody J, DiGioia III AM, et al (eds): Computer and Robotic Assisted Hip and Knee Surgery. New York, Oxford University Press, 2004, pp 43–48.
10. Del Schutte H Jr, Lipman AJ, Bannar SM, et al: Effects of acetabular abduction on cup wear rates in total hip arthroplasty. J Arthroplasty 13:621–626, 1998.
11. Paterno SA, Lachiewicz PF, Kelley SS: The influence of patient-related factors and the position of the acetabular component on the rate of dislocation after total hip replacement. J Bone Joint Surg Am 79:1202–1210, 1997.
12. Kennedy JG, Rogers WB, Soffe KE, et al: Effect of acetabular component orientation on recurrent dislocation, pelvic osteolysis, polyethylene wear, and component migration. J Arthroplasty 13:530–534, 1998.
13. Lewinnek GE, Lewis JL, Tarr R, et al: Dislocations after total hip-replacement arthroplasties. J Bone Joint Surg Am 60:217–220, 1978.
14. Kalteis T, Handel M, Bathis H, et al: Grifka imageless navigation for the insertion of the acetabular component in total hip arthroplasty: Is it as accurate as CT based navigation? J Bone Joint Surg Br 88:163–168, 2006.
15. Parratte S, Argenson JN: Validation and usefulness of a computer-assisted cup-positioning controlled study system in total hip arthroplasty. A prospective, randomized, controlled study. J Bone Joint Surg Am 89:494–499, 2007.
16. Leenders T, Vandevelde D, Mahieu G, Nuyts R: Reduction in variability of acetabular cup abduction using computer assisted surgery: A prospective and randomized study. Comput Aided Surg 7:99–106, 2002.
17. Wixson RL, MacDonald MA: Total hip arthroplasty through a minimal posterior approach using imageless computer-assisted hip navigation. J Arthroplasty 20(7 suppl 3):51–56, 2005.
18. Haaker RG, Tiedjen K, Ottersbach A, et al: Comparison of conventional versus computer-navigated acetabular component insertion. J Arthroplasty 22:151–159, 2007.
19. Schwieger K, Hille E, Morlock MM, et al: Comparison of robotic-assisted and manual implantation of a primary total hip replacement: A prospective study. J Bone Joint Surg Am 85:1470–1478, 2003.
20. Nogler M, Polikeit A, Wimmer C, et al: Primary stability of a robodoc implanted anatomical stem versus manual implantation. Clin Biomech (Bristol, Avon) 19:123–129, 2004.
21. Ritter MA, Faris PM, Keating EM, Meding JB: Postoperative alignment of total knee replacement. Its effect on survival. Clin Orthop Relat Res (299):153–156, 1994.
22. Merkow RL, Soudry M, Insall JN: Patellar dislocation following total knee replacement. J Bone Joint Surg Am 67:1321, 1985.

23. Whiteside LA, Arima J: The anteroposterior axis for femoral rotational alignment in valgus total knee arthroplasty. Clin Orthop Relat Res (321):168–172, 1995.

24. Kinzel V, Ledger M, Shakespeare D: Can the epicondylar axis be defined accurately in total knee arthroplasty? Knee 12:293–296, 2005.

25. Jerosch J, Peuker E, Philipps B, Filler T: Interindividual reproducibility in perioperative rotational alignment of femoral components in knee prosthetic surgery using the transepicondylar axis. Knee Surg Sports Traumatol Arthrosc 10:194–197, 2002.

26. Jenny JY, Boeri C: Low reproducibility of the intra-operative measurement of the transepicondylar axis during total knee replacement. Acta Orthop Scand 75:74–77, 2004.

27. Siston RA, Gioric NJ, Goodman SB, Delp SL: Surgical navigation for total knee arthroplasty: A perspective. J Biomech 40:728–735, 2007.

28. Chin PL, Yang KY, Yeo SJ, Lo NN: Randomized control trial comparing radiographic total knee arthroplasty implant placement using computer navigation versus conventional technique. J Arthroplasty 20:618–626, 2005.

29. Chauhan SK, Scott RG, Breidahl W, Beaver RJ: Computer-assisted knee arthroplasty versus a conventional jig-based technique. A randomised, prospective trial. J Bone Joint Surg Br 86:372–377, 2004.

30. Matziolis G, Krocker D, Weiss U, et al: A prospective, randomized study of computer-assisted and of implant alignment and rotation conventional total knee arthroplasty. Three-dimensional evaluation. J Bone Joint Surg Am 89:236–243, 2007.

31. Stockl B, Nogler M, Rosiek R, et al: Navigation improves accuracy of rotational alignment in total knee arthroplasty. Clin Orthop Relat Res (426):180–186, 2004.

32. Victor J, Hoste D: Image-based computer-assisted total knee arthroplasty leads to lower variability in coronal alignment. Clin Orthop Relat Res (428):131–139, 2004.

33. Kalairajah Y, Cossey AJ, Verrall GM, et al: Are systemic emboli reduced in computer-assisted knee surgery? A prospective, randomised, clinical trial. J Bone Joint Surg Br 88:198–202, 2006.

34. Kalairajah Y, Simpson D, Cossey AJ, et al: Blood loss after total knee replacement: Effects of computer-assisted surgery. J Bone Joint Surg Br 87:1480–1482, 2005.

35. Keene G, Simpson D, Kalairajah Y: Limb alignment in computer-assisted minimally-invasive unicompartmental knee replacement. J Bone Joint Surg Br 88:44–48, 2006.

36. Bauwens K, Matthes G, Wich M, et al: Navigated total knee replacement. A meta-analysis. J Bone Joint Surg Am 89:261–269, 2007.

37. Sikorski JM: Computer-assisted revision total knee replacement. J Bone Joint Surg Br 86:510, 2004.

38. Decking R, Markmann Y, Fuchs J, et al: Leg axis after computer-navigated total knee arthroplasty: A prospective randomized trial comparing computer-navigated and manual implantation. J Arthroplasty 20:282–288, 2005.

39. Bathis H, Perlick L, Tingart M, et al: Alignment in total knee arthroplasty: A comparison of computer-assisted surgery with the conventional technique. J Bone Joint Surg Br 86-B:683–687, 2004.

40. Widmer KH, Grutzner PA: Joint replacement-total hip replacement with CT based navigation. Injury 35(suppl 1):S-A84–A89, 2004.

41. Nabeyama R, Matsuda S, Miura H, et al: The accuracy of image-guided knee replacement based on computed tomography. J Bone Joint Surg Br 86:366–371, 2004.

42. Kalteis T, Handel M, Herold T, et al: Greater accuracy in positioning of the acetabular cup by using an image-free navigation system. Int Orthop 29:272–276, 2005.

How Do You Make a Diagnosis of an Infected Arthroplasty?

ALEXANDER SIEGMETH, MD, FRCS (TR & ORTH), DONALD S. GARBUZ, MD, MHSC, FRCSC, AND BASSAM A. MASRI, MD, FRCSC

Infection after a total hip or knee arthroplasty is an uncommon but serious complication with significant impact. Although the postoperative infection rate has decreased from 9% to 1% to 2%, large centers still treat a significant number of patients with infected arthroplasties every year. With the aging population and also younger patients demanding joint replacement procedures, the problem is likely to increase over the years to come.

Rational methods to prevent and diagnose infection must be established. Diagnosing an infection after a joint replacement can be straightforward in the acute postoperative period but challenging if it occurs months or years later. Accurate diagnosis is therefore important to avoid erroneous surgery.

Aseptic loosening is currently the most common diagnosis leading to a revision arthroplasty. However, infection must be excluded in all cases. The consequences of failing to correctly diagnose an infection will have serious consequences on outcome of the revision procedure, with reinfection occurring in most cases. The purpose of this chapter is to outline the various diagnostic options and to evaluate their accuracy based on the best evidence available in the literature.

OPTIONS

History and clinical examination are an important first step in diagnosing a prosthetic infection. Preoperative investigations include blood tests, aspiration, radiographs, and nuclear medicine techniques. Intraoperative tests include analysis of synovial fluid, Gram staining, histologic analysis of a frozen section, or intraoperative cultures.

EVIDENCE

History and Clinical Examination

No study has investigated solely the sensitivity and specificity of history and clinical examination to accurately diagnose a prosthetic infection. However, Spangehl and colleagues[1] correctly diagnosed 27 of 35 infected total hip arthroplasties with history and examination alone (Level I). All 35 infections were later confirmed with positive intraoperative cultures. Acute onset of pain, systemic illness, and sinus formation were the most commonly found signs and symptoms. No studies comment on the value of history and examination in correctly diagnosing an infected knee arthroplasty. History and physical examination are useful because they give you an initial index of suspicion or a pretest likelihood of infection. Further diagnostic testing simply changes the pretest likelihood of disease. As such, a patient who presents with a low likelihood of infection based on history and physical examination, will require much more stringent criteria to clearly diagnose infection. However, a patient who presents with florid signs and symptoms of infection will require much less stringent criteria for the confirmation of infection. This is an application of Bayes' theorem in probability theory, and this is why it is important to understand how to apply the various tests that are discussed in the context of the initial encounter with the patient, namely, the history and physical examination.

Preoperative Hematologic Tests

White Blood Cell Count. Obtaining a white blood cell count (WBC) is a routine preoperative investigation that is of little diagnostic value. In a prospective study (Level I evidence), Spangehl and colleagues[1] evaluated the diagnostic accuracy to correctly diagnose an infection in 202 hips. With a value of more than 11.0×10^9 WBC/L considered to be a positive result indicating infection, they found a sensitivity of 0.20 and a specificity of 0.96. The positive predictive value, however, was only 0.54, and the negative predictive value 0.85. Di Cesare and coworkers[2] (Level IV) undertook a prospective, case–control study of 58 patients undergoing reoperation. Seventeen were diagnosed as having a prosthetic infection. The sensitivity of WBCs was 0.47, and the specificity was 1.00. The positive predictive value was 1.00, and the negative predictive value was 0.82. In a retrospective case series (Level IV evidence), Canner and coauthors[3] note a low prevalence of increased WBC counts in patients with an infected total joint arthroplasty. Therefore, based on the evidence, WBC count is of limited use, except when the pretest probability is high.

Erythrocyte Sedimentation Rate and C-Reactive Protein. The erythrocyte sedimentation rate (ESR) is a measure of erythrocyte rouleaux formation, which occurs whenever an inflammatory condition is present. C-reactive protein (CRP) is an acute-phase protein synthesized in the liver. As with all acute-phase reactants, CRP level is increased in many inflammatory, infectious, and some neoplastic conditions. Spangehl and colleagues[1] (Level I) prospectively analyzed the ESR and CRP level in 171 and 142 revision hip arthroplasties. ESR had a sensitivity of 0.82, specificity of 0.85, positive predictive value of 0.58, and negative predictive value of 0.95. CRP had a sensitivity of 0.96, specificity of 0.92, positive predictive value of 0.74, and negative predictive value of 0.99. If both tests were negative (ESR <30 mm/hr, CRP <10 mg/L), the probability of infection was zero. When both tests were positive, the probability of infection was 0.83. Virolainen and researchers[4] (Level IV) also conclude that combined ESR and CRP are of value in the preoperative evaluation. For ESR, Di Cesare and coworkers[2] (Level IV) found a sensitivity of 1.0 and specificity of 0.56. CRP had a sensitivity of 0.95 and specificity of 0.76.

Greidanus and investigators[5] (Level I) evaluated 145 patients presenting for revision total knee arthroplasty for the presence of infection using the ESR and CRP. The ESR and CRP were obtained at the time of clinical assessment before definitive revision total knee arthroplasty. All patients had undergone preoperative aspiration for culture and had intraoperative periprosthetic tissue sent for bacterial culture. A diagnosis of infection was established for 45 of 151 knees that underwent revision total knee arthroplasty (prevalence, 0.298). The ESR (sensitivity, 0.93; specificity, 0.83; likelihood ratio positive, 5.81; accuracy, 0.86) and CRP (sensitivity, 0.91, specificity, 0.86; likelihood ratio positive, 6.89; accuracy, 0.86) had excellent diagnostic test performance. Combination testing of ESR and CRP together increases overall sensitivity to 0.95 for the diagnosis of infection. In this study, using receiver operating characteristics curves, the optimal cut point for ESR was found to be 22.5 mm/hr, and that of CRP was found to be 13.5 mg/L.

Serum Interleukin-6. Interleukin-6 (IL-6) is a factor produced by monocytes and macrophages. It functions as a hepatocyte-stimulating factor and induces the production of acute-phase reactants. Wirtz and coworkers[6] established that it returns to normal after total joint arthroplasties. Di Cesare and coworkers[2] (Level III) selected 58 patients who underwent a revision procedure and measured the IL-6 levels before and after surgery. Seventeen of the 58 patients were infected as determined after surgery with intraoperative cultures. The sensitivity of IL-6 was 1.0, the specificity was 0.95, the positive predictive value was 0.89, and the negative predictive value was 1.00. However, this study was done on a small and selected sample, and further large studies (Levels I and II) are needed to determine the value of IL-6 in accurately detecting infection before surgery.

Polymerase Chain Reaction. Polymerase chain reaction (PCR) is a molecular technique that allows the production of large quantities of DNA from one DNA molecule. Through this amplification, it enables the detection of rare RNA and DNA sequences. Various genetic diseases and infections can be diagnosed with PCR. Panousis and investigators[7] (Level II) conducted a prospective study of 92 cases undergoing a revision arthroplasty (76 hips, 16 knees) to evaluate the efficacy of PCR sampled intraoperatively from joint aspirate before capsulotomy to detect a prosthetic infection. The authors used a combination of ESR, CRP, preoperative aspiration, and intraoperative cultures to determine the presence or absence of infection. PCR yielded a high false-positive rate. The sensitivity was 92%, the specificity was 74%, the positive predictive value was 34%, and the negative predictive value was 98%.

NUCLEAR MEDICINE TECHNIQUES

Bone scans have traditionally been used to evaluate painful arthroplasties. The main problems encountered were the inability of a positive test to distinguish between infection, aseptic loosening, and impending fractures. Furthermore, many of these studies remain positive in asymptomatic prostheses for up to 2 years after surgery.

In a prospective study of 50 painful total hip arthroplasties, Reinartz and colleagues[8] (Level III) compared the value of technetium-99 triple-phase bone scan (TPBS) with 18-fluorodeoxyglucose (FDG) positron emission tomography (PET) in differentiating between infection and aseptic loosening. The sensitivity and specificity for the technetium scan to differentiate between a prosthetic infection and aseptic loosening was 0.68 and 0.68, and for the PET scan was 0.94 and 0.95. The sensitivity and specificity for the technetium scan to detect a pathologic process was 0.79 and 0.88, respectively, and of the PET 0.94 and 0.97, respectively. In contrast, Stumpe and coauthors[9] (Level II) compared PET, TPBS, and conventional radiography in the ability to differentiate between infection and aseptic loosening in 35 patients with painful hip replacements. The authors conclude that FDG-PET and TPBS had a similar diagnostic accuracy. Pill and investigators[10] (Level II) compared FDG-PET with [111]indium-white blood cell imaging in 92 patients with painful total hip arthroplasties. The specificity of both investigations to differentiate between infection and aseptic loosening was comparable (93% and 95%). However, FDG-PET yielded a significantly higher sensitivity (95% vs. 50%).

Preoperative Invasive Test

Preoperative Fluid Aspiration and Tissue Sampling. Spangehl and colleagues[1] analyzed the diagnostic accuracy of image-guided aspiration and tissue sampling in 180 patients undergoing a revision hip arthroplasty. Patients who were taking antibiotics were excluded from this study. The results of the initial aspiration showed a sensitivity of 0.86, a specificity of 0.94, a positive predictive value of 0.67, and a negative predictive value of 0.98. In five hips, repeat aspirations were performed because the initial results were inconsistent with the clinical presentation. This improved the diagnostic accuracy of the aspiration. This suggests that aspiration alone is not sufficient for the diagnosis because of the risk for false-positive and -negative results. For this reason, in low-probability cases, the authors suggest that if the ESR and the CRP are not suggestive of infection, an aspiration is not necessary. If, however, the pre-test probability is high, an aspiration in addition to the ESR and the CRP is required, particularly if the ESR and CRP are normal. In all cases, an aspiration is required to confirm the diagnosis of infection if the ESR or the CRP level is increased.

Williams and colleagues[11] (Level II) compared open capsular biopsy with needle aspiration in 273 consecutive total hip arthroplasties before revision surgery. Sensitivity and specificity of the 2 modalities were comparable (0.83 vs. 0.80 and 0.90 vs. 0.94, respectively). The authors conclude that both methods are reliable in differentiation between septic and aseptic loosening, but open biopsy offers no advantages over needle aspiration.

Sadiq and coworkers[12] (Level II) report on the diagnostic accuracy of open core biopsy to detect a prosthetic infection in 159 total hip and knee arthroplasties before a revision arthroplasty. This showed a sensitivity of 88%, a specificity of 91%, and an accuracy of 89% considering the final diagnosis. This suggests no advantage over less invasive techniques.

Trampuz and investigators[13] (Level II) analyzed the synovial fluid leukocyte count and differential obtained by arthrocentesis in 133 patients with a painful total knee arthroplasty. Using intraoperative cultures, they diagnosed aseptic failure in 99 patients and a prosthetic infection in 34 patients. A leukocyte count of more than 1.7×10^3 μL had a sensitivity of 94% and a specificity of 88%. A differential of more than 65% neutrophils had a sensitivity of 97% and a specificity of 98%. Notably, the absolute cell count is much lower than that seen in septic arthritis of an unreplaced joint. The differential count is of much greater importance. Whenever the neutrophil proportion is more than 65%, the likelihood of infection is high.

Intraoperative Tests

The definitive diagnosis of whether an arthroplasty is infected is made at surgery. Macroscopic evaluation of the operative site with the presence of pus is usually only of value in the acute situation. Chronic infections can present with inflamed tissues without any pus. This may look no different from cases affected by severe osteolysis because of polyethylene wear. For this reason, intraoperative diagnostic tests are required. These include frozen sections and intraoperative cultures.

Frozen Section. Frozen sections are particularly helpful when clinical suspicion is high but preoperative tests were negative or equivocal. For example in patients with inflammatory disease (rheumatoid arthritis), ESR or CRP can be high in the absence of infection. Preoperative aspiration can also be false negative or false positive. Spangehl and colleagues[1] evaluated frozen sections in 202 hips using the criteria of Mirra.[14] They considered a specimen infected if any single high-power field contained at least five stromal neutrophils. The analysis of the frozen section compared with the final histologic result had a sensitivity of 0.80, a specificity of 0.94, a positive predictive value of 0.74, and a negative predictive value of 0.96.

Using more stringent criteria (more than 10 polymorphonuclear leucocytes per high-power field), Bandit and coworkers[15] studied 121 revision total joint arthroplasties. They compared a positive frozen section with intraoperative cultures as the gold standard. For frozen section, the sensitivity was 0.6, the specificity was 0.93, the positive predictive value was 0.67, and the negative predictive value was 0.93. Therefore, using more stringent criteria lowers the sensitivity, making it possible to miss certain infections, without significantly increasing the specificity. Therefore, we recommend the use of more than 5 polymorphonuclear leucocytes per high-power field as the cut point instead of more than 10.

Intraoperative Cultures. In the absence of other factors, intraoperative cultures remain the gold standard to which all other investigations are compared. Unless the patient is already taking antibiotics, they should provide the definitive diagnosis in most patients with infection at the site of joint replacement. Spangehl and colleagues[1] analyzed specimens from 180 hips undergoing revision hip replacement. They took at least three intraoperative samples from obviously inflamed tissues. Infection was diagnosed if more than one third of all specimens was positive (2/3 or 3/3 samples); the sensitivity was 0.94, specificity was 0.97, positive predictive value was 0.77, and negative predictive value was 0.99. Atkins and researchers[16] (Level II) performed a prospective study of 297 revision hip and knee arthroplasties. The authors conclude that if three or more specimens out of five were positive, the sensitivity was 66% and the specificity was 99.6%.

RECOMMENDATIONS

No one diagnostic test is available today to make the definitive diagnosis of a chronically infected arthroplasty. Diagnosis starts with a thorough history and examination. Patients with an infected arthroplasty often describe pain unrelated to activity and not relieved by rest. Often the pain has been present since the initial operation, although different in character. There may be a history of a slow-healing wound after surgery or prolonged redness and swelling. Serial radiographs can show rapid loosening over months rather than years, as would be typical for aseptic loosening. Scalloping and osteolysis can be present but are more often absent.

Serologic investigations are performed in every patient with pain at the site of an arthroplasty. White blood cell count, CRP level, and ESR are routine. In the absence of any clinical suspicion and with a normal CRP level and a normal ESR, an infection can be safely excluded and no other tests are required. An aspiration with or without a synovial biopsy is warranted if either the CRP level or ESR is increased, and/or if there is clinical suspicion for an infection. If the first aspirate is negative, a repeat aspiration is warranted. It is also important to wait as long as possible after antibiotics are stopped to reduce the potential for a false-negative result, although in such a situation, a negative aspirate does not necessarily exclude the diagnosis of infection, and more imaging such as a serial bone/indium scan or a PET scan may be warranted. At the end of the day, the surgeon has to exercise substantial judgment in the interpretation of the battery of tests and has to apply Bayes' theorem before a definitive diagnosis may be made. An intraoperative frozen section is potentially helpful to aid in the diagnosis of such difficult cases. Intraoperative cultures (at least three samples from different locations taken with clean instruments) are mandatory in all revision cases. Some authors recommend withholding prophylactic antibiotics before obtaining these cultures; however, there is no high-level evidence to warrant such a practice. In straightforward cases where infection has been ruled out, and the probability of infection is low, the advantage of withholding antibiotics is not high enough to overshadow the increased risk for postoperative infection related to the lack of prophylactic antibiotics before the skin incision. For this reason, when we believe that infection has been ruled out, we administer prophylactic antibiotics. Of course, in cases where infection cannot be easily conclusively ruled out and the presurgical probability of infection is still reasonably high, we prefer to withhold preoperative antibiotics and to give them only after the intraoperative cultures have been taken. This way, if there is an unexpected positive culture results, the patient can be treated with 6 weeks of intravenous antibiotics after surgery[17] (Level V). Table 91–1 provides a summary of the evidence.

TABLE 91–1. Summary of the Evidence

STATEMENT	LEVEL OF EVIDENCE/ GRADE OF RECOMMENDATION	REFERENCES
1. Preoperative levels of ESR and CRP are highly sensitive and specific to exclude infection.	A	1–4
2. PCR has a low specificity to diagnose an infection.	B	6
3. Nuclear medicine techniques are sensitive but not specific. FDG-PET is superior to TPBS.	B	7–9
4. Preoperative joint aspiration and tissue sampling is sensitive and specific especially if repeated.	A, B	1, 10–12
5. Intraoperative frozen section is specific but not sensitive. The positive predictive value is low.	A, B	1, 14
6. Intraoperatively obtained cultures from at least three different locations are highly sensitive and specific.	A, B	1, 15

CRP, C-reactive protein; ESR, erythrocyte sedimentation rate; FDG, 18-fluorodeoxyglucose; PCR, polymerase chain reaction; PET, positron emission tomography; TPBS, triple-phase bone scan.

REFERENCES

1. Spangehl MJ, Masri BA, O'Connell JX, et al: Prospective analysis of preoperative and intraoperative investigations for the diagnosis of infection at the sites of two hundred and two revision total hip arthroplasties. J Bone Joint Surg Am 81A:672–682, 1999.
2. Di Cesare PE, Chang E, Preston CF, et al: Serum interleukin-6 as a marker of periprosthetic infection following total hip and knee arthroplasty. J Bone Joint Surg Am 87A:1921–1927, 2005.
3. Canner GC, Steinberg ME, Heppenstall RB, et al: The infected hip after total hip arthroplasty. J Bone Joint Surg Am 66A:1393–1399, 1984.
4. Virolainen P, Lahteenmaki, Hiltunen A, et al: The reliability of diagnosis of infection during revision arthroplasties. Scand J Surg 91:178–181, 2002.
5. Greidanus NV, Masri BA, Garbuz DS, et al.: Use of erythrocyte sedimentation rate and c-reactive protein level to diagnose infection before revision total knee arthroplasty. a prospective evaluation. J Bone Joint Surg Am 89:1409-1416, 2007.
6. Wirtz DC, Heller KD, Miltner O, et al: Interleukin 6: A potential inflammatory marker after total joint replacement. Int Orthop 24:194–196, 2000.

7. Panousis K, Grigoris P, Butcher I, et al: Poor predictive value of broad range PCS for the detection of arthroplasty infection in 92 cases. Acta Orthop Scand 76:341–346, 2005.
8. Reinartz P, Mumme T, Hermanns B, et al: Radionuclide imaging of the painful hip arthroplasty. J Bone Joint Surg Br 87-B:465–470, 2005.
9. Stumpe KD, Notzli HP, Zanetti M: FDP PET for differentiation of infection and aseptic loosening in total hip replacements: Comparison with conventional radiography and three phase bone scintigraphy. Radiology 231:333–341, 2004.
10. Pill SG, Parvizi J, Tang PH, et al: Comparison of fluorodeoxyglucose positron emission tomography and [111]indium-white blood cell imaging in the diagnosis of periprosthetic infection of the hip. J Arthroplasty 21(suppl 2):91–97, 200.
11. Williams JL, Norman P, Stockley I: The value of hip aspiration versus tissue biopsy in diagnosing infection before exchange hip arthroplasty surgery. J Arthroplasty 19:582–586, 2004.
12. Sadiq S, Wootton JR, Morris CA, et al: Application of core biopsy in revision arthroplasty for deep infection. J Arthroplasty 20:196–201, 2005.
13. Trampuz A, Hanssen AD, Osmon DR, et al: Synovial fluid leukocyte count and differential for the diagnosis of prosthetic knee infection. Am J Med 117:556–562, 2004.
14. Mirra JM, Amstutz HC, Matos M, et al: The pathology of the joint tissues and its clinical relevance in prosthesis failure. Clin Orthop 117:221–240, 1976.
15. Bandit DM, Kaufer H, Hartford JM: Intraoperative frozen section analysis in revision total joint arthroplasty. Clin Orthop Relat Res 401:230–238, 2002.
16. Atkins BL, Athanasou N, Deeks JJ, et al: Prospective evaluation of criteria of microbiological diagnosis of prosthetic-joint infection at revision arthroplasty. J Clin Microbiol 36:2932–2939, 1998.
17. Tsukayama DT, Estrada R, Gustilo RB: Infection after total hip arthroplasty. A study of the treatment of one hundred and six infections. J Bone Joint Surg Am 78:512–523, 1996.

SPORTS MEDICINE TOPICS

Chapter 92

Are Anterior Cruciate Ligament Injuries Preventable?

Warren R. Dunn, MD, MPH

The anterior cruciate ligament (ACL) is the most commonly injured ligament in the body. Disruption of the ACL is particularly common in athletic populations and among military personnel. There may be as many as 200,000 ACL injuries occurring in the United States each year. ACL deficiency leading to instability is associated with secondary meniscal and articular cartilage injury increasing the risk for gonarthrosis. ACL reconstruction is commonly performed to restore stability to the knee. It is estimated that more than 100,000 ACL reconstructions are performed annually in the United States, costing in excess of $2 billion.

Female individuals are two to six times more likely to injure the ACL compared with male individuals playing identical sports at similar levels. ACL reconstructions are performed most commonly in high-school- and college-aged individuals; however, ACL reconstruction in this active age group compared with older individuals is twice as common for female than male individuals, further supporting the findings of others that female individuals are at increased risk for ACL injury.[1]

Given the increasing incidence of ACL injury, together with the costly surgery to restore stability and lengthy rehabilitation involved to recover, this is an apt condition for both primary and tertiary preventive measures.[2] Primary prevention aims to reduce the incidence of ACL tears, whereas tertiary prevention targets a reduction in complications from the injury such as secondary injury of the knee or subsequent graft failure. Most of the research in this area has focused on primary prevention. Sex differences in lower extremity kinematics and neuromuscular control are some of the biomechanical factors that may contribute to increased risk for ACL injury in female individuals. In fact, differences in lower extremity kinematics have been shown in female individuals while just walking compared with age- and activity-level–matched male individuals.[3]

OPTIONS

The Henning Program was one of the first training interventions described for the prevention of ACL injury.[4] Henning viewed more than 500 videos of ACL injuries and concluded that the overwhelming majority of the injuries occurred without contact. In female basketball players, he notes that the most common noncontact injury mechanisms were planting and cutting, straight knee landing, and 1-step stopping with an extended knee. Based on these observations, the Henning Program focused on avoiding these positions and supplanting them with an accelerated rounded turn, bent-knee landing, and a 3-step stop with the knees flexed, respectively. This type of training has been expanded by others and could be generally categorized as a technique-movement awareness program.

Various types of intervention programs have been described to decrease ACL injury. These programs attempt to influence the neuromuscular kinetic chain through awareness, strengthening, flexibility, agility, proprioceptive, and plyometric training to reduce injury risk. However, two main types of preventive ACL programs have been put forward and investigated with more rigorous study design, specifically proprioception-balance training and plyometric-agility training. Proprioceptive-balance programs are intended to improve balance and increase coordination through exercises such as balancing on unstable surfaces and single-leg tasks with or without simultaneous tasks with the upper extremities. Plyometric-agility training focuses on improving dynamic stability and technique during sport-related tasks. These training programs typically involve landing, jumping, and decelerating in various positions at different intensity levels.

EVIDENCE

The knee ligament injury prevention (KLIP) training program is a low-intensity plyometric training program applicable for broad use in any active population.[5] The KLIP emphasizes landing mechanics with neuromuscular control at landing. Irmischer and colleagues[5] randomized 28 active college-age female individuals to a KLIP or control group, and showed that a 9-week KLIP program improved landing mechanics and decreased peak vertical impact force, as well as the rate of force displacement.

Nine studies of adequate design for potential casual inference, eight Level II studies,[6–13] and one Level I study[14] have investigated ACL prevention training programs; the characteristics of these studies are listed in Table 92–1. The results of the individual studies are listed in Figure 92–1 together with a forest plot graphically displaying the point estimates on a common scale. These studies are clinically and

TABLE 92–1. Characteristics of Anterior Cruciate Ligament Prevention Studies

AUTHOR (YEAR OF PUBLICATION)	DESIGN (LOE)	TRAINING PROGRAM	n	SPORT	INTERVENTIONS SEX	INTERVENTIONS n	CONTROL SPORT	CONTROL SEX
Caraffa et al. (1996)[6]	Cohort (II)	PB: using a BAPS board	300	Soccer	M	300	Soccer	F
Hewett et al. (1999)[7]	Cohort (II)	PA: plyometric jump training emphasizing technique, strength, power, agility, maximum vertical jump height	185 97 84	Volleyball Soccer Basketball	F F F	81 193 189 209 225	Volleyball Soccer Basketball Soccer Basketball	F F F M M
Hewett total			366			897		
Heidt et al. (2000)[8]	RCT (II)	PA: plyometric, strength, flexibility, technique training, and awareness of risky positions	42	Soccer	F	258	Soccer	F
Soderman et al. (2000)[9]	RCT (II)	PB: using a balance board	121	Soccer	F	100	Soccer	F
Myklebust (2003)[10]	Cohort (II)	PB: using foam mats and balance board, awareness training on landing technique	855 (1999–2000 season) 850 (2000–2001 season)	Handball Handball	F F	942 (1998–1999 control season)	Handball	F
Mandelbaum et al. (2005)[11]	Cohort (II)	PA: 20 prepractice warm-up of stretching, strengthening, plyometrics, and agility training	1885	Soccer	F	3818	Soccer	F
Petersen et al. (2005)[12]	Cohort (II)	PB: using foam mats and balance board, awareness training on landing technique, Henning principles	134	Handball	F	142	Handball	F
Olsen et al. (2005)[14]	RCT (I)	PB: using foam mats and balance board, awareness training on landing technique	808 150	Handball Handball	F M	778 101	Handball Handball	F M
Olsen total			958			879		
Pfeiffer et al. (2006)[13]	Cohort (II)	PA: "KLIP" program: plyometrics with landing technique and run-deceleration mechanics	191 189 197	Basketball Soccer Volleyball	F F F	319 244 299	Basketball Soccer Volleyball	F F F
Pfeiffer total			577			862		

KLIP, knee ligament injury prevention; LOE, level of evidence; PA, plyometric-agility; PB, proprioceptive-balance; RCT, randomized, controlled trial.

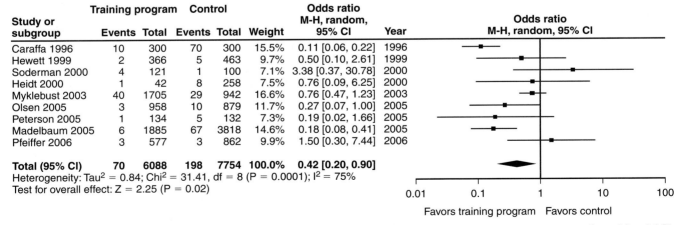

Study or subgroup	Training program Events	Training program Total	Control Events	Control Total	Weight	Odds ratio M-H, random, 95% CI	Year
Caraffa 1996	10	300	70	300	15.5%	0.11 [0.06, 0.22]	1996
Hewett 1999	2	366	5	463	9.7%	0.50 [0.10, 2.61]	1999
Soderman 2000	4	121	1	100	7.1%	3.38 [0.37, 30.78]	2000
Heidt 2000	1	42	8	258	7.5%	0.76 [0.09, 6.25]	2000
Myklebust 2003	40	1705	29	942	16.6%	0.76 [0.47, 1.23]	2003
Olsen 2005	3	958	10	879	11.7%	0.27 [0.07, 1.00]	2005
Peterson 2005	1	134	5	132	7.3%	0.19 [0.02, 1.66]	2005
Madelbaum 2005	6	1885	67	3818	14.6%	0.18 [0.08, 0.41]	2005
Pfeiffer 2006	3	577	3	862	9.9%	1.50 [0.30, 7.44]	2006
Total (95% CI)	**70**	**6088**	**198**	**7754**	**100.0%**	**0.42 [0.20, 0.90]**	

Heterogeneity: $Tau^2 = 0.84$; $Chi^2 = 31.41$, df = 8 (P = 0.0001); $I^2 = 75\%$
Test for overall effect: Z = 2.25 (P = 0.02)

Favors training program   Favors control

FIGURE 92–1. Forest plot showing the effect of anterior cruciate ligament (ACL) prevention programs on the odds of ACL injury. Studies are ordered according to the year of publication, with the number of events (ACL injury) given for each group. *Blue square* and *horizontal line* represent the odds ratio and 95% confidence intervals of the studies. *Diamond* denotes the combined odds ratio with its 95% confidence interval.

methodologically heterogeneous with a significant test for statistical heterogeneity (P = 0.0001). A random-effects model was developed in Review Manager 5[15] using the method of DerSimonian–Laird to calculate an overall pooled estimate of effect (odds ratio [OR], 0.42; 95% confidence interval [CI], 0.20–0.90) to account for between-study variation (heterogeneity). Considerable differences have been found in the type and frequency of training programs used, the study populations at risk, method of diagnosing ACL injury, and study designs. To that end, it is not surprising that the findings of these studies are not all compatible, and the pooled estimate of effect should be viewed with caution. Indeed, future studies should heed the advice of Padua and Marshall,[1] who have pointed out that it is imperative that future studies adopt a standardized method of verifying and reporting the incidence of ACL injury with a clear definition of exposure.

Based on a number-needed-to-treat analysis, Grindstaff and coworkers[16] pooled the results of 5 studies to estimate, for a competitive season, that it would take 89 subjects participating in a neuromuscular control training program to prevent 1 ACL injury (95% CI, 66–139).

Hewett and investigators[17] performed a meta-analysis to estimate the overall effect of injury prevention programs on the odds of ACL injury and reported a protective pooled OR of 0.40 (95% CI, 0.26–0.62). The meta-analysis in this review differs from that of Hewett et al.[17] in its methodology; specifically, Hewett et al.[17] pooled the results of six studies under the fixed-effect assumption of homogeneity. The meta-analysis in the current review includes several additional studies and accounts for the heterogeneity with a more conservative random-effects model.

AREAS OF UNCERTAINTY

The available published evidence regarding preventive training programs is primarily Level II[17] (Fair Evidence), save for Olsen and researchers'[14] Level I trial (Good Evidence). Based on this classification schema of evidence, a B grade of recommendation supports the use of training programs utilizing plyometric-agility or proprioception-balance exercises, or both, to reduce the incidence of ACL injuries. Many of the studies used a multidimensional approach (incorporating injury awareness, proprioception-balance, plyometric-agility); however, the specific aspects of these training programs that result in risk reduction are not entirely transparent, such as the relative contributions and/or interactions between the different components. Other areas of uncertainty include: (1) Is there a dose response to the intervention? In other words, is there a minimum amount necessary to be effective, and/or does more participation in a training program lead to further risk reduction? (2) Is there a temporal relation that is important and is it sport specific (preseason, in season, postseason)? (3) What is the duration of the effect?

TABLE 92–2. Summary of Recommendations

RECOMMENDATION	LEVEL OF EVIDENCE	GRADE OF RECOMMENDATION	REFERENCES
Neuromuscular training programs reduce the incidence of anterior cruciate ligament injury.	8 Level II studies 1 Level I study	B	5–12 13

REFERENCES

1. Padua DA, Marshall SW: Evidence supporting ACL-injury-prevention exercise programs: A review of the literature. Ath Ther Today 11:11–23, 2006.
2. Griffin LY, Albohm MJ, Arendt EA, et al: Understanding and preventing noncontact anterior cruciate ligament injuries: A review. Am J Sports Med 34:1512–1532, 2006.
3. Hurd WJ, Chmielewski TL, Axe MJ, et al: Differences in normal and perturbed walking kinematics between male and female athletes. Clin Biomech 19:465–472, 2004.
4. Griffin L: Prevention of Noncontact ACL Injuries. Rosemont, IL, American Academy of Orthopaedic Surgeons, 2001, p 93.
5. Irmischer BS, Harris C, Pfeiffer RP, et al: Effects of a knee ligament injury prevention exercise program on impact forces in women. J Strength Cond Res 18:703–707, 2004.
6. Caraffa A, Cerulli G, Projetti M, et al: Prevention of anterior cruciate ligament injuries in soccer. A prospective controlled study of proprioceptive training. Knee Surg Sports Traumatol Arthrosc 4:19–21, 1996.
7. Hewett TE, Lindenfeld TN, Riccobene JV, et al: The effect of neuromuscular training on the incidence of knee injury in female athletes. A prospective study. Am J Sports Med 27:699–706, 1999.
8. Heidt RS Jr, Sweeterman LM, Carlonas RL, et al: Avoidance of soccer injuries with preseason conditioning. Am J Sports Med 28:659–662, 2000.
9. Soderman K, Werner S, Pietila T, et al: Balance board training: Prevention of traumatic injuries of the lower extremities in female soccer players? A prospective randomized intervention study. Knee Surg Sports Traumatol Arthrosc 8:356–363, 2000.
10. Myklebust G, Engebretsen L, Braekken IH, et al: Prevention of anterior cruciate ligament injuries in female team handball players: A prospective intervention study over three seasons. Clin J Sport Med 13:71–78, 2003.
11. Mandelbaum BR, Silvers HJ, Watanabe DS, et al: Effectiveness of neuromuscular and proprioceptive training program in preventing anterior cruciate ligament injuries in female athletes: 2-year follow-up. Am J Sports Med 33:1003–1010, 2005.
12. Petersen W, Braun C, Bock W, et al: A controlled prospective case control study of a prevention training program in female

team handball players: The German experience. Arch Orthop Trauma Surg 125:614–621, 2005.

13. Pfeiffer RP, Shea KG, Roberts D, et al: Lack of a knee ligament injury prevention program on the incidence of noncontact anterior cruciate ligament injury. J Bone Joint Surg Am 88:1769–1774, 2006.

14. Olsen OE, Myklebust G, Engebretsen L, et al: Exercises to prevent lower limb injuries in youth sports: Cluster randomized controlled trial. BMJ 330:449, 2005.

15. Review Manager (RevMan) [Computer program]. Version 5.0. Copenhagen, The Nordic Cochrane Centre, The Cochrane Collaboration, 2007.

16. Grindstaff TL, Hammill RR, Tuzson AE, et al: Neuromuscular control training programs and noncontact anterior cruciate ligament injury rates in female athletes: A numbers-needed-to-treat analysis. J Athl Train 41:450–456, 2006.

17. Hewett TE, Ford KR, Myer GD: Anterior cruciate ligament injuries in female athletes: Part 2, a meta-analysis of neuromuscular interventions aimed at injury prevention. Am J Sports Med 34:490–498, 2006.

Chapter 93

Autograft Choice in Anterior Cruciate Ligament Reconstruction: Should It Be Patellar Tendon or Hamstring Tendon?

Daniel Whelan, MD, MSc, FRCS(C), Katie N. Dainty, MSc, CRPC, Denise Chan, BSc, MBT, and Nicholas G. Mohtadi, MSc

The optimal graft choice for reconstruction of the deficient anterior cruciate ligament (ACL) remains controversial. Graft options currently in use include autogenous or autologous patellar tendon, ipsilateral patellar tendon, hamstring tendons (double or quadruple strand), quadriceps tendon (with or without patellar bone), xenografts, and synthetic replacements or augmentations. Autograft tissue currently is the most common source for grafts worldwide, with the main choices being the patellar tendon and hamstring tendons (semitendinosus and gracilis). The advantages and disadvantages of both these popular autografts have been discussed extensively in the literature. Both the quadruple-strand hamstring and bone patellar tendon grafts have demonstrated more than adequate load to failure and single pull strengths with multiple fixation configurations when biomechanically compared with native ACLs.[1-3] Patellar tendon grafts have traditionally been favored for their robust strength, relative ease of operative fixation, and the potential for bone-to-bone ingrowth after implantation. Hamstring tendons are a relatively newer graft choice and have become popular for the relative ease and low morbidity of their harvest.

In the clinical research realm, most early investigations of ACL reconstruction were retrospective case series using a single graft or comparative retrospective cohorts. Such observational data were prone to the limitations of bias and confounding. More recently, however, several randomized trials have been published comparing outcomes.

Because of the dramatic increase in published trials on ACL graft choice in the last 4 years, a systematic review of published randomized, Level I evidence was undertaken. The objective in writing this chapter was to synthesize this evidence, in a narrative fashion, to obtain inference with respect to graft rerupture, postreconstruction laxity, and incidence of complications after ACL reconstruction with either bone–patellar tendon–bone (BPTB) or quadruple-strand hamstring autografts.

A comprehensive search of electronic publication databases (MEDLINE, EMBASE, and the Cochrane Central Register of Controlled Trials) was done to identify relevant studies. Bibliographies from relevant publications found electronically were hand-examined for further potential inclusions. A title review was also done for presentations and posters in the proceedings of three major orthopedic meetings (the American Academy of Orthopaedic Surgery, the International Society of Arthroscopy, Knee Surgery and Orthopaedic Sports Medicine, and the Canadian Orthopaedic Association).

Eighteen studies were identified by the search criteria as prospective, randomized comparisons with patients being allocated to receive one of the two specified autografts. Seven of these were subsequently excluded because group assignment was not specified as being *strictly* by random allocation (birth date/year randomization was accepted, however, because this did not have the potential for manipulation).[4-10] Three investigations were further eliminated because they used two-strand hamstring grafts (versus four).[11-13] One investigation reported outcome data recorded at 12 months (vs. 24 months).[14] Another study utilized a novel hamstring graft preparation (including a bone block) that was not believed to be a standard technique.[15] The remaining six investigations met the full criteria for eligibility and were included in the final analysis.[16-21]

The cumulative sample from the 6 investigations was 483 patients, 235 having received BPTB grafts and 248 having received quadruple-strand hamstring grafts. The studies typically included patients of similar age ranges (14–59 years). None of the studies included skeletally immature patients. The sex distribution favored male individuals. The proportion of acute (<3 months) versus chronic ACL injuries was difficult to determine from the information provided in each study, as was the presence of associated meniscal, chondral, or ligamentous pathology at the time of reconstruction.

TECHNICAL CONSIDERATIONS

The majority of the studies used "aperture fixation" with interference screws for graft fixation on both the femoral and tibial sides of the joint. Metal screws were the preferred fixation for both grafts in the earlier studies, with a trend to bioabsorbable screws for fixation of soft-tissue grafts in more recent investigations. Two studies used extracortical fixation with either plate or endobutton (Smith & Nephew, Andover, Massachusetts, USA) fixation on the femoral side for hamstring grafts.[17,18] Maletis and coworkers[19] used bioabsorbable screws on both the femoral and tibial sides; this is the only study to use identical fixation for both grafts. None of the studies specified the tension at which the grafts were fixed. The flexion angle of the knee at the time of fixation was inconsistently reported and varied from hyperextension to up to 70 degrees of flexion. Rehabilitation protocols were similar, as were follow-up schedules.

JOINT LAXITY

All reconstructions were performed endoscopically through single tibial incisions. Instrumented laxity measurements utilizing the KT-1000 arthrometer were common to all 6 studies; however, the forces at which the knees were tested (89 vs. 134 N vs. maximum manual) and the method of reporting (side-to-side difference vs. proportion of patients with mild/moderate/gross laxity) varied. Despite these differences, no statistically significant differences in terms of instrumented laxity between the 2 grafts were found in any of the individual studies. A trend existed toward increased side-to-side laxity with hamstring tendon grafts in all 6 studies; however, the differences were often small (<3 mm) and of uncertain clinical significance.

CLINICAL OUTCOMES

Strength and range of motion were inconsistently reported among the studies. Although early follow-up (<1 year) often demonstrated strength differences, no consistent trends were noted across the studies for either graft in terms of flexion and extension strength at 2 years after reconstruction. Maletis and coworkers[19] found persistent flexion weakness in the hamstring group and persistent quadriceps weakness in the patellar tendon group, but the deficits were small and of uncertain clinical significance. Similarly, although extension deficits were seen early in the BPTB group in several studies, the groups usually equilibrated at 2-year follow-up. In 2 studies, the extension deficit persisted.[17,20]

Two studies demonstrated a statistically significant proportion of patients in the hamstring group with an abnormal pivot shift examination at final follow-up.[17,19] The severity of the pivot shift (i.e., a "glide" vs. an overt subluxation) was specified in only 1 study, and no patients demonstrated more than a grade 1 (glide).[19] No differences were found between the grafts with respect to the one-leg hop test in the studies that reported this outcome.

FUNCTIONAL OUTCOMES

None of the investigations used a validated measure of health-related quality of life. The majority of the studies reported activity ratings and clinical composite measures that included some index of patient satisfaction. One study included the 36-Item Short Form Health Survey (SF-36), a generic measure of health-related quality of life, as part of the postoperative assessment.[19] A significant increase in physical function occurred between years 1 and 2 after ACL reconstruction in both groups. No differences were demonstrated between the grafts at 2 years.

The Lysholm score is a 100-point scoring system for examining a patient's knee-specific symptoms including mechanical locking, instability, pain, swelling, stair climbing, and squatting.[22] Lysholm scores were used to assess outcome in 5 of the 6 studies. Significant improvement was found from preoperative to postoperative scores in all of these studies. No significant differences were noted in the Lysholm scores between the 2 grafts. Similarly, Tegner scores, a patient-reported measure of activity level, improved from preoperative to postoperative assessments in five studies and did not show a statistical difference between the grafts at final assessment. In 1 study, more patients were able to return to their preoperative activity level with a BPTB graft.[19]

Knee-specific composite scores were frequently used to assess outcomes. These scores combine objective physician-assessed clinical data with subjective functional data obtained from patients. No differences were seen between the grafts in any of the studies utilizing the Cincinnati knee score or the International Knee Documentation Committee (IKDC) scores (both composite and subjective components).

COMPLICATIONS

Anterior knee pain is an important outcome after ACL reconstruction. Anterior knee pain was variably assessed among the group of studies, with some investigators reporting the incidence of anterior knee pain and others providing patient-reported scores or "knee walking/kneeling" ability. In all the investigations, knee pain was significantly greater after patellar tendon grafts were used. The incidence of knee pain before reconstruction was inconsistently reported.

Graft failure, rerupture, or both were poorly defined among the five studies. Twelve failures (5 BPTB, 11 hamstring) were reported before the 2-year final follow-up examination for an overall rate of 3.3%. No difference was reported in the rate of early failure between the two grafts.

Septic joint infections were rare with five reported from the six investigations (1%). Three cases resolved with arthroscopic lavage, administration of intravenous antibiotics, and retention of the original graft. In two cases, a staged revision reconstruction was necessary. No difference was seen in the rate of deep infection for the two grafts. Superficial infections were inconsistently reported, as were the rates of deep venous thrombosis, pretibial numbness, and arthrofibrosis.

VALIDITY/QUALITY ASSESSMENT

Despite the fact that these investigations were all randomized studies, from an epidemiologic perspective, the quality of the trials was variable. All six studies were relatively small. Only two studies specified a primary outcome of interest and performed an a priori sample size calculation accordingly. Loss to follow-up was poorly reported and not accounted for in any of the analyses. Neither post hoc power calculations nor calculation of confidence intervals was used in any of the studies, all of which failed to show major differences between the two grafts.

DISCUSSION

Utilizing only Level I, strictly randomized data, researchers found no major differences between the two grafts with respect to laxity, patient-assessed outcomes, or subjective scores (Table 93–1). The finding of a persistent pivot shift in a greater proportion of patients with hamstring reconstruction in 2 studies is an important observation. Both anterior knee pain and kneeling pain were experienced by more patients after BPTB grafts in all studies. The trials were international, including 4 Scandinavian, 2 American, and 1 Australian trial. The study group was young, active, and predominantly male. This would be consistent with the average patient requesting ACL reconstruction in the North American population.

In summarizing existing evidence, limitations are introduced by the heterogeneity and quality of the individual studies. In terms of heterogeneity, although the individual study designs and sample populations were similar—all were randomized trials conducted in young, active, predominantly male populations—the technical aspects of graft harvest, fixation, and tensioning were variable and may have introduced potentially important differences in graft survival and function at 2 years. Variations in epidemiologic quality among the individual trials might have led to overestimation or underestimation of treatment effects. Publication bias might have played a role in the original literature search because only 1 foreign language study was identified.[8]

Although this review has provided some insight into autograft selection, many unanswered questions remain regarding ACL reconstruction. There is a complete lack of data in the literature to guide decision making as to the optimal timing of ACL reconstruction. No Level I investigations compare acute ACL reconstruction (performed within 3 months of injury) with chronic reconstructions. Furthermore,

in the Level I investigations that were included in this review, no attempts were made to stratify randomization based on prognostic indicators such as concomitant cartilage, ligament or meniscal injury, the presence of ligamentous hypermobility, or body mass index. Such stratification could provide important prognostic information regarding these factors and guide future research initiatives.

Several previous reviews have been previously published comparing these 2 grafts with inconsistent findings. A "review of reviews" was undertaken by Poolman and coworkers[23] to investigate the reasons for the discordant findings. Eleven such reviews were identified in that investigation, with 3 favoring the patellar tendon graft for stability and 6 favoring the hamstring graft to prevent anterior knee pain. The quality of the individual reviews was highly variable and believed to be the most significant reason for the differences in their findings.

Limitations are imposed on this analysis because of inconsistent reporting of the outcome measures across the investigations and the lack of validated, patient-based measures of function. Although we suspect from these data that neither graft has a propensity for *failure* outright, a definitive conclusion on superiority awaits functional data at longer-term follow-up. The finding of a trend toward increased incidence of anterior knee pain with patellar tendon grafts should be interpreted in light of the fact that few studies record whether this pain preceded the reconstruction. Furthermore, the association of the increase in laxity (as assessed by the pivot shift examination) seen with hamstring grafts and patient function or sport participation is unknown.

The breadth of research on ACL reconstruction is expanding and evolving. The literature is plentiful, but its impact is weakened by underpowered investigations. A place exists for a large, multicenter trial to definitively explore this question with long-term functional outcomes; however, further small investigations are unnecessary and, we would suggest, an inefficient use of time and resource.

This brief narrative review is intended to provide the surgeon with up-to-date data, which can be used to appropriately educate his or her patients in the consent process before ACL reconstruction. Furthermore, this work represents the beginnings of a more extensive analysis that will appear in the Cochrane database. A wealth of data can be derived from this sample of Level I randomized trials on ACL reconstruction. Further inference may be possible with the raw data from each study and/or a formal meta-analysis as per the Cochrane database methodology. The Cochrane review will attempt to provide overall estimates of treatment effect via statistical pooling of study data. Definitive information, however, can come only from a large randomized trial with long-term functional data as a primary end point. Table 93–2 provides a summary of recommendations.

TABLE 93–1. Level of Evidence

STUDY	SIZE (N)	LOE	CHARACTERISTICS/RESULTS/CONCLUSIONS
Ejerhed et al. (2003)[16]	71 (34 PT, 37 HS)	I	*Study characteristics:* 24-month minimum follow-up 2 lost to follow-up (1 PT, 1 HS) 3 early failures (1 PT, 2 HS) *Results:* More patients could "knee walk" in HS group Equivalent Lysholm, Tegner, laxity, IKDC scores *Conclusions:* No significant difference for laxity Anterior knee pain greater in PT group
Feller and Webster (2003)[17]	65 (31 PT, 34 HS)	I	*Study characteristics:* 36-month minimum follow-up 6 lost to follow-up (4 PT, 2 HS) 1 early failure (PT) *Results:* More kneeling pain in PT group Extension deficits in PT group KT values greater in HS group More patients with pivot in HS group Equivalent Cincinnati score, IKDC score, return to activity *Conclusions:* Both grafts give satisfactory function Increased morbidity in PT group Increased laxity in HS group Increased femoral tunnel width in HS group
Jansson et al. (2003)[18]	PRCT: 99 (51 PT, 48 HS)	I	*Study characteristics:* 21-month minimum follow-up 16 lost to follow-up (13 PT, 3 HS) 4 early failures (4 HS) Extracortical femoral fixation in HS group *Results:* Equivalent KT 1000 Arthrometer (Medmetric Corp, San Diego, California, USA) IKDC, Lysholm, Tegner scores Equivalent Kujala patellofemoral score *Conclusions:* Both techniques improve performance Equal results for both groups
Laxdal et al. (2005)[21]	134* (40 PT, 39 HS)	I	*Study characteristics:* Average 26 months of follow-up 9 lost to follow-up (total only) 5 early failures (1 PT, 4 HS) Third randomized group: two-strand HS *Results:* Knee walking worse in PT group *Conclusions:* Less discomfort with knee walking in HS group No differences for laxity and function
Maletis et al. (2007)[19]	99 (46 PT, 53 HS)	I	*Study characteristics:* Average 24 months of follow-up 2 lost to follow-up (2 HS) 1 early failure (HT) Identical fixation for both grafts *Results:* Equivalent Lysholm, IKDC, Tegner scores Fewer with jumping difficulty in PT group More return to preinjury Tegner score in PT group Stronger extension in HS group Fewer with kneeling difficulty in HS group *Conclusions:* Good outcomes with both grafts Subtle differences may help guide graft choice
Shaieb et al. (2002)[20]	82 (41 PT, 41 HS)	I	*Study characteristics:* Average 33 months of follow-up 12 lost to follow-up 4 early failures (2 HS, 2 PT) Similar fixation for both grafts *Results:* Equivalent Lysholm score, KT, return to activity More knee pain and stiffness in PT group *Conclusions:* Both grafts gave good outcomes Both grafts performed similarly Fewer in HS group had pain and stiffness

*Three groups randomized, two hamstring groups (two and four strands). Only four-strand results considered.
HS, hamstring; IKDC, International Knee Documentation Committee; LOE, level of evidence; PRCT, prospective, randomized, control trial; PT, patellar tendon.

TABLE 93–2. Summary of Recommendations

STATEMENT	LEVEL OF EVIDENCE	GRADE OF RECOMMENDATION
1. Anterior cruciate ligament reconstruction with either bone–patellar tendon–bone or quadruple-strand hamstring tendon autograft provides restoration of knee stability, alleviation of knee-specific symptoms, and improvement in generic health-related quality of life versus preoperative assessment.	I	A
2. No statistically significant differences were found between bone–patellar tendon–bone autografts and quadruple-strand hamstring tendon autografts with respect to knee laxity and functional outcome at up to 2 years after surgery.	I	A
3. An increased incidence on anterior knee pain and kneeling pain after anterior cruciate ligament reconstruction with bone–patellar tendon–bone autograft versus hamstring tendon autograft was reported at up to 2 years after surgery.	I	A
4. In patients for whom kneeling is an occupational requirement or for whom the ability to kneel without pain is a significant part of cultural, religious, or sports participation, a quadruple-strand hamstring autograft has advantages over bone–patellar tendon–bone autograft for reconstruction of the anterior cruciate ligament.	I	A

REFERENCES

1. Noyes FR, Butler DL, Grood ES, et al: Biomechanical analysis of human ligament grafts used in knee-ligament repairs and reconstructions. J Bone Joint Surg Am 66A:344–352, 1984.
2. Woo SL, Kanamori A, Zeminski J, et al: The effectiveness of reconstruction of the anterior cruciate ligament with hamstrings and patellar tendon. A cadaveric study comparing anterior tibial and rotational loads. J Bone Joint Surg Am 84-A:907–914, 2002.
3. Woo SL, Chan SS, Yamaji T: Biomechanics of knee ligament healing, repair and reconstruction. J Biomech 30:431–439, 1997.
4. Aglietti P, Giron F, Buzzi R, et al: Anterior cruciate ligament reconstruction: Bone-patellar tendon-bone compared with double semitendinosus and gracilis tendon grafts. A prospective, randomized clinical trial. J Bone Joint Surg Am 86-A:2143–2155, 2004.
5. Aglietti P, Buzzi R, De Biase P, Zacherotti G: A comparison between patellar tendon and doubled semitendonosis/gracilis for ACL reconstruction: A minimum 5 year follow up. J Sports Traumatol Rel Res 19:57–68, 1997.
6. Aune AK, Holm I, Risberg MA, et al: Four-strand hamstring tendon autograft compared with patellar tendon-bone autograft for anterior cruciate ligament reconstruction—a randomized study with two-year follow-up. Am J Sports Med 29:722–728, 2001.
7. Eriksson K, Anderberg P, Hamberg P, et al: A comparison of quadruple semitendinosus and patellar tendon grafts in reconstruction of the anterior cruciate ligament. J Bone Joint Surg Br 83-B:348–354, 2001.
8. Ropke M, Becker R, Urbach D, Nebelung W: Semitendinosus tendon vs patellar ligament—clinical results after reconstruction of the ACL. Unfallchirurg 104:312–316, 2001.
9. Sajovic M, Vengust V, Komadina R, et al: A prospective, randomized comparison of semitendinosus and gracilis tendon versus patellar tendon autografts for ACL reconstruction. Am J Sports Med 34:1933–1940, 2006.
10. Zaffagnini S, Maracci M, Lo Presti M, et al: Prospective and randomized evaluation of ACL reconstruction with three techniques: A clinical and radiographic evaluation at five years follow up. Knee Surg Sports Traumatol 14:1060–1069, 2006.
11. Anderson AF, Snyder RB, Lipscomb AB: Anterior cruciate ligament reconstruction—a prospective randomized study of three surgical methods. Am J Sports Med 29:272–279, 2001.
12. Beynnon B, Johnson RJ, Fleming BC, et al: Anterior cruciate ligament replacement: Comparison of bone-patellar tendon-bone grafts with two-strand hamstring grafts. A prospective, randomized study. J Bone Joint Surg Am 84-A:1503–1513, 2002.
13. O'Neill DB: Arthroscopically assisted reconstruction of the anterior cruciate ligament: A prospective randomized analysis of three techniques. J Bone Joint Surg Am 78:803–813, 1996.
14. Beard DJ, Anderson JL, Davies S, et al: Hamstrings versus patellar tendon for ACL reconstruction: A randomized controlled trial. Knee 8:45–50, 2001.
15. Matsumoto A, Yoshiya S, Muratsu M, et al: A comparison of bone patellar tendon bone and bone hamstring bone autografts for ACL reconstruction. Am J Sports Med 34:213–219, 2006.
16. Ejerhed L, Kartus J, Sernert N, et al: Patellar tendon or semitendinosus tendon autografts for anterior cruciate ligament reconstruction? A prospective randomized study with a two-year follow-up. Am J Sports Med 31:19–25, 2003.
17. Feller JA, Webster KE: A randomized comparison of patellar tendon and hamstring tendon anterior cruciate ligament reconstruction. Am J Sports Med 31:564–573, 2003.
18. Jansson KA, Linko E, Sandelin J, Harilainen A: A Prospective randomized study of patellar versus hamstring tendon autografts for anterior cruciate ligament reconstruction. Am J Sports Med 31:12–18, 2003.
19. Maletis GB, Cameron SL, Tengan JJ, et al: A prospective randomized study of anterior cruciate ligament reconstruction. A comparison of patellar tendon and quadruple strand semitendonosis/gracilis tendons fixed with bioabsorbable interference screws. Am J Sports Med 35:385–394, 2007.
20. Shaieb MD, Kan DM, Chang S, et al: A prospective randomized comparison of patellar tendon versus semitendinosus and gracilis tendon autografts for anterior cruciate ligament reconstruction. Am J Sports Med 30:214–220, 2002.
21. Laxdal G, Kartus J, Hansson L, et al: A prospective randomized comparison of bone patellar tendon bone and hamstring grafts for ACL reconstruction. Arthroscopy 21:34–42, 2005.
22. Lysholm J, Gilquist J: Evaluation of knee ligament surgery results with special emphasis on the use of a scoring scale. Am J Sports Med 10:150–153, 1982.
23. Poolman RW, Aboulai JAK, Conter HJ, Bhandari M: Overlapping systematic reviews of ACL reconstruction comparing hamstring autograft with bone patellar tendon bone autograft: Why are they different? J Bone Joint Surg Am 89:1542–1552, 2007.

Is There a Role for Arthroscopy in the Treatment of Knee Osteoarthritis?

CHRISTOPHER C. DODSON, MD AND ROBERT G. MARX, MD, MSc, FRCSC

Arthroscopy was first described to treat osteoarthritis (OA) of the knee by Burman and coauthors[1] in 1934. Over the past several decades, arthroscopic debridement of the degenerative knee has become a commonly performed orthopedic procedure. Despite its popularity, the exact role of arthroscopy in treating OA is controversial. Older, primarily uncontrolled cohort studies have suggested that arthroscopy has a variety of benefits in patients with early OA.[2–6] However, a more recent study has suggested that the placebo effect may be responsible for the benefit related to arthroscopic treatment.[7] The variety of arthroscopic procedures, the retrospective nature of the majority of published studies, and the lack of control subjects probably adds even more confusion as to which patients will benefit from arthroscopy.[8]

Additional prospective, randomized, controlled studies are needed to try and define the role of arthroscopic debridement in the treatment of OA of the knee. This is essential because it would allow for a greater efficiency in the management of these patients; those who would benefit from surgery can be indicated, whereas those who would not can be spared the unnecessary expense and operative risk of a surgical procedure. In the meantime, it is important to analyze the current literature in an effort to determine which patients are most likely to benefit from arthroscopy. The goal of this chapter is to summarize the current literature in an effort to determine whether there is, in fact, a role for arthroscopy in the treatment of OA.

OPTIONS

Numerous treatment options are available for the patient with OA of the knee. Generally speaking, nonoperative treatments are indicated initially, followed by surgical options if the former are not effective. The degree of OA in the involved knee also plays a role in the decision-making process.

Nonoperative management begins with activity modification, physical therapy, and a trial of anti-inflammatory medications. Many patients will often experience significant relief after intra-articular corticosteroid injections and hyaluronate injections. It is important to note that the degree of pain relief, as well as how long it lasts, can be varied.[9]

Surgical management includes arthroscopic debridement and lavage, osteotomies to correct deformities, unicompartmental arthroplasty, and total knee arthroplasty. Osteotomy is indicated in younger patients with deformity and degenerative changes on one side of the knee. Unicompartmental arthroplasty is reserved for patients who have degenerative changes in primarily 1 compartment, good motion, knee stability, and no significant deformity. Finally, total knee arthroplasty is indicated in older patients with significant degenerative changes and multicompartment involvement of the knee. The role of arthroscopy in the osteoarthritic knee is not clear.

EVIDENCE

Several studies have been conducted in an effort to examine the effectiveness of arthroscopy in treating OA of the knee (Table 94–1). However, after conducting an evidence-based review of the current literature, we found only 1 study that contained Level I evidence. This study, by Moseley and colleagues,[7] was a prospective, randomized, placebo-controlled trial of 180 patients with OA who were assigned to receive arthroscopic debridement, arthroscopic lavage, or placebo surgery. Their inclusion criteria included: (1) age < 75 years, (2) OA as defined by the American College of Rheumatology, (3) knee pain despite at least 6 months of conservative management, and (4) no arthroscopy performed on the knee in the previous 2 years. The severity of OA was assessed radiographically and graded from 1 to 4. The scores from all 3 compartments were added for a total of 0 to 12. Of note, patients were excluded for severe deformity, for a score of more than 9 on the scale, or if there was a medical contraindication. Patients and assessors of outcome were blinded to the treatment group assignment, and outcomes were assessed at multiple points over a 24-month period with the use of 5 self-reported scores. The authors conclude that the outcomes after arthroscopic lavage or arthroscopic debridement were no better than those after a placebo procedure.

TABLE 94–1. Recent studies with their respective levels of evidence regarding the treatment of knee osteoarthritis with arthroscopy

STUDY	DESIGN	CASES *(N)*	LEVEL OF EVIDENCE	POSITIVE RESULTS
Moseley et al.[7]	Prospective, randomized, placebo controlled	180	I	No difference between arthroscopic group and placebo group
Dervin et al.[8]	Retrospective case series	126	IV	44%
Jackson and Rouse[12]	Retrospective case series	68	IV	95%
Chang et al.[13]	Prospective comparative	32	II	44%
Aaron et al.[14]	Cross-sectional cohort	122	II	65%
Jackson and Dieterichs[16]	Retrospective case series	121	IV	84%
Matsusue and Thomson[17]	Retrospective case series	68	IV	84%
McGinley et al.[18]	Retrospective case series	77	IV	67%

Several details about this study require a more in-depth evaluation because they are certainly relevant to the authors' conclusion that surgical intervention provided no benefit compared with placebo surgery. Forty-four percent of the eligible participants declined to participate in the study, which creates a selection bias; that is, it is possible that the patients who declined to participate had lower grades of OA and, therefore, might have experienced the best outcome.[10] In addition, the presence or absence of joint effusion was not reported. This is significant because some of the indications for knee arthroscopy, such as loose bodies or meniscal tears, can be manifested clinically by a joint effusion. Finally, the method of grading OA may lead to conflicting results. For example, a patient with one severely arthritic compartment may receive the same score as a patient with mild arthritis in all three compartments. These patients are probably not comparable clinically and would most likely have different outcomes after surgical intervention. Despite these criticisms, this investigation is still the only Level I study that addresses the role of arthroscopy in OA; therefore, the authors' conclusion should be acknowledged and taken into account when treating these patients.

Patients with symptomatic OA of the knee have a reported incidence rate of meniscal tears in up to 91% of magnetic resonance imaging (MRI) scans.[11] Some surgeons have proposed that patients who have pain secondary to clinically significant meniscal tears will benefit from arthroscopic mensical debridement. Dervin and investigators,[8] in a Level IV study, attempted to elicit preoperative factors that would predict a successful outcome after arthroscopy for OA of the knee. They conclude that three variables were significantly associated with clinical improvement: the presence of medial joint line tenderness, a positive Steinman test, and the presence of an unstable meniscal tear at arthroscopy. Jackson and Rouse,[12] in a Level IV study, reported 95% good to excellent results obtained with arthroscopic partial meniscectomy for clinically significant meniscal tears in the setting of substantial OA. Although Chang and colleagues[13] (Level II) conclude that patients with OA did not experience consistent relief after arthroscopy, they do point out that the subset of patients with anterior two-thirds medial mensical tears and any lateral meniscal tears did improve sig-

nificantly. It can be difficult to determine which meniscal tears are clinically significant; many authors will use the term *mechanical symptoms,* which includes locking and catching, and generally refers to unstable mensical tears. Some authors have attempted to determine whether mechanical symptoms are a prognostic factor associated with a positive outcome after arthroscopic debridement. The results have been mixed. Chang and colleagues[13] conclude that patients with mechanical symptoms tended to benefit, whereas Aaron and coworkers[14] (Level II) and Livesley and coauthors[15] found that the type of symptoms did not predict outcome. The term *mechanical symptoms* has a different meaning for different clinicians. Mechanical locking, which is when the knee becomes suddenly stuck in one position requiring manipulation that allows the knee to suddenly unlock, generally indicates the presence of a loose body or an unstable flap of meniscus or articular cartilage. Arthroscopy reliably eliminates this phenomenon even in the presence of arthritis. However, arthritis symptoms may not be relieved by the procedure. Lastly, the term *mechanical symptoms* is not specific to this type of locking.

Several authors have proposed that patients with low-grade OA can have substantial and long-lasting improvement after knee arthroscopy, whereas patients with high-grade OA fare less well. For example, Jackson and Dieterichs,[16] in a Level IV study, note 91% excellent results at 4 to 6 years after debridement for knees in which degenerative change was limited to fibrillation, which they rate as stage 2. When the disease progressed to fragmentation of the cartilage (stage 3), results deteriorated to 77% fair or good. Aaron and coworkers[14] and Livesley and coauthors[15] note similar trends: Patients with low grades of OA had acceptable pain relief that lasted up to 3 years, while patients with higher grades of OA had significantly worse results. Aaron and coworkers[14] also note that patients who had a joint space of 3 mm or larger on radiographs improved after arthroscopic debridement, whereas those with a joint space less than 2 mm rarely had a substantial relief of symptoms. It is fair to say that joint space directly correlates with the varying stages of OA; therefore, this finding supports the notion that patients with mild OA or larger joint spaces have better outcomes than those with higher grades of OA or smaller joint spaces. Matsusue and

Thomson[17] (Level IV) stratified their results of meniscal tear debridement based on coexisting degenerative changes within the involved compartment. They found that patients with early degenerative changes, classified as grade I or II, had 87% excellent results, whereas only 7% of the patients with grade III or IV changes experienced an excellent result. Finally, McGinley and coworkers[18] (Level IV) note that greater than 80% grade 4 changes within a single compartment was a risk factor for total knee arthroplasty within 2 years. Although it is difficult to compare and contrast these different studies, because many of the investigators used a different system for grading the severity of OA, there certainly seems to be a trend toward patients with early OA having better outcomes than those with advanced OA.

In a Level V article, Stuart and Lubowitz[19] propose that loose bodies within the knee joint is another prognostic factor associated with a positive result after arthroscopy in patients with OA. However, we have been unable to find data to support this statement. Aaron and coworkers[14] were unable to find an association between having loose bodies and a good result after arthroscopy, although only 9 of 122 patients in their study were identified as such.

Patients with fixed varus or valgus deformity, particularly valgus deformity, have consistently demonstrated poor results after arthroscopic debridement.[14,20] Likewise, patients with bilateral disease are considered poor candidates and were reported to undergo total knee arthroplasty at a greater rate (64%) when compared with a similar group of patients with unilateral disease (33%).[18]

GUIDELINES

The orthopedic surgeon has many tools to treat OA of the knee, one of which is arthroscopy. It is understandable why arthroscopic debridement is so commonly performed; it is relatively safe, is an outpatient procedure, and does not preclude later definitive surgery. Unfortunately, a consensus on the role of arthroscopy in the treatment of OA still has not been established. Some patients may benefit from arthroscopy, but the challenge remains identifying which patients are likely to benefit and which ones will not.

It is important for the clinician to keep in mind that OA of the knee is not a single entity but encompasses a spectrum of pathology. It is important for future investigations to stratify the severity of OA based on functional disability and radiographs. In addition, the specifics of physical examination and clinical symptoms should also be carefully documented. These factors are instrumental in developing guidelines to determine the type of surgical candidates who will experience predictable relief after arthroscopy.

Future studies, preferably with Level I or II evidence, will need to be conducted in an effort to determine indications, or lack thereof, for arthroscopic debridement of the osteoarthritic knee. These studies should be prospective, randomized, and have a high percentage of patient follow-up. In addition, the results should be categorized by history, physical examination, presence of loose bodies, presence of meniscal tears, and degree of OA present both radiographically and by intraoperative visualization. This will help in identifying subgroups that are amenable to arthroscopic debridement and those that are not.

RECOMMENDATIONS

Currently, insufficient evidence-based data are available to definitively recommend specific indications for the use of arthroscopy in the treatment of OA. Many of the prospective randomized studies in the literature lack stratification of arthritis severity, have poor enrollment, and have a small sample size. Other studies are retrospective in nature, lack randomization or a control group, have a selection bias, and lack a quantifiable outcome measure between groups. However, despite these limitations, we do believe that there is a role for arthroscopy in select patients with knee OA.

The senior author's (R.G.M.) current indications for arthroscopic surgery for patients with OA of the knee includes either patients who have clear mechanical locking as described earlier, or patients who have not responded successfully to conservative management, including at least non-steroidal anti-inflammatory drugs or acetaminophen as appropriate, chondroitin, and glucosamine, as well as physical therapy, and who also have mechanical symptoms (i.e., locking), meniscal tears confirmed by MRI that are believed to be symptomatic based on patient history and physical examination, mild arthritis as defined by a joint space of 3 mm or larger, and persistent pain with a mild deformity (i.e., varus < 10 degrees). We believe that arthroscopic debridement should generally not be performed in patients who have severe arthritis as defined by a joint space of less than 2 mm, fixed limb malalignment (>10 degrees), particularly valgus knees, and bilateral disease. Although we do not believe that the natural history of the arthritis can be significantly altered by arthroscopy, associated conditions such as new onset of pain from a meniscal tear or locking caused by a loose body can often be treated by arthroscopy in an arthritic knee with good results. Patients should be counseled that the degree of arthritis is probably best assessed intraoperatively, and that their clinical outcome will often depend on the severity of cartilage lesions that are seen during the arthroscopy procedure. As a result, it may not be possible to truly estimate the likelihood of success until after the operation.

Lastly, we counsel patients that arthritis symptoms tend to worsen over the long term, and that this is what they can expect over years in the future after arthroscopy in this setting. Table 94–2 provides a summary of recommendations.

TABLE 94–2. Grades of Recommendation for Summaries or Reviews of Orthopedic Surgical Studies

STATEMENTS	LEVEL OF EVIDENCE/GRADE OF RECOMMENDATION
1. Knee arthroscopy for symptomatic meniscal tears in the setting of osteoarthritis	C
2. Arthroscopic debridement for knee pain in the setting of osteoarthritis	I
3. Knee arthroscopy for loose body removal in the setting of osteoarthritis	C

REFERENCES

1. Burman MS, Finkelstein H, Mayer L: Arthroscopy of the knee joint. J Bone Joint Surg Am 16A:255–268, 1934.
2. Baumgaertner MR, Cannon WD Jr, Vittori JM, et al: Arthroscopic debridement of the arthritic knee. Clin Orthop Relat Res 253:197–202, 1990.
3. McLaren AC, Blokker CP, Fowler PJ: Arthroscopic debridement of the knee for osteoarthrosis. Can J Surg 34:595–598, 1991.
4. Ogilvie-Harris DJ, Fitsialos DP: Arthroscopic management of the degenerative knee. Arthroscopy 7:151–157, 1991.
5. Rand JA: Arthroscopic management of degenerative meniscus tears in patients with degenerative arthritis. Arthroscopy 1:253–258, 1985.
6. Yang SS, Nisonson B: Arthroscopic surgery of the knee in the geriatric patient. Clin Orthop Relat Res (316):50–58, 1995.
7. Moseley JB, O'Malley K, Petersen NJ, et al: A controlled trial of arthroscopic surgery for osteoarthritis of the knee. N Engl J Med 347:81–88, 2002.
8. Dervin GF, Stiell IG, Rody K, et al: Effect of arthroscopic debridement for osteoarthritis of the knee on health-related quality of life. J Bone Joint Surg Am 85:10–19, 2003.
9. Leopold SS, Redd BB, Warme WJ, et al: Corticosteroid compared with hyaluronic acid injections for the treatment of osteoarthritis of the knee. A prospective, randomized trial. J Bone Joint Surg Am 85A:1197–1203, 2003.
10. Siparsky P, Ryzewicz M, Peterson B, et al: Arthroscopic treatment of osteoarthritis of the knee. Clin Orthop Relat Res (455):107–112, 2007.
11. Bhattacharyya T, Gale D, Dewire P, et al: The clinical importance of meniscal tears demonstrated by magnetic resonance imaging in osteoarthritis of the knee. J Bone Joint Surg Am 85:4–9, 2003.
12. Jackson RW, Rouse DW: The results of partial meniscectomy in patients over 40 years of age. J Bone Joint Surg Br 64:481–485, 1982.
13. Chang RW, Falconer J, Stulberg SD, et al: A randomized controlled trial of arthroscopic surgery versus closed-needle joint lavage for patients with osteoarthritis of the knee. Arthritis Rheum 36:289–296, 1993.
14. Aaron RK, Skolnick AH, Reinert SE, et al: Arthroscopic debridement for osteoarthritis of the knee. J Bone Joint Surg Am 88:936–943, 2006.
15. Livesley PJ, Doherty M, Needoff M, et al: Arthroscopic lavage of osteoarthritic knees. J Bone Joint Surg Br 73:922–926, 1991.
16. Jackson RW, Dieterichs C: The results of arthroscopic lavage and debridement of osteoarthritic knees based on the severity of degeneration: A 4-to-6 year symptomatic follow-up. Arthroscopy 19:13–20, 2003.
17. Matsusue Y, Thomson NL: Arthroscopic partial medial meniscectomy in patients over 40 years old: A 5 to 11 year follow-up study. Arthroscopy 12:39–44, 1996.
18. McGinley BJ, Cushner FD, Scott WN: Debridement arthroscopy: 10-year follow-up. Clin Orthop Relat Res 367:190–194, 1999.
19. Stuart MJ, Lubowitz JH: What, if any, are the indications for arthroscopic debridement of the osteoarthritic knee? Arthroscopy 22:238–239, 2006.
20. Harwin SF: Arthroscopic debridement for osteoarthritis of the knee: Predictors of patient satisfaction. Arthroscopy 15:142–146, 1999.

Chapter 95

What Are Effective Therapies for Anterior Knee Pain?

Jenny McConnell, B App Sci (Phty), Grad Dip, Man Ther, M Biomed Eng

Anterior knee pain or patellofemoral (PF) pain is one of the commonest conditions presenting to clinicians involved in the management of sports injuries.[1,2] Prospective cohort studies report incidence rates of 7% to 15% in sporting and general populations.[3–6]

Currently, the cause of patellofemoral pain (PFP) is not known, but patients present with stereotypical symptoms, namely, anterior knee pain aggravated by flexed knee activities, both loaded, such as climbing stairs and squatting, and unloaded, such as sitting with the knee flexed ("moviegoer's" knee).

SOURCES OF PAIN

Much speculation had been made about the source of PFP, but evidence is mounting that the richly innervated infrapatellar fat pad could be a significant player.[7,8] A recent study by Bennell and colleagues,[9] in which the fat pad of asymptomatic individuals was injected with hypotonic saline, confirmed the finding that the fat pad can be a potent source of knee pain symptoms that are not just confined to the infrapatellar region but can refer to the proximal thigh as far as the groin. In addition, the lateral retinaculum seems to be responsible for some PF symptoms because numerous studies demonstrate nerve damage in the lateral retinaculum of patients with PFP, including nerve fibrosis, neuroma formation, and increased number of myelinated and unmyelinated nerve fibers with a predominant nociceptive component.[10–12]

Factors Predisposing to Patellofemoral Pain

Several factors predisposing an individual to PFP have been identified, ranging from overuse and training errors to faulty biomechanics. Structural causes of PFP are divided into intrinsic and extrinsic causes. Intrinsic structural factors are uncommon and relate to dysplasia of the patella or femoral trochlea and the position of the patella relative to the trochlea. Extrinsic structural faults are reported to cause a lateral tracking of the patella.[1,13,14] The extrinsic factors include increased Q angle, hamstrings and gastrocnemius muscle tightness, abnormal foot pronation, and quadriceps muscle dysplasia.

The Q angle, representing the line of pull of the rectus femoris muscle, has long been the benchmark of orthopedic surgeons to indicate PF function. Its value is widely debated in the literature, with many authors questioning the diagnostic relevance of the static Q angle, suggesting the dynamic Q angle has greater relevance.[1,15,16] The dynamic Q angle is affected by the position of the hip from above and the foot below during weight-bearing activities. The alignment of the hip and the foot is particularly critical at 30 degrees of knee flexion when the patella should be engaging in the trochlea. Many individuals with PFP have "squinting" patellae and an associated internal rotation of the femur, which has been hypothesized to cause tightness in the tensor fascia latae muscle and weakness of the gluteus medius muscle. Evidence in the literature of poor hip and pelvic control is limited, although there is some support that the hip abductor and rotator strength is decreased in individuals with PFP sufferers.[17–19] However, others claim that hip abductor and external rotator strength is no different in PFP subjects and healthy control subjects.[20] In addition, soft-tissue flexibility of various structures in the lower limb such as iliotibial band, hamstrings, gastrocnemius, and anterior hip structures has been suggested as being a factor in PFP syndrome, but the findings are quite disparate.

Abnormal foot biomechanics such as excessive, prolonged, or late pronation, which alters tibial and even entire lower limb rotation at varying times through range, has been proposed to adversely affect PF joint mechanics.[15,21,22] Intrinsic and extrinsic causes of abnormal foot position exist. The intrinsic causes relate to static foot postures such as forefoot and rearfoot varus and valgus. The extrinsic causes relate to the foot being lateral to the weight-bearing line, such as genu valgus and internal rotation of the femur, or the weight being borne on the lateral aspect of the foot, such as tibial varum. However, one research group has conflicting conclusions about the influence of foot pronation in subjects with PFP, suggesting that statically increased rearfoot varus may be a contributing factor in PFP,[23] whereas dynamically, individuals with PFP do not demonstrate excessive foot pronation or tibial internal rotation compared with asymptomatic individuals.[24]

The most common cause of PFP cited in the literature is quadriceps muscle weakness particularly of the vastus medialis oblique (VMO). Ideally, the synergistic relation between the VMO and vastus lateralis (VL) should maintain the alignment of the patella in the femoral trochlea, especially in the first 30 degrees of knee flexion, before the patella is fully engaged in the trochlea. It has been proposed that this balanced activation of the VMO and VL is disrupted in patients with PFPS. The issue of whether the disruption is in part a motor control dysfunction has been investigated by Mellor and Hodges,[25] who found that synchronization of motor unit action potentials is reduced in subjects with PFP (38%) compared with control subjects (90%). However, the evidence to support an imbalance in the activation of the vasti (either decreased activation of VMO or enhanced activation of VL) is contentious.[26–29] Differences in methodology (particularly with respect to the use of electromyography [EMG]) and the inherent heterogeneity in the PFPS population may account for some of the inconsistencies in study results.

Although there is inconclusive evidence to support or refute an imbalance in the magnitude of vasti activation in patients with PFPS, disrupted activation of the vasti may take the form of delayed activation of the VMO relative to the VL. It has been hypothesized that the VMO, which has a smaller cross-sectional area than the VL, must receive a feed-forward enhancement of its excitation level to track the patellar optimally.[30,31] Many studies that have examined individuals with PFPS have supported this hypothesis, by demonstrating that the EMG activity and reflex onset time of the VMO relative to the VL is delayed, when compared with asymptomatic individuals.[32–34] However, the issue remains controversial in the literature, with some studies demonstrating no differences in EMG onsets,[27,28,35,36] but a more recent study by Cowan and colleagues[34] found that although the majority of subject with PFP have a delayed onset of VMO relative to VL on a stair-stepping task (67% concentrically, 79% eccentrically), there were still some subjects whose VMO preceded VL activation. In addition, these investigators found that some of the control subjects (no history of PFP) exhibited a delayed onset of the VMO relative to the VL (46% concentrically and 52% eccentrically) on the stair-stepping task. Cowan and colleagues'[34] study may clarify some of the discrepancies found in the literature with regards to timing. The stratification of the groups occurs only when there are sufficient subject numbers to tease out the difference. Some of the earlier studies may not have a statistical significance because the power calculations had not been done and there were too few subjects.

Individuals with PFP not only demonstrate a delay in the onset of VMO relative to the VL but also relative to the prime mover (tibialis anterior and soleus, respectively) after postural perturbation where subjects were required to rock back on their heels or go up on their toes in response to a light stimulus.[37] In control subjects, the VMO preceded the prime mover and was activated with the VL.[37] This feed-forward strategy used by the central nervous system to control the patella can be restored by physical therapy rehabilitation strategies directed at altering muscle recruitment in functional movements.[38]

TREATMENT

PFP is not a self-limiting condition, so it is important to identify strategies that will alleviate the symptoms of this often chronic condition. The majority of patients with PFP respond to nonoperative (physical therapy) management, which aims to not only improve patellar tracking through active (quadriceps or VMO retraining) and passive (realignment procedures such as tape, brace, stretching) interventions but also improve lower-limb mechanics both proximally by pelvic muscle training and distally by enhancing foot function with orthotics or muscle training. Initially, the clinician needs to be able to significantly reduce the patient's symptoms. This is often achieved by taping or bracing the patella. One group of investigators suggests that bracing may even prevent the development of PFP in athletic individuals.[39]

Patellar taping should unload painful structures to enable the patient to be pain-free while doing activities. Theoretically, using tape could also provide a sustained stretch of the tight lateral structures, making use of the creep phenomenon, which occurs when a constant low load is applied to viscoelastic material such as the lateral retinacular tissues. Length of soft tissues can be increased with sustained stretching, and the magnitude of increased displacement is dependent on the duration of the applied stretch,[40] although there have been no studies to show changes in retinacular tissue length after taping.

Short-term pain reduction does occur with patellar taping and bracing[41–45] (Level of Evidence I), and research continues to focus on mechanisms to explain this pain relief. Two randomized, clinical trials did not find any benefits of using a medial glide tape while doing physical therapy in addition to physical therapy intervention.[46,47] The problem with both these studies is that the beneficial effect of tape was not established, and the tape was applied only for the physical therapy session, not while the individuals were doing other potentially painful weight-bearing activities.

A few studies have evaluated the effects of patellar taping and bracing on radiographic patellar alignment in patients with PFPS with conflicting results. Although improvements have been noted in some studies,[48] other studies failed to find radiologic evidence of changed patellar position.[43] A number of factors including different measurement procedures (weight bearing vs. non–weight bearing), taping techniques, and subject attributes may contribute to the disparate results.

Although no evidence has been reported that patellar tape can change the activation magnitude of the VMO or VL,[49] there is evidence that taping the patella can alter the onset timing of the VMO relative to the VL during stair ambulation.[50,51] Cowan and colleagues[50] used a randomized, crossover design in which participants with PFPS were required to complete the stair-stepping task under 3 experimental conditions: no tape, therapeutic tape, and control tape (Level of Evidence I). During the stair-stepping task, the application of the therapeutic tape was found to alter the temporal characteristics of VMO and VL activation, whereas the control tape had no effect. Taping the patella has also been shown to significantly increase isokinetic quadriceps torque,[41,42] as well as knee extensor moments and power during a vertical jump and lateral step up.[52]

In addition to taping the patella, taping the lateral thigh has been proposed as a technique to improve the balance of VL and VMO activity. The tape is applied firmly in a horizontal direction across the VL muscle belly and the midthigh level to inhibit the activity of VL. This premise has been investigated only in asymptomatic individuals in whom it was found that inhibitory tape significantly reduced the EMG activity of VL compared with no tape or placebo tape in a stair descent task.[53]

There seems to be consensus in the literature that bracing and/or taping that provides immediate pain relief should be used as an adjunct to treatment in conjunction with muscle retraining. VMO retraining to restore the dynamic stability of the patella is one of the mainstays of PFP rehabilitation programs. Traditionally, open chain exercises have been proposed to improve quadriceps muscle imbalance. There are 3 main open kinetic chain exercises: (1) isometric knee extension, (2) inner range knee extension (terminal or short-arc knee extension), and (3) straight leg raises. All 3 utilize knee flexion less than 30 degrees to minimize PF joint contact stress. The available evidence suggests that the VMO is not preferentially activated compared with VL during isometric knee extension, inner range quadriceps, or straight leg raises, regardless of the hip rotation bias.[54–57] In fact, all studies that evaluate both the straight leg raise and isometric quadriceps setting have shown less EMG activity in the single-joint extensors during a straight leg raise (even when resistance is applied) than during the isometric quadriceps setting exercise. The addition of hip rotation (internal or external) does not appear to have a beneficial effect on the activation of VMO.[56,57] Mixed results have been reported regarding the addition of hip adduction on the relative activation of VMO and VL, with some authors finding that hip adduction enhances the VMO/VL ratio,[58] whereas others found no benefit.[54,55]

However, there is increasing evidence that weight bearing or closed chain training is effective in preferentially activating the vasti. Stensdotter and colleagues[59] found in asymptomatic subjects that closed chain knee extension promoted a more simultaneous onset of EMG activity of the 4 different muscle portions of the quadriceps compared with open chain. In open chain, rectus femoris had the earliest EMG onset, whereas the VMO was activated last with smaller amplitude than in closed chain. These authors conclude that closed kinetic chain exercise promotes a more balanced initial quadriceps activation than open kinetic chain exercise. This supports the finding of Escamilla and coworkers,[60] who found that open kinetic chain exercises produced more rectus femoris activity, with closed chain exercises

producing more vasti activity. Closed kinetic training allows simultaneous training not only of the vasti but also the gluteals and trunk muscles to control the limb position in weight bearing.

A stable pelvis minimizes unnecessary stress on the knee. Training of the gluteus medius (posterior fibers) decreases hip internal rotation and the consequent valgus vector force that occurs at the knee. However, the evidence supporting the effect of hip muscle training alone on PFP symptoms is quite limited, with most studies being single-case studies with no long-term follow-up.[61,62] If the patient exhibits internal rotation and adduction of the femur during weight-bearing activities, indicating poor gluteal control, it has been suggested that taping the gluteals may improve the stability of the pelvis. Kilbreath and coworkers[63] recently demonstrated improved hip extension in a group of stroke patients after gluteal taping. The subjects who had experienced a stroke between 2 and 11 years ago walked at 2 different speeds (self-selected and fast) under three different conditions (control, therapeutic, and placebo tape). With the therapeutic tape in situ, subjects went from 3 degrees of hip flexion in the control situation to 11-degree extension in self-selected walking speed and 8 degrees in fast walking. No difference was found with placebo tape. The authors conclude that the shortened gluteal musculature could work more effectively and improve hip extension. Further research needs to be done to validate the use of gluteal tape to improve pelvic stability in patients with PFP.

Some promising evidence in the literature has evaluated the pain-reducing effect of orthotics in subjects with PFP who exhibit excessive pronation.[64–66] Both hard and soft orthotics are effective in relieving symptoms but do not have much effect in changing foot or lower limb alignment, so the mechanism of pain reduction remains unknown (Level of Evidence III).[67] Appropriate flexibility exercises are often included in the treatment regimen. Only 1 study has examined the effectiveness of a stretching program to decrease PFP symptoms.[68] Peeler and Anderson[68] recently found that after 3 weeks of quadriceps muscle stretching in weight bearing that there was a significant reduction in PFP (Level of Evidence III).

What is evident from the literature is that no one treatment is effective for PFP because it is a multifactorial problem that requires a multimodal approach. Strong evidence has been recorded in the literature that a McConnell-based physical therapy program is successful in managing PFP.[69,70] This includes patellar taping, patellar mobilizations, specific quadriceps and gluteal exercises often with biofeedback, and stretching for the anterior hip structures and hamstrings. A robust, randomized, placebo-controlled clinical trial of a McConnell-based physical therapy program in 71 patients with PFP demonstrated that the physical therapy group responded significantly better to treatment and had greater improvements in average pain, worst pain, and functional activities (Level of Evidence I). The physical therapy treatment changed the onset timing of VMO relative to VL

TABLE 95–1. Identifying Effective Therapies for Anterior Knee Pain

AUTHOR (YEAR OF PUBLICATION)	DESCRIPTION	LEVEL OF EVIDENCE OF PRIMARY QUESTION	TOPIC AND CONCLUSIONS
Crossley et al. (2002)[69]	Prospective, double-blind, randomized trial of McConnell-based physiotherapy program vs. placebo physiotherapy treatment for patellofemoral pain	I	71 patients randomized to physiotherapy or placebo group. Subjects and assessor blinded to group allocation; improved pain (VAS) and function in the patients in the McConnell-based physiotherapy group; change maintained at 3-month follow-up; longer-term follow-up not done as placebo group crossed over
Cowan et al. (2001)[50]	Prospective, double-blind, randomized trial of McConnell-based physiotherapy program vs. placebo physiotherapy treatment for patellofemoral pain	I	71 patients randomized to physiotherapy or placebo group; subjects and assessor blinded to group allocation; improved EMG onset timing of medial quads in the patients in the McConnell-based physiotherapy group
Clark et al. (2000)[46]	Prospective, randomized trial comparing exercise, taping, and education; exercise and education; taping and education; and education alone	I	81 patients with patellofemoral pain in an observer-blinded, prospective, factorial design, randomized, controlled trial showed that patients who exercised were significantly more likely to be discharged at 3 months than nonexercising patients, and these benefits were maintained at 1 year
Whittingham et al. (2004)[70]	Prospective, randomized trial comparing daily patella taping and exercise group or exercise alone group	I	24 patients randomized to either combination of daily patella taping and exercises group or exercise alone group; 4 weeks of daily patella taping and exercises was superior to exercise alone in improving pain and function in individuals with patellofemoral pain syndrome; no long-term follow-up
Witvrouw et al. (2000)[33]	Prospective study to evaluate the efficacy of open versus closed kinetic chain exercises in the nonoperative management of patellofemoral pain	II	60 patients were randomized into a 5-week program that consisted of only closed kinetic chain exercises or only open kinetic chain exercises; both groups experienced a statistically significant decrease in pain and an increase in functional performance; no long-term follow-up
Peeler and Anderson (2007)[68]	Pretest/post-test control group design to determine whether a 3-week static stretching program would increase quadriceps muscle flexibility in subjects with PJPS	III	83 subjects completed a 3-week static quadriceps stretching program; after the stretching program, a significant improvement in flexibility was detected for both groups, and the PJPS group reported a significant decrease in knee pain and improved joint function, but changes in quadriceps flexibility were poorly correlated with changes in knee pain and function
Saxena and Haddad (2003)[65]	Retrospective review of patients diagnosed with patellofemoral pain syndrome and fitted with semiflexible orthotics	III	102 patients treated for patellofemoral pain syndrome with semiflexible foot orthoses showed a decrease in pain; no control or placebo group, not randomized, and no long-term follow-up
Mascal et al. (2003)[61]	Case report of management of patellofemoral pain targeting hip, pelvis, and trunk muscle function	IV	2 patients with patellofemoral pain treated with hip, trunk, and pelvic muscle exercises for 14 weeks; improvements in pain and function; no control or placebo group, long treatment period, no follow-up

EMG, electromyography; PJPS, patellofemoral joint pain syndrome; VAS, visual analog pain scale.

during stair-stepping and postural perturbation tasks. At baseline in both the placebo and treatment groups, the VMO came on significantly later than the VL. After treatment, there was no change in muscle onset timing of the placebo group, but in the physiotherapy group, the onset of VMO and VL occurred simultaneously during concentric activity, and VMO preceded VL during eccentric activity.[39,71]

CONCLUSION

PFP is a multifactorial problem where it seems the symptoms are most likely to be arising from the fat pad or lateral retinaculum, which are highly nociceptive structures. A multimodal physical therapy program is effective. This consists of taping or bracing to relieve pain, performing weight-bearing exercises for the quadriceps and the gluteals, stretching the quadriceps in weight bearing, stretching the tight anterior hip structures, and in some cases, using orthotics. Table 95–2 provides a summary of recommendations for the management of PFP.

TABLE 95–2. Summary of Recommendations

RECOMMENDATION	LEVEL OF EVIDENCE/ GRADE OF RECOMMENDATION
1. Patients with patellofemoral pain respond well to a McConnell-based multimodal physical therapy program.	A
2. Patients with patellofemoral pain achieve short-term relief from pain by taping, bracing, or both.	A
3. Vastus medialis oblique is best activated together with the other vasti in weight-bearing positions.	B
4. Open chain exercises do not preferentially activate the VMO.	B
5. Soft or hard orthotics can relieve the symptoms of PFP in patients with excessive pronation.	B
6. Hip exercises alone may help patients with PFP.	I
7. Stretching the quadriceps in weight bearing may help PFP symptoms.	C

PFP, patellofemoral pain; VMO, vastus medialis oblique.

REFERENCES

1. Fulkerson J, Hungerford D: Disorders of the Patellofemoral Joint, 2nd ed. Baltimore, Williams & Wilkins, 1990.
2. Lutter L: The knee and running. Clin Sports Med 4:685–698, 1985.
3. Almeida S, Williams KM, Shaffer RA, et al: Epidemiological patterns of musculoskeletal injuries and physical training. Med Sci Sports Exerc 31:1176–1182, 1999.
4. Heir T, Glomsaker P: Epidemiology of musculoskeletal injuries among Norwegian conscripts undergoing basic military training. Scand J Med Sci Sports 6:186–191, 1996.
5. Jones BH, Cowan DN, Tomlinson JR, et al: Epidemiology of injuries associated with physical training among young men in the army. Med Sci Sports Exerc 25:197–203, 1993.
6. Milgrom C, Kerem E, Finestone A, et al: Patellofemoral pain caused by overactivity. A prospective study of risk factors in infantry recruits. J Bone Joint Surg Am 73A:1041–1043, 1991.
7. Dye SF, Vaupel GL, Dye CC: Conscious neurosensory mapping of the internal structures of the human knee without intraarticular anaesthesia. Am J Sports Med 26:773–777, 1998.
8. Witonski D, Wagrowska-Danielewicz M: Distribution of substance-P nerve fibers in the knee joint of patients with anterior knee pain. A preliminary report. Knee Surg Sports Traumatol Arthrosc 7:177–183, 1999.
9. Bennell K, Hodges P, Mellor R, et al: The nature of anterior knee pain following injection of hypertonic saline into the infrapatellar fat pad. J Orthop Res 22:116–121, 2004.
10. Fulkerson JP, Tennant R, Jaivin JS, et al: Histological evidence of retinacular nerve injury associated with patellofemoral malalignment. Clin Orthop Relat Res 197:196–205, 1985.
11. Sanchis-Alfonso V, Rosello-Sastre E: Immunohistochemical analysis for neural markers of the lateral retinaculum in patients with isolated symptomatic patellofemoral malalignment. Am J Sports Med 28:725–731, 2000.
12. Bierdert R, Lobenhoffer P, Lattermann C, et al: Free nerve endings in the medial and posteromedial capsuloligamentous complexes: Occurences and distribution. Knee Surg Sports Traumatol Arthrosc 8:68–72, 2000.
13. Goodfellow J, Hungerford D, Zindel M: Patellofemoral joint mechanics & pathology. J Bone Joint Surg Br 58B:287–299, 1976.
14. Gresalmer R, McConnell J: The Patella. Gaithersburg, MD, Aspen, 1998.
15. Powers CM: The influence of altered lower-extremity kinematics on patellofemoral joint dysfunction: A theoretical perspective. J Orthop Sports Phys Ther 33:639–646, 2003.
16. McConnell J: The physical therapist's approach to patellofemoral disorders. Clin Sports Med 21:363–387, 2002.
17. Brindle TJ, Mattacola C, McCrory J: Electromyographic changes in the gluteus medius during stair ascent and descent in subjects with anterior knee pain. Knee Surg Sports Traumatol Arthrosc 244–251, 2003.
18. Ireland ML, Willson JD, Ballantyne BT, et al: Hip strength in females with and without patellofemoral pain. J Orthop Sports Phys Ther 33:671–676, 2003.
19. Robinson RL, Nee RJ: Analysis of hip strength in females seeking physical therapy treatment for unilateral patellofemoral pain syndrome. J Orthop Sports Phys Ther 37:232–238, 2007.
20. Piva SR, Goodnite EA, Childs JD: Strength around the hip and flexibility of soft tissues in individuals with and without patellofemoral pain syndrome. J Orthop Sports Phys Ther 35:793–801, 2005.
21. Buchbinder R, Naparo N, Bizzo E: The relationship of abnormal pronation to chondromalacia patellae in distance runners. J Am Podiatr Assoc 69:159–161, 1979.
22. Tiberio D: The effect of excessive subtalar joint pronation on patellofemoral mechanics: A theoretical model. J Orthop Sports Phys Ther 9:160–165, 1987.
23. Powers CM, Maffucci R, Hampton S: Rearfoot posture in subjects with patellofemoral pain. J Orthop Sports Phys Ther 22:155–160, 1995.
24. Powers CM, Chen PY, Reischl SF, Perry J: Comparison of foot pronation and lower extremity rotation in persons with and without patellofemoral pain. Foot Ankle Int 23:634–640, 2002.
25. Mellor R, Hodges PW: Motor unit synchronization is reduced in anterior knee pain. J Pain 6:550–558, 2005.
26. Boucher JP, King MA, Lefebvre R, et al: Quadriceps femoris muscle activity in patellofemoral pain syndrome. Am J Sports Med 20:527–532, 1992.
27. Morrish GM, Woledge RC: A comparison of the activation of muscles moving the patella in normal subjects and in patients with chronic patellofemoral problems. Scand J Rehabil Med 29:43–48, 1997.
28. Powers CM, Landel RF, Perry J: Timing and intensity of vastus muscle activity during functional activities in subjects with and without patellofemoral pain. Phys Ther 76:946–955, 1996.
29. Souza DR, Gross M: Comparison of vastus medialis obliquus: Vastus lateralis muscle integrated electromyographic ratios between healthy subjects and patients with patellofemoral pain. Phys Ther 71:310–320, 1991.
30. Grabiner MD, Koh TJ, Draganich LF: Neuromechanics of the patellofemoral joint. Med Sci Sports Exerc 26:10–21, 1994.
31. Wickiewicz TL, Roy RR, Powell PL, et al: Muscle architecture of the human lower limb. Clin Orthop Relat Res 179:275–283, 1983.
32. Voight M, Weider D: Comparative reflex response times of the vastus medialis and the vastus lateralis in normal subjects with extensor mechanism dysfunction. Am J Sports Med 19:131–137, 1991.
33. Witvrouw E, Lysens R, Bellemans J, et al: Intrinsic risk factors for the development of anterior knee pain in an athletic population. A two year prospective study. Am J Sports Med 28:480–489, 2000.
34. Cowan SM, Bennell KL, Hodges PW, et al: Delayed onset of electromyographic activity of vastus medialis obliquus relative to vastus lateralis in subjects with patellofemoral pain syndrome. Arch Phys Med Rehabil 82:183–189, 2001.
35. Karst GM, Willet GM: Onset timing of electromyographic activity in the vastus medialis oblique and vastus lateralis

muscles in subjects with and without patellofemoral pain syndrome. Phys Ther 75:813–823, 1995.

36. Grabiner MD, Koh MA, Andrish JT: Decreased excitation of vastus medialis oblique and vastus lateralis in patellofemoral pain. Eur J Exp Musculoskel Rese 1:33–39, 1992.

37. Cowan SM, Hodges PW, Bennell KL, et al: Altered vastii recruitment when people with patellofemoral pain syndrome complete a postural task. Arch Phys Med Rehabil 83:989–995, 2002.

38. Cowan S, Bennell K, Hodges P, et al. Simultaneous feedforward recruitment of the vasti in untrained postural tasks can be restored by physical therapy. J Orthop Res 21:553–558, 2003.

39. Van Tiggelen D, Witvrouw E, Roget P, et al: Effect of bracing on the prevention of anterior knee pain—a prospective randomized study. Knee Surg Sports Traumatol Arthrosc 12:434–439, 2004.

40. Taylor D, Dalton J, Seaber A: Visco-elastic properties of muscle-tendon units. The biomechanical effect of stretching. Am J Sports Med 18:300, 1990.

41. Conway A, Malone T, Conway P: Patellar alignment/tracking alteration: Effect on force output and perceived pain. Isokinet Exerc Sci 2:9–17, 1992.

42. Handfield T, Kramer J: Effect of McConnell taping on perceived pain and knee extensor torques during isokinetic exercise performed by patients with patellofemoral pain syndrome. Physiotherapy Canada 39–44, 2000.

43. Worrell T, Ingersoll CD, Bockrath-Pugliese K, et al: Effect of patellar taping and bracing on patellar position as determined by MRI in patients with patellofemoral pain. J Athl Train 33:16–20, 1998.

44. Selfe J, Richards J, Thewlis D, Kilmurray S: The biomechanics of step descent under different treatment modalities used in patellofemoral pain. Gait Posture 27:258–263, 2008.

45. Powers CM, Ward SR, Chen YJ, et al: Effect of bracing on patellofemoral joint stress while ascending and descending stairs. Clin J Sport Med 14:206–214, 2004.

46. Clark DI, Downing N, Mitchell J, et al: Physiotherapy for anterior knee pain: A randomised controlled trial. Ann Rheum Dis 59:700–704, 2000.

47. Kowall MG, Kolk G, Nuber GW, et al: Patellar taping in the treatment of patellofemoral pain. A prospective randomized study. Am J Sports Med 24:61–66, 1996.

48. Herrington L: The effect of corrective taping of the patella on patella position as defined by MRI. Res Sports Med 14:215–223, 2006.

49. Cowan SM, Hodges PW, Crossley KM, Bennell KL: Patellar taping does not change the amplitude of electromyographic activity of the vasti in a stair stepping task. Br J Sports Med 40:30–34, 2006.

50. Cowan SM, Bennell KL, Crossley KM, et al: Physiotherapy treatment changes motor control of the vastii in patellofemoral pain syndrome (PFPS): A randomised, double-blind, placebo controlled trial. Med Sci Sports Exerc 33:S89, 2001.

51. Gilleard W, McConnell J, Parsons D: The effect of patellar taping on the onset of vastus medialis obliquus and vastus lateralis muscle activity in persons with patellofemoral pain. Phys Ther 78:25–32, 1998.

52. Ernst G P, Kawaguchi J, Saliba E: Effect of patellar taping on knee kinetics of patients with patellofemoral pain syndrome. J Orthop Sports Phys Ther 29:661–667, 1999.

53. Tobin S, Robinson G: The effect of McConnell's vastus lateralis inhibition taping technique on vastus lateralis and vastus medialis obliquus activity. Physiotherapy 26:173–183, 2000.

54. Karst GM, Jewett PD: Electromyographic analysis of exercises proposed for differential activation of medial and lateral quadriceps femoris muscle components. Phys Ther 73:286–299, 1993.

55. Cuddeford T, Williams AK, Medeiros JM: Electromyographic activity of the vastus medialis oblique and vastus lateralis muscles during selected exercises. J Man Manip Ther 4:10–15, 1996.

56. Cerny K: Vastus medialis oblique/vastus lateralis muscle activity ratios for selected exercises in persons with and without patellofemoral pain syndrome. Phys Ther 75:672–682, 1995.

57. Mirzabeigi E, Jordan C, Gronley JK, et al: Isolation of the vastus medialis oblique muscle during exercise. Am J Sports Med 27:50–53, 1999.

58. Hodges P, Richardson CA: The influence of isometric hip adduction on quadriceps femoris activity. Scand J Rehabil Med 25:57–62, 1993.

59. Stensdotter AK, Hodges PW, Mellor R, et al: Quadriceps activation in closed and in open kinetic chain exercise. Med Sci Sports Exerc 35:2043–2047, 2003.

60. Escamilla RF, Fleisig GS, Zheng N, et al: Biomechanics of the knee during closed kinetic chain and open kinetic chain exercises Med Sci Sports Exerc 30:556–569, 1998.

61. Mascal CL, Landel R, Powers C: Management of patellofemoral pain targeting hip, pelvis, and trunk muscle function: 2 case reports. J Orthop Sports Phys Ther 33:647–660, 2003.

62. Cibulka MT, Threlkeld-Watkins J: Patellofemoral pain and asymmetrical hip rotation. Phys Ther 85:1201–1207, 2005.

63. Kilbreath SL, Perkins S, Crosbie J, McConnell J: Gluteal taping improves hip extension during stance phase of walking following stroke. Aust J Physiother 52:53–56, 2006.

64. Eng JJ, Pierrynowski MR: Evaluation of soft foot orthotics in the treatment of patellofemoral pain syndrome. Phys Ther 73:62–68, 1993.

65. Saxena A, Haddad J: The effect of foot orthoses on patellofemoral pain syndrome. J Am Podiatr Med Assoc 93:264–271, 2003.

66. Johnston LB, Gross MT: Effects of foot orthoses on quality of life for individuals with patellofemoral pain syndrome. J Orthop Sports Phys Ther 34:440–448, 2004.

67. Nester CJ, van der Linden ML, Bowker P: Effect of foot orthoses on the kinematics and kinetics of normal walking gait. Gait Posture 17:180–187, 2003.

68. Peeler J, Anderson JE: Effectiveness of static quadriceps stretching in individuals with patellofemoral joint pain. Clin J Sport Med 17:234–241, 2007.

69. Crossley K, Bennell K, Green S, et al: Physical therapy for patellofemoral pain: A randomized, double-blinded, placebo-controlled trial. Am J Sports Med 30:857–865, 2002.

70. Whittingham M, Palmer S, Macmillan F: Effects of taping on pain and function in patellofemoral pain syndrome: A randomized controlled trial. J Orthop Sports Phys Ther 34:504–510, 2004.

71. Cowan SM, Bennell KL, Crossley KM, et al: Physical therapy alters recruitment of the vasti in patellofemoral pain syndrome. Med Sci Sports Exerc 34:1879–1885, 2002.

Chapter 96

What Is the Best Treatment for Chondral Defects in the Knee?

Tom Minas, MD, MS and Andreas H. Gomoll, MD

Damage to the articular cartilage comprises a spectrum of disease entities ranging from single, focal chondral defects to more advanced degenerative disease. Long implicated in the subsequent development of osteoarthritis, focal chondral defects result from various causative factors. Patients are approximately evenly split in reporting a traumatic versus an insidious onset of symptoms; athletic activities are the most common inciting event associated with the diagnosis of a chondral lesions.[1] Traumatic events and developmental causative agents such as osteochondritis dissecans (OCD) predominate in younger age groups. Several large studies have found high-grade chondral lesions (Outerbridge grades III and IV) in 5% to 11% of younger patients (<40 years) and up to 60% of older patients.[1-3] The most common locations for these defects are the medial femoral condyle (up to 32%) and the patella,[2,3] and most are detected incidentally during meniscectomy or anterior cruciate ligament reconstruction.[1,4] Notably, despite this relatively high incidence, many of these defects are incidental in nature and asymptomatic. It is agreed that articular cartilage lesions have no spontaneous repair potential and a propensity to worsen with time. Even though the natural history is still not completely understood, those involved in cartilage repair agree that one must look for background factors that predispose to the formation of these defects—malalignment and compartment overload of the tibiofemoral or patellofemoral compartments, joint laxity, contracture, meniscal insufficiency, and of course, genetic predisposition to osteoarthritis—for which to date clinical, biological, or genetic markers are lacking. Therefore, various techniques have evolved to stimulate defect repair or overtly replace these defects. The high costs and extensive rehabilitation associated with many of these procedures necessitate careful evaluation to establish their respective clinical and cost-effectiveness.

The field of cartilage repair is a recent development within orthopedic surgery with techniques that continue to evolve. Although there are no formal treatment algorithms that have been agreed on and validated by prospective comparative trials of the emerging techniques, practice-based algorithms have been recommended based on existing evidence and by matching patient characteristics to treatment efficacy and risks. High-quality outcomes research is necessary to provide a better understanding of the efficacy of these procedures and to enable physicians to properly indicate treatment.

This chapter provides an overview of the existing techniques and supporting data in an attempt to guide surgeons in their indications for the treatment of cartilage defects of the knee.

OPTIONS

Before the development of modern bioengineering techniques, orthopedists were restricted to procedures that aimed to palliate the effects of chondral lesions or attempted to stimulate a healing response initiated from the subchondral bone resulting in the formation of fibrocartilage to fill the defect. Simple arthroscopic lavage and debridement of lesions has been used since the 1940s in an effort to reduce symptoms resulting from loose bodies and cartilage flaps, and it is a common first-line treatment, especially for coincidental defects. Marrow stimulation techniques (MST), such as abrasion arthroplasty, drilling, and microfracture, attempt to induce a reparative response by perforation of the subchondral bone after radical debridement of damaged cartilage and removal of the tide mark "calcified" zone to enhance the integration of repair tissue. The resultant blood clot, and the primitive mesenchymal cells contained within, may differentiate into a fibrocartilaginous repair tissue that fills the defect. Unlike hyaline cartilage, this fibrocartilage largely consists of type I collagen and is mechanically less stable and less durable.[5] The pluripotential marrow-derived cells may also form bone, another mode of MST-related failure that is increasingly becoming recognized.[6] Although closely related, MSTs vary by the degree of trauma to the subchondral bone, which has been recognized as a factor in the failure of these techniques. Abrasion arthroplasty (or also abrasion chondroplasty) decorticated the superficial subchondral bone with a bur to expose the more porous bone below but also destabilized the subchondral bone with the risk for fracture. Drilling utilizes small drill bits or K-wires to perforate the subchondral bone, which can result in heat necrosis; microfracture avoids this issue by using special awls (microfracture or Steadman awls). Currently, most surgeons have abandoned the older methods in favor of microfracture, which is usually performed in an all-arthroscopic fashion.

Restorative cartilage repair techniques such as autologous chondrocyte implantation (ACI) introduce chondrogenic cells into the defect area, resulting in the formation of a repair tissue that more closely resembles the collagen type-II rich hyaline cartilage. The original technique of ACI was developed in the 1980s[7] and has been used in the United States to treat more than 10,000 patients since its approval by the U.S. Food and Drug Administration (FDA) in 1997. ACI is indicated for the treatment of medium to large chondral defects with no or shallow associated osseous deficits. It originally received FDA approval for application in the femoral condyle (medial, lateral, and trochlea) but has also been used successfully to treat patellar defects. ACI in its current form is a two-stage procedure with an initial arthroscopic cartilage biopsy, followed by a staged reimplantation through an arthrotomy. The next generation ACI-c (collagen-covered) technique was developed to reduce the reoperation rate because of hypertrophy of the periosteal patch used to cover the defect. This was achieved by substitution of periosteum with a collagen membrane, frequently consisting of a porcine type-I/III collagen bilayer membrane. The latest generation of ACI, termed MACI *(membrane associated),* cultures the chondrocytes directly on the aforementioned collagen membrane, which is then implanted arthroscopically or through a mini-open approach with fibrin glue or limited suturing.

Cartilage replacement techniques include osteochondral autograft and allograft transfers, such as the osteochondral autograft transfer system (OATS; Arthrex, Naples, FL), mosaicplasty (Smith & Nephew, Andover, MA), and mega-OATS techniques. Osteochondral autograft transplantation is used to address small to medium defects (1–4 cm²), often with associated bone loss. Osteochondral cylinders are harvested from lesser marginal weight-bearing areas of the knee joint and press-fitted into the prepared defect. Commonly, multiple cylinders have to be transplanted to fill larger defects. Osteochondral autografting is limited by the amount of cartilage that can be harvested without violating the weight-bearing articular surface.[8] The main advantage lies in its autogenicity, avoidance of disease transmission, immediate graft availability through harvesting of the patient's own tissue, and decreased cost of this single-stage procedure.

The treatment of chondral defects with fresh osteochondral allografts has garnered significant attention because of its potential to restore and resurface even extensive areas of damaged cartilage and bone. Osteochondral allograft transplantation is used predominantly in the treatment of large and deep osteochondral lesions resulting from OCD, osteonecrosis, and traumatic osteochondral fractures, but it can also be used to treat peripherally uncontained cartilage and bone defects. Furthermore, osteochondral allografting presents a viable salvage option after failure of other cartilage resurfacing procedures. The main advantages over autograft transplantation are the ability to closely match the curvature of the articular surface

by harvesting the graft from a corresponding location in the donor condyle, the ability to transplant large grafts, and the avoidance of donor-site morbidity. The main concerns with allograft transplantation are failure to incorporate with subchondral collapse and the risk for disease transmission (estimated at 1 in 1.6 million for the transmission of HIV[9]).

EVIDENCE

Table 96–1 provides an overview of cartilage repair studies. Table 96–2 provides a summary of treatment recommendations and respective levels of evidence for chondral defects in the knee.

Microfracture

Most studies show good outcomes in 60% to 80% of patients. Several studies have tried to define the indications for microfracture in regards to patient and defect characteristics. Kreuz and Erggelet[10] have demonstrated improved results in patients younger than 40 years, both in regard to validated scores and to magnetic resonance imaging (MRI) findings of better fill and quality. They also demonstrated a worsening between the 18- and 36-month follow-up scores for all patients in the older age group and for younger patients with patellofemoral defects (Level of Evidence II). In another study, the same authors report on the association between outcomes and defect locations, and found the best outcomes in femoral condyle lesions, whereas those in the patella group fared the worst (Level II).[11] Other authors have described better results in smaller lesions, body mass index less than 30, and shorter duration between onset of symptoms and start of treatment (Level IV).[6,12,13]

Autologous Chondrocyte Implantation

Several long-term case series have reported good-to-excellent results in 70% to 90% of patients after ACI in the knee, depending on the location (patella and femoral condyle) or the clinical series (Level IV).[14,15] Bentley and colleagues[16] compared ACI-c with mosaicplasty in a prospective randomized controlled trial (RCT), showing good and excellent results (Cincinnati score) in 88% of patients with ACI, but only 69% of mosaicplasties. All 5 patellar mosaicplasties were considered failures (Level I). In a similar study by Horas and coworkers,[17] mosaicplasty performed significantly better than ACI. Biopsies were obtained from a subgroup of patients and uniformly revealed fibrous tissue in all defects treated with ACI. This study, however, was limited by the use of nonstandard cell-culturing facilities (Level I).

In a prospective RCT comparing ACI-p (periosteum-covered) with ACI-c, (Gooding and coworkers[18] found no statistically significant differences in the clinical outcome, but a reoperation

TABLE 96–1. Overview of Cartilage Repair Studies

STUDY AUTHOR	DESIGN (LEVEL OF EVIDENCE)	FOLLOW-UP INTERVAL (NO. OF CASES)	PATIENT POPULATION	PATIENT AGE (DEFECT SIZE)	TREATMENT GROUPS	RESULTS
Kreuz et al.[10]	Prospective (II)	3 yr (70 patients)	Grade 3 and 4 chondral defects treated with microfracture	30 and 39 yr (average, 2.2 cm²)	Patient age: <40	All groups improved significantly; younger patients improved more. Older patients and patellofemoral lesions in younger patients worsened between 18 and 36 months.
Kreuz et al.[11]	Prospective (II)	3 yr (70 patients)	Grade 3 and 4 chondral defects treated with microfracture	40 yr (average, 2.2 cm²)	Defect locations: femoral condyle, trochlea, tibia, patella	All groups improved significantly, most in the femoral condyle group; results decreased between 18 and 36 months.
Mithoefer et al.[6]	Case series (IV)	41 mo (48 patients)	Grade 3 and 4 chondral defects treated with microfracture	41 yr (median, 2.8 cm²)	N/A	Significant improvement until 24 months after surgery, then deterioration. Poor fill on MRI correlated with poor outcome. BMI > 30 associated with poor fill and outcome.
Blevins et al.[12]	Case series (IV)	3.7 yr (140 patients)	Grade 3 and 4 chondral defects treated with microfracture	26 and 38 yr (average, 2.2 cm²)	Activity status: High-level vs. recreational athletes	Both groups with significant improvements. On second-look arthroscopy, no improvement in lesion grade in 8% of high-level and 35% of recreational athletes.
Peterson et al.[15]	Case series (IV)	4.2 yr (condyle) 2.7 yr (multiple lesions) (101 patients)	Grade 3 and 4 chondral defects treated with ACI	32 yr (condyle) 35 yr (multiple lesions) (average, 4.2/4.6 cm²)	N/A	Good and excellent results in 92% of femoral condyle lesions, 67% of multiple lesions, 89% of OCD, 65% of patellar lesions. Graft failure in 7 of 101 patients.
Bartlett et al.[19]	RCT (I)	12 mo (91 patients)	Grade 3 and 4 chondral defects	34 yr (average, 6 cm²)	ACI technique: ACI-c, MACI	No statistically significant differences between groups. Better outcomes in patients younger than 35 years and with symptoms for less than 50 months. Reoperation rate for graft hypertrophy in 9% of ACI-c and 6% of MACI.
Gooding et al.[18]	RCT (I)	24 mo (68 patients)	Grade 3 and 4 chondral defects	31 yr (average, 4.5 cm²)	ACI technique: ACI-p, ACI-c	Good and excellent results (Cincinnati score) in 74% of ACI-c and 67% of ACI-p, but dissimilar defect locations: 61% of lesions treated with ACI-p were patellar, whereas only 20% of those treated with ACI-c were in this location. Reoperation rate for graft hypertrophy was 36% in ACI-p and 0% for ACI-c.

Study	Level	Follow-up (patients)	Defect	Age	Technique	Results
Bentley et al.[16]	RCT (I)	19 mo (100 patients)	Grade 3 and 4 chondral defects	31 yr (average, 4.7 cm²)	Cartilage repair technique: ACI-c, mosaicplasty	Good and excellent results (Cincinnati score) in 88% of ACI and 69% of mosaicplasty patients. All 5 patellar mosaicplasties failed. No graft hypertrophy in patients with ACI (collagen membrane used).
Knutsen et al.[20]	RCT (I)	2 yr (80 patients)	Grade 3 and 4 chondral defects	33 yr (average, 5 cm²)	Cartilage repair technique: ACI, microfracture	No statistically significant differences between the groups at 2 years, except SF-36, which was better in microfracture group. Patients younger than 30 years and more active (Tegner score >4) did better, regardless of treatment. Defects larger than 4 cm² fared worse with microfracture, no similar effect was seen with ACI.
Gudas et al.[23]	RCT (I)	37 mo (57 patients)	Grade 3 and 4 chondral defects	24 yr (average, 2.8 cm²)	Cartilage repair technique: microfracture, OATS	Good and excellent results in 96% of OATS and 52% of microfracture patients. Return to sports in 93% of OATS and 52% of microfracture patients. Microfracture significantly worse in lesions >2 cm², and results deteriorated after 12 months. Both groups showed better results in patients younger than 30 years.
Gross et al.[24]	Case series (IV)	10 yr (127 patients)	Osteochondral defects of the femur and tibia	27 yr (femur) 43 yr (tibia)	N/A	Survivorship of 95% at 5 years, 80% to 85% at 10 years, and 65% to 74% at 15 years.
Gortz and Bugbee[25]	Case series (IV)	4.5 yr (43 patients)	Osteochondral defects of the femur	35 yr (average, 5.9 cm²)	N/A	88% had good and excellent results.

ACI, autologous chondrocyte implantation; ACI-c, collagen-covered autologous chondrocyte implantation; ACI-p, periosteum-covered autologous chondrocyte implantation; BMI, body mass index; MACI, membrane-associated autologous chondrocyte implantation; MRI, magnetic resonance imaging; N/A, not available; OATS, osteochondral autograft transfer system; OCD, osteochondritis dissecans; RCT, randomized, controlled trial; SF-36, 36-Item Short Form Health Survey.

TABLE 96–2. Treatment Recommendations and Respective Level of Evidence

RECOMMENDATION	LEVEL OF EVIDENCE/GRADE OF RECOMMENDATION
1. Microfracture treatment shows better results in smaller defects (<2–4 cm²).	B
2. Microfracture treatment shows best results in femoral condyle lesions.	B
3. Microfracture treatment results in better outcomes in younger patients (<30–40 years old).	B
4. Microfracture treatment results in better outcomes in patients with BMI <30.	C
5. ACI, microfracture, or mosaicplasty result in outcomes superior to each other.	I
6. Shorter duration of symptoms before cartilage repair results in better outcomes.	B
7. The use of a collagen membrane in place of a periosteal patch for ACI reduces the reoperation rate for graft hypertrophy.	A
8. ACI-c and MACI have comparable outcomes.	A
9. Osteochondral defects are amenable to osteochondral allograft transplantation.	B

ACI, autologous chondrocyte implantation; ACI-c collagen-covered autologous chondrocyte implantation; BMI, body mass index; MACI, membrane-associated autologous chondrocyte implantation.

rate for symptomatic graft hypertrophy of 36% in the periosteal covered group versus 0% with the collagen membrane (Level I). Bartlett and coauthors[19] presented a prospective RCT comparing the advanced techniques ACI-c and MACI, and reported no statistically significant differences between the groups. They also found improved outcomes in patients younger than 35 years and with pre-operative symptoms for less than 50 months (Level I).[19] Knutsen compared ACI with microfracture and found no significant differences. The 36-Item Short Form Health Survey (SF-36) improved more in the microfracture group, and the authors hypothesized whether this could be because of the more invasive nature of ACI. Furthermore, the authors observed better results in younger (<30 years) and more active (Tegner scale score >4) patients. Defects larger than 4 cm² fared worse than smaller lesions after microfracture treatment; no such effect was seen after ACI (Level I).[20]

Graft hypertrophy resulting in mechanical symptoms such as clicking and popping occurs in up to 25% to 30% of patients, typically 7 to 9 months after the procedure,[21] and can be addressed with arthroscopic debridement of the hypertrophic tissue. Newer techniques such as ACI-c and MACI have decreased the rate of symptomatic graft hypertrophy to less than 10% (Level I).[19]

Osteochondral Autograft Transplantation

Patients treated with osteochondral autograft transplantation experienced good-to-excellent results in approximately 90% of condylar lesions, 80% of tibial defects, and 70% of trochlear lesions.[22] The treatment of patellar defects remains controversial, with some groups reporting almost universal failure in this location.[16] Gudas and investigators[23] compared OATS with microfracture in a group of athletes, and demonstrated good and excellent results in 96% of patients treated with OATS versus 52% with microfracture. Rate of return to sports was 93% with OATS and 52% with microfracture. Microfracture had significantly worse results in lesions larger than 2 cm², and results started to deteriorate after the 12-month examination. Both groups showed better results in patients younger than 30 years (Level I).[23]

Osteochondral Allograft Transplantation

Gross reported on a large series of fresh osteochondral allografts for the treatment of predominately traumatic distal femoral and proximal tibial defects. Survivorship analysis demonstrated intact and well-functioning grafts (Hospital for Special Surgery score >70) in 95% of patients at 5 years, which decreased to 80% to 85% at 10 years and 65% to 74% at 15 years (Level IV).[24] Gortz and Bugbee[25] report good and excellent results in 88% of 43 fresh osteochondral allografts of the distal femur at an average follow-up time of 4.5 years (Level IV).

Summary

Summarizing the conclusions of the reviewed literature, both microfracture and osteochondral autograft transfer are appropriate treatment options for defects smaller than 4 cm². Evidence exists that autograft transfer allows faster and more likely return to sports for athletes, and this technique should therefore be considered in this population. Both techniques have limitations in larger defects because of diminished results with microfracture and donor-site morbidity in autograft transfer. Therefore, ACI and allograft transplantation should be considered for the treatment of lesions larger than 4 cm². Both have demonstrated similar results but have specific risks and benefits: Allograft transplantation is uniquely suited for the treatment of uncontained or deep osteochondral lesions but is limited by the scarcity of fresh grafts and the risk for disease transmission from the donor. ACI is not associated with either limitation and can be used for defects of any size and location. Good evidence has been reported that the use of collagen membranes in place of periosteal patches for ACI reduces the risk of reoperation with otherwise equivalent clinical outcome and should, therefore, be recommended as far as allowed by the local regulatory organizations (collagen membranes are not FDA-approved for use in ACI in the United States).

AREAS OF UNCERTAINTY

Study Design and Indications

Symptomatic chondral defects are relatively rare in a clinical practice; therefore, a surgeon must have a large tertiary referral practice to develop clinical expertise in this area. A large difference must exist in the treatment outcomes to have an adequately statistically powered study to compare treatments for a rare problem such as a chondral defect. However, the time end points must also be established in this field because any fibrocartilage repair may do well in the first 3 years, then the tissue and the clinical results will deteriorate. Consequently, not only is an adequately powered study necessary, but an appropriate length of follow-up to determine durability of the repair and the prevention of degenerative joint disease also is needed. Therefore, a multicenter prospective randomized study is necessary to recruit adequately.

Several authors have conducted studies comparing different repair techniques such as microfracture, mosaicplasty, and ACI with conflicting results. These studies are often compromised by the very nature of the procedures they were designed to investigate; for example, ACI as a cell-based therapy is dependent on a sophisticated cell-culturing process. The cell-culturing process requires phenotypic validation, cell viability assessment, and sterility process validation according to the FDA, GLP (Good Laboratory Practices), and GMP (Good Manufacturing Practices) to ensure sterile, safe, phenotypically stable cell implantation; however, not all authors utilize standardized and approved laboratory facilities.

The technical skill factor and "learning curve" for the ACI procedure and multiple osteochondral grafting technique is crucial. These procedures are challenging. Some studies have used multiple surgeons performing few surgeries, which may compromise the clinical outcomes. This is another appealing facet of the microfracture technique; its technical ease of performance to most parts of the knee joint may bias against a comparative study using ACI or mosaicplasty, for which technical perfection is a must to obtain a good clinical result.

Furthermore, it is unlikely that every chondral defect is amenable to every available treatment, but rather that there will be differences depending on the exact defect size and location. Therefore, even well-designed, prospective RCTs attempting to compare treatment options for a wide range of defects are bound to yield conflicting results.

To formulate better treatment guidelines, investigators must first assess each treatment option on its own to ascertain which type of defect it is most efficacious in. The success rates and clinical outcomes may then be established from these well-performed prospective clinical cohorts. A range of patient characteristics, defect location, and size will thus be established. Each defect will have one or several associated treatment options. We will then be able to conduct well-designed, adequately powered, ethically sound, comparative studies. These will be true Level I evidence-based outcome studies that will help guide treatments for our patients and provide data for evidence-based treatment algorithms. Only then will we be able to properly design trials that compare the efficacy of treatment options for the same type of defect.

Engebretsen evaluated the quality of cartilage repair studies in an update[26] to a previous publication[27] and commented on this subject:

> The increased focus on methodology in major journals by marking original articles with a level-of-evidence is highly appreciated. However, we would like to emphasize the fact that randomized controlled trials can have serious design flaws (i.e., not using independent reviewers, no statistical power analysis, not using an adequate randomization procedure, not accounting for eligible subjects not included in study), and therefore be rated as level-of-evidence II. We would also like to draw the reader's attention to the fact that several well performed case series (level-IV evidence) score very well on the CMS. These studies largely take into consideration multiple aspects of good methodological quality such as independent investigator, sufficient number of patients, well-described rehabilitation protocol, validated outcome measures and so forth, and are mainly lacking in not having a control group. We therefore recommend the reader to not entirely dismiss articles marked level-IV evidence, yet themselves assess the methodological quality of the paper when interpreting the results (for example using a grading system like the CMS).

We also agree with their recommendation that inclusion and exclusion criteria should be well-established, validated outcome measures for cartilage injuries should be used, and outcome assessment be made by an independent investigator, ideally by the patient without assistance.

BACKGROUND FACTORS

With the exception of clearly traumatic defects, most cartilage defects do not exist in isolation, but rather are associated with other pathologic entities. Careful evaluation can often identify structural abnormalities, such as malalignment, patellar instability, or insufficiency of the ligamentous and meniscal structures. The presence of these associated abnormalities introduces an additional layer of variability into studies because of the reproducibility of assessing background factors between surgeons and treating these before or concomitantly with the treatment of the chondral defect varies. To date, this correlation has not been firmly established. The disappointing early results of cartilage repair have been explained by the failure to properly diagnose and correct these associated bony and ligamentous abnormalities; for example, in early studies of patellar defects treated with ACI alone, good and excellent results were found in only one third of patients.[7] Later studies, however, identified patellar maltracking as an important associated abnormality, and concurrent use of a corrective osteotomy led to 71% good or excellent results.[28] These reports emphasize the importance of a thorough patient evaluation to correctly identify and treat all associated abnormalities to ensure the long-term success of chondral repair.

GUIDELINES

No guidelines based on comparative trials for the treatment of articular cartilage defects have been developed. Our preferred treatment algorithm is outlined in the following section.

RECOMMENDATIONS

We do not treat asymptomatic chondral defects at this time because the possibility to worsen patient's condition exists. Existing techniques currently do not report excellent results of more than 90%, and the natural history and progression of a chondral defect remains unknown for any given individual. Careful longitudinal follow-up in this situation is recommended to the patient with annual clinical examination for progressive crepitus and effusion. High-resolution MRI scan is performed to evaluate for potential defect size progression; conventional standing anteroposterior and flexion posteroanterior radiographs help to assess the overall cartilage space. Counseling regarding weight control and avoidance of impact loading sports is recommended. If the patient becomes symptomatic or there is progression in defect size, then surgery is recommended after the risks and benefits are discussed and an informed consent obtained. This is based on the most appropriate treatment from the guidelines that follow.

The background factors for the cartilage defect are evaluated with clinical examination and long alignment radiographs. The authors perform a corrective osteotomy to the neutral mechanical axis without overcorrection for any defects larger than 2 cm² if there is 2 degrees or more of mechanical varus or valgus, and correct any patellar maltracking through an anteromedialization of the tibial tubercle (Level II).

Single full-thickness chondral defects of the weight-bearing femoral condyles and trochlea of less than 10 mm in diameter are amenable to osteochondral autograft transfer (OATS or mosaicplasty). Occasionally, in a large knee, two plugs will be used to repair a lesion of 15 mm in diameter (Level IV). This technique has the advantages of a single-stage procedure, transfer of mature hyaline cartilage into the defect, and a comparatively uncomplicated postsurgical recovery. Donor-site morbidity is acceptable with use of a single plug. The donor sites are frequently "backfilled" with synthetic Calcium Sulfate-PLA/PGA copolymer (OBI TruFit plugs; Smith & Nephew) (Level V). Drains are used after surgery to prevent hemarthrosis and arthrofibrosis (Level V). Defects of the patella and tibial plateau should not be managed with this technique because the cartilage thickness mismatch between donor site (average, 2 mm) and patella (average, 5–7 mm) results in incongruities, resorption, and failure. Osteochondral autograft transfer may be performed arthroscopically but must be a precise fit—flush to the surface and orthogonally placed; hence miniarthrotomy for accurate placement should be considered if there is any concern for graft placement by arthroscopy.

Defects of the weight-bearing condyles, tibia, trochlea, and patella of 1 to 2 cm² are also amenable to microfracture with acceptable long-term results. The recovery and return to sports is longer than osteochondral autografting, and the success rate is less. However, microfracture is technically less challenging and can be applied to all locations within the knee. Long-term follow-up is necessary because the durability is less predictable and recurrent symptoms are common at 2 ½ to 5 years after surgery (Level I).

We prefer to treat defects larger than 2 cm² with ACI because of the good and predictable long-term results of this technique. Associated osseous defects deeper than 6 to 8 mm should be addressed with a bony procedure, either in a staged fashion with bone grafting followed by ACI 9 to 12 months later or with single-stage osteochondral allograft transplantation (mega-OATS) (Level IV).

Our primary indication for a fresh osteochondral allograft is a large, peripherally uncontained lesion, osteochondral defect with deep osseous component, avascular necrosis, or a previous ACI that has failed by fibrous repair. Otherwise, bone deficiency is not a contraindication for ACI if the defect is first bone grafted. The long-term results of ACI are superior to allograft, and for this reason, in a young person, our preference is a staged bone-cartilage repair with ACI (Level IV).

The field of cartilage repair is evolving. The relative efficacies of the differing techniques and their limitations are being elucidated through carefully conducted prospective cohorts to determine the best cartilage technique for any given defect, even though this study design does not afford the highest level of evidence. However, these studies will provide success and failure rates to subsequently design comparative, statistically well-powered, ethically just RCTs that will answer this question: "What is the best repair technique for this defect?" Currently, we can advocate an evidence-based algorithm for treatment based on patient and defect characteristics that will be cost-effective and sound.

REFERENCES

1. Aroen A, Loken S, Heir S, et al: Articular cartilage lesions in 993 consecutive knee arthroscopies. Am J Sports Med 32:211–215, 2004.
2. Curl WW, Krome J, Gordon ES, et al: Cartilage injuries: A review of 31,516 knee arthroscopies. Arthroscopy 13:456–460, 1997.
3. Hjelle K, Solheim E, Strand T, et al: Articular cartilage defects in 1,000 knee arthroscopies. Arthroscopy 18:730–734, 2002.
4. Piasecki DP, Spindler KP, Warren TA, et al: Intraarticular injuries associated with anterior cruciate ligament tear: Findings at ligament reconstruction in high school and recreational athletes. An analysis of sex-based differences. Am J Sports Med 31:601–605, 2003.
5. Nehrer S, Spector M, Minas T: Histologic analysis of tissue after failed cartilage repair procedures. Clin Orthop Relat Res (365):149–162, 1999.
6. Mithoefer K, Williams RJ 3rd, Warren RF, et al: The microfracture technique for the treatment of articular cartilage lesions in the knee. A prospective cohort study. J Bone Joint Surg Am 87:1911–1920, 2005.
7. Brittberg M, Lindahl A, Nilsson A, et al: Treatment of deep cartilage defects in the knee with autologous chondrocyte transplantation. N Engl J Med 331:889–895, 1994.
8. Garretson RB 3rd, Katolik LI, Verma N, et al: Contact pressure at osteochondral donor sites in the patellofemoral joint. Am J Sports Med 32:967–974, 2004.
9. Gitelis S, Cole BJ: The use of allografts in orthopaedic surgery. Instr Course Lect 51:507–520, 2002.
10. Kreuz PC, Erggelet C, Steinwachs MR, et al: Is microfracture of chondral defects in the knee associated with different results in patients aged 40 years or younger? Arthroscopy 22:1180–1186, 2006.
11. Kreuz PC, Steinwachs MR, Erggelet C, et al: Results after microfracture of full-thickness chondral defects in different compartments in the knee. Osteoarthritis Cartilage 14:1119–1125, 2006.
12. Blevins F. T, Steadman JR, Rodrigo JJ, Silliman J: Treatment of articular cartilage defects in athletes: An analysis of functional outcome and lesion appearance. Orthopedics 21:761–778, 1998.
13. Steadman JR, Briggs KK, Rodrigo JJ, et al: Outcomes of microfracture for traumatic chondral defects of the knee: Average 11-year follow-up. Arthroscopy 19:477–484, 2003.
14. Minas T: The role of cartilage repair techniques, including chondrocyte transplantation, in focal chondral knee damage. Instr Course Lect 48:629–643, 1999.
15. Peterson L, Minas T, Brittberg M, et al: Two- to 9-year outcome after autologous chondrocyte transplantation of the knee. Clin Orthop Relat Res (374):212–234, 2000.
16. Bentley G, Biant LC, Carrington RW, et al: A prospective, randomised comparison of autologous chondrocyte implantation versus mosaicplasty for osteochondral defects in the knee. J Bone Joint Surg Br 85:223–230, 2003.
17. Horas U, Pelinkovic D, Herr G, et al: Autologous chondrocyte implantation and osteochondral cylinder transplantation in cartilage repair of the knee joint. A prospective, comparative trial. J Bone Joint Surg Am 85-A:185–192, 2003.
18. Gooding CR, Bartlett W, Bentley G, et al: A prospective, randomised study comparing two techniques of autologous chondrocyte implantation for osteochondral defects in the knee: Periosteum covered versus type I/III collagen covered. Knee 13:203–210, 2006.
19. Bartlett W, Skinner JA, Gooding CR, et al: Autologous chondrocyte implantation versus matrix-induced autologous chondrocyte implantation for osteochondral defects of the knee: A prospective, randomised study. J Bone Joint Surg Br 87:640–645, 2005.
20. Knutsen G, et al: Autologous chondrocyte implantation compared with microfracture in the knee. A randomized trial. J Bone Joint Surg Am 86-A:455–464, 2004.
21. Micheli LJ, Browne JE, Erggelet C, et al: Autologous chondrocyte implantation of the knee: Multicenter experience and minimum 3-year follow-up. Clin J Sport Med 11:223–228, 2001.
22. Hangody L, Fules P: Autologous osteochondral mosaicplasty for the treatment of full-thickness defects of weight-bearing joints: Ten years of experimental and clinical experience. J Bone Joint Surg Am 85-A(suppl 2):25–32, 2003.
23. Gudas R, Kalesinskas RJ, Kimtys V, et al: A prospective randomized clinical study of mosaic osteochondral autologous transplantation versus microfracture for the treatment of osteochondral defects in the knee joint in young athletes. Arthroscopy 21:1066–1075, 2005.
24. Gross AE, Shasha N, Aubin P: Long-term followup of the use of fresh osteochondral allografts for posttraumatic knee defects. Clin Orthop Relat Res (435):79–87, 2005.
25. Gortz S, Bugbee WD: Allografts in articular cartilage repair. Instr Course Lect 56:469–481, 2007.
26. Jakobsen RB, Engebretsen L: An analysis of the quality of cartilage repair studies – an update. In ISAKOS Current Concepts Winter 2007. Edited, ISAKOS, 2007.
27. Jakobsen RB, Engebretsen L, Slauterbeck JR: An analysis of the quality of cartilage repair studies. J Bone Joint Surg Am 87:2232–2239, 2005.
28. Minas T, Bryant T: The role of autologous chondrocyte implantation in the patellofemoral joint. Clin Orthop Relat Res (436):30–39, 2005.

Chapter 97

Multiligament Knee Injury:
Should Surgical Reconstruction Be Acute or Delayed?

Jacquelyn Marsh, BHSc, Lyndsay Somerville, BSc, MSc,
J. Robert Giffin, MD, FRCSC, and Dianne Bryant, BSc, BA, MSc, PhD

Multiple ligament knee injuries involve rupture of at least 2 major ligaments of the knee usually involving 1 or both of the cruciates with or without injury to the collateral ligaments. Multiple knee ligament injuries are relatively rare and often the result of high-energy traumatic injuries. The optimal amount of time between injury and surgical intervention is controversial. Some argue for intervention in the acute stage, commonly defined as within 3 weeks of injury, whereas others have recommended delaying surgery a number of months depending on a variety of factors.[1-6]

We identified 16 articles; 7 studies compared acute with conservative treatment, and 9 studies compared acute with chronic surgical repair. The characteristics and levels of evidence of these studies are displayed in Table 97–1. There were no randomized trials, and only 1 study was prospective. Of the 9 studies that addressed acute versus chronic repair, 1 study[7] was excluded because it did not provide a direct comparison between the 2 cohorts. All studies included a variety of combinations of injured ligaments. The average sample size was 39 (range, 11–89). Studies were evaluated for methodologic quality according to a modified version of the Newstead–Ottawa Scale (NOS)[8]; a scale designed to assess the quality of nonrandomized studies (Table 97–2). Using this rating scale, each study is judged on 3 broad perspectives: the selection of study groups, the comparability of the groups, and the ascertainment of the outcome of interest. The maximum number of points is 8, which indicates a high-quality study. In general, the methodologic quality was poor; the maximum number of points awarded on the NOS was 6, and the majority of studies were awarded 3 points. The methodologic features of these studies are summarized in Table 97–3.

SUBJECTIVE OUTCOME MEASURES: A BRIEF DESCRIPTION

Functional Status

Five subjective functional outcome measures were common among studies: (1) Lysholm,[9] (2) International Knee Documentation Committee (IKDC),[10] (3) Meyer's Rating Scale,[11] (4) Knee Outcome Sur-

vey,[12] and (5) Hospital for Special Surgery.[13] A brief description of these outcome instruments follows.

The Lysholm scale is designed to document the patient's evaluation of function. It is a condition-specific outcome measure that contains 8 domains: limp, locking, pain, stair climbing, use of supports, instability, swelling, and squatting.[9] An overall score from 0 to 100 points is calculated, with 95 to 100 points indicating an excellent outcome; 84 to 94 points, a good outcome; 65 to 83 points, a fair outcome; and less than 65 points, a poor outcome. The instrument has face validity and acceptable construct and criterion validity, as well as test-retest reliability and adequate responsiveness.[14]

The IKDC scale has 2 versions. The older version included a subjective patient-rated assessment within a generally physician-rated form (now Knee Examination Form). The subjective portion included 2 patient-rated questions that ask, "How does your knee function?" and "How does your knee affect your activity level?" Patients provide a rating of normal (A), nearly normal (B), abnormal (C), or severely abnormal (D). The question with the lowest rating provides the score for that patient.[10,15] The latest version of the IKDC contains a separate form titled "The Subjective Knee Evaluation Form"[10] that is an 18-item, knee-specific questionnaire designed to detect changes in patients with a variety of knee conditions. The questions address 3 domains: physical symptoms (7 items), sports activities (10 items), and function before injury (1 item). The resulting total score is out of 100 possible points, which represents perfect knee function. This instrument has face validity and demonstrated construct validity, excellent test-retest reliability, and sensitivity to change.[10,15]

Meyers and coworkers[11] developed a rating scale to measure the functional ability of patients after treatment for knee dislocations. They defined "excellent" as the ability to return to work or previous level of activity without impairment and with a stable knee; "good" included having knee symptoms that did not preclude the patient's return to normal occupation and activities of daily living. In this classification, pain is present but is considered an annoyance, and symptoms of instability are unusual or minimal. A rating of

TABLE 97–1. Sample Characteristics of the Included Study

STUDY	INJURED LIGAMENTS	ACTIVITY AT INJURY	SAMPLE	GROUP SELECTION CRITERIA (USED TO ASCERTAIN PRESENCE/ABSENCE OF SELECTION BIAS)	SURGICAL PROCEDURES: LIGAMENTS	LENGTH OF FOLLOW-UP	TIME: INJURY TO SURGERY	LEVEL OF EVIDENCE
Almekinders and Logan[24]	14 ACL/PCL 5 MCL/LCL 12 not described	16 MVA 6 falls 9 other	26 males/ 5 females 32 yr (range, 15–76)	6 patients treated surgically 10 patients treated conservatively • Treatment selection based on surgeon's preference and experience • 15 lost to follow-up	4 patients had direct repair of all ligaments 2 patients had autograft reconstruction	Mean 40 mo	Within 2 weeks of injury	
Meyers et al.[11]	6 ACL/PCL 20 ACL/PCL/MCL 11 ACL/PCL/LCL 8 ACL/PCL/ LCL/MCL 4 ACL/LCL 1 ACL/MCL 2 LCL/MCL 1 not described	8 MVA 12 motorcycle 9 pedestrian vs. automobile 13 falls 6 miscella- neous 3 unknown 2 sports related	33 males/20 females Age range, 15–73 yr	20 patients treated surgically 13 patients treated conservatively • Selection criteria not described • 20 lost to follow-up	4 patients with at least one ligament repaired 16 patients with all ligaments repaired	>1 yr	Not described	
Richter et al.[19]	36 ACL/PCL/MCL 34 ACL/PCL/LCL 19 ACL/PCL/ LCL/MCL	56 MVA 17 sports 8 industrial 8 falls	69 males 20 females 33.5 yr (range, 15–76)	63 patients treated surgically 26 patients treated conservatively • Treatment selection based on general condition of the patient and associated injuries	37 ACL/PCL sutured 12 ACL/PCL fixed 11 ACL/PCL reconstructed 2 ACL reconstructed/PCL repaired 1 ACL repair/PCL reconstruction	Mean 8.2 yr (range, 2–25)	10.6 days (range, 0–140)	
Rios et al.[20]	2 ACL/PCL 11 ACL/PCL/MCL 9 ACL/PCL/LCL 4 ACL/PCL/ LCL/ MCL	19 MVA 3 sports 3 falls 1 fight	20 males/ 6 females 37 yr (range, 16–68)	21 patients treated surgically (all had no life-threatening conditions) 5 patients treated conservatively 4 surgery not recommended • 3 severe skeletal and visceral injuries • 1 *Pseudomonas* infection after bypass/severe popliteal artery disruption, causing necrosis of soleus and gastrocnemius muscles • 1 patient refused surgery	11 complete reconstruction of all damaged ligaments 3 either the ACL or PCL repaired 3 collateral ligament repair only 4 not described	Mean 36 months (range, 12–96) 5.6 days (range, 0–8)		

Continued

TABLE 97–1. Sample Characteristics of the Included Study—cont'd

STUDY	INJURED LIGAMENTS	ACTIVITY AT INJURY	SAMPLE	GROUP SELECTION CRITERIA (USED TO ASCERTAIN PRESENCE/ABSENCE OF SELECTION BIAS)	SURGICAL PROCEDURES: LIGAMENTS	LENGTH OF FOLLOW-UP	TIME: INJURY TO SURGERY	LEVEL OF EVIDENCE
Taylor et al.[25]	Not described	24 MVA / 6 sport related / 7 work related / 5 falls	31 males / 11 females / 36 yr (range, 8–77)	16 patients treated surgically • 10 surgery recommended • 4 open injuries • 2 irreducible dislocations • 3 had small fractures • 1 trapped lateral popliteal nerve • 3 primary repairs • 2 secondary procedures required • 1 Küntscher nail used for stabilization • 26 patients treated conservatively (knee reduced under general anesthesia, followed by casting)	Not described	Range 6 mo to 35 yr	Not described	
Werier et al.[18]	8 ACL/PCL/MCL/LCL / 14 ACL/PCL/MCL / 14 ACL/PCL/LCL / 1 ACL/MCL/LCL / 1 ACL/PCL	25 MVA / 4 sport injuries / 6 work related / 1 assault / 2 patients with bilateral ligament injury	28 males / 8 females / 32 yr (range, 17–85)	22 knees treated surgically / 16 knees treated conservatively • Treatment selection based on surgeon preference and presence of other injuries requiring surgery	19 ACL/PCL repair or reconstruction / 1 PCL repair or reconstruction / 2 not described	Mean 5 years (range, 18 mo to 10 yr)	Not described	
Wong et al.[21]	Not described	13 high velocity (MVA/falls) / 13 low velocity (jumping/twisting)	24 males / 2 females / 22 yr (range, 11–54)	15 patients treated surgically / 11 patients treated conservatively • Selection criteria not described	7 partial repair (suture repair of all disrupted ligaments or ACL reconstruction only) / 8 complete reconstruction (of all torn structures) • Closed immobilization (casting or with external fixation)	Median 33.5 mo (range, 6–144 mo)	Not described	
Harner et al.[6]	31 ACL/PCL/MCL/LCL	Not described	28.4 yr (range, 16–51)	19 acute / 12 chronic • Selection criteria not described	• Avulsed ligaments and tears of the medial collateral ligament were directly repaired • Complete tears of the cruciate and lateral collateral ligaments were reconstructed with fresh-frozen allograft tissue • Remaining injuries to the posterolateral structures were addressed by direct repair and/or allograft replacement	Mean 44 mo (range, 2–6 yr)	Acute: <3 weeks from injury Chronic: >3 weeks	

Study	Ligaments injured	Mechanism	Demographics	Treatment	Number/type reconstructed	Follow-up	Timing
Fanelli et al.[23]	19 ACL/PCL/PLC 9 ACL/PCL/MCL 6 ACL/PCL/ MCL/PLC 1 ACL/PCL	20 MVA 9 sports related 4 falls 1 industrial 1 pedestrian vs. automobile	26 males/9 females 35 yr	19 patients treated acutely 16 patients treated chronically • Selection criteria not described	35 ACL/PCL/MCL/PLC	Mean 24 mo (range, 24–120)	Not described
Karataglis et al.[2]	3 ACL/PCL/ LCL/PLC 1 ACL/PCL/ MCL/PLC 2 ACL/PCL/ MCL 9 ACL/PCL/ PLC 2 ACL/LCL/ PLC 1 ACL/MCL/ PLC/PLC 4 PCL/LCL/ PLC 3 ACL/PCL 1 ACL/MCL 7 PCL/PLC	16 MVA 14 sports 5 fall	27 males/8 females 35.1 yr (range, 17–60)	6 patients treated acutely • Patients had concomitant injuries that necessitated urgent surgical intervention • 29 patients treated chronically • Tertiary referral center with no trauma service	35 ACL/PCL/PLC/ MCL/LCL	Mean 40.3 mo (range, 12–124 mo)	Acute: within 3 weeks of injury Chronic: average 2.7 yr (range, 6 mo to 12 yr)
Liow et al.[3]	7 ACL/PCL/ LCL/PCL 5 ACL/PCL/MCL 6 ACL/LCL/PCL 1 PCL/LCL 2 ACL/PCL 1 PCL/MCL	12 sports 10 MVA	16 males/8 females 26.9 yr (range, 15–46)	8 knees treated acutely 14 knees treated chronically • Late referrals from outside regions	22 ACL/PCL/LCL/ MCL/PLC	Mean 32 mo (range, 11–77 mo)	Acute: <2 weeks Chronic: >6 months (range, 6–72 mo)
Noyes and Barber-Westin[5]	4 ACL/PCL/PLC 5 ACL/PCL/MCL 1 ACL/PCL/ MCL/PLC 1 ACL/PCL/ PLC	6 MVA 2 sports 2 hit by falling objects 1 industrial	10 males/1 female 27 yr (range, 17–42)	7 patients treated acutely 4 patients treated chronically • 2 had successful prior repairs of MCL • 2 had failed prior repair or reconstruction of ACL	11 ACL/PCL	Mean 4.5 yr (range, 2.5–6.9)	Acute: 14 days (range 7–28) Chronic: 22 mo (range, 13–31)
O'Donoghue[1]	Not described	Not described	Range 6–56 yr	44 patients treated acutely 36 patients treated chronically • Treatment selection based on surgeon preference	80 ACL/PCL/MCL/LCL	40 mo (range, 6 mo to 15 yr)	Acute: <2 weeks Chronic: >2 weeks
Tzurbakis et al.[22]	12 ACL/MCL 11 ACL/PCL/ PLC 25 ACL/PCL/ MCL/LCL	35 MVA 10 sports 2 work related 1 fall	41 males/7 females 28.6 yr (range, 16–40)	38 patients treated acutely 10 patients treated chronically • Selection criteria not described	Bony avulsed ligaments and acute tears of the posterolateral and posteromedial corner were repaired if possible Midsubstance tears of the cruciate ligaments and chronic cases were reconstructed with autografts	51.3 mo (range, 21.4–81.2 mo)	Acute: <3 weeks Chronic: >3 weeks
Wascher et al.[4]	7 ACL/PCL/MCL 6 ACL/PCL/PLC	6 MVA 5 sports 2 falls	27.5 yr (range, 14–51)	9 patients treated acutely 4 patients treated chronically • 1 patient with associated spine and abdominal injuries • 3 patients were late referrals	13 ACL/PCL reconstructed Different grafts for each patient	Mean 38.4 mo (range, 24–54)	Acute: <3 weeks Chronic: mean 11 mo (range, 1.5–17)

ACL, anterior cruciate ligament; LCL, lateral collateral ligament; MCL, medial collateral ligament; MVA, motor vehicle accident; PCL, posterior cruciate ligament; PLC, posterolateral complex.

TABLE 97–2. Newstead–Ottawa Scale

Selection

1. Representativeness of the acute cohort
   a. truly representative of average person with multiple ligament knee injury*
   b. somewhat representative of average person with multiple ligament knee injury*
   c. selected group, e.g., athletes, volunteers
   d. no description of the derivation of the acute cohort
2. Representativeness of the chronic (or conservative) cohort
   a. truly representative of average person with multiple ligament knee injury*
   b. somewhat representative of average person with multiple ligament knee injury*
   c. selected group, e.g., athletes, volunteers
   d. no description of the derivation of the chronic cohort
3. Allocation to group
   a. random allocation*
   b. surgeon preference
   c. no description of group allocation
4. Type of study
   a. prospective*
   b. retrospective

Comparability

1. Comparability of cohorts on the basis of the design or analysis
   a. study control subjects for age*
   b. study control subjects for any additional factor*
   c. no control group

Outcome

1. Assessment of outcome
   a. independent blind assessment*
   b. independent blind statistical analysis*
   c. nonblinded
   d. no description
2. Was follow-up long enough for outcomes to occur?
   a. yes (2+ years)*
   b. no
3. Adequacy of follow-up of cohorts
   a. complete follow-up—all subjects accounted for*
   b. subjects lost to follow-up unlikely to introduce bias (small number lost: >80% follow-up or description of those lost)*
   c. follow-up rate <80% and no description of those lost
   d. no statement

*Cohort studies: A study can be awarded a maximum of one star for each numbered item within the Selection and Outcome categories. A maximum of two stars can be given for Comparability.
From The Newcastle-Ottawa Scale (NOS). Assessing the quality of non-randomized studies in meta-analysis. Proceedings of the 3rd Symposium on Systematic Reviews: Beyond the Basics-Improving Quality and Impact. Oxford, St. Catherine's College, July 2000.

"fair" means the patient is performing all activities of daily living but has difficulty walking upstairs, walking on tiptoes, or running, and tends to avoid such activities. Finally, a "poor" functional rating is assigned to patients who cannot work and who are unable to perform daily activities.

The Knee Outcome Survey was developed to measure symptoms and functional limitations for patients with a variety of knee disorders, including ligamentous and meniscal injuries.[12] The Knee Outcome Survey consists of two scales, the Activities of Daily Living Scale and the Sports Activity Scale. The Activities of Daily Living Scale measures symptoms and functional limitations during activities of daily living. The score ranges from 0 to 100 points, with 100 points indicating an absence of symptoms and functional limitations during activities of daily living. The Activities of Daily Living Scale has been shown to be a reliable, valid, and responsive measure of symptoms and functional limitations during activities of daily living in individuals with a variety of knee injuries. The Sports Activity Scale measures symptoms and functional limitations experienced during sports activities. The Sports Activity Scale score ranges from 0 to 100 points, with 100 points representing the absence of symptoms and functional limitations during sports activities.[12]

Return to Activity

Two scales are used to measure patient activity level: (1) the Tegner Activity Level Scale and (2) the IKDC activity level scale. The Tegner Activity Level Scale rates the level of activity on a scale of 0 (off of work) to 10 (competitive contact sports).[16] The IKDC activity level scale measures return to activity on four levels: I is return to intensive activity, II is moderate activity, III is light activity, and IV is remain sedentary.

Ligament Stability

The overall IKDC Knee Examination Form assesses the function of the knee based on 4 factors: (1) subjective assessment, (2) symptoms, (3) range of motion (ROM), and (4) ligament examination. These factors are rated as normal (A), nearly normal (B), abnormal (C), and severely abnormal (D).[17] The overall final IKDC rating is based on group ratings for function, symptoms, ROM, and laxity. The worst problem area qualification defines the overall final qualification.

RESULTS

Lysholm Scale

Werier and colleagues[18] found that the average Lysholm scale score of 85 (95% confidence interval [CI], 80–90) in the reconstructed group was significantly greater than the average score of 69 (95% CI, 57–81) in those patients who were treated conservatively. When comparing the components of the Lysholm, the reconstructed group had a better ability to climb stairs and experienced less symptomatic instability. Similarly, Richter and investigators[19] found that the Lysholm score was significantly greater in those who underwent surgical treatment (78.3 ± 13.4) compared with those who had nonoperative treatment (64.8 ± 16.3).

International Knee Documentation Committee Subjective Score

Rios and coauthors[20] report the IKDC subjective score in terms of having excellent, good, fair, or poor results. The authors did not provide a definition of these classifications. The surgical group (*n* = 21) had

TABLE 97–3. Quality Characteristics of the Included Studies

STUDY	PROSPECTIVE OR RETROSPECTIVE	GREATER THAN 20% LOST TO FOLLOW-UP	ADEQUATE LENGTH OF FOLLOW-UP	ASSESSMENT OF OUTCOME BLINDED	COMPARABILITY OF COHORTS	QUALITY RATING	LEVEL OF EVIDENCE
Almekinders and Logan[24]	Retrospective	Yes	Yes	No/Yes*	No	2	III
Meyers et al.[11]	Prospective	Yes	Yes	No	Yes	2	II
Richter et al.[19]	Retrospective	No	Yes	Uncertain	No	3	III
Rios et al.[20]	Retrospective	No	Yes	Yes	No	4	III
Taylor et al.[25]	Retrospective	No	Yes	Uncertain	No	2	III
Werier et al.[18]	Retrospective	No	Yes	No	No	2	III
Wong et al.[21]	Retrospective	No	Yes	Uncertain	No	3	III
Fanelli et al.[23]	Prospective	No	Yes	Yes	Yes	6	II
Harner et al.[6]	Retrospective	No	Yes	No	Yes	6	III
Karataglis et al.[2]	Retrospective	No	Yes	Yes	No	3	III
Liow et al.[3]	Retrospective	No	Yes	Yes	No	4	III
Noyes and Barber-Westin[5]	Retrospective	No	Yes	Uncertain	No	2	III
O'Donoghue[1]	Retrospective	No	Yes	No	Yes	3	III
Tzurbakis et al.[22]	Retrospective	No	Yes	No	Yes	3	III
Wascher et al.[4]	Retrospective	No	Yes	No	Yes	3	III

*Some of the measured outcomes were blinded.

4 patients with excellent results and 10 patients with good results, whereas none of the patients in the conservatively managed group ($n = 5$) had excellent or good results. In a similar study, Wong and colleagues[21] found that operative patients had a significantly greater average IKDC score (75.8 ± 10.0) compared with the conservative group (63.7 ± 9.1), whose average was considered suboptimal.

Meyer's Rating Scale

According to the Meyer's Rating Scale, Meyers and researchers[11] found that of the 13 patients in the conservatively managed group, 10 reported poor functional outcome, 2 fair, and 1 good. Three patients in the surgical group ($n = 20$) were rated as poor, 3 fair, 11 good, and 3 excellent. The authors conclude that the surgical group had better outcomes after treatment compared with those patients who did not undergo ligament repair. Similarly, Rios and colleagues[20] reported that all of the patients in the conservatively managed group ($n = 5$) were reported to have fair or poor functional outcomes on the Meyer's scale, whereas only 2 patients were rated as fair and 2 as poor in the surgical group ($n = 21$). Sixteen patients in the surgical group had excellent or good results.

ACUTE VERSUS DELAYED RECONSTRUCTION

Lysholm Scale

Harner and colleagues[6] found that the 19 patients who underwent acute surgery had an average Lysholm score of 91 ± 7.0 points, compared with 80 ± 16.9 points for the 12 patients whose surgery was delayed. Although the acute group had a greater average score than the chronic group, this difference did not reach statistical significance. Similarly, Tzurbakis and coauthors[22] report a mean Lysholm score of 88.3 ± 11.9 for the acutely treated patients and a mean score of 81.7 ± 13.3 for the delayed group ($P > 0.05$). Similar differences were observed in Liow and investigators'

study[3] in which those patients who underwent surgery during the acute phase had better functional ratings (87; 95% CI, 81–91) than those patients who underwent late reconstruction (75; 95% CI, 53–100). All acutely treated knees had a Lysholm score of more than 80 compared with only 5 of the 14 (36%) knees with delayed treatment. Likewise, Wascher and coauthors[4] report a greater Lysholm score for patients treated acutely compared with chronic patients, with a mean score of 91.3 and 79.3, respectively. Finally, Fanelli and coauthors[23] report no statistically significant difference in the Lysholm score between acute and delayed treated knees; although no data were provided to support these conclusions.

International Knee Documentation Committee Patient Subjective Assessment

Tzurbakis and coauthors[22] report that 30 patients in the acutely treated group ($n = 38$) considered their knee to be normal or nearly normal. Only 5 of 10 patients treated in the delayed phase rated their knee as normal or nearly normal. This difference was statistically significant.

Meyer's Rating Scale

Harner and colleagues[6] report that 16 of 19 patients in the acute group had an excellent or good rating, and 3 had a fair rating. Of the 12 patients in the delayed group, 7 received an excellent or good rating, 2 received a fair rating, and 3 received a poor rating. The difference between the acute and delayed groups was not statistically significant. Similarly, Wascher and coauthors[4] found that 4 patients who underwent surgery in the acute phase ($n = 9$) had an excellent rating and 5 had a good outcome, whereas no patients were classified as fair or poor. In the delayed group ($n = 4$), 2 patients were rated as excellent, 1 rated as fair, and 1 rated as poor.

Knee Outcome Survey

One study[6] evaluated patients using the Knee Outcome Survey. The average score on the Activities of Daily Living scale for the acutely treated patients was 91 ± 6.4, and the patients who received delayed treatment had an average score of 84 ± 11.8. Despite the trend toward a better outcome in the acutely treated patients, this difference was not statistically significant. On the Sports Activity Scale, the patients in the acute group had a significantly greater average score (89 ± 10.3), compared with those in the delayed group (69 ± 27.9) points.

Using their own classification, Noyes and Barber-Westin[5] had all patients complete a separate rating of their perception of the overall outcome and knee condition, rated as poor, fair, good, very good, or normal. Three patients in the acute group ($n = 7$) rated their knees as normal; two patients rated as good, and two patients rated as poor. In the delayed group ($n = 4$), one patient rated their knee condition as very good, one patient as good, and two patients as fair. The authors conclude that the acute patients had better overall perceptions of their outcome compared with the chronic group.

Summary

All studies found that patients undergoing surgical treatment have better self-reported functional outcomes when compared with patients treated without surgery. All studies found that patients who underwent surgical treatment in the acute phase (<3 weeks after injury) experienced better self-reported functional outcomes when compared with patients whose surgery was delayed. For the majority of studies, however, the observed differences between groups were not statistically significant.

RETURN TO ACTIVITY

Acute versus Nonoperative

Richter and colleagues[19] report that patients who underwent surgical intervention returned to higher levels of activity (4.0) according to the Tegner Activity Scale compared with those who received nonoperative treatment (2.7). In this same study, the IKDC showed that significantly more patients in the surgical group returned to intense or moderate activities compared with the group managed without surgery.

Acute versus Delayed

According to the Tegner Activity score, Liow and investigators[3] found that 5 patients from the acute group ($n = 8$) had activity levels greater than 5, compared with 7 of the 14 patients who underwent delayed reconstruction. The mean Tegner level showed a trend toward the early reconstruction group returning to higher levels of activity than the late reconstruction group with average scores of 5 (range, 3–7) and

4.4 (range, 1–7), respectively. Fanelli and coauthors[23] also compared the results of the Tegner score between the acutely treated and delayed treatment patients. The authors conclude no statistically significant difference between acute and delayed treatment knees in their ability to return to activities after surgery. Noyes and Barber-Westin[5] found that of the four patients treated acutely, two patients had decreased work activities because of their knee condition, one had decreased work activities because of reasons unrelated to their knee, and two remained in the same occupation. Only one patient had returned to activity at follow-up. Three patients returned to occupations rated as light. All patients with delayed treatment had decreased their activities, sports and work-related activities, because of their knee condition.

Summary

In 1 study, patients who underwent surgical treatment returned to higher levels of activity when compared with those who did not have surgery. In general, the activity level of acutely treated patients was higher than for patients whose surgery was delayed; however, these differences were not large and did not reach statistical significance.

LIGAMENT STABILITY

Acute versus Non-operative

Richter and investigators[19] report that the proportion of patients who obtained a rating of nearly normal or normal (B) was significantly greater in those undergoing surgery (14/59) compared with those receiving nonoperative treatment (1/18).

Acute versus Delayed

Tzurbakis and coauthors[22] report that 27 of 35 patients in the acute group were graded as normal or nearly normal compared with 5 of the 9 patients in the delayed group. This difference was not statistically significant. From a possible 31 patients, Harner and colleagues[6] reported the final overall IKDC rating as nearly normal for 11 knees, abnormal for 12, and severely abnormal for 8. No knee received a normal overall IKDC rating. Ten of the 11 knees that received a nearly normal IKDC score had been treated acutely. An equal number of severely abnormal knees was reported in the acute and delayed groups. In a similar study, Liow and investigators[3] found no statistically significant difference in overall IKDC rating between patients who underwent reconstruction in either the acute or the delayed phase. They report that 3 of the 8 knees in the acute patients were rated as nearly normal, compared with 5 of the 14 knees that underwent delayed reconstruction. Of the patients who underwent surgical intervention in the acute phase, Wascher and coauthors[4] report four patients who rated their knees as nearly normal and four patients who gave a rating of abnormal. Of the patients in the delayed group, 2 knees were rated as nearly normal, one as abnormal, and one as severely abnormal.

Lachman Testing

Acute versus Non-operative. Werier and colleagues[18] reported the results of the Lachman test in 20 degrees of knee flexion. The Lachman test was classified as grade I (0–5 mm displacement), grade II (5–10 mm displacement), or grade III (>10 mm displacement).[18] A significantly greater number of individuals with a grade III Lachman were in the nonoperative group compared with the operative group.

Acute versus Delayed. Wascher and coauthors[4] measured the Lachman test with the knee in 20 degrees of flexion and reported that, in the acute group, 7 of 9 patients were normal, and 2 patients had 3 to 5 mm of anterior tibial translation. In the delayed group, 2 patients were graded as normal, and 2 patients had 3 to 5 mm of anterior translation. All patients in both groups had firm end points.

KT-1000 Arthrometer

Acute versus Non-operative. Two studies[19,24] used the KT-1000 arthrometer to measure cruciate ligament laxity. Almekinders and Logan[24] specifically looked at anteroposterior (AP) laxity of the knee. They defined abnormal AP laxity as 3-mm or more side-to-side difference when compared with the unaffected knee. The authors found that all patients in the nonoperative group had abnormal AP laxity compared with their contralateral knee, whereas only 2 of the 6 patients in the operative group experienced greater than 3 mm excursion. Similarly, Richter and investigators[19] examined cruciate ligament stability using KT arthrometer whereas performing the Lachman test (at 25 degrees of knee flexion) with 20 pounds of force. They report that, on average, patients treated without surgery had significantly greater translation (8.2 ± 3.4 mm) compared with the surgical group (5.1 ± 2.4 mm). Furthermore, in a similar study, Wong and investigators[21] report the mean AP tibial translation for the surgical group as 4.6 mm compared with 9.4 mm for the group managed without surgery.

Acute versus Delayed. Fanelli and coauthors,[23] Tzurbakis and coauthors,[22] and Mariani[8] all report no statistically significant difference in KT-1000 arthrometer measurement between acute and delayed cases in their respective studies. Similarly, Noyes and Barber-Westin[5] found that all but 1 patient in the acute group (*n* = 7) had less than a 3-mm difference in AP displacement testing compared with the contralateral knee. Two patients treated in the delayed phase (*n* = 4) had a less than 3-mm difference whereas 2 patients had greater than a 6-mm side-to-side difference. Similarly, Wascher and coauthors[4] report a mean side-to-side difference of 4.1 mm in the acute group compared with an average of 5.6 mm in the delayed treatment group. Conversely, Liow and in-

vestigators[3] reported that 6 of 8 acute ACL reconstructions had 3 to 5 mm difference compared with 9 of 14 delayed surgeries cases.

Summary

All studies demonstrated greater laxity (on average) in patients treated without surgery compared with patients treated with surgery. Although 2 studies showed slightly better results in acutely treated patients, the majority of the studies found no significant difference in ligament stability between acute and delayed treatment patients.

RANGE OF MOTION

Acute versus Nonoperative

Wong and colleagues[21] report the average ROM for the surgical patients to be 128 degrees compared with a mean of 137 degrees in the nonoperative patients. This difference was not statistically significant. There were significantly more flexion contractures in the surgical group. The authors emphasize the role of aggressive physiotherapy. Similarly, Richter and investigators[19] did not find a statistically significant difference in the proportion of patients with a deficit in either flexion or extension. In the surgical group, 29 of 59 patients that were managed had an extension deficit of 3 degrees or more, whereas 10 of 18 in the nonoperative group experienced this same deficit. Similarly, 44 patients in the surgical group and 16 patients in the nonoperative group had a flexion deficit of 3 degrees or more. Werier and colleagues'[18] study found that operative patients had a slightly smaller range of flexion at 120 degrees compared with the nonoperative treatment group at 130 degrees. In contrast, Almekinders and Logan's[24] study reported that ROM in the operative group was slightly better (129 ± 18 degrees) than in the nonoperative group (108 ± 22 degrees).

Acute versus Delayed

Harner and colleagues[6] found that total ROM was similar between patients who had undergone surgical treatment during the acute phase (128 ± 10 degrees) compared with those patients who underwent delayed surgery (129 ± 15 degrees). Similarly, Liow and investigators[3] report that the mean loss of extension in the acute group was 10 degrees compared with 7 degrees in the group that underwent late reconstruction. The acute group had a smaller loss of flexion (4 degrees) compared with the late reconstructions (8 degrees). Noyes and Barber-Westin[5] found that 5 of 7 patients treated during the acute phase had normal knee ROM, whereas all chronic patients (*n* = 4) had achieved normal knee ROM. Wascher and coauthors[4] found that the acute group had a mean ROM of 132.4 degrees, whereas for delayed patients, it was 125.8 degrees. Tzurbakis and coauthors[22] also found similar mean ROM between acute and chronic patients (129.5 ± 12.6 and 131.7 ± 12.3 degrees, respectively). They also report similar measures of mean flexion and extension losses between the acute and delayed patients.

Summary

Overall, the evidence does not show an important difference in ROM between patients treated with or without surgery, though patients treated without surgery tended to achieve a slightly greater ROM. Several investigators suggest that observed improvements in ROM might be credited to early rehabilitation rather than surgical treatment. Results were similar and not significantly different for patients treated acutely compared with patients whose surgery was delayed.

RADIOGRAPHIC OUTCOMES

Almekinders and Logan[24] used a blinded observer to rate the degenerative changes on plain radiograph. The overall score ranged from 0, no evidence of degenerative arthritis, to a maximum score of 10, severe degenerative arthritis. This study did not demonstrate any significant differences in the degenerative changes between the surgical and nonoperative treatment groups. Werier and colleagues[18] used the same rating scale and found that radiographic scores did not differ significantly between the 2 treatment groups. Fifty percent and 60% of the reconstructed and unreconstructed group, respectively, had completely normal radiographs. Richter and colleagues[19] used the Jager and Wirth radiologic scale to measure the degree of osteoarthritis in the affected knee. This scale ranges from grade 0 (no signs of osteoarthritis) to grade IV (severe osteoarthritis). The proportion of individuals with grade III or IV osteoarthritis was significantly greater in those who had a nonsurgical intervention compared with those who had surgery. This finding suggests that the use of a larger study may show a benefit to having surgery in terms of the subsequent development of osteoarthritis.

OTHER

Taylor and coworkers[25] assessed their patients on 3 factors—stability, pain, and movements—and classified each factor as either good, fair, or poor. They defined "good" as a stable, painless knee that had 90 degrees or greater flexion; "fair" as experiencing slight instability on straining, no pain, and range of flexion between 60 and 90 degrees; and "poor" as the remainder of patients. In contrast with the previous studies, Taylor and coworkers[25] found that the nonoperative patients achieved better function on the measured factors than the surgical group. In the conservative group of 26 patients, 18 were classified as good, 6 as fair, and two as poor compared with four good, 6 fair, and 6 poor in the operative group.

COMPLICATIONS

A common postoperative complication reported in the literature was knee joint stiffness. The evidence suggests that surgery during the acute phase is associated with a greater risk for motion loss or arthrofibrosis.[3,23] Liow and investigators[3] conclude that early repair or reconstruction of all injured ligaments may produce a better functional outcome and a more stable knee, but they also note that the risk for arthrofibrosis remains a concern in acutely treated patients. Fanelli and coauthors[23] made a similar suggestion that delaying surgery 2 to 3 weeks allows for swelling to decrease and offers a protected ROM. Noyes and Barber-Westin[5] and Wascher and coauthors[4] also note that acute reconstruction of the ligaments may increase the risk for postoperative arthrofibrosis; however, they stress the importance of aggressive rehabilitation to prevent this complication. Conversely, Harner and colleagues[6] found no increased joint stiffness in the acutely treated patients and advocate early ligament repair.

DISCUSSION

We conducted a systematic review of the literature to identify studies comparing surgical interventions with nonoperative interventions for multiple ligament knee injuries and studies comparing the outcomes of patients treated surgically in the acute phase (less than 3 weeks after injury) compared with patients whose surgery was delayed beyond the acute phase. In general, across a variety of outcomes and among studies, surgical intervention provided superior outcomes to patients treated without surgery. Furthermore, patients who underwent surgery within 3 weeks of injury did not appear to have better outcomes when compared with patients whose surgery was delayed. We must raise several cautions regarding the strength of the evidence in support of these conclusions. The remainder of this discussion focuses on these methodologic shortcomings and their potential influence on these findings.

Selection bias refers to a systematic difference between treatment groups in prognosis and subsequent responsiveness to the intervention as a result of the way they were chosen for participation in the study.[26] A randomized, controlled trial with adequate concealment of allocation protects against selection bias by ensuring that patient eligibility is determined before randomization so that clinician knowledge of treatment allocation cannot influence the decision whether to include or exclude a patient from the study. Our review did not identify any randomized studies. In fact, decisions about treatment, for the majority of studies, were left to the preference of the treating physician and were usually based on the presence or absence of concomitant injuries and the prognosis of the patient, almost certainly ensuring a selection bias. For example, Werier and colleagues[18] made the decision to perform operative repair based on the presence of injuries that required surgery (i.e., vascular injury, nerve injury), and Rios and coauthors[20] chose their nonoperative group based on the severity of concomitant injuries (i.e., patients were not fit for surgery). In this review, it was not possible to explore the magnitude of the bias introduced through selection strategies because no study was without methodologic flaws.

The proportion of patients lost to follow-up is another potential threat to the internal validity of a study. In general, a lost-to-follow-up rate of greater than 20% is considered to be a serious threat to the validity of the results because patients are rarely lost to follow-up for arbitrary reasons,[27] and there is a good possibility that those patients without complete follow-up have difference outcomes than patients with complete follow-up. In this review, 2 of the 15 eligible studies[11,24] reported a greater than 20% lost-to-follow-up rate.

One final methodologic feature that is important to maintaining the internal validity of the study is blinding of the data collector. Blinding is defined as concealment of group assignment from the patients, investigators, and/or outcome assessors in a trial.[27] Blinding reduces the potential influence on the measurement or interpretation of outcomes that conscious or unconscious opinions about the effectiveness of the intervention could potentially cause and reduces the potential for imbalances in cointerventions.[27] For example, in Richter and investigators'[19] study, 27 of 63 surgical patients also underwent a functional rehabilitation regimen in addition to their surgical intervention, but none of the conservatively managed patients received this program.

One further limitation of the studies included in this review was the lack of adequate power to make definitive conclusions about the effectiveness of treatment. None of the studies that we identified provided the details of their sample size calculation or included a discussion about power. None of the studies included information that would inform the interpretation of their results. Specifically, no study provided information about the magnitude of the between-groups difference that would constitute a minimally important difference. If the estimate of the treatment effect is accurate (i.e., the study is internally valid), the authors must also comment on the precision of their results by including CIs around their estimates. In addition, the authors should comment as to whether the CIs exclude with certainty the possibility of an important difference for studies with nonsignificant statistical findings, and for studies with significant statistical findings, the authors should comment as to whether the CIs exclude differences that patients/clinicians would consider unimportant.

Finally, it is important to note that there are important differences between studies that make it difficult to summarize the results. Specifically, the involved ligaments, concomitant injuries, patient function/pain before surgery, surgical procedure, and the type of postsurgical rehabilitation differed across studies. For example, Richter and investigators[19] report 43% of the surgical group participated in a functional rehabilitation program after surgery, whereas the others in this group and the nonoperative treatment group did not participate in this rehabilitation program. In addition, 19% of the nonoperative treatment group underwent an operative procedure on structures other than the cruciate ligaments. Noyes and Barber-Westin[5] also report that the patients in the delayed treatment group had significant symptoms and functional limitations before surgery, whereas none of the seven patients in the acute group had any knee symptoms before their injuries.

Finally, of the 16 studies identified in this review, 9 were published before the year 2000, and the oldest study was published in 1955. It is probable that surgical techniques have evolved and changed sufficiently over time to make it difficult to generalize the findings of older studies to what we might expect today; outcomes may be significantly different with newer surgical techniques compared with those used in the past.

RECOMMENDATIONS

Our systematic review of the literature failed to reveal a sound basis for the treatment algorithms or current "dogma" in caring for patients with multiligament knee injuries. However, methodologic shortcomings of these articles and their potential influence on reported outcomes are clearly related limitations in studying this patient population. The injuries remain relatively rare, and it is estimated that the average orthopedic surgeon will treat only 3 or 4 of these injuries during their entire career. It has been reported that incidence of these injuries is increasing because of several factors, including the expanded definition and the increase in the number of people participating in high-speed, risk-taking sports. Although awareness of multiligament knee injuries has improved dramatically, the definitive management of these complex injuries remains controversial because of the number of ligament injury patterns, varying degrees of concomitant injuries, differing patient function/pain before surgery, as well as the variety of surgical procedures and postsurgical rehabilitation protocols that have been recommended. Thus, it will likely take a much larger multicenter trial to ensure that patient enrollment is sufficient to power a study to be able to draw more definitive conclusions regarding best treatment for these patients. Table 97–4 provides a summary of recommendations.

Conclusion

The timing of surgical management for multiple ligament knee injuries remains controversial. There is a paucity of high-quality literature, and the majority of studies were underpowered. We recommend that larger studies with more rigorous methodology be conducted before definitive conclusions are made.

TABLE 97–4. Summary of Recommendations

STATEMENT	LEVEL OF EVIDENCE	GRADE OF RECOMMENDATION
1. In general, across a variety of outcomes, surgical intervention provides superior results versus conservative treatment after multiligament knee injury.	III	C
2. Early surgical reconstruction after multiligament knee injury (within 3 weeks) does NOT improve outcome versus delayed reconstruction.	III	C

REFERENCES

1. O'Donoghue DH: An analysis of end results of surgical treatment of major injuries to the ligaments of the knee. J Bone Joint Surg Am 37-A:1–13, 1955.
2. Karataglis D, Bisbinas I, Green MA, Learmonth DJ: Functional outcome following reconstruction in chronic multiple ligament deficient knees. Knee Surg Sports Traumatol Arthrosc 14:843–847, 2006.
3. Liow RY, McNicholas MJ, Keating JF, Nutton RW: Ligament repair and reconstruction in traumatic dislocation of the knee. J Bone Joint Surg Br 85:845–851, 2003.
4. Wascher DC, Becker JR, Dexter JG, Blevins FT: Reconstruction of the anterior and posterior cruciate ligaments after knee dislocation. Results using fresh-frozen nonirradiated allografts. Am J Sports Med 27:189–196, 1999.
5. Noyes FR, Barber-Westin SD: Reconstruction of the anterior and posterior cruciate ligaments after knee dislocation. Use of early protected postoperative motion to decrease arthrofibrosis. Am J Sports Med 25:769–778, 1997.
6. Harner CD, Waltrip RL, Bennett CH, et al: Surgical management of knee dislocations. J Bone Joint Surg Am 86:262–273, 2004.
7. Mariani PP, Margheritini F, Camillieri G: One-stage arthroscopically assisted anterior and posterior cruciate ligament reconstruction. Arthroscopy 17:700–707, 2001.
8. Anonymous: The Newcastle-Ottawa Scale (NOS). Assessing the quality of non-randomized studies in meta-analysis. Proceedings of the the 3rd Symposium on Systematic Reviews: Beyond the Basics-Improving Quality and Impact. Oxford, St. Catherine's College, July 2000.
9. Kocher MS, Steadman JR, Briggs KK, et al: Reliability, validity, and responsiveness of the Lysholm knee scale for various chondral disorders of the knee. J Bone Joint Surg Am 86-A:1139–1145, 2004.
10. Irrgang JJ, Ho H, Harner CD, Fu FH: Use of the International Knee Documentation Committee guidelines to assess outcome following anterior cruciate ligament reconstruction. Knee Surg Sports Traumatol Arthrosc 6:107–114, 1998.
11. Meyers MH, Moore TM, Harvey JP Jr: Traumatic dislocation of the knee joint. J Bone Joint Surg Am 57:430–433, 1975.
12. Irrgang JJ, Snyder-Mackler L, Wainner RS, et al: Development of a patient-reported measure of function of the knee. J Bone Joint Surg Am 80:1132–1145, 1998.
13. Mancuso CA, Sculco TP, Wickiewicz TL, et al: Patients' expectations of knee surgery. J Bone Joint Surg Am 83-A:1005–1012, 2001.
14. Kocher MS, Steadman JR, Briggs KK, et al: Reliability, validity, and responsiveness of the Lysholm knee scale for various chondral disorders of the knee. J Bone Joint Surg Am 86-A:1139–1145, 2004.
15. Irrgang JJ, Anderson AF, Boland AL, et al: Development and validation of the international knee documentation committee subjective knee form. Am J Sports Med 29:600–613, 2001.
16. Briggs KK, Kocher MS, Rodkey WG, Steadman JR: Reliability, validity, and responsiveness of the Lysholm knee score and Tegner activity scale for patients with meniscal injury of the knee. J Bone Joint Surg Am 88:698–705, 2006.
17. Hefti F, Muller W, Jakob RP, Staubli HU: Evaluation of knee ligament injuries with the IKDC form. Knee Surg Sports Traumatol Arthrosc 1(3-4):226–234, 1993.
18. Werier J, Keating JF, Meek RN: Complete dislocation of the knee—the long-term results of ligamentous reconstruction. Knee 5:255–260, 1998.
19. Richter M, Bosch U, Wippermann B, et al: Comparison of surgical repair or reconstruction of the cruciate ligaments versus nonsurgical treatment in patients with traumatic knee dislocations. Am J Sports Med 30:718–727, 2002.
20. Rios A, Villa A, Fahandezh J, et al: Results after treatment of traumatic knee dislocations: A report of 26 cases. J Trauma 55:489–494, 2003.
21. Wong CH, Tan JL, Chang HC, et al: Knee dislocations: A retrospective study comparing operative versus closed immobilization treatment outcomes. Knee Surg Sports Traumatol Arthrosc 12:540–544, 2004.
22. Tzurbakis M, Diamantopoulos A, Xenakis T, Georgoulis A: Surgical treatment of multiple knee ligament injuries in 44 patients: 2-8 years follow-up results. Knee Surg Sports Traumatol Arthrosc 14:739–749, 2006.
23. Fanelli GC, Edson CJ, Maish DR: Combined anterior/posterior cruciate ligament/medial/lateral side injuries of the knee. Sports Med Arthrosc 9:208–218, 2001.
24. Almekinders LC, Logan TC: Results following treatment of traumatic dislocations of the knee joint. Clin Orthop Relat Res (284):203–207, 1992.
25. Taylor AR, Arden GP, Rainey HA: Traumatic dislocation of the knee. A report of forty-three cases with special reference to conservative treatment. J Bone Joint Surg Br 54:96–102, 1972.
26. Bandolier on-line. Available at: http://www.jr2.ox.ac.uk/bandolier/aboutus.html. Accessed June 27, 2007.
27. Haynes RB, Sackett DL, Guyatt GH, Tugwell P: Clinical Epidemiology: How to Do Clinical Practice Research, 3rd ed. New York, Lippincott Williams & Wilkins, 2006.

Chapter 98

Should First-Time Shoulder Dislocators Be Stabilized Surgically?

Daniel Whelan, MD, MSc, FRCS(C)

DEFINING THE PROBLEM

The shoulder is a versatile complex of joints with a large functional range of motion. However, stability is sacrificed for this freedom of movement. The glenohumeral joint is a loosely opposed "ball-and-socket" type joint, and as such is the most commonly dislocated large joint in the body. The lifetime incidence of anterior shoulder dislocation has been reported to be 1% to 2% in the general population.[1,2] Recurrent instability after primary dislocation is a common problem.

After initial reduction of the joint, the traditional treatment for primary shoulder dislocations has been immobilization in a sling, with the arm in a position of adduction and internal rotation. The length of the immobilization period is controversial. A common recommendation is for 3 to 6 weeks in a sling to allow for early capsular healing followed by several months of rehabilitation including range-of-motion and strengthening exercises. Some authors have recommended abbreviated periods of immobilization, as short as 1 week, followed by early institution of therapy to promote restoration of a full range of motion.

The clinical course of patients after nonsurgical treatment has been investigated extensively. Of particular interest is the relatively high rate of recurrent instability in young patients. Estimates of the recurrence rate in this group have been reported to be anywhere between 17% and 96%.[2–10]

The anatomic abnormality associated with the majority of traumatic shoulder dislocations is the Bankart lesion—an avulsion of the anterior glenoid labrum and shoulder joint capsule at the insertion of the inferior glenohumeral ligament. The anterior capsulolabral complex is thought to be the major stabilizer of the shoulder to anterior subluxation. The frequency of recurrence, therefore, is postulated to be related to failure of this complex to heal in an anatomic position. Proponents of acute arthroscopic Bankart repair have emphasized that it is the ability to directly oppose and secure the lesion to its anatomic position at surgery that imparts immediate stability versus nonoperative methods. Early series of arthroscopic treatment of shoulder instability have shown it to be an effective modality in decreasing recurrence.[11,12]

Despite evidence in favor of arthroscopic stabilization, uncertainty still exists among the orthopedic community as to optimal timing of surgical intervention.[13,14] The cost, risk, and anxiety associated with surgery have caused some surgeons to adopt a strategy of "watchful neglect," allowing patients to demonstrate recurrent episodes of instability or dislocation before proceeding with an operative solution. Furthermore, although early surgery has the potential to result in a number of patients avoiding redislocation in the short term, the long-term functional benefits over a conservative approach are less well known.

This chapter attempts, via an evidence-based approach, to address whether early surgical intervention improves outcome after a primary shoulder dislocation. For the most part, this is a narrative overview of published investigations that describe results after conservative or arthroscopic treatments, or both, for first-time anterior shoulder dislocations. For the purposes of this review, the studies were divided into three categories: those reports describing primarily nonsurgical treatments, those describing arthroscopic treatments, and those designed as prospective comparative cohorts and/or randomized trials utilizing both surgical and nonsurgical treatment arms.

The specific patient population of interest for the review was young patients (<40 years old) who had sustained first-time, traumatic, anterior dislocations of the glenohumeral joint. These patients represent a group at high risk for recurrent dislocation and in whom treatment decisions are controversial. Studies pertaining to the methods of and issues regarding the reduction of shoulder dislocations were excluded. Also excluded were those investigations that included (or whose primary focus was) recurrent shoulder dislocations/instability, atraumatic dislocations, posterior dislocations, and multidirectionally unstable patients.

The concept of symptomatic recurrent instability merits further clarification. For the purposes of this review, patients were considered to have recurrent instability if the patient had sustained a subsequent (documented) dislocation or if the patient sought surgical intervention for symptoms of instability and/or subluxation, (but not necessarily dislocation) which he or she felt was intolerable. This definition excludes those patients who may have demonstrated clinical findings consistent with instability (most notably a positive apprehension test) but who did not wish to proceed with further intervention.

There were 43 potentially relevant study titles. More studies were identified secondarily on the basis of bibliographical reviews and hand searches of proceedings. Application of the study eligibility criteria eliminated 11 of the original titles, with 32 articles remaining for review: 13 describe primarily nonsurgical management, 9 describe arthroscopic interventions, 4 are observational studies that include the results for both surgically and nonsurgically treated patients, and 6 are randomized trials.

NONSURGICAL STUDIES

The natural history—or clinical course in the absence of active treatment (whether it be surgical or rehabilitative)—after anterior dislocation of the shoulder has been investigated extensively. Reports dating to the early part of the twentieth century highlight the recurrent nature of the problem.

In those reports predating 1990, retrospective (Level II, III, and IV) studies predominate.[4-6] These series are subject to the limitations of bias and confounding inherent in any investigation that relies on retrospectively collected data. Furthermore, most of these series include both primary and recurrent dislocators in the study sample. Perhaps the largest early series is that of Rowe and colleagues,[4] which reports on 488 patients with shoulder dislocations seen at Massachusetts General Hospital during the 20-year period from 1934 to 1954. Of the entire group, 398 (82%) were patients with primary dislocations with the remainder being recurrent. No information is provided as to immobilization or rehabilitative protocols prescribed for these patients. Although the inclusion of patients with recurrent instability makes it difficult to draw specific inferences on those patients with primary instability, Rowe was the first to document a relatively high recurrence rate (38%) after primary dislocation in a large series and to make conjectures about possible prognostic factors for recurrence including young age at initial dislocation and traumatic cause. Age was identified as the strongest single prognostic factor, with 83% of those patients younger than 20 years going on to further instability episodes.

In more recent investigations, there has been conflicting information as to the rate of recurrent instability and the optimum nonsurgical management. Henry and Genung[7] reported on a group of 121 first-time dislocators that was also reviewed retrospectively (Level II). A rate of recurrence of 85% to 90% was noted in these patients within 18 months of the injury; this was significantly greater than the previous reports of Rowe and others.[4] All patients in that study were younger than 32. Half of the group was immobilized in a sling for a variable period. Although randomization was not performed, equivalent rates of recurrent instability in immobilized and nonimmobilized patients led the authors to conclude that immobilization was of little benefit in reducing recurrence. Another Level III retrospective series of 124 patients by Simonet and Cofield[8] reports a lower overall rate of recurrence (33%), but again stresses the importance of age as a risk factor with more than 50% of

those patients younger than 40 years experiencing further instability.

Controversy as to the optimal rehabilitation program after first-time dislocation was introduced by both Aronen and Regan,[9] as well as Yoneda and co-workers,[10] who reported seemingly lower recurrence rates of 25% and 17.3%, respectively, with aggressive physical therapy. The former of these investigations was prospectively conducted on a small cohort of young male military cadets (*n* = 20)—a recognized "high-demand" population (Level IV). The authors used a rigorous rehabilitation protocol. Despite the fact that this protocol was described in detail, subsequent studies utilizing it on a similar population have failed to replicate the results.[11]

A prospective, multicenter cohort study was initiated in 1978 in a Swedish population (Level II). The results of this cohort have been published at 2-, 5-, and 10-year follow-up.[15-17] The group of 247 primary dislocations in patients between the ages of 12 and 40 years were quasi-randomized (on the basis of even or odd date of injury) to receive one of three methods of conservative treatment: sling and swathe for 3 weeks, sling for 1 week followed by restricted range of motion, or a "mixed" treatment for patients believed to be unfit for either of the first two arms. No significant differences were found in the rate of recurrent dislocations at 10 years after injury among the three groups. Overall, approximately 50% of the patients had experienced symptoms of instability at 10-year follow-up. Young age was again put forth as the single strongest predictor for recurrence. The presence of an associated fracture of the greater tuberosity was identified as protective. No association between recurrent instability and sex, handedness, or side of dislocation was identified. This Level I prognostic study represents the highest current level of evidence available regarding the natural history of anterior shoulder dislocations with long-term, prospectively collected data. This study has an impressively low loss to follow-up (3%) over the 10-year course.

A recently published study has suggested that immobilizing acutely dislocated shoulders in a position of relative external rotation reduced subsequent dislocation rates.[18] In a quasi-randomized prospective trial (Level II), Itoi and coauthors[18] demonstrate a 0% recurrence rate in 20 patients immobilized in external rotation versus a 30% recurrence rate in 20 patients immobilized in a sling at a mean follow-up of 15.5 months. Several randomized clinical trials are ongoing in Canada, the United States, and Australia to test this concept in a young at-risk population. The characteristics of the nonoperative studies are outlined in Table 98–1.

Arthroscopic Studies

The appearance in the literature of studies that address arthroscopic stabilization as a primary treatment modality for acute shoulder dislocations has been a relatively recent phenomenon. Before the

TABLE 98–1. Nonsurgical Management of Primary Dislocations: Study Characteristics

INVESTIGATION (YEAR OF PUBLICATION)	N	STUDY DESCRIPTION	LEVEL OF EVIDENCE	RECURRENCE RATE (%)
McGlaughlin and Cavallaro (1950)[5]	573	Retrospective series (primary and recurrent dislocators included)	II	50
Rowe (1956)[4]	398	Retrospective series (primary and recurrent dislocators included)	II	38*
Kazar and Relovsky (1969)[1]	760	Retrospective series (primary and recurrent dislocators included)	II	27
Kiviluoto et al. (1980)[6]	226	Retrospective series (primary and recurrent dislocators included)	IV	13*†
Henry and Genung (1982)[7]	121	Retrospective (primary dislocators); variable protocols; no immobilization (51%), slings with or without swathes (49%)	IV	88 (<32 yr)*
Simonet and Cofield (1984)[8]	124	Retrospective; 82% immobilized for average 3 weeks	IV	33
Aronen and Regan (1984)[9]	20	Prospective (therapeutic) cohort; sling × 3 weeks, THEN structured rehabilitation	IV	25 (all <22 yr)
Yoneda et al. (1982)[10]	104	Retrospective; sling and swathe × 5 weeks, THEN graduated ROM	IV	17.3 (average, 21 yr)
Hovelius (1987)[16]	257	Prospective (prognostic) cohort; sling × 1 week (52%) vs. sling and swathe 3 weeks	II	44*
Hoelen et al. (1990)[3]	168	Not specified		26
Kralinger et al. (2002)[19]	180	Sling × 3 weeks, no ER > 0 × 6 weeks, therapy		29.4
Itoi et al. (2003)[18]	40	Quasi-randomized trial; ER brace × 3 weeks vs. sling × 3 weeks	I	ER brace: 0 sling: 30
teSlaa et al. (2004)[20]	105	Unspecified (retrospective)	IV	26

*No difference in rate of recurrence for immobilized versus nonimmobilized patients.
†56% in patients <20 years; greater frequency of redislocation with *shorter* period of immobilization.
ER, external rotation.

advent of arthroscopy, operative management was usually considered only after a patient had demonstrated symptomatic recurrent instability. Arthroscopic stabilization has become increasingly popular for the treatment of shoulder instability because it offers potential advantages over formal open techniques including improved cosmesis, superior intra-articular visualization, and minimized disruption of the anterior soft tissues. Specifically, in the setting of a primary dislocation, the decreased morbidity offered by the arthroscopic approach—combined with the acuity of the Bankart lesion and its amenability to repair in this state—have made it an especially attractive option to surgeons who recognize the potential for recurrent instability with traditional nonoperative treatments.

The risk for recurrence after arthroscopic stabilization has been reported in several series, which are summarized in Table 98–2. Unfortunately, few reports distinguish between acute and recurrent dislocations

when presenting the results of these primarily retrospective series. In addition, a variety of different arthroscopic stabilization techniques is used in these studies, each with its own associated surgical "learning curve" and spectrum of complications. Identifying surgical complications and deriving estimates of patient satisfaction (beyond recurrence) from historical chart review is problematic. Keeping this in mind, it would still seem that the incidence of recurrent instability is tangibly reduced with early arthroscopic repair. Inferences beyond that are difficult.

Early *diagnostic* arthroscopy without stabilization has also been suggested to be useful in reducing the rate of recurrent shoulder instability. In two prospective studies, patients underwent arthroscopic lavage only.[21,22] The rationale for this procedure was both diagnostic and therapeutic. In removing intra-articular clot and debris, investigators suggest acute arthroscopic lavage allows the Bankart lesion to heal in

TABLE 98–2. Acute Arthroscopic Management of Primary Dislocations: Study Characteristics

INVESTIGATION (YEAR OF PUBLICATION)	N	STUDY DESCRIPTION	LEVEL OF EVIDENCE	RECURRENCE RATE (%)
Wheeler et al. (1989)[11]	9	Retrospective case series; staple capsulorraphy	IV	22
Uribe and Hechtman (1993)[12]	11	Retrospective case series; transglenoid sutures	IV	9
Arciero et al. (1995)[24]	25	Retrospective case series; bioabsorbable tacks	IV	5
Mole et al. (1996)[21]	21	Retrospective case series; arthroscopic lavage	IV	28.5
Salmon and Bell (1998)[25a]	17	Retrospective case series; transglenoid sutures	IV	17
Valentin et al. (1998)[25]	15	Retrospective case series; transglenoid sutures	IV	13
Boszotta and Helperstorfer (2000)[26]	72	Retrospective case series; transglenoid sutures	IV	6.9
teSlaa et al. (1995)[22]*	31	Retrospective case series; arthroscopic lavage	IV	55
Pienovi et al. (2003)[27]	31	Retrospective case series; transglenoid sutures	IV	12.9

*Investigation reported in abstract only.

an anatomically reduced position. Mole and colleagues[21] performed arthroscopic lavage on 30 patients within 4 days of an initial dislocation. Of the 21 (70%) patients available for follow-up at 24 months, 6 (28.5%) developed recurrent instability. teSlaa and co-workers[20] performed arthroscopy on 31 patients within 10 days of a first-time dislocation. At 5-year follow-up, 12 patients (38.7%) had sustained a recurrent dislocation, and a total of 17 patients (55%) had described at least 1 episode of symptomatic subluxation during the study period. From the results of this study, and that of Mole and colleagues,[21] the evidence of benefit with isolated arthroscopic lavage would seem to be weak.

Surgical complications were infrequent in the arthroscopic series reviewed. Traditionally, the rate of reported complications in large series of arthroscopic stabilizations for *recurrent* instability has also been low.[23] Complications were generally of low morbidity, ranging from stiffness (mildly decreased external rotation >30 degrees) in the involved shoulder to a surgical infection ($n = 1$) requiring repeat debridement and intravenous antibiotics. The overall complication rate for all the arthroscopic stabilizations reviewed was less than 1%. This is consistent with previous reports of complications after similar procedures for recurrent glenohumeral instability.[23]

Further characteristics of the arthroscopic series included in this review are presented in Table 98–2. Over time, recurrence rates have generally decreased without a corresponding increase in the incidence of complications. This is due in part to the increasing familiarity of surgeons with arthroscopic procedures, as well as refinements of the technique and equipment. Methods utilizing suture anchors are now the standard because the anterior labrum can be most securely approximated in an anatomic fashion with these devices.

COMPARATIVE STUDIES

Nonrandomized (Observational) Studies

In an effort to improve the quality of evidence in favor of acute arthroscopic stabilization, prospective trials were initiated at several U.S. military academies.[28,29] Investigators from these institutions had previously published series of both conservatively and arthroscopically treated first-time dislocations and were,

in their own words, biased to the merits of the arthroscopic approach. In separate trials, Wheeler[11] and Deberardino[29] prospectively evaluated cohorts of patients, all male military cadets, who were allowed to choose between conservative or arthroscopic treatment. Similarly, a recent Turkish study reports on 2 groups of arthroscopically stabilized and conservatively treated attendees at a military academy.[30] Again, these patients were allowed to choose their own treatment. All of these trials demonstrate a strong benefit with arthroscopic stabilization in limiting subsequent symptomatic instability. Inferences as to the true benefit of arthroscopy, however, are weakened by the potential for selection bias in the absence of randomization. A fourth prospective study, this one conducted on South American rugby players, reiterates the finding of significantly lower incidence of symptomatic instability with surgical intervention.[31] All the aforementioned investigations, although observational, have significance in the literature because they introduced the concept of acute surgical stabilization of the dislocated shoulder as a viable treatment alternative, thereby paving the way for the randomized trials that were to come. The characteristics of comparative, non-randomized investigations are discussed in Table 98–3.

Randomized Studies

Criticism fell on the aforementioned military trials both for failure to randomize and for a lack of generalizability. The military cadet population was seen as an extremely high-demand group of patients whose significant risk for recurrent instability may not reflect that seen in the general civilian population. A randomized trial was subsequently conducted in a military population. Bottoni and colleagues[32] reported the results of 24 cadets quasi-randomly allocated (on the basis of social insurance number) to receive arthroscopic stabilization ($n = 14$) versus nonoperative treatment ($n = 10$). Of those patients available for follow-up at an average of 36 months from the time of dislocation, recurrent instability was seen in 75% of the nonoperative group as compared with only 11% (1/9) of the arthroscopic group. Unequal group sizes may reflect the strictly nonrandom nature of treatment allocation.

TABLE 98–3. Comparative, Nonrandomized Investigations: Study Characteristics

INVESTIGATION (YEAR OF PUBLICATION)	N (n groups)	STUDY DESCRIPTION	LEVEL OF EVIDENCE	RECURRENCE RATE (%)†
Arciero et al. (1994)[28]	36 (15 C, 21 A)	Prospective (therapeutic) cohort study; sling × 4 weeks vs. arthroscopic staple	II	Sling: 80 Arthroscopy: 14
DeBerardino et al. (2001)[29]	54 (6 C, 48 A)	Prospective (therapeutic) cohort study; sling × 3 weeks vs. arthroscopic tack	II	Sling: 67 Arthroscopy: 12
Larrain et al. (2001)[31]	46 (18 C, 28 A)	Prospective (therapeutic) cohort study; sling × 3 weeks vs. transglenoid sutures or anchors	II	Sling: 96 Arthroscopy: 4
Yanmis et al. (2003)[30]	62 (32 C, 30 A)	Prospective (therapeutic) cohort study; sling × 3 weeks vs. arthroscopic tack	II	Sling: 38 Arthroscopy: 0

A, arthroscopic stabilization; C, conservative therapy.

TABLE 98–4. Comparative, Randomized Investigations: Study Characteristics

INVESTIGATION (YEAR OF PUBLICATION)	N (n groups)	STUDY DESCRIPTION	LEVEL OF EVIDENCE	RECURRENCE RATE (%)
Sandow (1995)[33]	20 (10 C, 10 A)	Randomized trial; sling × 4 weeks vs. arthroscopic tacks	I	C: 50 A: 10
Jakobsen et al. (2007)[34]	76 (39 C, 37 A)	Randomized trial; sling × 1 week vs. *open* stabilization	I	C: 51 A: 3
Wintzell et al. (1999)[35]	30 (15 C, 15 A)	Randomized trial; immediate vs. arthroscopic lavage	I	C: 60 A: 20
Bottoni et al. (2002)[32]	24 (12 C, 9 A)	Randomized trial; sling × 4 weeks vs. arthroscopic tacks	I	C: 75 A: 11
Kirkley et al. (1999)[36]	40 (21 C, 19 A)	Randomized trial; sling × 3 weeks vs. arthroscopic transglenoid sutures	I	C: 47 A: 16

A, arthroscopic stabilization; C, conservative therapy.

Two other randomized investigations comparing surgical interventions with conservative treatment for primary shoulder dislocators have been conducted. Sandow[33] has provisionally reported on 20 patients, all of whom were younger than 26 years, randomized to receive arthroscopic stabilization with a bioabsorbable tack versus sling immobilization for 4 weeks. Recurrence was significantly lower in the surgical group with only 1 of 10 patients demonstrating symptomatic instability (10%) versus 5 of 10 (50%) in the sling group. In the only investigation that included patients who underwent acute open stabilization, Jakobsen and coworkers[34] also found a significantly lower rate of redislocation with patients randomized to surgery (1/37; 2.7%) versus those immobilized in a sling for 1 week followed by therapy (20/39; 51%). This randomized trial includes prospectively collected data out to 10 years after dislocation.

On the suggestion that arthroscopic lavage may reduce recurrence, Wintzell and researchers[35] conducted a randomized trial to compare this treatment with sling immobilization. Arthroscopic lavage was performed within 10 days of dislocation in 15 patients. Another 15 patients (with no specific randomization scheme described) were given an optional sling for 1 week and encouraged to move the shoulder freely. At the 2-year follow-up examination, 3 (20%) of the patients in the lavage group had redislocated versus 9 (60%) in the nonoperative group.

Kirkley and coworkers[36] performed a randomized clinical trial on civilian patients. Forty patients younger than 30 years were allocated, on the basis of a permuted block, computer-generated, randomization scheme, to receive sling immobilization (n = 21) or undergo acute arthroscopic stabilization (n = 19) after first-time dislocation. The rate of recurrence at the 2-year follow-up was significantly lower in the arthroscopic group (47% vs. 15.9%). This study had few, if any, deficiencies with its design or analysis and remains the highest level of evidence in support of early arthroscopic stabilization to reduce recurrence. Secondary outcomes included validated general and disease-specific quality-of-life measurement tools. A preliminary analysis of patient-based outcomes at 2-year follow-up suggested a statistically higher level of function in those patients who underwent early arthroscopy. The *clinical* significance of the 15% difference in disease-specific outcome at final follow-up favoring the patients treated arthroscopically is unclear. This is due in part to the relative "newness" of the outcome measure used and the fact that function was considered a secondary outcome (therefore, the study may not have been adequately powered to show a clinically significant difference in function). Nonetheless, the results have important implications. If acute arthroscopy serves only to reduce early recurrence rates, with no significant long-term functional benefit, then an approach that optimizes conservative treatment may provide the greatest overall benefit to patients, whereas simultaneously limiting potential complications. The characteristics of all the comparative and/or randomized investigations are summarized in Table 98–4.

For the purposes of statistical pooling, weights were assigned to each study on the basis of sample size. A relative risk estimate of 0.35 (95% confidence interval, 0.18–0.65) confirms a strong benefit, based on the highest level of available evidence, with early arthroscopic treatments in reducing the risk for recurrent shoulder instability after first-time dislocation. None of the randomized studies identified any significant limitations in range of motion or strength after arthroscopic procedures. Unfortunately, each of the randomized trials identified used different outcome tools to report functional status or health-related quality of life, or both, thereby precluding a formal synthesis of the data. Only one perioperative complication, a septic joint after arthroscopic stabilization, was reported in the combined populations of the three trials (n = 89) for an overall complication rate of 1.1%.

CONCLUSIONS

Prognosis after First-Time Dislocation

The true rate of recurrent instability after primary anterior glenohumeral dislocation remains imprecise, with series reporting estimates that range from 17% to 90%. With few exceptions, most reports would suggest the rate of recurrent dislocation or symptomatic subluxation, or both, in young patients approaches 50%. Greater rates have been demonstrated in series with larger proportions of younger patients, males, and active military recruits. Even in the absence of recurrent instability, prospectively collected, disease-specific, health-related quality-of-life data suggest patients demonstrate prolonged functional deficits after a primary dislocation.[37] Age has been repeatedly demonstrated as the most significant prognostic factor in predicting recurrence. Recently, teSlaa and coworkers[20] have attempted to quantify this risk based on the odds ratio of recurrence with various age distributions. They suggest the risk for recurrence decreases by a factor of 0.09 (9%) with each additional year of patient age at the time of initial dislocation.

The presence of associated fractures was of variable prognostic significance in the development of recurrent instability. Fractures of the greater tuberosity seem to impart a protective effect that is independent of age and the degree of shoulder stiffness (associated with fracture immobilization).[19] Fractures of the humeral head (Hill–Sachs lesion) and anterior glenoid rim (the bony Bankart lesion) are suggested to increase the risk for recurrence; however, the difficulty of diagnosing and quantifying these lesions, particularly in retrospective studies, has made a definitive association elusive.

Interestingly, neither activity level nor participation in sports has been definitively shown to be associated with an increased risk for recurrence. Similarly, associations have not been demonstrated with recurrence rate and sex, side of dislocation, or hand dominance. The presence of generalized ligamentous laxity or hypermobility has not previously been investigated for an association with recurrent instability after a primary dislocation.

Role of Nonoperative Treatment

The optimal conservative management strategy after first-time shoulder dislocation remains unknown. Rehabilitation strategies have generally not been effective in reducing the rate of recurrent instability. Aronen and Reagan's[9] and Yoneda and coworkers'[10] reports, which describe recurrence rates on the order of 20%, are seemingly anomalous. Similarly, traditional immobilization devices such as a sling and/or sling and swathe have not altered the natural history after first-time dislocation. A relatively large prospective cohort with long-term follow-up (Level I prognostic evidence) has demonstrated equivalent recurrence rates with sling immobilization versus early range of motion and therapy.[17] Preliminary results from a small randomized trial have suggested merit in a novel immobilization strategy positioning the affected limb in external rotation.[18]

Role of Arthroscopy

The optimal arthroscopic technique has yet to be determined. Recent advances have included the use of suture anchors, a more anatomic approach to reconstructing the Bankart lesion, and improved surgical instrumentation to make the surgery less technically demanding. These advances, together with more clearly defined operative indications, have realized decreasing recurrence rates in more recent series describing acute arthroscopic stabilizations. Currently, there are limited data to support the use of acute arthroscopic lavage without stabilization.

A dramatic benefit was demonstrated with early open or arthroscopic stabilization in reducing recurrence rate after acute dislocations.[34,36] Several questions remain to be answered, however. The presence or absence of recurrent instability cannot be considered an appropriate surrogate for functional outcome. Patients may not experience a subsequent dislocation solely because of discontinuation of the activities that put them at risk. This point underpins the importance of assessing patient function as a primary outcome when conducting future investigations. The lack of a universally accepted, instability-specific outcome tool has made this difficult in the past. The introduction of the Western Ontario Shoulder Instability Index (WOSI), a tool with proven reliability, responsiveness, and validity, may make the assessment of patient-based functional outcomes after dislocation more consistent in the future.[38]

Debate over the role of early arthroscopy continues in the orthopedic community. Despite the relatively high level of evidence in support of this approach, some surgeons remain reluctant to expose patients to the risk, cost, and anxiety of surgery after a single dislocation episode. Kirkley and coworkers'[38] trial demonstrates that, although arthroscopy definitively reduces recurrence in the short term, functional benefits may not be as substantial. If we assume that function is not significantly improved with arthroscopy, then methods to reduce recurrence with nonoperative treatment may be the best approach. Itoi and coauthors'[18] trial suggests immobilization of the affected shoulder in a position of external rotation may be one such method.

As with any systematic review, the strength of inference is only as good as the quality of the primary studies and the scientific rigor with which the review was conducted. Meta-analyses that pool data from nonrandomized studies are subject to all of the limitations of the primary studies. Thus, combining the results of nonrandomized studies may result in a biased pooled estimate of effect that reflects the biases inherent to the observational studies.[39] The estimates of treatment effect described in the current review were generated from pooling only randomized investigations and, therefore, may be more reflective of the true benefits imparted by early arthroscopic intervention over traditional nonoperative methods.

The Cochrane group has published a review of surgical versus nonsurgical treatments for acute anterior shoulder dislocations (January 2004). The current review and the published Cochrane review were conducted independently and are similar in their findings with respect to the benefit of acute arthroscopic stabilization. Whereas the scope of the current review is broad, including all literature on the orthopedic management of primary shoulder dislocations, the Cochrane review has included only five randomized investigations that directly compare surgical versus nonsurgical interventions.[40]

Implications for Practice

Symptomatic recurrent instability after first-time anterior shoulder dislocation can be significantly reduced with early arthroscopic stabilization. The improvements in long-term quality of life and shoulder function after arthroscopic stabilization are uncertain.

Implications for Research

Although early arthroscopic intervention reduces recurrence, it may be that arthroscopic lavage without stabilization is sufficient. A randomized investi-

gation comparing arthroscopic lavage versus lavage with stabilization is indicated to resolve this issue.

There is relatively good evidence to suggest that modifications in the conservative treatment of primary traumatic anterior shoulder dislocation, specifically immobilization of the affected shoulder in external rotation, may improve on historically reported recurrence rates. Furthermore, this approach may provide equivalent functional outcomes without exposing patients to the risk, anxiety, and cost of surgery.

Future trials comparing arthroscopic and conservative treatments for first-time shoulder dislocation must include validated functional outcome measures as primary end points and be planned with a priori sample sizes sufficient to demonstrate clinically important differences in these outcomes. Such trials would optimally be conducted on groups of patients from the general population (vs. military or other homogenous populations) to improve the generalizability of the inferences that can be made. Table 98–5 provides a summary of recommendations.

TABLE 98–5. Summary of Recommendations

STATEMENT	LEVEL OF EVIDENCE	GRADE OF RECOMMENDATION
1. Recurrent instability after primary anterior shoulder dislocation is common. Age is a strong prognostic indicator for recurrence. Greater tuberosity fractures may be protective.[17]	I: Good evidence	NA
2. Arthroscopic stabilization after a primary anterior shoulder dislocation reduces episodes of recurrent instability versus sling immobilization.[36]	I: Good evidence	A
3. Open stabilization after primary anterior shoulder dislocation reduces episodes of recurrent instability versus nonoperative treatment.[34]	I: Good evidence	A
4. Arthroscopic stabilization after primary anterior shoulder dislocation improves functional outcome scores at early postoperative follow-up (<24 months); long-term benefits are unknown.[37]	I: Good Evidence	A
5. Immobilization of the affected shoulder in a position of external rotation after primary anterior shoulder dislocation reduces episodes of recurrent instability versus traditional sling immobilization.[18]	II: Fair evidence	B
6. Arthroscopic lavage immediately after primary anterior shoulder dislocation reduces episodes of recurrent instability versus sling immobilization.[35]	II: Fair evidence	B
7. Sling immobilization for up to 3 weeks after primary anterior shoulder dislocation likely does *not* reduce episodes of recurrent instability versus early motion rehabilitation protocols.[17]	II: Fair evidence	B

NA, not applicable

REFERENCES

1. Kazar B, Relovsky E: Prognosis of primary dislocations of the shoulder. Acta Orthop Scand 40:216–224, 1969.
2. Hovelius L: Incidence of shoulder dislocations in Sweden. Clin Orthop Relat Res (166):127–131, 1982.
3. Hoelen MA, Burgers AMJ, Rozing PM: Prognosis of primary anterior shoulder dislocation in young adults. Arch Orthop Trauma Surg 110:51, 1990.
4. Rowe CR: Prognosis in dislocations of the shoulder. J Bone Joint Surg [Am] 38-A:957–977, 1956.
5. McGlaughlin HL, Cavallaro WU: Primary anterior dislocation of the shoulder. Am J Surg 80:615, 1950.
6. Kiviluoto O, Pasila M, Sundholm JA: Immobilization after primary dislocation of the shoulder. Acta Orthop Scand 51:915, 1980.
7. Henry JH, Genung JA: Natural history of glenohumeral dislocation revisited. Am J Sports Med 10:135–137, 1982.
8. Simonet WT, Cofield RH: Prognosis in anterior shoulder dislocation. Am J Sports Med 12:19–21, 1984.
9. Aronen JG, Regan K: Decreasing the incidence of recurrence of first time anterior shoulder dislocations with rehabilitation. Am J Sports Med 12:283–291, 1984.
10. Yoneda B, Webb RP, MacIntosh DL: Conservative treatment of shoulder dislocations in young males. J Bone Joint Surg Br 64-B:254, 1982.
11. Wheeler JH, Ryan JB, Arciero RA, Molinari RN: Arthroscopic versus nonoperative treatment of acute shoulder dislocations in young athletes. Arthroscopy 5:213–217, 1989.
12. Uribe JW, Hechtman KS: Arthroscopically assisted repair of acute bankart lesion. Orthopedics 16:1019–1023, 1993.
13. Arciero RA: Acute arthroscopic bankart repair? Knee Surg Sports Traumatol Arthrosc 8:127–128, 2000.
14. Eriksson E: Should first-time traumatic shoulder dislocations undergo an acute stabilization procedure? Knee Surg Sports Traumatol Arthrosc 11:61–62, 2003.

15. Hovelius L, Eriksson K, Fredin H, et al: Recurrences after initial dislocation of the shoulder. J Bone Joint Surg Am 65-A:343–349, 1983.

16. Hovelius L: Anterior dislocation of the shoulder in teenagers and young adults: Five year prognosis. J Bone Joint Surg Am 69-A:393–399, 1987.

17. Hovelius L, Augustini BG, Fredin H, et al: Primary anterior dislocation of the shoulder in young patients: A ten year prospective study. J Bone Joint Surg Am 78-A:1677–1684, 1996.

18. Itoi E, Hatakeyama Y, Kido T, et al: A new method of immobilization after traumatic anterior dislocation of the shoulder: A preliminary study. J Shouler Elbow Surg 12:413–416, 2003.

19. Kralinger FS, Golser K, Wischatta R, et al: Predicting recurrence after primary shoulder dislocation. Am J Sport Med 30:116–120, 2002.

20. teSlaa RL, Wijffels PJM, Brand R, Marti K: The prognosis following acute primary glenohumeral dislocation. J Bone Joint Surg Br 86-B:58–64, 2004.

21. Mole D, Coudane H, Rio B, et al: The role of arthroscopy during the first episode of anteromedial luxation of the shoulder: Lesion assessment and recurrence factors. J Traumatol Sport 13:20–24, 1996.

22. teSlaa RL, Ritt M, Jansen BRH: A prospective arthroscopic study of acute initial anterior shoulder dislocation in the young [abstract]. Proceedings of the Sixth International Conference on Surgery of the Shoulder. Helsinki, June 1995.

23. Green MR, Christensen MD: Arthroscopic versus open Bankart procedures: A comparison of early morbidity and complications. Arthroscopy 9:371–374, 1993.

24. Arciero RA, Taylor DC, Snyder RJ, et al: Arthroscopic bioabsorbable tack stabilization of initial anterior shoulder dislocations: A preliminary report. Arthroscopy 11:410–417, 1995.

25. Valentin A, Winge S, Engstrom B: Early arthroscopic treatment of primary anterior shoulder dislocation. A follow-up study. Scand J Med Sci Sports 8:405–410, 1998.

25a. Salmon JM, Bell SN: Arthroscopic stabilization of the shoulder for acute primary dislocations using a transglenoid suture technique. Arthroscopy 14(2):143–147, 1998

26. Boszotta H, Helperstorfer W: Arthroscopic transglenoid suture repair for initial anterior shoulder dislocation. Arthroscopy 16:462–470, 2000.

27. Pienovi A, Quevedo L, Orive AG: Arthroscopic treatment of the first shoulder dislocation [abstract]. AAOS Annual Meeting. New Orleans, 2003.

28. Arciero RA, Wheeler JH, Ryan JB, McBride JT: Arthroscopic Bankart repair versus nonoperative treatment for acute, initial anterior shoulder dislocations. Am J Sports Med 22:589–594, 1994.

29. DeBerardino TM, Arciero RA, Taylor DC, Uhorchak JM: Prospective evaluation of arthroscopic stabilization of acute, initial anterior shoulder dislocations in young athletes. Am J Sports Med 29:586–592, 2001.

30. Yanmis I, Tunay S, Komurcu M, et al: The outcomes of acute arthroscopic repair and conservative treatment following first traumatic dislocation of the shoulder joint in young patients. Ann Acad Med Singapore 32:824–827, 2003.

31. Larrain MV, Botto GJ, Montenegro HJ, et al: Arthroscopic repair of acute traumatic anterior shoulder dislocations in young athletes. Arthroscopy 17:373–377, 2001.

32. Bottoni CR, Wilckens JH, DeBerardino TM, et al: A prospective, randomized evaluation of arthroscopic stabilization versus nonoperative treatment in patients with acute, traumatic, first-time shoulder dislocations. Am J Sports Med 30:576–580, 2002.

33. Sandow MJ: Arthroscopic repair for primary shoulder dislocation: A randomized clinical trial. J Bone Joint Surg Br 77-B:(supp I):67, 1995.

34. Jakobsen BW, Johannsen HV, Suder P, Søjbjerg JO: Primary repair versus conservative treatment of first-time traumatic anterior dislocation of the shoulder: A randomized study with 10-year follow-up. Arthroscopy 23:118–123, 2007.

35. Wintzell G, Haglund-Akerlind Y, Nowak J, et al: Arthroscopic lavage with nonoperative treatment for traumatic primary anterior shoulder dislocation: A two-year follow-up of a prospective randomized study. J Shoulder Elbow Surg 8:399–402, 1999.

36. Kirkley A, Griffen S, Richards C, et al: Prospective randomized clinical trial comparing the effectiveness of immediate arthroscopic stabilization versus immobilization and rehabilitation in first traumatic anterior dislocation of the shoulder. Arthroscopy 15:507–514, 1999.

37. Kirkley A, Werstine R, Ratjek A, Griffen S: Prospective randomized clinical trial comparing the effectiveness of immediate arthroscopic stabilization versus immobilization and rehabilitation in first traumatic anterior dislocations of the shoulder: Long-term evaluation. Arthroscopy 21:55–63, 2005.

38. Kirkley A, Griffen S, McLintock H, Ng L: The development and evaluation of a disease specific quality of life measurement tool for shoulder instability: The Western Ontario Shoulder Instability Index (WOSI). Am J Sports Med 26:764–772, 1998.

39. Concata J, Shah N, Horwitz RI: Randomized, controlled trials, observational studies, and the hierarchy of research design. N Engl J Med 342:1887–1892, 2000.

40. Handoll HHG, Almaiyah MA, Rangan A: Surgical versus nonsurgical treatment for acute anterior shoulder dislocation (Review). Cochrane Database Syst Rev (1):CD004325, 2004.

Chapter 99

Open versus Arthroscopic Repair for Shoulder Instability: What's Best?

ROBERT LITCHFIELD, MD, FRCSC AND FINTAN SHANNON, MD

Shoulder dislocations are a common sports injury, especially in contact sports such as hockey,[1,2] rugby,[3,4] and all forms of football,[5,6] but also in sports associated with falls, such as skiing,[7,8] and in sports in which shoulder movements are integral to the game, such as tennis, badminton, swimming, and baseball.[3,9,10] Most of these dislocations involve anterior dislocation,[3,7,8,11–15] during which the glenohumeral joint actually is disrupted. In some, the dislocation reduces itself spontaneously.[16] Other patients require manual reduction, often requiring anesthesia. Immediate conservative management after reduction may consist of a sling, more to alleviate pain and worry than to protect the joint, and avoidance of sporting activities for an extended time, possibly associated with analgesics, physiotherapy, or both; but the research on the acute management of shoulder dislocations is quite inconclusive,[17] and there is extreme variability in clinical practice.[18–20]

Irrespective of how shoulder dislocations are managed immediately after injury,[21] the risk for redislocating a shoulder is high without surgical repair, in some series approaching 90%, especially in younger athletes.[2,21] Conservative management, including the use of a sling in the short term and physiotherapy, is of uncertain benefit[21] and may actually increase this risk by delaying more definitive treatment.[22] Consequently, surgery commonly is considered, especially for those who are young and those wanting to return to athletic activities.

Currently, the surgical options can be classified broadly into open surgical repair and arthroscopic repair; however, ongoing debate rages regarding which is most effective for the treatment of shoulder dislocations, which has led to two meta-analyses and a further published review of the literature.[23–25] Certainly, early investigators seemed to identify either no difference between the approaches or some superiority of open surgery, but this conclusion largely was based on a single outcome: joint stability. Despite these early results, the arthroscopic repair of shoulder instability seems to have gathered momentum since the late 1990s.[24,25] This chapter is a review of the relatively limited comparative evidence, examining not only joint stability, but also several other outcomes of clinical interest. Note that these comparisons all are relatively recent, the first publication having been in 1996.[26]

SURGICAL OPTIONS

As stated earlier, the surgical options can be divided broadly into those performed via open surgery and those performed arthroscopically, but there is a variety of techniques that can be utilized within each approach. This especially appears to be true with arthroscopic shoulder repair, possibly because this approach is newer, and hence more in its evolutionary phase.[24,25] Some of the initial arthroscopic approaches included staple capsulorrhaphy, transglenoid suturing, bioabsorbable tack fixation, suture anchor fixation with capsular plication, and the combined use of intra-articular and extra-articular Suretac sutures.[26–41] More recently, most surgeons utilize a suture anchor system with or without knot tying. This variety, in itself, makes it difficult to compare between studies, and between the arthroscopic and open surgery approaches.

OUTCOMES OF INTEREST

Because there has been variability in the surgical approaches used, there also has been considerable variability in the outcomes measured. Virtually all investigators who have assessed open or arthroscopic repair alone or relative to each other have utilized *recurrent instability* as an outcome, and often as the primary outcome. However, how recurrent instability is defined has differed, some including a positive apprehension sign as an indicator of instability. No other single outcome has spanned all studies, but several investigators have adopted the use of validated multidimensional instruments, especially the shoulder-specific (joint-specific) evaluation instruments called the *Rowe Rating Scale,*[26,29,31,33,35–38,40] which initially was called the *Rating Sheet for Bankart Repair,* and the *Constant Score.*[28,31,33,35,37,38] Other shoulder-specific summation scores that have been utilized are the *modified Rowe Rating Scale,*[28] the *American Shoulder and Elbow Surgeons (ASES) Standardized Shoulder Assessment Form,*[39,41] and the *University of California Los Angeles (UCLA) Shoulder Rating Scale.*[26,36] Kirkley and colleagues'[43] *Western Ontario Shoulder Instability (WOSI)* scale, another instrument used in one of the comparative studies,[42] offers the advantage of being a disease-specific, rather than just a joint-specific, instrument, in that it specifically evaluates shoulder function in patients with shoulder instability. Like the Rowe and Constant scales, each of these instruments generates a summation score, often expressed as a percentage, which is derived from evaluations of individual parameters, such as pain, function, range of motion (ROM), strength, and stability, though which parameters are included, and how they are weighted varies from scale to scale. Some investigators also have compared the open and arthroscopic approaches with respect to the *change in summation score* from preoperative baseline to final evaluation.

Another summation score that has been used is the *36-Item Short Form Health Survey* (SF-36),[27] an instrument with several subscales to evaluate self-perceived patient well-being. The SF-36 is not specific to any joint or to any 1 medical or surgical condition; as such, it allows for comparison between conditions, which can be useful if one wishes to determine the relative worth of treatment of 1 condition versus another.

More individual outcomes of interest include the *apprehension sign*; the requirement for *further surgical procedures* on the involved shoulder; joint *ROM*, especially external rotation when the shoulder is abducted and forward flexion; *loss of joint ROM,* relative to presumed premorbid baseline or "normal" ROM; *pain severity,* for example, as rated on a visual analogue scale; the *rate and time to return to athletic activities*; the *rate and time to return to prior athletic activities*; the *rate and time to return to contact or so-called collision athletic activities*; and *radiographic evidence of cystic change or drill holes*. No article has reported on all these outcomes, or even the majority, again making interstudy comparisons difficult.

REVIEW OF OUTCOMES

Instability

As shown in Table 99–1, the earliest studies comparing arthroscopic repair of shoulder instability with the long-established open approach demonstrated superiority of the latter[26,29,40] (Level III). For example, among 12 patients undergoing open repair and 15 arthroscopy, Geiger and coworkers[29] identified a 44% rate of instability among those who had undergone arthroscopy but no instances of instability in those who had had open surgery ($P < 0.05$). Similarly, in the studies by Guanche and researchers[26] (Level III) and Steinbeck and Jerosch[40] (Level II), the rates of instability were 33% and 17% in those who had had arthroscopy versus 8% and 6% in the open surgery group, respectively. Though clinically appreciable, these latter 2 differences did not achieve statistical significance. Nonetheless, these 3 studies were among the 6 included in the meta-analysis published by Freedman and colleagues[24] in 2004 and the 11 studies included in the meta-analysis performed by Mohtadi and coworkers[25] in 2005, both of which

conclude that open is superior to arthroscopic repair, in terms of instability rates (Level III).

Later studies have been much less consistent. A few studies have uncovered some advantage of open surgery, such as Rhee and colleagues[37] (25% arthroscopy vs. 13% open; $P < 0.05$), Hubbell and coworkers[30] (60% vs. 0%; $P < 0.05$), Cole and coauthors[27] (24% vs. 16%; P value not significant [NS]), Karlsson and researchers[33] (15% vs. 10%; P value NS), and Sperber and investigators[38] (23% vs. 13%; P value NS) (Level III). In contrast, several other studies revealed no difference at all between the 2 surgical approaches,[28,31,35,36,39,42] and 1 study actually demonstrated a clinically impressive, albeit not statistically significant, difference in favor of arthroscopy (6% arthroscopy vs. 24% open; P value NS) (Level III). In some instances, no cases of postrepair instability were identified in either group.[28,35,39]

As stated earlier, 1 problem interpreting these data is that instability has not been consistently defined. For example, Kartus and colleagues[35] limited the designation of instability to shoulder dislocation, which clearly might have reduced the numbers this group considered unstable versus other investigative teams that included a positive apprehension sign. Nonetheless, what is apparent is that it is less clear now that open repair provides a lower risk for instability than it may have been 1 decade ago, possibly because of improved arthroscopic techniques and equipment, and increased experience among surgeons. It also is apparent, and quite understandable, that the results of arthroscopy are quite operator dependent.

Apprehension

Because a positive apprehension sign generally is indicative of shoulder instability, it is reasonable to expect that the presence of apprehension would parallel that of instability. But how sensitive and specific the apprehension sign is as an indicator of joint instability is a question that must be considered, as well as its level of intrarater and inter-rater reliability. Moreover, few current studies have examined the reliability, sensitivity, and specificity of most orthopedic signs,[44] and some evidence suggests that the inter-rater reliability of the apprehension sign (the rate at which different examiners agree that the same shoulder is either stable or unstable) may be as low as 50%, which is no better than the flip of a coin.[45]

In Geiger and coworkers'[29] study, the rates for shoulder instability were 17% and 6% for postarthroscopy and open repair, respectively, and a positive apprehension sign was detected in 30% and 6%, suggesting that almost half the patients with arthroscopy with positive apprehension signs were found not to have any other evidence of instability (Level III). In this study, the former intergroup difference, for instability, failed to achieve statistical significance, but the latter difference, for a positive apprehension sign, did. Concern exists regarding that, in several other studies, the presence of a positive apprehension sign was deemed enough for the investigators to consider the joint unstable, and the presence or absence of a positive apprehension sign per se was not reported.

Summation Scores

As stated earlier, the Rowe Shoulder Scale was the most commonly used summation instrument,[23,26,27,29,31,33,35–38,40] followed by the Constant Score,[28,31,33,35,37,38] with both scores often reported using an ordinal scale; for example, scores of 90% or greater might be categorized as an "excellent" result, scores from 75 to 89 a "good" result, scores from 51 to 74 "fair," and scores of 50 or less "poor." Consequently, the most commonly reported result has been the percentage of patients who achieved a good-to-excellent result, when combining the various parameters included in the instrument. With the Rowe Scale, these parameters are function, pain severity, joint stability, and ROM[28]; with the Constant Score, they are pain, function, ROM, and strength[28] (Level I). Interestingly, the tendency toward joint instability being more common among those who had undergone arthroscopic repair has not been reflected in either the Rowe or Constant scores, despite joint stability being a parameter in the Rowe Scale. For example, with the possible exception of the study by Geiger and coworkers,[29] in no study was there a statistically significant intergroup difference using either scale. In Geiger and coworkers'[29] study, 83% in the open group were assigned a postoperative functional rating of good to excellent, compared with only 50% in the arthroscopy group ($P = 0.05$) (Level III); however, it is not clear whether these ratings were based solely on the Rowe score, some combination of the Rowe score and a joint instability rating, or some other factor(s). If one assumes that Geiger's group did base their good-to-excellent rating solely on the Rowe score, then the overall average percentage of good-to-excellent ratings based on Rowe scores across the 10 studies that reported this parameter using this ordinal scale was 88% for open repair and 86% for arthroscopy, and the overall weighted average percentage (weighted by the number of subjects per group per study) of good-to-excellent ratings was 82% for the open group versus 77% for those who received arthroscopic repair ($\chi^2 = 1.83$; $P = 0.17$, NS) (Table 99–2). Excluding Geiger and coworkers'[29] study, the percentages are 88% versus 90% overall and 78% versus 79% weighted, respectively, which, again, is not a statistically significant difference (Level III). Constant scores actually trend toward favoring arthroscopy, with 94% in the arthroscopy group receiving good-to-excellent ratings versus 89% in the subjects with open repair; but again, this difference is not statistically significant ($\chi^2 = 1.48$; $P = 0.20$, NS) (see Table 99–2). Moreover, caution should be exercised interpreting the coalesced data because different investigative teams

defined the various ordinal categories differently. For example, in 1 study, any Rowe score from 75 to 89 was considered good,[31] but in another study, only scores from 81 to 90 were so designated, with scores from 70 to 80 considered fair[35]; in these same two studies, a "poor" result was defined as less than 50 and less than 70, respectively.

No summation instrument besides the Rowe or Constant scores has been utilized in a published comparison between open and arthroscopic shoulder repair more than twice; therefore, combining data across studies either cannot be done or would yield an insufficient number of subjects to be meaningful. However, with the exception of the UCLA Shoulder Rating Scale score being greater in the arthroscopy group in a single study,[36] where a higher score corresponds to a better result, no statistically significant differences have been noted with any scale.

Range of Motion

As equivocal as the data are with respect to virtually every other outcome, the evidence for shoulder ROM is reasonably clear. Joint shoulder ROM or loss of ROM was reported as a separate outcome in 10 of the comparison studies,[26–30,33,35,38,39,42] most often referring to external rotation with the shoulder abducted and forward flexion.

In no study was ROM in any plane superior in the open surgery group. Conversely, a statistically significant advantage of arthroscopic repair was identified by 6 investigative teams, and this was noted both with external rotation[30,33,35,42] and forward flexion[26,27,30] (Level III). This discrepancy favoring arthroscopic repair was evident even in Guanche and researchers'[26] study, in which arthroscopy was associated with greater than a 33% rate of instability and fewer than half of patients with arthroscopy were deemed to have had a "good" or "excellent" result,[29] and Hubbell and coworkers'[30] study, in which 60% versus 0% of the patients with arthroscopy developed recurrent instability (Level III). Despite these seemingly poor results among the patients with arthroscopy, at least in terms of stability, nonetheless, there was a mean of 5.1 degrees of forward flexion lost in those undergoing open repair versus just a 1.0-degree loss in the arthroscopy group in the former study ($P = 0.02$)[29]; and 45% of the patients with open surgery versus 0% after arthroscopy suffered a loss of external rotation in the latter study ($P < 0.05$).[30]

In 2001, Kailes and Richmond[32] published an article comparing arthroscopic versus open repair of shoulder instability using *expected value decision analysis* (Level III). Basing their analysis on no study published after 1997, and hence emphasizing data generally favoring open versus arthroscopic repair and studies generally examining 1 approach versus the other, rather than comparative studies, these authors predicted a rate of recurrent instability among those receiving arthroscopic repair at 35%

TABLE 99–1. Published Studies Comparing Open versus Arthroscopic Repair of Shoulder Instability

| INVESTIGATORS (YEAR OF PUBLICATION) | STUDY DESIGN | LEVEL OF EVIDENCE | CASES (N) | | DURATION OF FOLLOW-UP | ARTHROSCOPIC TECHNIQUE | PRIMARY OUTCOME(S) |
			OPEN REPAIR	ARTHROSCOPY			
Guanche et al. (1996)[26]	Retrospective	III	12	15	Minimum 17 mo (range, 17–42)	Transglenoid sutures (10) Suture anchor (5)	Recurrent instability (subluxation, dislocation) Apprehension on PE
Geiger et al. (1997)[29]	Retrospective	III	18	16	Minimum 15 mo (15–44)	Transglenoid sutures	Recurrent instability (subluxation, dislocation)
Steinbeck and Jerosch (1998)[40]	Prospective, nonrandom	II	32	30	Mean 38 mo (24–60)	Transglenoid sutures	Recurrent instability (subluxation, dislocation) Apprehension
Kartus et al. (1998)[35]	Prospective, semirandom (patients choose procedure)	II	18	18	Median 28, 31 mo (18–46)	Intra-articular and extra-articular Suretac sutures	Recurrent instability Poor Rowe score Poor Constant score
Jorgensen et al. (1999)[31]	Prospective semirandom (selection per home address)	II	20	21	Median 36 mo (30–52)	Transglenoid sutures Anterior capsular plication	None stated
Cole and Warner (2000)[23]	Prospective, nonrandom Treatment based on EUA/ arthroscopy	II	22	37	Mean 54 mo (27–72)	Transfixing Suretac (2–3)	Recurrent instability (subluxation, dislocation) Apprehension
Karlsson et al. (2001)[33]	Prospective, nonrandom (?)	II	53	66	Medians 36, 28 mo (24–63)	Suretac fixators	Recurrent instability (subluxation, dislocation)

VALIDATED OUTCOME TOOL	RESULTS	CONCLUSIONS	METHODOLOGIC CONCERNS
UCLA	Recurrent instability: 33% arthroscopy vs. 8% open (NS)	Open stabilization superior	Longer mean interval between injury and surgery in arthroscopy group
Rowe	Apprehension: arthroscopy 40% vs. open 8% ($P < 0.05$) Good-to-excellent result (Rowe): 83% open, 47% arthroscopy ($P = 0.06$, NS) Further surgery required: 27% arthroscopy vs. 0% open ($P = 0.05$) Loss of forward flexion: 5.4 degrees open vs. 1.0 degrees arthroscopy ($P = 0.02$)		
Rowe	Recurrent instability: 44% arthroscopy vs. 0% open ($P < 0.05$) Good-to-excellent result: 83% open vs. 50% arthroscopy ($P = 0.05$) Returned to work or primary sport: 89% open vs. 53% arthroscopy ($P = 0.02$) Mean ROM: arthroscopy 92 degrees vs. open 89 degrees (NS)	Open stabilization superior	
Rowe	Recurrent instability: 17% arthroscopy vs. 6% open (NS) Apprehension: 30% arthroscopy vs. 6% open ($P < 0.05$) Good-to-excellent result (Rowe): 91% open, 80% arthroscopy (NS)	Open stabilization slightly superior	Group assignment based on arthroscopy findings; selection bias
Rowe	No cases of recurrent dislocations in either group	Arthroscopy superior	Longer mean interval between first injury and surgery in open group (60 vs. 24 mo)
Constant	Good-to-excellent Rowe score: 100% arthroscopy, 83% open (NS) Good-to-excellent Constant score: 89% arthroscopy, 78% open (NS) Abducted external rotation: 83 degrees arthroscopy, 65 degrees open ($P < 0.05$) Radiographic evidence of drill holes or cysts: 56% open vs. 23% arthroscopy ($P < 0.05$)		Lack of recurrent instability in any group suggests lack of generalizability of subjects
Rowe	Instability: 10% in each group	Approaches comparable except better ROM and cosmesis with arthroscopy	Longer mean interval between injury and surgery in arthroscopy group
Constant	Rowe (arthroscopy: 93%, open: 95%) and Constant (arthroscopy: 83%; open: 79%) scores similar Failure to regain original function: 35% open vs. 33% arthroscopy ROM less in open group (no statistical analysis done)		
SF-36	Failures: 24% arthroscopy vs. 18% open (NS)	Treatment should be based on EUA plus scope	Heterogenous pathology
Rowe	Good-to-excellent (Rowe): 76% arthroscopy vs. 77% open (NS)		Treatment based on EUA plus Capsule/GHL morphology
ASES	ASES and SF-36 scores similar ROM (forward flexion) less in open group ($P < 0.05$) 75% in each group returned to the same sport		
Rowe	Instability: 15% arthroscopy vs. 10% open (NS)	Approaches comparable	Nonrandom group assignment
Constant	Rowe score: 93% arthroscopy vs. 89% open (NS) Constant score: 91% Arthroscopy vs. 89% open (NS) Abducted external rotation: 90% arthroscopy vs. 80% open ($P < 0.05$)	External rotation better with arthroscopy	

TABLE 99–1. Published Studies Comparing Open versus Arthroscopic Repair of Shoulder Instability—cont'd

INVESTIGATORS (YEAR OF PUBLICATION)	STUDY DESIGN	LEVEL OF EVIDENCE	CASES (N)		DURATION OF FOLLOW-UP	ARTHROSCOPIC TECHNIQUE	PRIMARY OUTCOME(S)
			OPEN REPAIR	ARTHROSCOPY			
Sperber et al. (2001)[38]	Prospective, random	II	26	30	24 mo	Biodegradable tacks	Recurrent instability
Kim et al. (2002)[36]	Retrospective case–control	III	30	59	Mean 39 mo	Anchors, capsular plication and proximal shift	Recurrent instability
Hubbell et al. (2004)[30]	Retrospective	III	20	30	Min 60 mo (no range)	Transglenoid sutures	None stated
Fabbriciani et al. (2004)[28]	Prospective, randomized	I	30	30	2 yr	SCOI technique	Constant score
Wang et al. (2005)[41]	Retrospective case–control	III	22	20	2 yr	Bankart repair	Instability Costs
Sperling et al. (2005)[39]	Retrospective case–control Patients all ≥50 yr old	III	6	5	Mean 6.5 yr	?	Recurrent instability
Bottoni et al. (2006)[42]	Prospective RCT	II	29	32	Minimum 24 mo (24–48)	Suture anchor (0–6)	Recurrent instability (subluxation, dislocation) Ability to return to full military duties
Rhee et al. (2006)[37]	Retrospective, nonrandom Athletes in contact sports	IV	32	16	Mean 72 mo (30–136)		Recurrent instability (subluxation, dislocation)

ASES, American Shoulder and Elbow Surgeons; EUA, examination under anesthesia; GHL=glenohumeral ligaments; MDI, multidirectional instability; NS, not significant; PE, physical exam; RCT, randomized, controlled trial; ROM, range of motion; SCOI, Southern California Orthopedic Institute; SF-36, 36-Item Short Form Health Survey; UCLA, University of California Los Angeles; WOSI, Western Ontario Shoulder Instability.

VALIDATED OUTCOME TOOL	RESULTS	CONCLUSIONS	METHODOLOGIC CONCERNS
Rowe	Instability: 23% arthroscopy vs. 13% open (NS)	Approaches comparable	Rowe and Constant data only provided for stable shoulders
Constant	Rowe score among stable shoulders: 100% arthroscopy vs. 98% open (NS) Constant score among stable shoulders: 100% arthroscopy vs. 95% open (NS) Loss of abducted external rotation: 9 degrees arthroscopy vs. 10 degrees open (NS)		
Rowe	Instability: 10% in each group	Approaches comparable	Nonrandom group assignment
UCLA	Good-to-excellent: 91% arthroscopy vs. 87% open (NS) Rowe ($P = 0.04$) and UCLA ($P = 0.03$) scores greater in the arthroscopy group No other differences		
None	Postoperative instability: 60% arthroscopy vs. 0% open ($P < 0.05$) Reoperation required: 27% arthroscopy vs. 0% open ($P < 0.05$) Some loss of external rotation: 45% Open group vs. 0% Arthroscopy ($p < 0.05$) Mean degrees of external rotation lost: Open group 8o Return to collision sports: Open 35% vs. Arthroscopy 30% (NS)	Open procedure better for athletes in contact sports Arthroscopy better if external rotation important	Included first time and MDIs
Constant	Instability: not reported in either group	Approaches comparable	
Modified Rowe	Constant score: 97% arthroscopy vs. 94% open (NS) Improvement in Constant score from baseline: 23% arthroscopy vs. 20% open (NS) Modified Rowe: 91% arthroscopy vs. 87% open (NS) Constant ROM score: 39.6 arthroscopy vs. 37.8 open ($P = 0.02$)	Arthroscopy may yield greater ROM	
ASES1	Instability: 24% open vs. 6% arthroscopy (NS) ASES scores similar Overall costs greater for open procedure because of required postoperative admission	Approaches comparable Arthroscopy less expensive	Retrospective, nonrandom study Small samples
ASES1	Instability: not reported in either group ASES: 98% open vs. 87% arthroscopy (NS) Mean shoulder elevation: 178 degrees open vs. 174 degrees arthroscopy (NS) External rotation: 72 degrees arthroscopy vs. 70 degrees open (NS)	Approaches comparable in patients 50 yr old	Small sample Retrospective, nonrandom study
WOSI	Failure: 3% ($n = 1$) in each group WOSI scores similar ROM less in open group (NS)	Approaches comparable	Generalizability of military population Heterogenous pathology No standard arthroscopy technique
Rowe	Instability: 25% arthroscopy vs. 13% open ($P = 0.04$)	Open procedure better for athletes in contact sports	Retrospective, nonrandom
Constant	No other differences		

TABLE 99–2. Rowe and Constant Scores in Patients after Arthroscopic versus Open Repair of Shoulder Instability

STUDY (YEAR OF PUBLICATION)	OPEN REPAIR		ARTHROSCOPIC REPAIR	
	N	GOOD TO EXCELLENT	N	GOOD TO EXCELLENT
Rowe Scores				
Guanche et al. (1996)[26]	12	83%	15	47%
Geiger et al. (1997)[29]	18	83%	16	50%
Steinbeck and Jerosch (1998)[40]	32	91%	30	80%
Kartus et al. (1998)[35]	18	83%	18	100%
Jorgensen et al. (1999)[31]	20	95%	21	90%
Cole and Warner (2000)[23]	22	77%	37	76%
Karlsson et al. (2001)[33]	53	89%	66	93%
Sperber et al. (2001)[38]	26	98%	30	100%
Kim et al. (2002)[36]	30	87%	59	91%
Fabbriciani et al.* (2004)[28]	30	87%	30	91%
Rhee et al. (2006)[37]	32	N/A	16	N/A
Total	261		322	
Average		88%		86%
Weighted average		82%		77%
Constant scores				
Kartus et al. (1998)[35]	18	78%	18	89%
Jorgensen et al. (1999)[31]	20	79%	21	83%
Karlsson et al. (2001)[33]	53	89%	66	91%
Sperber et al. (2001)[38]	26	95%	30	100%
Fabbriciani et al. (2004)[28]†	30	94%	30	97%
Rhee et al. (2006)[37]	32	N/A	16	N/A
Total	147		165	
Average		87%		92%
Weighted average		88%		92%

*Unclear whether Rowe Scale used to determine good-to-excellent designation.
†Modified Rowe scale used.
N/A, not available.

versus just 5% in the open surgery group. However, they also estimate that 40% of those undergoing open repair would lose shoulder ROM versus just 10% for arthroscopy. Their predictions for were identical for all other outcomes, including minor complication rate (2%), major complication rate (2%), time decrement for rehabilitation and minor complications (4.5 and 3.0 months, respectively), functional decrement for major complications,[25] utility of stability without recurrences (1.0 out of 1), utility of recurrent instability (0.4 out of 1), and disutility of decreased ROM (0.1 out of 1).[32]

Other Outcomes

As stated previously, no other outcome has been reported in any more than a few studies, making comparisons between open and arthroscopic repair difficult for these parameters. In studies in which shoulder dislocations, subluxations, and/or instability were found to be more common in the arthroscopy group, a return to sports and especially to contact sports was less likely in this group as well.[29,30] Conversely, when there was no intergroup difference in the rate of instability, there similarly was no difference in the rate of return to athletics or other previous activities.[27,31] One study[35] examined for the radiographic presence of either drill holes or cysts, the implication

being that these represent damage to bone; these abnormalities were statistically more common in the open group (56% vs. 23%; $P < 0.05$) (Level II). The only 2 studies that evaluated costs, 1 in the United States[41] and 1 in Germany,[46] both discovered that arthroscopic repair of the unstable shoulder was significantly less costly, largely because of the reduced need for postoperative hospitalization after arthroscopic versus open procedures.

One outcome that is conspicuously missing from studies is subscapularis weakness, which could be different in the 2 groups, because of significant muscle disruption that occurs with the open procedure that generally is not an issue with arthroscopy. In 1 study, 12 patients with shoulder instability who underwent arthroscopic stabilization were compared with 10 who underwent open surgery and 12 healthy control subjects[47] (Level III). Whereas none of the patients with arthroscopy exhibited any subscapularis weakness after surgery, such weakness was noted in 7 of the 10 patients who underwent open surgery ($P < 0.05$), and magnetic resonance imaging revealed evidence of subscapularis muscle atrophy in the latter group as well. Another study demonstrated that the subscapularis weakness that occurs after open capsular shift lasts an average of almost 9 weeks, but that all patients had regained full strength within 20 weeks.[48] This difference may be 1 of the reasons behind the slightly higher Constant scores exhibited by patients with arthroscopy, because strength is 1 of the 4 major subscales.

SUMMARY OF LITERATURE

What is most clear about the relative effectiveness of arthroscopic versus open surgical repair of shoulder instability is that the data provide no clear answers. In general, it appears that open surgery may be more effective at reducing the likelihood of recurrent instability, which, in turn, may affect the rate at which injured athletes can return to their prior sport, especially if collisions are involved.

However, that difference may be disappearing, or may already have disappeared, as arthroscopic techniques and equipment, and the experience and skills of surgeons with respect to arthroscopic shoulder procedures advance. Conversely, the evidence is reasonably clear that arthroscopy yields better ROM of the involved shoulder. Costs also appear to be less with arthroscopy, largely because there is less of a need for postoperative hospitalization. Beyond that, a review of other outcomes, including various summation scores, either reveals no difference or a tendency to favor the arthroscopic approach; and data on subscapularis strength, which may be significantly worse in the open surgery group, largely are absent.

RECOMMENDATIONS

Since the late 1980s, there has been a dramatic shift from open to arthroscopic surgery in the shoulder. It is obvious that the scope is here to stay; fortunately, improvements in instrumentation, visualization, fluid management, and implant materials have made arthroscopic procedures easier, more efficient, and reliable. I favor nonmetallic anchoring devices to prevent inadvertent trauma to the articular cartilage. Many anchors now come with new generation permanent suture materials that are abrasion resistant and extremely strong; these new sutures make the shoulder arthroscopic procedure easier to perform, and allow for a more secure repair and perhaps more progressive rehabilitation.

The learning curve for shoulder stabilization surgery is not short and should not be encouraged for surgeons performing infrequent shoulder-stabilizing surgeries. Skills training is available through many societies and organizations, and is an essential part of obtaining and maintaining safe and effective techniques. Many of the surgical steps required to perform an arthroscopic stabilization can be practiced outside the operating room, for example, arthroscopic knot-tying techniques, suture passing, management strategies, and safe and effective portal placement. As with any procedure, patient selection is important. Ideal

patients for arthroscopic stabilization would have a soft-tissue Bankart lesion because large glenoid rim fractures might compromise the ability to stabilize the joint. If the status of the glenoid is uncertain on the plain films, then a CT scan with three-dimensional reconstruction is recommended. If at the time of scope the inferior glenohumeral ligaments have avulsed off the humeral neck, the so-called HAGL (humeral avulsion glenohumeral ligaments) lesion, then this is best managed through an open approach (Level V). Athletes involved with throwing or overhead sports such as tennis and volleyball are good candidates for an arthroscopic approach because it is easier to maintain external rotation and sport function. Young athletes with an acute anterior dislocation should be informed about the option of surgical stabilization even after a single dislocation to prevent ongoing instability, as well as the subsequent soft-tissue and bone injury associated with multiple recurrences. The surgeon must avoid overconstraining the shoulder joint whether the surgery is performed open or arthroscopic because most patients would choose instability over stiffness and loss of function. Severe motion loss is strongly correlated with arthritis of the glenohumeral joint. Table 99–3 provides a summary of recommendations.

TABLE 99–3. Summary of Recommendations

STATEMENT	LEVEL OF EVIDENCE/GRADE OF RECOMMENDATION	REFERENCES
1. Traumatic unidirectional anterior shoulder instability can be safely treated with an arthroscopic or open stabilization technique.	B	23,31,35 38, 40, 42
2. Arthroscopic approaches are more likely to maintain shoulder external rotation.	B	28, 30, 31, 33
3. Open stabilization procedures are better for athletes involved in contact sports.	B	30,37
4. An arthroscopic stabilization may be more cost effective than an open procedure.	B	41

REFERENCES

1. Gerberich SG, Finke R, Madden M, et al: An epidemiological study of high school ice hockey injuries. Childs Nerv Syst 3:59–64, 1987.
2. Hovelius L: Shoulder dislocation in Swedish ice hockey players. Am J Sports Med 6:373–377, 1978.
3. Hazmy CH, Parwathi A: Sports-related shoulder dislocations: A state-hospital experience. Med J Malaysia 60(suppl C):22–25, 2005.
4. Brooks JH, Fuller CW, Kemp SP, Reddin DB: Epidemiology of injuries in English professional rugby union: Part 2 training Injuries. Br J Sports Med 39:767–775, 2007.
5. Pagnani MJ, Dome DC: Surgical treatment of traumatic anterior shoulder instability in American football players. J Bone Joint Surg Am 84-A:711–715, 2002.
6. Roberts SN, Taylor DE, Brown JN, et al: Open and arthroscopic techniques for the treatment of traumatic anterior shoulder instability in Australian rules football players. J Shoulder Elbow Surg 8:403–409, 1999.
7. Kocker MS, Feagin JA Jr: Shoulder injuries during alpine skiing. Am J Sports Med 24:665–669, 1996.
8. Weaver JK: Skiing-related injuries to the shoulder. Clin Orthop Relat Res 216:24–28, 1987.
9. Perry J: Anatomy and biomechanics of the shoulder in throwing, swimming, gymnastics, and tennis. Clin Sports Med 2:247–270, 1983.
10. Bak K, Faunø P: Clinical findings in competitive swimmers with shoulder pain. Am J Sports Med 25:254–260, 1997.
11. Hazmy CH, Parwathi A: The epidemiology of shoulder dislocation in a state-hospital: A review of 106 cases. Med J Malaysia 60(suppl C):17–21, 2005.
12. Hoelen MA, Burgers AM, Rozing PM: Prognosis of primary anterior shoulder dislocation in young adults. Arch Orthop Trauma Surg 110:51–54, 1990.
13. Hovelius L: Incidence of shoulder dislocation in Sweden. Clin Orthop Relat Res 166:127–131, 1982.
14. Owens BD, Duffey ML, Nelson BJ, et al: The incidence and characteristics of shoulder instability at the United States Military Academy. Am J Sports Med 35:1168–1173, 2007.
15. Simonet WT, Melton LJ 3rd, Cofield RH, Ilstrup DM: Incidence of anterior shoulder dislocation in Olmsted County, Minnesota. Clin Orthop Relat Res 186:186–191, 1984.
16. Saragaglia D, Picard F, Le Bredonchel T, et al: [Acute anterior instability of the shoulder: Short- and mid-term outcome after conservative treatment] [In French]. Rev Chir Orthop Reparatrice Appar Mot 87:215–220, 2001.
17. Handoll HH, Hanchard NC, Goodchild L, Feary J: Conservative management following closed reduction of traumatic anterior dislocation of the shoulder. Cochrane Database Syst Rev 25: CD004962, 2006.
18. Chong M, Karataglis D, Learmonth D: Survey of the management of acute traumatic first-time anterior shoulder dislocation among trauma clinicians in the UK. Ann R Coll Surg Engl 88:454–458, 2006.
19. Buss DD, Lynch GP, Meyer CP, et al: Nonoperative management for in-season athletes with anterior shoulder instability. Am J Sports Med 32:1430–1433, 2004.
20. te Slaa RL, Wijffels MP, Marti RK: Questionnaire reveals variations in the management of acute first time shoulder dislocations in the Netherlands. Eur J Emerg Med 10:58–61, 2003.
21. Chalidis B, Sachinis N, Dimitriou C, et al: Has the management of shoulder dislocation changed over time? Int Orthop 31:385–389, 2007.
22. Kirkley A, Werstine R, Ratjek A, Griffen S: Prospective randomized clinical trial comparing the effectiveness of immediate arthroscopic stabilization immobilization and rehabilitation in first traumatic anterior dislocations of the shoulder: Long-term evaluation. Arthroscopy 21:55–63, 2005.
23. Cole BJ, Warner JJP: Arthroscopic versus open bankart repair for traumatic anterior shoulder instability. Clin Sports Med 19:19–48, 2000.
24. Freedman KB, Smith AP, Romeo AA, et al: Open Bankart repair versus arthroscopic repair with transglenoid sutures or bioabsorbable tacks for recurrent anterior instability of the shoulder: A meta-analysis. Am J Sports Med 32:1520–1527, 2004.
25. Mohtadi NGH, Bitar IJ, Sasyniuk TM, et al: Arthroscopic versus open repair for traumatic anterior shoulder instability: A meta-analysis. Arthroscopy 21:652–658, 2005.
26. Guanche CA, Quick DC, Sodergren KM, Buss DD: Arthroscopic versus open reconstruction of the shoulder in patients with isolated Bankart lesions. Am J Sports Med 24:144–148, 1996.
27. Cole BJ, L'Insalata J, Irrgang J, Warner JJP: Comparison of arthroscopic and open anterior shoulder stabilization: A two to six-year follow-up study. J Bone Joint Surg Am 82:1108–1114, 2006.
28. Fabbriciani C, Milano G, Demontis A, et al: Arthroscopic versus open treatment of Bankart lesion of the shoulder: A prospective randomized study. Arthroscopy 20:456–462, 2004.
29. Geiger DF, Hurley JA, Tovey JA, Rao JP: Results of arthroscopic versus open suture repair. Clin Orthop Relat Res 337:111–117, 1997.
30. Hubbell JD, Ahmad S, Bezenoff LS, et al: Comparison of shoulder stabilization using arthroscopic transglenoid sutures versus open capsulolabral repair. A 5-year minimum follow-up. Am J Sports Med 32:650–654, 2004.
31. Jorgensen U, Svend-Hansen H, Bak K, Pedersen I: Recurrent post-traumatic anterior shoulder dislocation—open versus arthroscopic repair. Knee Surg Sports Traumatol Arthrosc 7:118–124, 1999.
32. Kailes SB, Richmond JC: Arthroscopic vs. open Bankart reconstruction: A comparison using expected value decision analysis. Knee Surg Sports Traumatol Arthrosc 9:379–385, 2001.
33. Karlsson J, Magnusson L, Ejerhed L, et al: Comparison of open and arthroscopic stabilization for recurrent shoulder dislocation in patients with a Bankart lesion. Am J Sports Med 29:538–542, 2001.
34. Karnezis IA, Sarangi PP: Arthroscopic repair versus open surgery for shoulder instability. J Bone Joint Surg Am 83A:952, 2001.
35. Kartus J, Ejerhed L, Funck E, et al: Arthroscopic and open shoulder stabilization using absorbable implants. A clinical and radiographic comparison of two methods. Knee Surg Sports Traumatol Arthrosc 6:181–188, 1998.
36. Kim SH, Ha KI, Kim SH: Bankart repair in traumatic anterior shoulder instability: Open versus arthroscopic technique. Arthroscopy 18:755–763, 2002.
37. Rhee YG, Ha JH, Cho NS: Anterior shoulder stabilization in collision athletes: Arthroscopic versus open bankart repair. Am J Sports Med 34:979–985, 2006.
38. Sperber A, Hamberg P, Karlsson J, et al: Comparison of an arthroscopic and an open procedure for posttraumatic instability of the shoulder: A prospective, randomized multicenter study. J Shoulder Elbow Surg 10:105–108, 2001.
39. Sperling JW, Duncan SMF, Torchia ME, et al: Bankart repair in patients aged fifty years or greater: Results of arthroscopic and open repairs. J Shoulder Elbow Surg 14:111–113, 2005.
40. Steinbeck J, Jerosch J: Arthroscopic transglenoid stabilization versus open anchor suturing in traumatic anterior instability of the shoulder. Am J Sports Med 26:373–378, 1998.
41. Wang C, Ghalambor N, Zarins B, Warner JJP: Arthroscopic versus open Bankart repair: Analysis of patient subjective outcome and cost. Arthroscopy 21:1219–1222, 2005.
42. Bottoni CR, Smith EL, Berkowitz MJ, et al: Arthroscopic versus open shoulder stabilization for recurrent anterior instability: A prospective randomized clinical trial. Am J Sports Med 34:1730–1737, 2006.
43. Kirkley A, Griffen S, McLintock H, Ng L: The development and evaluation of a disease-specific quality of life measurement tool for shoulder instability. The Western Ontario Shoulder Instability Index (WOSI). Am J Sports Med 26:764–772, 1998.
44. Hegedus EJ, Goode A, Campbell S, et al: Physical examination tests of the shoulder: A Systematic Review with Meta-analysis of Individual Tests. Br J Sports Med 42:80–92, 2008.
45. Tzannes A, Murrell GA: Clinical examination of the unstable shoulder. Sports Med 32:447–457, 2002.

46. Bohnsack M, Brinkmann T, Ruhman O, et al: [Open versus arthroscopic shoulder stabilization. An analysis of the treatment costs] [In German]. Orthopade 32:654–658, 2003.

47. Scheibel M, Nikulka C, Dick A, et al: Structural integrity and clinical function of the subscapularis musculotendinous unit after arthroscopic and open shoulder stabilization. Am J Sports Med 35:1153–1161, 2007.

48. Slabaugh MA, Bents RT, Tokish JM, et al: Timing of return of subscapularis function in open capsular shift patients. J Shoulder Elbow Surg 16:544–547, 2007.

Tears of rotator cuff can be repaired by open or mini-open surgery, or arthroscopically. Codman first described open repair in 1911. Charles Neer is credited with describing the most commonly performed open technique in which acromioplasty with or without resection of the lateral end of clavicle is performed, a bone trough is made at the articular margin for reattachment of the cuff, and transosseous sutures are placed through bone tunnels. Complex sutures are possible because of the open exposure. The advent of a mini-open technique was largely in response to the most important shortcoming of open repair, the necessity for deltoid detachment. In the mini-open technique, the acromioplasty is done arthroscopically, and the cuff repaired through a smaller deltoid-splitting incision. Most recently, advances have allowed the passage of sutures arthroscopically and, therefore, an all arthroscopic rotator cuff repair procedure.

The advantages of minimally invasive surgery over more invasive techniques are generally recognized. With minimal soft-tissue violation, pain and tissue damage are minimized, reducing analgesic use and potentially allowing early discharge from hospital and return of function. The risk for stiffness, which is common after open surgery, may be minimized. In addition, it has been suggested that the use of the arthroscope, when repairing the rotator cuff, offers specific advantages. It not only spares the deltoid from potential detachment, it provides enhanced visualization of the tear and associated pathology. Tear geometry and edge mobility are better appreciated when observed arthroscopically. Intra-articular pathology of the biceps tendon, labrum, and articular cartilage, which could affect decision making, can be assessed. Concerns about arthroscopic repair include inadequate visualization because of bleeding, fluid extravasation, difficulty in passing sutures, suture failure, and a steep learning curve. Arguably, advances in technology and technique have addressed all but the last of these concerns. The cost of arthroscopic surgery in terms of time and equipment remains a concern. This chapter analyzes the evidence available to support decision making in rotator cuff repair surgery.

PREFERENCES—A MATTER OF CHOICE

No Level I or II full manuscript published reports of studies favor 1 type of repair over another. Mohtadi and Hollingshead[46] compared open with mini-open

repairs in a randomized, controlled trial and found no difference in disease-specific quality-of-life outcomes at 1 year (only available Level I evidence on rotator cuff repair). Most of the evidence in the literature is Level III with patients compared retrospectively. These articles often report a surgeon's transition from an open to a less invasive technique. The open cases serve as a control group for the newer technique.[1-5] Such studies are generally poorly controlled and subject to the multiple types of bias inherent in retrospective studies. Retrospective Level IV studies, where cohorts are studied after a particular surgery and analyzed without any comparator group, are most common and are ill-equipped to compare one technique over another.

A surgeon's preferences are largely dictated by the training the surgeon has received. In agreement with elsewhere in surgery, there appears to be a general trend toward less invasive procedures. The patient choice, however, is clear. Sperling and colleagues[6] demonstrate an overwhelming 92% patient preference for arthroscopic shoulder surgery compared with open. Patients anticipated superior functional outcomes and less morbidity with arthroscopic surgery. Moreover, a significant number of patients would prefer to avoid surgery if the only option was an open procedure. In the consumer-driven society of today, patient preferences at least partially explain the trend from open to mini-open, and ultimately to arthroscopic cuff repair.

Assessment of the success of cuff repairs is problematic. Historically, success was measured using relatively crude, nonvalidated assessments of clinical parameters, sometimes assigning a score or groupings such as good or excellent. Modern studies more often use functional outcome measures in which the patients assess their symptoms and ability to function using validated, specially designed questionnaires. There has also been a move recently to look at success in terms of the integrity of the repair using imaging methods such as magnetic resonance imaging (MRI) or ultrasound. This difference in the way success is measured makes it difficult to compare studies and particularly to compare new and old repair techniques. In general, most authors have reported clinical improvement after all types of cuff repairs. Since Codman's first description in 1911, many surgeons have reported good results with open repairs. Ellman,[7] Hawkins,[8] Cofield[9], and others report in early articles 72% to 87% good to excellent results on the basis of improvement in pain, function, and strength (Level IV). More recently, Klepps,[10] Mellado,[11] and Bishop and others[12] have shown 71% to 90% good functional results. Whereas Mellado and coworkers[11] used the UCLA score (and postoperative MRI studies), others have used American Shoulder and Elbow Surgeons (ASES) and Constant scores. Functional outcome scores of arthroscopic repairs are similar. Burkhart and coauthors,[13,14] Gartsman and coworkers,[15] Youm and researchers,[16] and Bishop and others[12] (ASES and Constant) have reported 80% to 93% satisfaction rates using UCLA and Constant scores (Level IV).

Studies of early arthroscopic repairs suggest greater re-tear rates than with open surgery. Improvements in implants and evolution of technique now are reported to produce intact cuffs as often as open repairs. Verma and coworkers[17] found a 25% re-tear rate after both mini-open and arthroscopic repairs at 2-year ultrasound follow-up (Level III). Boileau and coauthors[18] report a 29% recurrence rate on computed tomography (CT). Fuchs[43], and Goutalier[44] found a 10% to 30% re-tear rate for small and medium tears with greater rates for massive tears. In the largest multicenter study published to date, Flurin et al.[19] assessed 576 arthroscopically repaired cuffs with MRI or CT arthrogram. Seventy-five percent showed no dye leakage compared with a mean of 69% for all published series in the literature for open repairs (Level IV). The authors conclude that arthroscopic repairs yield intact cuffs as often as open repairs. Previously, Gerber and colleagues[20] had provided a useful reference point, reporting an MRI-proven recurrent defect in 40% of open repairs of massive tears in 32 shoulders compared with 22% for arthroscopic repairs in 49 shoulders, which included multiple tendon tears[21] (Level III). Lafosse[41] reports a 12% failure rate on 105 cuffs repaired arthroscopically; 70% of these tears were large or massive.

Verma and coworkers,[17] Bishop and others[12] have found that good functional results are possible in the absence of a watertight repair. Irrespective of the technique used, however, there is evidence that intact repairs correlate with better functional results. In 1991, Harryman[45] suggested that clinical results after open repair correlate with cuff integrity based on ultrasound. Though he found significant satisfaction rates in terms of motion, strength, and pain relief even in the presence of recurrent defects, better results were seen with intact cuffs. Gerber and colleagues[20] found that patients who had a re-tear (on MRI) showed less improvement than those who had intact repairs.

COUNTERARGUMENTS

Exposure/Visualization—Seeing Is Believing!

Codman proposed a saber-cut incision in the earliest known description of rotator cuff repair. Since then, anterior, posterior, and extensile approaches have been described. Neer popularized anterior acromioplasty to relieve rotator cuff impingement. All traditional open approaches involve detachment of the deltoid from the acromion to varying degrees. Although the majority of authors recommend minimal deltoid dissection, large and massive tears often require extensive exposure, placing the deltoid attachment at risk. Burkhart and coauthors[22] highlight another theoretical disadvantage of open repair. They hypothesize that "open exposure places undue focus on medial-to-lateral transfer of the torn cuff edge to the greater tuberosity bone trough. Because the surgeon's visualization is limited medially, all the efforts are directed at somehow to bring the cuff to the bone bed. This approach ignores the tear morphology and ultimately results in a repair with greater tension on bone tendon interface. Such repairs are more likely to fail". Since Burkhart and coauthors'[22] work on tear morphology and progression, open repairs have tried to address this issue.

Arthroscopic surgery starts with glenohumeral examination. The superior labrum, the long head of the biceps, and joint surfaces are evaluated for coexisting pathology. Bursoscopy allows examination of the subacromial space (need for acromioplasty), cuff tear morphology, medial retraction, and mobility of cuff edges. The acromioclavicular joint can be assessed and resected, if warranted. Appropriate releases (anterior or posterior) and margin convergence sutures can be planned with more accuracy because of the enhanced visualization.

REPAIR STRENGTH

The strength of a tendon repair ultimately depends on several links in the chain of the repair. The links include the suture-bone interface, suture strength, suture-tendon interface, and the cuff tissue itself. Much of the recent scientific work has focused on strengthening the materials that are implanted, leaving the cuff tissue as the weakest link over which we currently have no control.

Traditionally, open repairs have used transosseous sutures. Gerber and colleagues[23] showed that bone itself provides a poor fixation point. In 8 of 16 shoulders, transosseous fixation failed by the sutures pulling out of the bone early in the postoperative course. This is more relevant in the poor quality osteoporotic bone encountered in the elderly. Though the authors did not test bone anchors, they recommend that transosseous bone fixation must be supplemented with a cortical bone augmentation device. Craft and coworkers[24] compared 4 suture anchors with transosseous repairs and found equal initial fixation strength. Reed and coauthors[25] found that anchor repair was significantly stronger than transosseous sutures irrespective of bone quality. Chhabra and investigators,[26] in a cadaver study, found that double-loaded anchors provide stronger fixation than transosseous repair in the immediate postoperative period.

Though most of these studies tested sutures and repair strength by ultimate load to failure, Hecker and coauthors[27] suggest that this may not be the best way to assess suture security because it may not reflect the real clinical situation. Barber and colleagues[28] echoed this and argued that cyclic load testing is more appropriate. Cyclic loading occurs with repeated arm motion, applying a modest force on the repair. They tested 4 commonly used absorbable anchors on human cadaveric humeri. After cyclical load testing, they found that none of the anchors showed signs of failure. In addition, Burkhart and coauthors[22] have shown that cyclic loading can cause failure with sutures cutting through bone in transosseous repairs.

With the use of new polyblend "super sutures," the weakest link has all but shifted to the tendon tissue. Cummins and Murrell,[29] Gartsman,[30] and others have shown that the new sutures hardly ever break, and the failure to load strength far exceeds 200 N for the commonly used No. 2 sutures compared with Ethibond or other commonly used sutures.

Tendon tissue quality and the suture-tendon interface are the only remaining areas of concern in achieving a stable and durable repair. Whereas the former is beyond the surgeon's control, the latter can be favorably influenced by more complex suture configurations. Complex suture passes such as the Mason Allen configuration are believed to yield the strongest interface[38]. Because these are difficult to pass arthroscopically, this has provided an argument for superior strength of open repairs. Arthroscopy advocates have countered by demonstrating nearly the same construct strength with subtle modifications, which are possible to do arthroscopically.[31–33] Burkhart and Brady,[34] on the other hand, have advocated simple suture configuration with double-loaded anchors. In a biomechanical study, they calculated that maximal load per suture does not exceed 37.7 N if double-loaded anchors are placed 1 cm apart. Simple suture configurations are enough to withstand this load.

REHABILITATION AND RECOVERY

Gerber and colleagues[23] and others have found that most of the failures occur in the early postoperative period. Thus, irrespective of type of repair, it needs to be protected in the first 4 to 10 weeks. The type of rehabilitation is usually based on the size of tear and tissue quality. After the initial protection period, many authors[1,13] have observed an earlier return to functional range of motion after arthroscopic repair.

COMPLICATIONS

Deltoid detachment and atrophy have been reported to occur in 3% to 18% of open rotator cuff repairs. Similarly, infection has affected the result in 1% to 3% of open repairs.[35] Recovery of motion in the early postoperative period (first 3 months) after open repairs usually lags behind arthroscopic repairs, though results in terms of range of motion are comparable at 1 year.[1,5] As discussed earlier, re-tear as a complication in small and moderate tears is reportedly similar for arthroscopic and open repairs, but some studies have suggested that there may be a greater incidence of re-tear in arthroscopic repair of massive tears.[12] Nho found 6 cases of subacromial impingement in the mini-open group compared with 1 in the arthroscopic group that needed repeat surgery. Overall, he found 14 complications in 473 patients (prevalence rate, 3%) in the arthroscopic group compared with 27 complications in 411 patients (prevalence rate, 6.6%) in mini-open group.

RECOMMENDATIONS

Arthroscopic surgery is the choice of most of our patients. It permits better visualization and detects coexisting pathology, which allows a planned and systematic approach to management. The repair construct is strong and can withstand physiologic loads. The complication rate is low, though there may be an increased incidence of re-tears in massive tears. Fortunately, functional outcomes even in these cases are generally improved and the most recent reports suggest that, as techniques improve, equivalent or even better results are being achieved in large tears repaired arthroscopically. Besides, recent reports of Flurin, Cole, and Lafosse show better or equivalent results in large or massive tears repaired arthroscopically. In fact, literature comparison of 2 types of repair at various points of time since the earlier 1990s shows a distinct trend of continuously improving results with arthroscopic repairs. Cost concerns have not been specifically studied for rotator cuff repairs; however, Wang and coworkers[36] and Bohnsack and coauthors,[37] in separate studies, found cost of arthroscopic Bankart repair to be less than that of open surgery.

Barring a greater incidence of complications in the case of open repairs, no single factor in the published literature overwhelmingly favors one technique over another. The trend is toward arthroscopic repair as the least invasive technique because it is in many surgical procedures. Based on largely Level III/IV evidence available, it is our opinion that arthroscopic cuff repair seems to be a superior technique in skilled hands. However, the absence of Level I studies prevents us from making a grade A recommendation. Our recommendation is, therefore, a grade C recommendation in favor of arthroscopic rotator cuff repair. Prospective, randomized multi-center trials are currently being conducted by groups such as JOINTS Canada and should provide more definitive answers in the near future. Tables 100–1 and 100–2 provide a summary of recommendations and levels of evidence.

TABLE 100–1. Levels of Evidence for Studies on Arthroscopic Rotator Cuff Repair

AUTHOR (YEAR OF PUBLICATION)	DESCRIPTION	EVIDENCE	CONCLUSION
Nho et al. (2007)[40]	Systematic review of arthroscopic rotator cuff repair and mini-open rotator cuff repair	Level III: systematic review of literature	No technique recommended over other. Slightly higher rate of complication in mini-open group.
Cole et al. (2007)[35]	Arthroscopic rotator cuff repair: prospective functional outcome and repair integrity at minimum 2-year follow-up	Level IV: prospective study of 49 consecutive repairs with MRI	Overall failure rate is 22%, mostly in tears involving infraspinatus.
Lafosse et al. (2007)[41]	The outcome and structural integrity of arthroscopic rotator cuff repair with use of the double-row suture anchor technique	Level IV: prospective study of 105 consecutive repairs with CT/MRA	Arthroscopic repair with double-row suture anchor technique results in a much lower rate of failure than has previously been reported in either open or arthroscopic repair methods.
Liem et al. (2007)[42]	Clinical outcome and tendon integrity of arthroscopic versus mini-open supraspinatus tendon repair: an MRI-controlled matched-pair analysis	Level III: retrospective, therapeutic, comparative study	In isolated supraspinatus tears, arthroscopic rotator cuff repair produces excellent clinical results and equivalent tendon integrity compared with mini-open repair.
Flurin et al. (2005)[19]	Arthroscopic repair of cuff tears: a multicentric retrospective study of 576 cases with anatomic assessment		75% intact tears compared with a mean of 69% for all published series in the literature for open repairs
Gerber et al. (2000)[20]	The results of repair of massive tears of the rotator cuff	Prospective analysis	60% of tears are intact, functionally better than persistent defects.
Severud et al. (2003)[1]	All-arthroscopic versus mini-open rotator cuff repair	Retrospective outcome study	Surgery times are comparable. Patients regain motion faster in the first 12 weeks with the all-arthroscopic technique. A steep learning curve is present.

CT, computed tomography; MRA, magnetic resonance angiography; MRI, magnetic resonance imaging.

TABLE 100–2. Summary of Recommendations

STATEMENT	LEVEL OF EVIDENCE/GRADE OF RECOMMENDATIONS
Rotator cuff repair should be performed arthroscopically.	C

REFERENCES

1. Severud EL, Ruotolo C, Abbott DD, et al: All-arthroscopic versus mini-open rotator cuff repair: A long-term retrospective outcome comparison. Arthroscopy 19:234–238, 2003.
2. Ide J, Maeda S, Takagi K: A comparison of arthroscopic and open rotator cuff repair. Arthroscopy 21:1090–1098, 2005.
3. Kang L, Henn RF, Tashjian RZ, et al: Early outcome of arthroscopic rotator cuff repair: A matched comparison with mini-open rotator cuff repair. Arthroscopy 23:573–582, e1–e2, 2007.
4. Yamaguchi K, Ball CM, Galatz LM: Arthroscopic rotator cuff repair transition from mini-open to all-arthroscopic. Clin Orthop Relat Res (390):83–94, 2001.
5. Baker CL, Liu SH: Comparison of open and arthroscopically assisted rotator cuff repairs. Am J Sports Med 23:99–104, 1995.
6. Sperling JW, Smith AM, Cofield RH, et al: Patient perceptions of open and arthroscopic shoulder surgery. Arthroscopy 23:361–366, 2007.
7. Ellman H, Hanker G, Bayer M: Repair of the rotator cuff. End-result study of factors influencing reconstruction. J Bone Joint Surg Am 68:1136–1144, 1986.
8. Hawkins RJ, Misamore GW, Hobeika PE: Surgery for full-thickness rotator-cuff tears. J Bone Joint Surg Am 67:1349–1355, 1985.
9. Cofield RH: Rotator cuff disease of the shoulder. J Bone Joint Surg Am 67:974–979.
10. Klepps S, Bishop J, Lin J, et al: Prospective evaluation of the effect of rotator cuff integrity on the outcome of open rotator cuff repairs. Am J Sports Med 32:1716–1722, 2004.
11. Mellado JM, Calmet J, Olona M, et al: Surgically repaired massive rotator cuff tears: MRI of tendon integrity, muscle fatty degeneration, and muscle atrophy correlated with intraoperative and clinical findings. AJR Am J Roentgenol 184:1456–1463, 2005.
12. Bishop J, Klepps S, Lo IK, et al: Cuff integrity after arthroscopic versus open rotator cuff repair: A prospective study. J Shoulder Elbow Surg 15:290–299, 2006.
13. Burkhart SS, Danaceau SM, Pearce CE Jr: Arthroscopic rotator cuff repair: Analysis of results by tear size and by repair technique—margin convergence versus direct tendon-to-bone repair. Arthroscopy 17:905–912, 2001.
14. Burkhart SS, Barth JR, Richards DP, et al: Arthroscopic repair of massive rotator cuff tears with stage 3 and 4 fatty degeneration. Arthroscopy 23:347–354, 2007.

15. Gartsman GM, Khan M, Hammerman SM: Arthroscopic repair of full-thickness tears of the rotator cuff. J Bone Joint Surg Am 80:832–840, 1998.
16. Youm T, Murray DH, Kubiak EN, et al: Arthroscopic versus mini-open rotator cuff repair: A comparison of clinical outcomes and patient satisfaction. J Shoulder Elbow Surg 14:455–459, 2005.
17. Verma NN, Dunn W, Adler RS: All-arthroscopic versus mini-open rotator cuff repair: A retrospective review with minimum 2-year follow-up. Arthroscopy 22:587–594, 2006.
18. Boileau P, Brassart N, Watkinson DJ, et al. Arthroscopic repair of full-thickness tears of the supraspinatus: Does the tendon really heal? J Bone Joint Surg Am 87:1229–1240, 2005.
19. Flurin PH, Landreau P, Gregory T. Arthroscopic repair of full-thickness cuff tears: a multicentric retrospective study of 576 cases with anatomical assessment. Rev Chir Orthop Reparatrice Appar Mot 91(S8):31-42, 2005. [Article in French]
20. Gerber C, Fuchs B, Hodler J: The results of repair of massive tears of the rotator cuff. J Bone Joint Surg Am 82:505–515, 2000.
21. Deleted in proof.
22. Burkhart SS, Danaceau SM, Pearce CE Jr: Arthroscopic rotator cuff repair: Analysis of results by tear size and by repair technique—margin convergence versus direct tendon-to-bone repair. Arthroscopy 17:905–912, 2001.
23. Gerber C, Schneeberger AG, Perren SM, et al: Experimental rotator cuff repair. A preliminary study. J Bone Joint Surg Am 81:1281–1290, 1999.
24. Craft DV, Moseley JB, Cawley PW, et al: Fixation strength of rotator cuff repairs with suture anchors and the transosseous suture technique. J Shoulder Elbow Surg 5:32–40, 1996.
25. Reed SC, Glossop N, Ogilvie-Harris DJ: Full-thickness rotator cuff tears. A biomechanical comparison of suture versus bone anchor techniques. Am J Sports Med 24:46–48, 1996.
26. Chhabra A, Goradia VK, Francke EI, et al: In vitro analysis of rotator cuff repairs: A comparison of arthroscopically inserted tacks or anchors with open transosseous repairs. Arthroscopy 21:323–327, 2005.
27. Hecker AT, Shea M, Hayhurst JO, et al: Pull-out strength of suture anchors for rotator cuff and Bankart lesion repairs. Am J Sports Med 21:874–879, 1993.
28. Barber FA, Coons DA, Ruiz-Suarez M: Cyclic load testing of biodegradable suture anchors containing 2 high-strength sutures. Arthroscopy 23:355–360, 2007.
29. Cummins CA, Murrell GA: Mode of failure for rotator cuff repair with suture anchors identified at revision surgery J Shoulder Elbow Surg 12:128–133, 2003.
30. Gartsman GM: All arthroscopic rotator cuff repairs. Orthop Clin North Am 32:501–510, 2001.
31. Sileo MJ, Ruotolo CR, Nelson CO, et al: A biomechanical comparison of the modified Mason-Allen stitch and massive cuff stitch in vitro. Arthroscopy 23:235–240, 240.e1–2, 2007.
32. Schlegel TF, Hawkins RJ, Lewis CW, et al: An in vivo comparison of the modified Mason-Allen suture technique versus an inclined horizontal mattress suture technique with regard to tendon-to-bone healing: A biomechanical and histologic study in sheep. J Shoulder Elbow Surg. 16:115–121, 2007.
33. Klinger HM, Steckel H, Spahn G, et al: Biomechanical comparison of double-loaded suture anchors using arthroscopic Mason-Allen stitches versus traditional transosseous suture technique and modified Mason-Allen stitches for rotator cuff repair. Clin Biomech (Bristol, Avon) 22:106–111, 2007.
34. Burkhart SS, Brady PC: A Cowboy's Guide to Advanced Shoulder Arthroscopy. Philadelphia, Lippincott Williams & Wilkins, 2006, pp 34–35.
35. Cole BJ, McCarty LP 3rd, Kang RW, et al: Arthroscopic rotator cuff repair: prospective functional outcome and repair integrity at minimum 2-year follow-up. J Shoulder Elbow Surg 16(5):579–585, 2007.
36. Herrera MF, Bauer G, Reynolds F, et al: Infection after mini-open rotator cuff repair. J Shoulder Elbow Surg 11(6):605–608, 2002.
37. Wang C, Ghalambor N, Zarins B, et al: Arthroscopic versus open Bankart repair: analysis of patient subjective outcome and cost. Arthroscopy 21(10):1219–1222, 2005.
38. Bohnsack M, Brinkmann T, Rühmann O, et al: Open versus arthroscopic shoulder stabilization. An analysis of the treatment costs. Orthopade 32(7):654–658, 2003.
39. Burkhart SS, Diaz Pagan JL, Wirth MA, et al: Cyclic loading of anchor-based rotator cuff repairs: confirmation of the tension overload phenomenon and comparison of suture anchor fixation with transosseous fixation. Arthroscopy 13(6):720–724, 1997.
40. Nho SJ, Shindle MK, Sherman SL et al: Systematic Review of Arthroscopic Rotator Cuff Repair and Mini-Open Rotator cuff repair. J Bone Joint Surg Am 89:127–136, 2007.
41. Lafosse L, Brozska R, Toussaint B et al: The outcome and structural integrity of arthroscopic rotator cuff repair with use of the double-row suture anchor technique. J Bone Joint Surg Am 89(7):1533–1541, 2007.
42. Liem D, Bartl C, Lichtenberg S: Clinical outcome and tendon integrity of arthroscopic versus mini-open supraspinatus tendon repair: a magnetic resonance imaging-controlled matched-pair analysis. Arthroscopy 23(5):514–521, 2007.
43. Fuchs B, Gilbart MK, Hodler J: Clinical and structural results of open repair of an isolated one-tendon tear of the rotator cuff. Arthroscopy 23(5):514–521, 2007.
44. Goutallier D, Postel JM, Gleyze P, Leguilloux P: Influence of cuff muscle fatty degeneration on anatomic and functional outcomes after simple suture of full-thickness tears. J Shoulder Elbow Surg 12(6):550–554, 2003.
45. Harryman DT 2nd, Mack LA, Wang KY: Repairs of the rotator cuff. Correlation of functional results with integrity of the cuff. J Bone Joint Surg Am 73(7):982–989, 1991.
46. Mohtadi NG, Hollingshead SK, et al: A randomized clinical trial comparing open to arthroscopic acromioplasty with mini-open rotator cuff repair for full-thickness rotator cuff tears: disease-specific quality of life outcome at an average 2-year follow-up. Am J Sports Med 36(6):1043–1051, 2008.

Subject Index